ALZHEIMER'S DISEASE PATHOGENESIS-CORE CONCEPTS, SHIFTING PARADIGMS AND THERAPEUTIC TARGETS

Edited by **Suzanne De La Monte**

Alzheimer's Disease Pathogenesis-Core Concepts, Shifting Paradigms and Therapeutic Targets
Edited by Suzanne De La Monte

Published by InTech

Janeza Trdine 9, 51000 Rijeka, Croatia

Publishing Process Manager Petra Zobic

Technical Editor Teodora Smiljanic

Cover Designer InTech Design Team

Additional hard copies can be obtained from orders@intechopen.com

Alzheimer's Disease Pathogenesis-Core Concepts, Shifting Paradigms and Therapeutic Targets, Edited by Suzanne De La Monte
p. cm.
978-953-307-690-4

For EU product safety concerns:
IN TECH d.o.o., Prolaz Marije Krucifikse Kozulić 3, 51000 Rijeka, Croatia,
info@intechopen.com or visit our website at intechopen.com.

Meet the editor

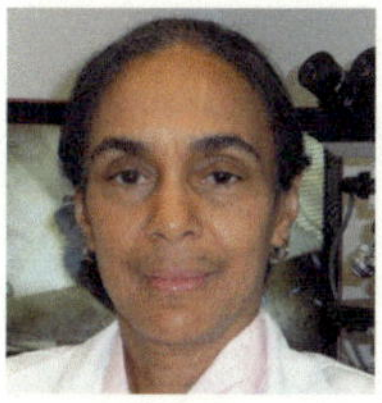

Dr. Suzanne M. de la Monte, M.D., M.P.H. is Professor of Neuropathology, Neurology, and Neurosurgery at the Rhode Island Hospital and the Alpert Medical School of Brown University, Providence, RI. She received her undergraduate degree from Cornell University, Ithaca, N.Y., M.D. from the Weill College of Medicine at Cornell University, and masters in public health (M.P.H.) from the Blumberg School of Public Health at Johns Hopkins University, Baltimore, MD. Dr. de la Monte completed her residency in Anatomical Pathology and fellowship in Pediatric Pathology at The Johns Hopkins Hospital, and a fellowship in Neuropathology at the Massachusetts General Hospital. She received postdoctoral research training at the Massachusetts General Hospital. Currently, Dr. de la Monte directs research on the role of insulin resistance as a mediator of neurodegeneration in relation to Alzheimer's disease, alcoholism, obesity, diabetes, and development. Her research led to the provocative concept that Alzheimer's is "Type 3 Diabetes".

Contents

Preface

Alzheimer's disease is the most common cause of dementia in modern industrialized and high technology-driven cultures, and it is rapidly spreading to poorer nations throughout the world. For years, research on Alzheimer's was focused on gene mutations and polymorphisms in large kindred or selected populations. Those studies championed the roles of either, amyloid deposition and neurotoxicity, or intra-neuronal accumulations of abnormally phosphorylated tau as the principal mediators of neurodegeneration. For some time, only two major camps were recognized: one for the "Tau-ists", and the other for the "β-APP-tists". Soldiers in each camp vigorously defended their own turf, and every square-inch of newly gained ground, fighting off all major as well as minor threats. Such divisive approaches ended up being counter-productive. Eventually, a cease fire was called, and a new era of collaboration and exchange arrived. Fortunately, even during those intellectually lean years, new and distinct concepts about the pathogenesis of Alzheimer's disease began to emerge and gain steam. To some extent, the flourishing of alternative concepts, including the roles of oxidative stress, mitochondrial dysfunction, metal toxicities, cerebrovascular disease, and immune/inflammatory responses as mediators of neurodegeneration, was inspired by the facts that: 1) the most important risk factor for developing Alzheimer's is aging; and 2) over 90% of Alzheimer cases exhibit sporadic rather than familial occurrences. More recently, interest in the contributions of diabetes mellitus, obesity and insulin resistance as causal or contributing factors in the pathogenesis of Alzheimer's disease has grown considerably. Although much of the current research is still heavily focused on the direct and indirect roles of amyloid- and phosphorylated tau-mediated neurotoxicity and neurodegeneration, the field has broadened and the paradigm depicting the path toward Alzheimer's has shifted to accommodate newer and more diverse concepts. This book, "Alzheimer's Disease Pathogenesis: Core Concepts, Shifting Paradigms, and Therapeutic Targets" is an exciting work because the collection of chapters provides insight into the full range of concepts that are now under serious consideration with regard to the pathogenesis of Alzheimer's disease. This book is unusual in that it provides current information within each of the sub-disciplines, and therefore will satisfy the needs and interests of both newcomers to the field, and specialized experts interested in understanding concepts and approaches to Alzheimer's that are distinct from their own.

The Overview section contains two chapters that summarize and review the standard features of Alzheimer's pathology, epidemiology, genetics, and pathophysiology. This is an excellent section for reviewing the basics and the basis for which therapeutic and diagnostic approaches have already been developed and are currently under investigation. The second section, "Amyloid and Tau Mediated Neurotoxicity and Neurodegeneration" provides a well-balanced series of 7 chapters that explain how amyloid deposits and fibrils are generated from amyloid precursor protein, including the enzymes, biochemical, and molecular mediators of the process, the pathogenesis of Tau pathology, and how oligomers of both amyloid and tau fibrils contribute to the pathogenesis and progression of Alzheimer's disease. The first two chapters in this section provide excellent accounts of the expression and function amyloid precursor protein (APP) and the processing and cleavage of APP to amyloid beta. The authors explain the biochemical and pathological mechanisms that drive amyloid beta accumulation in Alzheimer's. Dr. Santos provides a very clear and informative discussion of how amyloid precursor protein is processed, and current concepts concerning the mechanisms by which amyloid-beta accumulates in plaques, fibrils, and oligomers. The chapter by Dr. Ueno extends these concepts, providing a thorough and highly topical account of the structure and function of the blood-brain barrier, information that is needed to understand problems that must be overcome for effective treatment of neurodegenerative diseases. In addition, the chapter provides insight the role the abnormal blood-brain barrier plays in mediating amyloid-beta accumulation in the brain, including the mechanisms of increased periphery-to-brain influx, and impaired clearance from brain to periphery. The discussion by Professor Sergeant is quite novel in its description of how amyloid and tau fibrils can spread within a system or circuitry in the brain via microvesicular bodies, somewhat reminiscent of how Prions are thought to propagate disease from one part of the brain to another. Tau pathology and how it evolves and contributes to the neurodegeneration cascade are covered in the chapter by Dr. Garcia-Sierra. The final two chapters enlighten the readers about the roles of oligomers and prefibrillar aggregates of amyloid and tau as mediators of neurotoxicity and neurodegeneration. The information provided is sufficient for the reader to gain an excellent grasp of the field. These chapters are particularly important because the mechanisms of neurotoxicity and neurodegeneration that the authors detail are linchpins of current hypotheses that connect amyloid and tau pathology to other conceptual frameworks of Alzheimer's disease pathogenesis.

The third section, "Abnormalities in Signal Transduction and Gene Regulation" addresses the core abnormalities in Alzheimer's from the perspective that aberrations in intracellular signaling mechanisms, neurotransmitter and neurotrophin expression, and gene regulation mediate neurodegeneration, including tau and amyloid pathology. The first chapter in this section is concerned with the role of increased glycogen synthase kinase 3β (GSK-3β) activation as a mediator of both aberrant tau phosphorylation and amyloid fibril formation. Since aberrant activation of GSK-3 β can promote both tau and amyloid pathology, it could serve as a therapeutic target in

AD. These points are discussed. The second chapter in this section also takes a unifying approach in considering the role of Pin1 as a protective molecule for selectively phosphorylating tau and amyloid precursor protein (APP) in strategic sites that reduce neurotoxic fibril formation and attendant neuronal death/degeneration. The role of neurotrophin dysfunction in the pathogenesis of cognitive impairment harkens back to much earlier days when interest in neurotransmitter deficiency and impaired neurotrophin functions as mediators of Alzheimer's was topical. Devising ways to supply more neurotrophins or improve the sensistive of neurotrophin receptors could help address the problem of failing neural plasticity with Alzheimer's disease progression. Finally, the analysis of micro-RNAs in relation to Alzheimer's is cutting edge. The authors illustrate how this relatively new approach to determining how gene expression could be altered in the absence of mutation can now be applied to the study of Alzheimer's disease. Awareness that epigenetic modifications of gene expression could mediate some of the abnormalities in Alzheimer's brains, opens the door to examining other means of epigenetic gene dysregulation or suppression in the pathogenesis of neurodegeneration.

The section, "Oxidative Stress, Reactive Oxygen Species, and Heavy Metals" is critical because, irrespective of whatever hypothesis one chooses to investigate, consideration must be given to the role of oxidative injury because it is a highly consistent feature of Alzheimer's as well as other neurodegenerative diseases. Mitochondria are the powerhouse of all cells, and mitochondrial dysfunction is a feature of Alzheimer's. The lead-off chapter summarizes mitochondrial pathology, pathophysiology, and gene/DNA abnormalities that have been recognized for decades as features of Alzheimer's. Although the causes are not known, they nonetheless drive injury and neurodegeneration. The next two chapters emphasize the importance of oxidative stress and injury as major factors contributing to the disruption in neuronal structure and neurotransmitter homeostasis. The chapters shed light on the concept that, given the broad importance of oxidative stress as a mediator or propagator of Alzheimer's, it could serve as both a biomarker of disease status, and a target for therapy. The final two chapters in this section pertain to the potential pathogenic role of redox transition heavy metals, particularly copper and iron. Besides being found within Alzheimer brain lesions, redox metals may mediate their toxic effects by promoting protein aggregation and misfolding, resulting in toxic accumulation in brain. The chapter contributed by Dr. Burbano highlights the potential contributions of increased exposure to metal contaminants in the environment as a mediator of sporadic Alzheimer's.

The section, "Metabolic Derangements: Glucose, Insulin, and Diabetes", is extremely exciting and topical because it provides a compelling argument that brain insulin resistance is at the core of Alzheimer's, and that our current epidemics of obesity, diabetes, and body insulin resistance are part and parcel with the Alzheimer's epidemic. The first two chapters give succinct accounts for how insulin resistance contributes to virtually every aspect of Alzheimer's and in fact could be the root cause in sporadic cases. Besides the epidemiology and experimental data that support this hypothesis, the chapters by Drs. Bosco and de la Monte demonstrate how impairments in insulin signaling and glucose metabolism mediate brain energy deficits, oxidative stress, amyloid deposition, and tau pathology. The chapter by Dr. de la Monte takes the concept one step further by connecting insulin resistance diseases to environmental toxin exposures, i.e. nitrosamines, and lifestyle choices, i.e. obesity. Of course, glucose utilization and energy metabolism are dependent upon availability of micronutrients, particularly the neural B vitamins, but also others that have anti-oxidant and neuroprotective actions. This topic is discussed in the final chapter in this section. The information included in this section highlights opportunities for preventative and therapeutic intervention, as well as diagnostics.

Because the field of Alzheimer's research has broadened, seemingly peripheral concepts are making their way toward center stage. The contribution of vascular disease and low-flow states is important because as many as 40% of individuals with Alzheimer's progress due to cerebral ischemia. This problem could be caused by microvascular disease stemming from diabetes and/or hypertension. Some newer concepts, such as autophagy, are extensions from other fields in biology and shown to have relevance to Alzheimer's pathogenesis. The chapters on plasmalogen and gangliosies are of interest because they attend to the white matter pathology in Alzheimer's; a subject that has been greatly ignored despite evidence for substantial fiber loss even in the very early stages of disease. The concept that neurotransmitter deficits, particularly reductions in acetylcholine, mediate cognitive impairment in Alzheimer's is alive and well. Re-attending to this problem with the goal of improving the effectiveness of cholinesterase inhibitors is timely and critical for enhancing the level and duration of treatment responses in the future.

The final section, Potential Therapeutic Strategies" deliberately juxtaposes concepts on potential therapeutic strategies to address the three core mediators of Alzheimer's disease: 1) Tau and amyloid neurotoxicity; 2) oxidative stress; and 3) brain insulin resistance. Although the ultimate objectives are to cure or prevent progression of Alzheimer's, the conceptual framework that guides the strategy differs for each of the arguments. Drugs targeting the aggregation, fibrillization, and oligomer accumulation and toxicity, including the use of immunotherapy, would attack the molecular and structural lesions in Alzheimer's. Although these approaches still dominate, they may not be sufficient to undermine the causes of those lesions. On the other and, if those lesions mediate neurodegeneration, we must understand how to reduce their burden in the brain. The chapter by Professor Kayed provides an excellent discussion on this topic. The chapter by Professor Yadav aptly deals with the problems of amyloid toxicity, oxidative stress and metal toxicity utilizing an in silico drug design point of view. This approach is state-of-the art and it is very much worthwhile to grasp this topic which is presented in excellent format, including a large number of illustrations. Finally, to control or cure problems caused by brain insulin resistance and deficiency, many approaches have been used including, insulin therapy, insulin sensitizer agents, and anti-diabetes drugs, all of which have been at least partially effective in different clinical trials, but limited by side-effects and sometimes, marginal degrees of efficacy. However, the potential use of incretin hormones, particularly glucagon-like peptide-1 (GLP-1) as a neuroprotective agent is potentially very exciting because GLP-1 promotes insulin secretion, is safe, and has similar positive effects on brain energy metabolism, plasticity, and cognitive function as insulin. GLP-1 was shown to have significant therapeutic effects in mouse models of Alzheimer's. In addition, there are already commercially available GLP-1 analogs that are used clinically. This topic is very well discussed by Dr. Holscher. The findings from the experimental use of incretin treatments with regard to rescuing Alzheimer's disease support the concept that the underlying basis for Alzheimer's is somehow integrally tied to insulin resistance in the brain. However, the honest truth is that effective management and treatment of Alzheimer's will ultimately rely on multi-pronged therapies that target up-stream, mid-stream, and down-stream mediators of disease. "Alzheimer's Disease Pathogenesis: Core Concepts, Shifting Paradigms, and Therapeutic Targets" is an excellent singe-volume resource that provides more than ample information on each of the topics mentioned. Readers and scholars will find the material informative and provocative.

Suzanne M. de la Monte, MD, MPH
Professor of Neuropathology, Neurology, and Neurosurgery,
Lifespan Academic Institutions-Rhode Island Hospital,
Warren Alpert School of Medicine at Brown University, Providence, RI,
USA

Part 1

Overview

1

Alzheimer´s Disease – The New Actors of an Old Drama

Mario Álvarez Sánchez, Carlos A. Sánchez Catasús, Ivonne Pedroso Ibañez, Maria L. Bringas and Arnoldo Padrón Sánchez
International Center of Neurological Restoration
Cuba

1. Introduction

Alzheimer's Disease is the most common neurodegeneration and the prototype of this group of diseases. Now threatens to become an epidemy with a predictable and profound impact.

In 1906 Alois Alzheimer brilliantly defined the clinicopathologic syndrome that now bears his name to relate the progression of cognitive impairment to pathological anatomic findings wich remains as the markers of the disease: amyloid plaques and neurofibrillary tangles. After more than a hundred years since its description, especially in the last two decades new interesting clues have been revealed to understanding the basic mechanisms of disease. This research highlights the discovery of genes in familial and sporadic forms, the description in detail of the beta amyloid cascade and tau protein metabolism and a better understanding of the role of vascular factors, inflammation, brain resistance to insulin and the recent and intriguing findings about the role of the prion receptors and prion like mechanisms in the development of disease. Thus, new actors earn role in the pathophysiology of an ancient drama: Alzheimer’s disease.

This chapter discusses these topics with the assurance that in the coming years will be the basis for the development of new diagnostic tools and more effective treatments.

2. Pathology

2.1 Macroscopic

Alzheimer's disease (AD) is characterized by a global involvement, bilateral and symmetrical in both hemispheres with cortical predominance. There is reduced transparency and fibrosis of the leptomeninges and subarachnoid large gaps remains in the spaces left between the cerebral sulci. When the meninges are removed we can see a pale brain with weight decrease of approximately 800 to 1000g from 1300 to 1700g in the normal adult. There is greater involvement of the association areas (fronto temporal and parietal) and to a lesser degree of primary motor and sensory areas. The most affected region is the mesial temporal lobe and especially the entorhinal cortex. The increase of the ventricles is secondary to parenchymal loss. A recent neuroimage-based quantitative meta-analysis revealed that early AD affects structurally the hippocampal regions (figures 1.A and 1.B), while functionally affects the inferior parietal lobules (figures 1.C and 1.D), which might be

caused by regional amyloid deposits and by disconnection from the hippocampus through disruption of the cingulum bundle (Schroeter et al., 2009).
Although not define the disease, there is usually involvement of the subcortical white matter leukoaraiosis as well as small infarcts and atherosclerotic changes in large arteries.

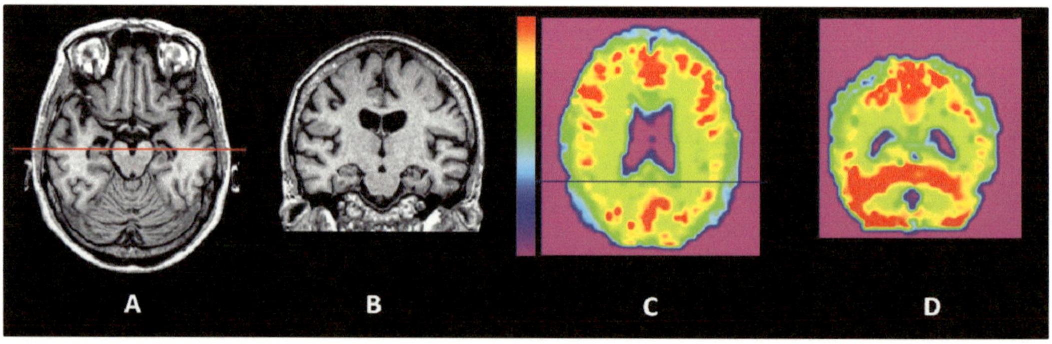

Fig. 1. Brain MRI (Magnetic Resonance Imaging) and perfusion SPECT (Single Photon Emission Computed Tomography) images of a patient with AD in early stage examined in our institution (female, age= 66 years, Mini Mental State Examination (MMSE)=22); all images are oriented in the radiological convention. A) Axial view of high resolution MRI image (T1) showing brain atrophy, particularly in the hippocampus bilaterally; B) Coronal slice at the level of the red line show in the axial view; C) ^{99m}Tc-ECD SPECT image using a double-head system and corrected for partial volume effect (corrected for atrophy), showing regional hypoperfusion in the parietal regions, particularly in the angular gyrus bilaterally; and D) Coronal slice at the level of the blue line show in the axial view C. For comparison see figure 2 with similar images of a clinically healthy subject.

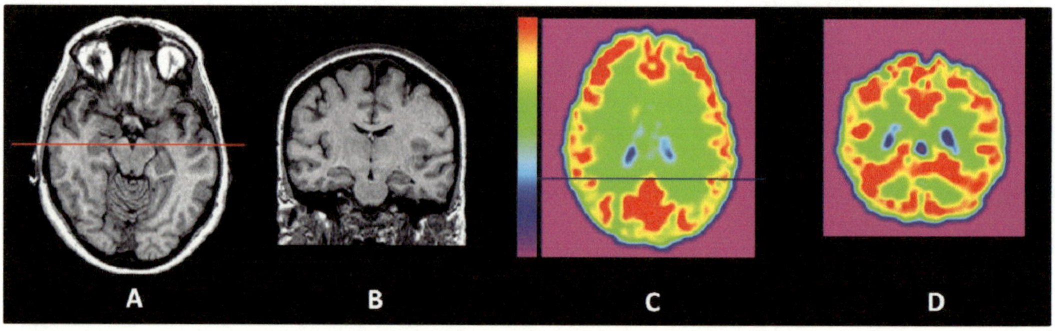

Fig. 2. Brain MRI and perfusion SPECT images of a clinically healthy subject (female, age= 64 years, MMSE=30). A) to D) are similar images show in figure 1.

There are atypical or asymmetric forms where the degeneration and atrophy is restricted to one lobe or cerebral hemisphere. A series of cases shows that these phenotypes are not as infrequent as it is supposed (Alladi et al., 2007). The pathology of AD is a common substrate in the Posterior Cortical Atrophy, Non Fluent Progressive Aphasia and Cortico Basal Degeneration although is rare in others such as Semantic Dementia and Fronto Temporal Dementia. In the case of Non Fluent Progressive Aphasia most cases corresponds with typical findings of AD.

2.2 Microscopic

Corroborate the findings described above. It were also observed important changes such as subcortical neuronal depopulation of the nucleus basalis of Meynert, raphe nuclei, the nucleus ceruleus, amygdala, and white matter lesions. The two typical lesions that define AD are senile plaques and neurofibrillary tangles:

2.2.1 Senile Plaques (SP)

Observed in the interstice, between neurons. They measure between 20 and 100 microns and consist of a core which principal component is beta amyloid (βA). This core is surrounded by a nest formed by degenerating neurites, activated microglia and astrocytes. Other substances that conform the SP are the alpha-synuclein (principal not amyloid component), alpha 1 antichymotrypsin, alpha 2 macroglobulin, apolipoprotein E, ubiquitin and the presenilins. Degenerative neurons are also distinguished around but not in contact with the plaques. According his appearance they are classified as:

a. Difuse. Formed by a delicate network of fine filaments of amyloid fibrils without degenerate neurites. Center and its boundaries are not well defined.
b. Primitive. Are the most common. They are characterized by disordered extracellular Aβ deposits wich are poorly or not fibrillar. Center is not well defined but the borders are more accurate.
c. Classic. Also called neuritic plaques, amyloid have a center surrounded by a crown composed of reactive astrocytes, microglia and dystrophic neurites corresponding to dendrites and degenerate axons.
d. Burns. Present only a condensed central amyloid. It has no cellular components.

These forms represent different developmental stages of the plaques, beginning with the accumulation of diffuse amyloid, then it is organized and defined, by associating the immune response. Finally, the cellular elements disappear.

The SP are relatively rare in limbic structures and neocortex and are more visible in frontal temporal and occipital regions, while respecting the primary sensorimotor areas. They can be found in the brains of people without cognitive deficits, but to a lesser extent (Table 1). Higher concentrations are criteria for pathological diagnosis of AD.

Age (years)	Amount
Less than 50	Less than 5
Between 50 and 65	Less than 9
Between 66 and 75	Less than 11
More than 75	Less than 16

Table 1. Amount of Senile Plaques (SP) per mm3 with 200x augmentation.

We can now follow the progression of βA in vivo deposits using Carbon-11-Pittsburgh Compound B Positron Emission Tomography (PIB-PET) which correlates with the number of SP. This technique shows a broader distribution in both normal subjects and patients with AD. One study (Engler et al., 2006) compared the PIB-PET signal between healthy controls and patients with AD found that was higher in patients. Unexpectedly, the most notable

difference was found in the striatum. Other regions with significant differences were the frontal, temporal and occipital lobes. By repeating the test after two years, there was only one significant difference in the occipital cortex of patients with AD. The PIB-PET signal change did not correlate with the progression of cognitive impairment suggesting that, after an initial period, βA deposits stabilizes.
Some familiar forms as mutations of presenilin 1 that cause variant-AD have atypical SP that coexists with the usual. There are Cotton Wool plaques, non cored and devoid of dystrophic neurites. The distribution is also uncommon, presenting high concentrations in the interhemispheric motor cortex representing the lower extremities, which is consistent with early-onset spasticity that often accompanies memory and visuospatial disorders (Koivunen et al., 2008).

2.2.2 Neuro-fibrillary tangles (NFT)

Neurons present an accumulation of flame-shaped inclusions and sometimes form a elongated basket around the nucleus. The inclusions are basophils to the hematoxylin and eosin and strongly stained with silver stains. The inclusions fill the cytoplasm, particularly in the soma and apical dendrite causing neuronal death mainly by apoptosis. Finally there are only remnants of the cytoskeleton, such as ghosts´ nodules.
Development of new staining techniques to visualize phosphorylated Tau protein (Tau-p) while they are soluble, in early states called pre-fibrillar, is the basis for classification according to the developmental stages of Braak, which suggested changes in the pathological diagnostic criteria (figure 3).
The NFT is distributed in very characteristics areas as the entorhinal and perirhinal allocortex, CA1 region of hippocampus and the amygdala. Also found in the nucleus basalis of Meynert, Temporal isocortex (areas 20 and 21 of Brodmann) and the rest of the hippocampal structures. The NFT coincide with the SP in fronto temporal regions but their presence is lower in not limbic structures.
Recent studies in patients with AD show that less than one third of cases had a "pure" disease, being more frequent association of SP and NFT with vascular lesions (50%) or Lewy bodies (20 %).

2.2.3 Vascular changes

Over 80% of patients have cerebral amyloid angiopathy, which affects the pial vessels of the brain and especially the capillaries, which become refined, atrophic, fragmented and distorted. Endothelial basement membrane is thickened and disrupted, with amyloid deposits and collagen which is associated with an inflammatory response that includes the vascular endothelium, perivascular microglia, pericytes and astrocytes, interfering with the functioning of the blood-brain barrier (BBB) (Bowman et al., 2007).
The muscular layer shows segmentary contractions and peripheral vascular plexus is impaired or absent. Often these changes are accompanied by ischemic or hemorrhagic lesions.
A meta-analysis included 5 studies and 450 patients (Cordonnier and van der Flier, 2011) finds that in 23% of cases are characterized by microbleeding with focal leakage of hemosiderin from small abnormal blood vessels. Microbleedings prevalence is higher in AD patients than in subjects with mild cognitive impairment, while in the general population is

rare. The microbleedings are distributed in cortico-subcortical regions predominantly in the occipital lobe, a pattern shared with amyloid angiopathy (Zlokovic, 2008).

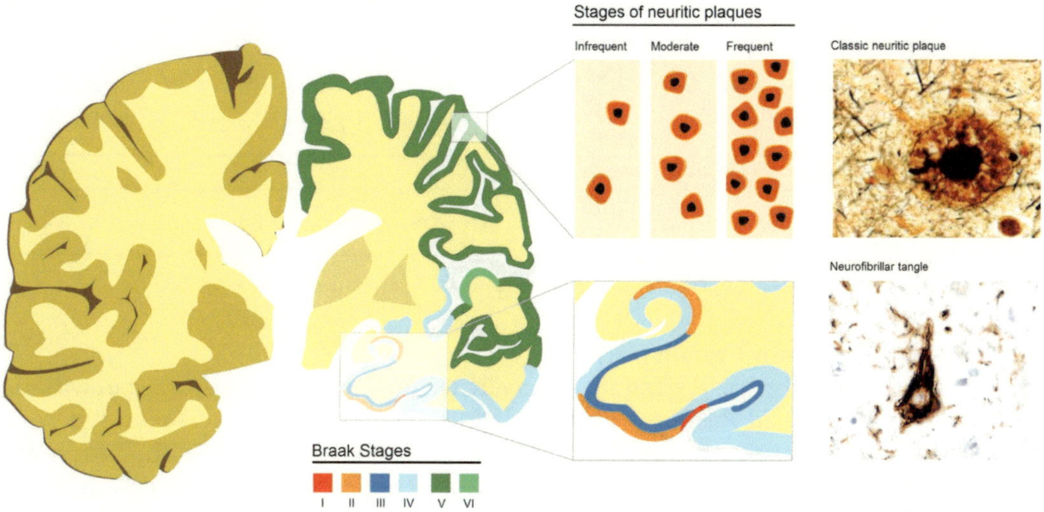

Fig. 3. Schematic representation of a hemisphere of a normal subject (left) and a hemisphere of a person with AD (right). A scale of colors represent the Braak´s NFT stages. The first stages are entorhinal (I and II) with absent or mild symptoms. Stages III and IV are called limbic and are associated with memory deficit (which influences the intellectual reserve) and subtle changes of personality. In cortical stages (V and VI) adding further deterioration in neocortical regions with the reverse pattern of myelination, affecting primarily the association areas and finally the primary areas. The stages of senile plaques are represented in the top.

2.2.4 Other less specific findings include

- Inclusions and pigments: Lipofuscin, Hirano bodies (actin) and Lewy bodies (alpha synuclein).
- Granulovacuolar degeneration: The presence of intra-neuronal vacuoles (3 to 5 microns) that can be associated or not with NFT. It is mostly found in the hippocampus.
- Other: satellitosis, neuronofagia and fragmentation are stages of neuronal death mediated by glia.

3. Genetics

The AD is an entity with genetic and clinical heterogeneity. There are familial and sporadic forms (Table 2).

3.1 Familial AD

The familial AD forms are relatively rare, less than 10% and have an autosomal dominant pattern. The debut occur at an early age (Early Onstet AD or EAOD), characterized by cognitive impairment associated with other neurological signs such as spasticity, motor control disorders, ataxia and seizures.

Debut	Chromosome	Herency	Product
Early Onset Alzheimer Disease (EOAD)			
28-50	14	Autosomal Dominant	Presenilin 1
40-50	1	Autosomal Dominant	Presenilin 2
55-65	21	Autosomal Dominant	amyloid precursor protein (APP)
Late Onset Alzheimer Disease (LOAD)			
Later or never	19	Autosomal Recesive	Apolipoprotein E4

Table 2. Relation between genotype and phenotype in Alzheimer´s Disease (AD)

3.1.1 Amyloid Precursor Protein (APP)

The first advances in the understanding of genetic factors related to the AD began with the discovery of the Amyloid Precursor Protein (APP) in brain of carriers of Down syndrome with cognitive impairment. The gene encoding this protein is located in the 21q21 locus and is inherited in an autosomal dominant pattern of early onset. More than 32 missense mutations have now been described in 85 families.

The APP gene encodes by alternative splicing. The larger form is a polypeptide of 770 amino acids. Alternative splicing of exon 7 encoding the Kurnitz domain and exon 8 encoding the OX-2 antigen wich is a polypeptide of 695 amino acids that predominate and other of 751, less frequent. So far their function is unknown, although presumably involved in the regulation of neuronal plasticity and signal transduction.

3.1.2 Presenilin 1 (PSEN1)

Presenilin (PSEN) is the major component of the gamma-secretase. The Locus of PSEN1 was found on chromosome 14q24.2. The PSEN1 is a polytopic membrane protein that forms the catalytic center of the gamma-secretase complex. Other functions independent of βA are the acidification of vacuoles by the addition of ATPase, required for autophagy, calcium regulation and stimulation of neuronal growth and survival (Pimplikar et al., 2010).

Depending on the PSEN1 mutation type may be an increase or decrease in the production of beta-amyloid. Missense mutations of PSEN1 have full penetrance and are the most common cause of early-onset familial AD, between 25-65 years, causing the more severe clinical forms.

3.1.3 Presenilin 2 (PSEN2)

The locus is located on 1q42.13. PSEN2 is expressed in a variety of tissues including the brain, primarily in neurons. Their mutations are rare and only 14 variants have been described in six families.

3.1.4 Apolipoprotein E epsilon (APOE-ε)

The role of variations in the gene APOE-ε on chromosome 19q13.2 as a risk factor for late onset AD has been demonstrated. Its variations are associated with both late-onset familial AD and 20% of sporadic AD.

This gene has multiple alleles: E2, E3 and E4. In both, normal subjects and AD patients the least common is E2 and the most common is E3, but in subjects with AD the E4 allele has a frequency almost equal to E3. In its heterozygous composition APOE-ε4 gene increases the risk four times, with onset between 5 and 10 years earlier.

In subjects homozygous for APOE-ε 4, the risk is increased fifteen times with onset between 10 and 20 years earlier. It is noteworthy that 42% of patients with LOAD have not alleles APOE-ε 4 as its absence does not rule out the disease.

Under normal conditions, APOE is produced predominantly in astrocytes, whereas under stress neurons are the main source. APOE participates in the distribution and metabolism of cholesterol and triglycerides. APOE-ε 4 is less efficient than E2 and E3 variants for the reuptake and efflux of cholesterol in neurons and astrocytes. On the other hand, APOE-ε4 is more efficient for the aggregation of beta-amyloid.

3.2 Sporadic AD

Sporadic forms have onset of symptoms later, over 60 years (LOAD). A large proportion of these cases have a family history of dementia suggesting a strong genetic component. On the other hand, the history of a first degree relative diagnosed with AD increase the risk of AD from two to seven times.

Attempts to demonstrate associations between genetic variations and sporadic AD others than APOE-ε4 has been inconsistent and rarely replicated. This scenario has been changing over the past three years with the results of studies of Genome Wide Association Studies (GWAS).

An article that reviews 15 GWAS (Bertram et al., 2010) confirms once again the relevance of the APOE gene variations as the most important risk factor in sporadic AD. At the same time new candidate genes have begun to emerge. Among the most notable are genes involved in beta-amyloid metabolism: Ataxin1 (ATX1), Siglec33 (CD33), Clusterin aka Apolipoprotein J (CLU-APOJ), Complement Component (3b/4b) receptor 1 (CR1); regulators of Tau phosphorylation: GRB2-Associated Binding Protein 2 (GAB2) and modulators of synaptic transmission as Protocadherin11 X linked (PCDH11X) and Inositol Phosphatydil Clathrin Assembly Binding Protein (PICALM).

However, it is appropriate to remember that these new variants increase the risk only from 0.10 to 0.15 times suggesting that, rather than the independent effect should be referred to the impact of gene networks. Overall, mutations in APOE and new variants described and confirmed could justify up to 50% of cases of sporadic AD.

Neuro Image Alzheimer's Disease Initiative (ADNI) extends the capacity of association between genetic variants and phenotypes of the AD because provides data from neuroimaging and other biomarkers. One of the most interesting findings of this study is the linear relationship between the number of alleles PICALM G and thinning of the entorhinal cortex, an effect that is independent of APOE variants (Saykin et al., 2010).

4. Pathogenesis

Traditionally attention has focused on the typical lesions and its primary components: the βA of the SP and tau protein in the NFT, examining the impact that the accumulation of these compounds in different parts of the brain tissue. Currently the research focus has shifted to the initial and solubles states of both metabolic pathways: amyloid cascade and tau phosphorylation, trying to unravel the relationship between them and their earlier effects.

4.1 Amyloid beta metabolism

The βA is a small peptide fragment of a transmembrane protein called amyloid precursor protein (APP). This protein is found in cytoplasmic membranes, endosomal and Golgi system of the nervous system and blood cells. Both the APP and its products, including the βA can also be located in mitochondria. Certain isoforms of APP have a domain protease inhibitor Kunitz regulating the coagulation cascade. In normal subjects the βA peptide is fragmented by a protein alpha-secretase which divides into two segments forming nexin II modulator action of coagulation and the βA of 16 amino acid peptide highly soluble.

This βA peptide binds to alpha 2 macroglobulin, which signals the proteins to be degraded and form a βA-A2M complex that binds to a protease. The product of these interactions is reintroduced into the nerve cell to adhere to them first through A2M for the membrane receptor that is common to LDL and APOE.

There is an alternative way that is the complete detachment of the peptide βA 40 to 42 amino acids. This occurs by the action of beta-secretase BACE (division 1) and gamma-secretase (split 40-42). The gamma secretase is composed of four segments: presenilin, nicastrin, APH-1 PEN2 and presenilin, the active site. βA 1-42 segments are more difficult to degrade and tend to aggregate to form oligomers (OM). Monomers do not produce damage, however, since dimers formed are capable of causing cell death mediated by microglia.

Although OM can be composed of aggregates of 2 to 100 peptides, the most frequents are the compounds for 3 to 7 segments. Unlike the SP, which are usually away from the regions of greatest damage, the OM has a wider distribution and can cause functional and structural changes in regions typically affected in AD, for example the entorhinal cortex and CA1, respecting initially CA3 and Cerebellum. Synapse loss and cognitive impairment correlates well with the concentration of OM, but not with SP. On the other hand, the OM may diminish or even abolish Long Term Potentiation (LTP), an effect that is selective because it does not affect Excitatory Post Synaptic Potential (EPSP) or Long Term Depression (LTD).

Apparently these changes in electrical activity are mediated by prion receptors PrPc, molecules with which the OM have a high affinity. Indeed, blocking these receptors with anti-PrPc antibodies can reverse the behavioral and learning disorders in experimental models of AD in mice (Chung et al., 2010). Larger aggregates called Proto fibrils (PF) are also able to induce toxicity and cell death, however, these molecules are less stable (Klein, 2002).

Apolipoprotein J (APOJ) secreted by astrocytes may prevent the formation of PF, but not of OM, in fact facilitates their aggregation by increasing the substrate and serve as a chaperone. Interestingly, Clum-APOJ mutations are well replicated as risk factors in GWAS studies.

Finally, the formation of insoluble fibrils, whose center is composed of 1-42 βA which is then added βA 1-40, accumulates in the interstice where suffers the loss of helical conformation (alpha helix) to adopt a beta sheet conformation, very difficult to degrade. These complexes achieve stability by association with several proteins, including SAP (Serum Amyloid Component) very stable and only degradable in the liver and accompanying amyloid deposits from any source (Figure 4A). The presence of these bodies cause the activation of the immune system, especially the microglia, which perpetuate the inflammation and injury by free radicals.

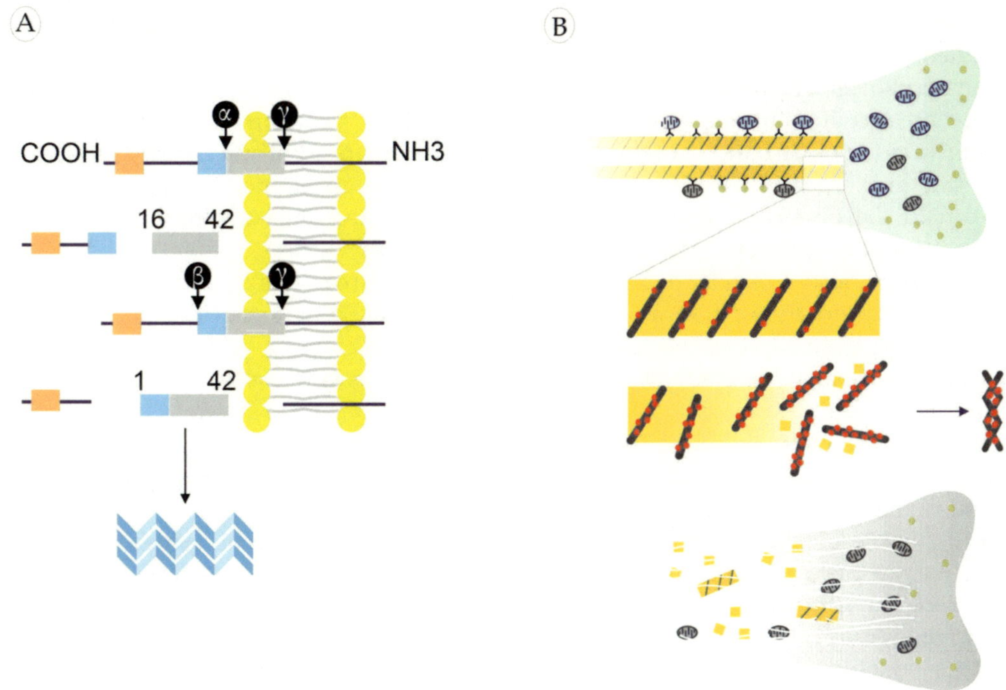

Fig. 4. A) The amyloid beta is part of a transmembrane protein whose end is intracellular NH3 and extracellular COOH. Cleavage by alpha and gamma secretases produces a peptide 16-42 very soluble and easily degradable. The alternative cleavage by beta and gamma secretases produces insoluble 1-42 peptide, then added in formation of folded sheets, very difficult to degrade.
B). Tau proteins are part of the microtubule-associated proteins. The hyperphosphorylation of these proteins causes a disruption of the cytoskeleton engaging features such as maintaining the structure and intracellular transport. Hyperphosphorylated tau proteins forming paired helices very difficult to degrade. This eventually leads to neuronal death and depopulation.

4.2 Neurofibrillary metabolism

The NFT are mainly composed of paired helical filaments formed by hyperphosphorylated tau protein. They are also formed by other proteins such as MAP2 (predominantly in dendrites), ubiquitin, and βA peptides, supporting the theory of amyloidogenesis as a primary lesion.

Tau proteins predominate in axons and form the group of MAP (Microtubule Associated Protein) interacting with microtubules during cell movement and transport assembling or disassembling the microtubules depending on whether there lengthening or shortening of the extensions, especially in axons. Recent research has found that tau proteins are also located in the dendrites, although in a much lower concentration. Here are involved in cytoskeletal functions and signal transduction by facilitating the activity of protein tyrosine kinase FYN (FYN), which phosphorylates the 2B subunit of N-Methyl-D-aspartate (NMDA) receptors, mediating their interaction with Protein Posinaptic Density (PSD-95). This interaction is critical for the efficiency of the synapse and in its absence there is a decrease of experimental seizures (Ittner et al., 2010).

Tau hyperphosphorylation has several effects. First results in their haste and self-aggregation forming, in the case of AD paired helical filaments that impede axonal transport. On the other hand, Tau-p have a greater affinity for FYN and thereby increase its concentration in the dendrites. This leads to a shift in the concentration of Tau protein from the axon to the dendrites, finally occupying the soma and breaking the cell dynamics leading eventually apoptotic neurodegeneration (figure 4 B).

An interesting question is why does the progression and spread of Tau-p follows a route so stereotyped as proposed in the anatomical and pathological Braak´s stages?

In our view there are two possible answers:

1. This pattern shows a gradient of susceptibility to increasing exposure to an aggressor factor. In this case the obvious candidate would be the OM. However, as we have seen, after a first phase, the deposition rate of βA and PIB-PET load stabilizes, while the spread and damage induced by Tau-p continues at the same time that the neuronal loss and cognitive impairment
2. Tau-p molecules and their aggregates do not require external factors, but these formations have a prion-like behavior. Tau-p are seeds that can penetrate the cell and recruit Tau functional molecules making them hyper-phosphorylated forms. Thus continues the cycle of aggregation and spreading the damage to other areas.

The latter possibility seems to be reinforced by an experimental model that achieved with very small concentrations of Tau-p and in a short time, a degree of infection similar to that observed in tissues of patients with AD (prion-like dissemination). (Clavaguera et al., 2009;Guo and Lee, 2011).

4.3 Relationship between Tau and βA metabolism

A complex problem is determining which is the primary lesion and the relationship between them. There are some facts that suggest that the primary is the βA accumulation. For example, βA accumulation precedes the presence of NFT. Also been achieved KO mice that produce accumulation βA with all the features of these lesions without neurofibrillary tangles. These mice have cognitive deficits comparable to that human AD. Moreover, the demonstration of tau protein as a basis for degenerations with dementia that occur (Frontotemporal dementia and parkinsonism linked to chromosome 17; Progressive Supranuclear Palsy and Pick's dementia) in the absence of SP, support the protagonism of the NFT.

A very interesting hypothesis has been proposed by Ittner and Gotz, called "Tau Axis Hypothesis" (Ittner and Gotz, 2011). Here suggest that the presence of Tau protein in the dendrite is essential for OM mediated toxicity. In fact, in experimental models the absence of interaction Tau-FYN prevents the development of cognitive, behavioral disorders or neuronal degeneration induced by OM. On the other hand, increasing the concentration of OM increases the phosphorylation of Tau protein, which moves them to the dendrites and increases its affinity for FYN, closing a vicious circle.

4.4 Vascular factors

The frecuent presence of vascular lesions in patients with AD and the results of epidemiological studies suggest that vascular risk factors increase the likelihood of suffering

from AD and once established, accelerate the progression of cognitive impairment. The most important are hypertension, advanced age, atherosclerosis, homocystinemia, hyperlipidemia, metabolic syndrome and obesity. Cerebral vascular lesions, especially lacunar infarcts increase to double the risk of AD (Ott et al., 1999).
It also showed that cerebral hypoperfusion precedes onset of clinical dementia and that the reduction in cerebral blood flow (CBF) occurs before cognitive impairment and hippocampal atrophy. This is consistent with results achieved by our group.
The Nun Study (Snowdon et al., 1997) relates the number of vascular lesions with the severity of Alzheimer's disease by showing that individuals with one or two lacunar infarctions had a greater cognitive deterioration than individuals who had no stroke, regardless of the number of neurofibrillary tangles in the cortex.
Experimental studies in rodents have shown that chronic cerebral hypo-perfusion and transient cerebral ischemia increases the production of amyloid peptide precursor, beta amyloid protein and the accumulation of hyperphosphorylated Tau protein, which simulates the changes of Alzheimer's disease. However, these conditions of intense ischemia are not present in normal subjects or patients with AD.
The beta amyloid peptide has a vasoconstrictor effect, which could be related to the early decrease in CBF and the narrowing of the average diameter capillary. In AD the mean diameter capillary is decreased, which is associated with cognitive impairment even before the accumulation of SP and NFT.
In the AD there is an increase of Advanced Glycation End products (AGE) that accumulate on the walls of blood vessels. In addition, the concentrations of AGE receptors (RAGE) are several times increased in vessels, microglia and neurons. The binding of βA to RAGE in the luminal membrane of the BBB leads to the peripheral βA input in to the brain followed by binding to neurons. Increased RAGE becomes a pro-inflammatory signal that activates microglia (Zlokovic, 2008).
Low density lipoprotein receptor related protein 1 (LRP) is a member of the family of LDL and a major clearance receptor for βA at the BBB. LRP concentrations decline with age and are particularly low in the elderly and patients with AD.
BBB dysfunction is early and confirmed by a series of morphological changes such as reducing the number of mitochondria, tight junctions, loss of pericytes and the presence of pinocytotic in cerebral microvessels.
In a clinical study showed the BBB impairement in 22% of patients with AD (Bowman et al., 2007). The rate of damage progression was measured by concentrations of albumin in Cerebrospinal Fluid (CSF) and correlated with worsening of cognitive performance.
Cholinergic nuclei, dramatically affected in AD, have a regulatory effect on CBF, particularly groups of the substantia innominata and the Nuclei basalis magnocellularis (SI / NBM). In healthy volunteers who were given Scopolamine, the CBF decreased from 20%.
The opposite effect was found in an experimental study where chronic deep electrical stimulation of the region SI / NBM produced a sustained increase in CBF in basal ganglion and Cortex, particularly in fronto parietal regions.

4.5 Cerebral insulin resistance

Insulin in the brain plays an important role in regulating metabolism, and alterations in activity are directly related to metabolic diseases such as obesity, diabetes or metabolic syndrome. In the mammalian brain, insulin induces anorexia, weight loss and regulates the hypothalamic control of food intake.

The insulin receptor (IR) is a glycoprotein of 300 to 400 kDa, formed by two identical alpha chains located in the extracellular region and two beta subunits that end within the cytosol, the beta chains have intrinsic tyrosine kinase activity. The IR is found in higher concentrations in neurons when compared with the glial cells. The IR is distribuited at the brain structures in different densities, they expression have proved at the olfactory bulb, hypothalamus, pituitary, choroid plexus, thalamus, piriform cortex, hippocampal formation, amygdaloid nuclei, prefrontal cortex and cerebellum. The IR largest concentrations are at the level of the olfactory bulb, hypothalamus, hippocampus and cerebellum. The IR is widely found in the synapses, especially in the dendritic tree where it regulates neurotransmitter release and the recruitment of receptors.

Within the brain, function of Insulin / Insulin like Growth Factor (IGF) include stimulation of neuronal and oligodendroglial survival, growth factor, regulation of mitochondrial function and energy metabolism, expression of Tau and acetylcholine transferase.

The IGF2 is abundantly expressed in the hippocampus. Recent research shows that IGF2 plays an essential role in the regulation of LTP and memory consolidation, one of the cognitive functions affected in early stages of AD (Chen et al., 2011).

The search for an association between insulin metabolism and AD brain has been extensively investigated in recent years. The starting point takes place in epidemiological studies wich strongly indicate that diabetes mellitus (DM) is a risk factor for AD. A closer look identifies insulin resistance as risk factor independent of changes in blood sugar levels. In people with insulin resistance and cognitive impairment without DM there is a reduction in the rate of cerebral glucose utilization. This pattern is also different in people with DM type 2 or pre DM during the execution of cognitive tasks, suggesting that insulin resistance could be taken as an early marker of AD (Baker et al., 2011).

Unlike the vascular brain disease that affects mainly CA1, a region highly susceptible to ischemia, insuline resistance selectively damaged the entorhinal cortex, one of the first areas involved in AD.

Biochemical and genetic data show that insulin degrading enzyme (IDE) is involved in insulin and Aβ homeostasis. The expression and activity of IDE is significantly decreased in AD brains compared with age-matched controls. In addition, IDE and Aβ are deposited in SP and vessels, indicating a gross conformational change by post-translational mechanisms. These changes in the distribution and activity of IDE may result in hormone resistance, insufficient degradation of insulin and Aβ, formation of Aβ oligomers and neurodegeneration.

The possibility that the AD is the result of a selective insulin resistance in the brain has been proposed by de la Monte et al. with solid clinical and experimental arguments that crystallize into a new concept: the DM type 3 (de la Monte and Wands, 2008).

In post mortem studies of brains affected by AD were significant decreases in concentrations of Insulin and Insulin like Growth Factor (IGF). By comparing the expression of IGF with Braak´s stages shows that the involvement is early and progressive decline increasingly as they progress Braak´s stages, what is more remarkable for IGF1.

Streptozocin experimental models in rats lead to a selective reduction of the expression of insulin / IGF in the brain without changing peripheral levels of glucose or insulin. In these animals are changes similar to the AD such as increased BA, Tau phosphorylation, neurodegeneration and gliosis and decreased genes associated with neurons,

oligodendroglia, and acetyl choline transferase, while increase genes related to microglia and inflammation (de la Monte and Wands, 2008).
Other factors that may have some weight in neuronal loss and progression of damage are: the development of inflammatory changes, damage to mitochondria, the energy imbalance, the increased production of free radicals, the problems of calcium metabolism, the toxicity of some elements such as aluminum, inefficient autophagy and suppression of neurogenesis.

5. Clinical expression

As we have seen, there are many factors which interact and are interwoven pathways, increasing the capacity of injury in different brain areas, which is expressed as a progressive cognitive deficit, which begins as a disorder of recent memory and then progresses to affect in advanced stages, the majority of brain functions. Each pathway described above can be added to the final damage but there are two main theories that justify the initial cognitive deficits of AD, these are: The "Theory of cortical disconnection" and "Cholinergic theory".

5.1 Theory of cortical disconnection

Neurofibrillary tangles in the entorhinal cortex, wich is the cortical portal of the hippocampus, are distributed in layers II, which together with the layer III form the perforant pathway to the hippocampus and the layer IV receiving eference from the hippocampus. In this way hippocampus is isolated from the neocortex. This adds to the deficit of glutamate and other neuropeptides such as neuropeptide Y, oxytocin, vasopressin and somatostatin in the association cortices adding a cortico-cortical disconnection that correlates with aphasia, apraxia and agnosia, as well as visuospatial and executives disorders. At first the degeneration is slight and apparently can be offset by the cognitive reserve, however, as neurodegeneration progresses, this mechanism is not sufficient. The techniques of functional magnetic resonance imaging at 7 Tesla can define in vivo the degree of atrophy of specific regions of the hippocampus (Kerchner et al., 2010)..

5.2 Cholinergic theory

In advanced stages there is a decrease of over 90% of the activity of acetylcholinesterase which identifies a dramatic impairment of the cholinergic system in this disease. This causes early and progressive memory affection. One study suggests that progression of cholinergic deficit is not linear but at an early stage levels rise, falling years later. This is similar to what occurs with serotonin (Dekosky et al., 2002).
The selective degeneration of the nucleus basalis of Meynert, principal cholinergic eference to neocortex and septal nuclei and diagonal band of Broca, subcortical cholinergic eference, especially to the hippocampus, cause a progressive anterograde memory. Some authors hypothesize that the clinical expresion of depression needs some indemnity of cholinergic pathways, close to normal levels, which occurs only in initial stages.
As mentioned before, there is evidence of early changes in regional CBF, which could be related to the degeneration of cholinergic population that has a regulatory effect. This is known as the cholinergic-vascular theory.
As part of a research project in our institution (International Center of Neurological Restauration-CIREN), and with the collaboration of other Cubans institutions, we compared the global cerebral blood flow (gCBF) in absolute units (ml/min/100 g) at resting state

between 38 controls and 40 amnestic MCI subjects, both groups with similar demographic and vascular risk factors (limited). We explored also a possible association between gCBF and cognitive function, after controlling for age, gender, level of education and global brain atrophy (quantified on 3D T1-weighted MRI images). gCBF was measured by spectral analysis of radionuclide angiography, which is a simple and non-invasive method for the quantification of gCBF (Murase et al., 1999;Van et al., 2001) and linearly correlated with gCBF measured by using PET (Takasawa et al., 2004). Our results show a significant decrease of gCBF in the MCI group as compared with controls ($p < 0.05$, Mann-Whitney U Test, figure 5).

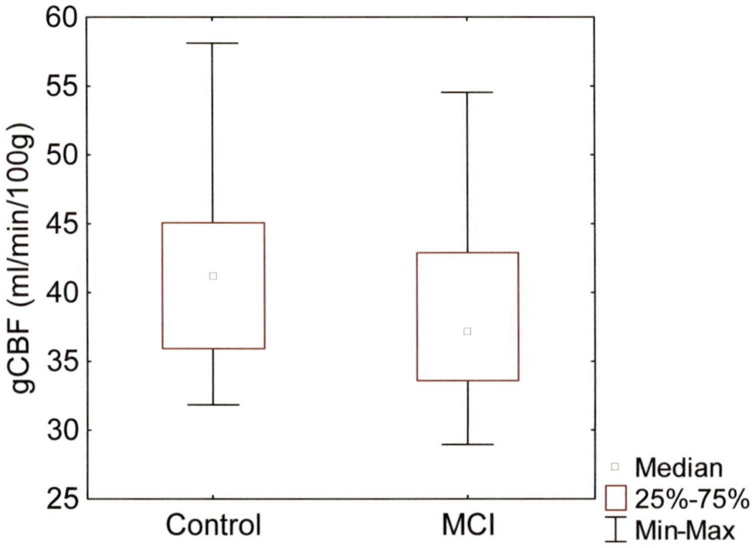

Fig. 5. MCI group show less gCBF than control group.

We also found in the MCI group a direct association between gCBF and semantically unrelated word-pairs learning (immediate recall) as measured by the hard-word pairs learning score of the Wechsler memory scale (Spearman $R = 0.46$, $p < 0.005$, figure 6), after removing the effects of age, gender, level of education and global brain atrophy (standardized z_scores). Control subjects show no association.

Interestingly, other domains of cognitive function (attention, episodic memory, working memory, verbal fluency, praxis and executive function) show no association with gCBF. Thus verbal learning is probably more sensitive than other cognitive functions in MCI patients, particularly semantically unrelated word-pairs learning. Many studies have reported very early deficits in associative memory in MCI patients, which is the ability to associate unrelated items presented together during the encoding phase, or to associate one item to its spatial or visual context (Belleville et al., 2008).

The decrease of gCBF observed in our MCI group cannot be explained by a clear vascular cause, related to demographic variables or brain atrophy. One possible explanation of our findings could be to assume a gradual reduction of cholinergic vasodilatory innervations of cerebral blood vessels as a result of a gradual cholinergic deficit originating in the basal forebrain, which also affect learning and memory (Schliebs and Arendt, 2006). This assumption is supported by previous studies (Claassen and Jansen, 2006;Farkas and Luiten, 2001).

A way to confirm a gradual reduction of regional vasodilatory innervations in the MCI state would be to study the cerebrovascular reserve and find out the connection with cognitive decline. This study will be the subject of further research. Perhaps a more complete evaluation of this topic could be the combined studies in the same MCI subjects (or equivalent animal model) of cerebral blood flow and direct measurements of cholinergic activity and plaque formation (for example, using PET imaging). Recent studies suggest an interaction between vascular, cholinergic and "amyloid β" hypotheses of AD.

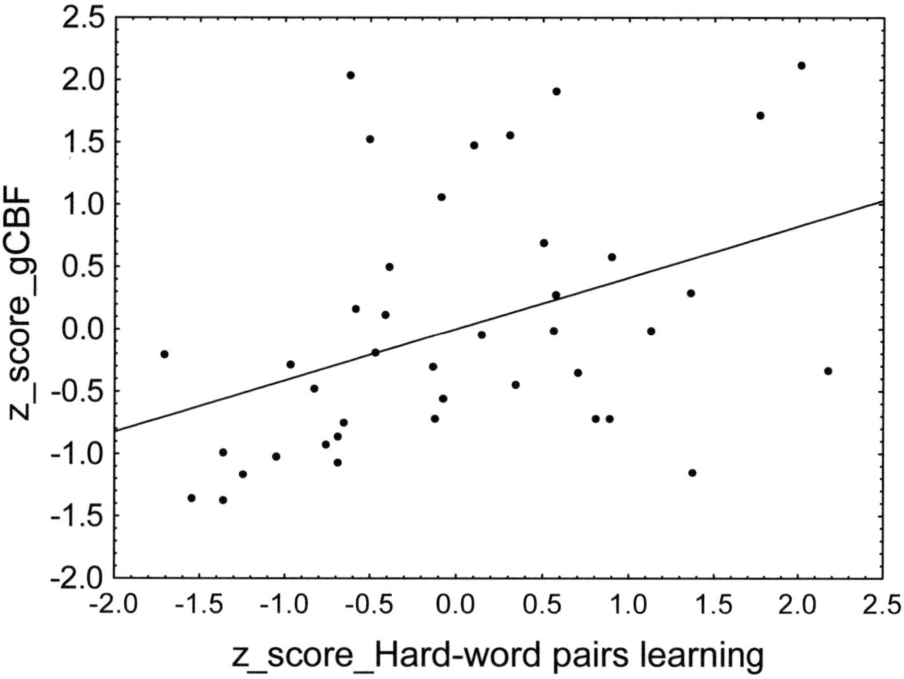

Fig. 6. There is a positive correlation between gCBF and semantically unrelated word-pairs learning in the MCI group.

5.3 Role of others neurotransmitters

Other neurotransmitter imbalances better explain the non-cognitive symptoms. As mentioned, there is a greater involvement of the raphe nuclei, the nucleus ceruleus and a relative sparing of the substantia nigra.

Serotonin deficit. It is related to depressive symptoms as well as obsession, compulsion and aggression. This is observed both in AD and in normal people. A study with Fluoro-benzamidoethylpiperazine-PET shows that in Mild Cognitive Impairment patients exists up-regulation of hippocampal serotonin, apparently as a compensatory mechanism. Once the AD is stablished, serotonin levels falls. (Truchot et al., 2007).

Noradrenaline deficit. It is also observed associated with depression and psychomotor agitation. With this neurotransmitter occurs something unique because although there is a depoblaction of nucleus ceruleus (where there are Lewy bodies), there is a cortical noradrenergic hyperactivity, which is attributed to an increased sensitivity and the production of cortical noradrenaline. The increased sensitivity is observed in the prefrontal cortex and in the hippocampus. However, the increased concentration of noradrenaline is only found in the prefrontal cortex. In cases of depression there is noradrenaline decrease, while those with agitation there is an increase.

Relative dopamine preservation. This causes an imbalance choline / dopamine with the relative increase of the latter, a substrate of observed hallucinations, sleep disorders and psychosis. In 30% of AD patients there is a decrease of dopamine with the presence of a parkinsonian syndrome. However, the preservation of posture and gait to advanced stages is a characteristic of cortical dementia.

6. Conclusions

Currently there are notable advances in understanding the basic mechanisms of AD. This has allowed the design of biomarkers of the disease in vivo wich are able to define its presence, with a high degree of sensitivity and specificity, even before establishing the cognitive deficits characteristic of this entity. This has led to reconsider the diagnostic criteria and include diagnostic tools such as PIB-PET, Magnetic Resonance and Cerebrospinal Fluid (Dubois et al., 2007).

This extends the time for preventive or early intervention, using new treatments designed to block the damage in the early stages of the cascade of events. The prevention of risk factors and the use of new drugs such as fibrillar aggregation inhibitors, intranasal insulin and anti-PrPc antibodies promise to change the current scenario, dominated by discrete symptomatic treatment gains.

7. References

Alladi, S., J. Xuereb, T. Bak, P. Nestor, J. Knibb, K. Patterson, and J. R. Hodges, 2007, Focal cortical presentations of Alzheimer's disease: Brain, v. 130, no. Pt 10, p. 2636-2645.

Baker, L. D., D. J. Cross, S. Minoshima, D. Belongia, G. S. Watson, and S. Craft, 2011, Insulin resistance and Alzheimer-like reductions in regional cerebral glucose metabolism for cognitively normal adults with prediabetes or early type 2 diabetes: Arch.Neurol., v. 68, no. 1, p. 51-57.

Belleville, S., S. Sylvain-Roy, B. C. de, and M. C. Menard, 2008, Characterizing the memory changes in persons with mild cognitive impairment: Prog.Brain Res., v. 169, p. 365-375.

Bertram, L., C. M. Lill, and R. E. Tanzi, 2010, The genetics of Alzheimer disease: back to the future: Neuron, v. 68, no. 2, p. 270-281.

Bowman, G. L., J. A. Kaye, M. Moore, D. Waichunas, N. E. Carlson, and J. F. Quinn, 2007, Blood-brain barrier impairment in Alzheimer disease: stability and functional significance: Neurology, v. 68, no. 21, p. 1809-1814.

Chen, D. Y., S. A. Stern, A. Garcia-Osta, B. Saunier-Rebori, G. Pollonini, D. Bambah-Mukku, R. D. Blitzer, and C. M. Alberini, 2011, A critical role for IGF-II in memory consolidation and enhancement: Nature, v. 469, no. 7331, p. 491-497.

Chung, E., Y. Ji, Y. Sun, R. J. Kascsak, R. B. Kascsak, P. D. Mehta, S. M. Strittmatter, and T. Wisniewski, 2010, Anti-PrPC monoclonal antibody infusion as a novel treatment for cognitive deficits in an Alzheimer's disease model mouse: BMC.Neurosci., v. 11, p. 130.

Claassen, J. A., and R. W. Jansen, 2006, Cholinergically mediated augmentation of cerebral perfusion in Alzheimer's disease and related cognitive disorders: the cholinergic-vascular hypothesis: J.Gerontol.A Biol.Sci.Med.Sci., v. 61, no. 3, p. 267-271.

Clavaguera, F. et al., 2009, Transmission and spreading of tauopathy in transgenic mouse brain: Nat.Cell Biol., v. 11, no. 7, p. 909-913.

Cordonnier, C., and W. M. van der Flier, 2011, Brain microbleeds and Alzheimer's disease: innocent observation or key player?: Brain, v. 134, no. Pt 2, p. 335-344.

de la Monte, S. M., and J. R. Wands, 2008, Alzheimer's disease is type 3 diabetes-evidence reviewed: J.Diabetes Sci.Technol., v. 2, no. 6, p. 1101-1113.

Dekosky, S. T., M. D. Ikonomovic, S. D. Styren, L. Beckett, S. Wisniewski, D. A. Bennett, E. J. Cochran, J. H. Kordower, and E. J. Mufson, 2002, Upregulation of choline acetyltransferase activity in hippocampus and frontal cortex of elderly subjects with mild cognitive impairment: Ann.Neurol., v. 51, no. 2, p. 145-155.

Dubois, B. et al., 2007, Research criteria for the diagnosis of Alzheimer's disease: revising the NINCDS-ADRDA criteria: Lancet Neurol., v. 6, no. 8, p. 734-746.

Engler, H. et al., 2006, Two-year follow-up of amyloid deposition in patients with Alzheimer's disease: Brain, v. 129, no. Pt 11, p. 2856-2866.

Farkas, E., and P. G. Luiten, 2001, Cerebral microvascular pathology in aging and Alzheimer's disease: Prog.Neurobiol., v. 64, no. 6, p. 575-611.

Guo, J. L., and V. M. Lee, 2011, Seeding of normal tau by pathological tau conformers drives pathogenesis of Alzheimer-like tangles: J.Biol.Chem..

Ittner, L. M., and J. Gotz, 2011, Amyloid-beta and tau--a toxic pas de deux in Alzheimer's disease: Nat.Rev.Neurosci., v. 12, no. 2, p. 65-72.

Ittner, L. M. et al., 2010, Dendritic function of tau mediates amyloid-beta toxicity in Alzheimer's disease mouse models: Cell, v. 142, no. 3, p. 387-397.

Kerchner, G. A., C. P. Hess, K. E. Hammond-Rosenbluth, D. Xu, G. D. Rabinovici, D. A. Kelley, D. B. Vigneron, S. J. Nelson, and B. L. Miller, 2010, Hippocampal CA1 apical neuropil atrophy in mild Alzheimer disease visualized with 7-T MRI: Neurology, v. 75, no. 15, p. 1381-1387.

Klein, W. L., 2002, Abeta toxicity in Alzheimer's disease: globular oligomers (ADDLs) as new vaccine and drug targets: Neurochem.Int., v. 41, no. 5, p. 345-352.

Koivunen, J. et al., 2008, PET amyloid ligand [11C]PIB uptake shows predominantly striatal increase in variant Alzheimer's disease: Brain, v. 131, no. Pt 7, p. 1845-1853.

Murase, K., T. Inoue, H. Fujioka, Y. Ishimaru, A. Akamune, Y. Yamamoto, T. Mochizuki, and J. Ikezoe, 1999, An alternative approach to estimation of the brain perfusion index for measurement of cerebral blood flow using technetium-99m compounds: Eur.J.Nucl.Med., v. 26, no. 10, p. 1333-1339.

Ott, A., R. P. Stolk, H. F. van, H. A. Pols, A. Hofman, and M. M. Breteler, 1999, Diabetes mellitus and the risk of dementia: The Rotterdam Study: Neurology, v. 53, no. 9, p. 1937-1942.

Pimplikar, S. W., R. A. Nixon, N. K. Robakis, J. Shen, and L. H. Tsai, 2010, Amyloid-independent mechanisms in Alzheimer's disease pathogenesis: J.Neurosci., v. 30, no. 45, p. 14946-14954.

Saykin, A. J. et al., 2010, Alzheimer's Disease Neuroimaging Initiative biomarkers as quantitative phenotypes: Genetics core aims, progress, and plans: Alzheimers.Dement., v. 6, no. 3, p. 265-273.

Schliebs, R., and T. Arendt, 2006, The significance of the cholinergic system in the brain during aging and in Alzheimer's disease: J.Neural Transm., v. 113, no. 11, p. 1625-1644.

Schroeter, ML., Stein, T., Maslowski N. and Neumann J., 2009, Neural correlates of Alzheimer's disease and mild cognitive impairment: A systematic and quantitative meta-analysis involving 1351 patients. NeuroImage, v. 47, p. 1196–1206.

Snowdon, D. A., L. H. Greiner, J. A. Mortimer, K. P. Riley, P. A. Greiner, and W. R. Markesbery, 1997, Brain infarction and the clinical expression of Alzheimer disease. The Nun Study: JAMA, v. 277, no. 10, p. 813-817.

Takasawa, M. et al., 2004, Spectral analysis of 99mTc-HMPAO for estimating cerebral blood flow: a comparison with H2(15)O PET: Ann.Nucl.Med., v. 18, no. 3, p. 243-249.

Truchot, L. et al., 2007, Up-regulation of hippocampal serotonin metabolism in mild cognitive impairment: Neurology, v. 69, no. 10, p. 1012-1017.

Van, L. K., F. Dumont, M. Koole, and R. Dierckx, 2001, Non-invasive methods for absolute cerebral blood flow measurement using 99mTc-ECD: a study in healthy volunteers: Eur.J.Nucl.Med., v. 28, no. 7, p. 862-872.

Zlokovic, B. V., 2008, New therapeutic targets in the neurovascular pathway in Alzheimer's disease: Neurotherapeutics., v. 5, no. 3, p. 409-414.

2

Pathophysiology of Late Onset Alzheimer Disease

Ahmet Turan Isik[1] and M. Refik Mas[2]
[1]*Bezmialem Vakif University, Faculty of Medicine, Department of Geriatric Medicine, Istanbul,*
[2]*9 Eylul University, Faculty of Medicine, Department of Internal Medicine, Izmir*
Turkey

1. Introduction

As the world population has aged, the number of people affected by Alzheimer Disease is rapidly increasing in the world. It is important for clinicians to recognize early signs and symptoms of dementia and to note potentially modifiable risk factors and early disease markers.

Accumulation of Aβ peptides may be the key event in pathogenesis of AD. The exact mechanism by which Aβ peptide deposition induces neurotoxicity is unclear, but it appears the oxidative stress plays an important role. Oxidative stress is extensive in AD and Aβ peptides stimulate oxidative stress by both direct and indirect mechanisms. Aβ peptides by themselves may act as enzymes and can bind to mitochondrial proteins resulting in the generation of free radicals. Furthermore, Aβ peptides generate oxidative stress via neuroinflammation. Considerable evidence has supported that neuroinflammation is associated with AD pathology. In addition, in AD, vascular injury and parenchymal inflammation perpetuate the cycle of protein aggregation and oxidation in the brain, and diffuse pathological changes include cerebral amyloid angiopathy, affecting more than 90% of patients with Alzheimer's disease, capillary abnormalities, disruption of the blood-brain barrier, and large-vessel. In addition, it was reported that clearance of Aβ along diseased perivascular channels and through the blood-brain barrier is impeded in AD atheroma and that deregulation of Aβ transport across the capillary blood–brain barrier is caused by the imbalanced expression of low-density lipoprotein receptor-related proteins and receptors for advanced glycation end products. Besides, insulin resistance and hyperinsulinemia are implicated in a number of pathophysiological processes related to AD. It was demonstrated that reduced brain insulin signaling is associated with increased tau phosphorylation and Aβ levels in a streptozotocin induced model of diabetes mellitus. Moreover, insulin promotes the release of intracellular Aβ in neuronal cultures and accelerates Aβ trafficking to the plasma membrane. In addition, impaired insulin or insulin like growth factor-1 (IGF-1) signaling can result in the hyper-phosphorylation of tau, which can cause cell death mediated by apoptosis, mitochondrial dysfunction or necrosis and promote oxidative stress, which contributes to the neurodegeneration cascade and leads to dementia-associated behavioral and cognitive deficits.

In shortly, the current pathophysiological approach to LOAD are based on a number of common mechanisms of neurodegeneration, such as accumulation of abnormal proteins, mitochondrial dysfunction and oxidative stress, impaired insulin signaling, calcium homeostasis dysregulation, early synaptic disconnection and late apoptotic cell death. Aging itself is associated with mild cognitive deterioration, probably due to subtle multifactorial changes resulting in a global decrease of a functional brain reserve.

2. Pathophysiology of late onset Alzheimer disease

As the world population has aged, dementia has become a common diagnosis in aging populations and the numbers will increase in the forthcoming years. Nowadays, the number of people affected by Alzheimer Disease (AD) is rapidly increasing in the world. AD is an age-related progressive neurodegenerative disorder presented by memory loss and severe cognitive decline (Isik & Bozoglu, 2010).

AD is characterized by extensive atrophy of the brain caused by a series neuropathologic change, including neuronal loss, intracellular neurofibrillary tangles (NFTs) made up of Tau protein, extracellular senile plaques formed by β-amyloid (Aβ) and synaptic loss (Ballatore et al., 2007 & Haass Selkoe, 2007). Amyloid plaques and NFT result from an aberration in deposition of the Aβ peptide and the hyperphosphorylated tau protein, respectively, and these depositions lead to neuronal loss and neurotoxicity in the brain affected by AD (Isik, 2010). However, plaques and NFTs are not unique to AD, as these same structural changes occur with normal aging and in many others neurodegenerative disorders (Jackson-Siegal, 2005). Great confusion existed as to whether the dementia often observed in normal aging and AD were the same or different entities. It took nearly a century to define that the plaques were composed primarily of a specific peptide initially named A4 and today referred to as Aβ and that tangles are composed primarily of hyperphosphorylated forms of tau, a microtubule-associated protein. Tau is a protein known to stabilize microtubules present primarily in axonal processes and involved in axonal transport of subcellular components. The abnormal phosphorylation of this microtubule-related protein leads to molecular protein structures called paired helical filaments (PHFs), which constitute the ultrastructural core of the microscopic structures recognized as NTFs. Most contemporary research on the molecular basis of the disease has focused chiefly on these two proteins, and the causality of the disease has been attributed to either or both of these proteins. For a while, the two camps of thought were humorously referred to as the Baptists (for Aβ) and the Taoists (for tau) (Cuello, 2007). A distinguishing feature of AD is that the plaques and NFTs are localized to areas in the brain corresponding to the clinical symptoms. Although the development of plaques and NFTs eventually leads to a noticeable clinical condition, the process is thought to start years before the initial onset of symptoms (Jackson-Siegal, 2005).

3. Risk factors

Great number of nongenetic risk factors have been identified or proposed for the sporadic form of the disease. Of these, unequivocally, aging is the most relevant. To define between the AD and aging, that AD might reflect a continuum of the brain aging can be proposed. In other words, given the opportunity, every individual should eventually succumb to AD. This view can be supported by the undeniable fact that aging is the most important of the nongenetic risk factors as shown by the ever growing incidence of AD with aging. On the other hand, the prevalent notion is that the incidence of AD is influenced by a multitude of risks factors in addition to aging, which might act in a cooperative manner. The extent of the life span could also be regulated by the genetic background interacting with environmental as well as lifestyle aspects. The role of genetics in determining the life span is complex and paradoxical. In short, the prevalent view is that for the sporadic form of AD, it is not necessarily all in the genes but rather interplay with the life experience of that particular individual. The molecular mechanisms of brain aging remain elusive. Several molecular events are suspects in the age-related downfall of brain function, which might be linked to the earlier appearance of AD. Some researchers have paid attention to low levels of vitamin B complex and the plasma elevation of homocysteine, as being responsible for age-related cognitive deficits and unleashing the AD pathology (Cuello, 2007). Furthermore, our results demonstrated that replacement and close follow up of vitamin B12 deficiency are crucial in the elderly population regardless of any disturbance in the hematological parameters (Bozoglu et al., 2010).

While early onset AD is almost genetically based, there are no specific gene mutations that are associated with inheritance of the disease in late onset AD (LOAD). The expression of the apolipoprotein E (ApoE) 4 allele is one of the risk factors identified for LOAD. In the central nervous system, ApoE is synthesized by astrocytes, microglia, and, to a lesser extent, by neurons. The role of ApoE in LOAD pathogenesis is not fully elucidated, but it has been suggested that ApoE is very important in trafficking of amyloid β (Aβ) peptide. In addition, apolipoprotein J (clusterin), an amyloid β-peptide chaperone, TOMM40, a transporter of proteins across the mitochondrial membrane, and Sortillin-related receptor, which functions to partition amyloid precursor protein away from β-secretase and γ-secretase, are recently discovered proteins encoded by the risk genes for LOAD. However, it was reported that higher plasma concentrations of clusterin correlate significantly with the presence and severity of AD but doesn't correlate with the risk for onset of the disease (Schrijvers et al, 2011).

In addition to nonmodifiable genetic risk factors, potentially modifiable factors, such as hypertension, diabetes mellitus, hyperlipidemia, hyperhomocysteinemia, coronary and peripheral artery diseases, alcohol, smoking, obesity, levels of physical or mental activity, levels of education, and environmental exposures have been investigated to identify risk factors for LOAD. Furthermore, it has been reported that risk index methods including these risk factors provide a practical, flexible, and objective framework for identifying the optimal combination of measures for identification of high-risk individuals for prevention and early intervention efforts. Despite the personal and social burden of LOAD, our understanding of the genetic predisposition to LOAD and the contribution of other risk factors remains limited. More importantly, there are few data to explain the overall risks and benefits of prevention strategies or their impact on risk modification (Isik, 2010; Querfurth & La Ferla, 2010).

4. Pathogenesis

The amyloid material was initially thought to be systemically derived from serum proteins and characterized as a short peptide (9). Aβ peptides are natural products of metabolism consisting of 36 to 43 amino acids. Monomers of Aβ40 are more prevalent than the aggregation-prone and damaging Aβ42 species. β-amyloid peptides originate from proteolysis of the amyloid precursor protein (APP) lodged in cell membranes by the sequential enzymatic actions of beta-site amyloid precursor protein–cleaving enzyme 1 (BACE-1), a β-secretase, and γ-secretase, a protein complex with presenilin 1 at its catalytic core (Cuello, 2007). In this process the release of Aβ peptides is achieved by the consecutive action of a β-secretase cleaving APP at the N-terminal site of the Aβ domain, followed by its cleavage at the γ-secretase site at the C-terminal end, thus generating Aβ fragments of diverse lengths, but typically of 40 and 42 amino acids in length. The longer peptide, Aβ 1-42, is more neurotoxic and more prone to aggregation and amyloidogenic. The β- and γ-secretases have been identified and cloned. Two proteins are currently recognized with β-secretase functions. They are named BACE 1 and 2, of which BACE 1 appears to be more important for the development of the AD pathology (Vassar & Citron, 2000). The β-secretases release a large peptide which in biochemical jargon is referred to as C99, containing both the Aβ motif and another motif defined as AICD (APP internal C-terminal domain). The γ-secretase site is more complex. Initially, it was proposed that presenilins (mutations of which were already known to cause familial forms of AD) were the actual γ-secretase. Today, there is consensus that the γ-secretase site is composed of an ensemble of proteins, some of which might be responsible for the modulation of the APP-catalytic activity preselinins 1 and 2. This complex has the peculiarity of being capable of a catalytic action in the fairly hydrophobic milieu of cell and organelle membranes (Cuello, 2007).The catalytic activity of the γ-secretase action is ultimately responsible for the liberation of the amyloidogenic Aβ peptide and the AICD fragment (Wolfe, 2006). AICD is suspected to either act as a transcription factor or be involved in cell signaling mechanisms in the CNS, however, its actual biological significance is still being debated (Cuello, 2007). Finally, an imbalance between production and clearance, and aggregation of peptides, causes Aβ to accumulate, and this excess may be the initiating factor in Alzheimer's disease. This idea, called the "amyloid hypothesis," is based on studies of genetic forms of AD, including Down's syndrome, and evidence that Aβ42 is toxic to cells (Querfurth & La Ferla, 2010).

Amyloid plaques, together with NFTs, occur in AD and other neurodegenerative disorders, in addition to normal aging (Guillozet et al., 2003). The number of NFTs is a pathologic marker of the severity of AD. The major component of the tangles is an abnormally hyperphosphorylated and aggregated form of tau. Normally an abundant soluble protein in axons, tau promotes assembly and stability of microtubules and vesicle transport. Hyperphosphorylated tau is insoluble, lacks affinity for microtubules, and self-associates into paired helical filament structures. Enzymes that add and those that remove phosphate residues regulate the extent of tau phosphorylation (8). These NFTs have a clear-cut temporal and topographic distribution across brain areas as the disease progresses. The best staging of such structures has been provided by Braak and Braak (Braak H& Braak E, 1998). Interestingly, the earliest Braak stage is the occurrence of NFTs in the entorhinal cortex in the absence of an obvious deposition of Aβ material in this brain region. This observation has been used as an argument to dissociate tau from Aβ pathology in AD. The causal relation between these two molecular pathologies remains uncertain (Cuello, 2007).

The amyloid cascade hypothesis posits that Aβ triggers Tau pathology, but the details of this relationship are still poorly understood. Accumulation of Aβ peptides may be the key event in the pathogenesis of AD and experimental models have suggested that exposure of neurons to Aβ is toxic and elicits abnormal changes in Tau (Garg et al., 2011). Although new imaging techniques and powerful animal models have helped understanding the time course and the mechanisms of the lesions, the relationship between Aβ accumulation and tau pathology is still badly understood and the mechanism of LOAD continues to be debated (4). In some studies, the changes in Tau were ascribed to a toxic Tau fragment of 17 kD generated by calpain cleavage and located in the N-terminal half of Tau, but other N-terminal parts of Tau were reported to be toxic as well. In these cases, the toxicity could be triggered by Aβ, but there was no apparent relationship to the aggregation of Tau. By contrast, studies on other cleavage reactions had shown that truncation of Tau in the C terminal domain by caspase-3 or by lysosomal proteases could generate Tau fragments with a high tendency for aggregation (Garg et al., 2011).

Data obtained by electron microscopy and immunocytochemical and biochemical analysis on synaptic marker proteins in AD biopsies and autopsies indicate that synaptic loss in the hippocampus and neocortex is an early event and the major structural correlate of cognitive dysfunction. From all cortical areas analyzed, the hippocampus appears to be the most severely affected by the loss of synaptic proteins, while the occipital cortex is affected least. Although the cause for this failure is still unknown, recent evidence indicates a link between plastic synaptic changes and control of differentiation and cell cycle-repression within a neuron (Arendt, 2009). In mild Alzheimer's disease, there is a reduction of about 25% in the presynaptic vesicle protein synaptophysin (Querfurth & La Ferla, 2010) and there is evidence that living neurons lose their synapses in AD. Furthermore, synaptic function is impaired in living neurons, as demonstrated by decrements in transcripts related to synaptic vesicle trafficking (Coleman & Yao, 2003).

The exact mechanism by which Aβ peptide deposition induces neurotoxicity is unclear, but it appears that oxidative stress plays an important role. Besides, Aβ is a potent mitochondrial poison, especially affecting the synaptic pool. In AD, exposure to Aβ inhibits key mitochondrial enzymes in the brain and in isolated mitochondria. Cytochrome c oxidase is specifically attacked. Consequently, electron transport, ATP production, oxygen consumption, and mitochondrial membrane potential all become impaired (Querfurth & La Ferla, 2010). Consequently, oxidative stress is extensive in AD, and Aβ peptides stimulate oxidative stress by both direct and indirect mechanisms. Aβ peptides by themselves may act as enzymes and can bind to mitochondrial proteins, resulting in the generation of free radicals (Lustbader et al., 2004; Newman et al., 2007) Aβ peptides also generate oxidative stress via neuroinflammation. Considerable evidence has supported the hypothesis that neuroinflammation is associated with AD pathology (Newman et al., 2007).

Interestingly, AD was speculated as the brain equivalent of non-insulin-dependent diabetes mellitus (Hoyer, 1998; Craft et al., 2000). It was demonstrated that reduced brain insulin signaling is associated with increased tau phosphorylation and Aβ levels in a Streptozotocin induced model of diabetes mellitus, and also insulin promotes the release of intracellular Aβ in neuronal cultures and accelerates Aβ trafficking to the plasma membrane. Similarly, Intravenous insulin infusion also raised plasma Aβ42 levels in patients with AD but not in normal adults, an effect that was exaggerated in patients with AD with higher body mass indexes. In addition, impaired insulin or IGF-1 signaling can result in the hyper-phosphorylation of tau, which can cause cell death mediated by apoptosis, mitochondrial dysfunction or necrosis and promote oxidative stress, which contributes to the neurodegeneration cascade, and leads to dementia-associated behavioral and cognitive deficits. For this reason, it seems that insulin resistance causes Tau phosphorylation and neurofibrillary tangle formation and increased beta amyloid aggregation in late onset AD (1). In a recent study, Zhao and Townsend are demonstrated that insulin resistance and Aβ disrupt common signal transduction cascades including the insulin receptor family/Phosphoinositide 3-kinase/Akt/Glycogen synthase kinase-3(GSK3) pathway. They reported that both disease processes contribute to overlapping pathology, thereby compounding disease symptoms and progression (Zhao & Townsend, 2009). Besides, Proctor and Gray reported that GSK3β over activity leads to an increase in levels of Aβ plaques and tau tangle (Weller et al., 2009).The age-associated decline in the metabolic rate and utilization of glucose by the frontal cortex imply that insulin resistance can cause executive dysfunctions in older people, not only global cognitive impairment. Insulin resistance may cause decreased cortical glucose utilization especially in hippocampus and entorhinal cortex and also increased oxidative stress with advanced glycation end-products. In humans, raising plasma insulin levels through intravenous infusion increased cerebrospinal fluid levels of the Aβ 42 peptide; this effect was exacerbated by age. That insulin may interfere with Aβ degradation via its regulation of the metalloprotease insulin-degrading enzyme (IDE) may also be an important mechanism in late-onset AD that the Aβ clearance rather than Aβ production may be of special importance. Actually, the Aβ-degrading capacity of IDE in the Alzheimer Disease brains is about 50% of that of control brains, but insulin degradation decreases by about 30% only. Decreased IDE mRNA and IDE activity have been found in the hippocampus of late-onset AD brains; however, in neurons adjacent to senile plaques, IDE is up-regulated (Isik & Bozoglu, 2010).

Furthermore, in AD, vascular injury and parenchymal inflammation perpetuate the cycle of protein aggregation and oxidation in the brain, and diffuse pathologic changes include cerebral amyloid angiopathy, affecting more than 90% of patients with AD, capillary abnormalities, disruption of the blood-brain barrier, and large-vessel channels (Querfurth & La Ferla, 2010; Price et al., 2001). It has also been reported that clearance of Aβ along diseased perivascular channels and through the blood-brain barrier is impeded in AD atheroma, (Deane & Zlokovic, 2007) and that deregulation of Aβ transport across the capillary blood–brain barrier is caused by the imbalanced expression of low-density lipoprotein receptor-related proteins and receptors for advanced glycation end products (Price et al., 2001; Proctor & Gray 2010).

The calcium hypothesis of AD proposes that activation of the amyloidogenic pathway remodels the neuronal Ca(2+) signalling pathways responsible for cognition by enhancing the entry of Ca(2+) and/or the release of internal Ca(2+) by ryanodine receptors or InsP(3) receptors. The specific proposal is that Ca(2+) signalling remodelling results in a persistent elevation in the level of Ca(2+) that constantly erases newly acquired memories by enhancing the mechanism of long-term depression. Neurons can still form memories through the process of long term potentiation, but this stored information is rapidly removed by the persistent activation of long-term depression. Further dysregulation in Ca(2+) signalling will then go on to induce the neurodegeneration that characterizes the later stages of dementia (Berridge, 2010).

Finally, the current pathophysiologic approach to LOAD is based on a number of common mechanisms of neurodegeneration, including accumulation of abnormal proteins, mitochondrial dysfunction, and oxidative stress, impaired insulin signaling, calcium homeostasis dysregulation, early synaptic disconnection, and late apoptotic cell death. Aging itself is associated with mild cognitive deterioration, probably due to subtle multifactorial changes resulting in a global decrease of functional brain reserve.

5. References

Arendt T (2009) Synaptic degeneration in Alzheimer's disease. Acta Neuropathol. 118:167-179.

Ballatore C, Lee VM & Trojanowski JQ (2007) Tau-mediated neurodegeneration in Alzheimer's disease and related disorders. Nat. Rev. Neurosci. 8: 663-672.

Berridge MJ (2010) Calcium Signalling and Alzheimer's Disease.Eur J Physiol. 459:441-449.

Braak H & Braak E (1998) Argyrophilic grain disease: Frequency of occurrence in different age categories and neuropathological diagnostic criteria. Journal of Neural Transmission. 105:801-819.

Bozoglu E, Isik AT, Doruk H, Kilic S (2010) The Effects of Early Vitamin B12 Replacement Therapy on The Cognitive and Functional Status of Elderly Subjects. Bulletin of Clinical Psychopharmacology. 20:115-119.

Craft S, Asthana S, Schellenberg G & et al. (2000) Insulin effects on glucose metabolism, memory, and plasma amyloid precursor protein in Alzheimer's disease differ according to apolipoprotein-E genotype. Ann NY Acad Sci. 903: 222-228.

Coleman PD & Yao PJ (2003) Synaptic slaughter in Alzheimer's disease. Neurobiol Aging. 24:1023–1027.

Cuello AC (2007) Overview of the Alzheimer's Disease Pathology and Potential Therapeutic Targets. Eds: Cuello AC. Pharmacological Mechanisms in Alzheimer's Therapeutics, Springer, Canada, 1-27.

Deane R & Zlokovic BV (2007) Role of the blood-brain barrier in the pathogenesis of Alzheimer's disease. Curr Alzheimer Res. 4:191–197.

Garg S, TimmT, Mandelkow E, Mandelkow E & Wang Y (2011) Cleavage of Tau by calpain in Alzheimer's disease: the quest for the toxic 17 kD fragment. Neurobiology of Aging. 32:1-14.

Glenner GG & Wong CW (1984) Alzheimer's disease and Down's syndrome: Sharing of a unique cerebrovascular amyloid fibril protein. Biochemical and Biophysical Research Communications. 12:1131-1135.

Guillozet AL, Weintraub S, Mash DC & Mesulam MM (2003) Neurofibrillary tangles, amyloid and memory in aging and mild cognitive impairment. Arch Neurol. 60:729-736.

Haass C & Selkoe DJ (2007) Soluble protein oligomers in neurodegeneration: lessons from the Alzheimer's amyloid beta-peptide. Nat. Rev.Mol. Cell Biol. 8, 101–112

Hoyer S (1998) Is sporadic Alzheimer disease the brain type of non-insulin dependent diabetes mellitus? A challenging hypothesis. J Neural Transm. 105: 415-422.

Isik AT (2010) Late onset Alzheimer's disease in older people. Clinical Interventions in Aging. 5:307-311.

Isik AT & Bozoglu E (2010) Chapter 20-Insulin resistance in Alzheimer disease: Eds: Aucoin L, Prideux T:Handbook of Type 1 Diabetes Mellitus: Etiology, Diagnosis, and Treatment, Nova Science, Hauppauge NY.

Jackson-Siegal J (2005) Our current understanding of the pathophysiology of Alzheimer's Disease. Adv Stud Pharm. 2(4):126-135.

Lustbader JW, Cirilli M & Lin C (2004) ABAD directly links Abeta to mitochondrial toxicity in Alzheimer's disease. Science. 304:448-452.

Newman M, Musgrave FI & Lardelli M (2007) Alzheimer disease: Amyloidogenesis,the presenilins and animal models. Biochimica Biophysica Acta. 1772:285-297.

Querfurth HW & La Ferla FM (2010) Mechanisms of Disease:Alzheimer's Disease. N Engl J Med. 362;4:329-344.

Price JM, Chi X, Hellermann G & Sutton ET (2001) Physiological levels of beta-amyloid induce cerebral vessel dysfunction and reduce endothelial nitric oxide production. Neurol Res. 23:506–512.

Proctor CJ & Gray DA (2010) GSK3 and p53 is there a link in Alzheimer's disease? Molecular Neurodegeneration. 5(7);1-15.

Schrijvers EM, Koudstaal PJ, Hofman A & Breteler MM (2011) Plasma clusterin and the risk of Alzheimer Disease. JAMA. 305:1322-1326.

Vassar R & Citron M (2000) Abeta-generating enzymes: Recent advances in beta and gamma-secretase research. Neuron. 27:419-422.

Weller RO, Boche D & Nicoll JAR (2009). Microvasculature changes and cerebral amyloid angiopathy in Alzheimer's disease and their potential impact on therapy. Acta Neuropathol. 118:87–102.

Wolfe MS (2006) The gamma-secretase complex: Membrane-embedded proteolytic ensemble. Biochemistry. 45:7931-7939.

Zhao WQ & Townsend M (2009) Insulin resistance and amyloidogenesis as common molecular foundation for type 2 diabetes and Alzheimer's disease. Biochimica et Biophysica Acta, 1792: 482-496.

Part 2

Amyloid and Tau Mediated Neurotoxicity and Neurodegeneration

3

Expression and Cerebral Function of Amyloid Precursor Protein After Rat Traumatic Brain Injury

Tatsuki Itoh[1], Motohiro Imano[2], Shozo Nishida[3], Masahiro Tsubaki[3], Shigeo Hashimoto[4], Akihiko Ito[1] and Takao Satou[1,5,6]

[1]*Department of Pathology, Kinki University Faculty of Medicine,*
[2]*Department of Surgery, Kinki University Faculty of Medicine,*
[3]*Kinki University Faculty of Pharmaceutical Sciences,*
[4]*Department of Pathology, PL Hospital,*
[5]*Division of Hospital Pathology, Hospital of Kinki University Faculty of Medicine,*
[6]*Division of Sports Medicine, Institute of Life Science, Kinki University,*
Japan

1. Introduction

The β-amyloid protein derived from amyloid precursor protein (APP) (Goldgaber et al., 1987; Robakis et al., 1987) is a major component of senile plaque, and β-amyloid protein deposits in Alzheimer disease (AD) (Masters et al., 1985; Selkoe et al., 1986) are thought to be produced by alternative processing of APP (Golde et al., 1992). Therefore, the overexpression of APP is an important factor in the neuronal degeneration of AD (Murakami et al., 1998). The expression of APP has also been shown to increase in swollen axons and neuronal perikarya after neuronal injury, including ischemia (Stephenson et al., 1992) and stab injury (Otsuka et al., 1991). As the pathological findings in dementia pugilistica mimic those in AD (Roberts et al., 1990), it has been posited that traumatic brain injury (TBI) is an epidemiological risk factor for AD (Schofield et al., 1997; DeKosky et al., 2007), although other genetic factors, which include the apoE genotype, might act additively (Nicoll et al., 1995; DeKosky et al., 2007). These findings suggest that the overexpression of APP after TBI may potentiate Alzheimer disease pathology. However, the chronological changes in APP expression have not been evaluated after TBI. Furthermore, the function of APP has not been evaluated after TBI.
In this study,

1. we immunohistochemically investigated chronogical changes in cellular sources and levels of APP production compared to that of mRNA for APP as assessed by RT-PCR in the rat brain following traumatic brain injury.
2. In addition, we investigated the function of APP by assessing water maze and morphological changes following direct infusion of the anti-APP antibody into the damaged brain region following TBI.

2. Materials and methods

2.1 Surgical procedure

Male Wistar rats (8–9 weeks old, 200–250g in weight) were anesthetized by intraperitoneal pentobarbital (50mg/kg) injection. The scalp was incised on the midline and the skull was exposed. A 2–2.5mm hole was drilled (1 mm posterior, + 1 mm right lateral to bregma) in the right parietal calvaria. Brain injury above the dura mater was then induced with a pneumatic control injury device (Itoh et al., 2005; Itoh et al., 2007; Itoh et al., 2009) at an impact velocity of 4m/sec (impact tip diameter of 1mm; fixed impact deformation of 2mm depth from the cerebral surface) (Itoh et al., 2005; Itoh et al., 2007; Itoh et al., 2009). Control rats were subjected to a sham operation, but no cortical penetration injury was inflicted. The contralateral hemisphere was not used as a control, since that area may have been affected by the impact. Rats were placed in a heated cage to maintain their body temperature at 37°C during the recovery from anesthesia.

2.2 Anti-APP antibody infusion

The drug infusion protocol was as previously described (Green-Sadan et al., 2003). Immediately, after TBI, the animals were placed in a stereotactic frame and fitted with a brain infusion cannula (Alzet brain infusion kit 3, 1mm, Alzet, San Diego, CA, USA). The cannula was implanted with the tip inserted into the damaged brain region (1 mm posterior, + 1 mm right lateral to bregma). The cannula was secured with dental cement. A micro-osmotic pump (Model 2001; rate of 1µl/h, Alzet), filled with 300 µl infusion volume kept 37°C, was implanted subcutaneously in the neck and connected to the infusion cannula. Rats received an infusion of either anti-APP antibody (IgG2a isoform, 1µg/ml; anti-APP antibody group; Chemicon, Temecula, CA, USA) diluted in sterilized phosphate buffer saline (0.1M PBS, pH 7.4–7.5; n=20) or sterilized PBS only (PBS group; n=20) for seven days immediately after TBI. For the control of the Morris water maze experiments, ten animals with no operation (sham operation group, no injury) were also collected. In sham operation group, a micro-osmotic pump was implanted subcutaneously in the neck without infusion cannula. Moreover, sham operation group was used only the behavioural experiments. As probe and the extent of APP antibody infusion test, although data not shown in this study, we investigated that the extent of APP antibody diffusion with Evans blue using the osmotic pump and confirmed Evans blue extended whole brain from center of infusion area.

2.3 Morris water maze experiments

A circular, thermostatically regulated, dark gray PVC-plastic water tank (180cm wide, 45cm deep, filled with tap water at 22±1°C), located in the center of the testing room and surrounded by extra-maze cues, was used in the spatial learning task. A constant asymmetrical array of lamps and pictures served as cues for spatial orientation. A circular dark gray platform (15cm wide) submerged 1cm below the water surface served as a platform. The platform was placed in the center of one of the quadrants, i.e., the target quadrant, of the water maze (Elvander et al., 2004). The experiments were monitored using a digital TV system connected to a computer (Elvander et al., 2004). Training took place between 8:00a.m. and 3:00p.m. during seven consecutive days. Each daily training session consisted of four trials with a 120s cutoff time, followed by 30s rest on the platform. Memory was tested in fifteen animals from each of the anti-APP antibody group and the PBS group, and in ten sham operation group animals, starting at day one and continued up to seven days after TBI/sham operation.

2.4 Immunohistochemistry

1, 3, 7, 30 and 90 days after TBI and after the last the Morris water maze test at seven days, rats from each group were perfused intracardially with 300ml of PBS followed by 300ml of 4% paraformaldehyde (PFA; pH 7.4–7.5) in PBS. The brains were then removed and stored in PFA for three days, before the maximum size of the lesion was sliced into serial coronal sections (50µm thick) using a microslicer (Dousaka EM, Kyoto, Japan).

Sections were treated with 3% H_2O_2 in Tris-buffered saline (TBS; 0.1M Tris-HCl, pH 7.5, 0.15M NaCl) containing 0.1% Triton X-100 (TBS-T) for 30min. Next, the sections were washed three times with TBS-T, blocked with 3% bovine serum albumin (BSA; Sigma-Aldrich, St. Louis, MO, USA) in TBS-T for 30min, and incubated with a mouse monoclonal anti- microtubule associate protein-2 (MAP-2) antibody as a marker of neuronal cell (1:10000 dilution; Sigma-Aldrich), a mouse monoclonal anti-neurofilament (NF) antibody as a marker of neuronal cell (1:10000 dilution; DAKO, Glostrup, Denmark), a rabbit polyclonal anti-Glial Fibrillary Acidic Protein (GFAP) antibody (1:10000 dilution; DAKO, Glostrup, Denmark), a mouse monoclonal anti-APP antibody (1:1000 dilution; Chemicon, Temecula, CA, USA) or a mouse monoclonal anti-CD11b antibody as a marker of microglia/macrophage (1:1000 dilution; Chemicon, Temecula, CA, USA) overnight at room temperature. Following extensive washing, the sections were further incubated with a HISTIFINE Rat-PO (multi)-kit (Nichirei, Osaka, Japan), consisting of a mixed solution of peroxidase-conjugated anti-mouse and rabbit IgG as the secondary antibody, for 60min at room temperature. The HISTIFINE Rat-PO kits contained preabsorbed rat serum, and showed very minimal non-specific binding by rat serum in injured rat tissues. Labeling was visualized using diaminobenzidine (DAB; Vector Peroxidase Substrate Kit; Vector Laboratories, Burlingame, CA, USA) for 5min, and the sections were counterstained with hematoxylin.

For TUNEL-staining at three days after TBI, the brains from five rats in each of the anti-APP antibody group and the PBS group were collected as above. Sections were used for TUNEL-staining, a marker of apoptosis. TUNEL-staining was performed using an *in situ* Apoptosis Detection Kit (TaKaRa Biochemicals Co., Kyoto, Japan) according to the manufacturer's instructions. Sections were treated with Proteinase K for 10min, followed by treatment with 3% H_2O_2 in TBS-T for 30min. Next, the sections were washed three times with TBS-T, and incubated with a TdT Enzyme Labeling solution for 90min at room temperature. Labeling was visualized using DAB. The controls for the TUNEL stains were performed without enzyme. Furthermore, to investigate TUNEL-positive cells phenotype, MAP-2 or GFAP immunofluorescence staining was performed following TUNEL-staining. Sections were treated with Proteinase K for 10min. Next, the sections incubated with a fluorescein isothiocyanate (FITC)-conjugated TdT Enzyme Labeling solution for 90min at room temperature. Next, the sections were washed extensively and incubated with an anti-MAP-2 antibody (1:300 dilution; Sigma) or anti-GFAP antibody (1:300 dilution; DAKO) overnight at room temperature. Following extensive washing, the sections were further incubated with Alexa Flour 555 anti-mouse IgG (for anti-MAP-2 antibody) or rabbit IgG (for anti-GFAP antibody, 1:300 dilution; BD Biosciences Pharmingen, San Diego, CA) for 80 min at room temperature. Subsequently, the sections were observed using a confocal laser-scanning microscope (LSM5 PASCAL; Carl Zeiss Jena GmbH, Jena, Germany).

2.5 Quantification

To determined the number of APP -positive neurites and cells, MAP-2-, GFAP-, or TUNEL-positive cells, each DAB-positive cells around the damaged area (cortex) without white matter after TBI were observed and DAB-labeled cells were counted in three serial sections (each section was 50 μm in thickness) under a Nikon E 1000M microscope (Nikon Corporation, Tokyo, Japan) using a 20x objective. To determine the measured area of DAB-positive cells, an image of the measured area was captured under the Nikon E 1000M microscope at 1x magnification using a CCD camera (ACT-2U; Nikon Corporation). The measured area in each image was traced and measured using a computer (Power Macintosh G3; Apple Computers, Cupertino, CA) and the NIH Image 1.6 software (NIH, Bethesda, MD). The number of DAB-positive cells was expressed as positive cell number/100μm^3.

2.6 Double-immunofluorescence staining

Each serial section was washed with TBS-T, blocked with 3% BSA in TBS-T for 30 min, and incubated with a polyclonal rabbit anti-APP antibody (1:300 dilution; Chemicon) overnight at room temperature. Following extensive washing, the sections were further incubated with a polyclonal rhodamine-conjugated anti-rabbit IgG antibody (1:300 dilution; DAKO) for 80 min at room temperature. Next, the APP-stained sections were washed extensively and incubated with a monoclonal mouse anti-NF antibody (1:300 dilution; DAKO), a marker for neurons and nerve fiver; a monoclonal mouse anti-MAP-2 antibody (1:300 dilution; Sigma), a marker for neurons; a monoclonal mouse anti-CD11b antibody (1:300 dilution; AbD Serotec, Raleigh, NC), a marker for macrophages/microglia or a monoclonal mouse anti-GFAP antibody (1:300 dilution; DAKO), a marker for astroglia overnight at room temperature. Following extensive washing, the sections were further incubated with a polyclonal fluorescein isothiocyanate (FITC)-conjugated anti-mouse IgG antibody (1:300 dilution; DAKO) for 80 min at room temperature. Subsequently, the sections were observed by fluorescence microscopy (Nikon E-800; Nikon, Tokyo, Japan).

2.7 Reverse transcription-polymerase chain reaction (RT-PCR)

The mRNA expression levels were investigated by RT-PCR at 1 to 90 days after TBI. Five rats were used for each time point. Briefly, total RNA was isolated from an area of the cerebral cortex (without the corpus callosum and hippocampus) with a diameter of 2 mm from the center of the lesion using RNA-Bee (Tel-Test Inc., Friendswood, TX) and redissolved in water, before the concentration was determined photometrically using the wavelength ratio of 260 nm/280 nm. The two oligonucleotide primers used for APP mRNA were: (accession No X07648): sense primer: 5 '-GGA TGC GGA GTT CGG ACA TG -3 'antisense primer: 5 '-GTT CTG CAT CTG CTC AAA G -3 'Rat glyceraldehyde-3-phosphate dehydrogenase (GAPDH) (CLONTECH, No5507, BD Biosciences Pharmingen, San Diego, CA) was used as an internal control.

RT-PCR was performed using an mRNA PCR Kit (TaKaRa Biochemicals Co., Kyoto, Japan) according to the manufacturer's instructions. RT was performed at 42°C for 25 min, followed by heat inactivation at 99°C for 5 min. PCR amplification was carried out in a PCR EXPRESS (Hybaid US, Franklin, MA) for 30 cycles of 2 min at 94°C, 30 s at 94°C, 30 s at 55°C and 1.5 min at 72°C. The final step was extended to 5 min at 72°C. After separation by electrophoresis in 1.5% agarose gels, the products were stained with ethidium bromide and located by fluorescence using UV light (3UV Transilluminator; UVP, Upland, CA). Bio Max 1D TM1.5.1 (Kodak, Tokyo, Japan) was used to evaluate the band intensities of the PCR bands. The signals were normalized to the corresponding GAPDH signal in the same RNA sample.

2.8 Enzyme-linked immunosorbent assay (ELISA) for APP

The APP protein levels after TBI were investigated by ELISA using extracts of the TBI area. Five rats were used for each time point. Briefly, brain tissue from the above-described TBI area was isolated at each time point, and homogenized (10% w/v) in homogenizing buffer (PBS containing 0.25 mol/L sucrose, 5 mmol/L ethylene glycol bis(2-aminoethyl ether)-tetraacetic acid (EGTA), 25 μg/ml leupeptin, 25 μg/ml aprotinin) at 4°C using a hand homogenizer. After treatment of the homogenates with ultrasonic waves at 4°C for 100 s and centrifugation at 20,000 *g* for 30 min at 4°C, the resulting supernatants were collected. The protein concentrations of the supernatants were determined using a DC Protein Assay Kit (Bio-Rad Laboratories, Hercules, CA) according to the manufacturer's instructions, and then adjusted to 1 μg/μl. The brain tissue samples were stored at -80°C until analysis by ELISA. ELISAs were performed as previously described. Briefly, flat-bottomed microtiter plates (type H for ELISA; Sumitomo Bakelite Co., Tokyo, Japan) were coated with a rabbit polyclonal anti-APP antibody (diluted to 0.5 μg/ml in PBS containing 3% BSA (PBS-B); Chemicon) and blocked with 300 μl of PBS containing 3% BSA, 1% sucrose and 0.05% Tween 20 for 120 min at room temperature. The plates were then washed three times with PBS containing 0.05% Tween 20 (PBS-T). Recombinant APP (Chemicon) was serially diluted with PBS-B (0.001-12 ng/ml) and used to construct a standard curve. Aliquots (100 μl) of the diluted samples were incubated in the wells at 4°C overnight. After washing, 100 μl of a mouse monoclonal anti-APP antibody (1:10000 dilution in PBS-B; Chemicon) was added to each well and incubated for 2 h at room temperature. After washing, 100 μl of simple-stain MAX-PO (mouse)-kit (Nichirei) consisting of a peroxidase-conjugated anti-mouse IgG was added to each well. Color development was carried out using an Enzyme Reaction Kit Type T (Sumitomo Bakelite Co., Tokyo, Japan), and the absorbances at 490 nm were measured using a microplate reader (Model 3550UV; Bio-Rad Laboratories). The detection limit of the assay for APP was 0.005 ng/ml. The measurements were made in duplicate.

2.9 Area measurement of damaged brain region

To determine the area of the damage region at seven days after TBI, after the last the Morris water maze five rats per group were collected as above, and the anteroposterior of the maximum size of the lesion was sliced into forty serial coronal sections (50μm thick). Anteroposterior sections 1–40 were stained with hematoxylin and eosin (HE). Images of the HE stain in the forty anteroposterior serial sections were captured using a Nikon E 1000M microscope at 1X magnification and a CCD camera. The area of the damaged region in each image was traced and measured by computer, and the average area of the damaged region calculated over the forty serial sections.

2.10 Statistical analysis

Water maze data were expressed as mean±SE. Data were analyzed using ANOVA and Fisher's PLSD-test (Stat View®; SAS Institute Inc, Cary, NC. USA). Other data were expressed as mean±SD and analyzed using ANOVA. $p<0.05$ was considered statistically significant.

3. Results

3.1 Double-immunofluorescence of amyloid precursor protein (APP) and neurofilament (NF), microtubule-associated protein-2 (MAP-2), glial fibrillary acidic protein (GFAP) or CD11b

The neuronal or microglial localizations of APP protein in the cortical traumatic injured rats at 1 day, 3 days and 7 days post-lesion are illustrated (Fig.1-3). Neurons, astroglia or microglia were identified by immunohistochemical staining using anti-NF, anti-MAP-2, and anti-GFAP or anti-CD11b, respectively. Double labeling immunohistochemistry with anti-

NF (Fig. 1A) and anti-APP (Fig. 1B) antibodies clearly demonstrated the co-localization of NF and APP proteins in swollen and dystrophic nerve fibers at 1day after TBI (Fig. 1C). At 7 days after cortical traumatic injury, MAP-2-positive nerve cell cytoplasm (Fig. 1D) was positive for APP (Fig. 1E&F).

Anti-GFAP (Fig. 2A) or anti-CD11b (Fig. 2D) and anti-APP (Fig. 2B&E) antibodies did not demonstrate co-localization in the same cells at 3 days after cortical traumatic injury (Fig. 2C&F). At 7 days after traumatic injury, a few CD11b-positive cells (Fig. 2G) expressed weakly positive APP immunoreactivity (Fig. 2H&I).

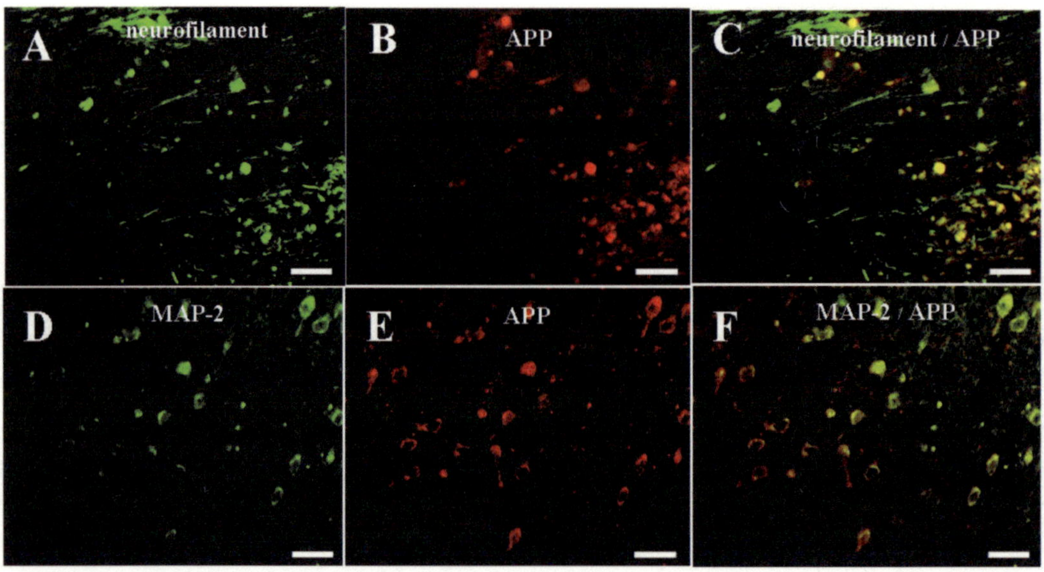

Fig. 1. Double-immunofluorescence staining of localized neurofilaments (A) or MAP-2 (D) and APP (B, E) around the damaged area after traumatic brain injury. At 1 day after injury, damaged dystrophic and swollen neurites (A, green) in the cortex were APP-positive (B, red). The merged image (C) of panels (A) and (B) reveals colocalization of these proteins (yellow). At 7 days after injury, neurons near the injured portion were positive for MAP-2 (D, green) and APP (E, red). The merged image (F) of panels (D) and (E) reveals colocalization of these proteins (yellow). Scale bar = 50 μm.

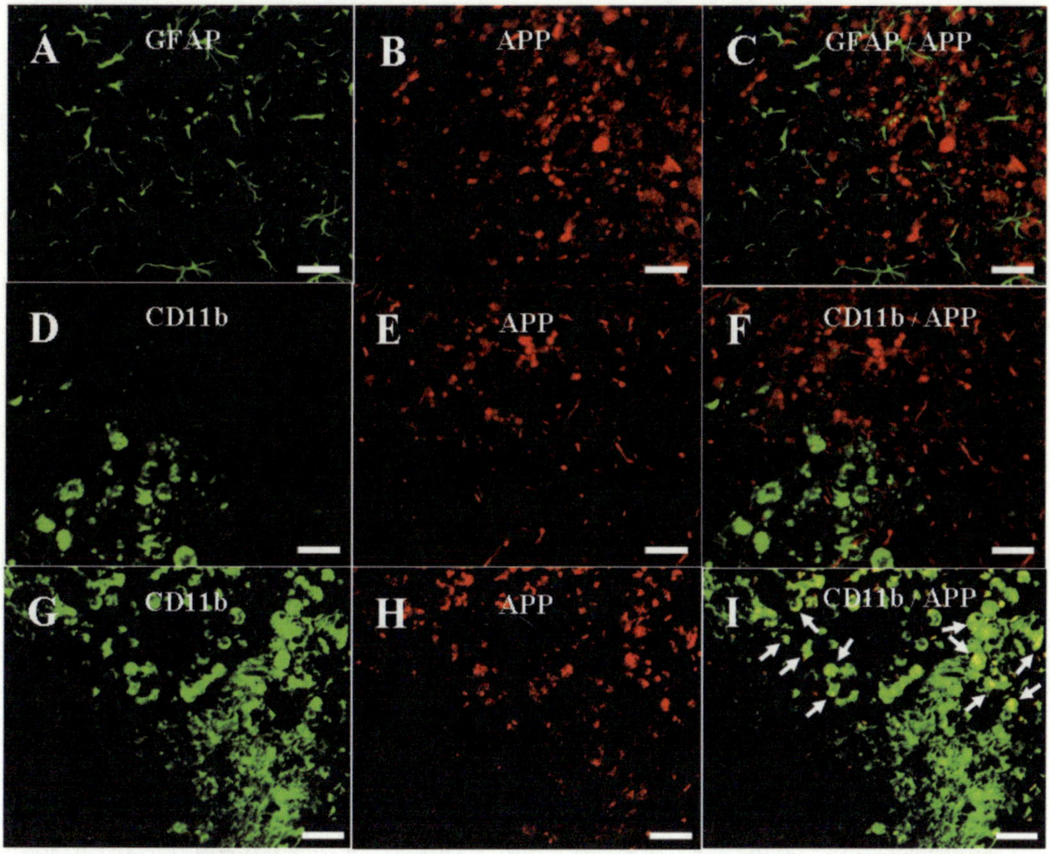

Fig. 2. Double-immunofluorescence staining for GFAP (A) or CD11b (D, G) and APP (B, E, H) around the damaged area after traumatic brain injury. At 3 days after the injury, GFAP-immunopositive (A, green) and APP-immunopositive (B, red) cells are observed. The merged image (C) of panels (A) and (B) does not show any colocalization. At 3 days after the injury, CD11b-immunopositive (D, green) and APP-immunopositive (E, red) cells are observed. The merged image (F) of panels (D) and (E) does not show any colocalization. However, at 7 days after the injury, CD11b-immunopositive (G, green) and APP-immunopositive (H, red) cells are colocalization (I, arrows). Scale bar = 50 µm.

3.2 Immunostaining and APP-immunopositive cell and neurites count after TBI

There were many APP-positive damaged swollen and dystrophic neurites at 1 day after TBI (Fig. 3A). At 7 days after TBI, there were many APP-positive neurons and a few APP-positive damaged swollen and dystrophic neurites (Fig. 3B). However, there were no APP-immunopositive cells and fivers in the sham-operated cerebral cortex (Fig. 3C). The number of APP-positive neurites ($p<0.001$, Fig. 3D) and cells ($p<0.001$, Fig. 3E) was increased in the cortex as early as 1 day following injury, with the elevation becoming significant from 1 day to 90 days($p<0.001$, Fig. 3E). There were no such changes in the sham group (Fig. 3D&E).

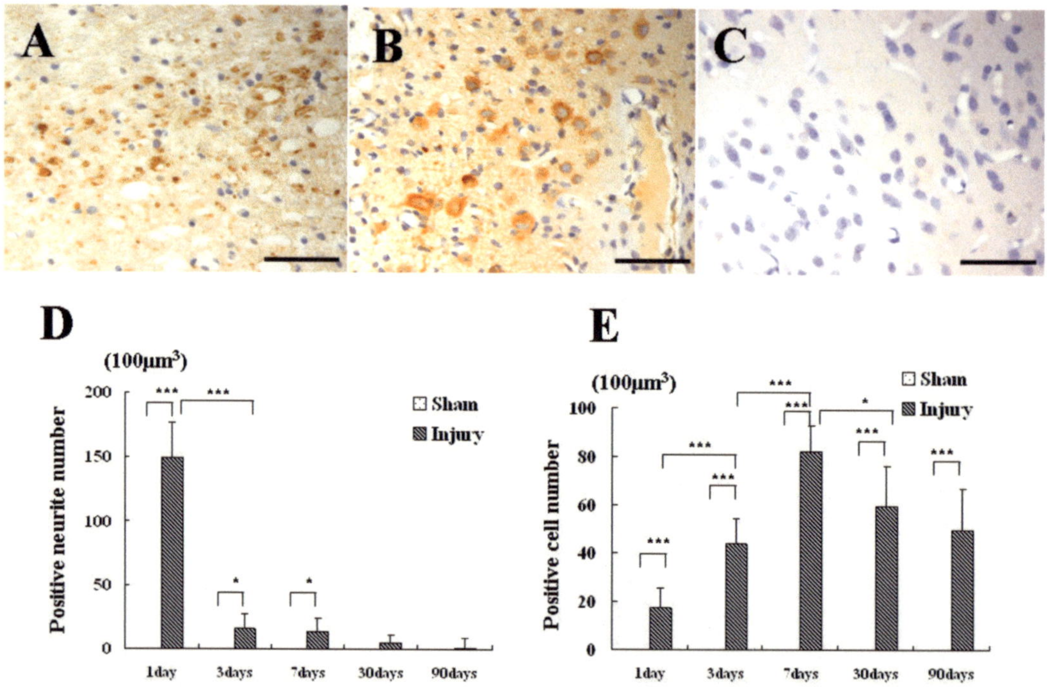

Fig. 3. Immunostaining for APP around the damaged cerebral cortex after traumatic brain injury. At 1 day after injury, there are many APP-positive damaged dystrophic and swollen neurites (A). At 7 days after injury, there are many APP-positive neurons and a few APP-positive damaged dystrophic and swollen neurites (B). However, the sham-operated control cortex does not contain any APP staining or APP-immunopositive cells (C). Scale bar = 50 μm. Graph showing the numbers of APP-immunopositive neurites (D) and cells (E) around the damaged cerebral cortex after traumatic rat brain injury. The results are shown as the mean ± SD. *$P < 0.05$, ***$P < 0.001$, $n = 5$.

3.3 RT-PCR analysis of APP

As determined by RT-PCR, the mRNA levels for APP were elevated after cortical injury. The APP transcript level displayed an increase in the cortex as early as 1 day following injury, with the elevation becoming significant between 1 day and 30 days and returning to the control level by 90 days (p<0.05, Fig. 4A) . One peak of elevation was determined between 1 day and 30 days after injury. There were no such changes in the sham group (Fig. 4A).

3.4 APP protein in brain tissue after TBI

As determined by ELISA, the levels of APP were elevated after cortical injury. ELISA demonstrated a pattern similar to that showing by RT-PCR. APP levels displayed an increase in the injured side as early as 1 day following injury, with the elevation becoming significant between 1 day and 90 days (p<0.001, Fig. 4B). One peak of elevation was determined between 1 day and 90 days after injury (Fig. 4B). There were no such changes in the sham group (Fig. 4B).

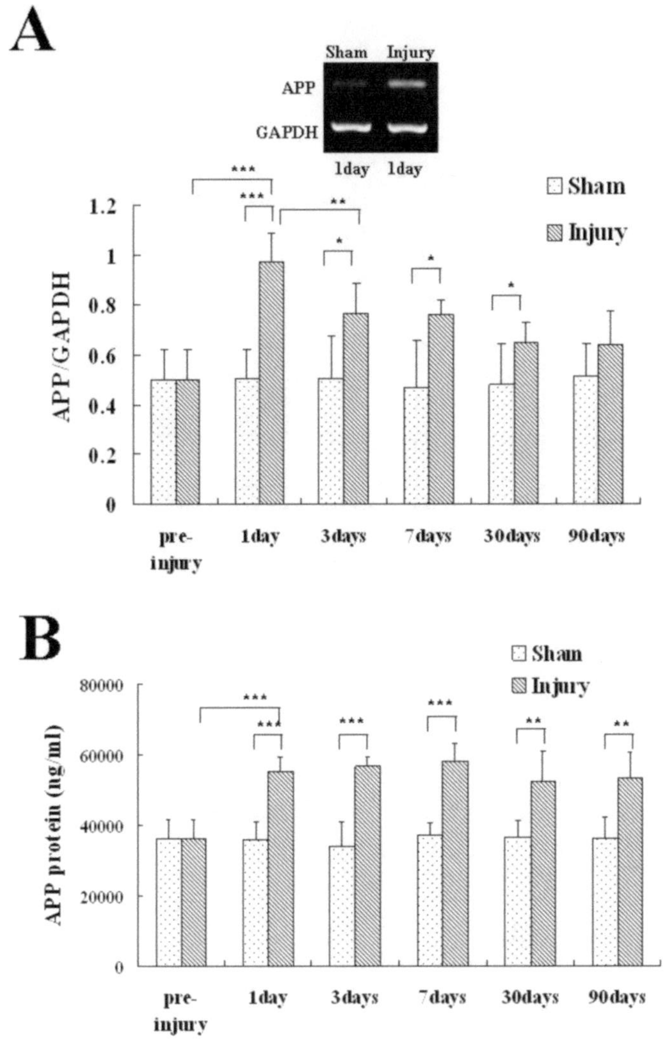

Fig. 4. Graphs show the optical density units of ethidium bromide-stained RT-PCR products for APPmRNA expression (A) and the level of APP protein (B) after traumatic brain injury. The results are shown as the mean ± SD. *$P < 0.05$, **$P < 0.01$, ***$P < 0.001$, $n = 5$.

3.5 Water maze experiments

When compared with the sham operation group, the arrival time to platform was significantly increased at seven days after TBI in the PBS group (p<0.001, Fig. 5). However, at seven days after TBI, the arrival time to platform was significantly decreased in the anti-APP antibody group versus the PBS group (p<0.001, Fig. 5), and was not different from the sham operation group at seven days after TBI (Fig. 5).

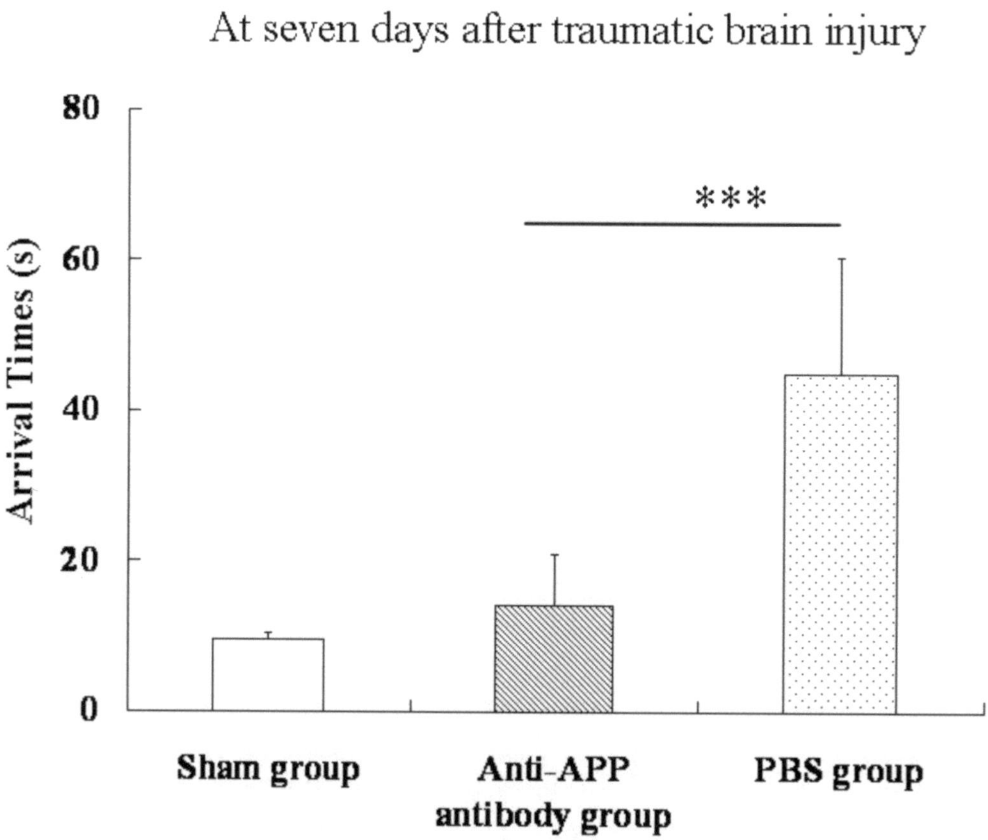

Fig. 5. The effect of anti-APP antibody on cerebral function at seven days after TBI. Anti-APP antibody (1μg/ml) or PBS was infused over seven days by osmotic pump (1μl/hr). The sham operation group had no injury. The effects of treatment group on arrival time to platform are shown. Values represent mean±SE (n=10/group). PBS group *vs.* anti-APP antibody group *vs.* sham operation group. ***$p<0.001$

3.6 Area of the damaged brain region after TBI

HE images of the damaged brain region at seven days after TBI can be seen in Figure 6A-B. The area of the damaged brain region was significantly decreased in the anti-APP antibody group versus the PBS group ($p<0.001$, Fig. 6C).

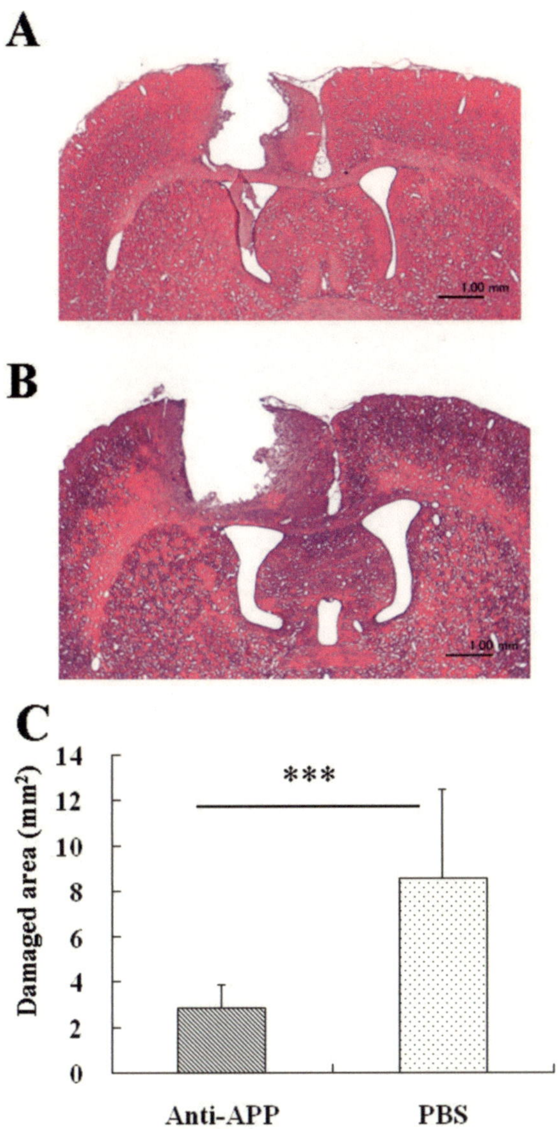

Fig. 6. The size of the damaged brain region at seven days after TBI. HE stains show the anti-APP antibody group (1μg/ml) (A) and the PBS group (B). Scale bar = 1mm. (C) Measurement results of each group (n=5/group). Anti-APP antibody group *vs.* PBS group. $^{***}p<0.001$.

3.7 Immunostaining and GFAP-immunopositive cell counts after TBI

Immunostaining results for GFAP expression and the numbers of GFAP-positive cells around the damaged brain region at seven days after TBI can be seen in Figure 7A-E. In the anti-APP antibody group there were many larger GFAP-positive cells with GFAP staining in their cytoplasm and long elongated projections around the damaged region (Fig 7. A-B). Furthermore, there were many GFAP-positive fibers that formed glial scars after TBI, and these fibers were enriched at the damaged brain region (Fig. 7A). In contrast, in the PBS group there were only a few small GFAP-positive cells which possessed a small GFAP-positive cytoplasm and a few projections (Fig. 7C-D). There was a significant increase in the number of GFAP-positive cells in the anti-APP antibody group versus the PBS group (p<0.001, Fig. 7E).

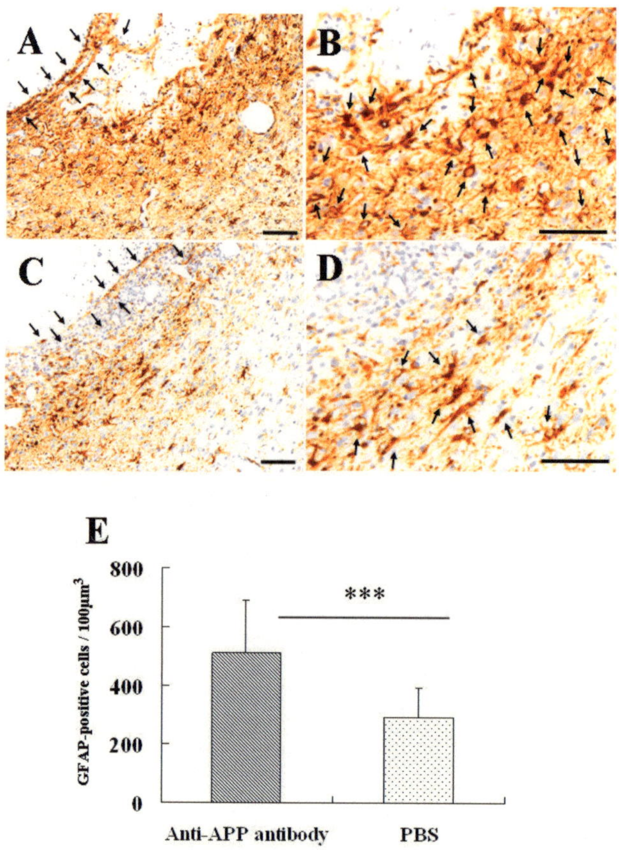

Fig. 7. GFAP expression around the damaged region at seven days after TBI. Note that there were many glial scars (A, arrows) and many large GFAP-positive cells and projections (B, arrows) in the anti-APP antibody group (1μg/ml; A: low power, B: high power), while glial scars (C, arrows), only a few small GFAP-positive cells, and a few projections (D, arrows) were observed in the PBS group (C: low power, D: high power). Scale bar = 50μm. (E) Number of GFAP-positive cells in each group (n=10/group). Anti-APP antibody group *vs.* PBS group. ***p<0.001.

3.8 Immunostaining and MAP-2-immunopositive cell counts after TBI

Immunostaining results for MAP-2 expression and the numbers of MAP-2-positive cells around the damaged region at seven days after TBI can be seen in Figure 8A-C. In the anti-APP antibody group there were many large MAP-2-positive nerve cells (cytoplasm stained) and MAP-2-positive fibers (Fig. 8A). In contrast, in the PBS group there were only a few small MAP-2-positive cells which possessed a small MAP-2-immunopositive cytoplasm and a few MAP-2-positive fibers (Fig. 8B). There was a significant increase in the number of MAP-2-positive cells in the anti-APP antibody group versus the PBS group ($p<0.001$, Fig. 8C).

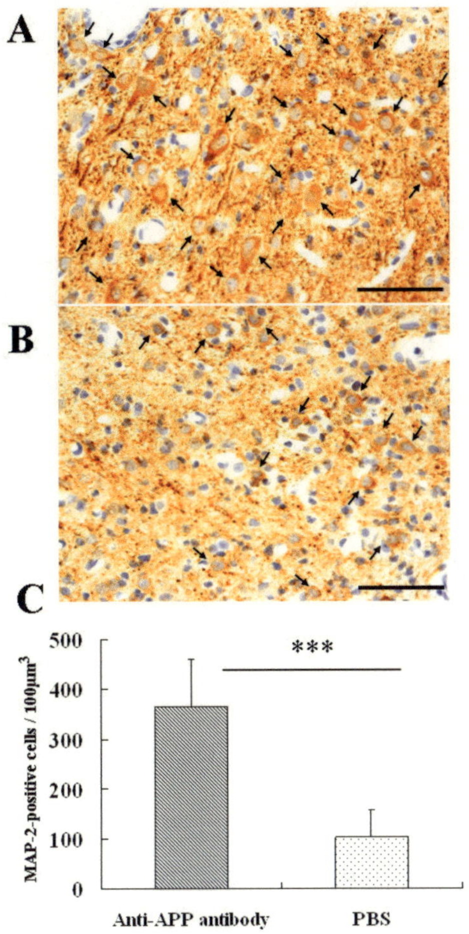

Fig. 8. MAP-2 expression around the damaged region at seven days after TBI. Note that numerous large MAP-2-positive cells and fibers were observed in the anti-APP antibody group (1μg/ml; A, arrows), while only a few small MAP-2-positive cells and a few fibers were observed in the PBS group (B, arrows). Scale bar = 50μm. (C) The number of MAP-2-positive cells in each group (n=10/group). Anti-APP antibody group *vs*. PBS group. ***$p<0.001$.

3.9 TUNEL-staining and TUNEL-positive cells counts after TBI

TUNEL-staining results and the numbers of TUNEL-positive cells around the damaged region at three days after TBI can be seen in Figure 9A-E. In the anti-APP antibody group there were only a few TUNEL-positive cells which possessed a small cytoplasm, such as glial cells, or a large cytoplasm, such as neural cells (Fig. 9A). In contrast, in the PBS group there were many TUNEL-positive cells which possessed small or large cytoplasm's (Fig. 9B). Furthermore, Almost TUNEL-positive cells in PBS group colocalize with the MAP-2 staining (Fig. 9C). A few TUNEL-positive cells in PBS group colocalize with the GFAP staining (Fig. 9D). In addition, the number of TUNEL-positive cells in the anti-APP antibody group was significantly decreased versus the PBS group ($p<0.001$, Fig. 9E).

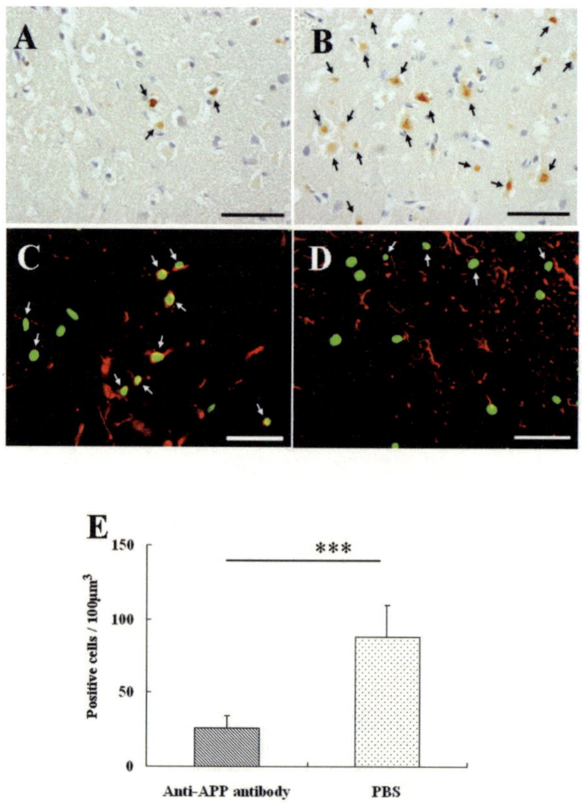

Fig. 9. TUNEL-staining around the damaged region at three days after TBI. Note that there were only a few TUNEL-positive cells, which possessed small or large cytoplasms, in the anti-APP antibody group (1μg/ml; A, arrows), while many small or large cytoplasm TUNEL-positive cells were observed in the PBS group (B, arrows). (C) and (D) were indicated TUNEL-staining (green) and MAP-2 (C, red) or GFAP (D, red) immunofluorescence staining in PBS group. Many TUNEL-positive (C, green) cells showed MAP-2-immunopositive (C, red). A few TUNEL-positive (D, green) cells showed GFAP-immunopositive (D, red). The merged image of TUNEL- and MAP-2- or GFAP-positive cells showed arrows (C&D). Scale bar = 50μm. (E) Number of TUNEL-positive cells in each group (n=5/group). Anti-APP antibody group *vs.* PBS group. ***$p<0.001$.

4. Discussion

The hypothesis that head trauma is a risk factor associated with subsequent development of Alzheimer disease is based on the neuropathology of dementia (Roberts 1988; Roberts et al., 1994). Some reports have shown that the expression of APP is enhanced by various forms of brain injury, including traumatic (Otsuka et al., 1991), chemical (Nakamura et al., 1992) , and ischemic injury (Stephenson et al., 1992). Further, the overexpression of APP suggests the possibility of an Alzheimer disease-like pathology after traumatic brain injury (Rumble et al., 1989). Previously, the appearance of APP in the brain during pathological events was usually attributed to its synthesis by neurons, macrophages, microglia or astrocytes (Otsuka et al., 1991). However, APP was synthesized by neurons, as showing by immunohistochemical, ELISA and RT-PCR obtained performed in this study. In the present report, double labeling immunohistochemistry with anti-NF or anti-MAP-2 and anti-APP antibodies demonstrated the co-localization. Furthermore, we showed that the expression of APP in neurons and neurites was significantly increased in the cerebral cortex after traumatic brain injury. It has been pointed out that increased APP immunoreactivity occurrs in damaged axons due to disturbance of fast anterograde axonal transport (Koo et al., 1990)by destroyed cytoskeletal proteins, including neurofilaments (Posmantur et al., 1994) and MAP-2 (Taft et al., 1992). These results suggested that APP synthesis was increased from the early phase after brain injury and it lasted for a long period during the experiment. In the present study, the mRNA and protein levels for APP were elevated after TBI. It was previously reported that APP mRNA and protein levels were increased in neurons after TBI (Van den Heuvel et al., 1999; Ciallella et al., 2002). Furthermore, expression of APP was increased in neurons after ischemia and axonal injury (Stephenson et al., 1992; Xie et al., 2003). Taken together, these results suggest that APP is synthesized by neurons, rather than glial cells and macrophages/microglia, after TBI. In future studies, it will be necessary to further clarify the cell type producing APP after TBI.

TBI occurs as the result of a direct mechanical insult to the brain, and induces degeneration and death in the central nervous system (CNS) (Chirumamilla et al., 2002; Rice et al., 2003). Following the initial mechanical insult, secondary pathways are activated that contribute to the ischemic damage induced by circulatory disturbance, blood-brain barrier disruption and excitotoxic damage (Kawamata et al., 1995; Azbill et al., 1997; Xiong et al., 1997). The expression of APP has also been shown to increase in swollen axons and neuronal perikarya after neuronal injuries, including ischemia (Stephenson et al., 1992) and stab injuries (Otsuka et al., 1991). CNS disorders can be caused by the widespread neuronal and axonal degeneration induced by TBI (Chirumamilla et al., 2002; Rice et al., 2003). Taken together, these results suggest that APP leaks out from damaged and necrotic axons and neuronal cytoplasm after TBI. In the present study, CD11b-positive cells were colocalized with APP protein at 7 days after TBI. It appeared that macrophages/microglia engulfed and digested the APP that leaked from axons and neurons during this phase. Therefore, at 7 days after TBI, both neurons and macrophages/microglia expressed APP.

The overexpression of APP suggests the possibility of an Alzheimer disease-like pathology after TBI (Rumble et al., 1989; Itoh et al., 2009). Previously, the appearance of APP in the brain during pathological events was usually attributed to its synthesis by neurons, macrophages, microglia, or astrocytes (Otsuka et al., 1991). Sun *et al.* reported that overproduction of APP induced expression of the apoptosis-related Fas antigen in cultured neural, astrocytes, and microglia (Sun et al., 2004). Furthermore, APP induced nitric oxide synthetase (iNOS) and nitric oxide (NOS) production, and induced neural and glial cell apoptosis(Sun et al., 2004). In the present study, a continuous infusion of the anti-APP antibody infusion inhibited neural and glial apoptotic cell death at three days after TBI. This neuroprotection was associated with numerous GFAP-positive cells and glial scars, suggesting that the anti-APP antibody inhibited APP-induced glial cell apoptosis.

It was previously reported that APP which was expressed on the cell membrane of cultured cortical neural cells controlled intracellular Ca^{2+} entry (Bouron et al., 2004). Intracellular entry of Ca^{2+} activates Ca^{2+}-dependent signal pathways and can induce neural cell death. Additionally, choline acetyltransferase (ChAT) activity was decreased in the frontal cortex and hippocampus of APP 695 transgenic mice, an Alzheimer model overexpressing APP, and increased the number of apoptotic neurons(Feng et al., 2004). These APP 695 transgenic mice exhibit increased learning and memory impairment (Feng et al., 2004). In the present study, in the anti-APP antibody group there was an increase in the number of MAP-2-positive cells and a reduction in the arrival time to platform versus the PBS group. These data suggested that the anti-APP antibody increased ChAT activity and inhibited neural degeneration induced by overproduced APP in the frontal cortex and hippocampus after TBI, while cerebral function may be improved. As such, measurement of ChAT activity in the anti-APP antibody and the PBS groups after TBI will form the basis of future research.

Recent evidence suggests that APP, a ubiquitously expressed, highly conserved integral membrane glycoprotein, is not only a sensitive marker of axonal injury (Gentleman et al., 1993; Blumbergs et al., 1995), but may also have an important functional role following TBI. APP is upregulated acutely in injured neurons and reactive astrocytes following TBI (Pierce et al., 1996; Van den Heuvel et al., 1999), and this upregulation has been associated with increase hippocampal cell death (Murakami et al., 1998). Although the mechanisms leading to cell death are unknown, as the precursor to the neurotoxic Aβ protein, the conversion of APP to Aβ may have detrimental effects including an increased risk for development of Alzheimer's disease (Chen et al., 2004). Indeed, there are numerous clinical studies demonstrating substantial Aβ deposition and the formation of amyloid plaques (Smith et al., 2003; Ikonomovic et al., 2004). Furthermore, following TBI in the rat there is an increased β-secretase enzyme expression (BACE 11) that could potentially facilitate Aβ production (Blasko et al., 2004), a direct link between increase APP levels and increased Aβ deposition and toxicity (Stone et al., 2002).

In contrast to the potential deleterious effects of APP, an early acute rise in APP during the reparative phase of injury has resulted in the hypothesis that APP may actually serve a neuroprotective function (Van Den Heuvel et al., 2004). APP has been shown to be both beneficial and detrimental depending on its method of posttranslational processing within cells. The beneficial, secreted α form of APP (sAPPα) is generated by α-secretase cleavage, whereas the secreted APPβ (sAPPβ) and deleterious Aβ are generated from cleavage by β- and γ-secretases (Hardy 1997). sAPPα has been reported to have many neuroprotective and neurotrophic functions within the central nervous system (CNS) (Mattson et al., 1993); for instance, sAPPα administration reduced neuronal injury and improved functional outcome following rat TBI (Thornton et al., 2006). The α-secretase pathway is a non-amyloidogenic pathway in which the majority of APP is normally processed (Suh and Checler 2002), while after brain injury the β- and γ-secretase pathways are activated and are responsible for producing the toxic sAPPβ (Matrone et al., 2008; Sola Vigo et al., 2008) and Aβ (Mills and

Reiner 1999; Stone et al., 2002; Blasko et al., 2004). For instance, sAPPβ was shown to induce apoptotic cell death in PC 12 cells and neuronal degeneration in rat hippocampal neurons (Matrone et al., 2008; Sola Vigo et al., 2008). Nakagawa et al. reported that the APP overexpression of ST6Gal-1 in Neuro2 enhanced producing sAPP and the level of the extracellular sAPP β form is increased the level of sAPPα form(Nakagawa et al., 2006). In AD brain, increase of the extracellular sAPP beta level could affect the pathology of AD(Nakagawa et al., 2006). In the present study, anti-APP antibody treatment resulted in a reduction of neuronal and glial apoptotic cell death and recovery of memory and learning function to sham operation group levels, after TBI. These data suggest that toxic sAPPβ is produced more than sAPPα after TBI, and that toxic sAPPβ may be responsible for the neuronal and glial cell degeneration and death. Additionally, overproduction of sAPPβ after brain injury may facilitate Aβ production and deposition.

In the adult CNS, TBI results in a rapid response from resident astrocytes, a process often referred to as reactive astrocytosis or glial scarring (Davies et al., 1999; Jurynec et al., 2003). Glial scars have been reported to inhibit neurite elongation of damaged neurons and axonal regeneration, and thus prevent functional recovery (Davies et al., 1999; Jurynec et al., 2003). Furthermore, neurite outgrowth of cultured rat hippocampal neurons was found to be inhibited by glial scars *in vitro* (Rudge and Silver 1990). However, gliosis and glial scars protect against secondary insults that contribute to the ischemic damage induced by circulatory disturbance, blood-brain barrier disruption, excitotoxic damage, and free radicals (Pekny and Nilsson 2005). Moreover, reactive astrocytes secrete neurotrophic factor (NTF), nerve growth factor (NGF), and extracellular matrix which induce axonal outgrowth and regeneration of the neural network (Bechmann and Nitsch 2000; Deller et al., 2000). In addition, the formation of glial scars prevents leakage of secreted factors, and separates non-damaged areas from damaged areas, thereby maintaining normal CNS homeostasis (Silver et al., 1997; Gallo and Chittajallu 2001). Therefore, although the role of gliosis and glial scars in neuronal regeneration after brain injury remains controversial, the results from the present study suggest that gliosis and glial scars after TBI might be beneficial.

The results from the present study also demonstrated that infusion of the anti-APP antibody into the damaged region following TBI inhibited degeneration of neuronal and glial cells induced by overproduced APP after brain injury, with a significant reduction in injury size. This may be attributed a protective effect of the anti-APP antibody against neural and glial cell death induced by overproduced APP after TBI.

5. Conclusion

In conclusion, the results of the present study have demonstrated that TBI induces long-term increases in APP overexpression in the neuronal perikarya and neurites. In addition, endogenous overproduced APP after TBI inhibited astrocyte activity around the damaged brain region and induced neural cell degeneration. On the basis of these findings, we speculate that overexpression of APP after TBI is related to Alzheimer type dementia, and is an important risk factor for this disease.

6. Acknowledgments

The authors thank Mari Yachi and Emi Watanabe for technical assistance.

7. References

Azbill, R. D., Mu, X., Bruce-Keller, A. J., et al. (1997). Impaired mitochondrial function, oxidative stress and altered antioxidant enzyme activities following traumatic spinal cord injury. *Brain Res*, Vol.765, No.2, (September 2007), pp.283-290, ISSN 0006-8993.

Bechmann, I., & Nitsch, R. (2000). Involvement of non-neuronal cells in entorhinal-hippocampal reorganization following lesions. *Ann N Y Acad Sci*, Vol.911, (September 2007), pp.192-206, ISSN1749-6632.

Blasko, I., Beer, R., Bigl, M., et al. (2004). Experimental traumatic brain injury in rats stimulates the expression, production and activity of Alzheimer's disease beta-secretase (BACE-1). *J Neural Transm*, Vol.111, No.4, (September 2007), pp.523-536, ISSN 1435-1463.

Blumbergs, P. C., Scott, G., Manavis, J., et al. (1995). Topography of axonal injury as defined by amyloid precursor protein and the sector scoring method in mild and severe closed head injury. *J Neurotrauma*, Vol.12, No.4, (September 2007), pp.565-572, ISSN 1557-9042.

Bouron, A., Mbebi, C., Loeffler, J. P., et al. (2004). The beta-amyloid precursor protein controls a store-operated Ca2+ entry in cortical neurons. *Eur J Neurosci*, Vol.20, No.8, (September 2007), 2071-2078, ISSN 1460-9568.

Chen, X. H., Siman, R., Iwata, A., et al. (2004). Long-term accumulation of amyloid-beta, beta-secretase, presenilin-1, and caspase-3 in damaged axons following brain trauma. *Am J Pathol*, Vol.165,No. 2, (September 2007), pp.357-371, ISSN 0002-9440.

Chirumamilla, S., Sun, D., Bullock, M. R., et al. (2002). Traumatic brain injury induced cell proliferation in the adult mammalian central nervous system. *J Neurotrauma*, Vol.19, No. 6, (September 2007), pp.693-703, ISSN 1557-9042.

Ciallella, J. R., Ikonomovic, M. D., Paljug, W. R., et al. (2002). Changes in expression of amyloid precursor protein and interleukin-1beta after experimental traumatic brain injury in rats. *J Neurotrauma*, Vol.19, No.12, (September 2007), pp.1555-1567, ISSN 1557-9042.

Davies, S. J., Goucher, D. R., Doller, C., et al. (1999). Robust regeneration of adult sensory axons in degenerating white matter of the adult rat spinal cord. *J Neurosci*, Vol.19, No.14, (September 2007), pp.5810-5822, ISSN 1529-2401.

DeKosky, S. T., Abrahamson, E. E., Ciallella, J. R., et al. (2007). Association of increased cortical soluble abeta42 levels with diffuse plaques after severe brain injury in humans. *Arch Neurol*, Vol.64, No.4, (March 2008), pp.541-544, ISSN 0003-9942.

Deller, T., Haas, C. A., & Frotscher, M. (2000). Reorganization of the rat fascia dentata after a unilateral entorhinal cortex lesion. Role of the extracellular matrix. *Ann N Y Acad Sci*, Vol.911, (September 2007), pp.207-220, ISSN 0077-8923.

Elvander, E., Schott, P. A., Sandin, J., et al. (2004). Intraseptal muscarinic ligands and galanin: influence on hippocampal acetylcholine and cognition. *Neuroscience*, Vol.126, No.3, (September 2007), pp.541-557, ISSN 0306-4522.

Feng, Z., Chang, Y., Cheng, Y., et al. (2004). Melatonin alleviates behavioral deficits associated with apoptosis and cholinergic system dysfunction in the APP 695 transgenic mouse model of Alzheimer's disease. *J Pineal Res*, Vol.37, No.2, (September 2007), pp.129-136, ISSN 0742-3098.

Gallo, V., & Chittajallu, R. (2001). Neuroscience. Unwrapping glial cells from the synapse: what lies inside? *Science*, Vol.292, No.5518, (September 2007), pp.872-873, ISSN 0036-8075.

Gentleman, S. M., Nash, M. J., Sweeting, C. J., et al. (1993). Beta-amyloid precursor protein (beta APP) as a marker for axonal injury after head injury. *Neurosci Lett*, Vol.160, No.2, (September 2007), pp.139-144, ISSN 0304-3940.

Golde, T. E., Estus, S., Younkin, L. H., et al. (1992). Processing of the amyloid protein precursor to potentially amyloidogenic derivatives. *Science*, Vol.255, No.5045, (September 2007), pp.728-730, ISSN 0036-8075.

Goldgaber, D., Lerman, M. I., McBride, O. W., et al. (1987). Characterization and chromosomal localization of a cDNA encoding brain amyloid of Alzheimer's disease. *Science*, Vol.235, No.4791, (September 2007), pp.877-880, ISSN 0036-8075.

Green-Sadan, T., Kinor, N., Roth-Deri, I., et al. (2003). Transplantation of glial cell line-derived neurotrophic factor-expressing cells into the striatum and nucleus accumbens attenuates acquisition of cocaine self-administration in rats. *Eur J Neurosci*, Vol.18, No.7, (September 2007), pp2093-2098, ISSN 1460-9568.

Hardy, J. (1997). Amyloid, the presenilins and Alzheimer's disease. *Trends Neurosci*, Vol.20, No.4, (September 2007), pp.154-159, ISSN 0166-2236.

Ikonomovic, M. D., Uryu, K., Abrahamson, E. E., et al. (2004). Alzheimer's pathology in human temporal cortex surgically excised after severe brain injury. *Exp Neurol*, Vol.190, No.1, (September 2007), pp.192-203, ISSN 0041-4886.

Itoh, T., Satou, T., Hashimoto, S., et al. (2005). Isolation of neural stem cells from damaged rat cerebral cortex after TBI. *Neuroreport*, Vol.16, No.15, (September 2007), pp.1687-1691, ISSN 0959-4965.

Itoh, T., Satou, T., Nishida, S., et al. (2007). Immature and mature neurons coexist among glial scars after rat traumatic brain injury. *Neurol Res*, Vol.29, No.7, (December 2010), pp.734-742, ISSN 0161-6412.

Itoh, T., Satou, T., Nishida, S., et al. (2009). Expression of amyloid precursor protein after rat traumatic brain injury. *Neurol Res*, Vol.31, No.1, (December 2010), pp.103-109, ISSN 0161-6412.

Jurynec, M. J., Riley, C. P., Gupta, D. K., et al. (2003). TIGR is upregulated in the chronic glial scar in response to central nervous system injury and inhibits neurite outgrowth. *Mol Cell Neurosci*, Vol.23, No.1, (September 2007), pp.69-80, ISSN 1044-7431.

Kawamata, T., Katayama, Y., Hovda, D. A., et al. (1995). Lactate accumulation following concussive brain injury: the role of ionic fluxes induced by excitatory amino acids. *Brain Res*, Vol.674, No.2, (September 2007), pp.196-204, ISSN 0006-8993.

Koo, E. H., Sisodia, S. S., Archer, D. R., et al. (1990). Precursor of amyloid protein in Alzheimer disease undergoes fast anterograde axonal transport. *Proc Natl Acad Sci U S A*, Vol.87, No.4, (September 2007), pp.1561-1565, ISSN 0027-8424.

Lewen, A., Li, G. L., Olsson, Y., et al. (1996). Changes in microtubule-associated protein 2 and amyloid precursor protein immunoreactivity following traumatic brain injury in rat: influence of MK-801 treatment. *Brain Res*, Vol.719, No.1-2, (September 2007), pp.161-171, ISSN 0006-8993.

Masters, C. L., Multhaup, G., Simms, G., et al. (1985). Neuronal origin of a cerebral amyloid: neurofibrillary tangles of Alzheimer's disease contain the same protein as the amyloid of plaque cores and blood vessels. *Embo J*, Vol.4, No.11, (September 2007), pp.2757-2763, ISSN 0261-4189.

Matrone, C., Di Luzio, A., Meli, G., et al. (2008). Activation of the amyloidogenic route by NGF deprivation induces apoptotic death in PC12 cells. *J Alzheimers Dis*, Vol.13, No.1, (September 2007), pp.81-96, ISSN 1387-2877.

Mattson, M. P., Cheng, B., Culwell, A. R., et al. (1993). Evidence for excitoprotective and intraneuronal calcium-regulating roles for secreted forms of the beta-amyloid precursor protein. *Neuron*, Vol.10, No.2, (September 2007), pp.243-254, ISSN 0896-6273.

Mills, J., & Reiner, P. B. (1999). Regulation of amyloid precursor protein cleavage. *J Neurochem*, Vol.72, No.2, (September 2007), pp.443-460, ISSN 0022-3042.

Murakami, N., Yamaki, T., Iwamoto, Y., et al. (1998). Experimental brain injury induces expression of amyloid precursor protein, which may be related to neuronal loss in the hippocampus. *J Neurotrauma*, Vol.15, No.11, (September 2007), pp.993-1003, ISSN 1557-9042.

Nakagawa, K., Kitazume, S., Oka, R., et al. (2006). Sialylation enhances the secretion of neurotoxic amyloid-beta peptides. *J Neurochem*, Vol.96, No.4, (December 2010), pp.924-933, ISSN 0022-3042.

Nakamura, Y., Takeda, M., Niigawa, H., et al. (1992). Amyloid beta-protein precursor deposition in rat hippocampus lesioned by ibotenic acid injection. *Neurosci Lett*, Vol.136, No.1, (September 2007), pp.95-98, ISSN 0304-3940.

Nicoll, J. A., Roberts, G. W., & Graham, D. I. (1995). Apolipoprotein E epsilon 4 allele is associated with deposition of amyloid beta-protein following head injury. *Nat Med*, Vol.1, No.2, (September 2007), pp.135-137, ISSN 0065-1311.

Otsuka, N., Tomonaga, M., & Ikeda, K. (1991). Rapid appearance of beta-amyloid precursor protein immunoreactivity in damaged axons and reactive glial cells in rat brain following needle stab injury. *Brain Res*, Vol.568, No.1-2, (September 2007), pp.335-338, ISSN 0006-8993.

Pekny, M., & Nilsson, M. (2005). Astrocyte activation and reactive gliosis. *Glia*, Vol.50, No.4, (September 2007), pp.427-434.

Pierce, J. E., Trojanowski, J. Q., Graham, D. I., et al. (1996). Immunohistochemical characterization of alterations in the distribution of amyloid precursor proteins and beta-amyloid peptide after experimental brain injury in the rat. *J Neurosci*, Vol.16, No.3, (September 2007), pp.1083-1090, ISSN 1529-2401.

Posmantur, R., Hayes, R. L., Dixon, C. E., et al. (1994). Neurofilament 68 and neurofilament 200 protein levels decrease after traumatic brain injury. *J Neurotrauma*, Vol.11, No.5, (September 2007), pp.533-545, ISSN 1557-9042.

Rice, A. C., Khaldi, A., Harvey, H. B., et al. (2003). Proliferation and neuronal differentiation of mitotically active cells following traumatic brain injury. *Exp Neurol*, Vol.183, No2, (September 2007), pp.406-417, ISSN 0014-4886.

Robakis, N. K., Ramakrishna, N., Wolfe, G., et al. (1987). Molecular cloning and characterization of a cDNA encoding the cerebrovascular and the neuritic plaque amyloid peptides. *Proc Natl Acad Sci U S A*, Vol.84, No.12, (September 2007), pp.4190-4194, ISSN 0027-8424.

Roberts, G. W. (1988). Immunocytochemistry of neurofibrillary tangles in dementia pugilistica and Alzheimer's disease: evidence for common genesis. *Lancet*, Vol.2, No.8626-8627, (September 2007), pp.1456-1458, ISSN 0140-6736.

Roberts, G. W., Allsop, D., & Bruton, C. (1990). The occult aftermath of boxing. *J Neurol Neurosurg Psychiatry*, Vol.53, No.5, (September 2007), pp.373-378, ISSN 0027-8424.

Roberts, G. W., Gentleman, S. M., Lynch, A., et al. (1994). Beta amyloid protein deposition in the brain after severe head injury: implications for the pathogenesis of Alzheimer's disease. *J Neurol Neurosurg Psychiatry*, Vol.57, No.4, (September 2007), pp.419-425, ISSN 0027-8424.

Rudge, J. S., & Silver, J. (1990). Inhibition of neurite outgrowth on astroglial scars in vitro. *J Neurosci*, Vol.10, No.11, (September 2007), pp.3594-3603, ISSN 1529-2401.

Rumble, B., Retallack, R., Hilbich, C., et al. (1989). Amyloid A4 protein and its precursor in Down's syndrome and Alzheimer's disease. *N Engl J Med*, Vol.320, No.22, (September 2007), pp.1446-1452, ISSN 1553-4406.

Schofield, P. W., Tang, M., Marder, K., et al. (1997). Alzheimer's disease after remote head injury: an incidence study. *J Neurol Neurosurg Psychiatry*, Vol.62, No.2, (September 2007), pp.119-124, ISSN 0022-3050.

Selkoe, D. J., Abraham, C. R., Podlisny, M. B., et al. (1986). Isolation of low-molecular-weight proteins from amyloid plaque fibers in Alzheimer's disease. *J Neurochem*, Vol.46, No.6, (September 2007), pp.1820-1834, ISSN 0022-3042.

Silver, I. A., Deas, J., & Erecinska, M. (1997). Ion homeostasis in brain cells: differences in intracellular ion responses to energy limitation between cultured neurons and glial cells. *Neuroscience*, Vol.78, No.2, (September 2007), pp.589-601, ISSN 0077-8923.

Smith, D. H., Uryu, K., Saatman, K. E., et al. (2003). Protein accumulation in traumatic brain injury. *Neuromolecular Med*, Vol.4, No.1-2, (September 2007), pp.59-72, ISSN 1535-1084.

Sola Vigo, F., Kedikian, G., Heredia, L., et al. (2008). Amyloid-beta precursor protein mediates neuronal toxicity of amyloid beta through Go protein activation. *Neurobiol Aging*, Vol.30, No.9, (September 2007), pp.1379-1392, ISSN 0197-4587.

Stephenson, D. T., Rash, K., & Clemens, J. A. (1992). Amyloid precursor protein accumulates in regions of neurodegeneration following focal cerebral ischemia in the rat. *Brain Res*, Vol.593, No.1, (September 2007), pp.128-135, ISSN 0006-8993.

Stone, J. R., Okonkwo, D. O., Singleton, R. H., et al. (2002). Caspase-3-mediated cleavage of amyloid precursor protein and formation of amyloid Beta peptide in traumatic axonal injury. *J Neurotrauma*, Vol.19, No.5, (September 2007), pp.601-614, ISSN 1557-9402.

Suh, Y. H., & Checler, F. (2002). Amyloid precursor protein, presenilins, and alpha-synuclein: molecular pathogenesis and pharmacological applications in Alzheimer's disease. *Pharmacol Rev*, Vol.54, No.3, (September 2007), pp.469-525, ISSN 0362-1642.

Sun, K. H., Sun, G. H., Su, Y., et al. (2004). Acidic-rich region of amyloid precursor protein induces glial cell apoptosis. *Apoptosis*, Vol.9, No.6, (September 2007), pp.833-841, ISSN 1360-8185.

Taft, W. C., Yang, K., Dixon, C. E., et al. (1992). Microtubule-associated protein 2 levels decrease in hippocampus following traumatic brain injury. *J Neurotrauma*, Vol.9, No.3, (September 2007), pp.281-290, ISSN 1557-9042.

Thornton, E., Vink, R., Blumbergs, P. C., et al. (2006). Soluble amyloid precursor protein alpha reduces neuronal injury and improves functional outcome following diffuse traumatic brain injury in rats. *Brain Res*, Vol.1094, No.1, (September 2007), pp.38-46, ISSN 0006-8993.

Van den Heuvel, C., Blumbergs, P. C., Finnie, J. W., et al. (1999). Upregulation of amyloid precursor protein messenger RNA in response to traumatic brain injury: an ovine head impact model. *Exp Neurol*, Vol.159, No.2, (September 2007), pp.441-450, ISSN 0014-4886.

Van Den Heuvel, C., Donkin, J. J., Finnie, J. W., et al. (2004). Downregulation of amyloid precursor protein (APP) expression following post-traumatic cyclosporin-A administration. *J Neurotrauma*, Vol.21, No.11, (September 2007), pp.1562-1572, ISSN 1557-9042.

Xie, Y., Yao, Z., Chai, H., et al. (2003). Potential roles of Alzheimer precursor protein A4 and beta-amyloid in survival and function of aged spinal motor neurons after axonal injury. *J Neurosci Res*, Vol.73, No.4, (September 2007), pp.557-564, ISSN 1097-4547.

Xiong, Y., Gu, Q., Peterson, P. L., et al. (1997). Mitochondrial dysfunction and calcium perturbation induced by traumatic brain injury. *J Neurotrauma,* Vol.14, No.1, (September 2007), pp.23-34, ISSN 1557-9042.

4

Key Enzymes and Proteins in Amyloid-Beta Production and Clearance

Cecília R A Santos[1], Isabel Cardoso[2,3] and Isabel Gonçalves[1]
[1]*University of Beira Interior- Health Sciences Research Centre, Covilhã*
[2]*Escola Superior de Tecnologia da Saúde do Porto, Instituto Politécnico do Porto, Vila Nova de Gaia,*
[3]*Molecular Neurobiology Unit, IBMC- Instituto de Biologia Molecular e Celular, Porto, Portugal*

1. Introduction

Last century, in 1907, Alois Alzheimer first described the disease that now bears his name, relating a 54-year-old female case with presenile dementia. Alzheimer's disease (AD), an irreversible progressive neurodegenerative disorder, is actually the most common form of dementia. AD affects more than 24 million people all over the world, and is predicted to double every 20 years, becoming one of the medical burdens of our days. More than 90% of AD cases are sporadic late-onset, and have a complex idiopathic aetiology. The small number of early onset AD cases, is related to hereditary monogenic defects, and has provided important clues for understanding the AD pathology (Bertram, et al. 2007). Although the available drugs are able to delay the symptoms and progression of the disease and to positively influence the quality of life of the patients, at present there is still no cure for AD.

AD is characterized clinically by progressive decline in cognitive function and neuropatologically by the presence of neuropil threads and neuron loss, in addition to the molecular hallmarks of neurofibrillar tangles and neuritic (or senile) plaques in the brain. Neuritic plaques are extracellular amyloid deposits found abundantly in the hippocampus, in the neocortex and in the amygdala of AD brains. These pathological brain changes may occur 20 to 30 years prior to the onset of the clinical symptoms and the symptomatic phase of AD can last from 5 to 12 years (DeKosky and Marek 2003). The extracellular neuritic plaque deposits of amyloid were first investigated by (Glenner and Wong 1984), when they purified microvascular amyloid deposits from AD brains, and provided a partial sequence of a 4kDa subunit protein, that they named amyloid-beta (Aβ) peptide. Around the same time, the hyperphosphorylated tau (p-tau), a microtubule assembly protein, was identified as the main constituent of the neurofibrillar tangles (NFTs) that accumulate inside many neurons in AD brains (Grundke-Iqbal, et al. 1986). Amyloid deposition and neurofibrillar tangles, occur with some frequency in brains of young adults with Down's syndrome (Schochet, et al. 1973). The discovery that amyloid deposits in the brain from Down syndrome were composed of Aβ peptide (Glenner and Wong 1984), as well as the cloning of the beta amyloid precursor protein (APP), with its localization to the chromosome 21

(Korenberg, et al. 1989), led the scientists to search AD-causing mutations in the APP gene. Since that, several mutations associated with familial early onset forms of AD have been described, either in the APP gene (Kowalska 2003) or in preselin 1 (PS1) or preselin 2 (PS2) genes (Bertram et al. 2007). Either PS1 or PS2 can be the catalytic subunit of γ-secretase, which is the final endoprotease in the pathways that generate the Aβ peptide (see section 2). All these findings led to the amyloid cascade hypothesis, articulated by John Hardy and others (Hardy and Higgins 1992), in which the accumulation of Aβ peptide, generated from the proteolytic cleavage of APP in the brain, could trigger a complex downstream cascade that results in the symptoms of AD. This hypothesis states that gradual accumulation and aggregation of the hydrophobic Aβ peptide initiates a cascade that leads to synaptic alterations, astrocytic and microglial activation, the modification of the soluble tau protein into insoluble paired helical filaments, and progressive neuronal loss associated with multiple neurotransmitter deficiencies and cognitive failure (Hardy and Selkoe 2002). The cascade hypothesis suggests that stopping or slowing formation of the Aβ plaques would delay the onset of the disease symptoms. Aβ is found in the extracellular fluids of the brain, including cerebrospinal fluid (CSF), and in the interstitial fluid surrounding neurons and glial cells in brain lobes (Seubert, et al. 1992; Vigo-Pelfrey, et al. 1993). Over the last years, several key proteins have been described as being implicated in Aβ production and clearance, but further elucidation of the mechanisms involved in the process will be important for identifying new potential therapies to reduce Aβ accumulation and combat AD. This book chapter reviews the production of Aβ from APP and the proteins involved in its degradation and clearance .

2. Generation of amyloid beta peptides

The β amyloid precursor protein, APP, takes a central position in AD pathogenesis, as it is processed by the sequential action of β- and γ-secretase, generating the Aβ peptide, which is deposited as amyloid plaques in brains of AD individuals. APP is an integral membrane protein, with a large N-terminal extracellular domain and a short C-terminal cytoplasmatic domain, which is expressed ubiquitously in neuronal and non-neuronal cells.
The human APP gene is located on chromosome 21 (Korenberg et al. 1989) and alternative splicing results in protein isoforms of various lengths: two isoforms predominant in non-neuronal tissues (751- and 770-), and the 695-amino acid form, that is the predominant isoform in neurons (Kang and Muller-Hill 1990). APP belongs to a protein family that includes APP-like protein 1 (APLP1) and 2 (APLP2) (Eggert, et al. 2004), a group of type-I transmembrane proteins that are processed in the same fashion. APP is hydrolyzed into different fragments (Figure 1) during its intracellular trafficking, and these metabolites mediate various functions (Haass 2004; Haass and Selkoe 1993). APP is first cleaved by either α- or β-secretase at the α- or β-sites, respectively, which lie in the extracellular domain of the APP. These proteases compete for APP, originating: soluble APPα (sAPPα, for α-secretase) or soluble APPβ (sAPPβ, for β-secretase), which are released to the extracellular space, and a membrane anchored C-terminal end (C83 for α-secretase or C99 for β-secretase). Subsequently, in the lipid bilayer, γ-secretase acts in the C-terminal end, C83 or C99. The γ-cleavage of C83 generates the APP intracellular domain (AICD), with 6kDa, and the N-terminal peptide with 3kDa (p3) into the extracellular space. γ-cleavage of C99, in a specific sequence (Aβ domain) generates Aβ peptide and the AICD. This pathway of APP processing by β-secretase followed by γ-secretase leading to Aβ peptide is called the

amyloidogenic pathway. Aberrant and/or cumulative Aβ production, have been postulated to be the main etiological basis of AD. The alternative pathway of APP processing by α-secretase followed by γ-secretase, in which no Aβ is formed, is termed nonamyloidogenic pathway.

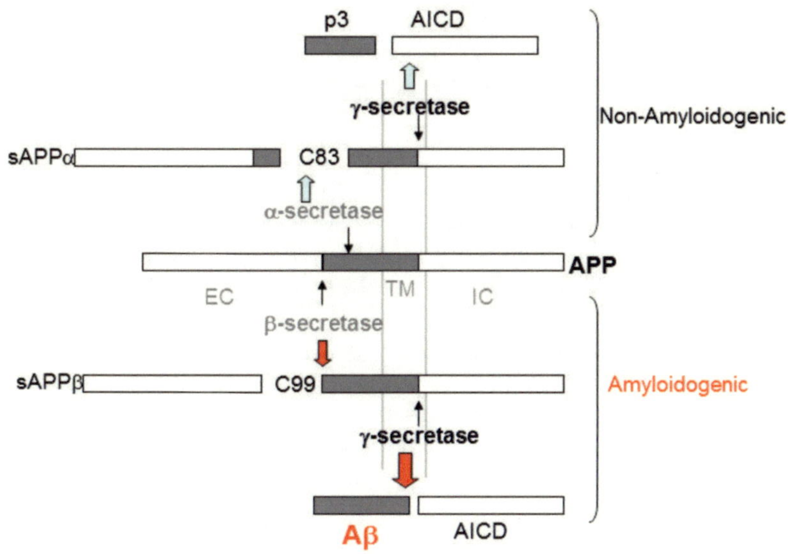

Fig. 1. Schematic diagram of APP processing (not drawn in scale). TM-transmembrane;EC-extracelular; IC- intracellular

Aβ is a ~4kDa peptide with 38 to 43 amino acids, depending on the site of γ-secretase cleavage. Aβ peptide is normally produced by cells and under physiological conditions there are two major species: Aβ40 and Aβ42. The major species produced is Aβ40 and corresponds to 90% of the total Aβ peptide. The minor species produced, Aβ42, is more prone to aggregation due to two additional hydrophobic amino acids, and therefore it is the predominant species accumulated in AD brain plaques.

A number of proteins influence the subcellular trafficking itinerary of APP and β-secretase between the cell surface, endosomes and the Trans-Golgi-Network (TGN). APP is synthesized in the endoplasmic reticulum (ER) and is transported through the Golgi apparatus to the TGN, where the highest concentration is found in steady state neurons (Greenfield, et al. 1999). From TGN, the APP can be transported, in TGN-derived vesicles, to cell surface where it is either cleaved by α-secretase to produce sAPPα, or internalized via the endosomal-lysosomal pathway (Caporaso, et al. 1994). The Aβ peptide is generated either in the ER and TGN (Greenfield et al. 1999), as in the endosomal/lysosomal system (Haass and Selkoe 1993). Available evidence suggests that co-residence of APP and β-secretase in the endosomal compartments promotes amyloidogenesis. Retrograde transport of APP, out of the endosome to the TGN, reduces Aβ production, while APP routed to, and kept at the cell surface, enhances its non-amyloidogenic processing (Tang 2009).

Very little is known about the physiological function of APP and its proteolytic products. APP knockout mice (KO) are viable and fertile, showing a slight abnormal phenotype

(Dawson, et al. 1999). APLP1 and APLP2 KO mice are also viable and fertile, but APP/APLP2 and APLP1/APLP2 double null mice and APP/APLP1/APLP2 triple null mice show early postnatal lethality (Heber, et al. 2000; von Koch, et al. 1997). APP/APLP1 double null mice are viable, suggesting redundant functions of amyloid precursor protein family members (Heber et al. 2000). Putative suggested roles for APP include trafficking, neurotrophic signalling, control of cell adhesion, neuritic outgrowth and synaptogenesis, apoptosis and transcription regulation (Zheng and Koo 2006). As APP is proteolysed in the cell, the net effect of full-length APP on cellular activity may be a combination of the function of its proteolytic products, depending on the proportion levels of each of them.

2.1 Alpha-secretase

APP is cleaved by α-secretase in the center of Aβ domain, precluding Aβ peptide generation, and a soluble domain of APP is released: sAPPα. Three related proteases, all from the ADAM family, had been suggested to exert the α-secretase activity: ADAM-9, ADAM-10 and ADAM-17 (Asai, et al. 2003). Like full length APP, members of the ADAM family (a desintegrin and metalloprotease family) are type-I transmembrane proteins, possessing both potential adhesion and protease domains. Several studies suggested α-secretase activity for ADAM-9. However, as RNAi of ADAM-9 has no effect in sAPPα generation (Kuhn, et al. 2010), ADAM-9 seems to be involved only in regulated α-cleavage and not in constitutive α-secretase activity. Different studies strongly suggest that ADAM-10 is the main constitutive α-secretase that is active at the cell surface (Lammich, et al. 1999) (Jorissen, et al. 2010), but there may exist some functional redundancy in α-cleavage by the ADAM protease family. ADAM-17 is an 824 amino acid polypeptide containing a secretory signal sequence, a desintegrin domain and a metalloprotease domain, that also seems to be involved in regulated α-secretase activity (Merlos-Suarez, et al. 2001).

sAPPα has important roles in neuronal plasticity/survival, stem cell proliferation in CNS, and is able to rescue the abnormalities of APP deficient mice, indicating that most of APP´s physiological function is mediated by sAPPα (Zhang, et al. 2011).

2.2 Beta-secretases: BACEs

β-secretase cleavage is the first critical step in the APP amyloidogenic pathway, and increased β-secretase activity levels have been correlated with brain Aβ deposition in late onset AD patients (Li, et al. 2004). Aβ peptide is generated from APP by a sequential two-step proteolytic process involving β- and γ-secretases (Haass 2004), being BACE 1 (β-site APP cleaving enzyme 1) the major β-secretase in the cell (Vassar, et al. 1999). BACE1 is a member of the pepsin family of aspartyl proteases, and its activity on APP generates the membrane bound C-terminal fragment (CTFβ or C99). BACE1 requires acidic environment for optimal activity and cleaves APP at the known β-site locations, Asp1 and Glu11. Overexpression of BACE1 induces cleavage of APP at β-sites and is mainly found in the early Golgi, late Golgi/early endosomes and endosomes with acidic environment. BACE1 is also found at the cell surface (Huse, et al. 2002; Vassar et al. 1999).

BACE2 is an additional β-secretase, mapped in 21q22.3 region (Solans, et al. 2000), that also cleaves β-secretase substrates. However, BACE2 expression in neurons is lower than BACE1 (Bennett, et al. 2000). BACE1 null mice died in the first weeks and those that survived, were smaller, presented hyperactive behaviour, were affected by hypomyelination of peripheral nerves and had altered neurological behaviours such as elevated pain sensitivity

(Dominguez, et al. 2005). BACE2 KO mice are healthy overall, while a deficiency of both BACE1 and BACE2 enhanced the BACE1 KO lethality phenotype, suggesting functional redundancy (Dominguez et al. 2005).
Cathepsin B has been proposed as another β-secretase. Although its inhibition has been found to reduce Aβ production, its physiological activity is not well established (Hook, et al. 2009).

2.3 The gamma secretase complex

γ-secretase is a protein complex, of high molecular weight, responsible for the membrane cleavage of the APP C-terminal remnants after cleavage by either α- or β-secretase (C83 and C99, respectively). The cleavage of C83 and C99 by γ-secretase generates p3 and the Aβ peptide, respectively. In addition to C83 and C99 peptides, several non-APP substracts are cleaved by γ-secretase and all of them are type-I transmembrane proteins that require ectodomain shedding as a prerequisite to γ-secretase cleavage (Haapasalo and Kovacs 2011). γ-secretase complex comprises four core components which include: presenilin (PS1 or PS2), nicastrin, anterior pharynx-defective-1 (APH-1), and presenilin enhancer-2 (PEN2) (Kimberly and Wolfe 2003; Takasugi, et al. 2003). All of these four core components of γ-secretase are necessary for the enzymatic activity of the complex. PS1 and PS2 are two presenilin homologs, and several mutations in the corresponding genes have been described as the major cause of familial AD cases (Bertram et al. 2007). Different kinds of experimental evidences suggest that presenilins are transmembrane proteins with crucial catalytic roles in γ-secretase activity (Zhang et al. 2011). Nicastrin, other component of γ-secretase, is a type-I transmembrane glycoprotein considered the scaffolding protein of the complex (Vassar and Citron 2000). Finally, the other two components of γ-secretase are: APH-1, that interacts with nicastrin to form a stable intermediate in the early assembly stages of the complex and PEN-2, that regulates PS endoproteolysis (Vassar and Citron 2000). Besides the four components of γ-secretase complex, some factors, playing a modulatory role, have been described. Example of that is CD147 that when down regulated increases Aβ production and TMP21/p23 that regulates γ-cleavage (Zhang et al. 2011).
Experimental evidences support the idea that γ-secretase resides in ER, Golgi-TGN, endosomes and intermediate compartments, most of which (except TGN) do not correspond to the main localizations of APP (Cupers, et al. 2001).

3. Enzymes and peptides involved in amyloid-beta degradation and clearence

The clearance of Aβ in the human central nervous system (CNS), is roughly 8% of total production per hour. It is controlled by Aβ degradation in the brain and by its efflux from the CNS to the peripheral circulation through the blood-brain barrier or the blood-cerebrospinal fluid barrier (Zlokovic 2004). The high clearance of Aβ is in part due to the presence of cryptidases in several cellular compartments and reduction of Aβ degradation by these enzymes may be implicated in the progression of AD cases. Aβ accumulation, and the concomitant formation of amyloid plaques observed in AD brains occurs in the extracellular space. It is also in this compartment, that Aβ can be degraded by cell surface and/or secreted cryptidases, such as insulin degrading enzyme and neprylisin. The subcellular distribution of Aβ degrading cryptidases is a strong indicator that Aβ degradation can be controlled at multiple subcellular compartments, such as the mitochondria, ER, Golgi, endosomes and lisossomes (Malito, et al. 2008).

In the brain, Aβ metabolism is mainly regulated by the activity of neprilysin (NEP) and insulin-degrading enzyme (IDE), but presequence peptidase, endothelin converting enzyme (ECE), angiotensin-converting enzyme (ACE), the uPA/tPA- plasmin system and matrix metalloproteinases are also involved in the process (Table 1). In addition, some proteins as transthyretin (TTR), gelsolin, alpha2-macroglobulin and apolipoprotein E do also play an important role in Aβ clearance and degradation. Some of them do actually have a direct function in Aβ catabolism such as TTR, plasmin, and gelsolin, which have the capacity to cleave the peptide, others because their interaction with Aβ enable its degradation or prevent its neurotoxicity as it is the case of alpha-2-macroglobulin and apolipoprotein E (Table 2).

Enzymes	Function	Brain distribution	References
IDE	Hydrolises peptide bonds of Aβ40 and Aβ42	Neurons, microglia, endothelial cells, choroid plexus epithelial cells	(Bora et al. 2010; Bora and Prabhakar 2010; Malito et al. 2008)
NEP	Hydrolises peptide bonds of Aβ42	Neurons, microglia, endothelial cells, choroid plexus epithelial cells	(Malito et al. 2008; Meilandt et al. 2009)
PreP	Hydrolises peptide bonds of Aβ40 and Aβ42 in mitochondria		(Falkevall et al. 2006)
ECE	Hydrolises peptide bonds of Aβ40 and Aβ42	Neurons, astrocytes, endothelial cells	(Miners et al. 2008b)
ACE	Converts Aβ42 to Aβ40 Cleaves Aβ40	Neurons, endothelial cells, choroid plexus epithelial cells	(Miners et al. 2008a; Zou et al. 2007)
Plasmin	Degrades aggregated and non-aggregated Aβ40 and Aβ42 Inhibits Aβ fibrillogenesis	Neurons, microglia	(Tucker et al. 2002; Tucker et al. 2000b)
MMP-2	Hydrolises peptide bonds of Aβ40 and Aβ42 Beta-secretase activity	Microglia, astrocytes, Schwann cells	(Miners et al. 2008a)
MMP-9	Hydrolises peptide bonds of Aβ40 and Aβ42 and aggregated Aβ fibrils	Neurons, endothelial cells	(Miners et al. 2008a; Yan et al. 2006)

Table 1. Functions and brain distribution of key enzymes in Aβ clearance.

Key players	Function	Brain distribution	References
TTR	Hydrolises peptide bonds of Aβ40 and Aβ42, and aggregated Aβ oligomers and fibrils	choroid plexus epithelial cells meninges	(Costa et al. 2008; Schwarzman et al. 1994)
Gelsolin	Inhibits fibrillization of Aβ and defibrillates preformed fibrils	Oligodendrocytes, microglia, choroid plexus epithelial cells	(Chauhan et al. 2008; Ray et al. 2000)
Alpha-2 macroglobulin	Aβ carrier, binds Aβ protecting it from proteolysis, reduces Aβ aggregation and fibril formation	astroglia	(Du et al. 1998; Du et al. 1997)
Apo E	Binds Aβ enhancing the proteolytic activity of NEP, and IDE	Astrocytes, neurons, microglia	(Jiang et al. 2008)
MT-2	Diminishes Aβ binding to TTR Prevents copper mediated aggregation of Aβ	Cortical neurons	(Chung et al. 2010; Martinho et al. 2010)
MT-3	Increases Aβ binding to TTR Inhibits formation of Aβ aggregates	Cortical neurons	(Irie and Keung, 2001, 2003; Martinho et al. 2010)

Table 2. Functions and brain distribution of key proteins in Aβ clearance.

3.1 IDE – Insulin degrading enzyme

Insulin degrading enzyme (IDE) is a ~ 110 kDa zinc-containing metalloendopeptidase that degrades monomeric forms of Aβ peptides and insulin, which has also high nanomolar affinity for other substrates with different sequences and structures. The common features of IDE substrates are that they are all amyloidogenic in nature. So, besides Aβ and insulin, IDE also cleaves, insulin-like growth factor 2, atrial natriuretic peptide, bradykinin, endorphin, and glucagon. However, *in vivo* relevance of this degrading activity has only been demonstrated for Aβ and insulin (Malito et al. 2008). Interestingly, patients with type 2 diabetes are under an increased risk of AD. In addition, Aβ is a direct competitive inhibitor of insulin binding and action, and this is a likely justification for the increased levels of Aβ observed in insulin resistant AD patients (Xie, et al. 2002). This dual effect of IDE stresses the importance of the development of inhibitors and activators of its activity for the treatment of diabetes and AD, respectively.

The first evidences of the capacity of IDE to degrade Aβ were reported by Kurochkin and Goto (1994) who identified a protein of 110,000 Da present in cytosol fractions from rat brain and liver that cross-linked to ^{125}I-labeled synthetic Aβ. A few years later IDE was actually identified as the main soluble Aβ degrading enzyme in human brain and in neuronal cell cultures, where its action takes places in the extracellular milieu (McDermott and Gibson 1997). Besides its ability to degrade Aβ, IDE activity is also associated with oligomerization of synthetic Aβ at physiological levels in the conditioned media of cultured cells (Qiu, et al. 1998). In addition, evidence that membrane-associated and secreted IDE isoforms carry out the degradation and clearance of Aβ secreted by neurons and microglia was provided a couple of years later (Bertram, et al. 2000).

IDE is composed of four homologous domains that share 15–24% sequence similarity. These domains form two functional N- and C-terminal domains that are joined by an extended 28 amino acid residue loop, creating a large catalytic chamber which can accommodate substrates of the order of 6 kDa. Substrate binding is assisted by the C-terminal domain and, its hydrolysis occurs at the N-terminal domain (Li, et al. 2006). The active site of IDE encompasses the His-Glu-aa-aa-His sequence and requires zinc. IDE enzyme hydrolyses several peptide bonds of both Aβ40 and Aβ42, but is particularly efficient at hydrolysing the Lys28-Gly29 peptide bond followed by the Phe19-Phe20 and His14-Gln15 bonds of these substrates (Bora, et al. 2010; Bora and Prabhakar 2010).

IDE is expressed by cortical and subcortical neurons, and has been detected in the cytoplasm of the three major components of the vascular wall: endothelial cells, pericytes and smooth muscle cells (Dorfman, et al. 2010; Gao, et al. 2004). IDE is also expressed towards the apical surface of the choroid plexus tissue where its inhibition leads to disrupted metabolism of Aβ and its concurrent accumulation at the blood-CSF barrier (Behl, et al. 2009). Besides the cytoplasm, IDE is found in endosomes, on the cell surface, and in the extracellular milieu. The type of cell in the nervous system expressing IDE establishes whether it is secreted or associated with the cell surface. Primary mouse microglia and the BV-2 cell line are found to secrete IDE, but in primary hippocampal neurons and differentiated PC12 cells only membrane associated IDE has been found. IDE is also present in mitochondria, and in the dendrites of neurons (Malito et al. 2008).

Evidence that IDE activity in AD brains is reduced compared to age-matched controls has been giving support to the hypothesis that reduced IDE activity may contribute to Aβ accumulation in the brain (Perez, et al. 2000). For example, membrane-bound IDE protein concentrations and activity decrease during the conversion from mild cognitive impairment (MCI) to mild-severe AD in the hippocampus, which correlates negatively with brain Aβ42 content in MCI and in AD brain (Zhao, et al. 2007). Still, other studies indicate that IDE may be less important in the process of Aβ clearance (Wang, et al. 2010). There is also evidence that in transgenic mice brain, Aβ plaques induce cortical mRNA and protein levels of IDE in parallel with increased Aβ40 and Aβ42 production, suggesting a positive feedback regulatory mechanism of Aβ regulation (Vepsalainen, et al. 2008).

3.2 NEP – Neprilysin

Neprilysin (NEP) is a 90–110 kDa plasma membrane glycoprotein of the neutral zinc metalloendopeptidase family. It consists of a short N-terminal cytoplasmic tail, a single transmembrane helix and a large C-terminal extracellular ectodomain. The ectodomain of neprilysin is largely made of α-helices with six disulfide bridges and at least three N-glycosylation sites. The ectodomain encompasses the catalytic site, with the conserved HExxH motif necessary for zinc coordination and a proteolytic chamber (Malito et al. 2008). NEP is widely expressed in several tissues such as the brush-border of intestinal and kidney epithelial cells, neutrophils, thymocytes, lung, prostate, testes, and brain. In the brain, it is expressed on the plasma membranes of neurons, pre- and post-synaptically, and is most abundant in the nigrostriatal pathway, and in brain areas vulnerable to amyloid plaque deposition, such as the hippocampus (Wang, et al. 2006). It is also expressed in the tunica media and endothelium of cortical and leptomeningeal blood vessels where it participates in the regulation of the vascular tone, and in pyramidal neurons. NEP is also involved in the regulation of neuropeptide signalling (Dorfman et al. 2010; Miners, et al. 2008b).

NEP has been implicated in the degradation of Aβ. It degrades Aβ42 *in vivo,* and when NEP is inhibited, Aβ degradation in rat hippocampus is blocked with a concomitant increase of Aβ42 plaques in this brain region, and in the cortical region outside the hippocampus. In addition, the capacity to degrade Aβ42 of exogenous origin is severely compromised in NEP knockout homozygote mice in which the levels of Aβ40 and Aβ42 remain very high. These studies are corroborated by correlative studies in patients with sporadic AD and healthy age matched controls. Overexpression of NEP in brains of human amyloid precursor protein (hAPP) transgenic mice decreases overall Aβ levels and amyloid plaque burdens by 50% and effectively prevented early Aβ deposition in the neocortex and hippocampus. However, it did not reduce levels of Aβ oligomers or improved deficits in spatial learning and memory. The differential effect of NEP on plaques and oligomers suggests that NEP-dependent degradation of Aβ affects plaques more than oligomers and that these structures may form through distinct assembly mechanisms (Meilandt, et al. 2009). Moreover, the expression of NEP on the surface of leukocytes, trough lentivirus transplantation of bone marrow cells, reduced soluble brain Aβ levels by ~30% and lowered the accumulation of Aβ peptides by 50–60% when transplantation was performed at both young and early adult age. This peripheral NEP expression reduced amyloid dependent performance deficits of these animals in the Morris Water Maze (Guan, et al. 2009). *Ex-vivo* gene delivery of a soluble form of NEP, via fibroblasts, into transgenic APP mice also demonstrated increased clearance of plaques. Interestingly, mRNA and protein levels of NEP can be induced by intracranial injections of Aβ42, which also reduced the accumulation of amyloid plaques (Malito et al. 2008). Microglia from old PS1-APP mice, but not from younger mice, have a twofold to fivefold decrease in expression of NEP, compared with their littermate controls (Hickman, et al. 2008). Despite all the evidence sustaining the proteolytic action of NEP on Aβ, the molecular basis of the interaction between NEP and Aβ remains largely unexplained because the volume of the proteolytic chamber of NEP is about half the size of Aβ (Malito et al. 2008).

3.3 Presequence peptidase

Presequense peptidase (PreP) is a 110 kDa metalloprotease, ubiquitously expressed, but with higher abundance in heart and skeletal muscle. It is responsible for degradation of targeting peptides, which have been cleaved off inside the mitochondrial matrix after protein import, but it also cleaves other unstructured peptides up to 65 amino acids (Stahl, et al. 2002). More recently, PreP was shown to completely degrade Aβ40 and Aβ42, which are present in mitochondria. More relevance is added to this action of PreP as it has been shown that hPreP is actually the only protease responsible for degradation of Aβ in the mitochondria (Falkevall, et al. 2006) and Aβ-induced mitochondrial toxicity has been associated with AD (Tillement, et al. 2011).

Human PreP consists of 4 domains, creating two halves connected by a hinge region. The two halves can create a large catalytic chamber of 10 000 Å where Aβ fits. The inverted zinc-binding motif is located in the N-terminal region, but also includes residues located in the C-terminal half, about 800 amino acids distant from the zinc-binding motif (Johnson, et al. 2006). Unlike IDE, PreP cannot degrade insulin, making PreP a better therapeutic agent candidate than IDE as its use would preclude deleterious side effects associated with the degradation of insulin. Another interesting feature of PreP is that its proteolytic activity against Aβ is abolished under oxidizing conditions, probably due to the formation of a disulphide bridge between Cys90 and Cys527 that inhibits the substrate from entering the catalytic chamber. These findings indicate a possible inhibition of hPreP under elevated ROS production in mitochondria implicated in AD, and might therefore be relevant in this disease (Alikhani, et al. 2009).

3.4 ECE – Endothelin converting enzyme

Endothelin-converting enzymes 1 and 2 (ECE-1 and ECE-2) were originally implicated in the processing of pro-hormone forms of endothelin. They are type II integral membrane zinc metalloendopeptidases that are primarily localized to the endothelium throughout the human vasculature. They share common catalytic substrates and are responsible for cleaving big endothelins to produce potent vasoconstrictor endothelins (Miners, et al. 2008a; Miners et al. 2008b).

ECE sequences and domain organization are similar to NEP's and are also capable of degrading Aβ *in vitro* and *in vivo* (Eckman, et al. 2001). Homozygous knockouts for ECE-1 are lethal and heterozygous animals show an increased amount of Aβ40 and Aβ42 in the brain. Homozygous ECE-2 knockout mice show a gene dose dependent increase of both forms of Aβ in the brain as well (Eckman, et al. 2006; Eckman, et al. 2003).

ECE-1 is present in neurons, specifically in pyramidal neurons of the hippocampus and layer V of the neocortex, and to a less extent in astrocytes (Sluck, et al. 1999). In mice, ECE-2 is largely confined to the brain; in the rat brain, ECE-1 occurs in the cerebrovascular endothelium, whereas ECE-2 is predominantly neuronal, with special incidence on hippocampal pyramidal neurons (Miners et al. 2008a; Miners et al. 2008b).

There is evidence of significant decrease in ECE-2 gene expression in AD patients (Weeraratna, et al. 2007). The contribution of ECE-1 to the accumulation of Aβ or reduction in local microvascular blood flow in AD seems to be detrimental, with abnormal production of ET-1 being more likely to reflect Aβ -mediated upregulation of ECE-2 (Palmer, et al. 2010).

3.5 ACE – Angiotensin-converting enzyme

Angiotensin-converting enzyme (ACE) is a membrane-bound zinc metalloprotease expressed in blood vessels throughout the body. ACE is extremely important for the regulation of fluid homeostasis and blood pressure. It converts angiotensin I to the potent vasoconstrictor angiotensin II. Within the brain, ACE has been detected in cortical pyramidal neurons and in the cerebral vasculature. Its highest levels occur in circumventricular organs, such as the subfornical organ, area postrema, and the median eminence but was detected in other areas such as the caudate nucleus, putamen, substantia

nigra pars reticularis, nucleus of the solitary tract, dorsal motor nucleus, median preoptic nucleus, and choroid plexus in rat, human, rabbit, sheep and monkey (Miners et al. 2008a).
ACE has two homologous domains, each having a functional active site. The N-domain of ACE is responsible for converting Aβ42 to Aβ40, whereas the angiotensin-converting activity is found predominantly in the C-domain of ACE. N-linked glycosylation is essential for both Aβ42 to Aβ40 conversion and angiotensin-converting activities and protects ACE from proteolysis (Zou, et al. 2009).
The first correlations between ACE and AD were found in 1985 by Zubenko and colleagues (Zubenko, et al. 1985) who showed that the CSF of patients with moderate degrees of senile dementia of the AD type exhibited about half the ACE activity of age and sex-matched control individuals, raising the possibility that ACE activity in the CSF could be an index of AD. In a posterior study, however, no differences in ACE activity in the CSF were found between AD patients and age matched controls raising some controversy on this issue (Konings, et al. 1993), but other studies reported reduced activity of ACE in the parietal cortex of AD brains (Ichai, et al. 1994).
ACE was found to significantly inhibit Aβ aggregation in 2001 (Hu, et al. 2001). The inhibition of aggregation was specifically blocked by preincubation of ACE with an ACE inhibitor, lisinopril. ACE degraded Aβ by cleaving Aβ40 at the site Asp(7)-Ser(8). Compared with Aβ40, aggregation and cytotoxic effects of the degradation products Aβ-(1-7) and Aβ-(8-40) peptides were reduced or virtually absent. These findings led to the hypothesis that previous associations of ACE genotype with AD susceptibility (Farrer, et al. 2000; Hu, et al. 1999; Isbir, et al. 2001; Yang, et al. 2000) could rely on its capacity to degrade Aβ and prevent the accumulation of amyloid plaques *in vivo*. Besides Aβ40 degradation, cellular expression of ACE also promotes degradation of naturally secreted Aβ42, and leads to the clearance of both species (Hemming and Selkoe 2005). In addition, ACE also converts Aβ42 to Aβ40 which is less neurotoxic (Zou, et al. 2007).
Pharmacological inhibition of ACE with a widely prescribed drug, captopril, promotes the accumulation of cell-derived Aβ in the media of APP expressing cells and questions if prescribed ACE inhibitors against hypertension could elevate cerebral Aβ levels in humans (Hemming and Selkoe 2005). To address this question the ACE inhibitor captopril was administered to two lines of APP transgenic mice presenting low or high levels of Aβ with associated plaque deposition. In both models, captopril did not affect cerebral Aβ levels nor plaque deposition or peripheral Aβ levels (Hemming, et al. 2007).
Epidemiological data obtained from a male population, however, suggests that angiotensin receptor blockers are more efficient in reducing the incidence and progression of AD and dementia compared with ACE inhibitors or other cardiovascular drugs (Li, et al. 2010). However, there are strong indications that ACE inhibitors may reduce the risk for and progression of dementias (Shah, et al. 2009). Still, these effects remain rather controversial, and prescription of ACE inhibitors against hypertension should be regarded with caution (Hajjar, et al. 2008; Kehoe and Wilcock 2007; Shah et al. 2009). Alternatively, ACE inhibitors could be designed to specifically target the angiotensin-converting C-domain, without inhibiting the Aβ42 to Aβ40-converting activity of ACE or increasing neurotoxic Aβ42 (Zou et al. 2009).

3.6 uPA/tPA-plasmin system

Plasmin is a serine protease generated from the proteolytic cleavage of inactive plasminogen, by tissue-type (tPA) or by urokinase-type plasminogen activator (uPA). In the brain, plasminogen is synthesized in neurons, whereas uPA and tPA expression can be induced in neurons as well as in microglia. This system is involved in many normal neural functions, such as neuronal plasticity, learning, and memory (Wang et al. 2006; Zhao and Pei 2008).

uPA and tPA are induced by Aβ treatment in primary rat embryonic cortical cultures *in vitro* as well as in a murine model of Aβ accumulation *in vivo* (Tucker, et al. 2000b). In addition, it plasmin degrades both non-aggregated and aggregated Aβ40 (Tucker, et al. 2000a), and also degrades Aβ42, preventing Aβ42 aggregation into beta-pleated sheet structures (Exley and Korchazhkina 2001). Plasmin also inhibits Aβ toxicity, reduces Aβ deposition *in vitro,* and inhibits Aβ fibrillogenesis (Tucker, et al. 2002). The anti-amyloidogenic effect of plasmin is further enhanced by its capacity to increase the processing of human APP, and efficiently degrading secreted amyloidogenic and non-amyloidogenic APP fragments. Consistent with these observations, brains from AD patients contain reduced levels of plasmin (Ledesma, et al. 2000). Moreover, Aβ injected into the hippocampus of mice lacking either tPA or plasminogen persists causing activation of microglial cells and neuronal damage. Conversely, Aβ injected into wild-type mice is rapidly cleared and does not cause neuronal degeneration (Melchor, et al. 2003). Assembly of Aβ42, on the other hand, seems to promote the up-regulation of the tPA/plasminogen proteolytic system, which can modulate the deposition of amyloid plaques *in vivo,* in a negative feedback mechanism (Lee, et al. 2007).

3.7 Matrix metalloproteinases

Matrix metalloproteinases (MMPs) are zinc- and calcium dependent endopeptidases, produced by neurons and glial cells. Metalloproteinase 2 (MMP-2) can be detected in the walls of some blood vessels and scattered white matter glia. Metalloproteinase 3 (MMP-3) is present in and around some neurons and within occasional amyloid plaques, and metalloproteinase 9 (MMP-9) is present in many neurons.

MMP-2 and MMP-9 all have Aβ-degrading activity *in vitro,* although the Aβ degrading activity of these MMPs has not received so much attention *in vivo.* However MMP-2 and MMP-9 activity are elevated in homogenates of hippocampal tissue from AD brains, and several cell types (glial, neuronal and vascular) up-regulate endogenous MMP-2 -3 and -9 expression in response to Aβ stimulation (Deb and Gottschall 1996; Miners et al. 2008b; Gottschall 1996).

MMP-2 also known as gelatinase A/type IV collagenase/matrix hydrolyses Aβ40 and Aβ42 peptides at Lys 16-Leu 17, at Leu 34-Met 35, and Met 35-Val 36 peptide bonds (Roher, et al. 1994). Besides its Aβ degrading activity, MMP-2 has also beta-secretase activity (LePage, et al. 1995). In AD brains, MMP-2 is present in the reactive microglia located in the center of senile plaques, and in Schwann cells (Yamada, et al. 1995). Aβ stimulates the expression and activation of MMP-2 to a large extent due to the increased expression of membrane type-1 (MT1)-MMP expression, the primary MMP-2 activator (Jung, et al. 2003).

There seems to be a complex regulation of MMP2 expression by oligomeric Aβ in astrocytes. Oligomeric Aβ directly down-regulates MMP2 expression and activation in astrocytes. However, it also induces the production of pro-inflammatory cytokines which stimulate production of MMP2 (Li, et al. 2011).

Increased MMP-9 immunolabelling has been detected in neurons of AD patients, as well as in neurofibrillary tangles, plaques and blood vessel walls, but not in granular neurons or glial cells. MMP-9 is also detected in the vicinity of extracellular amyloid plaques (Backstrom, et al. 1996). MMP-9, unlike ECE-1, NEP and IDE, is capable of cleaving aggregated Aβ fibrils (Miners et al. 2008b). It cleaves Aβ at several sites, predominantly at Leu34-Met35 within the membrane-spanning domain (Backstrom et al. 1996; Yan, et al. 2006). The presence of the apoE4 significantly dampens Aβ-induced MMP-9 in primary cultures of rat astrocytes. This effect may affect Aβ clearance and promote Aβ deposition in AD brains (Guo, et al. 2006). There is also evidence that reduction of Aβ levels through the action of MMP-9 may also result from the direct processing of cell surface APP with an alpha-secretase like activity, substantially reducing the levels of secreted Aβ peptide (Talamagas, et al. 2007).

Aged APP/presenilin 1 mouse astrocytes surrounding amyloid plaques, showed enhanced expression of MMP-2 and MMP-9. Astrocyte-conditioned medium obtained from these animals degraded Aβ, producing several small fragments. In the brains of MMP-2 and MMP-9 KO mice, significant increases in the Aβ levels were found in comparison to wild-type controls. This study reinforces previous *in vitro* evidences that MMP-2 and -9 may contribute to extracellular brain Aβ clearance through the degradation of Aβ (Yin, et al. 2006).

Several MMPs polymorphisms have been examined in relation to the risk of developing dementia with controversial results (Baig, et al. 2008; Helbecque, et al. 2007; Reitz, et al. 2008; Reitz, et al. 2010). MMPs may also be considered potential plasmatic and cerebrospinal fluid markers of AD as the levels of MMP-3 in the plasma and CSF of AD patients was found higher than in controls, whereas MMP-2 was significantly decreased in CSF but unchanged in plasma (Horstmann, et al. 2010).

3.8 Transthyretin

Transthyretin (TTR) is a 55 kDa homotetrameric protein secreted mainly by the liver and choroid plexus into the plasma and CSF, respectively (Soprano, et al. 1985). The name "transthyretin" discloses its dual physiological role as a carrier for thyroid hormones (Woeber and Ingbar 1968) and retinol, the latter through the binding to retinol-binding protein (Goodman 1985). TTR plasma concentration is age dependent and in healthy newborns it is about half of that in adults (Stabilini, et al. 1968; Vahlquist, et al. 1975), varying from 20 to 40 mg/ dL. In spite of the low TTR levels in CSF (~2 mg/ dL), the choroid plexus is presented as the major site of TTR expression, expressed as a ratio of tissue/mass, corresponding to a 30-fold higher than that found in plasma and represents 20% of the total CSF proteins (Weisner and Kauerz 1983).

Over a hundred TTR mutations have been associated with Familial Amyloid Polyneuropathy (FAP), some of which are very common in Portuguese patients, such as the valine at position 30 substituted by a methionine (TTR V30M) (Saraiva, et al. 1984), others provide a very aggressive phenotype, such as the TTR L55P (Jacobson, et al. 1992). Curiously, TTR T119M was described as an example of a non-aggressive mutation that inclusively has a protective role against the disease (Almeida, et al. 2000).

The first report that associates TTR to Aβ and AD as a protective molecule is from Schwarzman et al. who describes the capacity of normal CSF to inhibit amyloid formation and concluded that TTR was the major Aβ binding protein in the CSF, that could also decrease the aggregation state of the peptide and its toxicity (Schwarzman, et al. 1994). Prior to this finding, TTR was found associated to senile plaques, NFTs and microangiopathic lesions (Shirahama, et al. 1982). The sequestration hypothesis was raised suggesting that normally produced Aβ is sequestered by certain extracellular proteins, thereby preventing amyloid formation and Aβ cytotoxicity; when sequestration fails amyloid formation occurs (Schwarzman and Goldgaber 1996). The observation that TTR is reduced in the CSF of AD patients further supported the idea of a TTR protective role in this pathology (Serot, et al. 1997). Authors also observed a decrease in TTR levels with age which could be related to the epithelial atrophy in the choroid plexus. Along time several reports described TTR decrease in CSF of AD patients (Davidsson, et al. 2002; Serot et al. 1997; Gloeckner, et al. 2008; Hansson, et al. 2004) although it remains unclear whether this reduction is restricted to AD, or on the contrary is common to other neurodegenerative disorders (Chiang, et al. 2009). It is also uncertain if the TTR decrease in the CSF happens early in disease development (or even before symptoms appears) or if it is a latter event, and thus studies involving patients with mild cognitive impairment (MCI) and early-staged probable AD patients are needed.

Other studies using a transgenic model of *Caenorhabditis elegans* expressing Aβ42 supported a TTR role in AD as administration of TTR rescued the neurodegeneration observed in this model (Link 1995). Mammalian models used to recapitulate AD features were never completely successful as AD transgenic mice did not show NFTs and demonstrate little or no neuronal cell loss (Holcomb, et al. 1998; Hsiao, et al. 1996; Irizarry, et al. 1997a; Irizarry, et al. 1997b; Stein and Johnson 2002). However, in some of the models, animals showed increased TTR expression in the hippocampus (Stein and Johnson 2002); TTR was then described to be a survival gene (Stein and Johnson 2002) and although this work is controversial because TTR expression is thought to be confined to the choroid plexus and meninges (in the case of the brain), authors further showed that when a chronic infusion of an antibody against TTR was applied into the hippocampus of mice expressing human APP, an increase of Aβ, tau phosphorylation, neuronal loss and apoptosis were observed (Stein, et al. 2004). Underlying these observations is, according to authors, sAPPα that leads to increased expression of protective genes, such as TTR, to confer neuroprotection (Stein et al. 2004). Other studies, using transgenic APP mice hemizigous for endogenous TTR showed accelerated Aβ deposition (Choi, et al. 2007), while double transgenic mice for APP and TTR presented lower deposition (Buxbaum, et al. 2008). However, in other models, TTR was described to have the opposite effect and was associated with increased vascular Aβ deposition (Wati, et al. 2009).

Regarding the nature of TTR/Aβ interaction, different researchers confirmed TTR binding to Aβ (Carro, et al. 2002; Liu and Murphy 2006; Costa, et al. 2008) not only to the monomer but also to Aβ oligomers and fibrils, raising the hypothesis that TTR may be involved in the formation of senile plaques (Costa et al. 2008); TTR was also able to inhibit and to disrupt Aβ fibrils. However, which TTR conformation binds Aβ peptide is still controversial. Du Murphy et al. showed that TTR tetramers interact preferably with Aβ aggregates rather than Aβ monomers enhancing Aβ aggregation, whereas TTR monomers arrest Aβ aggregate growth (Du and Murphy 2010). On the other hand, studies by Costa et al. (Costa et al. 2008) showed that soluble Aβ binds to different TTR variants correlating negatively with the amyloidogenic potential of the TTR mutant. Thus, TTR119M presented the highest affinity to Aβ, contrarily to what was observed by Du and Murphy (Du and Murphy 2010). Other

studies also indicated a different relation between TTR variant/amyloidogenic potential and binding to the peptide, with amyloidogenic mutants binding less to Aβ peptide and inhibiting less its aggregation (Schwarzman, et al. 2004). In this work it was also shown that TTRs were functional tetramers. Hence, other studies are necessary to completely understand the nature of the TTR/Aβ interaction, concerning both Aβ and TTR species involved. Structural analysis, obtained from computer-assisted modeling (Schwarzman et al. 2004) predicted the existence of an Aβ binding domain on the surface of each TTR monomer; residues 30-60, especially the 38-42 region of TTR seemed to be the key structure of the Aβ binding domain (Schwarzman and Goldgaber 1996; Schwarzman, et al. 2005). Du and Murphy, identified the A strand, in the inner β-sheet of TTR, as well as the EF helix, as regions of TTR that are involved with Aβ association (Du and Murphy 2010).
The discussion on the TTR interaction with Aβ and consequent inhibition of aggregation and toxicity reduction raised the hypothesis that mutations in the TTR gene or conformational changes in the protein induced by aging, could affect the sequestration properties. A study was conducted with the aim of identifying mutations in the TTR gene in the AD population but no correlation was found (Palha, et al. 1996). Finally, and concerning the mechanism underlying TTR protective role in AD, Costa and colleagues found that TTR is able to proteolytically process Aβ peptide (Costa et al. 2008). Regarding TTR ability to degrade Aβ, several cleavage sites were identified and the newly generated Aβ peptides shown to have decreased amyloidogenic potential, when compared to the full length counterpart (Costa et al. 2008); TTR is also able to degrade aggregated forms of the peptide and inhibition of the TTR activity resulted in increased Aβ fibril formation (Costa et al. 2008).

3.9 Gelsolin

Gelsolin can be found both as an intrinsic cytoplasmic protein and as a secreted protein in plasma and CSF (Kwiatkowski, et al. 1985). Intracellular gelsolin regulates actin polymerization by binding to actin, and it also caps and breaks the actin filaments (Janmey, et al. 1985; Matsumoto, et al. 2003). Secreted (plasma/CSF) and intracellular gelsolin originate from the alternative splicing of a single gene, but their disulphide structure is different with recognised functional implications. All of the five cysteine (Cys) residues present in human cytoplasmic gelsolin are free thiols, whereas in plasma/CSF gelsolin, three Cys residues are free thiols and the other two Cys residues are disulfide-linked (Wen, et al. 1996). The five free thiol groups are likely to confer anti-oxidant properties to the molecule. Secreted gelsolin has an extension of 25 amino acids at its N-terminal, which is absent in the cytoplasmic form (Chauhan, et al. 2008).
Gelsolin found in the CSF may originate from oligodendrocytes or microglia (Chauhan et al. 2008). It was also suggested that choroid plexus may be responsible for the presence of gelsolin in CSF (Matsumoto et al. 2003), where it may have also an important function counteracting the neurotoxicity of Aβ (Antequera, et al. 2009; Vargas, et al. 2010).
Plasma and cytosolic gelsolin both bind Aβ and the Aβ -gelsolin complex exists in the plasma and in the cytosol (Chauhan, et al. 1999; Ji, et al. 2008). Both inhibit the fibrillation of Aβ, and defibrillate preformed fibrils (Ray, et al. 2000). In addition it has been demonstrated that when administered to transgenic mouse models of AD reduces the Aβ40/Aβ42 and the amyloid load (Hirko, et al. 2007; Matsuoka, et al. 2003). Therefore, gelsolin may also be looked as a potential therapeutic agent against AD.

3.10 Alpha2-macroglobulin

Alpha2-macroglobulin (a2M) is a 720 kDa soluble glycoprotein composed of four identical 180 kDa subunits, each encoded by a single-copy gene on human chromosome 12. Each subunit contains at least five binding sites: the bait region, the internal thiol ester, the receptor binding site, the Aβ binding site, and the zinc binding site. The bait region, the internal thiol ester and the receptor binding site are crucial for the activation and internalization of a2M. The bait region binds any known protease. The four bait regions in the tetramer are in close contact and get cleaved by the bound proteases, triggering activation of a2M. This conformational change results in the exposure of the four thiol esters, and of the four receptor binding sites, to the extracellular environment. The receptor binding site of each monomer, a 27 residue consensus sequence located at their C-terminal tail, will then bind to the receptor and mediate the internalization of the complex. The Aβ binding site is located between the bait and the receptor binding regions of each monomer (Borth 1992; Du, et al. 1997; Hughes, et al. 1998; Kovacs 2000).

Binding to Aβ42 occurs with high affinity (Kd= 3.8×10^{-10} M) and protects the peptide from proteolysis by exogenous trypsin, suggesting that a2M may function as a carrier protein for Aβ and may serve to regulate clearance of Aβ from such tissues as the brain (Du et al. 1997; Hughes et al. 1998). a2M co-incubated with Aβ significantly reduces aggregation and fibril formation *in vitro*, and cultured fetal rat cortical neurons are less vulnerable to the toxic actions of Aβ following pretreatment with a2M, being likely that a2M has the capacity to keep Aβ in a soluble state, preventing fibril formation and associated neurotoxicity (Du, et al. 1998). a2M also inhibits both Aβ fibril formation and Aβ -induced cytotoxicity in PC12 cells (Monji, et al. 2000). The inhibition of the formation of amyloid fibrils are probably due to the interaction of a2M with prefibrillar species to maintain the solubility of Aβ (Yerbury, et al. 2009), and therefore their aggregation state in the extracellular milieu. In addition, Qiu et al described a serine protease that binds to a2M to form a stable high molecular weight complex capable of efficiently cleaving Aβ (Qiu, et al. 1996). This serine protease-a2M complex was capable of proteolytically digesting both Aβ40 and Aβ42, resulting in disruption of the central region of the peptide (residues 10–35), which is believed to mediate the conformational change that underlies Aβ self-aggregation (Qiu et al. 1996).

a2M is also a physiological ligand for the low-density lipoprotein receptor-related protein (LRP) abundantly expressed in the CNS. The a2M/Aβ complexes can be degraded by glioblastoma cells and fibroblasts via LRP, but the degradation of free Aβ must be mediated via an LRP-independent pathway. These results suggest that LRP can function as a clearance receptor for Aβ via a2M (Narita, et al. 1997). The effect of self-aggregation and LRP-1 ligands on the elimination of human Aβ 40 from the rat brain across the blood-brain barrier has been investigated recently. In the first instance it was demonstrated that the elimination rate of ^{125}I hAβ40 dimer was 92.7% decreased compared to the ^{125}I hAβ40 monomer. When pre-incubated with LRP-1 ligands, such as activated a2M, apolipoprotein E2 (apoE2), apoE3, apoE4, and lactoferrin, the elimination of ^{125}I hAβ40) was reduced. There seems that dimerization and LRP-1-ligand complex formation prevents the elimination of Aβ40 from the brain across the blood-brain barrier (Ito, et al. 2007).

There is also an over-representation of a common a2M polymorphism, Val1000 (GTC)/Ile1000 (ATC) in AD patients, which correlates with an increase in Aβ burden (Kovacs 2000; Liao, et al. 1998), further sustaining the importance of a2M in Aβ clearance.

3.11 Apolipoprotein E

From all the proteins and peptides associated with AD and amyloid beta metabolism, apolipoprotein E (ApoE) is probably the most thoroughly studied, and several recent reviews give excellent and comprehensive overviews about its structure and function (Zhong and Weisgraber 2009a, b), and the pathways in which it is involved in AD (Kim, et al. 2009), either Aβ dependent or Aβ independent (Huang 2010; Mahley, et al. 2006). Therefore, this section will just give a brief overview about ApoE and will focus only on its association with AD via Aβ dependent pathways.

ApoE is a 34,2 kDa glycoprotein containing 299 amino acids. The protein contains two structural domains that are responsible for different functions of apoE. The amino-terminal domain (residues 1-191) contains the lipoprotein receptor binding region (residues 136-150), and the carboxyl-terminal domain (residues 216-299) contains the major lipoprotein (lipid) binding domain.

There are three common isoforms of ApoE, ApoE2, ApoE3 and ApoE4, which are encoded by three alleles (e2, e3 and e4, respectively) of a single gene. Sequence differences among the ApoE isoforms reside only on amino acids 122 or 158 which may be cysteine or arginine, but are sufficient to determine significant functional consequences (Huang 2010; Mahley et al. 2006).

ApoE4 is the major known genetic risk factor for AD and as much as 65–80% of all AD patients are ApoE4 carriers. This allele is over-represented in late-onset familial AD in several populations and in late-onset sporadic AD (Farrer, et al. 1997). In addition, as the number of Apo E alleles increases, the risk of onset of AD also increases while the age of onset decreases; as the number of ApoE4 alleles increases from 0 to 2, the risk of developing late-onset AD increases from 20% to 90%, and the mean age of onset decreases from 84 to 68 years (Corder, et al. 1993; Frangione, et al. 1996). The N and C terminal domains of ApoE interact in ApoE4 (called domain interaction), which is mediated by the formation of a salt bridge between Arg-61 in the N- terminus and Glu-255 in the C- terminus of ApoE4. This interaction might be the molecular basis for the detrimental effects of ApoE4 in AD pathogenesis (Huang 2010).

ApoE is expressed in several organs but is mainly expressed in the liver, followed by the brain. Non-neuronal cells, mainly astrocytes and to some extent microglia, are the major cell types that express apoE in the brain (Boyles, et al. 1985; Pitas, et al. 1987). Neurons also produce ApoE under certain conditions, particularly in response to brain injury (Boschert, et al. 1999) .

ApoE (E2 and E3) are important for the distribution of lipids among cells throughout the body and within the CNS, where the principal apolipoproteins are, and where they transport lipids and cholesterol for cell repair and neurite outgrowth. These properties are not shared by Apo E4 which seems to counteract the features of Apo E2 and ApoE3 with detrimental effects (Mahley et al. 2006).

ApoE is also essential for astrocytes to bind, internalize and degrade Aβ deposits (Koistinaho, et al. 2004). ApoE binds Aβ with high affinity. It was demonstrated that lipid-free ApoE4 and ApoE3 form stable complexes with Aβ, with ApoE4 being more effective in the formation of the complex, but inducing a pathological β-sheet conformational change in Aβ ((Wisniewski and Frangione 1996). This interaction requires the N-terminal and the C-terminal domains, and there are strong indications that the interaction is affected by the lipid content (Weisgraber and Mahley 1996).

ApoE, but not ApoE4 plays a role in facilitating the proteolytic clearance of soluble Aβ from the brain. The endolytic degradation of Aβ peptides within microglia by NEP and related enzymes is dramatically enhanced by ApoE. Similarly, Aβ degradation extracellularly by IDE is facilitated by ApoE. The capacity of ApoE to promote Aβ degradation is dependent upon the ApoE isoform and its lipidation status. The enhanced expression of lipidated ApoE, through the activation of liver X receptors, stimulates Aβ degradation (Jiang, et al. 2008).

In contrast, Apo E4 inhibits Aβ clearance and stimulates Aβ deposition (Huang, et al. 2004). It also enhances Aβ production and potentiates Aβ induced chromosomal leakage and apoptosis (Mahley and Huang 2006). In addition, ApoE4 enhances Aβ42 oligomer induced toxicity (Manelli, et al. 2007). Taken together these observations sustain the effects of ApoE4 in the enhancement of the overall Aβ burden via interaction with the peptide.

3.12 Metallothioneins 2 and 3

Metallothioneins (MTs) were discovered as cadmium binding proteins in equine kidney cortex. MTs is a generic name for a superfamily of low molecular weight cysteine- and metal-rich proteins with high affinity for divalent metals, such as zinc, cadmium and copper with four major isoforms, MT-1 to MT-4, identified in humans. They occur in all living organisms from the simplest forms of life, such as prokaryotes to the most complex, such as higher plants and vertebrate animals. It is clear that MTs are multipurpose proteins with unquestionable metal binding and anti-oxidant properties. In addition, there is increasing evidence that MT-1 and MT-2 (MT-1/2), and MT-3 display such diverse physiological actions as inhibition of pro-apoptotic mechanisms, enhancement of cell survival, tissue regeneration, and have anti-inflammatory properties. Concurrent with this wide array of functions, MT-1/2 have been implicated in neuroprotection and neurodegeneration, and particularly in AD (Hidalgo, et al. 2009; Penkowa, et al. 2006).

It is interesting that a considerable body of work has related an increase of MT-1/2 brain levels with aging and AD. In AD patients elevated levels of cytokines and IL-1 may induce MT-1/2 production in astrocytes. Studies in animal models of AD, showed that the MT-1/2 levels were higher, when compared to WT mice, while MT-3 levels were unaltered or reduced, suggesting that these proteins may have a relevant role in providing long term protection against inflammation (Hidalgo et al. 2009). This up-regulation of MT-1/2 in animal models of AD may have detrimental consequences in Aβ clearance as MT-2 diminishes the binding of TTR to Aβ (Martinho, et al. 2010). Considering TTR an Aβ scavenger as explained above, a less efficient removal of Aβ would be expected when MT-2 levels are increased, and this appears to be the case in AD. Furthermore, inhibition of homeodomain interacting protein kinase 2 activity in AD patients, might be involved in p53 misfolding, most likely through MT-2A upregulation (Lanni, et al. 2010). In addition, it was also shown that MT-2A may also prevent copper-mediated Aβ aggregation and neurotoxicity, by a mechanism which primarily involves a specific metal exchange interaction between Zn7.MT-2A and Cu(2).Aβ, and subsequent inhibition of H_2O_2 generation (Chung, et al. 2010). Furthermore, a metal swap between Zn7.MT-3 and soluble and aggregated Aβ1–40–Cu(II) abolishes ROS production and related cellular toxicity (Meloni, et al. 2008).

These studies relating metal exchange and Aβ aggregation, conducted to a recent interest in the use of metal-chelation drugs as a potential therapy for AD. For example, the administration of the copper and zinc chelating drug, clioquinol, prevents plaque formation in transgenic AD mice (Hegde, et al. 2009).

Since the discovery of MT-3 as a growth inhibitory factor, with reduced expression levels in AD brains compared to age-matched controls, several studies provide evidence that MT-3 is related to the aetiology of AD. Some studies indicate that MT-3 may potentially promote the clearance of Aβ plaques, while others show an opposite trend or even no differences (Howells, et al. 2010). MT-3 alone antagonizes the toxic effect of Aβ because it inhibits the formation of SDS-resistant Aβ aggregates, thereby protecting cortical neurons from its toxic effects. Both the full-length and the N-terminal domain of MT-3 promote neuron survival at low concentrations but inhibited it at high concentrations. These observations suggest that the anti- Aβ activity of MT-3 is different from its neuronal growth inhibitory activity. Other possible mechanisms underlying the protection of MT-3 from Aβ toxicity may be related to its interaction with TTR by improving its Aβ degrading capacity (Martinho et al. 2010).

4. Conclusion

The extracellular neuritic plaque deposits of amyloid found in AD brains contain Aβ, and according to the amyloid cascade hypothesis, the accumulation of Aβ peptide, can trigger gradual synaptic alterations, astrocytic and microglial activation, and modification of the soluble tau protein into insoluble paired helical filaments, with progressive neuronal loss and cognitive failure (Hardy and Selkoe 2002). The cascade hypothesis suggests that stopping or slowing formation of the Aβ plaques would delay the onset of the disease symptoms. Therefore, it is crucial to thoroughly elucidate the regulation of Aβ production and clearance to design new and effective therapies against AD.

APP, takes a central position in AD pathogenesis, as Aβ arises from its proteolytic cleavage through the sequential action of β- and γ-secretase. APP is first cleaved by either α- or β-secretase at the α- or β-sites, respectively, which lie in the extracellular domain of APP. These proteases originate: soluble APPα (sAPPα, for α-secretase) or soluble APPβ (sAPPβ, for β-secretase), which are released to the extracellular space, and a membrane anchored C-terminal end (C83 for α-secretase or C99 for β-secretase). γ-cleavage of C99, generates the Aβ peptide. This pathway is known as the amyloidogenic pathway. Misregulation of all the intervenients in this process may lead to Aβ accumulation. If APP cleavage by β-secretase or γ-cleavage of C99 is more effective than α-secretase, then the all process shifts into the accumulation of Aβ. Also if APP synthesis is enhanced, as it is the case of several mutated forms of APP associated with early onset AD, the production of Aβ is also increased with similar results (Ertekin-Taner 2007). So, alterations in APP synthesis and processing by both secretases, or downstream in the γ-secretase complex action, may account for more severe forms of disease. Another good example of that are the mutations associated with presenilins 1 and 2 , which are part of the γ-secretase complex, known to be responsible for early onset inherited forms of AD (Ertekin-Taner 2007).

Once Aβ has been produced, other important players come into action (Figure 2). These are all the enzymes and proteins that, either by directly cleaving Aβ into less harmful peptides or making them more prone to proteolysis or less susceptible to aggregation through protein-protein interactions, will reduce the Aβ load in vulnerable areas of the brain.

Reduced degradation of Aβ by proteases is generally accepted to enhance plaque pathology in AD brains, and may depend on several factors such as decreased mRNA expression or decreased protein levels or activity, either in the brain cortex, hippocampus or in brain microvessels; and post-translational modifications, such as oxidation and deposition of the enzymes in the diseased brain with consequent loss of its native structure and functionality (Dorfman et al, 2010.).

IDE and NEP are well accepted as Aβ degrading enzymes, but although few studies compare the relative contribution of each of these enzymes to the overall Aβ load, NEP seems to be the major protease involved in Aβ degradation. In transgenic mice models of familial AD, over-expression of IDE or NEP prevents amyloid plaque pathology and consequent early death (Leissring, et al. 2003) indicating that degradation of Aβ by these metalloproteinases may be of high therapeutic interest for AD patients. A recent study carried out in AD patients showed that, NEP mRNA, protein levels, and activity are decreased compared to normal controls without any cognitive impairment. In these patients IDE activity was unchanged, though mRNA levels increased. In the same study ECE-1 expression or activity in AD brains was not different from age-matched controls. Correlation analyses suggested that NEP expression was correlated with Aβ accumulation and clinical diagnosis, being lower in AD than in controls, whereas no correlations of IDE and ECE-1 with Aβ levels or clinical diagnosis has been found. These findings provide additional support for NEP as the major protease involved in Aβ degradation (Wang et al. 2010).

Age is the major risk factor for AD. Aβ -synthesizing enzyme activities increase with age, coinciding with declining soluble Aβ and increasing insoluble Aβ (Miners, et al, 2008b.). In addition, there is an overall ageing-related down regulation of Aβ degrading proteases which is particularly relevant for NEP but not for IDE in transgenic Tg2576 mice brains (Dorfman et al., 2010). Nevertheless further studies assessing the relative contribution of each of these enzymes , IDE, NEP, Prep, ECE, ACE and plasmin are necessary to understand why the system redundancy is not always effective, and which of these enzymes may be more adequate as candidate therapeutic targets.

Regarding proteins with the capacity to degrade Aβ or of interfering in the process, TTR is probably the most promising, with potential as a biomarker of the disease and even as a putative therapeutic agent. The literature shows that TTR plays an important role in the modulation of Aβ aggregation and toxicity. The use of TTR as a sera biomarker for diagnosis purposes in AD patients should also be explored, with obvious advantages, for both patients and researchers, and there are already indications that sera TTR is decreased in AD patients when compared to age-matched controls (Han et al., 2011). Moreover, it is important to investigate the factors that affect TTR/A-Beta binding and/or TTR alterations that lead to its decreased in AD, such as protein oxidation (Biroccio et al., 2006). Further studies are necessary to unravel the mechanism underlying TTR protective role in AD, to establish if TTR decline is a cause or consequence of disease, and the cellular pathways involved.

Other proteins as gelsolin, a2M and Apo E counteract Aβ deposition through interactions with the peptide, but apparently none of them seem to have the capacity to cleave the peptide. In general these proteins bind Aβ and the effects of these interactions translate into preventing Aβ fibrillation, and eventually on disaggregation of pre-existent fibrils (gelsolin and a2M); binding of enzymes conferring them the capacity to degrade Aβ (a2M) or may enhance the capacity of Aβ proteases, as NEP and IDE to cleave Aβ (ApoE). MT ½ and MT3 bind TTR affecting its capacity to cleave Aβ and prevent metal associated Aβ aggregation or inhibit their formation.

The scientific achievements acquired over the past decade on all the pathways and key players involved in the amyloid cascade will hopefully contribute to the development of more adequate therapies against AD in a closer future.

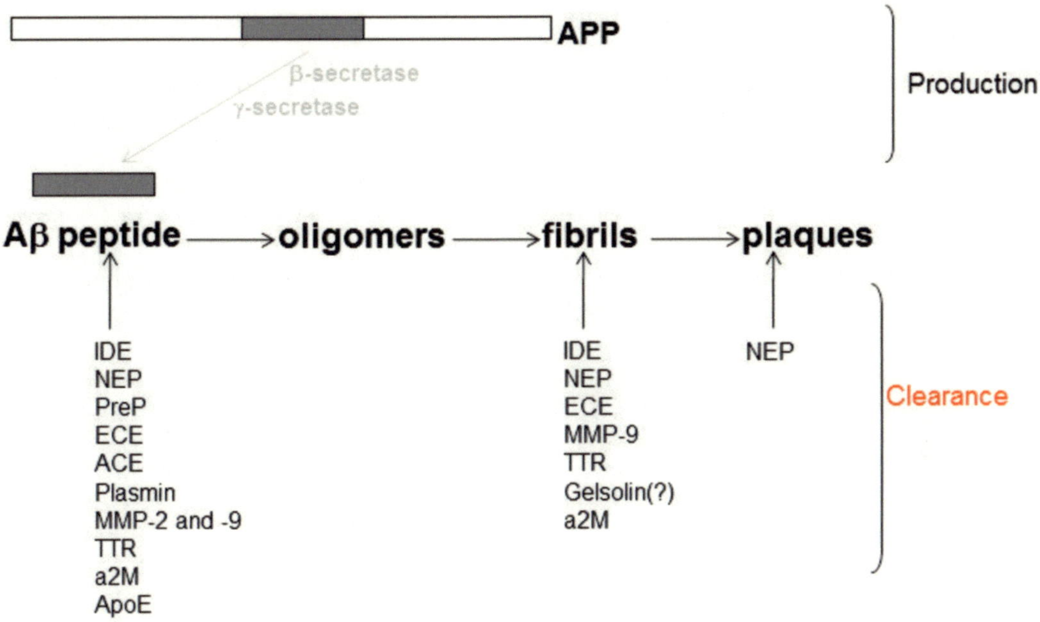

Fig. 2. Schematic diagram depicting APP processing: key proteins in amyloid-beta production and clearance (not drawn in scale). IDE- Insulin degrading enzyme; NEP- Neprilysin; PreP- Presequence peptidase; ECE –Endothelin-converting enzyme; ACE- Angiotensin-converting enzyme; MMP- Matrix metalloproteinase; TTR-Transthyretin; a2M- Alpha2-macroglobulin; ApoE- apolipoprotein E.

5. Acknowledgments

Portuguese Foundation for Science and Technology (FCT) research grants PTDC/SAU-NMC/114800/2009 and POCI/SAU-NEU/64593/2006, by COMPETE (Programa operacional Temático Factores de Competitividade) and POCI 2010 (Programa Operacional Ciência e Inovação 2010), respectively, with the participation of the European Communitarian Fund FEDER

6. References

Alikhani N, Ankarcrona M & Glaser E 2009 Mitochondria and Alzheimer's disease: amyloid-beta peptide uptake and degradation by the presequence protease, hPreP. *J Bioenerg Biomembr* 41 447-451.

Almeida MR, Alves IL, Terazaki H, Ando Y & Saraiva MJ 2000 Comparative studies of two transthyretin variants with protective effects on familial amyloidotic polyneuropathy: TTR R104H and TTR T119M. *Biochem Biophys Res Commun* 270 1024-1028.

Antequera D, Vargas T, Ugalde C, Spuch C, Molina JA, Ferrer I, Bermejo-Pareja F & Carro E 2009 Cytoplasmic gelsolin increases mitochondrial activity and reduces Abeta burden in a mouse model of Alzheimer's disease. *Neurobiol Dis* 36 42-50.

Asai M, Hattori C, Szabo B, Sasagawa N, Maruyama K, Tanuma S & Ishiura S 2003 Putative function of ADAM9, ADAM10, and ADAM17 as APP alpha-secretase. *Biochem Biophys Res Commun* 301 231-235.

Backstrom JR, Lim GP, Cullen MJ & Tokes ZA 1996 Matrix metalloproteinase-9 (MMP-9) is synthesized in neurons of the human hippocampus and is capable of degrading the amyloid-beta peptide (1-40). *J Neurosci* 16 7910-7919.

Baig S, Kehoe PG & Love S 2008 MMP-2, -3 and -9 levels and activity are not related to Abeta load in the frontal cortex in Alzheimer's disease. *Neuropathol Appl Neurobiol* 34 205-215.

Behl M, Zhang Y & Zheng W 2009 Involvement of insulin-degrading enzyme in the clearance of beta-amyloid at the blood-CSF barrier: Consequences of lead exposure. *Cerebrospinal Fluid Res* 6 11.

Bennett BD, Babu-Khan S, Loeloff R, Louis JC, Curran E, Citron M & Vassar R 2000 Expression analysis of BACE2 in brain and peripheral tissues. *J Biol Chem* 275 20647-20651.

Bertram L, Blacker D, Mullin K, Keeney D, Jones J, Basu S, Yhu S, McInnis MG, Go RC, Vekrellis K, et al. 2000 Evidence for genetic linkage of Alzheimer's disease to chromosome 10q. *Science* 290 2302-2303.

Bertram L, McQueen MB, Mullin K, Blacker D & Tanzi RE 2007 Systematic meta-analyses of Alzheimer disease genetic association studies: the AlzGene database. *Nat Genet* 39 17-23.

Biroccio A, Del Boccio P, Panella M, Bernardini S, Di Ilio C, Gambi D, Stanzione P, Sacchetta P, Bernardi G, Martorana A, Federici G, Stefani A, Urbani A. Differential post-translational modifications of transthyretin in Alzheimer's disease: a study of the cerebral spinal fluid. Proteomics. 2006 Apr;6(7):2305-13.

Biroccio A, Del Boccio P, Panella M, Bernardini S, Di Ilio C, Gambi D, Stanzione P, Sacchetta P, Bernardi G, Martorana A, Federici G, Stefani A, Urbani A. Differential post-translational modifications of transthyretin in Alzheimer's disease: a study of the cerebral spinal fluid. Proteomics. 2006 Apr;6(7):2305-13. Bora RP, Ozbil M & Prabhakar R 2010 Elucidation of insulin degrading enzyme catalyzed site specific hydrolytic cleavage of amyloid beta peptide: a comparative density functional theory study. *J Biol Inorg Chem* 15 485-495.

Bora RP & Prabhakar R 2010 Elucidation of interactions of Alzheimer amyloid beta peptides (Abeta40 and Abeta42) with insulin degrading enzyme: a molecular dynamics study. *Biochemistry* 49 3947-3956.

Borth W 1992 Alpha 2-macroglobulin, a multifunctional binding protein with targeting characteristics. *FASEB J* 6 3345-3353.

Boschert U, Merlo-Pich E, Higgins G, Roses AD & Catsicas S 1999 Apolipoprotein E expression by neurons surviving excitotoxic stress. *Neurobiol Dis* 6 508-514.

Boyles JK, Pitas RE, Wilson E, Mahley RW & Taylor JM 1985 Apolipoprotein E associated with astrocytic glia of the central nervous system and with nonmyelinating glia of the peripheral nervous system. *J Clin Invest* 76 1501-1513.

Buxbaum JN, Ye Z, Reixach N, Friske L, Levy C, Das P, Golde T, Masliah E, Roberts AR & Bartfai T 2008 Transthyretin protects Alzheimer's mice from the behavioral and biochemical effects of Abeta toxicity. *Proc Natl Acad Sci U S A* 105 2681-2686.

Caporaso GL, Takei K, Gandy SE, Matteoli M, Mundigl O, Greengard P & De Camilli P 1994 Morphologic and biochemical analysis of the intracellular trafficking of the Alzheimer beta/A4 amyloid precursor protein. *J Neurosci* 14 3122-3138.

Carro E, Trejo JL, Gomez-Isla T, LeRoith D & Torres-Aleman I 2002 Serum insulin-like growth factor I regulates brain amyloid-beta levels. *Nat Med* 8 1390-1397.

Chauhan V, Ji L & Chauhan A 2008 Anti-amyloidogenic, anti-oxidant and anti-apoptotic role of gelsolin in Alzheimer's disease. *Biogerontology* 9 381-389.

Chauhan VP, Ray I, Chauhan A & Wisniewski HM 1999 Binding of gelsolin, a secretory protein, to amyloid beta-protein. *Biochem Biophys Res Commun* 258 241-246.

Chiang HL, Lyu RK, Tseng MY, Chang KH, Chang HS, Hsu WC, Kuo HC, Chu CC, Wu YR, Ro LS, et al. 2009 Analyses of transthyretin concentration in the cerebrospinal fluid of patients with Guillain-Barre syndrome and other neurological disorders. *Clin Chim Acta* 405 143-147.

Choi SH, Leight SN, Lee VM, Li T, Wong PC, Johnson JA, Saraiva MJ & Sisodia SS 2007 Accelerated Abeta deposition in APPswe/PS1deltaE9 mice with hemizygous deletions of TTR (transthyretin). *J Neurosci* 27 7006-7010.

Chung RS, Howells C, Eaton ED, Shabala L, Zovo K, Palumaa P, Sillard R, Woodhouse A, Bennett WR, Ray S, et al. 2010 The native copper- and zinc-binding protein metallothionein blocks copper-mediated Abeta aggregation and toxicity in rat cortical neurons. *PLoS One* 5 e12030.

Corder EH, Saunders AM, Strittmatter WJ, Schmechel DE, Gaskell PC, Small GW, Roses AD, Haines JL & Pericak-Vance MA 1993 Gene dose of apolipoprotein E type 4 allele and the risk of Alzheimer's disease in late onset families. *Science* 261 921-923.

Costa R, Ferreira-da-Silva F, Saraiva MJ & Cardoso I 2008 Transthyretin protects against A-beta peptide toxicity by proteolytic cleavage of the peptide: a mechanism sensitive to the Kunitz protease inhibitor. *PLoS One* 3 e2899.

Cupers P, Bentahir M, Craessaerts K, Orlans I, Vanderstichele H, Saftig P, De Strooper B & Annaert W 2001 The discrepancy between presenilin subcellular localization and gamma-secretase processing of amyloid precursor protein. *J Cell Biol* 154 731-740.

Davidsson P, Westman-Brinkmalm A, Nilsson CL, Lindbjer M, Paulson L, Andreasen N, Sjogren M & Blennow K 2002 Proteome analysis of cerebrospinal fluid proteins in Alzheimer patients. *Neuroreport* 13 611-615.

Dawson GR, Seabrook GR, Zheng H, Smith DW, Graham S, O'Dowd G, Bowery BJ, Boyce S, Trumbauer ME, Chen HY, et al. 1999 Age-related cognitive deficits, impaired long-term potentiation and reduction in synaptic marker density in mice lacking the beta-amyloid precursor protein. *Neuroscience* 90 1-13.

Deb S & Gottschall PE 1996 Increased production of matrix metalloproteinases in enriched astrocyte and mixed hippocampal cultures treated with beta-amyloid peptides. *J Neurochem* 66 1641-1647.

DeKosky ST & Marek K 2003 Looking backward to move forward: early detection of neurodegenerative disorders. *Science* 302 830-834.

Dominguez D, Tournoy J, Hartmann D, Huth T, Cryns K, Deforce S, Serneels L, Camacho IE, Marjaux E, Craessaerts K, et al. 2005 Phenotypic and biochemical analyses of BACE1- and BACE2-deficient mice. *J Biol Chem* 280 30797-30806.

Dorfman VB, Pasquini L, Riudavets M, Lopez-Costa JJ, Villegas A, Troncoso JC, Lopera F, Castano EM & Morelli L 2010 Differential cerebral deposition of IDE and NEP in sporadic and familial Alzheimer's disease. *Neurobiol Aging* 31 1743-1757.

Du J & Murphy RM 2010 Characterization of the interaction of beta-amyloid with transthyretin monomers and tetramers. *Biochemistry* 49 8276-8289.

Du Y, Bales KR, Dodel RC, Liu X, Glinn MA, Horn JW, Little SP & Paul SM 1998 Alpha2-macroglobulin attenuates beta-amyloid peptide 1-40 fibril formation and associated neurotoxicity of cultured fetal rat cortical neurons. *J Neurochem* 70 1182-1188.

Du Y, Ni B, Glinn M, Dodel RC, Bales KR, Zhang Z, Hyslop PA & Paul SM 1997 alpha2-Macroglobulin as a beta-amyloid peptide-binding plasma protein. *J Neurochem* 69 299-305.

Eckman EA, Adams SK, Troendle FJ, Stodola BA, Kahn MA, Fauq AH, Xiao HD, Bernstein KE & Eckman CB 2006 Regulation of steady-state beta-amyloid levels in the brain by neprilysin and endothelin-converting enzyme but not angiotensin-converting enzyme. *J Biol Chem* 281 30471-30478.

Eckman EA, Reed DK & Eckman CB 2001 Degradation of the Alzheimer's amyloid beta peptide by endothelin-converting enzyme. *J Biol Chem* 276 24540-24548.

Eckman EA, Watson M, Marlow L, Sambamurti K & Eckman CB 2003 Alzheimer's disease beta-amyloid peptide is increased in mice deficient in endothelin-converting enzyme. *J Biol Chem* 278 2081-2084.

Eggert S, Paliga K, Soba P, Evin G, Masters CL, Weidemann A & Beyreuther K 2004 The proteolytic processing of the amyloid precursor protein gene family members APLP-1 and APLP-2 involves alpha-, beta-, gamma-, and epsilon-like cleavages: modulation of APLP-1 processing by n-glycosylation. *J Biol Chem* 279 18146-18156.

Ertekin-Taner N 2007 Genetics of Alzheimer's disease: a centennial review. *Neurol Clin* 25 611-667, v.

Exley C & Korchazhkina OV 2001 Plasmin cleaves Abeta42 in vitro and prevents its aggregation into beta-pleated sheet structures. *Neuroreport* 12 2967-2970.

Falkevall A, Alikhani N, Bhushan S, Pavlov PF, Busch K, Johnson KA, Eneqvist T, Tjernberg L, Ankarcrona M & Glaser E 2006 Degradation of the amyloid beta-protein by the novel mitochondrial peptidasome, PreP. *J Biol Chem* 281 29096-29104.

Farrer LA, Cupples LA, Haines JL, Hyman B, Kukull WA, Mayeux R, Myers RH, Pericak-Vance MA, Risch N & van Duijn CM 1997 Effects of age, sex, and ethnicity on the association between apolipoprotein E genotype and Alzheimer disease. A meta-analysis. APOE and Alzheimer Disease Meta Analysis Consortium. *Jama* 278 1349-1356.

Farrer LA, Sherbatich T, Keryanov SA, Korovaitseva GI, Rogaeva EA, Petruk S, Premkumar S, Moliaka Y, Song YQ, Pei Y, et al. 2000 Association between angiotensin-converting enzyme and Alzheimer disease. *Arch Neurol* 57 210-214.

Frangione B, Castano EM, Wisniewski T, Ghiso J, Prelli F & Vidal R 1996 Apolipoprotein E and amyloidogenesis. *Ciba Found Symp* 199 132-141; discussion 141-135.

Gao W, Eisenhauer PB, Conn K, Lynch JA, Wells JM, Ullman MD, McKee A, Thatte HS & Fine RE 2004 Insulin degrading enzyme is expressed in the human cerebrovascular endothelium and in cultured human cerebrovascular endothelial cells. *Neurosci Lett* 371 6-11.

Glenner GG & Wong CW 1984 Alzheimer's disease and Down's syndrome: sharing of a unique cerebrovascular amyloid fibril protein. *Biochem Biophys Res Commun* 122 1131-1135.

Gloeckner SF, Meyne F, Wagner F, Heinemann U, Krasnianski A, Meissner B & Zerr I 2008 Quantitative analysis of transthyretin, tau and amyloid-beta in patients with dementia. *J Alzheimers Dis* 14 17-25.

Goodman DS 1985 Retinoids and retinoid-binding proteins. *Harvey Lect* 81 111-132.

Gottschall PE 1996 beta-Amyloid induction of gelatinase B secretion in cultured microglia: inhibition by dexamethasone and indomethacin. *Neuroreport* 7 3077-3080.

Greenfield JP, Tsai J, Gouras GK, Hai B, Thinakaran G, Checler F, Sisodia SS, Greengard P & Xu H 1999 Endoplasmic reticulum and trans-Golgi network generate distinct populations of Alzheimer beta-amyloid peptides. *Proc Natl Acad Sci U S A* 96 742-747.

Grundke-Iqbal I, Iqbal K, Tung YC, Quinlan M, Wisniewski HM & Binder LI 1986 Abnormal phosphorylation of the microtubule-associated protein tau (tau) in Alzheimer cytoskeletal pathology. *Proc Natl Acad Sci U S A* 83 4913-4917.

Guan H, Liu Y, Daily A, Police S, Kim MH, Oddo S, LaFerla FM, Pauly JR, Murphy MP & Hersh LB 2009 Peripherally expressed neprilysin reduces brain amyloid burden: a novel approach for treating Alzheimer's disease. *J Neurosci Res* 87 1462-1473.

Guo S, Wang S, Kim WJ, Lee SR, Frosch MP, Bacskai BJ, Greenberg SM & Lo EH 2006 Effects of apoE isoforms on beta-amyloid-induced matrix metalloproteinase-9 in rat astrocytes. *Brain Res* 1111 222-226.

Haapasalo A & Kovacs DM 2011 The Many Substrates of Presenilin/gamma-Secretase. *J Alzheimers Dis.*

Haass C 2004 Take five--BACE and the gamma-secretase quartet conduct Alzheimer's amyloid beta-peptide generation. *EMBO J* 23 483-488.

Haass C & Selkoe DJ 1993 Cellular processing of beta-amyloid precursor protein and the genesis of amyloid beta-peptide. *Cell* 75 1039-1042.

Hajjar IM, Keown M, Lewis P & Almor A 2008 Angiotensin converting enzyme inhibitors and cognitive and functional decline in patients with Alzheimer's disease: an observational study. *Am J Alzheimers Dis Other Demen* 23 77-83.

Han SH, Jung ES, Sohn JH, Hong HJ, Hong HS, Kim JW, N DL, Kim M, Kim H, Ha HJ, Kim YH, Huh N, Jung MW, Mook-Jung I. 2011 Human Serum Transthyretin Levels Correlate Inversely with Alzheimer's Disease. J Alzheimers Dis.

Hansson SF, Puchades M, Blennow K, Sjogren M & Davidsson P 2004 Validation of a prefractionation method followed by two-dimensional electrophoresis - Applied to cerebrospinal fluid proteins from frontotemporal dementia patients. *Proteome Sci* 2 7.

Hardy J & Selkoe DJ 2002 The amyloid hypothesis of Alzheimer's disease: progress and problems on the road to therapeutics. *Science* 297 353-356.

Hardy JA & Higgins GA 1992 Alzheimer's disease: the amyloid cascade hypothesis. *Science* 256 184-185.

Heber S, Herms J, Gajic V, Hainfellner J, Aguzzi A, Rulicke T, von Kretzschmar H, von Koch C, Sisodia S, Tremml P, et al. 2000 Mice with combined gene knock-outs reveal essential and partially redundant functions of amyloid precursor protein family members. *J Neurosci* 20 7951-7963.

Hegde ML, Bharathi P, Suram A, Venugopal C, Jagannathan R, Poddar P, Srinivas P, Sambamurti K, Rao KJ, Scancar J, et al. 2009 Challenges associated with metal chelation therapy in Alzheimer's disease. *J Alzheimers Dis* 17 457-468.

Helbecque N, Cottel D, Hermant X & Amouyel P 2007 Impact of the matrix metalloproteinase MMP-3 on dementia. *Neurobiol Aging* 28 1215-1220.

Hemming ML & Selkoe DJ 2005 Amyloid beta-protein is degraded by cellular angiotensin-converting enzyme (ACE) and elevated by an ACE inhibitor. *J Biol Chem* 280 37644-37650.

Hemming ML, Selkoe DJ & Farris W 2007 Effects of prolonged angiotensin-converting enzyme inhibitor treatment on amyloid beta-protein metabolism in mouse models of Alzheimer disease. *Neurobiol Dis* 26 273-281.

Hickman SE, Allison EK & El Khoury J 2008 Microglial dysfunction and defective beta-amyloid clearance pathways in aging Alzheimer's disease mice. *J Neurosci* 28 8354-8360.

Hidalgo J, Chung R, Penkowa M, Vašák M. 2009 Structure and function of vertebrate metallothioneins, in"Metallothioneins and Related Chelators", Vol. 5 of 'Metal Ions in

Life Sciences'; Sigel, A., Sigel, H., Sigel, R.K.O., Eds. (2009) The Royal Society of Chemistry, Cambridge, UK, pp 279-317.

Hirko AC, Meyer EM, King MA & Hughes JA 2007 Peripheral transgene expression of plasma gelsolin reduces amyloid in transgenic mouse models of Alzheimer's disease. *Mol Ther* 15 1623-1629.

Holcomb L, Gordon MN, McGowan E, Yu X, Benkovic S, Jantzen P, Wright K, Saad I, Mueller R, Morgan D, et al. 1998 Accelerated Alzheimer-type phenotype in transgenic mice carrying both mutant amyloid precursor protein and presenilin 1 transgenes. *Nat Med* 4 97-100.

Hook VY, Kindy M, Reinheckel T, Peters C & Hook G 2009 Genetic cathepsin B deficiency reduces beta-amyloid in transgenic mice expressing human wild-type amyloid precursor protein. *Biochem Biophys Res Commun* 386 284-288.

Horstmann S, Budig L, Gardner H, Koziol J, Deuschle M, Schilling C & Wagner S 2010 Matrix metalloproteinases in peripheral blood and cerebrospinal fluid in patients with Alzheimer's disease. *Int Psychogeriatr* 22 966-972.

Howells C, West AK & Chung RS 2010 Neuronal growth-inhibitory factor (metallothionein-3): evaluation of the biological function of growth-inhibitory factor in the injured and neurodegenerative brain. *Febs J* 277 2931-2939.

Hsiao K, Chapman P, Nilsen S, Eckman C, Harigaya Y, Younkin S, Yang F & Cole G 1996 Correlative memory deficits, Abeta elevation, and amyloid plaques in transgenic mice. *Science* 274 99-102.

Hu J, Igarashi A, Kamata M & Nakagawa H 2001 Angiotensin-converting enzyme degrades Alzheimer amyloid beta-peptide (A beta); retards A beta aggregation, deposition, fibril formation; and inhibits cytotoxicity. *J Biol Chem* 276 47863-47868.

Hu J, Miyatake F, Aizu Y, Nakagawa H, Nakamura S, Tamaoka A, Takahash R, Urakami K & Shoji M 1999 Angiotensin-converting enzyme genotype is associated with Alzheimer disease in the Japanese population. *Neurosci Lett* 277 65-67.

Huang Y 2010 Abeta-independent roles of apolipoprotein E4 in the pathogenesis of Alzheimer's disease. *Trends Mol Med* 16 287-294.

Huang Y, Weisgraber KH, Mucke L & Mahley RW 2004 Apolipoprotein E: diversity of cellular origins, structural and biophysical properties, and effects in Alzheimer's disease. *J Mol Neurosci* 23 189-204.

Hughes SR, Khorkova O, Goyal S, Knaeblein J, Heroux J, Riedel NG & Sahasrabudhe S 1998 Alpha2-macroglobulin associates with beta-amyloid peptide and prevents fibril formation. *Proc Natl Acad Sci U S A* 95 3275-3280.

Huse JT, Liu K, Pijak DS, Carlin D, Lee VM & Doms RW 2002 Beta-secretase processing in the trans-Golgi network preferentially generates truncated amyloid species that accumulate in Alzheimer's disease brain. *J Biol Chem* 277 16278-16284.

Ichai C, Chevallier N, Delaere P, Dournaud P, Epelbaum J, Hauw JJ, Vincent JP & Checler F 1994 Influence of region-specific alterations of neuropeptidase content on the catabolic fates of neuropeptides in Alzheimer's disease. *J Neurochem* 62 645-655.

Irie, Y., and Keung, W. M. (2001) Metallothionein-III antagonizes the neurotoxic and neurotrophic effects of amyloid beta peptides. Biochem Biophys Res Commun 282, 416-420

Irie, Y., and Keung, W. M. (2003) Anti-amyloid beta activity of metallothionein-III is different from its neuronal growth inhibitory activity: structure-activity studies. Brain research 960, 228-234

Irizarry MC, McNamara M, Fedorchak K, Hsiao K & Hyman BT 1997a APPSw transgenic mice develop age-related A beta deposits and neuropil abnormalities, but no neuronal loss in CA1. *J Neuropathol Exp Neurol* 56 965-973.

Irizarry MC, Soriano F, McNamara M, Page KJ, Schenk D, Games D & Hyman BT 1997b Abeta deposition is associated with neuropil changes, but not with overt neuronal loss in the human amyloid precursor protein V717F (PDAPP) transgenic mouse. *J Neurosci* 17 7053-7059.

Isbir T, Agachan B, Yilmaz H, Aydin M, Kara I, Eker D & Eker E 2001 Interaction between apolipoprotein-E and angiotensin-converting enzyme genotype in Alzheimer's disease. *Am J Alzheimers Dis Other Demen* 16 205-210.

Ito S, Ohtsuki S, Kamiie J, Nezu Y & Terasaki T 2007 Cerebral clearance of human amyloid-beta peptide (1-40) across the blood-brain barrier is reduced by self-aggregation and formation of low-density lipoprotein receptor-related protein-1 ligand complexes. *J Neurochem* 103 2482-2490.

Jacobson DR, McFarlin DE, Kane I & Buxbaum JN 1992 Transthyretin Pro55, a variant associated with early-onset, aggressive, diffuse amyloidosis with cardiac and neurologic involvement. *Hum Genet* 89 353-356.

Janmey PA, Chaponnier C, Lind SE, Zaner KS, Stossel TP & Yin HL 1985 Interactions of gelsolin and gelsolin-actin complexes with actin. Effects of calcium on actin nucleation, filament severing, and end blocking. *Biochemistry* 24 3714-3723.

Ji L, Chauhan A & Chauhan V 2008 Cytoplasmic gelsolin in pheochromocytoma-12 cells forms a complex with amyloid beta-protein. *Neuroreport* 19 463-466.

Jiang Q, Lee CY, Mandrekar S, Wilkinson B, Cramer P, Zelcer N, Mann K, Lamb B, Willson TM, Collins JL, et al. 2008 ApoE promotes the proteolytic degradation of Abeta. *Neuron* 58 681-693.

Johnson KA, Bhushan S, Stahl A, Hallberg BM, Frohn A, Glaser E & Eneqvist T 2006 The closed structure of presequence protease PreP forms a unique 10,000 Angstroms3 chamber for proteolysis. *EMBO J* 25 1977-1986.

Jorissen E, Prox J, Bernreuther C, Weber S, Schwanbeck R, Serneels L, Snellinx A, Craessaerts K, Thathiah A, Tesseur I, et al. 2010 The disintegrin/metalloproteinase ADAM10 is essential for the establishment of the brain cortex. *J Neurosci* 30 4833-4844.

Jung SS, Zhang W & Van Nostrand WE 2003 Pathogenic A beta induces the expression and activation of matrix metalloproteinase-2 in human cerebrovascular smooth muscle cells. *J Neurochem* 85 1208-1215.

Kang J & Muller-Hill B 1990 Differential splicing of Alzheimer's disease amyloid A4 precursor RNA in rat tissues: PreA4(695) mRNA is predominantly produced in rat and human brain. *Biochem Biophys Res Commun* 166 1192-1200.

Kehoe PG & Wilcock GK 2007 Is inhibition of the renin-angiotensin system a new treatment option for Alzheimer's disease? *Lancet Neurol* 6 373-378.

Kim J, Basak JM & Holtzman DM 2009 The role of apolipoprotein E in Alzheimer's disease. *Neuron* 63 287-303.

Kimberly WT & Wolfe MS 2003 Identity and function of gamma-secretase. *J Neurosci Res* 74 353-360.

Koistinaho M, Lin S, Wu X, Esterman M, Koger D, Hanson J, Higgs R, Liu F, Malkani S, Bales KR, et al. 2004 Apolipoprotein E promotes astrocyte colocalization and degradation of deposited amyloid-beta peptides. *Nat Med* 10 719-726.

Konings CH, Kuiper MA, Scheltens P, Grijpma AM, van Pelt W & Wolters EC 1993 Re-evaluation of cerebrospinal fluid angiotensin-converting enzyme activity in patients with 'probable' Alzheimer's disease. *Eur J Clin Chem Clin Biochem* 31 495-497.

Korenberg JR, Pulst SM, Neve RL & West R 1989 The Alzheimer amyloid precursor protein maps to human chromosome 21 bands q21.105-q21.05. *Genomics* 5 124-127.

Kovacs DM 2000 alpha2-macroglobulin in late-onset Alzheimer's disease. *Exp Gerontol* 35 473-479.

Kowalska A 2003 Amyloid precursor protein gene mutations responsible for early-onset autosomal dominant Alzheimer's disease. *Folia Neuropathol* 41 35-40.

Kuhn PH, Wang H, Dislich B, Colombo A, Zeitschel U, Ellwart JW, Kremmer E, Rossner S & Lichtenthaler SF 2010 ADAM10 is the physiologically relevant, constitutive alpha-secretase of the amyloid precursor protein in primary neurons. *EMBO J* 29 3020-3032.

Kurochkin IV & Goto S 1994 Alzheimer's beta-amyloid peptide specifically interacts with and is degraded by insulin degrading enzyme. *FEBS Lett* 345 33-37.

Kwiatkowski DJ, Janmey PA, Mole JE & Yin HL 1985 Isolation and properties of two actin-binding domains in gelsolin. *J Biol Chem* 260 15232-15238.

Lammich S, Kojro E, Postina R, Gilbert S, Pfeiffer R, Jasionowski M, Haass C & Fahrenholz F 1999 Constitutive and regulated alpha-secretase cleavage of Alzheimer's amyloid precursor protein by a disintegrin metalloprotease. *Proc Natl Acad Sci U S A* 96 3922-3927.

Lanni C, Nardinocchi L, Puca R, Stanga S, Uberti D, Memo M, Govoni S, D'Orazi G & Racchi M 2010 Homeodomain interacting protein kinase 2: a target for Alzheimer's beta amyloid leading to misfolded p53 and inappropriate cell survival. *PLoS One* 5 e10171.

Ledesma MD, Da Silva JS, Crassaerts K, Delacourte A, De Strooper B & Dotti CG 2000 Brain plasmin enhances APP alpha-cleavage and Abeta degradation and is reduced in Alzheimer's disease brains. *EMBO Rep* 1 530-535.

Lee JY, Kweon HS, Cho E, Byun HR, Kim DH, Kim YH, Han PL & Koh JY 2007 Upregulation of tPA/plasminogen proteolytic system in the periphery of amyloid deposits in the Tg2576 mouse model of Alzheimer's disease. *Neurosci Lett* 423 82-87.

Leissring MA, Farris W, Chang AY, Walsh DM, Wu X, Sun X, Frosch MP & Selkoe DJ 2003 Enhanced proteolysis of beta-amyloid in APP transgenic mice prevents plaque formation, secondary pathology, and premature death. *Neuron* 40 1087-1093.

LePage RN, Fosang AJ, Fuller SJ, Murphy G, Evin G, Beyreuther K, Masters CL & Small DH 1995 Gelatinase A possesses a beta-secretase-like activity in cleaving the amyloid protein precursor of Alzheimer's disease. *FEBS Lett* 377 267-270.

Li NC, Lee A, Whitmer RA, Kivipelto M, Lawler E, Kazis LE & Wolozin B 2010 Use of angiotensin receptor blockers and risk of dementia in a predominantly male population: prospective cohort analysis. *BMJ* 340 b5465.

Li P, Kuo WL, Yousef M, Rosner MR & Tang WJ 2006 The C-terminal domain of human insulin degrading enzyme is required for dimerization and substrate recognition. *Biochem Biophys Res Commun* 343 1032-1037.

Li R, Lindholm K, Yang LB, Yue X, Citron M, Yan R, Beach T, Sue L, Sabbagh M, Cai H, et al. 2004 Amyloid beta peptide load is correlated with increased beta-secretase activity in sporadic Alzheimer's disease patients. *Proc Natl Acad Sci U S A* 101 3632-3637.

Li W, Poteet E, Xie L, Liu R, Wen Y & Yang SH 2011 Regulation of matrix metalloproteinase 2 by oligomeric amyloid beta protein. *Brain Res.*

Liao A, Nitsch RM, Greenberg SM, Finckh U, Blacker D, Albert M, Rebeck GW, Gomez-Isla T, Clatworthy A, Binetti G, et al. 1998 Genetic association of an alpha2-macroglobulin (Val1000lle) polymorphism and Alzheimer's disease. *Hum Mol Genet* 7 1953-1956.

Link CD 1995 Expression of human beta-amyloid peptide in transgenic Caenorhabditis elegans. *Proc Natl Acad Sci U S A* 92 9368-9372.

Liu L & Murphy RM 2006 Kinetics of Inhibition of beta-Amyloid Aggregation by Transthyretin. *Biochemistry* 45 15702-15709.

Mahley RW & Huang Y 2006 Apolipoprotein (apo) E4 and Alzheimer's disease: unique conformational and biophysical properties of apoE4 can modulate neuropathology. *Acta Neurol Scand Suppl* 185 8-14.

Mahley RW, Weisgraber KH & Huang Y 2006 Apolipoprotein E4: a causative factor and therapeutic target in neuropathology, including Alzheimer's disease. *Proc Natl Acad Sci U S A* 103 5644-5651.

Malito E, Hulse RE & Tang WJ 2008 Amyloid beta-degrading cryptidases: insulin degrading enzyme, presequence peptidase, and neprilysin. *Cell Mol Life Sci* 65 2574-2585.

Manelli AM, Bulfinch LC, Sullivan PM & LaDu MJ 2007 Abeta42 neurotoxicity in primary co-cultures: effect of apoE isoform and Abeta conformation. *Neurobiol Aging* 28 1139-1147.

Martinho A, Goncalves I, Cardoso I, Almeida MR, Quintela T, Saraiva MJ & Santos CR 2010 Human metallothioneins 2 and 3 differentially affect amyloid-beta binding by transthyretin. *Febs J* 277 3427-3436.

Matsumoto N, Kitayama H, Kitada M, Kimura K, Noda M & Ide C 2003 Isolation of a set of genes expressed in the choroid plexus of the mouse using suppression subtractive hybridization. *Neuroscience* 117 405-415.

Matsuoka Y, Saito M, LaFrancois J, Gaynor K, Olm V, Wang L, Casey E, Lu Y, Shiratori C, Lemere C, et al. 2003 Novel therapeutic approach for the treatment of Alzheimer's disease by peripheral administration of agents with an affinity to beta-amyloid. *J Neurosci* 23 29-33.

McDermott JR & Gibson AM 1997 Degradation of Alzheimer's beta-amyloid protein by human and rat brain peptidases: involvement of insulin-degrading enzyme. *Neurochem Res* 22 49-56.

Meilandt WJ, Cisse M, Ho K, Wu T, Esposito LA, Scearce-Levie K, Cheng IH, Yu GQ & Mucke L 2009 Neprilysin overexpression inhibits plaque formation but fails to reduce pathogenic Abeta oligomers and associated cognitive deficits in human amyloid precursor protein transgenic mice. *J Neurosci* 29 1977-1986.

Melchor JP, Pawlak R & Strickland S 2003 The tissue plasminogen activator-plasminogen proteolytic cascade accelerates amyloid-beta (Abeta) degradation and inhibits Abeta-induced neurodegeneration. *J Neurosci* 23 8867-8871.

Meloni G, Sonois V, Delaine T, Guilloreau L, Gillet A, Teissie J, Faller P & Vasak M 2008 Metal swap between Zn7-metallothionein-3 and amyloid-beta-Cu protects against amyloid-beta toxicity. *Nat Chem Biol* 4 366-372.

Merlos-Suarez A, Ruiz-Paz S, Baselga J & Arribas J 2001 Metalloprotease-dependent protransforming growth factor-alpha ectodomain shedding in the absence of tumor necrosis factor-alpha-converting enzyme. *J Biol Chem* 276 48510-48517.

Miners JS, Ashby E, Van Helmond Z, Chalmers KA, Palmer LE, Love S & Kehoe PG 2008a Angiotensin-converting enzyme (ACE) levels and activity in Alzheimer's disease, and relationship of perivascular ACE-1 to cerebral amyloid angiopathy. *Neuropathol Appl Neurobiol* 34 181-193.

Miners JS, Baig S, Palmer J, Palmer LE, Kehoe PG & Love S 2008b Abeta-degrading enzymes in Alzheimer's disease. *Brain Pathol* 18 240-252.

Monji A, Yoshida I, Tashiro K, Hayashi Y, Matsuda K & Tashiro N 2000 Inhibition of A beta fibril formation and A beta-induced cytotoxicity by senile plaque-associated proteins. *Neurosci Lett* 278 81-84.

Narita M, Holtzman DM, Schwartz AL & Bu G 1997 Alpha2-macroglobulin complexes with and mediates the endocytosis of beta-amyloid peptide via cell surface low-density lipoprotein receptor-related protein. *J Neurochem* 69 1904-1911.

Palha JA, Moreira P, Wisniewski T, Frangione B & Saraiva MJ 1996 Transthyretin gene in Alzheimer's disease patients. *Neurosci Lett* 204 212-214.

Palmer JC, Kehoe PG & Love S 2010 Endothelin-converting enzyme-1 in Alzheimer's disease and vascular dementia. *Neuropathol Appl Neurobiol* 36 487-497.

Penkowa M, Tio L, Giralt M, Quintana A, Molinero A, Atrian S, Vasak M & Hidalgo J 2006 Specificity and divergence in the neurobiologic effects of different metallothioneins after brain injury. *J Neurosci Res* 83 974-984.

Perez A, Morelli L, Cresto JC & Castano EM 2000 Degradation of soluble amyloid beta-peptides 1-40, 1-42, and the Dutch variant 1-40Q by insulin degrading enzyme from Alzheimer disease and control brains. *Neurochem Res* 25 247-255.

Pitas RE, Boyles JK, Lee SH, Foss D & Mahley RW 1987 Astrocytes synthesize apolipoprotein E and metabolize apolipoprotein E-containing lipoproteins. *Biochim Biophys Acta* 917 148-161.

Qiu WQ, Borth W, Ye Z, Haass C, Teplow DB & Selkoe DJ 1996 Degradation of amyloid beta-protein by a serine protease-alpha2-macroglobulin complex. *J Biol Chem* 271 8443-8451.

Qiu WQ, Walsh DM, Ye Z, Vekrellis K, Zhang J, Podlisny MB, Rosner MR, Safavi A, Hersh LB & Selkoe DJ 1998 Insulin-degrading enzyme regulates extracellular levels of amyloid beta-protein by degradation. *J Biol Chem* 273 32730-32738.

Ray I, Chauhan A, Wegiel J & Chauhan VP 2000 Gelsolin inhibits the fibrillization of amyloid beta-protein, and also defibrillizes its preformed fibrils. *Brain Res* 853 344-351.

Reitz C, van Rooij FJ, de Maat MP, den Heijer T, Hofman A, Witteman JC & Breteler MM 2008 Matrix metalloproteinase 3 haplotypes and dementia and Alzheimer's disease. The Rotterdam Study. *Neurobiol Aging* 29 874-881.

Reitz C, van Rooij FJ, Soares HD, de Maat MP, Hofman A, Witteman JC & Breteler MM 2010 Matrix metalloproteinase 3 haplotypes and plasma amyloid beta levels: the Rotterdam Study. *Neurobiol Aging* 31 715-718.

Roher AE, Kasunic TC, Woods AS, Cotter RJ, Ball MJ & Fridman R 1994 Proteolysis of A beta peptide from Alzheimer disease brain by gelatinase A. *Biochem Biophys Res Commun* 205 1755-1761.

Saraiva MJ, Birken S, Costa PP & Goodman DS 1984 Family studies of the genetic abnormality in transthyretin (prealbumin) in Portuguese patients with familial amyloidotic polyneuropathy. *Ann N Y Acad Sci* 435 86-100.

Schochet SS, Jr., Lampert PW & McCormick WF 1973 Neurofibrillary tangles in patients with Down's syndrome: a light and electron microscopic study. *Acta Neuropathol* 23 342-346.

Schwarzman AL & Goldgaber D 1996 Interaction of transthyretin with amyloid beta-protein: binding and inhibition of amyloid formation. *Ciba Found Symp* 199 146-160; discussion 160-144.

Schwarzman AL, Gregori L, Vitek MP, Lyubski S, Strittmatter WJ, Enghilde JJ, Bhasin R, Silverman J, Weisgraber KH, Coyle PK, et al. 1994 Transthyretin sequesters amyloid beta protein and prevents amyloid formation. *Proc Natl Acad Sci U S A* 91 8368-8372.

Schwarzman AL, Tsiper M, Gregori L, Goldgaber D, Frakowiak J, Mazur-Kolecka B, Taraskina A, Pchelina S & Vitek MP 2005 Selection of peptides binding to the amyloid b-protein reveals potential inhibitors of amyloid formation. *Amyloid* 12 199-209.

Schwarzman AL, Tsiper M, Wente H, Wang A, Vitek MP, Vasiliev V & Goldgaber D 2004 Amyloidogenic and anti-amyloidogenic properties of recombinant transthyretin variants. *Amyloid* 11 1-9.

Serot JM, Christmann D, Dubost T & Couturier M 1997 Cerebrospinal fluid transthyretin: aging and late onset Alzheimer's disease. *J Neurol Neurosurg Psychiatry* 63 506-508.

Seubert P, Vigo-Pelfrey C, Esch F, Lee M, Dovey H, Davis D, Sinha S, Schlossmacher M, Whaley J, Swindlehurst C, et al. 1992 Isolation and quantification of soluble Alzheimer's beta-peptide from biological fluids. *Nature* 359 325-327.

Shah K, Qureshi SU, Johnson M, Parikh N, Schulz PE & Kunik ME 2009 Does use of antihypertensive drugs affect the incidence or progression of dementia? A systematic review. *Am J Geriatr Pharmacother* 7 250-261.

Shirahama T, Skinner M, Westermark P, Rubinow A, Cohen AS, Brun A & Kemper TL 1982 Senile cerebral amyloid. Prealbumin as a common constituent in the neuritic plaque, in the neurofibrillary tangle, and in the microangiopathic lesion. *Am J Pathol* 107 41-50.

Sluck JM, Lin RC, Katolik LI, Jeng AY & Lehmann JC 1999 Endothelin converting enzyme-1-, endothelin-1-, and endothelin-3-like immunoreactivity in the rat brain. *Neuroscience* 91 1483-1497.

Solans A, Estivill X & de La Luna S 2000 A new aspartyl protease on 21q22.3, BACE2, is highly similar to Alzheimer's amyloid precursor protein beta-secretase. *Cytogenet Cell Genet* 89 177-184.

Soprano DR, Herbert J, Soprano KJ, Schon EA & Goodman DS 1985 Demonstration of transthyretin mRNA in the brain and other extrahepatic tissues in the rat. *J Biol Chem* 260 11793-11798.

Stabilini R, Vergani C, Agostoni A & Agostoni RP 1968 Influence of age and sex on prealbumin levels. *Clin Chim Acta* 20 358-359.

Stahl A, Moberg P, Ytterberg J, Panfilov O, Brockenhuus Von Lowenhielm H, Nilsson F & Glaser E 2002 Isolation and identification of a novel mitochondrial metalloprotease (PreP) that degrades targeting presequences in plants. *J Biol Chem* 277 41931-41939.

Stein TD, Anders NJ, DeCarli C, Chan SL, Mattson MP & Johnson JA 2004 Neutralization of transthyretin reverses the neuroprotective effects of secreted amyloid precursor protein (APP) in APPSW mice resulting in tau phosphorylation and loss of hippocampal neurons: support for the amyloid hypothesis. *J Neurosci* 24 7707-7717.

Stein TD & Johnson JA 2002 Lack of neurodegeneration in transgenic mice overexpressing mutant amyloid precursor protein is associated with increased levels of transthyretin and the activation of cell survival pathways. *J Neurosci* 22 7380-7388.

Takasugi N, Tomita T, Hayashi I, Tsuruoka M, Niimura M, Takahashi Y, Thinakaran G & Iwatsubo T 2003 The role of presenilin cofactors in the gamma-secretase complex. *Nature* 422 438-441.

Talamagas AA, Efthimiopoulos S, Tsilibary EC, Figueiredo-Pereira ME & Tzinia AK 2007 Abeta(1-40)-induced secretion of matrix metalloproteinase-9 results in sAPPalpha release by association with cell surface APP. *Neurobiol Dis* 28 304-315.

Tang BL 2009 Neuronal protein trafficking associated with Alzheimer disease: from APP and BACE1 to glutamate receptors. *Cell Adh Migr* 3 118-128.

Tillement L, Lecanu L & Papadopoulos V 2011 Alzheimer's disease: effects of beta-amyloid on mitochondria. *Mitochondrion* 11 13-21.

Tucker HM, Kihiko-Ehmann M & Estus S 2002 Urokinase-type plasminogen activator inhibits amyloid-beta neurotoxicity and fibrillogenesis via plasminogen. *J Neurosci Res* 70 249-255.

Tucker HM, Kihiko-Ehmann M, Wright S, Rydel RE & Estus S 2000a Tissue plasminogen activator requires plasminogen to modulate amyloid-beta neurotoxicity and deposition. *J Neurochem* 75 2172-2177.

Tucker HM, Kihiko M, Caldwell JN, Wright S, Kawarabayashi T, Price D, Walker D, Scheff S, McGillis JP, Rydel RE, et al. 2000b The plasmin system is induced by and degrades amyloid-beta aggregates. *J Neurosci* 20 3937-3946.

Vahlquist A, Rask L, Peterson PA & Berg T 1975 The concentrations of retinol-binding protein, prealbumin, and transferrin in the sera of newly delivered mothers and children of various ages. *Scand J Clin Lab Invest* 35 569-575.

Vargas T, Antequera D, Ugalde C, Spuch C & Carro E 2010 Gelsolin restores A beta-induced alterations in choroid plexus epithelium. *J Biomed Biotechnol* 2010 805405.

Vassar R, Bennett BD, Babu-Khan S, Kahn S, Mendiaz EA, Denis P, Teplow DB, Ross S, Amarante P, Loeloff R, et al. 1999 Beta-secretase cleavage of Alzheimer's amyloid precursor protein by the transmembrane aspartic protease BACE. *Science* 286 735-741.

Vassar R & Citron M 2000 Abeta-generating enzymes: recent advances in beta- and gamma-secretase research. *Neuron* 27 419-422.

Vepsalainen S, Hiltunen M, Helisalmi S, Wang J, van Groen T, Tanila H & Soininen H 2008 Increased expression of Abeta degrading enzyme IDE in the cortex of transgenic mice with Alzheimer's disease-like neuropathology. *Neurosci Lett* 438 216-220.

Vigo-Pelfrey C, Lee D, Keim P, Lieberburg I & Schenk DB 1993 Characterization of beta-amyloid peptide from human cerebrospinal fluid. *J Neurochem* 61 1965-1968.

von Koch CS, Zheng H, Chen H, Trumbauer M, Thinakaran G, van der Ploeg LH, Price DL & Sisodia SS 1997 Generation of APLP2 KO mice and early postnatal lethality in APLP2/APP double KO mice. *Neurobiol Aging* 18 661-669.

Wang DS, Dickson DW & Malter JS 2006 beta-Amyloid degradation and Alzheimer's disease. *J Biomed Biotechnol* 2006 58406.

Wang S, Wang R, Chen L, Bennett DA, Dickson DW & Wang DS 2010 Expression and functional profiling of neprilysin, insulin-degrading enzyme, and endothelin-converting enzyme in prospectively studied elderly and Alzheimer's brain. *J Neurochem* 115 47-57.

Wati H, Kawarabayashi T, Matsubara E, Kasai A, Hirasawa T, Kubota T, Harigaya Y, Shoji M & Maeda S 2009 Transthyretin accelerates vascular Abeta deposition in a mouse model of Alzheimer's disease. *Brain Pathol* 19 48-57.

Weeraratna AT, Kalehua A, Deleon I, Bertak D, Maher G, Wade MS, Lustig A, Becker KG, Wood W, 3rd, Walker DG, et al. 2007 Alterations in immunological and neurological gene expression patterns in Alzheimer's disease tissues. *Exp Cell Res* 313 450-461.

Weisgraber KH & Mahley RW 1996 Human apolipoprotein E: the Alzheimer's disease connection. *FASEB J* 10 1485-1494.

Weisner B & Kauerz U 1983 The influence of the choroid plexus on the concentration of prealbumin in CSF. *J Neurol Sci* 61 27-35.

Wen D, Corina K, Chow EP, Miller S, Janmey PA & Pepinsky RB 1996 The plasma and cytoplasmic forms of human gelsolin differ in disulfide structure. *Biochemistry* 35 9700-9709.

Wisniewski T & Frangione B 1996 Molecular biology of brain aging and neurodegenerative disorders. *Acta Neurobiol Exp (Wars)* 56 267-279.

Woeber KA & Ingbar SH 1968 The contribution of thyroxine-binding prealbumin to the binding of thyroxine in human serum, as assessed by immunoadsorption. *J Clin Invest* 47 1710-1721.

Xie L, Helmerhorst E, Taddei K, Plewright B, Van Bronswijk W & Martins R 2002 Alzheimer's beta-amyloid peptides compete for insulin binding to the insulin receptor. *J Neurosci* 22 RC221.

Yamada T, Yoshiyama Y, Sato H, Seiki M, Shinagawa A & Takahashi M 1995 White matter microglia produce membrane-type matrix metalloprotease, an activator of gelatinase A, in human brain tissues. *Acta Neuropathol* 90 421-424.

Yan P, Hu X, Song H, Yin K, Bateman RJ, Cirrito JR, Xiao Q, Hsu FF, Turk JW, Xu J, et al. 2006 Matrix metalloproteinase-9 degrades amyloid-beta fibrils in vitro and compact plaques in situ. *J Biol Chem* 281 24566-24574.

Yang JD, Feng G, Zhang J, Lin ZX, Shen T, Breen G, St Clair D & He L 2000 Association between angiotensin-converting enzyme gene and late onset Alzheimer's disease in Han chinese. *Neurosci Lett* 295 41-44.

Yerbury JJ, Kumita JR, Meehan S, Dobson CM & Wilson MR 2009 alpha2-Macroglobulin and haptoglobin suppress amyloid formation by interacting with prefibrillar protein species. *J Biol Chem* 284 4246-4254.

Yin KJ, Cirrito JR, Yan P, Hu X, Xiao Q, Pan X, Bateman R, Song H, Hsu FF, Turk J, et al. 2006 Matrix metalloproteinases expressed by astrocytes mediate extracellular amyloid-beta peptide catabolism. *J Neurosci* 26 10939-10948.

Zhang YW, Thompson R, Zhang H & Xu H 2011 APP processing in Alzheimer's disease. *Mol Brain* 4 3.

Zhao J & Pei G 2008 Evoking plasmin for beta-amyloid clearance. *Cell Res* 18 803-804.

Zhao Z, Xiang Z, Haroutunian V, Buxbaum JD, Stetka B & Pasinetti GM 2007 Insulin degrading enzyme activity selectively decreases in the hippocampal formation of cases at high risk to develop Alzheimer's disease. *Neurobiol Aging* 28 824-830.

Zheng H & Koo EH 2006 The amyloid precursor protein: beyond amyloid. *Mol Neurodegener* 1 5.

Zhong N & Weisgraber KH 2009a Understanding the association of apolipoprotein E4 with Alzheimer disease: clues from its structure. *J Biol Chem* 284 6027-6031.

Zhong N & Weisgraber KH 2009b Understanding the basis for the association of apoE4 with Alzheimer's disease: opening the door for therapeutic approaches. *Curr Alzheimer Res* 6 415-418.

Zlokovic BV 2004 Clearing amyloid through the blood-brain barrier. *J Neurochem* 89 807-811.

Zou K, Maeda T, Watanabe A, Liu J, Liu S, Oba R, Satoh Y, Komano H & Michikawa M 2009 Abeta42-to-Abeta40- and angiotensin-converting activities in different domains of angiotensin-converting enzyme. *J Biol Chem* 284 31914-31920.

Zou K, Yamaguchi H, Akatsu H, Sakamoto T, Ko M, Mizoguchi K, Gong JS, Yu W, Yamamoto T, Kosaka K, et al. 2007 Angiotensin-converting enzyme converts amyloid beta-protein 1-42 (Abeta(1-42)) to Abeta(1-40), and its inhibition enhances brain Abeta deposition. *J Neurosci* 27 8628-8635.

Zubenko GS, Volicer L, Direnfeld LK, Freeman M, Langlais PJ & Nixon RA 1985 Cerebrospinal fluid levels of angiotensin-converting enzyme in Alzheimer's disease, Parkinson's disease and progressive supranuclear palsy. *Brain Res* 328 215-221.

5

Transporters in the Blood-Brain Barrier

Masaki Ueno, Toshitaka Nakagawa and Haruhiko Sakamoto
Faculty of Medicine, Kagawa University
Japan

1. Introduction

The mammalian brain restricts the entrance of ions and solutes circulating in the bloodstream by two cellular barriers, namely, the blood-brain barrier (BBB) and blood-cerebrospinal fluid (CSF) barrier (Brightman et al., 1970; Ballabh, 2004). The BBB is built up by a monolayer of endothelial cells (ECs) lining the brain capillaries that restricts the movement of small polar molecules and macromolecules between the blood and the brain interstitial fluid (Reese & Karnovsky, 1967; Brightman & Reese, 1969; Vorbrodt, 1988). The endothelial barrier is supplemented with capillary pericytes that share the basement membrane with the ECs. Moreover, perivascular end-feet of the astrocyte almost totally cover the abluminal surface of the microvascular basement membrane. The blood-CSF barrier is built up by a monolayer of epithelial cells of the choroid plexus separating the blood from the CSF. This blood-CSF epithelial barrier is of great functional importance because the fenestrated endothelium of the choroid plexus capillaries is leaky and permeable to blood-borne solutes. Although the choroid plexus is traditionally considered the major component of the blood-CSF barrier, a similar barrier is formed by the functional complexes between the arachnoid cells. This barrier is also important because substances passing into the stroma of the choroid plexus after intravenous presentation may find their way into the CSF by crossing the ependyma adjacent to the root of the choroid plexus; this is as described as a "functional leak" by Brightman et al. (1970), while van Deurs (1978) denies the existence of this functional leak. These barriers maintain a constant chemical environment within the central nervous system (CNS), which is optimal for the function of neurons.

The brain capillaries were characterized morphologically as the site of the BBB by Reese and Karnovsky (1967) after introduction of electron microscopy and the use of horseradish peroxidase as a macromolecular tracer. Further ultrastructural studies (van Deurs, 1980; Brightman, 1989) revealed that the continuous endothelium of brain capillaries possesses several unique structural and functional features (Vorbrodt & Dobrogowska, 2003). First, the paracellular cleft between adjacent ECs is sealed by continuous strands of tight junctions (TJs). Second, the endocytic (pinocytic) and transcytotic activities are very low, and therefore, the transendothelial traffic of solutes (via plasmalemmal vesicles) is low. Third, the uptake of essential nutrients from the bloodstream into the brain interstitial fluid is selectively mediated through specific transport-related molecules such as receptors and carriers. Fourth, the presence of numerous mitochondria in the EC cytoplasm suggests a high metabolic activity and an energy-requiring function of these cells (Oldendorf et al.,

1977). In contrast, classical studies on the passage of tracers from the blood have demonstrated that the barrier function is defective or absent in certain regions of the brain, since these regions become stained by intravenously administered dyes (Brightman, 1989; Brightman & Tao-Cheng, 1993; Broadwell, 1992; Broadwell & Sofroniew, 1993). These regions have been described collectively as the circumventricular organs (CVOs), which comprise the median eminence, the neurohypophysis, the pineal gland, the organum vasculosum of the lamina terminalis, the subfornical organ, the subcommissural organ, and the area postrema. These are specialized tissues that are not typical of the CNS. The median eminence, one of the CVOs, is the site of the portal system of capillaries that receives the releasing hormones and transports them to the anterior pituitary. In addition, the CVOs contribute to transport from the bloodstream to the brain by bypassing the BBB (Broadwell, 1992a; Broadwell & sofroniew, 1993), while the BBB protects against the passive entrance of solutes circulating in the bloodstream. On the other hand, in order to selectively receive nutrients and essential molecules and discharge undesirable substances from the brain, there are several kinds of active transporters such as carrier-mediated, active efflux, ion, and receptor-mediated transporters in the BBB.

2. The transcytotic pathway in the BBB

2.1 The transendothelial pathways

Non-lipid-soluble micromolecules and macromolecules are capable of circumventing the "fluid-brain barrier" by intracellular routes related to three separate and distinct endocytic processes (Broadwell & Balin, 1988; Broadwell 1992b), namely, fluid-phase endocytosis, adsorptive endocytosis, and receptor-mediated endocytosis. First, fluid-phase endocytosis is a constitutive process for acquiring extracellular macromolecules and recycling of the plasma membrane. This internalization process occurs indiscriminantly and without binding to the cell surface (Broadwell & Balin, 1988). Second, adsorptive endocytosis concerns molecules such as lectins that bind to carbohydrate moieties on the cell surface (e.g., wheat germ agglutinin), and positively charged (cationized) molecules that bind to negatively charged cell surface components. Third, receptor-mediated endocytosis has been identified in clathrin-coated vesicles with the binding of a ligand (e.g., insulin, transferrin (Tf)) to a cell surface receptor specific for that ligand; the binding then triggers the internalization of the receptor-ligand complex. Clathrin-mediated endocytosis from the plasma membrane allows cells to internalize proteins and other biomolecules from their environment via specific receptors. Receptors are endocytosed by their capture in clathrin-coated vesicles budding from the plasma membrane. In addition, vesiculo-vacuolar organelle (VVO) (Kohn et al., 1992) and vesiculo-tubular structures (VTS) (Tagami et al., 1983; Lossinsky et al., 1983) have been suggested as transendothelial pathways for macromolecular extravasation.

Clathrin is the main scaffold protein of the coat formed by trimers, the so-called triskelions, that oligomerize both in vivo and in vitro to form polygonal clathrin cages (Keen et al., 1979; Liu et al., 2001). In receptor-mediated endocytosis, clathrin coats assemble on the cytoplasmic face of the plasma membrane forming pits that invaginate and pinch off the receptor-containing portion of the membrane to form clathrin-coated vesicles (Kirchhausen, 1999). One clathrin-independent route for endocytosis involves caveolae (small caves), which are specialized micro domains of the plasma membranes (Dautry-Varsat, 2001; Stan, 2002; Parton et al., 2006; Mehta & Malik, 2006). Caveolae are small flasked-shaped membrane invaginations that can be distinguished from coated pits by their size (50-80 nm diameter, compared to 100-110nm for coated pits). Caveolae are involved in many cellular functions, such as not only endocytosis but also signal transduction, mechano-transduction, potocytosis, and cholesterol trafficking. In addition, it is thought that endothelial caveolae are involved in capillary permeability via their participation in the transcytosis process. Supporting this role in endocytosis are several reports on the uptake of cholera toxin and also studies on SV40 virus internalization (Pelkmans et al., 2001; Pelkmans & Helenius, 2002). On the other hand, the involvement of caveolae in the transcytosis of macromolecules was recently questioned by the caveolin knockout mouse model (Drab et al., 2001). Hommelgaard et al. (2005) describe that most caveolae are stable microdomains at the cell surface and that only a small fraction of caveolae are constitutively internalized, leading to a quantitatively minor uptake of ligands and receptors. On the other hand, Pelkman and Zerial (2005) have shown the dynamic nature of caveolae trafficking. Using highly advanced techniques, it will be possible to determine whether or how the trafficking of caveolae from the apical to the basal side of the endothelium regulates endothelial permeability.

In contrast to normal microvessels, vessels that supply tumors are strikingly hyperpermeable to circulating macromolecules such as plasma proteins. Tracer studies have shown that macromolecules cross the tumor vascular endothelium by way of a cytoplasmic organelle, VVO. VVO is made up of grape-like clusters of interconnecting uncoated vesicles and vacuoles, bound by trilaminar unit membranes, that span the entire thickness of the vascular endothelium, thereby providing a potential trans-endothelial connection between the vascular lumen and the extravascular space (Kohn et al., 1992; Feng et al., 1996; Dvorak et al., 1996). Macromolecular tracers preferentially cross hyperpermeable tumor microvessels through VVOs. Study results indicate that VVOs provide a major pathway for the extravasation of circulating macromolecules across the endothelia of venules in response to several mediators and suggest that upregulated VVO function accounts for the well-known hyperpermeability of tumor blood vessels.

Based on morphologic evidence from studies of BBB injuries, some authors have discovered a unique EC system that fuses together forming transendothelial cell channels. Later, a similar EC was profiled as vesiculo-canalicular or VTS. The VTS was described originally in brain injury (Tagami et al., 1983), and subsequently considered by others to represent a possible structural mechanism for inflammatory or tumor cell transport across the BBB (Lossinsky et al., 1983; Azzarelli et al., 1984; Lossinsky et al., 1989; Nag, 1990; Lossinsky & Shivers, 2004).

2.2 Transporters in brain microvasculature (Figs. 1, 2, & 3)

The blood-to-brain influx transporters supply hydrophilic nutrients and other essential molecules such as glucose (Pardridge & Oldendorf, 1975), lactate/monocarboxylates (Cremer et al., 1979), and creatine (Ohtsuki et al., 2002). In addition, L-tyrosine, L-tryptophan, and L-histidine are precursors of neurotransmitters, and are transported from the blood to the brain via a Na^+-independent neutral amino acid transporter (system L) at the BBB (Ohtsuki & Terasaki, 2007). The system L is potentially important for drug delivery to the brain. L-Dopa is transported across the BBB by system L, and is ready biotransformed in the brain to dopamine (Gomes & Soares-da-Silva, 1999). On the other hand, there are several kinds of efflux transporters at the BBB such as ATP-binding cassette (ABC) transporters, organic anion transport (OAT) systems, aminoacid transport systems, and so

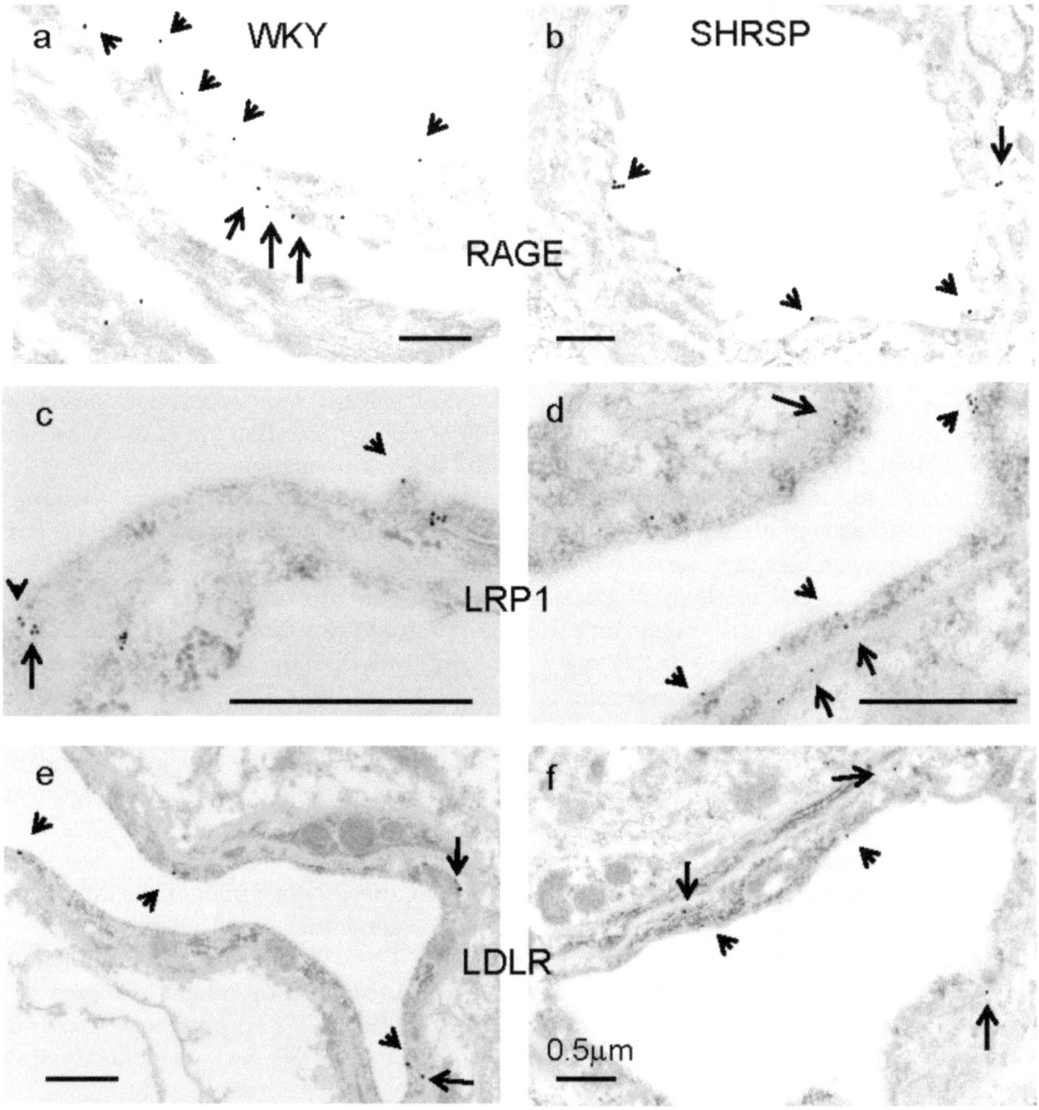

Fig. 1. Representative immunoelectron micrographic images of RAGE (a,b), LRP1 (c,d), and LDLR (e,f) are shown in the ECs of hippocampal vessels in Wistar-Kyoto (a,c,e) and SHRSP (b,d,f) rats. The rat brains were removed after perfusion with physiological saline and perfusion-fixed with 4% paraformaldehyde in 0.1M phosphate buffer (PB). The brain tissue was embedded in LR White resin after additional fixation in 1% glutaraldehyde in 0.1M PB for 1 hour. (a,b) Ultrathin sections were stained with goat anti-RAGE antibody (Santa Cruz Biotechnol), followed by incubation in a solution of anti-goat IgG antibody conjugated with colloidal gold particles of 25 nm diameter (Aurion), diluted with phosphate buffered saline (1:20), for 1 h at RT. (c,d) Ultrathin sections were stained with rabbit anti-LRP1 antibody (Santa Cruz), followed by incubation in a solution of anti-rabbit IgG antibody conjugated with colloidal gold particles of 10 nm diameter (Aurion), diluted with phosphate buffered saline (1:20), for 1 h at RT. (e,f) Ultrathin sections were stained with goat anti-LDLR antibody (Santa

Cruz), followed by incubation in a solution of anti-goat IgG antibody conjugated with colloidal gold particles of 25 nm diameter (Aurion), diluted with phosphate buffered saline (1:20), for 1 h at RT. The ultrathin sections were stained with uranyl acetate and Reynold's lead citrate, and were examined in a JEM-1200EX electron microcope (JEM, Tokyo, Japan). Labeling by 25, 10, or 25-nm gold particles conjugated with the antibody against RAGE, LRP1, or LDLR is found in the cytoplasm of the ECs including the luminal (arrowheads) and abluminal (arrows) membranes, and the basal lamina. Scale bars indicate 0.5 μm.

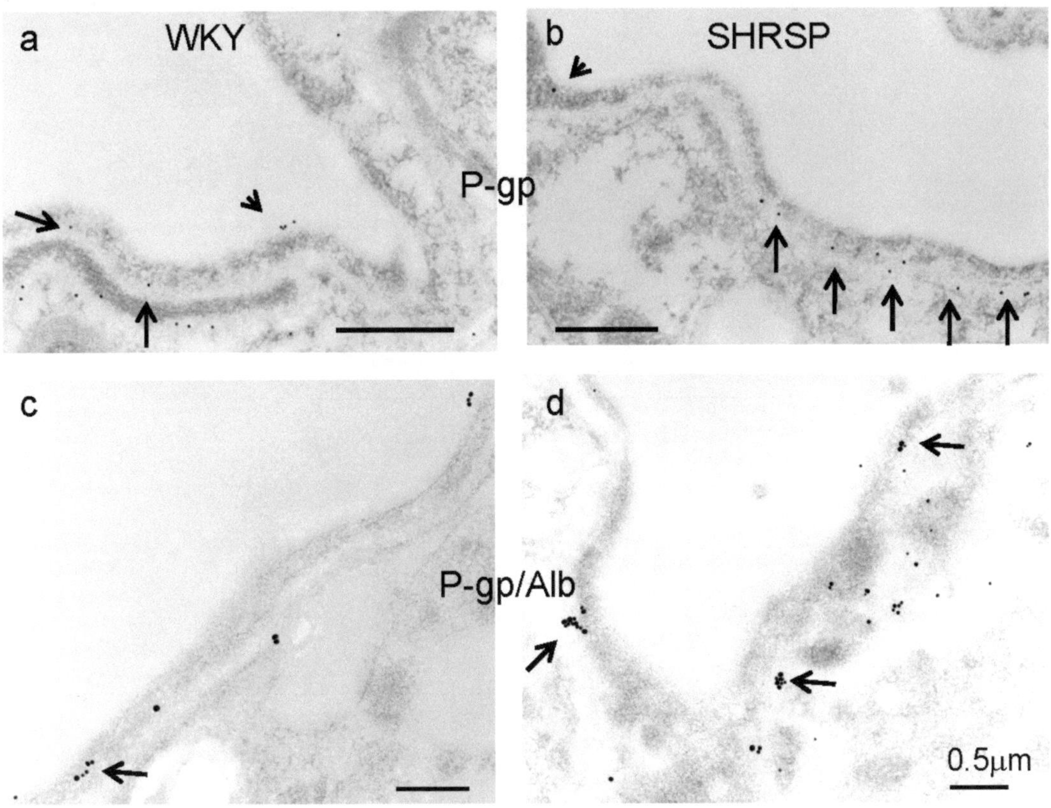

Fig. 2. Representative immunoelectron micrographic images of P-gp labelled by 10-nm gold particles (a-d) and albumin labelled by 15-nm gold particles (c,d) are shown in the ECs of hippocampal vessels in normotensive Wistar-Kyoto (WKY) (a,c) and stroke-prone spontaneously hypertensive rats (SHRSP) (b,d). The rat brains were processed as shown in Fig.1. (a,b) Ultrathin sections were stained with mouse anti-P-gp antibody (Abcam, Cambridge), followed by incubation in a solution of anti-mouse IgG antibody conjugated with colloidal gold particles of 10 nm diameter (EY Laboratories), diluted with phosphate buffered saline (1:20), for 1 h at RT. (c,d) Ultrathin sections were stained with first antibodies **against P-gp and albumin**, followed by incubation in a solution of second antibodies conjugated with colloidal gold particles of 10 or 15 nm diameter (EY Laboratories, CA, USA). The immunosignals for P-gp are frequently colocalized with those of serum albumin (c,d: arrows). The immunosignals of serum albumin in the basal lamina or perivascular areas represent increased vascular permeability. Scale bars indicate 0.5 μm.

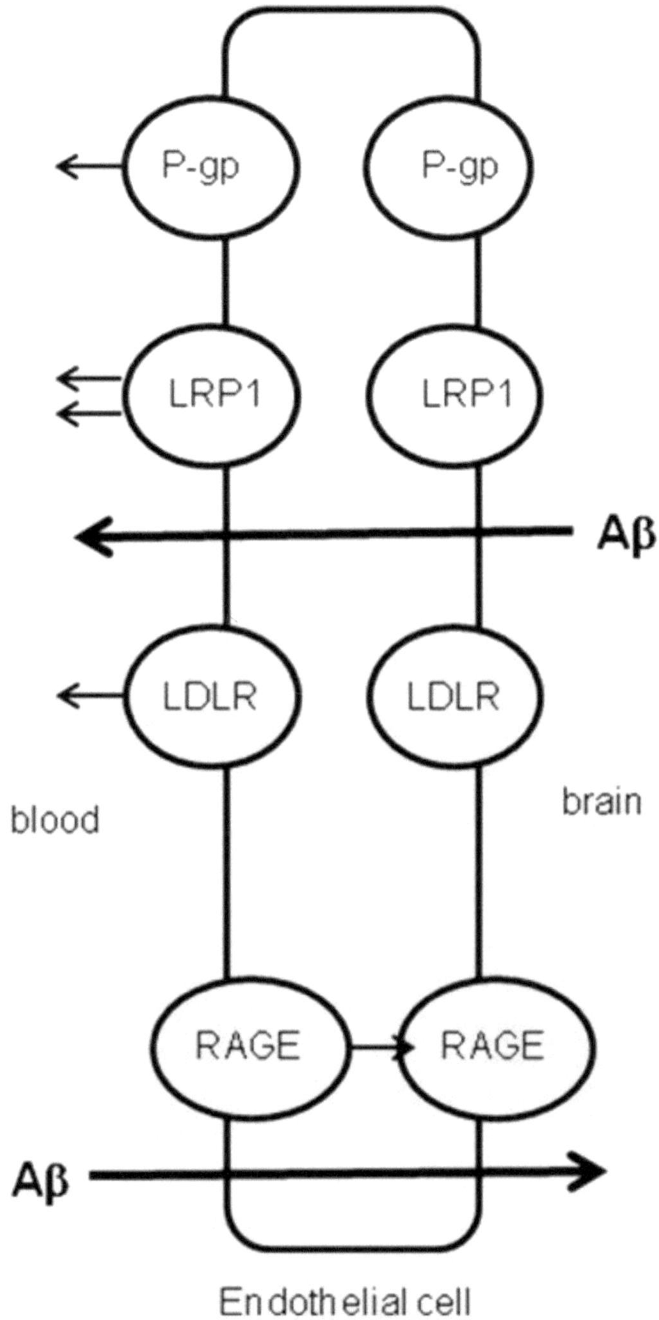

Fig. 3. Representative active efflux and influx transporters of Aβ proteins are shown according to data from **Figs. 1 & 2.**

Pgp, LRP1, and LDLR of efflux transporters are expressed on each membrane of the endothelial cytoplasm, while RAGE, the influx transporter, is also expressed on each membrane of the endothelial cytoplasm.

on (Ohtsuki & Terasaki 2007). Major representatives of the ABC efflux transporters are the multidrug resistance protein (MDR), multidrug resistance associated protein (MRP), and breast cancer resistance protein (BCRP) (Tamai & Tsuji, 2000). P-glycoprotein (P-gp), which belongs to the MDR family, preferentially transports cationic and/or zwitterionic compounds as substrates, whereas the MRP family preferentially transports anionic compounds, although there is some overlap between them (Hollo et al., 1996). Newly discovered categories of transporters are the OAT family, the organic cation transporter (OCT) family, the organic cation transporter novel type (OCTN)/carnitine transporter family (Bart et al., 2000; sekine et al., 2000), and the monocarboxylic acid transporter (MCT) family (Price et al., 1998), which is expected to be responsible for the transport of some organic anions from the brain to the EC and/or from the EC to the blood (Tamai & Tsuji, 2000). In addition, the concentrative nucleoside transporter, equilibrative nucleoside transporter subfamilies, and receptor-mediated transport systems such as the transferrin receptors and the scavenger receptors have also been detected in brain capillaries or brain capillary EC lines (Brett et al., 1993; de Boer et al., 2003).

(a) P-gp (Figs. 2 & 3)

The multidrug resistance efflux transporter P-gp was the plasma membrane protein first demonstrated in cancer cells by reducing intracellular levels of chemotherapeutic drugs (Ling, 1995). However, P-gp is also expressed in various normal tissues such as the liver, kidney, intestine, and brain, where it functions to protect the tissue against potentially toxic exogenous compounds (Bodo et al., 2003; Fromm, 2003; Schinkel & Jonker, 2003). In addition, it is known that P-gp is identified not only in normal epithelial cells with secretory/excretory functions but also in the ECs of capillary blood vessels in the brain (Schinkel et al., 1994) and the testis (Melaine et al., 2002). Until quite recently, P-gp in the brain had been thought to be primarily located in the apical (luminal) membrane of capillary ECs that form the BBB and to become part of the mechanisms involved in protecting the brain from xenobiotics (Schinkel, 1999; Bendayan et al., 2002; de Boer, 2003). A study using a new polyclonal antibody against P-gp (Schlachetzki & Pardridge, 2003) demonstrated dual expression of P-gp at astrocytes and the endothelium in normal primate brains. In addition, Bendayan et al. (2006) recently reported that P-gp localized to both the luminal and abluminal membranes of capillary ECs as well as in adjacent pericytes and astrocytes. We also confirmed the localization of P-gp to the luminal and abluminal membranes of cerebral ECs (Fig. 2). These authors reported that P-gp was distributed along the nuclear envelope, in the caveolae, cytoplasmic vesicles, Golgi complex, and rough endoplasmic reticulum. They stated that this glycoprotein might regulate drug transport processes in the CNS at both the cellular and subcellular levels.

P-gp substrates include not only a wide variety of antineoplastic agents but also many other hydrophobic compounds such as immunosuppressive agents, cardiac glycosides, opioid analgesics, antibiotics, pesticides, antiepileptics, antidepressants, and human immunodeficiency virus protease inhibitors (Schinkel & Jonker, 2003). Inhibition of P-gp can be achieved by antidepressants (Weiss et al., 2003), suggesting the possibility that the usage of a medicine together with an antidepressant may lead to an increase in the brain concentration of the medicine. It has also been shown that at clinically relevant doses given orally, oxytetracycline is able to saturate P-gp and, subsequently, the net absorption of other drugs increases (Schrickx & Fink-Gremmels, 2007). In addition, the large number of psychoactive drugs that are substrates of P-gp could be potentially involved in a significant number of drug-drug interactions related to P-gp. Because of overlapping substrates specificities between CYP3A4 and P-gp, many drug interactions may involve both CYP2A4 and P-gp (Linnet & Ejing, 2008). Therefore, it is important to distinguish CYP3A4-mediated inhibition from P-gp-mediated one in order to make appropriate interpretation of drug interaction data.

P-gp deficiency induces an undesirable effect on the brain. It has been hypothesized that Aβ proteins are deposited in periarterial interstitial fluid drainage pathways of the brain, contributing significantly to cerebral amyloid angiopathy in Alzheimer's disease (Weller et al., 1998). Vogelgesang et al. (2004) reported that Aβ deposition occurred first in arterioles, where P-gp expression was primarily low, and accordingly, the P-gp expression disappeared completely with the accumulation of Aβ proteins. In addition, Cirrito et al. (2005) reported that P-gp deficiency at the BBB increased amyloid-β deposition in a murine model of Alzheimer's disease, suggesting that P-gp normally discharges Aβ out of the brain or periarterial interstitial fluid, and that perturbation of Aβ efflux directly affects Aβ accumulation within the brain or perivascular areas. P-gp expression was increased in the BBB-damaged vessels of a stroke-prone hypertensive rat (Fig. 2). It is likely that the expression of P-glycoprotein increases as a temporary physiological compensatory response in BBB-damaged vessels to discharge intracerebral or periarterial undesirable substances from the brain. These findings suggest that endothelial P-gp contributes to efflux of undesirable substances from the brain or periarterial interstitial fluid. Concerning transendothelial transport of β-amyloid protein, the receptor for advanced glycation end products (RAGE) is thought to be a primary transporter of β-amyloid across the BBB into the brain from systemic circulation, while the low-density lipoprotein receptor-related protein (LRP)-1 mediates transport of β-amyloid out of the brain (Donahue et al., 2006; Zlokovic, 2005). RAGE versus LRP balance regulates Alzheimer amyloid β-peptide clearance through transport across the BBB (Deane et al., 2004). In addition, BBB efflux function of the P-gp transport system was decreased at later disease stages of Parkinson's disease, suggesting that the P-gp dysfunction contributes to neuronal damage due to increased accumulation of toxins such as insoluble α-synuclein (Bartels et al., 2008). According to a paper reported by Widder *et al.* (2007), the P-gp is a major exporter of oxidized glutathione and plays a crucial role in the genesis of multiple vascular abnormalities that accompany hypertension. Moreover, its presence is essential for the hypertensive response to angiotension II. These findings suggest that the increased expression of P-gp in vessels may directly induce the BBB damage. We showed the colocalization of P-gp with serum albumin (Figs. 2c, 2d), suggesting that the expression of P-gp is upregulated in the vessels with mild BBB damage.

(b) MRP

MRP1 is a member of the ATP-binding cassette superfamily and is expressed in non-P-gp expressing MDR cell lines (Cole et al., 1992). Of the MRP family, MRP1, MRP3, and MRP5 are expressed in the BBB (Kool et al., 1997; Huai-Yun et al., 1998; Regina et al., 1998). Since MRP is involved in extrusion of conjugated xenobiotics that may be harmful to the brain, some authors suggest that MRP1 and/or its closely related proteins are expressed at the luminal side of the brain capillaries (Kusuhara et al., 1998; Seethataman et al., 1998). However, this has not been proven experimentally.

(c) Scavenger receptors (Figs. 1a,b & 3)

Scavenger receptors are multifunctional receptors with a wide substrate specificity [98]. Particularly, the class A, type I scavenger receptor (SR-AI) and the class B, type I scavenger receptor (SB-BI) are expressed at endothelial cells of cerebral capillaries (de Vries et al., 1993; Silver & Tall, 2001; Goti et al., 2001). In addition, these receptors are widely expressed in mammalian tissues, particularly the liver, macrophages, endothelial cells, etc. This makes these receptors less suitable for targeting drugs to the brain. Their role at the BBB seems to be a very important one because the SR-AI receptor seems to be involved with neurodegenerative diseases. In addition, the SR-BI receptor has been shown to play a role in the transport of cholesteryl esters at the BBB. Malfunction of this receptor can also result in atherosclerotic events leading to neurodegenerative processes in the brain. Mackic et al. (1998) found binding of the soluble monomeric 1-40 amino acid peptide Alzheimer amyloid-beta (Aβ) at the SR-AI and the receptor for advanced glycation end products (RAGE) at endothelial cells of brain capillaries.

(d) Transporters of Aβ protein (Figs. 1, 2, & 3)

Concerning Aβ clearance in the brain, continuous removal of toxic substances such as Aβ-peptide species from the central nervous system is important for preventing their potentially neurotoxic accumulations in brain interstitial fluid (Deane et al., 2004). It has been suggested that vascular Aβ receptors are expressed in endothelial cells, transfer Aβ across the BBB into circulation, and thus mediate clearance of Aβ from the brain (Zlokovic, 2004, 2008a, 2008b). Alternatively, Aβ receptors may also mediate Aβ clearance via phagocytosis of Aβ by microglia and astrocytes. Both the low-density lipoprotein receptor (LDLR) and the LDLR-related protein 1 (LRP1) act as receptors for Aβ efflux (Fryer et al., 2005; Abdulkarim & Hameed, 2006; Sagare et al., 2007) (Figs. 1c, 1d, 1e, 1f & Fig. 3). LDLR also regulates apolipoprotein E (apoE) levels in the CNS and LDLR-deficient Alzheimer transgenic mice show increased cerebral Aβ deposition (Cao et al., 2006). The LDLR is an important apoE receptor that regulates human and murine apoE endocytosis and levels in the brain (Mahley, 1988). In addition, it has been clarified that the LDLR itself regulates the level of apoE in the CNS and LDLR deficiency causes an increase in murine apoE level (Sagare et al., 2007). Accordingly, it is likely that LDLR expression is inversely related with the level of apoE. Interestingly, the apoE displays antioxidant activity (Hayek et al., 1994; Miyata & Smith, 1996). LRP1 is a member of the LDLR family and functions both as a multi-functional scavenger and signaling receptor and as a transporter and metabolizer of cholesterol and apoE-containing lipoproteins (Herz & Marschang, 2003). LRP1 binds both ApoE/Aβ complexes and Aβ and regulates their clearance from brain to blood (Zlokovic, 2004; Shibata et al., 2000). Besides the LDLR family, some other potential Aβ-binding receptors have been identified. P-glycoprotein (multidrug resisitance 1, MDR1) (Lam et al., 2001), scavenger receptor CD36 (Coraci et al., 2002), the formylpeptide receptor-like-1 (FPRL1) (Le et al., 2001), and the transmembrane amyloid precursor protein (APP) itself (Lorenzo et al., 2000) also function as Aβ receptors.

In contrast, the RAGE binds Aβ proteins and transports them from blood to brain (Deane et al., 2003). It is thought that the RAGE versus LRP balance regulates Alzheimer Aβ-peptide clearance through transport across the BBB (Zlokovic, 2004) (Figs. 1a, 1b, 1c, 1d & Fig. 3). The net flux of Aβ into or out of the brain is the algebric sum of the inward flux and outward flux and presumably depends upon the density and activity of these receptors.

RAGE is a member of the immunoglobulin superfamily of cell surface molecules and engages diverse ligands relevant to distinct pathological processes (Schmidt et al., 1999). The RAGE ligands include not only Aβ proteins but also glycation products, termed advanced glycation end products (AGEs), which occur at sites of oxidant stress in diabetes and atherosclerosis. The AGEs diminish vascular barrier function in the ECs of diabetic vasculopathy (Wautier et al., 1996). The engagement of RAGE with AGEs is shown to elicit oxidative stress generation and subsequently evoke inflammatory responses in ECs, thus being involved in atherosclerosis (Schmidt & Stern, 2000). In addition, the exogenously administered soluble form of RAGE may capture and eliminate circulating AGEs, thus protecting against the AGE-induced vascular cell damage by acting as a decoy receptor for AGEs (Park et al., 1998). Accordingly, oxidative damage may be induced in conditions with excess AGEs or few RAGEs. Actually, concerning the localization of Aβ transporters in the rat ECs, the immunoreaction of LRP1, LDLR, P-gp, and RAGE is seen in the cytoplasm of the ECs including the luminal and abluminal membranes (Figs. 1, 2 & 3). It is likely that the localization may move to the other areas of the ECs or appear in another cell in pathological conditions. In vessels of normotensive rats without BBB damage, the immunosignals of P-gp are located in luminal and abluminal membranes of the ECs (Figs. 2a, 2c). In contrast, in vessels of hypertensive rats, which were reported to show mild BBB damage, more immunosignals of P-gp are located to abluminal membranes of the ECs and the basal lamina than in vessels of normotensive rats (Figs. 2b, 2d). In addition, the immunosignals of P-gp are frequently colocalized with those of albumin (Fig. 2c, 2d). These may be a response to discharge intracerebral or periarterial undesirable substances from the brain.

3. Glycocalyx in endothelial surface

The glycocalyx is a negatively charged, surface coat of proteoglycans, glycosaminoglycans, and adsorbed plasma proteins lining the luminal surface of the ECs (Luft, 1966). Some researchers have put forward the concept that the endothelial glycocalyx contributes to the vasculoprotective effects of the vessel wall (Nieuwdorp et al., 2005). This layer has also been shown to be involved in maintaining vascular permeability (Henry & Duling, 1999). The endothelial glycocalyx can be evaluated by measuring the binding capacity of cationized ferritin on the luminal endothelial surface. In addition, the glycocalyx harbours a wide array of enzymes that might contribute to its vasculoprotective effect. Extracellular superoxide dismutase, an enzyme that converts oxygen radicals to hydrogen peroxide, is bound to heparan sulphate proteoglycans within glycocalyx (Li et al., 1998). Damage to the glycocalyx is accompanied by increased shedding of extracellular superoxide dismutase, which is probably related to the decreased availability of heparan sulphate binding sites. The glycocalyx damage shifts the balance towards a pro-oxidant state. These observations are of particular interest because altered vascular permeability, attenuated nitric oxide bioavailability, and redox dysregulation are the earliest characteristics of atherogenesis (Libby, 2002). In addition, disappearance of the glycocalyx is expected to be followed by exposure of adhesion molecules on ECs and subsequent leukocyte rolling, tethering, and transmigration, which are critical in the course of atherogenesis (Mulivor & Lipowsky, 2002). This evidence suggests that intact glycocalyx is necessary for the maintenance of normal vascular function, and that disruption of glycocalyx by atherogenic stimuli increases the vascular vulnerability to atherogenesis. Moreover, it is known that endothelial glycocalyx is disturbed in various types of vascular diseases (Luft, 1966). It is also known that inflammation induces glycocalyx shedding (Mulivor & Lipowsky, 2002). One of the most common chemokines expressed in the CNS during inflammation is monocyte chemoattractant protein-1 (Mulivor & Lipowsky, 2002). High chemokine expression is found in many pathological settings accompanied by inflammation, providing a chemoattractant gradient for leukocyte influx to the brain (Murphy, 1994; Rollins, 1997).

4. Extracellular pathways bypassing the BBB

It is known that a blood-borne protein gaining extracellular access to non-BBB sites can move not only within the CSF of the subarachnoid space but also into the brain parenchyma adjacent to each of the leaky sites (Broadwell & Sofroniew, 1993). Once in the Virchow-Robin and superficial perivascular clefts, blood-borne protein is free to circulate in the perivascular tree throughout the CNS, conveyed by the pulsatile activity of beating arterioles, and for endocytosis by perivascular phagocytes (Roher et al., 2003). It is possible in experimental animals that blood-borne macromolecules escaping the subfornical organ, a BBB-free area, have ready access not only to the white matter of the corpus callosum (Broadwell & Sofroniew, 1993), but also to the hippocampus. In addition, a drainage pathway through the subarachnoid spaces of olfactory nerves from the brain to deep cervical lymph nodes has been proposed by Bradbury et al. (1981).

5. Potential pathway of blood-borne compounds into the brain

As mentioned above, the endothelial glycocalyx with extracellular enzymes covers the luminal surface of the ECs and accordingly works at the first line of the BBB. The ECs of brain capillaries are morphologically characterized by limited vesicular transcytosis and tight junctions. Enzymatic constituents in the endothelial cytoplasm of brain capillaries inactivate some substrates. The endothelial transcytosis in brain capillaries is limited to specific substrates because several kinds of influx and efflux transporters are located at the BBB. In these ways, the BBB impedes the influx of intravascular compounds from the blood to the brain. In order to work medicines on brain function, medicines should be transferred into the brain through the BBB, and the medicines entering the brain should be prevented from discharging into the blood by the transporters or modification by the enzymes. Various trials for medicines to pass the BBB into the brain parenchyma have been performed. Osmotic opening of TJs has been reported in several types of animal models (Neuwelt & Dahlborg, 1989), since the original reports by Broman and Olsson in the 1940s (Brosman & Olsson, 1948). It is likely that reversible opening of TJs would be useful for delivery of medicines into the brain. It is also known that the intra-arterial administration of alkylglycerols transiently increases the penetration of drugs and macromolecules across the BBB, suggesting that the administration of alkylglycerols could be a unique method for enhanced drug delivery to the brain and to brain tumors (Erdlenbruch et al., 2000; Lee et al., 2002). It is most likely that increased lipophilicity of drugs makes transportation into the brain easy. Compounds bound to lectins are thought to be easily transported by adsorptive vesicular transport. Enhanced vesicular transport can be used to deliver compounds into the brain. Transient inhibition of P-gp by medicines such as antidepressants may be useful for delivery of anticancer drugs into the brain. It is likely that the manipulation of P-gp will be useful for delivery of medicines in the brain with cerebrovascular diseases. The RAGE versus LRP balance regulates Alzheimer Aβ-peptide clearance through transport across the

BBB (Zlokovic, 2004). Accordingly, the influx/efflux of some substances is regulated under the expressions of these receptors. If a targeted region is situated near one of the circumventricular organs (CVOs), the delivery of medicines to that region could be achieved via CVO capillaries. There are extracellular pathways bypassing the BBB. Blood-borne proteins gaining extracellular access to non-BBB sites can move not only within the cerebrospinal fluid of the subarachnoid space, but also into the brain parenchyma adjacent to each of the leaky sites (Broadwell & Sofroniew, 1993). It is possible in experimental animals that blood-borne macromolecules escaping the subfornical organ, a BBB-free area, have ready access not only to the white matter of the corpus callosum (Broadwell & Sofroniew, 1993), but also to the hippocampus. A drainage pathway through the subarachnoid spaces of olfactory nerves from the brain to deep cervical lymph nodes has been also proposed by Bradbury et al. (1981). Accordingly, nasally inhaled medicines can affect parts of the brain through the subarachnoid spaces of olfactory nerves. In addition, it has been investigated in experimental animals whether the treatment of brain diseases is possible by using gene targeting technology that delivers the gene across the BBB after i.v. administration of nonviral formulation of the gene (Shi et al., 2001). In the experiment, the plasmid DNA was targeted to the brain with pegylated immunoliposomes using a targeting ligand such as an antibody to transferrin receptor or insulin receptor. Thus, detailed information on the BBB is necessary and useful to plan a strategy and develop therapies against various brain and vascular diseases.

6. Conclusion

The blood-brain barrier (BBB) not only impedes the influx of intravascular substances from blood to brain, but also promotes transport of substances from blood to brain or from brain to blood through several transport systems such as carrier-mediated transport, active efflux transport, ion transport, or receptor-mediated transport systems. The multidrug resistance transporter P-glycoprotein is an ATP-dependent efflux pump and contributes to efflux of many drugs such as anti-cancer drugs and undesirable substances such as amyloid-β (Aβ) proteins from the brain or periarterial interstitial fluid into the blood. The deficiency of P-glycoprotein, a representative efflux transporter of Aβ, at the BBB increases Aβ deposition in an Alzheimer disease mouse model. Continuous removal of toxic substances such Aβ-peptide species from the central nervous system is important for preventing their potentially neurotoxic accumulation in brain interstitial fluid. It has been suggested that vascular Aβ transporters in endothelial cells transfer Aβ across the BBB into circulation and thus mediate clearance of Aβ from the brain. The low-density lipoprotein receptor-related protein 1 (LRP1) is a major efflux transporter for Aβ. In addition, the low-density lipoprotein receptor (LDLR) may also act as Aβ receptors. In the central nervous system, LDLR also regulates the level of apolipoprotein E (apoE), which displays antioxidant activity. LDLR-deficient Alzheimer transgenic mice show increased cerebral Aβ deposition. Besides the LDLR family, some other potential Aβ-binding receptors have been identified. Scavenger receptor CD36, the formylpeptide receptor-like-1 (FPRL1), and the transmembrane amyloid precursor protein (APP) itself also function as Aβ receptors. In contrast, the receptor for advanced glycation end products (RAGE) binds Aβ proteins and transports them from blood to brain. It is thought that the influx versus efflux transporters balance regulates Alzheimer Aβ-peptide clearance through transport across the BBB. The RAGE ligands include not only Aβ proteins but also advanced glycation end products (AGEs), which occur at sites of oxidant stress in diabetes and atherosclerosis. The AGEs diminish vascular barrier function in the endothelium of diabetic vasculopathy. The net flux of Aβ into or out of the brain is the algebric sum of the inward flux and outward flux and presumably depends upon the density and activity of these receptors. Thus, Aβ clearance in the brain endothelial cells is an important function of the BBB. Dysfunction of the BBB with efflux and influx transporters of Aβ proteins may contribute to the pathogenesis of several kinds of degenerative neuronal dysfunction or disorders including Alzheimer's disease.

7. Acknowledgement

This research was supported by grant 22590958 from the Ministry of Education, Culture, Sports, Science and Technology of Japan (Masaki Ueno). We would like to thank Ms M. Kawauchi for technical assistance and Ms A. Kimura for editorial assistance.

Abbreviations: Aβ = amyloid-β, ABC = ATP-binding cassette, **AGEs = advanced glycation end products,** apoE = apolipoprotein E, AVP = arginine-vasopressin, BBB = blood-brain barrier, BCRP = breast cancer resistance protein, CNS = central nervous system, CSF = cerebrospinal fluid, CVO = circumventricular organ, DSIP = delta-sleep inducing peptide, EC = endothelial cell, LDLR = low-density lipoprotein receptor, LHRH = luteinizing-hormone releasing hormone, LRP1 = low-density lipoprotein receptor-related protein 1, MCT = monocarboxylic acid transporter, MDR = multidrug resistance protein, MRP = multidrug resistance associated protein, OAT = organic anion transporter, OCT = organic cation transporter, OCTN = organic cation transporter novel type, P-gp = P-glycoprotein, PTS = peptide transport system, RAGE = receptor for advanced glycation end product, Tf = transferrin, Tf-R = transferrin-receptor, TJ= tight junction, Tyr-MIF-1 = tyrosine melanocyte-stimulating inhibitory factor 1, VTS = vesiculo-vacuolar organelle, VVO = vesiculo-tubular structure

8. References

Abdulkarim, Y.; Hameed, Z. (2006). Is the LDL receptor involved in cortical amyloid protein clearance? *Neurochem. Res.*, 31, 839-847.

Azzarelli, B.; Mirkin, L.D.; Goheen, M.; Muller, J.; Crockett, C. (1984). The leptomeningeal vein. A site of re-entry of leukemic cells into the systemic circulation. *Cancer*, 54, 1333-1343.

Ballabh, P.; Braun, A.; Nedergaard, M. (2004). The blood-brain barrier: an overview. Structure, regulation, and clinical implications. *Neurobiol. Disease*, 16, 1-13.

Bart, J.; Groen, H.J.M.; Hendrikse, N.H.; van der Graaf, W.T.A.; Vaalburg, W.; de Vries, E.G.E. (2000). The blood-brain barrier and oncology: new insights into function and modulation. *Cancer Treat. Rev.*, 26, 449-462.

Bartels, A.L.; Willemsen, A.T.M.; Kortekaas, R.; de Jong, B.M.; de Vries, R.; de Klerk, O.; van Oostrom, J.C.H.; Portman, A.; Leenders, K.L. (2008). Decreased blood-barin barrier P-glycoprotein function in the progression of Parkinson's disease, PSp and MSA. *J. Neural. Transm.*, 115, 1001-1009.

Bendayan, R.; Lee, G.; Bendayan, M. (2002). Functional expression and localization of P-glycoprotein at the blood brain barrier. *Microsc. Res. Tech.*, 57, 365-380.

Bendayan, R.; Ronaldson, P.T.; Gingras, D.; Bandayan, M. (2006). In situ localization of P-glycoprotein (ABCB1) in human and rat brain. *J. Histochem. Cytochem.*, 54, 1159-1167.

Bodo, A.; Bakos, E.; Szeri, F.; Varadi, A.; Sarkadi, B. (2003). The role of multidrug transporters in drug availability, metabolism and toxicity. *Toxicol. Lett.*, 140-141, 133-143.

Brett, J.; Schmidt, A.M.; Zou, Y.S.; Yan, S.D.; Weidman, E.; Pinsky, D.J.; Neeper, M.; Przysiecki, M.; Shaw, A.; Migheli, A.; Stern, D.M. (1993). Survey of the distribution of a newly characterized receptor for advanced glycation end products in tissues. *Am. J. Pathol.*, 143, 1699-1712.

Bradbury, M.W.B.; Cserr, H.F.; Westrop, R.J. (1981). Drainage of cerebral interstitial fluid into deep cervical lymph of the rabbit. *Am. J. Physiol.*, 240, F329-F336.

Broman, T.; Olsson, O. (1948). The tolerance of cerebral blood vessels to a constrast medium of the diodrast group. *Acta Radiol. (Stockh)*, 30, 326-636.

Brightman, M.W.; Reese, T.S.; Feder, N. (1970). Assessment with the electron microscope of the permeability to peroxidase of cerebral endothelium and epithelium in mice and shrks. In: *Capillary permeability*, Crone C, Lassen NA, Eds.; Munksgaard: Copenhagen, pp 468-476.

Brightman, M.W.; Reese, T.S. (1969). Junctions between intimately apposed cell membranes in the vertebrate brain. *J. Cell Biol.*, 40, 648-677.

Brightman, M.W. (1989). The anatomic basis of the blood-brain barrier. In: *Implications of the Blood-Brain Barrier and Its Manipulation*, Neuwelt, E.A.; Ed; Vol. 1, Plenum Medical: New York, Vol. 1, pp. 53-83.

Brightman, M.W.; Tao-Cheng, J.H. (1993). Tight junctions of brain endothelium and epithelium. In: *The Blood-Brain Barrier*, Pardridge, W.M. Ed.; Raven Press: New York, pp. 107-125.

Broadwell, R.D.; Balin, B.J.; Salcman, M. (1988). Transcytotic pathway for blood-borne protein through the blood-brain barrier. *Proc. Natl. Acad. Sci. U.S.A.*, 85, 632636.

Broadwell, R.D. (1992a) Pathways into, through, and around the fluid-brain barrier. *NIDA Res. Monogr.*, **120**, 230-258.

Broadwell, R.D. (1992b). Pathways into, through, and around the fluid-brain barrier. *NIDA Res. Monogr.*, 120, 230-258.

Broadwell, R.D.; Sofroniew, M.V. (1993) Serum proteins bypass the blood-brain fluid barriers for extracellular entry to the central nervous system. *Exp. Neurol.*, 120, 245-263.

Cao, D.; Fukuchi, K.; Wan, H.; Kim, H.; Li, L. (2006). Lack of LDL receptor aggravates learning and amyloid deposits in Alzheimer transgenic mice. *Neurobiol. Aging*, 27, 1632-1643.

Cirrito, J.R.; Deane, R.; Fagan, A.M.; Sprinner, M.L.; Parsadanian, M.; Finn, M.B.; Jiang, H.; Prior, J.L.; Sagare, A.; Bales, K.R.; Paul, S.M.; Zlokovic, B.V.; Piwnica-Worms, D.; Hotzman, D.M. (2005). P-glycoprotein deficiency at the blood-brain barrier increases amyloid-β deposition in an Alzheimer disease mouse model. *J. Clin. Invest.*, 115, 3285-3290.

Cole, S.P.; Bhardwaj, G.; Gerlach, J.H.; Mackie, J.E.; Grant, C.E.; Almquist, K.C.; Stewart, A.J.; Kurz, E.U.; Duncan, A.M.; Deeley, R.G. (1992). Overexpression of a transporter gene in a multidrug-resistant human lung cancer cell line. *Science*, 258, 1650-1654.

Coraci, I.S.; Husemann, J.; Berman, J.W.; Hulette, C.; Dufour, J.H.; Campanella, G.K.; Luster, A.D.; Silverstein, S.C.; El-Khoury, J.B. (2002). CD36, a class B scavenger receptor, is expressed on microglia in Alzheimer's disease brains and can mediate production of reactive oxygen species in response to beta-amyloid fibrils. *Am. J. Pathol.*, 160, 101-112.

Cremer, J.E.; Cunningham, V.J.; Pardridge, W.M.; Braun, L.D.; Oldendorf, W.H. (1979). Kinetics of blood-brain barrier transport of pyruvate, lactate and glucose in sucking, weanling and adult rats. *J. Neurochem.*, 33, 439-445.

Dautry-Varsat, A. Clathrin-independent endocytosis. (2001). In: *Endocytosis*, Marsh, M. Ed.: Oxford University Press. Oxford, pp26-57.

de Boer, A.G.; van der Sandt, I.C.; Gaillard, P.J. (2003). The role of drug transporters at the blood-brain barrier. *Annu. Rev. Pharmacol. Toxicol.*, 43, 629-656.

de Vries, H.E.; Kuiper, J.; de Boer, A.G.; van Berkel, T.J.C.; Breimer, D.D. (1993). Characterization of the scavenger receptor on bovine cerebral endothelial cells in vitro. *J. Neurochem.*, 61, 1813-1821.

Deane, R.; Du, Y.S.; Submamaryan, R.K.; LaRue, B.; Jovanovic, S.; Hogg, E.; Welch, D.; Manness, L.; Lin, C.; Yu, J.; Zhu, H.; Ghiso, J.; Frangione, B.; Stern, A.; Schmidt, A.M.; Armstrong, D.L.; Arnold, B.; Liliensiek, B.; Nawroth, P.; Hofman, F.; Kindy, M.; Stern, D.; Zlokovic, B. (2003). RAGE mediates amyloid-β peptide transport across the blood-brain barrier and accumulation in brain. *Nat. Med.*, 9, 907 913.

Deane, R.; Wu, Z.; Zlokovic, B.V. (2004). RAGE (Yin) versus LRP (Yang) balance regulates Alzheimer amyloid β-peptide clearance through transport across the blood-brain barrier. *Stroke*, 35, 2628-2631.

Donahue, J.E.; Flaherty, S.L.; Johanson, C.E.; Duncan, III J.A.; Silverberg, G.D.; Miller, M.C.; Tavares, R.; Yang, W.; Wu, Q.; Sabo, E.; Hovanesian, V.; Stopa, E.G. (2006). RAGE, LRP-1, and amyloid-beta protein in Alzheimer's disease. *Acta Neuropathol.*, 112, 405-415.

Drab, M.; Verkade, P.; Elger, M.; Kasper, M.; Lohn, M.; Lauterbach, B.; Menne, J.; Lindschau, C.; Mende, F.; Luft, F.C.; Schedl, A.; Haller, H.; Kurzchalia, T.V. (2001). Loss of caveolae, vascular dysfunction, and pulmonary effects in caveolin-1 gene-disrupted mice. *Science*, 293, 2449-2452.

Dvorak, A.M.; Kohn, S.; Morgan, E.S.; Fox, P.; Nagy, J.A.; Dvorak, H.F. (1996). The vesiculo-vacuolar organelle (VVO): a distinct endothelial cell structure that provides a transcellular pathway for macromolecular extravasation. *J. Leukoc. Biol.*, 59, 100-115.

Erdlenbruch, B.; Jendrossek, V.; Eibl, H.; Lakomek, M. (2000). Transient and controllable opening of the blood-brain barrier to cytostatic and antibiotic agents by alkylglycerols in rats. *Exp. Brain Res.*, 135, 417-422.

Feng, D.; Nagy, J.A.; Hipp, J.; Dvorak, H.F.; Dvorak, A.M. (1996). Vesiculo-vacuolar organelles and the regulation of venule permeability to macromolecules by vascular permeability factor, histamine, and serotonin. *J. Exp. Med.*, 183, 1981-1986.

Fromm, M.F. (2003). Importance of P-glycoprotein for drug disposition in humans. *Eur. J. Clin. Invest.*, 33, 6-9.

Fryer, J.D.; DeMattos, R.B.; McCormick, L.M.; O'Dell, M.A.; Spinner, M.L.; Bales, K.R.; Paul, S.M.; Sullivan, P.M.; Parsadanian, M.; Bu, G.; Holtman, D.M. (2005). The low density lipoprotein receptor regulates the level of central nervous system and murine apolipoprotein E but does not modify amyloid plaque pathology in PDAPP mice. *J. Biol. Chem.*, 280, 25754-25759.

Gomes, P.; Soares-da-Silva, P. (1999). L-Dopa transport properties in an immortalized cell line of rat capillary cerebral endothelial cells. RBE4. *Brain Res.*, 829, 143-150.

Goti, D.; Hrzenjak, A.; Levak-Frank, S.; Frank, S.; van der Westhyzen, D.R.; Malle, E.; Sattler, W. (2001). Scavenger receptor class B type 1 is expressed in porcine brain capillary endothelial cells and contributes to selective uptake of HDL-associated vitamine E. *J. Neurochem.*, 76, 498-508.

Hayek, T.; Oiknine, J.; Brook, J.G.; Aviram, M. (1994). Increased plasma and lipoprotein and lipid peroxidation in APOE-deficient mice. *Biochem. Biophys. Res. Commun.*, 201, 1567-1574.

Henry, C.B.; Duling, B.R. (1999). Permeation of the luminal capillary glycocalyx is determined by hyaluronan. *Am. J. Physiol.*, 277, H508-H514.

Herz, J.; Marschang, P. (2003). Coaxing the LDL receptor family into the fold. *Cell*, 112, 289-292.

Hollo, Z.; Homolya, L.; Hegedus, T.; Sarkadi, B. (1996). Transport properties of the multidrug resistance-associated protein (MRP) in human tumor cells. *FEBS Lett.*, 383, 99-104.

Hommelgaard, A.M.; Roepstoff, K.; Vilhardt, F.; Torgersen, M.L.; Sandvig, K.; van Deurs, B. (2005). Caveolae: stable membrane domains with a potential for internalization. *Traffic*, 6, 720-724.

Huai-Yun, H.; Secrest, D.T.; Mark, K.S.; Carnev, D.; Braudquist, C.; Elmquist, W.F.; Miller, D.W. (1998). Expression of multidrug resistance-associated protein (MRP) in brain microvessel endothelial cells. *Biochem. Biophys. Res. Commun.*, 243, 816-820.

Keen, J.H.; Willingham, M.C.; Pastan, I.H. (1979). Clathrin-coated vesicles: isolation, dissociation and factor-dependent reassociation of clathrin baskets. *Cell*, 16, 303-312.

Kirchhausen T. (1999). Adaptors for clathrin-mediated traffic. *Annu. Rev. Cell Dev. Biol.*, 15, 705-732.

Kohn, S.; Nagy, J.A.; Dvorak, H.F.; Dvorak, A.M. (1992). Pathways of macromolecular tracer transport across venules and small veins. Structural basis for the hyperpermeability of tumor blood vessels. *Lab. Invest.*, 67, 596-607.

Kool, M.; de Haas, M.; Scheffer, G.L.; Scheper, R.J.; van Ejik, M.J.; Juijn, J.A.; Baas, F.; Borst, P. (1997). Analysis of expression of cMOAT (MRP2), MRP3, MRP4, and MRP5, homologues of the multidrug resistance-associated protein gene (MRP1), in human cancer cell lines. *Cancer Res.*, 57, 3537-3547.

Kusuhara, H.; Suzuki, H.; Naito, M.; Tsuruo, T.; Sugiyama, Y. (1998). Characterization of efflux transport of organic anions in mouse brain capillary endothelial cells. *J. Pharmacol. Exp. Ther.*, 285, 1260-1265.

Lam, F.C.; Liu, R.; Lu, P.; Shapiro, A.B.; Renoir, J.M.; Sharom, F.J.; Reiner, P.B. (2001). Beta-amyloid efflux mediated by P-glycoprotein. *J. Neurochem.*, 76, 1121-1128.

Le, Y.; Gong, W.; Tiffany, H.L.; Tumanov, A.; Nedospasov, S.; Shen, W.; Dunlop, N.M.; Gao, J.L.; Murphy, O.M.; Oppenheim, J.J.; Wang, J.M. (2001). Amyloid (beta) 42 activates a G-protein-couples chemoattractant receptor, FRP-like-1. *J. Neurosci.*, 21, RC123-RC127.

Lee, H.J.; Zhang, Y.; Pardridge, W.M. (2002). Blood-brain barrier disruption following the internal carotid arterial perfusion of alkyl glycerols. *J. Drug Target*, 463-467.

Li, Q.; Bolli, R.; Qiu, Y.; Tang, X.L.; Murphree, S.S.; French, B.A. (1998). Gene therapy with extracellular superoxide dismutase attenuates myocardial stunning in conscious rabbits. *Circulation*, 98, 1438-1448.

Libby, P. (2002). Inflammation in atherosclerosis. *Nature*, 420, 868-874.

Ling, V. (1995). P-glycoprotein: its role in drug resistance. *Am. J. Med.*, 99, 315-345.

Linnet, K.; Ejsing T.B. (2008). A review on the impact of P-glycoprotein on the penetration of drugs into the brain. Focus on psychotropic drugs. *Eur. Neuropsychopharmacol.*, 18, 157-169.

Liu, S.-H.; Mallet, W.G.; Brodsky, F.M. (2001). Clathrin-mediated endocytosis. In: *Endocytosis*, Marsh, M. Ed.; Oxford University Press: Oxford, pp.1-25.

Lorenzo, A.; Yuan, M.; Zhang, Z.; Paganetti, P.A.; Sturchler-Pierrat, C.; Staufenbiel, M.; Mautino, J.; Vigo, F.S.; Sommer, B.; Yankner, B.A. (2000). Amyloid beta interacts with the amyloid precursor protein: a potential toxic mechanism in Alzheimer's disease. *Nat. Neurosci.*, 3, 460-464.

Lossinsky, A.S.; Vorbrodt, A.W.; Wisniewski, H.M. (1983). Ultrastructural studies of vesicular and canalicular transport structures in the injured mammalian blood-brain barrier. *Acta Neuropathol.*, 61, 239-245.

Lossinsky, A.S.; Badmajew, V.; Robson, J.; Moretz, R.C.; Wisniewski, H.M. (1989). Sites of egress of inflammatory cells and horseradish peroxidase transport across the blood-brain barrier in a murine model of chronic relapsing experimental allergic encephalomyelitis. *Acta Neuropathol.*, 78, 359-371.

Lossinsky, A.S.; Shivers, R.R. (2004). Structural pathways for macromolecular and cellular transport across the blood-brain barrier during inflammatory conditions. Review. *Histol. Histopathol.*, 19, 535-564.

Luft, J.H. (1966). Fine structures of capillary and endocapillary layer as revealed by ruthenium red. *Fed. Proc.*, 25, 1773-1783.

Mackic, J.; Stins, M.; McComb, J.; Calero, M.; Ghiso, J.; Kim, K.; Yan, S.; Stern, D.; Schmidt, A.; Frangione, B.; Zlokovic, B. (1998). Human blood-brain barrier receptors for Alzheimer's amyloid-beta 1-40. Asymmetrical binding, endocytosis, and transcytosis at the apical side of brain microvascular endothelial monolayer. *J. Clin. Invest.*, 102, 734-743.

Mahley, R.W. (1988). Apolipoprotein E: cholesterol transport protein with expanding role in cell biology. *Science*, 240, 622-630.

Mehta, D.; Malik, A.B. (2006). Signaling mechanisms regulating endothelial permeability. *Physiol. Rev.*, 86, 279-367.

Melaine, N.; Lienard, M.-O.; Dorval, I.; Gaoscogne, C.L.; Lejeune, H.; Jegou, B. (2002). Multidrug resistance genes and P-glycoprotein in the testis of the rat, mouse, guinea pig, and human. *Biol. Reprod.*, 67, 1699-1707.

Miyata, M.; Smith, J. (1996). Apolippprotein E allele-specific antioxidant activity and effects on cytotoxicity insults and β-amyloid peptides. Nature Genet., 14, 55-61.

Mulivor, A.W.; Lipowsky, H.H. (2002). Role of glycocalyx in leukocyte-endothelial cell adhesion. *Am. J. Physiol. Heart Circ. Physiol.*, 282, H1282-H1291.

Murphy, P.M. (1994). The molecular biology of leukocyte chemoattractant receptors. *Annu. Rev. Immunol.*, 12, 593-633.

Nag, S. (1990). Presence of transendothelial channels in cerebral endothelium in chronic hypertension. *Acta Neurochir. Suppl. (Wien)*, 51, 335-337.

Neuwelt, E.A.; Dahlborg, S.A. (1989). Blood-brain barrier disruption in the treatment of brain tumors: Clinical implications. In: Implications of the blood-brain barrier and its manipulation. Neuwelt, E.A. Ed.; New York, Plenum Publishing Corp. Vol. II , pp. 195-261.

Nieuwdorp, M.; Meuwese, M.C.; Vink, H.; Hoekstra, J.B.L.; Kastelen, J.J.P.; Stroes, E.S.G. (2005). The endothelial glycocalyx: a potential barrier between health and vascular disease. *Curr. Opin. Lipidol.*, 16, 507-511.

Ohtsuki, S.; Tachikawa, M.; Takanaga, H.; Shimizu, H.; Watanabe, M.; Hosoya, K.; Terasaki, T. (2002). The blood-brain barrier creatine transporter is a major pathway for supplying creatine to the brain. *J. Cereb. Blood Flow Metab.*, 22, 1327-1335.

Ohtsuki, S.; Terasaki, T. (2007). Contribution of carrier-mediated transport systems to the blood-brain barrier as a supporting and protecting interface for the brain; importance for CNS drug discovery and development. *Pharm. Res.*, 24, 1745-1758.

Oldendorf, W.H.; Cornford, M.E.; Brown, W.J. (1977). The large apparent work capacity of the blood-brain barrier: a study of mitochondrial content of capillary endothelial cells in brain and other tissues of rat. *Ann. Neurol.*, 1, 409-417.

Pardridge, W.M.; Oldendorf, W.H. (1975). Kinetics of blood-brain transport of hexoses. *Biochim. Biophys. Acta.*, 382, 377-392.

Park, L.; Raman, K.G.; Lee, K.J.; Lu, Y.; Jr. Ferran, L.J.; Chow, W.S.; Stern, D.; Schmidt, A.M. (1998). Suppression of accelerated diabetic atherosclerosis by the soluble receptor for advanced glycation end products. *Nat. Med.*, 4, 1025-1031.

Parton, R.G.; Hanzal-Bayer, M.; Hancock, J.F. (2006). Biogenesis of caveolae: a structural model for caveolin-induced domain formation. *J. Cell Sci.*, 119, 787-796.

Pelkmans, L.; Kartenbeck, J.; Helenius, A. (2001). Caveolar endocytosis of simian virus 40 reveals a new two-step vesicular-transport pathway to the ER. *Nat. Cell Biol.*, 3, 473-483.

Pelkmans, L.; Helenius, A. (2002). Endocytosis *via* caveolae. *Traffic*, 3, 311-320.

Pelkmans, L.; Zerial, M. (2005). Kinase-regulated quantal assemblies and kiss-and-run recycling of caveolae. *Nature*, 436, 128-133.

Price, N.T.; Jackson, V.N.; Halestrap, A.P. (1998). Cloning and sequencing of four new mammalian monocarboxylate transporter (MCT) homologues confirms the existence of a transporter family with an ancient past. *Biochem. J.*, 329, 321-328.

Reese, T.S.; Karnovsky, M.J. (1967). Fine structural localization of a blood-brain barrier to exogenous peroxidase. *J. Cell Biol.*, 34, 207-217.

Regina, A.; Koman, A.; Piciotti, M.; El Hafny, B.; Center, M.S.; Bergmann, R.; Couranud, P.O.; Roux, F. (1998). MRP1 multidrug resistance-associated protein and P-glycoprotein expression in rat brain microvessel endothelial cells *J. Neurochem.*, 71, 705-715.

Roher, A.E.; Kuo, Y.-M.; Esh, C.; Knebel, C.; Weiss, N.; Kalback, W.; Luehrs, D.C.; Childress, J.L.; Beach, T.G.; Weller, R.O.; Kokjohn, T.A. (2003). Cortical and leptomeningeal cerebrovascular amyloid and white matter pathology in Alzheimer's disease. *Mol. Med.*, 9, 112-122.

Rollins, B.J. (1997). Chemokines. *Blood*, 90, 909-928.

Sagare, A.; Deane, R.; Bell, R.D.; Johnson, B.; Hamm, K.; Pendu, R.; Marky, A.; Lenting, P.J.; Wu, Z.; Zarcone, T.; Goate, A.; Mayo, K.; Perlmutter, D.; Coma, M.; Zhong, Z.; Zlokovic, B.V. (2007). Clearance of amyloid-β by circulating lipoprotein receptors. *Nat. Med.*, 13, 1029-1031.

Schinkel, A.H.; Smit, J.J.; van Tellingen, O.; Beijnen, J.H.; Wagennaar, E.W.; van Deemter, L.; Mol, C.A.; van der Valk, M.A.; Robanus-Maandag, E.C.; Riele, H.P.; Berns, A.J.M.; Borst, P. (1994). Distribution of the mouse mdr1a P-glycoprotein gene leads to a deficiency in the blood-brain barrier and to increased sensitivity to drugs. *Cell*, 77, 491-502.

Schinkel, A.H. (1999). P-glycoprotein, a gatekeeper in the blood-brain barrier. *Adv. Drug Deliv. Rev.*, 36, 179-194.

Schinkel, A.H.; Jonker, J.W. (2003). Mammalian drug efflux transporters of the ATP binding cassette (ABC) family: an overview. *Adv. Drug Deliv. Rev.*, 55, 3-29.

Schlachetzki, F.; Pardridge, W.M. (2003). P-glycoprotein and caveolin-1α in endothelium and astrocytes of primate brain. *Neuroreport*, 14, 2041-2046.

Schmidt, A.M.; Yan, S.D.; Wautier, J.-L.; Stern, D. (1999). Activation of receptor for advanced glycation end products. A mechanism for chronic vascular dysfunction in diabetic vasculopathy and atherosclerosis. *Circ. Res.*, 84, 489-497.

Schmidt, A.M.; Stern, D. (2000). Atherosclerosis and diabetes: the RAGE connection. *Curr. Atheroscler. Rep.*, 5, 430-436.

Schrickx, J.; Fink-Gremmels, J. (2007). P-glycoprotein-mediated transport of oxytetracycline in the Caco-2 cell model. *J. Vet. Pharmacol. Therap.*, 30, 25-31.

Seetharaman, S.; Barrand, M.A.; Maskell, L.; Scheper, R.J. (1998). Multidrug resistance-related transport proteins in isolated human brain microvessels and in cells cultures from these isolates. *J. Neurochem.*, 70, 1151-1159.

Sekine, T.; Cha, S.H.; Endou, H. (2000). The multispecific organic anion transporter (OAT) family. *Pflügers Arch. – Eur. J. Physiol.*, 440, 337-350.

Shi, N.; Zhang, Y.; Boado, R.J.; Pardridge, W.M. (2001). Brain-specific expression of an exogenous gene after i.v. administration. *Proc. Natl. Acad. U.S.A.*, 98, 12754-12759.

Shibata, M.; Yamada, S.; Kumar, M.; Calero, J.; Bading, B.; Frangione, D.; Holtzman, C.; Miller, C.; Strickland, D.; Ghiso, J.; Zlokovic, B. (2000). Clearance of Alzheimer's amyloid-ss(1-40) peptide from brain by LDL receptor-related protein-1 at the blood-brain barrier. *J. Clin. Invest.*, 106, 1489-1499.

Silver, D.L.; Tall, A.R. (2001). The cellular biology of scavenger receptor class B type 1. *Curr. Opin. Lipidol.*, 12, 497-504.

Stan, R.-V. (2002). Structure and function of endothelial caveolae. *Microsc. Res. Tech.*, 57, 350-364.

Tagami, M.; Kubota, A.; Sunaga, T.; Fujino, H.; Maezawa, H.; Kihara, M.; Nara, Y.; Yamori, Y. (1983). Increased transendothelial channel transport of cerebral capillary endothelium in stroke-prone SHR. *Stroke*, 14, 591-596.

Tamai, I.; Tsuji, A. (2000). Transporter-mediated permeation of drugs across the blood-brain barrier. J. *Pharm. Sci.*, 89, 1371-1388.

van Deurs, B. (1978). Microperoxidase uptake into the rat choroids plexus epithelium. *J. Ultrastruct. Res.*, 62, 168-180.

van Deurs, B. (1980). Structural aspects of brain barriers, with special reference to the permeability of the cerebral endothelium and choroidal epithelium. *Int. Rev. Cytol.*, 65, 117-191.

Vogelgesang, S.; Warzok, R.W.; Cascorbi, I.; Kunert-Keil, C.; Schroeder, E.; Kroemer, H.K.; Siegmund, W.; Walker, L.C.; Pahnke, J. (2004). The role of P-glycoprotein in cerebral amyloid angiopathy; implications for the early pathogenesis of Alzheimer's disease. *Curr. Alzheimer Res.*, 1, 121-125.

Vorbrodt, A.W. (1988). *Ultrastructural cytochemistry of blood-brain barrier endothelia in Prog. Histochem. Cytochem.*, Gustav Fisher Verlag: Stuttgart, New York, pp. 1-99.

Vorbrodt, A.W.; Dobrogowska, D.H. (2003). Molecular anatomy of intracellular junctions in brain endothelial and epithelial barriers: electron microscopist's view. *Brain Res. Rev.*, 42, 221-242.

Wautier, J.-L.; Zoukourian, C.; Chappey, O.; Wautier, M.-P.; Guillausseau, P.-J.; Cao, R.; Hori, O.; Stern, D.; Schmidt, A.M. (1996). Receptor-mediated endothelial cell dysfunction in diabetic vasculopathy. *J. Clin. Invest.*, 97, 238-243.

Weiss, J.; Gregor, S.-M.; Dormann, G.; Martin-Facklam, M.; Kerpen, C.J.; Ketabi-Kiyanvash, N.; Haefeli, W.E. (2003). Inhibition of P-glycoprotein by newer antidepressants. *J. Pharmacol. Exp. Ther.*, 305, 197-204.

Weller, R.O.; Massey, A.; Newman, T.A.; Hutchings, M.; Kuo, Y.-M.; Roher, A.E. (1998). Cerebral amyloid angiopathy: amyloid beta accumulates in putative interstitial fluid drainage pathways in Alzheimer's disease. *Am. J. Pathol.*, 153, 725-733.

Widder, J.D.; Guzik, T.J.; Mueller, C.F.H.; Clempus, R.E.; Schmidt, H.H.H.W.; Dikalov, S.I.; Griendling, K.K.; Jones, D.P.; Harrison, D.G. (2007). Role of the multidrug resistance protein-1 in hypertension and vascular dysfunction caused by angiotensin II. *Arterioscler. Thromb. Vasc. Biol.*, 27, 762-768.

Zlokovic, B.V. (2004). Clearning amyloid through the blood-brain barrier. *J. Neurochem.*, 89, 807-811.

Zlokovic, B.V. (2005). Neurovascular mechanisms of Alzheimer's neurodegeneration. *Trends Neurosci.*, 28, 202-208.

Zlokovic, B.V. (2008a). New therapeutic targets in the neurovascular pathway in Alzheimer's disease. *Neurotherapeutics*, 5, 409-414.

Zlokovic, B.V. (2008b). The blood-brain barrier in health and chronic neurodegenerative disorders. *Neuron*, 57, 178-201.

6

Contribution of Multivesicular Bodies to the Prion-Like Propagation of Lesions in Alzheimer's Disease

Valérie Vingtdeux[1], Luc Buée[2,3] and Nicolas Sergeant[2,3]
[1]Litwin-Zucker Research Center for the Study of Alzheimer's Disease, The Feinstein Institute for Medical Research
[2]Inserm, U837, Alzheimer & Tauopathies
[3]Univ Lille Nord de France, UDSL, Faculty of Medicine, Institute of Predictive Medicine and Therapeutic Research, Jean-Pierre Aubert Research Centre
[1]USA
[2,3]France

1. Introduction

Alzheimer's disease (AD) is a chronic developing dementing disease characterized by coexistence of two types of lesions, the parenchymal amyloid deposits and the intraneuronal neurofibrillary tangles. Amyloid deposits are composed of amyloid-beta peptides that derive from sequential cleavages of its precursor named amyloid protein precursor (APP). Neurofibrillary tangles (NFT) results from intraneuronal aggregation of abnormally modified microtubule-associated Tau proteins. A synergistic relationship between the two lesions may trigger the progression of the disease. Thus, starting in the entorhinal cortex and slowly progressing through temporal, frontal, parietal and occipital cortex, the progression of NFT is well correlated with clinical expression of the disease. However, little is known about the mechanism underlying spatiotemporal propagation of these lesions ultimately leading to the disease. A growing number of studies suggest a prion-like diffusion of amyloid deposits and NFT, which could even be extrapolate to several other neurodegenerative diseases. In the present chapter, we will develop the current hypotheses regarding the molecular and cellular mechanisms driving the development and spreading of Alzheimer's disease lesions involving multivesicular bodies.

2. Alzheimer's disease

Alzheimer's disease is a slow and progressive disease affecting the brain and characterized by the loss of superior cognitive functions leading to dementia and death. Two neuropathological brain lesions are found in the brain tissue and their presence is instrumental for providing a definite diagnosis of the disease, as firstly described by Alois Alzheimer (Alzheimer, 1911). Amyloid deposits are amorphous parenchymal deposits of β-sheet ordered proteinaceous material. Amyloid deposition is observed with aging, in Alzheimer's disease, Down's syndrome, Dementia with Lewy bodies and vascular dementia, all of which are aged-related neurodegenerative disorders. The major constituent of amyloid deposits is a small peptide of 39 to 43 amino acid residues, named Aβ for amyloid-beta peptide (Glenner and Wong, 1984), which derives from multiple and sequential cleavages of a larger precursor, named amyloid precursor protein (APP).

2.1 APP structure and metabolism

The amyloid precursor protein APP is encoded by a single *APP* gene located on the long arm of chromosome 21 at position 21q11.2 (Kang *et al.*, 1987; Goldgaber *et al.*, 1987). The gene span more than 170kb and is constituted of 19 exons (Yoshikai *et al.*, 1990). Alternative splicing generates seven isoforms but there is a single neuronal isoform in human adult brain that is composed of 695 amino acids (Konig *et al.*, 1991). APP is a transmembrane protein with a large extra membrane domain, a transmembrane domain, and a short cytosolic tail composed of 59 amino acids (Fig. 1). The exact role of APP remains elusive but many functions have been proposed, for example APP was suggested to be instrumental to iron cellular homeostasis (Duce *et al.*, 2010), to regulate intracellular transport, to be a cell surface receptor, and some fragments derived from the cleavage of APP are suggested to be neuroprotective or to promote axon outgrowth (Chasseigneaux *et al.*, 2011) whereas others are related to an ancestral immunological mechanism of defense and would have antibacterial peptide property (Soscia *et al.*, 2010). However, the full spectrum of APP functions remains to be elucidated.

2.2 APP cleavage by secretases and amyloid production

Proteolytic cleavage of APP brings into play sequential events involving first the liberation of its ectodomain either by α- or β-secretase activities. These cleavages generate carboxy-terminal fragments remaining anchored to the plasma membrane and they shed extracellular soluble fragments, both of which are playing a role in axon outgrowth *in vitro* (Chasseigneux *et al.*, 2011). The first cleavage to occur is mediated by α-secretase. This cleavage generates a soluble APP fragment α (sAPPα) and a carboxy-terminal α fragment composed of 83 amino acids (named C83 or CTFα). This cleavage takes place within the sequence of Aβ peptide thus precluding its formation. This pathway is therefore referred to as the non-amyloidogenic pathway. The α-secretase activity is carried by metalloproteases called ADAMs (for A Disintegrin And Metalloprotease). Several ADAM proteases with an α-secretase activity have been identified, including ADAM-17 or TACE (EC 3.4.24.86, peptidase family M12) (Buxbaum *et al.*, 1998), ADAM-10 (EC 3.4.24.81, peptidase family M12) (Lammich *et al.*, 1999 ; Lopez-Perez *et al.*, 2001), and ADAM-9 (EC 3.4.24.-) (Hotoda *et al.*, 2002; Koike *et al.*, 1999).

Alternatively to α-secretase, APP can be processed by β-secretase which can cleave at the first amino-terminal amino acid residue starting Aβ peptide sequence or at position 11, referred to as β'-cleavage. This β-cleavage generates a soluble fragment sAPPβ and a CTF comprised of 99 amino acids (C99 or CTFβ). This pathway is referred to as the amyloidogenic pathway. The protease responsible for both β- and β'-cleavage has been identified as BACE-1 (for β-site APP cleaving enzyme-1) (Memapsin 2, EC 3.4.23.46, peptidase family A1) (Hussain *et al.*, 1999 ; Lin *et al.*, 2000; Sinha *et al.*, 1999 ; Vassar *et al.*, 1999 ; Yan *et al.*, 1999). All APP-CTFs (CTFα, β' and β) can subsequently be cleaved at the juxtamembrane region by the γ-secretase. However, ectodomain cleavage of APP is mandatory to intramembrane γ-secretase proteolysis of APP-CTFs.

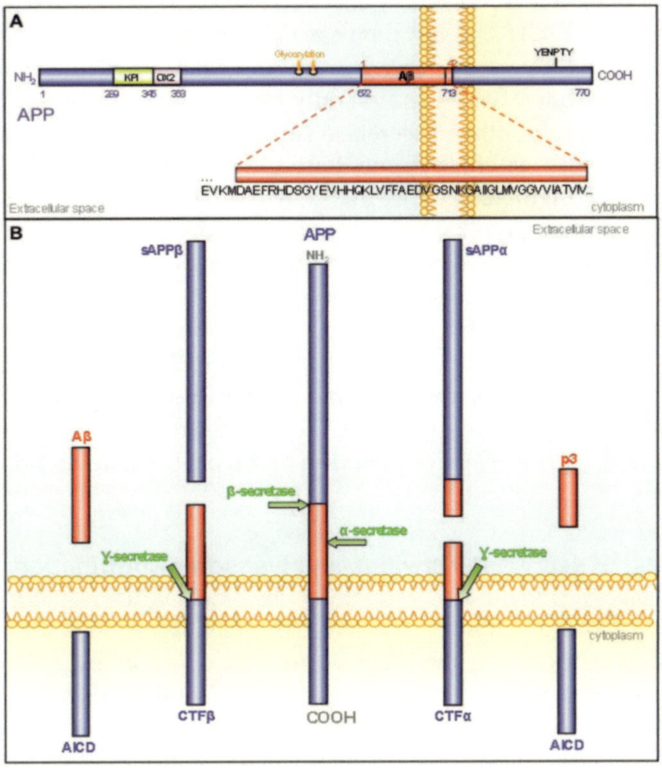

Fig. 1. *Amyloid protein precursor structure and metabolism.* (A) Schematic representation of APP structure. (B) APP processing by secretase activities. α- and β-secretase activities cleave APP in its extracellular domain to release respectively a soluble fragment sAPPα or sAPPβ in the extracellular space and generate carboxy-terminal fragments CTFα or CTFβ. These CTFs can subsequently be processed by γ-secretase to generate AICD and Aβ or p3.

The APP intracellular domain (AICD) is released from both CTFα and CTFβ. The γ-secretase cleavage of CTFβ represents the last step for Aβ production. The γ-secretase is a multiprotein complex composed of at least four proteins which are necessary and sufficient to form an active enzymatic complex (Edbauer *et al.*, 2003; Kimberly *et al.*, 2003 ; Takasugi *et al.*, 2003) which is composed of Presenilin (PS) (EC 3.4.23.-) (De Strooper *et al.*, 1998 ; Zhang *et al.*, 2000), Nicastrin (Esler *et al.*, 2002; Yu *et al.*, 2000), Aph-1 and Pen-2 (Bammens *et al.*, 2011; Francis *et al.*, 2002 ; Goutte *et al.*, 2002 ; Lee *et al.*, 2002 ; Steiner *et al.*, 2002; for review see Jorissen *et al.*, 2010). APP is not the unique γ-secretase substrate. This aspartyl protease belongs to the family of intramembrane-cleaving proteases, which also comprises the signal-peptide peptidases family of proteases (for review see Wolfe, 2010). Yet, more than 60 substrates of the γ-secretase have been characterized including APP (Jorissen *et al.*, 2010). Targeting the γ-secretase for drugs development that repress Aβ production is especially challenging due in part to the substrate-polyspecificity of this protease (For review see De Strooper *et al.*, 2010). However, recent data has shown that Gleevec/Imatinib, a tyrosine kinase inhibitor anti-cancer drug, could repress Aβ production without affecting γ-secretase cleavages of other substrates such as Notch (Netzer *et al.*, 2003; He at al., 2010). Noteworthy,

Aβ production and release is repressed by Gleevec but AICD, which is released also from γ-secretase cleavage of APP-CTFs, is not repressed. Thus, two products that are supposedly generated by a same γ-secretase protease can be oppositely regulated; one is reduced the other is increased. However, Aβ is generated only from CTFβ whereas AICD can be released from several APP-CTFs as for other γ-secretase substrates. This mechanism is also observed with alkalizing drugs such as chloroquine, bafilomycin A1 and NH_4Cl (Schrader-Fischer and Paganetti, 1996; Vingtdeux *et al.*, 2007; Eisele *et al.*, 2007), also referred to as lysomotropic drugs. Although, alkalizing drugs are known modifiers of intracellular and intravesicular pH, the molecular mechanism lowering Aβ production without modifying other γ-secretase substrate cleavages remain elusive. A mechanism has recently been proposed for Imatinib/Gleevec. Gleevec may repress the regulating function of a novel modulator of γ-secretase protease activity named GSAP (Gamma-Secretase Activating Protein) (He *et al.*, 2010). The substrate recognition of APP-CTFs is enhanced by GASP and consequently increases the production of Aβ. Gleevec represses GASP association to the γ-secretase complex leading to a selective lowering of Aβ production but not AICD or other γ-secretase substrates.

2.3 Cell localization of secretase activities and lysosome contribution

The α- and β-secretases are sheddases that release the extracellular domain of APP as well as several others type I transmembrane proteins. The cleavage and localization of enzyme activity is supposed to occur at the plasma membrane or in early endosomes. As for instance, BACE-1 resides within endosomes and APP endocytosis is a prerequisite for cleavage of APP by BACE1 and generation of Aβ (Ehehalt *et al.*, 2003; Vassar *et al.*, 1999; Walter *et al.*, 2001). BACE-1 optimal protease activity necessitates an acidic pH and acidification of endosome occurs during the route of endosomes to fuse with lysosomes where BACE1 is degraded (Koh *et al.*, 2005). Cleavage of APP-CTFs by γ-secretase can occur at several places in the cell (e.g. plasma membrane, endosomes…). Discrepancies exist regarding the cell localization of γ-secretase byproducts. Several APP metabolites including APP, APP-CTFs, Aβ and AICD have been shown to accumulate in multivesicular bodies following treatment of cells with alkalizing drugs (Verbeek *et al.* 2002; Vingtdeux *et al.*, 2007). Interestingly and similarly to Gleevec, these alkalizing drugs such as chloroquine, ammonium chloride, bafilomycin A1, block Aβ production without affecting AICD generation (Vingtdeux *et al.*, 2007). AICD can be released outside the cell and also inside the cell, reach the nucleus (Goodger *et al.*, 2009) where AICD may regulate gene expression (Pardossi-Piquard *et al.*, 2005). Interestingly, intracellular AICD may be generated from APP-CTFs produced from β-secretase (Belyaev *et al.*, 2010). However, further investigation is needed to determine whether there is one or several AICD and what is the function of AICD. For instance, BACE1 cleavage of APP and AICD derived from βCTF may contribute to learning, memory and neuronal plasticity (Ma *et al.*, 2007).

2.4 Neurofibrillary tangles and microtubule-associated Tau

Neurofibrillary tangles are characterized by intraneuronal accumulation of fibrillar material named paired helical filaments. Abnormally modified Tau proteins are the major components of this filamentous material. Tau proteins belong to the family of microtubule-associated proteins. A single gene, named *MAPT* located at position 17q21 encoded for several isoforms resulting from alternative splicing of exons 2, 3 and 10 in the human adult brain. Thus, they are six isoforms, half of which contains the exon-10 encoding sequence, two-third are having the exon 2 whereas the exon 3 is found in one-third of Tau isoforms. In the human brain, Tau proteins constitute a family of six isoforms (six mRNAs) that range from 352 to 441 amino acids. Their molecular weight ranges from 45 to 65 kDa when resolved on polyacrylamide gel electrophoresis in presence of sodium dodecyl sulfate (SDS-PAGE). The Tau isoforms differ from each other by the presence of either three (3R) or four repeat-regions (4R) in the carboxy-terminal (C-terminal) part of the molecule and the absence or presence of one or two inserts (29 or 58 amino acids) in the amino-terminal (N-terminal) part (Goedert *et al.*, 1989a; Goedert *et al.*, 1989b; Andreadis *et al.*, 1992). Each of these isoforms is likely to have particular physiological roles since they are differentially expressed during development. For instance, only one Tau isoform, characterized by 3R and no N-terminal inserts, is present during fetal stages, while the six isoforms (with one or two N-terminal inserts and 3 or 4R) are expressed during adulthood (Goedert and Jakes, 1990; Kosik *et al.*, 1989). Exons 2 and 3 are alternatively spliced in the brain whereas included in muscle (Leroy *et al.*, 2006). Thus, Tau isoforms are likely to have specific functions related to absence or presence of regions encoded by cassette exons 2, 3 and 10. Furthermore, the six Tau isoforms are not equally expressed in neurons. For example, Tau mRNAs containing exon 10 are not found in granular cells of the dentate gyrus (Goedert *et al.*, 1989a). Thus, Tau isoforms are differentially distributed in neuronal subpopulations.

Tau proteins bind microtubules through repetitive regions in their C-terminal part. These repetitive regions are the repeat domains (R1-R4) encoded by exons 9-12 (Lee *et al.*, 1989). The three (3R) or four copies (4R) are made of a highly conserved 18-amino acid repeat (Goedert *et al.*, 1989b, Himmler, 1989, Lee *et al.*, 1988, Lee *et al.*, 1989) separated from each other by less conserved 13- or 14-amino acid inter-repeat domains. Tau proteins are known to act as promoter of tubulin polymerization in vitro, and are involved in axonal transport (Brandt and Lee, 1993; Cleveland *et al.*, 1977a; Weingarten *et al.*, 1975). They have been shown to increase the rate of microtubule polymerization, and to inhibit the rate of depolymerization (Drechsel *et al.*, 1992). The 18-amino acid repeats bind to microtubules through a flexible array of distributed weak sites (Butner and Kirschner, 1991, Lee *et al.*, 1989). It has been demonstrated that adult Tau isoforms with 4R (R1-R4) are more efficient at promoting microtubule assembly than the fetal isoform with 3R (R1, R3-R4) (Butner and Kirschner, 1991; Goedert and Jakes, 1990; Gustke *et al.*, 1994). Interestingly, the most potent part to induce microtubule polymerization is the inter-region between repeats 1 and 2 (R1-R2 inter-region) and more specifically peptide 274KVQIINKK281 within this sequence. This R1-R2 inter-region is unique to 4R Tau (since it occurs between exons 9 and 10), adult-specific and responsible for differences in the binding affinities between 3R and 4R Tau (Goode and Feinstein, 1994). Recent evidence supports a role for the microtubule-binding domain in the modulation of the phosphorylation state of Tau proteins. A direct and competitive binding has been demonstrated between residues 224-236 (according to the numbering of the longest isoform) and microtubules on one hand, and residues 224-236 and protein phosphatase 2A (PP2A) on the other hand (Sontag *et al.*, 1999). As a consequence, microtubules could inhibit PP2A activity by competing for binding to Tau at the microtubule-binding domains. The lysine residue 280 is crucial for microtubule-binding of 4R Tau. This lysine is mutated in genetic form of FTDP-17 and promotes Tau aggregation in vitro and in vivo (Fischer *et al.*, 2007; Eckermann *et al.*, 2007). Much more recently, acetylation of Tau has been shown to regulate microtubule-binding of Tau (Min *et al.*, 2010; Cohen *et al.*, 2011). Histone acetyl transferase P300 or CREB-binding protein (CBP) and deacetylase SIRT1 or HDAC6 likely regulate the acetylation of Tau (Min *et al.*, 2010; Cohen *et al.*, 2011). Moreover, Tau-acetylation is suggested to promote Tau aggregation and is observed in animal models, Alzheimer's disease and brain tissues of patients with Tauopathies, at the exception of Pick's disease where Pick bodies are negative for acetylated lys-280 as well as phosphorylation at ser-262 (Cohen *et al.*, 2011; Sergeant *et al.*, 1997; Probst *et al.*, 1996). However, due to selective aggregation of 3R Tau in Pick's disease (Delacourte *et al.*, 1996; Sergeant *et al.*, 1997), acetylation of 3R Tau on another lysine residue cannot be precluded.

Besides its major microtubule-binding, -stabilizing, paralleled-ordering functions, Tau also has other functions. Tau proteins bind to spectrin and actin filaments (Carlier *et al.*, 1984, Correas *et al.*, 1990, Henriquez *et al.*, 1995, Selden and Pollard, 1983). Through these interactions, Tau proteins may allow microtubules to interconnect with other cytoskeletal components such as neurofilaments (Miyata *et al.*, 1986; Andreadis *et al.*, 1995) and may restrict the flexibility of the microtubules (Matus, 1990). There is also evidence that Tau proteins interact with cytoplasmic organelles. Such interactions may allow for binding between microtubules and mitochondria (Jung *et al.*, 1993). The Tau N-terminal projection domain also permits interactions with neural plasma membrane (Brandt *et al.*, 1995). Thus, Tau may act as a mediator between microtubules and plasma membrane. This interaction has been defined as involving a binding between the proline-rich sequence in the N-terminal part of Tau proteins and the SH3 domains of Src-family non-receptor tyrosine kinases, such as Fyn. Studies have determined that human Tau Tyr18 and Tyr29 are phosphorylated by the Src family tyrosine kinase Fyn (Lee *et al.*, 2004; Williamson *et al.*, 2002). The same proline-rich region of Tau proteins is likely involved in the interaction with phospholipase C-γ (PLC-γ) isozymes (Jenkins and Johnson, 1998; Hwang *et al.*, 1996). Hwang and colleagues have demonstrated in vitro that Tau proteins complex specifically with the SH3 domain of PLC-γ, and enhance its activity in the presence of unsaturated fatty acids such as arachidonic acid. These results suggest that in cells that express Tau proteins, receptors coupled to cytosolic phospholipase A2 may activate PLC-γ indirectly, in the absence of the usual tyrosine phosphorylation, through the hydrolysis of phosphatidylcholine to generate arachidonic acid (Jenkins and Johnson, 1998; Hwang *et al.*, 1996). Altogether, these data indicate that Tau proteins may also play a role in the signal transduction pathway involving PLC-γ (for review see Rhee, 2001). In line with this idea, recent data demonstrate that Tau is necessary for glutamatergic signaling (Ittner *et al.*, 2010).

2.5 The cortical brain spreading of neurofibrillary degeneration

With aging, neurofibrillary tangles are affecting the entorhinal cortex followed by the hippocampal formation. At this stage, no clear clinical symptoms are associated with the presence of these lesions and they are therefore considered as an aging-associated phenomenon. But this remains an open debate. Indeed, neuropathological as well as biochemical approaches show that Tau pathology of Alzheimer's disease spreads progressively, invariably, hierarchically, from the transentorhinal cortex to the whole neocortex, along cortico-cortical connections. The brain regions that are sequentially affected explain well the successive types of cognitive impairments that characterize the disease: amnesia following the entorhinal and hippocampal degeneration; aphasia, apraxia and agnosia with the involvement of the neocortex. Of course, amyloid and Tau pathology are present before the clinical symptoms, because neuronal plasticity is able to compensate at the first AD stages. Our studies show that Tau pathology is already distributed in the hippocampal formation and the temporal cortex at the "pre-clinical" stage of AD (Delacourte *et al.*, 1999, 2002).

PHF-Tau pathology, visualized as a triplet of abnormal Tau proteins, was systematically present in variable amounts in the entorhinal and hippocampal regions of non-demented patients aged over 75 years. When Tau pathology was found in other brain areas, it was always along a stereotyped, sequential, hierarchical pathway. The progression was categorized into 10 stages according to the brain regions affected: transentorhinal cortex (S1), entorhinal (S2), hippocampus (S3), anterior temporal cortex (S4), inferior temporal cortex (S5), mid temporal cortex (S6), polymodal association areas (prefrontal, parietal inferior, temporal superior) (S7), unimodal areas (S8), primary motor (S9a) or sensory (S9b, S9c) areas, and all neocortical areas (S10). Up to stage 6, the disease could be asymptomatic. In all cases of our study, stage 7 individuals with two polymodal association areas affected by Tau pathology were cognitively impaired. Since the neuropathological observation of this stereotype cortical brain progression of Tau pathology (Braak and Braak, 1991; Duyckaerts *et al.*, 1997) is the question of how does neurofibrillary degeneration is selective toward neuronal subpopulations of cortical brain layers III and V (Hof *et al.*, 1990) and progressively propagates through brain structures.

3. Multivesicular bodies and exosomes

3.1 Multivesicular bodies

During endocytosis, some of the extracellular components, such as viruses, ligands or diffusible factors and, part of the plasma membrane proteins are internalized and are either recycled to the cell surface via early endosomes and recycling endosomes or will be address through a set of vesicular compartments: early endosomes, late endosomes and finally delivered to lysosomes for degradation (for review see Gruenberg, 2009). Late endosomes are also known as multivesicular endosomes or multivesicular bodies (MVBs) (Gruenberg and Stenmark, 2004; Raposo and Marks, 2007) and are prerequisite before degradation of internalized material by fusion with lysosomes. Multivesicular bodies are large vesicles of several hundred nanometers that are characterized by numerous smaller intraluminal vesicles (ILVs) formed by the inward budding of the endosome limiting membrane. The formation of these intraluminal vesicles requires sequential steps and the contribution of complex multi molecular machinery named ESCRT for Endosomal Sorting Complex Required for Transport. The ESCRT machinery is composed of four ESCRT complexes (0, I, II and III) acting sequentially to sort cargo and to form a coated subdomain on endosomes that forms the ILVs (Fig. 2). The Vps27/Hrs-Hse1/STAM complex (ESCRT-0) is first recruited to the endosomes by binding PI(3)P and ubiquitinated cargos. ESCRT-0 then recruits ESCRT-I (composed of Tsg101/Vps23-Vps28-Vps37) to the membrane, where ESCRT-I interacts with ubiquitinated cargos via its Vps23 subunit. Then, ESCRT-I recruits ESCRT-II complex (composed of Vps22/Eap30-Vps25/Eap25-Vps36/Eap45), which in turn initiates the oligomerization of ESCRT-III complex (composed of Vps2/CHMP2-Vps20/CHMP6-Vps24/CHMP3-Snf7/Vps32/CHMP4). Finally, ESCRT-III recruits supplementary factors like Bro1 and Vsp4 AAA ATPase. Bro1 will recruit a deubiquitination enzyme whereas Vps4 AAA ATPase will work to break apart ESCRT-III and other ESCRT complexes, resulting in their dissociation from the membrane. Evidences for alternative pathways for cargos sorting into MVBs are emerging, which are independent of the ESCRT machinery but seems to depend on lipid composition of raft-based micro domains. Proper cholesterol levels in late endosomes generated by ORPs (oxysterol-binding protein-related proteins) are required for normal MVBs formation and MVB-mediated membrane protein degradation (Kobuna *et al.*, 2010).

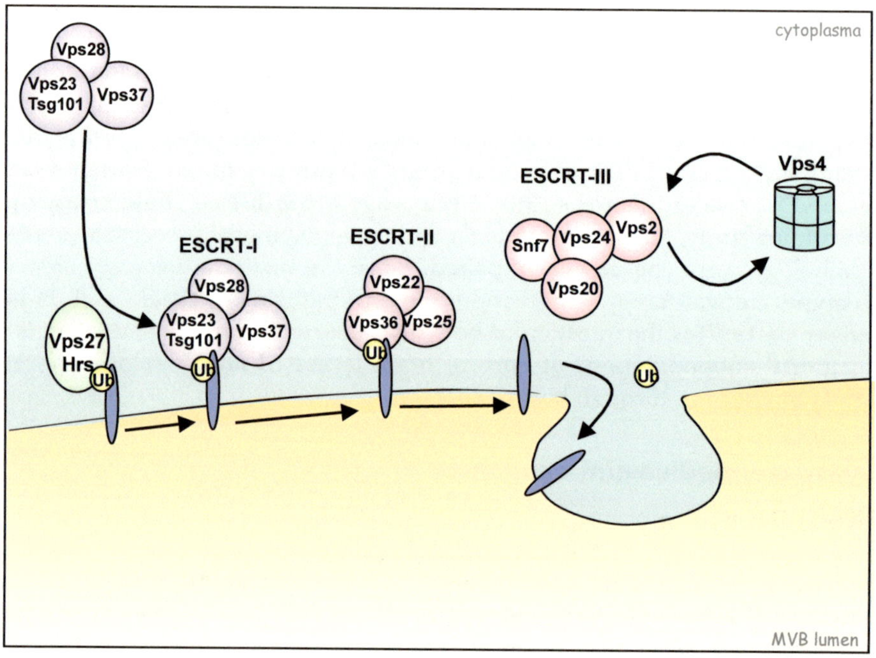

Fig. 2. *Model for the ubiquitin-dependent sorting of proteins by the ESCRT machinery.* The different ESCRT complexes act sequentially for the recognition and sorting of ubiquitinated transmembrane proteins into the internal vesicles of multivesicular bodies.

The phospholipid LBPA (lysobisphosphatidic acid) possessed the capacity to drive the formation of membrane invaginations within acidic liposomes. Alix controls this invagination process *in vitro* and the organization of LBPA-containing endosomes *in vivo* (Matsuo *et al.*, 2004). These micro domains also contain high concentrations of sphingolipids from which ceramide are formed. Ceramide induced the coalescence of small microdomains into larger domains, which promotes domain-induced budding. In addition ceramide cone-shapped structure might induce spontaneous negative curvature by creating an area difference between the membrane leaflets (Trajkovic *et al.*, 2008). Ubiquitination (Ub) is the main sorting signal for cargo entry into the vesicles that bud from the limiting membrane into the lumen of endosomes during the biogenesis of MVBs. A single Ub is sufficient to direct ILV targeting. Ub is recognized by an expanding cohort of endosomal proteins, which may act as Ub-sorting receptors responsible for binding and directing cargo toward ILVs like some ESCRT subunits, including Vps27/Hrs, Vps23/Tsg101 and Vps36/Eap45 (For review see: Piper and Katzmann, 2007). Many integral membrane proteins targeted for lysosomal degradation are ubiquitinated; however, non-ubiquitin sorting signals have also been described. Much less is known about non-Ub signals that sort proteins to ILVs; proteins which have been described to enter ILVs in an Ub-independent manner include Pmel17/Silver (Berson, 2003), TfR (Geminard, 2004), Nedd4 (Morita and Sundquist, 2004),

sna3 (McNatt, 2007; Oestreich 2007). Two motifs 'NTR' and 'PKD' located on the extracellular part of Pmel17 are responsible for its targeting into the internal vesicles of MVBs (Theos *et al.*, 2006) and COP9 signalosome (CSN)-associated protein CSN5 is involved in protein sorting into ILVs since siRNA of CSN5 causes a significant increase in both ubiquitinated and non-ubiquitinated proteins detected in exosomes (Liu *et al.*, 2009).
Genetic also supports the importance of functional MVB in neurological disease and frontotemporal dementia. Thus, the gene encoding the ESCRT-III subunit CHMP2B was found to be mutated in a form of frontotemporal dementia (Skibinski *et al.*, 2005) and amyotrophic lateral sclerosis (Cox *et al.*, 2010) suggesting that functional MVBs are required to prevent accumulation of abnormal proteins that can disrupt neural function and ultimately lead to neurodegeneration (Filimonenko *et al.*, 2007). Mutations in *CHMP2B* were first described in Danish and Belgian families but remain rare (Ghanim *et al.*, 2010). Mutations are supposed to lead to C-terminal truncation of CHMP2B. Brain tissue examination of patient with *CHMP2B* mutation showed enlarged vacuoles stained with a mannose-6-phosphate receptor antibody. The truncated protein impairs the fusion of endosome with lysosomes without obvious modification of protein sorting to MVB (Urwin *et al.*, 2010). Staining of tissue from Alzheimer disease patients with CHMP2B showed an accumulation of the protein in vesicular structures resembling GranuloVacuolar Degeneration (Yamazaki *et al.*, 2010; Funk *et al.*, 2011) suggestive of defective autophagic and endocytic pathways in Alzheimer disease. Thus, restoring or enhancing the lysosomal degradation and rates of autophagic protein turnover in a transgenic animal model of amyloid deposition can rescue the phenotype and decrease the amyloid burden (Yang *et al*, 2011). Together, a defective function of the endocytic pathway including MVB, autophagy and lysosome may certainly contribute to the development of Alzheimer disease.

3.2 Exosomes

Alternatively to their fusion with lysosomes for degradation of their contents, MVBs have been described to fuse with the plasma membrane and release their content in the extracellular space, the ILVs contained in the MVBs when released are known as exosomes. Exosomes have a size ranging from 40 to 100 nm and can be secreted by many cell types including neuronal cells (Faure J *et al.*, 2006; Rajendran *et al.*, 2006; Vingtdeux *et al.*, 2007; Lachenal *et al.*, 2010). Exosomes are isolated from the media of cultured cells. However, purification of exosomes is not trivial since membrane fragments or cell debris can easily contaminate exosome preparation. Due to their small size, exosomes are obtained after filtration on 0.22 μm filters and by a series of centrifugation and sucrose gradient (Raposo et al., 1996; Wubbolts *et al.*, 2003; Faure *et al.*, 2006; For review see Olver and Vidal, 2007). Further immunoisolation can be used (Wubbolts *et al.*, 2003). Several parameters should be evaluated to ascertain the purity of exosomes preparation. The first and likely most important characteristic is the observation of exosomes by transmission electron microscopy. Several proteins are also common to exosomes and described in exosomes preparation that originate from different sources (For review Vella *et al.*, 2008). Interestingly, several tetraspanins proteins are enriched in exosomes and may contribute to exosomes formation (De Gassart *et al.*, 2004; Wubbolts *et al.*, 2003). Tetraspanins are a growing family of transmembrane proteins with pleiotropic functions found associated with lipid-raft micro domains (for review Hemler *et al.*, 2005). Interestingly, tetraspanins CD81 and CD9, which are found in exosomes derived from B-cells (Wubblots *et al.*, 2003), are co-purified with the γ-secretase interactome. Absence of those tetraspanins induces a partial disruption of γ-secretase activity or reduces γ-secretase substrate interaction (Wakabayashi *et al.*, 2009). Although detailed molecular mechanisms remain unknown, together those results further support the idea that MVB and most possibly exosomes are important cellular compartments for APP metabolism regulation and that several γ-secretase regulators may act at this level.

Little is known about the requirements and regulation of MVBs fusion with the plasma membrane and the release of exosomes outside cells. Recently, in primary neuronal culture cell, release of exosomes by neurons was shown to be regulated by glutamatergic signaling (Lachenal *et al.*, 2010). Calcium ionophores stimulate exosomes release in some cell types suggesting that intracellular calcium levels also play a role in plasma membrane fusions event. The Rab family of GTPase proteins seems to be required for exosomes release. Rab11, a well-known regulator of endosomal recycling, has been linked to the control of exosomes release in K562a cells (Savina *et al.*, 2005). Silencing of five other Rab proteins, Rab2b, Rab9a, Rab5a, Rab27a and Rab27b inhibited exosomes secretion. Rab27a and Rab27b function in MVBs docking to the plasma membrane (Ostrowski *et al.*, 2010). Inhibition of Rab35 function leads to intracellular accumulation of endosomal vesicles and impairs exosomes secretion possibly by controlling the docking/tethering of endocytic vesicles with the plasma membrane (Hsu *et al.*, 2010). MVBs fate can be affected by macroautophagy (hereafter referred to as autophagy). During autophagy, parts of the cytoplasm and organelles are encapsulated in double-membrane vacuoles called autophagosomes, which eventually fuse with lysosomes for degradation (for review see Levine *et al.*, 2011). Under conditions that stimulate autophagy, MVBs are diverted to autophagic pathway with subsequent inhibition in exosomes secretion (Fader *et al.*, 2008). With regards to Tau, the autophagy-lysosomal pathway contributes to the degradation of Tau (Wang *et al.*, 2009).

How exosomes are processed in recipient cells is not yet fully understood. Exosomes are able to be endocytosed into the endosomal system of recipient cells. Once internalized, exosomes could fuse with the limiting membrane of endosomes to deliver their cytoplasmic content into the host cell cytoplasm. It is also possible that exosomes could directly fuse with the plasma membrane. Although their exact function remains to be discovered, within the extracellular space and in biological fluids such as urine or serum, exosomes have been proposed to participate in different physiological and/or pathological processes such as neurodegenerative diseases (for review see Vella *et al.*, 2008). They could be responsible not only for protein and lipids exchange between cells, but also for mRNA and microRNAs exchange (Valadi *et al.*, 2007). Exosome release and content may be regulated by cellular stress. Thus DNA damage and activation of p53 induce the expression of protein that will be included inside exosomes (Yu *et al.*, 2006). Exosomes may mediate a signal of cellular damage or stress. In the central nervous system, exosomes are proposed to constitute an intercellular communication system (for review see Mathivanan *et al.*, 2011). AICD and several APP metabolites are found in exosomes derived from primary neuronal cultured cells (Vingtdeux *et al.*, 2007) (Fig. 3). L1 CAM that is also processed by γ-secretase (Riedle *et al.*, 2009) is recovered in exosomes (Lachenal *et al.*, 2011). Although speculative, if several intracellular domains of proteins processed by γ-secretase are internalized and secreted within exosomes, the fusion of those exosomes with surrounding cells may regulate gene expression by those intracellular domains and therefore constitute a cell communication system.

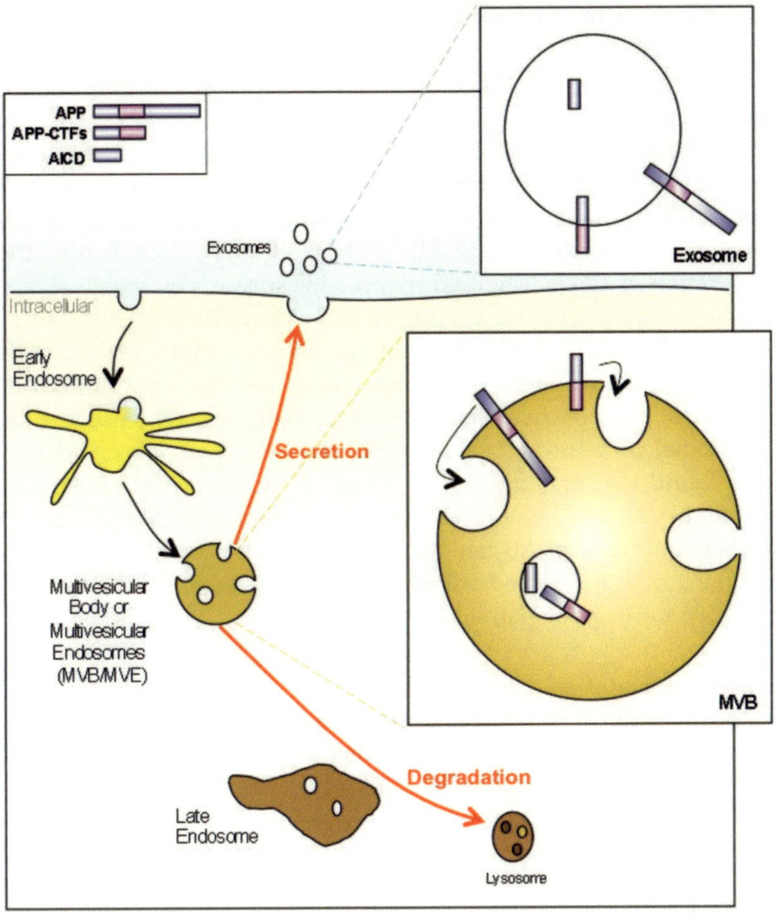

Fig. 3. *APP and its metabolites are present in multivesicular bodies and exosomes.* APP and APP-CTFs are internalized and directed into the internal vesicles of multivesicular bodies (MVB). At this point APP and its metabolites can either be degraded after the fusion of MVB with lysosomes or can be released in the extracellular space in association with exosomes consecutively to the fusion of MVB with the plasma membrane.

4. Prion-like propagation of amyloid and Tau pathology

Besides being a potential system of intercellular communication, exosomes are also known to be instrumental to the dissemination of pathogens, whether those are viruses or proteinaceous pathogens. The first pathological protein described associated with exosomes was the prion protein (PrP) (Fevrier *et al.*, 2004; Alais *et al.*, 2008). Prions diseases are fatal neurodegenerative disorders. They are associated with the conversion of the cellular prion protein (PrPc) into the scrapie PrP (PrPSc), an abnormal conformational state that tends to form amyloid deposits in brain tissue leading to dementia. Into its misfolded conformation the PrPSc is thought to be infectious (For review see Aguzzi and Rajendran, 2009). Recent findings revealed an unexpected role for exosomes in vehiculation of prions: exosomes from prion-infected neuronal cells have been demonstrated to be efficient initiators of prion propagation in uninfected recipient cells and, more importantly, to produce prion disease when inoculated into mice.

4.1 Amyloid propagation

Exosomal release instead of lysosomal processing might be of advantage to cells that have poor degradative capacities. In the context of AD, exosomes secretion could be a way to dispose of unwanted proteins. Indeed, maturation of autophagolysosomes and their retrograde transport are impeded in AD. The underlying mechanism behind the hypothesis that neurodegeneration in AD is triggered by proteins spread, cell-to-cell, throughout brain areas could be the shipping of toxic agents such as Aβ or Tau by exosomes. What at the beginning would be beneficial (to bypass a degradation system which is overwhelmed) could become the reason why there is propagation of the disease thorough the brain. Aβ peptides are released by cells in association with exosomes (Rajendra *et al.*, 2006) and interestingly, exosomal proteins such as Alix and flotillin-1 were observed around neuritic plaques, a lesion found in brains from AD patients (Rajendran *et al.*, 2006) suggesting that exosomes-associated Aβ could be involved in plaque formation. MVBs are an intracellular compartment where internalized Aβ can grow into fibrils thereby MVBs may also contribute to amyloid plaque formation (Friedrich *et al.*, 2010). Overall these results suggest that exosomes could play a role in the pathogenesis of AD.

4.2 Tau pathology propagation

The stereotype propagation scheme of neurofibrillary degeneration in AD is evidenced by neuropathological examination as well as biochemical analyses but until recently, hypotheses and experiments trying to address this question remained elusive. Neurofibrillary degeneration is following cortico-cortical connections therefore suggesting a loss of neurotrophic factor or a diffusible factor responsible for a cascade of molecular events leading to Tau aggregation and neuronal death. However, what is this propagating factor? What if Tau itself wouldn't be the "missing link"? Thus, recent data suggest that neurofibrillary degeneration cortical spreading could follow a transmissible prion-like process. In fact, aggregates of PHF-Tau were purified from a transgenic mice model of neurofibrillary degeneration. Intracranial injection of this preparation was done in a different mouse model, which overexpresses human Tau protein but does not display Tau pathology. Following the injection, development of a Tau pathology was observed. This pathology progressed from the injection site to neighboring brain structures, suggestive of a propagating mechanism (Clavaguera *et al.*, 2010). However, results show that PHF-Tau are sufficient to promote the transformation of normal human Tau into "pathological Tau" leading to the formation of neurofibrillary degeneration, the prototypical neuropathological lesion of Alzheimer disease. However, how an extracellular transmissible agent could reach the intracellular compartment to transform the normal protein remains an open question. Very recently, Frost and collaborators have shown using a cell-based system that extracellular Tau aggregates are internalized inside cells and promote the mis-folding and fibrillization of Tau (Frost *et al.*, 2009). Internalization of preformed Tau fibrils is facilitated by the use of a lipid-based protein delivery system (BioPorter®) and is likely mediated by endocytosis (Guo *et al.*, 2011). Moreover, in addition to transmissibility of Tau-fibril conformation, the internalized preformed fibrils reduce microtubule-stabilization suggesting a loss-of-function of normal Tau in infected cells. Although, the mechanisms of

Tau fibrils diffusion remain elusive *in vitro* and *in vivo* arguments strongly support the notion of prion-like transmissibility of Tau-PHF in Alzheimer's disease and possibly in other Tauopathies. There are some evidences suggesting that Tau may be secreted and secretion of Tau may differ depending of Tau isoform. Thus, Tau isoforms with exon 2 encoding sequence are likely not secreted and this exon 2 sequence is therefore suggested to repress Tau secretion (Kim *et al.*, 2010). However, it is not known how Tau is secreted, exosomes? Preliminary study suggests that Tau is not in the exosomes derived from primary embryonic neuronal culture cells (Fauré *et al.*, 2006). Further work is therefore needed to determine how Tau is secreted and by which cell-based mechanism. A good example of such a dilemma is fibroblast growth factor 2 that is a secreted growth factor without any signal peptide and that is also found in cell nucleus following its interaction with its cognate receptors (Meunier *et al.*, 2009). Tau is likely secreted and is also located into the nucleus following stress conditions (Sultan *et al.*, 2011). Tau secretion, as for Tau nuclear localization, may depend upon yet undefined conditions and therefore, contributions of MVB-exosomes pathways or autophagy-lysosomal pathways (Wang *et al.*, 2009) remain completely open. Recent data strongly suggest that both pathways are possibly interconnected (Sahu *et al.*, 2010). With regards to Tau, the degradation systems may bring insights for the potential routing of Tau to MVB-exosomes or autophagy lysosome pathway. In NFT or more generally in aggregates, Tau is found ubiquitinated, thus suggesting that Tau may be processed by the proteasome (David *et al.*, 2002). Ubiquitin-independent degradation system, such as the caspase or calpain cleavage of Tau have also been described (Berry *et al.*, 2003; Carrettiero *et al.*, 2009; Delobel *et al.*, 2005; Ding *et al.*, 2006; Ferreira *et al.*, 2011) The autophagy-lysosomal pathway contributes to the degradation of Tau via the chaperone-mediated autophagy (CMA) (Wang *et al.*, 2009; for review see Wang *et al.*, 2010). The CMA is a lysosome-mediated degradation system of cytosolic protein (for review see Arias *et al.*, 2010). This system implies the recognition of substrates by a complex of chaperones and translocation of substrates inside lysosomes for further degradation. The CMA malfunction has been connected to the development of several neurodegenerative diseases including Parkinson disease and Alzheimer Disease (Arias *et al.*, 2010). Although speculative and purely hypothetic, through the use of CMA, aggregates of proteins or even oligomers could reach the lysosome and due to their low sensitivity to degradation (e.g. Tau aggregates), the fusion of lysosome with other vesicular structures such as MVB could finally lead to the release of aggregates outside the cell and contribute to their propagation following neuronal connections. Alternatively, proteins such as Tau would normally be addressed to lysosome by the CMA system but a defective lysosome could be the place where oligomers are generated and thereafter route to MVB/exosome pathway. However, further work is definitely needed to get insights into these mechanisms.

5. How to explain the selective patterns of neurodegeneration in Tauopathies?

Conceptually, how could we imagine that prion-like spreading of misfolded proteins could reproducibly cause selective patterns of neurodegeneration and skipping nearby "less vulnerable" neuronal targets. That's certainly a major fundamental question to address, which to date remains with no clear answer even in prion disease. Why is the brain affected in prion diseases and no other organs? Why in this scheme of spatiotemporal spreading and propagation of lesions in Alzheimer disease and other tauopathies only selective neuronal subpopulations are affected. As for instance, affected neurons in Alzheimer disease essentially belong to the cholinergic system. One possibility would be that selectivity of propagation could follow neuronal circuitry through synaptic transmission. This is possible if exosomes are preferentially release at the synaptic junction, as suggested by Smalheiser (2007). They are strong evidences that exosomes are produced and secreted by neurons (Lachenal *et al.*, 2011). However, the demonstration derives from *in vitro* experiments using primary neuronal embryonic culture cells. Study of exosomes in tissue yet remains highly challenging. Consequently, little if not nothing is known about the cell localization of exosomes release and their propensity of diffusion *in vivo*. They are therefore other possibilities, such as the tunneling nanotubes (for review see Goedert *et al.*, 2010). Tunneling nanotubes are fine membrane channels that have recently been described in mammalian cells for communication between cells but also for cell-to-cell propagation of misfolded prion proteins (for review see Gerdes *et al.*, 2007; Gousset *et al.*, 2009). These tunneling nanotubes could also propagate other transmissible misfolded proteins but the question of selectivity of transmission remains however open. Coming back to exosomes and now considering that exosomes release and secretion is controlled and localized to pre- or post-synaptic locations then several hypotheses can be postulated. In both pre- and post-synaptic situations propagation through exosomes would be closely dependent upon neuronal connections, as far as the diffusion of exosomes is following a paracrine or "juxtacrine" rule of diffusion (Mathivanan *et al.*, 2010). Thus, only interconnected neurons would disseminate toxic species via exosomes. We can also imagine that exosomes originating from different type of neurons (e.g. cholinergic, GABAergic, glutamatergic…) and may contain specific membrane associated biomarkers. Intercellular communication mediated by exosomes may result from passive fusion of exosome membrane with the plasma membrane of the targeted cell or may use a ligand receptor system. In line with the latter system, the selectivity of intercellular communication could result from specific interaction between ligand and receptor. They are several examples that could illustrate a selectivity of propagation of exosomes using this ligand receptor selectivity. For instance, protocadherin is a cluster of 52 cadherin-like genes with a singular organization. The amino-terminal region of protocadherins is encoded by three sets of separate exons arranged in three clusters (alpha, beta and gamma). N-terminal encoding exons are spliced with one of three carboxy-terminal encoding exons. Alternative splicing generates an extraordinary diversity of protocadherin isoforms suggested to confer selective and specific intermolecular membrane-associated protein interactions (Wu et al., 2000; Wang et al., 2002). The second example is DSCAM, the Drosophila homolog of human Down syndrome cell adhesion molecule that belongs to the axonal guidance receptor family. Alternative splicing of DSCAM can generate as many as 38016 mRNA isoforms and therefore lead to expression of huge protein diversity (Schmucker *et al.*, 2000). More interestingly, one DSCAM protein isoform binds exactly to the same isoform but not a slightly different one, making the binding of DSCAM isoforms very stringent (Wojtowicz *et al.*, 2004). As for DSCAM, the selectivity of transmission pattern could be mediated following an axonal guidance-like system. In a very simplified view, axonal guidance is driven by equilibrium between attractive and repulsive signals through specific signaling pathways, allowing axonal growth and connection to its specific neuronal target (for review see Bashaw and Klein, 2011). Thus exosomes release from one type of cell will be attracted by its target cell and repulsed by surrounding cells. Altogether, examples provide could contribute to neuronal communication and propagation of misfolded proteins along specific identified neuronal circuitries. Although, all these hypotheses could be envisioned a better knowledge of the metabolism of exosomes in vitro and in vivo is necessary to address this problematic.

6. Conclusion

Among pathophysiological mechanisms of neurodegenerative diseases leading to intra or extracellular protein aggregates, a consensual mechanism support a common mechanism of prion-like propagation of mis-folded proteins. However, when this mechanism implies the propagation from cell-to-cell, cellular pathways incriminate remains poorly understood. A growing body of evidences suggests that the endocytic - multivesicular and exosomes pathways may be instrumental to this process. Much is known about the routing of proteins through those recycling or degradative pathway but much less is known about the contribution of those systems to the development of neurodegenerative diseases. However, this MBV-exosome system can be diverted from its physiological function as for instance to produce human immunodeficiency viral particles (Nguyen *et al.*, 2003; for review see Gould *et al.*, 2003). Following this hypothesis, the autophagy-lysosome and/or MVB-exosome pathways could also be diverted to deliver and propagate toxic oligomers or aggregates in neurodegenerative disease such as Alzheimer's disease. Blocking intracellular inclusion of those toxic species to this secretory pathway could also represent a potential therapeutic approach of neurodegenerative diseases such as Amyloidopathies, Tauopathies, Synucleopathies, all of which are sharing a "prion-like" propagation of toxic mis-folded proteins.

7. Acknowledgements

Our work is financially supported by the Association Française contre les Myopathies (AFM 14269, 15047), the ANR (BLAN 1114 01), the Centre National de la Recherche Scientifique (CNRS), the Institut National pour la Santé et la Recherche Médicale (INSERM), the French Ministry for Youth, National Education and Research and the Nord/Pas de Calais Region.

8. References

Addo, M. M., Yu, X. G., Rathod, A. et al. (2003) Comprehensive epitope analysis of human immunodeficiency virus type 1 (HIV-1)-specific T-cell responses directed against the entire expressed HIV-1 genome demonstrate broadly directed responses, but no correlation to viral load. *J Virol*, 77, 2081-2092.

Aguzzi, A. and Rajendran, L. (2009) The transcellular spread of cytosolic amyloids, prions, and prionoids. *Neuron*, 64, 783-790.

Alais, S., Simoes, S., Baas, D., Lehmann, S., Raposo, G., Darlix, J. L. and Leblanc, P. (2008) Mouse neuroblastoma cells release prion infectivity associated with exosomal vesicles. *Biol Cell*, 100, 603-615.

Altfeld, M., Addo, M. M., Rosenberg, E. S. et al. (2003) Influence of HLA-B57 on clinical presentation and viral control during acute HIV-1 infection. *AIDS*, 17, 2581-2591.

Altfeld, M., Addo, M. M., Shankarappa, R. et al. (2003) Enhanced detection of human immunodeficiency virus type 1-specific T-cell responses to highly variable regions by using peptides based on autologous virus sequences. *J Virol*, 77, 7330-7340.

Alzheimer, A. (1911) Uber eigenartige Krankheitsfalle des spateren Alters. *Zbl Ges Neurol Psych,* 4, 356–385.

Ambrose, J. A., Gould, R. B., Kurian, D. C., DeVoe, M. C., Pearlstein, N. B., Coppola, J. T. and Siegal, F. P. (2003) Frequency of and outcome of acute coronary syndromes in patients with human immunodeficiency virus infection. *Am J Cardiol,* 92, 301-303.

Andreadis, A., Broderick, J. A. and Kosik, K. S. (1995) Relative exon affinities and suboptimal splice site signals lead to non-equivalence of two cassette exons. *Nucleic Acids Res,* 23, 3585-3593.

Andreadis, A., Brown, W. M. and Kosik, K. S. (1992) Structure and novel exons of the human tau gene. *Biochemistry,* 31, 10626-10633.

Arias, E. and Cuervo, A. M. (2010) Chaperone-mediated autophagy in protein quality control. *Curr Opin Cell Biol.*

Bammens, L., Chavez-Gutierrez, L., Tolia, A., Zwijsen, A. and De Strooper, B. (2011) Functional and Topological Analysis of Pen-2, the Fourth Subunit of the {gamma}-Secretase Complex. *J Biol Chem,* 286, 12271-12282.

Bashaw, G.J. & Klein, R. (2010) Signaling from Axon Guidance Receptors. Cold Spring Harbor Perspectives in Biology 2, a001941-a001941.

Berry, R. W., Abraha, A., Lagalwar, S., LaPointe, N., Gamblin, T. C., Cryns, V. L. and Binder, L. I. (2003) Inhibition of tau polymerization by its carboxy-terminal caspase cleavage fragment. *Biochemistry,* 42, 8325-8331.

Berson, J. F., Theos, A. C., Harper, D. C., Tenza, D., Raposo, G. and Marks, M. S. (2003) Proprotein convertase cleavage liberates a fibrillogenic fragment of a resident glycoprotein to initiate melanosome biogenesis. *J Cell Biol,* 161, 521-533.

Braak, H. and Braak, E. (1991) Neuropathological stageing of Alzheimer-related changes. *Acta Neuropathol,* 82, 239-259.

Brandt, R. and Lee, G. (1993) Functional organization of microtubule-associated protein tau. Identification of regions which affect microtubule growth, nucleation, and bundle formation in vitro. *J Biol Chem,* 268, 3414-3419.

Brandt, R., Leger, J. and Lee, G. (1995) Interaction of tau with the neural plasma membrane mediated by tau's amino-terminal projection domain. *J Cell Biol,* 131, 1327-1340.

Butner, K. A. and Kirschner, M. W. (1991) Tau protein binds to microtubules through a flexible array of distributed weak sites. *J Cell Biol,* 115, 717-730.

Buxbaum, J. D., Liu, K. N., Luo, Y. et al. (1998) Evidence that tumor necrosis factor alpha converting enzyme is involved in regulated alpha-secretase cleavage of the Alzheimer amyloid protein precursor. *J Biol Chem,* 273, 27765-27767.

Carlier, M. F., Simon, C., Cassoly, R. and Pradel, L. A. (1984) Interaction between microtubule-associated protein tau and spectrin. *Biochimie,* 66, 305-311.

Carrettiero, D. C., Hernandez, I., Neveu, P., Papagiannakopoulos, T. and Kosik, K. S. (2009) The cochaperone BAG2 sweeps paired helical filament- insoluble tau from the microtubule. *J Neurosci,* 29, 2151-2161.

Chasseigneaux, S., Dinc, L., Rose, C., Chabret, C., Coulpier, F., Topilko, P., Mauger, G. and Allinquant, B. (2011) Secreted amyloid precursor protein beta and secreted amyloid precursor protein alpha induce axon outgrowth in vitro through Egr1 signaling pathway. *PLoS One,* 6, e16301.

Clavaguera, F., Goedert, M. and Tolnay, M. (2010) Induction and spreading of tau pathology in a mouse model of Alzheimer's disease. *Med Sci (Paris),* 26, 121-124.

Cleveland, D. W., Hwo, S. Y. and Kirschner, M. W. (1977) Purification of tau, a microtubule-associated protein that induces assembly of microtubules from purified tubulin. *J Mol Biol,* 116, 207-225.

Cohen, T. J., Guo, J. L., Hurtado, D. E., Kwong, L. K., Mills, I. P., Trojanowski, J. Q. and Lee, V. M. (2011) The acetylation of tau inhibits its function and promotes pathological tau aggregation. *Nat Commun,* 2, 252.

Correas, I., Padilla, R. and Avila, J. (1990) The tubulin-binding sequence of brain microtubule-associated proteins, tau and MAP-2, is also involved in actin binding. *Biochem J,* 269, 61-64.

Cox, L. E., Ferraiuolo, L., Goodall, E. F. et al. (2010) Mutations in CHMP2B in lower motor neuron predominant amyotrophic lateral sclerosis (ALS). *PLoS One,* 5, e9872.

David, D. C., Layfield, R., Serpell, L., Narain, Y., Goedert, M. and Spillantini, M. G. (2002) Proteasomal degradation of tau protein. *J Neurochem,* 83, 176-185.

de Gassart, A., Geminard, C., Hoekstra, D. and Vidal, M. (2004) Exosome secretion: the art of reutilizing nonrecycled proteins? *Traffic,* 5, 896-903.

De Strooper, B., Saftig, P., Craessaerts, K., Vanderstichele, H., Guhde, G., Annaert, W., Von Figura, K. and Van Leuven, F. (1998) Deficiency of presenilin-1 inhibits the normal cleavage of amyloid precursor protein. *Nature,* 391, 387-390.

De Strooper, B., Vassar, R. and Golde, T. (2010) The secretases: enzymes with therapeutic potential in Alzheimer disease. *Nat Rev Neurol,* 6, 99-107.

Delacourte, A., David, J. P., Sergeant, N. et al. (1999) The biochemical pathway of neurofibrillary degeneration in aging and Alzheimer's disease. *Neurology,* 52, 1158-1165.

Delacourte, A., Robitaille, Y., Sergeant, N. et al. (1996) Specific pathological Tau protein variants characterize Pick's disease. *J Neuropathol Exp Neurol,* 55, 159-168.

Delacourte, A., Sergeant, N., Champain, D., Wattez, A., Maurage, C. A., Lebert, F., Pasquier, F. and David, J. P. (2002) Nonoverlapping but synergetic tau and APP pathologies in sporadic Alzheimer's disease. *Neurology,* 59, 398-407.

Delobel, P., Leroy, O., Hamdane, M., Sambo, A. V., Delacourte, A. and Buee, L. (2005) Proteasome inhibition and Tau proteolysis: an unexpected regulation. *FEBS Lett,* 579, 1-5.

Ding, H., Matthews, T. A. and Johnson, G. V. (2006) Site-specific phosphorylation and caspase cleavage differentially impact tau-microtubule interactions and tau aggregation. *J Biol Chem,* 281, 19107-19114.

Draenert, R., Altfeld, M., Brander, C. et al. (2003) Comparison of overlapping peptide sets for detection of antiviral CD8 and CD4 T cell responses. *J Immunol Methods,* 275, 19-29.

Drechsel, D. N., Hyman, A. A., Cobb, M. H. and Kirschner, M. W. (1992) Modulation of the dynamic instability of tubulin assembly by the microtubule-associated protein tau. *Mol Biol Cell,* 3, 1141-1154.

Duyckaerts, C. and Hauw, J. J. (1997) Diagnosis and staging of Alzheimer disease. *Neurobiol Aging,* 18, S33-42.

Eckermann, K., Mocanu, M. M., Khlistunova, I. et al. (2007) The beta-propensity of Tau determines aggregation and synaptic loss in inducible mouse models of tauopathy. *J Biol Chem,* 282, 31755-31765.

Edbauer, D., Winkler, E., Regula, J. T., Pesold, B., Steiner, H. and Haass, C. (2003) Reconstitution of gamma-secretase activity. *Nat Cell Biol,* 5, 486-488.

Esler, W. P., Kimberly, W. T., Ostaszewski, B. L., Ye, W., Diehl, T. S., Selkoe, D. J. and Wolfe, M. S. (2002) Activity-dependent isolation of the presenilin- gamma -secretase complex reveals nicastrin and a gamma substrate. *Proc Natl Acad Sci U S A,* 99, 2720-2725.

Faure, J., Lachenal, G., Court, M. et al. (2006) Exosomes are released by cultured cortical neurones. *Mol Cell Neurosci,* 31, 642-648.

Feeney, M. E., Draenert, R., Roosevelt, K. A., Pelton, S. I., McIntosh, K., Burchett, S. K., Mao, C., Walker, B. D. and Goulder, P. J. (2003) Reconstitution of virus-specific CD4 proliferative responses in pediatric HIV-1 infection. *J Immunol,* 171, 6968-6975.

Feeney, M. E., Roosevelt, K. A., Tang, Y., Pfafferott, K. J., McIntosh, K., Burchett, S. K., Mao, C., Walker, B. D. and Goulder, P. J. (2003) Comprehensive screening reveals strong and broadly directed human immunodeficiency virus type 1-specific CD8 responses in perinatally infected children. *J Virol,* 77, 7492-7501.

Ferreira, A. and Bigio, E. H. (2011) Calpain-mediated tau cleavage: a mechanism leading to neurodegeneration shared by multiple tauopathies. *Mol Med.*

Fevrier, B., Vilette, D., Archer, F., Loew, D., Faigle, W., Vidal, M., Laude, H. and Raposo, G. (2004) Cells release prions in association with exosomes. *Proc Natl Acad Sci U S A,* 101, 9683-9688.

Filimonenko, M., Stuffers, S., Raiborg, C. et al. (2007) Functional multivesicular bodies are required for autophagic clearance of protein aggregates associated with neurodegenerative disease. *J Cell Biol,* 179, 485-500.

Fischer, D., Mukrasch, M. D., von Bergen, M., Klos-Witkowska, A., Biernat, J., Griesinger, C., Mandelkow, E. and Zweckstetter, M. (2007) Structural and microtubule binding properties of tau mutants of frontotemporal dementias. *Biochemistry,* 46, 2574-2582.

Francis, R., McGrath, G., Zhang, J. et al. (2002) aph-1 and pen-2 are required for Notch pathway signaling, gamma-secretase cleavage of betaAPP, and presenilin protein accumulation. *Dev Cell,* 3, 85-97.

Friedrich, R. P., Tepper, K., Ronicke, R., Soom, M., Westermann, M., Reymann, K., Kaether, C. and Fandrich, M. (2010) Mechanism of amyloid plaque formation suggests an intracellular basis of Abeta pathogenicity. *Proc Natl Acad Sci U S A,* 107, 1942-1947.

Frost, B., Jacks, R. L. and Diamond, M. I. (2009) Propagation of tau misfolding from the outside to the inside of a cell. *J Biol Chem,* 284, 12845-12852.

Funk, K. E., Mrak, R. E. and Kuret, J. (2011) Granulovacuolar degeneration (GVD) bodies of Alzheimer's disease (AD) resemble late-stage autophagic organelles. *Neuropathol Appl Neurobiol,* 37, 295-306.

Geminard, C., De Gassart, A., Blanc, L. and Vidal, M. (2004) Degradation of AP2 during reticulocyte maturation enhances binding of hsc70 and Alix to a common site on TFR for sorting into exosomes. *Traffic,* 5, 181-193.

Gerdes, H., Bukoreshtliev, N. & Barroso, J. (2007) Tunneling nanotubes: A new route for the exchange of components between animal cells. *FEBS Letters* 581, 2194-2201.

Ghanim, M., Guillot-Noel, L., Pasquier, F., Jornea, L., Deramecourt, V., Dubois, B., Le Ber, I. and Brice, A. (2010) CHMP2B mutations are rare in French families with frontotemporal lobar degeneration. *J Neurol,* 257, 2032-2036.

Glenner, G. G. and Wong, C. W. (1984) Alzheimer's disease and Down's syndrome: sharing of a unique cerebrovascular amyloid fibril protein. *Biochem Biophys Res Commun,* 122, 1131-1135.

Goedert, M. and Jakes, R. (1990) Expression of separate isoforms of human tau protein: correlation with the tau pattern in brain and effects on tubulin polymerization. *Embo J*, 9, 4225-4230.

Goedert, M., Spillantini, M. G., Jakes, R., Rutherford, D. and Crowther, R. A. (1989) Multiple isoforms of human microtubule-associated protein tau: sequences and localization in neurofibrillary tangles of Alzheimer's disease. *Neuron*, 3, 519-526.

Goedert, M., Spillantini, M. G., Potier, M. C., Ulrich, J. and Crowther, R. A. (1989) Cloning and sequencing of the cDNA encoding an isoform of microtubule-associated protein tau containing four tandem repeats: differential expression of tau protein mRNAs in human brain. *Embo J*, 8, 393-399.

Goedert, M., Clavaguera, F. & Tolnay, M. (2010) The propagation of prion-like protein inclusions in neurodegenerative diseases. *Trends in Neurosciences* 33, 317-325.

Goldgaber, D., Lerman, M. I., McBride, O. W., Saffiotti, U. and Gajdusek, D. C. (1987) Characterization and chromosomal localization of a cDNA encoding brain amyloid of Alzheimer's disease. *Science*, 235, 877-880.

Goode, B. L. and Feinstein, S. C. (1994) Identification of a novel microtubule binding and assembly domain in the developmentally regulated inter-repeat region of tau. *J Cell Biol*, 124, 769-782.

Gould, S. J., Booth, A. M. and Hildreth, J. E. (2003) The Trojan exosome hypothesis. *Proc Natl Acad Sci U S A*, 100, 10592-10597.

Gousset, K. et al. (2009) Prions hijack tunneling nanotubes for intercellular spread. *Nature* 11, 328-336.

Goutte, C., Tsunozaki, M., Hale, V. A. and Priess, J. R. (2002) APH-1 is a multipass membrane protein essential for the Notch signaling pathway in Caenorhabditis elegans embryos. *Proc Natl Acad Sci U S A*, 99, 775-779.

Gruenberg, J. (2009) Viruses and endosome membrane dynamics. *Curr Opin Cell Biol*, 21, 582-588.

Gruenberg, J. and Stenmark, H. (2004) The biogenesis of multivesicular endosomes. *Nat Rev Mol Cell Biol*, 5, 317-323.

Guo, J. L. and Lee, V. M. (2011) Seeding of normal tau by pathological tau conformers drives pathogenesis of Alzheimer-like tangles. *J Biol Chem*.

Gustke, N., Trinczek, B., Biernat, J., Mandelkow, E. M. and Mandelkow, E. (1994) Domains of tau protein and interactions with microtubules. *Biochemistry*, 33, 9511-9522.

Hemler, M. E. (2005) Tetraspanin functions and associated microdomains. *Nat Rev Mol Cell Biol*, 6, 801-811.

Henriquez, J. P., Cross, D., Vial, C. and Maccioni, R. B. (1995) Subpopulations of tau interact with microtubules and actin filaments in various cell types. *Cell Biochem Funct*, 13, 239-250.

Himmler, A., Drechsel, D., Kirschner, M. W. and Martin, D. W., Jr. (1989) Tau consists of a set of proteins with repeated C-terminal microtubule-binding domains and variable N-terminal domains. *Mol Cell Biol*, 9, 1381-1388.

Hof, P. R., Cox, K. and Morrison, J. H. (1990) Quantitative analysis of a vulnerable subset of pyramidal neurons in Alzheimer's disease: I. Superior frontal and inferior temporal cortex. *J Comp Neurol*, 301, 44-54.

Hotoda, N., Koike, H., Sasagawa, N. and Ishiura, S. (2002) A secreted form of human ADAM9 has an alpha-secretase activity for APP. *Biochem Biophys Res Commun*, 293, 800-805.

Hsu, C., Morohashi, Y., Yoshimura, S. et al. (2010) Regulation of exosome secretion by Rab35 and its GTPase-activating proteins TBC1D10A-C. *J Cell Biol,* 189, 223-232.

Hussain, I., Powell, D., Howlett, D. R. et al. (1999) Identification of a novel aspartic protease (Asp 2) as beta-secretase. *Mol Cell Neurosci,* 14, 419-427.

Hwang, S. C., Jhon, D. Y., Bae, Y. S., Kim, J. H. and Rhee, S. G. (1996) Activation of phospholipase C-gamma by the concerted action of tau proteins and arachidonic acid. *J Biol Chem,* 271, 18342-18349.

Ittner, L. M., Ke, Y. D., Delerue, F. et al. (2010) Dendritic function of tau mediates amyloid-beta toxicity in Alzheimer's disease mouse models. *Cell,* 142, 387-397.

Jenkins, S. M. and Johnson, G. V. (1998) Tau complexes with phospholipase C-gamma in situ. *Neuroreport,* 9, 67-71.

Jorissen, E. and De Strooper, B. (2010) Gamma-secretase and the intramembrane proteolysis of Notch. *Curr Top Dev Biol,* 92, 201-230.

Jung, D., Filliol, D., Miehe, M. and Rendon, A. (1993) Interaction of brain mitochondria with microtubules reconstituted from brain tubulin and MAP2 or TAU. *Cell Motil Cytoskeleton,* 24, 245-255.

Kang, J., Lemaire, H. G., Unterbeck, A., Salbaum, J. M., Masters, C. L., Grzeschik, K. H., Multhaup, G., Beyreuther, K. and Muller-Hill, B. (1987) The precursor of Alzheimer's disease amyloid A4 protein resembles a cell-surface receptor. *Nature,* 325, 733-736.

Kim, W., Lee, S. and Hall, G. F. (2010) Secretion of human tau fragments resembling CSF-tau in Alzheimer's disease is modulated by the presence of the exon 2 insert. *FEBS Lett,* 584, 3085-3088.

Kimberly, W. T., LaVoie, M. J., Ostaszewski, B. L., Ye, W., Wolfe, M. S. and Selkoe, D. J. (2003) Gamma-secretase is a membrane protein complex comprised of presenilin, nicastrin, Aph-1, and Pen-2. *Proc Natl Acad Sci U S A,* 100, 6382-6387.

Kobuna, H., Inoue, T., Shibata, M., Gengyo-Ando, K., Yamamoto, A., Mitani, S. and Arai, H. (2010) Multivesicular body formation requires OSBP-related proteins and cholesterol. *PLoS Genet,* 6.

Koike, H., Tomioka, S., Sorimachi, H. et al. (1999) Membrane-anchored metalloprotease MDC9 has an alpha-secretase activity responsible for processing the amyloid precursor protein. *Biochem J,* 343 Pt 2, 371-375.

Konig, G., Salbaum, J. M., Wiestler, O., Lang, W., Schmitt, H. P., Masters, C. L. and Beyreuther, K. (1991) Alternative splicing of the beta A4 amyloid gene of Alzheimer's disease in cortex of control and Alzheimer's disease patients. *Brain Res Mol Brain Res,* 9, 259-262.

Kosik, K. S., Orecchio, L. D., Bakalis, S. and Neve, R. L. (1989) Developmentally regulated expression of specific tau sequences. *Neuron,* 2, 1389-1397.

Lachenal, G., Pernet-Gallay, K., Chivet, M. et al. (2010) Release of exosomes from differentiated neurons and its regulation by synaptic glutamatergic activity. *Mol Cell Neurosci,* 46, 409-418.

Lammich, S., Kojro, E., Postina, R., Gilbert, S., Pfeiffer, R., Jasionowski, M., Haass, C. and Fahrenholz, F. (1999) Constitutive and regulated alpha-secretase cleavage of Alzheimer's amyloid precursor protein by a disintegrin metalloprotease. *Proc Natl Acad Sci U S A,* 96, 3922-3927.

Lee, G., Cowan, N. and Kirschner, M. (1988) The primary structure and heterogeneity of tau protein from mouse brain. *Science,* 239, 285-288.

Lee, G., Neve, R. L. and Kosik, K. S. (1989) The microtubule binding domain of tau protein. *Neuron,* 2, 1615-1624.

Lee, G., Thangavel, R., Sharma, V. M. et al. (2004) Phosphorylation of tau by fyn: implications for Alzheimer's disease. *J Neurosci,* 24, 2304-2312.

Leroy, O., Wang, J., Maurage, C. A., Parent, M., Cooper, T., Buee, L., Sergeant, N., Andreadis, A. and Caillet-Boudin, M. L. (2006) Brain-specific change in alternative splicing of Tau exon 6 in myotonic dystrophy type 1. *Biochim Biophys Acta,* 1762, 460-467.

Levine, B., Mizushima, N. and Virgin, H. W. (2011) Autophagy in immunity and inflammation. *Nature,* 469, 323-335.

Lin, X., Koelsch, G., Wu, S., Downs, D., Dashti, A. and Tang, J. (2000) Human aspartic protease memapsin 2 cleaves the beta-secretase site of beta-amyloid precursor protein. *Proc Natl Acad Sci U S A,* 97, 1456-1460.

Liu, Y., Shah, S. V., Xiang, X. et al. (2009) COP9-associated CSN5 regulates exosomal protein deubiquitination and sorting. *Am J Pathol,* 174, 1415-1425.

Lopez-Perez, E., Zhang, Y., Frank, S. J., Creemers, J., Seidah, N. and Checler, F. (2001) Constitutive alpha-secretase cleavage of the beta-amyloid precursor protein in the furin-deficient LoVo cell line: involvement of the pro-hormone convertase 7 and the disintegrin metalloprotease ADAM10. *J Neurochem,* 76, 1532-1539.

Martinez-Vicente, M., Talloczy, Z., Wong, E. et al. (2011) Cargo recognition failure is responsible for inefficient autophagy in Huntington's disease. *Nat Neurosci,* 13, 567-576.

Mathivanan, S., Ji, H. and Simpson, R. J. (2011) Exosomes: extracellular organelles important in intercellular communication. *J Proteomics,* 73, 1907-1920.

Matsuo, H., Chevallier, J., Mayran, N. et al. (2004) Role of LBPA and Alix in multivesicular liposome formation and endosome organization. *Science,* 303, 531-534.

Matus, A. (1990) Microtubule-associated proteins and the determination of neuronal form. *J Physiol (Paris),* 84, 134-137.

Meunier, S., Navarro, M. G., Bossard, C., Laurell, H., Touriol, C., Lacazette, E. and Prats, H. (2009) Pivotal role of translokin/CEP57 in the unconventional secretion versus nuclear translocation of FGF2. *Traffic,* 10, 1765-1772.

Min, S. W., Cho, S. H., Zhou, Y. et al. (2010) Acetylation of tau inhibits its degradation and contributes to tauopathy. *Neuron,* 67, 953-966.

Miyata, Y., Hoshi, M., Nishida, E., Minami, Y. and Sakai, H. (1986) Binding of microtubule-associated protein 2 and tau to the intermediate filament reassembled from neurofilament 70-kDa subunit protein. Its regulation by calmodulin. *J Biol Chem,* 261, 13026-13030.

Morita, E. and Sundquist, W. I. (2004) Retrovirus budding. *Annu Rev Cell Dev Biol,* 20, 395-425.

Nguyen, D. G., Booth, A., Gould, S. J. and Hildreth, J. E. (2003) Evidence that HIV budding in primary macrophages occurs through the exosome release pathway. *J Biol Chem,* 278, 52347-52354.

Nguyen, D. G., Booth, A., Gould, S. J. and Hildreth, J. E. (2003) Evidence that HIV budding in primary macrophages occurs through the exosome release pathway. *J Biol Chem,* 278, 52347-52354.

Oestreich, A. J., Aboian, M., Lee, J., Azmi, I., Payne, J., Issaka, R., Davies, B. A. and Katzmann, D. J. (2007) Characterization of multiple multivesicular body sorting determinants within Sna3: a role for the ubiquitin ligase Rsp5. *Mol Biol Cell,* 18, 707-720.

Olver, C. and Vidal, M. (2007) Proteomic analysis of secreted exosomes. *Subcell Biochem,* 43, 99-131.

Ostrowski, M., Carmo, N. B., Krumeich, S. et al. (2010) Rab27a and Rab27b control different steps of the exosome secretion pathway. *Nat Cell Biol,* 12, 19-30; sup pp 11-13.

Piper, R. C. and Katzmann, D. J. (2007) Biogenesis and function of multivesicular bodies. *Annu Rev Cell Dev Biol,* 23, 519-547.

Probst, A., Tolnay, M., Langui, D., Goedert, M. and Spillantini, M. G. (1996) Pick's disease: hyperphosphorylated tau protein segregates to the somatoaxonal compartment. *Acta Neuropathol,* 92, 588-596.

Rajendran, L., Honsho, M., Zahn, T. R., Keller, P., Geiger, K. D., Verkade, P. and Simons, K. (2006) Alzheimer's disease beta-amyloid peptides are released in association with exosomes. *Proc Natl Acad Sci U S A,* 103, 11172-11177.

Rajendran, L., Honsho, M., Zahn, T. R., Keller, P., Geiger, K. D., Verkade, P. and Simons, K. (2006) Alzheimer's disease beta-amyloid peptides are released in association with exosomes. *Proc Natl Acad Sci U S A,* 103, 11172-11177.

Raposo, G. and Marks, M. S. (2007) Melanosomes--dark organelles enlighten endosomal membrane transport. *Nat Rev Mol Cell Biol,* 8, 786-797.

Raposo, G., Nijman, H. W., Stoorvogel, W., Liejendekker, R., Harding, C. V., Melief, C. J. and Geuze, H. J. (1996) B lymphocytes secrete antigen-presenting vesicles. *J Exp Med,* 183, 1161-1172.

Rhee, S. G. (2001) Regulation of phosphoinositide-specific phospholipase C. *Annu Rev Biochem,* 70, 281-312.

Riedle, S., Kiefel, H., Gast, D., Bondong, S., Wolterink, S., Gutwein, P. and Altevogt, P. (2009) Nuclear translocation and signalling of L1-CAM in human carcinoma cells requires ADAM10 and presenilin/gamma-secretase activity. *Biochem J,* 420, 391-402.

Sahu, R., Kaushik, S., Clement, C. C. et al. (2011) Microautophagy of cytosolic proteins by late endosomes. *Dev Cell,* 20, 405-406.

Savina, A., Fader, C. M., Damiani, M. T. and Colombo, M. I. (2005) Rab11 promotes docking and fusion of multivesicular bodies in a calcium-dependent manner. *Traffic,* 6, 131-143.

Selden, S. C. and Pollard, T. D. (1983) Phosphorylation of microtubule-associated proteins regulates their interaction with actin filaments. *J Biol Chem,* 258, 7064-7071.

Sergeant, N., David, J. P., Goedert, M., Jakes, R., Vermersch, P., Buee, L., Lefranc, D., Wattez, A. and Delacourte, A. (1997) Two-dimensional characterization of paired helical filament-tau from Alzheimer's disease: demonstration of an additional 74-kDa component and age-related biochemical modifications. *J Neurochem,* 69, 834-844.

Sergeant, N., David, J. P., Lefranc, D., Vermersch, P., Wattez, A. and Delacourte, A. (1997) Different distribution of phosphorylated tau protein isoforms in Alzheimer's and Pick's diseases. *FEBS Lett,* 412, 578-582.

Sinha, S., Anderson, J. P., Barbour, R. et al. (1999) Purification and cloning of amyloid precursor protein beta-secretase from human brain. *Nature,* 402, 537-540.

Skibinski, G., Parkinson, N. J., Brown, J. M. et al. (2005) Mutations in the endosomal ESCRTIII-complex subunit CHMP2B in frontotemporal dementia. *Nat Genet,* 37, 806-808.

Smalheiser, N.R. (2007) Exosomal transfer of proteins and RNAs at synapses in the nervous system. *Biol Direct* 2, 35.

Schmucker, D., Clemens, J. C., Shu, H., Worby, C. A., Xiao, J., Muda, M., Dixon, J. E. and Zipursky, S. L. (2000) Drosophila Dscam is an axon guidance receptor exhibiting extraordinary molecular diversity. Cell, 101, 671-684.

Sontag, E., Nunbhakdi-Craig, V., Lee, G., Brandt, R., Kamibayashi, C., Kuret, J., White, C. L., 3rd, Mumby, M. C. and Bloom, G. S. (1999) Molecular interactions among protein phosphatase 2A, tau, and microtubules. Implications for the regulation of tau phosphorylation and the development of tauopathies. *J Biol Chem*, 274, 25490-25498.

Soscia, S. J., Kirby, J. E., Washicosky, K. J. et al. (2011) The Alzheimer's disease-associated amyloid beta-protein is an antimicrobial peptide. *PLoS One*, 5, e9505.

Steiner, H., Winkler, E., Edbauer, D., Prokop, S., Basset, G., Yamasaki, A., Kostka, M. and Haass, C. (2002) PEN-2 is an integral component of the gamma-secretase complex required for coordinated expression of presenilin and nicastrin. *J Biol Chem*, 277, 39062-39065.

Sultan, A., Nesslany, F., Violet, M. et al. (2011) Nuclear tau, a key player in neuronal DNA protection. *J Biol Chem*, 286, 4566-4575.

Takasugi, N., Tomita, T., Hayashi, I., Tsuruoka, M., Niimura, M., Takahashi, Y., Thinakaran, G. and Iwatsubo, T. (2003) The role of presenilin cofactors in the gamma-secretase complex. *Nature*, 422, 438-441.

Theos, A. C., Truschel, S. T., Tenza, D., Hurbain, I., Harper, D. C., Berson, J. F., Thomas, P. C., Raposo, G. and Marks, M. S. (2006) A lumenal domain-dependent pathway for sorting to intralumenal vesicles of multivesicular endosomes involved in organelle morphogenesis. *Dev Cell*, 10, 343-354.

Trajkovic, K., Hsu, C., Chiantia, S., Rajendran, L., Wenzel, D., Wieland, F., Schwille, P., Brugger, B. and Simons, M. (2008) Ceramide triggers budding of exosome vesicles into multivesicular endosomes. *Science*, 319, 1244-1247.

Urwin, H., Authier, A., Nielsen, J. E. et al. (2010) Disruption of endocytic trafficking in frontotemporal dementia with CHMP2B mutations. *Hum Mol Genet*, 19, 2228-2238.

Valadi, H., Ekstrom, K., Bossios, A., Sjostrand, M., Lee, J. J. and Lotvall, J. O. (2007) Exosome-mediated transfer of mRNAs and microRNAs is a novel mechanism of genetic exchange between cells. *Nat Cell Biol*, 9, 654-659.

Vassar, R., Bennett, B. D., Babu-Khan, S. et al. (1999) Beta-secretase cleavage of Alzheimer's amyloid precursor protein by the transmembrane aspartic protease BACE. *Science*, 286, 735-741.

Vella, L. J., Sharples, R. A., Nisbet, R. M., Cappai, R. and Hill, A. F. (2008) The role of exosomes in the processing of proteins associated with neurodegenerative diseases. *Eur Biophys J*, 37, 323-332.

Vingtdeux, V., Hamdane, M., Begard, S., Loyens, A., Delacourte, A., Beauvillain, J. C., Buee, L., Marambaud, P. and Sergeant, N. (2007) Intracellular pH regulates amyloid precursor protein intracellular domain accumulation. *Neurobiol Dis*, 25, 686-696.

Vingtdeux, V., Hamdane, M., Loyens, A. et al. (2007) Alkalizing drugs induce accumulation of amyloid precursor protein by-products in luminal vesicles of multivesicular bodies. *J Biol Chem*, 282, 18197-18205.

Wakabayashi, T., Craessaerts, K., Bammens, L. et al. (2009) Analysis of the gamma-secretase interactome and validation of its association with tetraspanin-enriched microdomains. *Nat Cell Biol*, 11, 1340-1346.

Wang, X., Su, H. & Bradley, A. (2002) Molecular mechanisms governing Pcdh-gamma gene expression: evidence for a multiple promoter and cis-alternative splicing model. *Genes & Development* 16, 1890-1905.

Wang, Y., Kruger, U., Mandelkow, E. and Mandelkow, E. M. (2011) Generation of tau aggregates and clearance by autophagy in an inducible cell model of tauopathy. *Neurodegener Dis,* 7, 103-107.

Wang, Y., Martinez-Vicente, M., Kruger, U., Kaushik, S., Wong, E., Mandelkow, E. M., Cuervo, A. M. and Mandelkow, E. (2009) Tau fragmentation, aggregation and clearance: the dual role of lysosomal processing. *Hum Mol Genet,* 18, 4153-4170.

Wang, Y., Martinez-Vicente, M., Kruger, U., Kaushik, S., Wong, E., Mandelkow, E. M., Cuervo, A. M. and Mandelkow, E. (2010) Synergy and antagonism of macroautophagy and chaperone-mediated autophagy in a cell model of pathological tau aggregation. *Autophagy,* 6, 182-183.

Weingarten, M. D., Lockwood, A. H., Hwo, S. Y. and Kirschner, M. W. (1975) A protein factor essential for microtubule assembly. *Proc Natl Acad Sci U S A,* 72, 1858-1862.

Williamson, R., Scales, T., Clark, B. R. et al. (2002) Rapid tyrosine phosphorylation of neuronal proteins including tau and focal adhesion kinase in response to amyloid-beta peptide exposure: involvement of Src family protein kinases. *J Neurosci,* 22, 10-20.

Wojtowicz, W. M., Flanagan, J. J., Millard, S. S., Zipursky, S. L. and Clemens, J. C. (2004) Alternative splicing of Drosophila Dscam generates axon guidance receptors that exhibit isoform-specific homophilic binding. Cell, 118, 619-633.

Wu, Q. & Maniatis, T. (2000) Large exons encoding multiple ectodomains are a characteristic feature of protocadherin genes. *Proc Natl Acad Sci USA* 97, 3124-3129.

Wubbolts, R., Leckie, R. S., Veenhuizen, P. T., Schwarzmann, G., Mobius, W., Hoernschemeyer, J., Slot, J. W., Geuze, H. J. and Stoorvogel, W. (2003) Proteomic and biochemical analyses of human B cell-derived exosomes. Potential implications for their function and multivesicular body formation. *J Biol Chem,* 278, 10963-10972.

Yamazaki, Y., Takahashi, T., Hiji, M., Kurashige, T., Izumi, Y., Yamawaki, T. and Matsumoto, M. (2010) Immunopositivity for ESCRT-III subunit CHMP2B in granulovacuolar degeneration of neurons in the Alzheimer's disease hippocampus. *Neurosci Lett,* 477, 86-90.

Yan, R., Bienkowski, M. J., Shuck, M. E. et al. (1999) Membrane-anchored aspartyl protease with Alzheimer's disease beta-secretase activity. *Nature,* 402, 533-537.

Yang, D. S., Stavrides, P., Mohan, P. S. et al. (2011) Reversal of autophagy dysfunction in the TgCRND8 mouse model of Alzheimer's disease ameliorates amyloid pathologies and memory deficits. *Brain,* 134, 258-277.

Yoshikai, S., Sasaki, H., Doh-ura, K., Furuya, H. and Sakaki, Y. (1990) Genomic organization of the human amyloid beta-protein precursor gene. *Gene,* 87, 257-263.

Yu, G., Nishimura, M., Arawaka, S. et al. (2000) Nicastrin modulates presenilin-mediated notch/glp-1 signal transduction and betaAPP processing. *Nature,* 407, 48-54.

Zhang, Z., Nadeau, P., Song, W., Donoviel, D., Yuan, M., Bernstein, A. and Yankner, B. A. (2000) Presenilins are required for gamma-secretase cleavage of beta-APP and transmembrane cleavage of Notch-1. *Nat Cell Biol,* 2, 463-465.

7

Pathological Stages of Abnormally Processed Tau Protein During Its Aggregation into Fibrillary Structures in Alzheimer's Disease

Francisco García-Sierra[1] et al.*
[1]*Department of Cell Biology, Center of Research and Advanced Studies of the National Polytechnic Institute*
[1]*México*

1. Introduction

Abnormal aggregation of tau protein within the cytoplasm of susceptible neurons has been considered one of the major hallmarks that define the neuropathology of Alzheimer's disease (AD) (Iqbal et al., 2010; Pritchard et al., 2011). At early stages of neuronal degeneration tau protein is accumulated in the form of early non-assembled aggregates that may alter the normal functioning of affected neurons (Hoozemans et al., 2009; Luna-Munoz et al., 2007). Nonfibrillar aggregation of tau protein as a pre-tangle state has been reported to occur early in the disease but also observed in nondemented very old individuals (Garcia-Sierra et al., 2000). Some studies have reported that oligomeric species of tau protein represent the toxic structures rather than fibrillary structures (Berger et al., 2007; Maeda et al., 2006), however few studies have analyzed and determined a positive correlation between the load of pre-tangle carrying neurons and the clinical symptoms of AD. Further alterations in neurons may occur when the soluble aggregates of tau become assembled into insoluble polymers referred to as paired helical filaments (PHFs) that may also obstruct the transit and distribution of intracellular components, modify the neuronal morphology and alter the cytoskeleton (Ballatore, Lee & Trojanowski, 2007; Kidd, 2006). These filaments progressively coalesce into neurofibrillary tangles (NFTs) which eventually lead to the neuronal death (Guo & Lee, 2011). It is generally accepted that in AD cases, the density of NFTs is the best correlate with the dementia score (Arriagada, Marzloff & Hyman, 1992; Gomez-Isla et al., 1997).

*Gustavo Basurto-Islas[1,3], Jaime Jarero-Basulto[1], Hugo C. Monroy-Ramírez[1], Francisco M. Torres Cruz[1], Hernán Cortés Callejas[1], Héctor M. Camarillo Rojas[1], Zdena Kristofikova[4], Daniela Ripova[4], José Luna-Muñoz[5], Raúl Mena[5], Lester I. Binder[6] and Siddhartha Mondragón-Rodríguez[1,2]
[1]*Department of Cell Biology, Center of Research and Advanced Studies of the National Polytechnic Institute, México*
[2]*Department of Physiology, University of Montreal, Canada*
[3]*Department of Neurochemistry, New York State Institute for Basic Research in Developmental Disabilities, USA*
[4]*Laboratory of Biochemistry and Brain Pathophysiology, Prague Psychiatric Center, Czech Republic*
[5]*Department of Neuroscience, Center of Research and Advanced Studies of the National Polytechnic Institute, México*
[6]*Department of Cell and Molecular Biology, Feinberg School of Medicine, Northwestern University, USA*

The description about the progression of the neurofibrillary pathology in AD has been proposed by Braak and Braak (Braak et al., 1993, 1996), which states that there is a stereotype in the appearance and distribution of NFTs along entorhinal, limbic and isocortical areas. It is well known that in AD, NFTs and dystrophic neurites (DNs) are mostly composed of tau protein which has undergone several posttranslational modifications such as abnormal phosphorylation, conformational changes and truncation (Du et al., 2007; Novak et al., 1991; Wischik et al., 1988a). In this regard, we have previously proposed that a continuous and specific pathway of conformational changes and truncation of tau protein is occurring during the maturation of NFTs (Binder et al., 2005; Guillozet-Bongaarts et al., 2005, Mondragon-Rodriguez et al., 2009).
The sum of our data support that not only the number of NFTs defines the progression of AD, but also the state of proteolysis of the C-terminus which is associated with conformational changes, i.e. structural modification along the tau molecule (Garcia-Sierra, Mondragon-Rodriguez & Basurto-Islas, 2008). In distinct populations of NFTs, the occurrence of mutually exclusive truncations at either acid aspartic-421 (Asp^{421}) or glutamic acid-391 (Glu^{391}) correlated well with the evolution of the disease (Basurto-Islas et al., 2008). This cascade of pathological molecular events may give a better correlation with the neuropathological progression of the disease. In our model of pathologic processing of tau we pointed out the existence of chimeric NFTs which are composed of diverse molecules of tau characteristically in different stages of proteolysis.

2. The neurofibrillary pathology of AD

The observed neuropathological changes in patients with AD are at least partly the result of the accumulation of NFTs (Fig. 1, arrows) and amyloid-β (Aβ) deposits (Aβ-plaques) (Fig. 1, asterisk) around the hippocampal area (Braak & Braak, 1994; Tseng, Kitazawa & LaFerla, 2004). However, the numeric correlation between Aβ-plaques and clinical symptoms in AD barely represents what is happening in the neurodegenerative process. Also the simple Aβ-accumulation *per se* is not the only etiological factor to trigger AD abnormalities (Lee et al., 2005). Cited studies explain why many aged individuals, despite the presence of high numbers of senile plaques, show little or no cognitive decline (Lee et al., 2004). With these data in mind, the belief that the Aβ-accumulation is a consequence rather that a cause is gaining more support. However, the pathology of the NFTs, mainly composed of tau protein, remains as a relevant criterion for the diagnosis of AD after death, because of the spatial correlation, albeit not perfect, between the number of NFTs and the clinical symptoms of this disease (Braak & Braak, 1991; Murayama & Saito, 2004). The support for this asseveration is mainly based on Braak's study, in which the occurrence and progression of NFTs along allocortical and isocortical areas was described (Braak & Braak, 1991).
This study evaluates the density and distribution of NFTs along the brain and classifies them into I, II, entorhinal; III, IV, limbic; and V, VI, neocortical stages. These three groups of stages correspond to normal cognition, cognitive impairment, and dementia (Braak & Braak, 1997). Note that this correlation is not sufficient to demonstrate a cause and effect relationship between NFTs and cognitive deficits. In this regard, the obvious question raised is why do brains of AD patients show the pathology of NFTs? Despite all the information available the answer is not even close to being addressed. However, a huge number of strategies focused on the mechanisms governing the aggregation of the tau protein into PHFs and NFTs (Kosik, Joachim & Selkoe, 1986) have attempted to address this. Those

efforts have been directed to unmask the mechanisms involved in tau dysregulation and its abnormal processing during AD (Kidd, 2006).

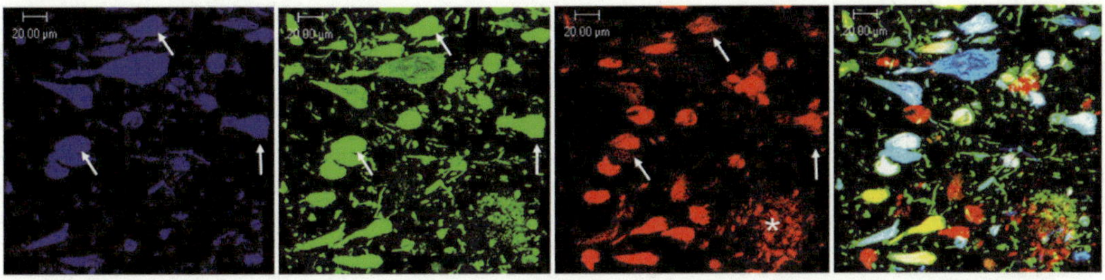

Fig. 1. Neurofibrillary pathology in the brain of patients with Alzheimer's disease. NFTs (arrows) are triple labeled with antibodies to tau protein (blue and green channels) and thiazin red (red channel). An amyloid-ß-core plaque is visualized in the red channel (asterisk). Neuropil threads are mostly observed in the green channel. Images taken from the hippocampus.

3. Abnormally processed tau protein is the major component of the neurofibrillary pathology in AD

There is a considerable amount of data consistent with the hypothesis that the aggregated state of tau could be functioning as a potential mediator to neurodegeneration, by either creating novel toxic species (*gain of function*) or by interfering with the normal function of the tau protein itself (*loss of function*) (Honson & Kuret, 2008). The aggregated state of tau interferes with the axonal transport, a result that further supports the crucial role of aggregated tau in the pathogenesis of AD (Stokin & Goldstein, 2006).

The growing facts showed that the aggregation certainly contributes to neurodegeneration, however the data also showed that the final aggregated state (NFTs) during AD, by bringing some compensatory properties, could exert a beneficial role (Congdon & Duff, 2008; Gotz et al., 2008). Despite this controversial fact, the aggregation debate has pointed out three posttranslational modifications as the key events; hyperphosphorylation, conformational changes, and cleavage, all of them taking place in the tau molecule and that are believed to promote the pathological and aggregated state of this protein (Chun & Johnson, 2007; Du et al., 2007; Yin & Kuret, 2006).

Aberrant phosphorylation of some sites as Ser^{262} has been proposed to play a crucial role in reducing the binding properties of the tau protein to the microtubules, driving the tubulin-unassociated tau protein to a soluble state that in turn could become an aggregated entity (Biernat et al., 1993; Gustke et al., 1992). Some reports had set the path for aberrant phosphorylation as a strong candidate promoting the formation of tau oligomers, and sequentially to the assembly into PHFs. Thus phosphorylation at sites such as $Ser^{396, 404}$ has been proposed to cause PHF structures in a model *in vitro* (Schaffer et al., 2008). Following the approaches *in vitro*, dysregulation of protein kinases and protein phosphatases that control tau phosphorylation has been reported (Mandelkow et al., 1992; Schaffer et al., 2008). However, some data came from the approach *in vitro* and do not necessarily reproduce the cytoplasmic conditions seen for tau protein in the disease. Nevertheless, it has long been reported that in the brains of AD patients the tau protein residing in the PHFs is abnormally phosphorylated at several residues, therefore, it has been concluded that this modification plays an important role during the formation of NFTs (Iqbal, del & Grundke-Iqbal, 2008; Wang, Grundke-Iqbal & Iqbal, 1996).

It has also been postulated that structural changes in the molecule of the tau protein can be caused by phosphorylation of specific residues, which then cause local modifications, which in turn transiently lead to extensive folding of the N-terminus (Luna-Munoz et al., 2005,2007). It was also suggested that phosphorylation at site Ser^{356} conditioned by the fourth microtubule-binding domain may be responsible for conformational changes of tau and self-aggregation (Du et al., 2007). Moreover, the conformational changes in this molecule have been proposed to mediate dimerization of tau and the subsequent formation of NFTs. The support for this hypothesis comes from the theory that the extreme ends of the tau protein may reduce the aggregating properties of the protein if they had an unfolded conformation (Gamblin, Berry & Binder, 2003a). Conformational changes in tau protein leading to its abnormal aggregation in the AD brain has been monitored by using conformational-dependent antibodies such as Alz-50, MC1, and Tau-66 (Carmel et al., 1996; Ghoshal et al., 2001; Jicha et al., 1997a). These antibodies, with discontinuous epitopes along the tau molecule, only recognize tau protein when these residues approach one another, which only occurs through the folding of the N–terminus over the repeated domains. This conformational alteration is mostly found when tau is abnormally aggregated into affected neurons in the brain of AD patients (Garcia-Sierra et al., 2003).

The cleavage of the tau protein has also been implicated in the abnormal processing of tau protein that contributes to its self-assembly into PHFs and increased toxicity (Gamblin et al., 2003b; Wischik et al., 1988b). It has been proposed that tau protein is a substrate of several intracellular proteases associated with the turnover of proteins such as cathepsins, calpains, and caspases (Gamblin et al., 2003b; Rissman et al., 2004; Wang et al., 2009; Yang & Ksiezak-Reding, 1995). Interestingly, cleavage of the tau protein is also related to apoptosis, because this action is specifically caused by caspase-3 generating a large truncated product preserving its N-terminus, but proteolytically truncated at the position Asp^{421} at the C-terminus (Fasulo et al., 2000; Gamblin et al., 2003b). This truncation was also involved with both nucleation and extension of tau fibrilization *in vitro* (Gamblin et al., 2003a; Rissman et al., 2004) and is closely related to toxicity in cell and animal models (Garcia-Sierra et al., 2008). The relevance of truncation of tau protein has also been demonstrated to have a positive correlation with the clinical symptoms of AD (Basurto-Islas et al., 2008).

Furthermore, it has been shown that cleavage and phosphorylation together can alter the tau microtubule interaction (Ding, Matthews & Johnson, 2006), however in a nonpathological role it was recently shown that phosphorylation at site Ser^{422} prevents cleavage of the tau protein at site Asp^{421} (Guillozet-Bongaarts et al., 2006).

To date both conformational changes and cleavage have been involved in the pathological processing of tau protein, which made them relevant candidates as potential therapeutic targets. The current scenario that attempts to elucidate how these posttranslational modifications interact with one another to drive the fibrillary aggregation of tau and the timing of occurrence along the evolution of AD disease still remains elusive. However, we believe that some answer could be gotten from the chronological characterization at the molecular level of the major lesions, the NFTs that correlate better with the cognitive impairment observed in AD patients. This approach may turn the present scenario into a more promising pathway to the understanding of the genesis and maturation of the NFTs.

4. Abnormal hyperphosphorylation of tau protein and its relationship to the pathology of the neurofibrillary tangle

In 1986, abnormally phosphorylated tau protein in the brains of AD patients was reported (Grundke-Iqbal et al., 1986b). Back then it was found that tau was a phosphodependent protein regulated via coordinated actions of kinases and phosphatases, which mostly preserve this protein in a low phosphorylated state in association with microtubules (Liu, Liang & Gong, 2006; Mandelkow et al., 1995). In AD, either dysregulation of phosphatases or upregulation of kinases such as calcium and calmodulin-dependent kinase II (CaM Kinase II), protein phosphatase 2A (PP2A), mitogen-activated protein kinase (ERK II), glycogen synthase Kinase-3β (GSK-3β), protein phosphatase-1 and -2C, p70 kinase, cyclic-AMP-dependent protein kinase, protein kinase C, and casein kinase II may lead to the formation of hyperphosphorylated tau protein (Avila, 2008; Iqbal & Grundke-Iqbal, 2008).

Moreover, in AD the tau protein is abnormally phosphorylated not only in those sites traditionally controlling its microtubule binding properties but more unconventional residues increase its phosphorylated state, such as Ser^{396} Ser^{214} and Ser^{262} (Biernat et al., 1993; Bramblett et al., 1993; Schneider et al., 1999). Additionally, it has been proposed that cytosolic-phosphorylated tau is able to recruit normal tau and MAP protein causing microtubule disruption (Alonso et al., 1997, 2001; Iqbal et al., 2008). Besides these modifications that lead to the loss of function of tau, hyperphosphorylation also causes the tau protein to self-aggregate into nonfibrillary or fibrillary aggregates that are not easily eliminated from the cytoplasm of altered neurons in AD. An increased phosphorylation of tyrosine residues was found to correlate to the formation of tau aggregates (Vega et al., 2005). Concomitantly from experiments *in vitro,* it is long been reported that pseudophosphorylation of tau protein increases its ability to polymerize (Alonso et al., 2001). When the process of tau aggregation was evaluated *in vitro* in the presence of methylglyoxal and acrolein (drugs that cause lipid peroxidation) the fibrilization was slightly enhanced in phosphorylated tau species (Kuhla et al., 2007).

Soluble aggregates composed of abnormally phosphorylated tau were isolated from the brains of AD patients and were referred to as the A68 fraction, because of its electrophoretic mobility compared to normal tau protein (Brion et al., 1991; Lee et al., 1991; Vincent & Davies, 1990). In accordance with these data, it was shown that tau protein in the PHFs, which are the main component of the NFTs, was abnormally hyperphosphorylated at several residues (Grundke-Iqbal et al., 1986b). At the neuropathological level, large amounts of NFTs seem to progress according to the evolution of AD with early invasion into those areas that start the neurofibrillary degeneration along the perforant pathway, correlating with the cognitive decline of patients with dementia (Garcia-Sierra et al., 2000). In agreement with these findings, CaM Kinase II that phosphorylates tau at site Ser^{416} was found to be closely related to the accumulation of tau in the soma of affected neurons in the brain of AD patients (Yamamoto et al., 2005). By using transgenic models, phosphorylation of tau was found to represent an essential modification that causes self-aggregation and abnormalities in the normal functioning of this protein (Delobel et al., 2008).

In contrast to pathological properties, some authors using polymerization models have suggested that abnormal phosphorylation of tau protein enhances, but does not trigger, fibrilization (Necula & Kuret, 2004). Other investigators have shown that abnormally phosphorylated tau protein residing in the PHFs can be released and rescued from this inactive state to recover normal functions, such as microtubule binding after dephosphorylation mainly caused by active phosphatases (Wang et al., 1998). Despite this controversy and noting its pathological role as a major issue, the phosphorylated state of tau protein has been associated with neurodegeneration in AD, likely by causing the impairment of the axonal transport, as was demonstrated in both the aggregated and nonaggregated state (Lapointe et al., 2008; Mandelkow et al., 2003). Accumulation of tau aggregates inside neurons may represent either a physical impediment for the cytoskeletal organization that affects the organelle transport or a recruiting structure that binds diverse molecular components in a nonspecific fashion. Despite the controversy about the toxicity of the nonaggregated state of the phosphorylated tau *versus* fibrillary structures as the major pathological players, the well-described NFTs remain as the stronger candidate.

5. Abnormal phosphorylation and conformational changes of tau protein during the formation and maturation of neurofibrillary tangles

In some neurodegenerative disorders it is well-known that the misfolding of linear proteins causes them to adopt conformations that may affect their normal functioning and cause them to self-aggregate. This is common for AD and prion diseases, in which proteins prone to folding attain an altered conformational state with properties that inevitably lead to cell death (Carrell & Gooptu, 1998; Soto, 1999). It is believed those conformational changes could cause the proteins to adopt an amyloid-conformation and finally to disease, although the mechanisms remain unknown (Kelly, 1996). It has been postulated that the conformational changes in tau protein could actually be driving a nucleation phenomenon similar to that occurring in the brain of AD patients (Fox, Harvey & Rossor, 1996).

The tau protein under physiological conditions has a random coil structure (Barghorn, Davies & Mandelkow, 2004; Sadqi et al., 2002), but in AD tau develops conformational changes that alter its normal function and increases its aggregation properties into a pathological ß-sheet conformation. Large amounts of this conformationally altered protein have been reported to aggregate during the progression of AD (Ghoshal et al., 2002). The mechanisms driving conformational changes are still elusive, however data referring to local alterations in the tau structure showed abnormal phosphorylation of specific residues as a major factor (Jicha et al., 1997b; Luna-Munoz et al., 2007). The description of the first conformational change discovered in the tau molecule was based on the characterization of the Tau-2 monoclonal antibody, which was developed by immunizing mice with tau protein purified from bovine brain (Papasozomenos & Binder, 1987) . When this antibody was tested against tau residing in PHFs purified from the brains of AD patients, immunoreactivity was stronger than that shown by human monomeric tau. From this result it was concluded that Tau-2 recognized a conformational shift occurring in polymeric tau that mimicked the original residue contained in bovine tau. The normal monomer of tau contains a proline residue in the site of the recognition of Tau-2, however during tau fibrilization this residue adopts a serine-like conformation that is now detected by this antibody. Following the same trend, immunization of mice was also done with brain extracts from AD patients, producing a new conformational antibody named Alz-50 (Wolozin et al., 1986). Immunoreactivity of this antibody was based on the extensive folding of the N-terminus of the tau molecule over the third microtubule-binding domain, which was revealed when the epitope mapping of this antibody reported a discontinuous sequence of recognition (residues 7-9 and 312-342) (Carmel et al., 1996). Thereafter the Alz-50 conformational antibody was described as a reliable marker of tau neuropathology in AD (Brady & Mufson, 1991; Hyman et al., 1988; Tourtellotte et al., 1990).

Since then, conformational changes have gained more attention from the AD-study community, which has proposed this modification to be related to transcriptional abnormalities during the genesis of tau protein in human brain neurons (Hyman, Augustinack & Ingelsson, 2005). In contrast, a variable role has been attributed to the Alz-50 conformation of tau protein because the normal activity of neurons was reported to take place in the presence of tau protein attaining the Alz-50 conformation (Salehi et al., 1995; van de Nes et al., 1998). These data are intriguing and crucial because the Alz-50 conformational change is present as an early event during the pathology of AD. Later there were claims that the Tau-66 antibody could recognize a discontinuous sequence (residues 155-244 and 305-314) in the tau molecule, which was developed by immunizing mice with three repeated domains of tau polymers assembled *in vitro* (Ghoshal et al., 2001).

Supporting the conformational change as a pathological event, different structures, called granulovacuolar, and fibrillar lesions that correlated with several determinations of episodic memory, were detected (Ghoshal et al.,1999, 2002). The epitopes of both conformational changes recognized by Alz-50 and Tau-66 partially overlap in a common region located at the third repeated domain, suggesting this part of the molecule as a relevant site for the protein folding. Local conformational changes in the repeat-domain region have also been reported (Du et al., 2007). The local and structural conformational changes adopted by the tau protein can be explained in part by phosphorylation of specific amino acids that change the charge and thermodynamic stability of an unfolded conformation. It has also been suggested that phosphorylation of the tau protein at site Thr^{231} precedes the Alz-50 conformational change (Luna-Munoz et al.,2005, 2007).

The main data about the relationship between phosphorylation and conformational changes come from AD tissue, which somehow yielded the question about how phosphorylation was able to generate those foldings in the proteins. By asking this question and by using two test proteins, cystatin and NtrC, it was reported that phosphorylation is able to change the free energy landscape, which in turn modifies the original structure by changing it into a folded conformation (Latzer, Shen & Wolynes, 2008). More related to AD, phosphorylation of Ser and Thr residues in the Pro-rich region of the tau protein causes this protein to have a polyproline II helix conformation (Bielska & Zondlo, 2006). The ability of tau to aggregate *in vitro* is increased once phosphorylation at the site Ser^{356} occurs. Additionally this phosphorylation favored a local conformation (Du et al., 2007). More recently, pseudophosphorylation *in vitro* of proline residues along the epitopes of AT8 and PHF1, two tau phosphodependent antibodies, caused the pathological conformation in the tau molecule that is recognized by the MC1 antibody (Jeganathan et al., 2008). So far the data set out clearly those phosphorylations are highly related to the conformational change seen during AD, though the time-course of the appearance of both events is not clear.

By attempting to determine the time-course by which phosphorylation of the tau protein and conformational changes are associated to one another in the authentic disease, we have analyzed the profile of the immunoreactivity of NFTs to tau antibodies that map the entire molecule and recognize both conformational changes and diverse phosphorylation residues during the progression of AD. Our data have shown a strong relationship between the Alz-50 conformational change and the phosphorylation of multiple residues in the tau molecule such as $Ser^{396, 404}$ (labeled by the AD2 antibody) at the C-terminus. Both events may occur in the same molecule of tau protein, which is shown by the close colocalization observed in a large number of NFTs. Other phosphorylation sites such as $Ser^{199, 202}$ Thr^{205}, Ser^{262}, and Ser^{422} were also linked to the Alz-50 conformation.

These observations demonstrated a close relationship between conformational changes and phosphorylation, with the latter as a possible cause of the folded state of the tau protein. These NFTs are the common neuropathological features during early stages of AD, in which most of these structures are composed of C-terminus intact tau protein (immunoreactive to Tau-46.1 antibody) and also having the Alz-50 conformational change (arrows in Fig. 2). The fibrillary state of these structures is clearly seen by the positive signal to TR, a fluorescent marker for a β-pleated sheet conformation as shown by already assembled PHFs (Mena et al., 1995). The light-blue to white pseudocolor of these structures observed in the merge channel of Fig. 2, indicates the existence of C-terminus intact and conformationally altered tau protein in an assembled state.

It can be also seen that some NFTs are only detected by TR (asterisks), which may imply that these structures have been further processed and both the Alz-50 conformation and the C-terminus of tau molecule are likely lost by proteolysis. Further, it can be seen that the neuritic component along the neuropil is also composed of C-terminus intact and conformationally altered tau protein, though the state of assembly does not yet show a fibrillary aggregation (thiazin-red negative). This result indicates a more delayed accumulation and processing of tau protein along this component. According to our data, we have found that most of these abnormal phosphorylation and conformational changes in the full-length tau protein occur in the early stages of AD.

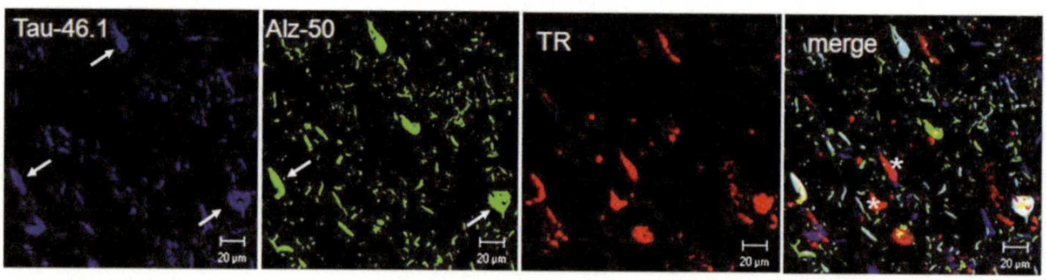

Fig. 2. The Alz-50 conformation of tau in NFTs is associated with preservation of the C-terminus. At early stages of AD, in most of the Alz-50 positive NFTs (green channel), tau preserves its extreme C-terminus intact (Tau-46.1 labeling). Arrows indicate the double labeling of these NFTs (note also the triple labeling with TR as a white pseudocolor in the merge channel). In more advanced NFTs these epitopes are missed and they are labeled only by TR (asterisk). Images taken from the hippocampus.

Maturation of NFTs has been associated with the transformation of morphology and composition of these structures (Garcia-Sierra et al., 2001). After the maturation of the early NFTs described above, we have observed that the tau protein in a fibrillary state is further processed to yield a new conformation as observed by using the conformationally dependent antibody Tau-66 (Garcia-Sierra et al., 2003; Ghoshal et al., 2001, 2002). At the intermediate stages of AD, early NFTs now progress from entorhinal areas to the hippocampal formation. The more advanced NFTs that follow the maturation process are recognized by the Tau-66 antibody, that in this case the N-folding conformation adopted by tau has also lost its extreme C-terminus. Although the adoption of the Tau-66 conformational change may imply the loss of some phosphorylated residues in the tau protein, the AD2 epitope ($pSer^{396, 404}$) is preserved at least in some NFTs.

Thus, it is clear that the Tau-66 conformational change is not associated with the full-length tau protein. As initially reported (Garcia-Sierra et al., 2003), we also found that both conformations of tau in the NFTs, the Alz-50 and the Tau-66, were mutually exclusive, because they were not synchronized along the time-course and area of distribution. Moreover, Alz-50 and Tau-66 never were colocalized in the same NFT. These data also support our proposal for the Alz-50 conformational changes as an early event, but more importantly also show the nonsynchronic stage of the neuropil pathology compared to the NFTs formation.

These particular changes in the tau molecule also occur in the temporal cortex. It has been reported that NFTs in this area display a laminar distribution occurring mostly in cortical layers II,III,V, and VI (Thangavel et al., 2008). These structures are also conformed of tau protein phosphorylated at several domains (Thangavel et al., 2008; Guillozet-Bongaarts et al., 2006) and some showing immunoreactivity to Alz-50 antibody (de la Monte et al., 1992).

Summarizing, during the progression of early and intermediate stages of AD, the discriminatory presence of each conformational event sets the dynamic behavior of tau during the maturation of NFTs, started by the N-terminus folding that is caused by the phosphorylation of specific domains. These time-dependent conformational changes also occur during the aggregation of the tau protein into the neuritic component, but not synchronized in time with those changes shown in the NFTs.

6. Cleavage of tau protein and the maturation of the NFTs

The pathologic processing of the tau protein, in which several residues are lost, has been attributed to intracellular proteolysis (Gamblin et al., 2003b; Novak, Kabat & Wischik, 1993; Rissman et al., 2004). The early biochemical analysis of the insoluble fraction of homogenates of the brain of AD patients revealed an enriched fraction of PHFs (Greenberg & Davies, 1990; Grundke-Iqbal et al., 1986a; Wischik et al., 1988b). When this fraction was completely digested using pronase, a minimum PHF-core remained as an insoluble protease-resistant fraction (Novak et al., 1993; Wischik et al., 1988b). The remaining PHF-core comprised a 12 kDa portion of the tau protein beginning in the vicinity of histidine-268 and containing the tubulin-binding domains.

This fragment ended at the site glutamic acid-391 (Glu^{391}) towards the extreme C-terminus (Novak, 1993,1994). No morphological differences were found between native PHFs and the remaining PHF-core when analyzed by electron microscopy, but the latter was antigenically deprived of the N- and C-termini commonly found in the tau protein during its early aggregation in AD (Wischik et al., 1995). Mice were immunized with this PHF-core fraction to develop the monoclonal antibody MN423 that specifically labeled the Glu^{391}-truncated residue in the tau protein (Novak et al., 1989, 1991, 1993). Validating the importance of the truncated tau protein at site Glu^{391}, correlation of this event with the NFT progression, and the clinical symptoms were demonstrated (Garcia-Sierra et al., 2001). Despite the promising alternative for the role of the Glu^{391} cleavage of tau during the formation of NFTs in AD, a limited relevance has been attributed to the cleavage because so far no intracellular proteases have been described to be responsible for this event. Even though the polymeric state of the Glu^{391}-cleaved tau inside the cytoplasm of affected neurons in AD has been associated with toxicity in vulnerable areas of the brain, such as those corresponding to the perforant pathway (Garcia-Sierra et al., 2001), it is well-documented that an abnormal proteolytic processing of proteins occurs as part of the aging process and cell death in several neurodegenerative diseases (Cotman et al., 2005; Newman et al., 2005; Rubinsztein, 2006). One of the most cited participants is a family of cysteine-aspartyl proteases, referred

to as caspases, that are reported to be active during apoptosis and have an increased expression in AD (Dickson, 2004; Rubinsztein, 2006).
Some other cleavage sites have been found in the tau protein, mainly occurring at the C-terminus residue aspartic acid-421 (Asp^{421}), for which caspase-3 was found mainly responsible for this action (Gamblin et al., 2003b; Horowitz et al., 2004). From the previous data we can see that the cleavage of the tau protein has been strongly related to the apoptosis process, which is also thought to contribute to the neurodegeneration during AD.

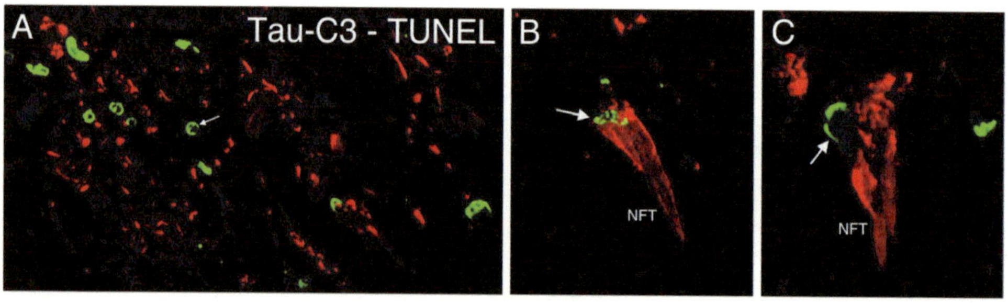

Fig. 3. Apototic nuclei are disseminated in the hippocampus of AD cases. Arrows in A indicate TUNEL-positive nuclei in cells lacking NFTs (neurofibrillary tangles). In panels B and C, two NFTs composed of Asp^{421}-truncated tau (positive to Tau-C3 antibody) are in close association with TUNEL-positive nuclei (arrows). Images obtained by confocal microscopy represent the merge channel of double labeling samples with TUNEL (green) and Tau-C3 antibody (red).

In the brain of AD patients, increased amount of cell undergoing apoptosis was reported in comparison to age-matched nondemented individuals (de la Monte, Sohn & Wands, 1997; Lucassen et al., 1997; Nagy & Esiri, 1997). Because apoptosis is characterized by several biochemical changes involving activation of proteolytic caspases, it was thought this mechanism could generate Asp^{421}-truncated tau *in situ*. By using the *in situ* cell death detection kit TUNEL (deoxynucleotydyl transferase dUTP end labeling), which detects apoptotic nuclei (Gold et al., 1994), we found mostly in the hippocampus of AD patients that a large population of neurons contained apoptotic nuclei in the absence of intracellular NFTs (arrows in panel A, Fig. 3). However in some specific populations of apoptotic neurons, NFTs composed of Asp^{421}-truncated tau were detected in the cytoplasmic space (Arrows in panels B and C, Fig.3).
However, some investigators have postulated that apoptosis during AD could also be a consequence instead of being the causal event (Dickson, 2004). A simple nonmathematic and chronological relationship between AD and apoptosis has been proposed suggesting that this process does not change or affect the course of AD (Zhu et al., 2006). In sum, the contradictory data about the apoptosis during AD and the discovery of proteolytic cleavage of the tau protein by multiple caspases raised the question whether or not these families of enzymes were also responsible for the truncation at Glu^{391}. However, neither caspases nor calpain (Newman et al., 2005) were directly associated with the formation of this truncated epitope. Despite the controversy about the genesis of the truncated species of tau protein, experiments *in vitro* corroborated that both truncated tau variants, the Asp^{421} and Glu^{391}, were able to polymerize at a faster rate than the normal C-terminus-intact tau protein (Abraha et al., 2000; Rissman et al., 2004). This result corroborated the

abnormal properties of the truncated tau protein compared to those of the wild-type molecule. For the Asp^{421} cleavage, it was found in the brain of AD patients by using a monoclonal antibody called Tau-C3, which was developed by immunization of mice with this truncated variant and proved to be specific for the Asp^{421} ending residue. By using this antibody further support for a relevant role of Asp^{421}-cleaved tau in AD was corroborated by the positive correlation found between the density of NFTs recognized by Tau-C3 and the neuropathological progression of the disease described by Braak and Braak (1991), and to the clinical severity of dementia (Basurto-Islas et al., 2008). Additionally, a close relationship to the presence of the Apolipoprotein-E (ε4) allelic variant was found in cases with an increased density of NFTs immunoreactive to the Tau-C3 antibody (Basurto-Islas et al., 2008).

7. Unified model of tau processing during the evolution of AD

All the previous evidence highlighted the important role for the cleavage of tau protein as a relevant mechanism leading to the well-described AD pathology. However, how these truncations could interact with another to determine the formation of the fibrillary pathology, and how they may affect conformational changes of the tau protein, are important questions that require further investigation. Trying to address these questions we turned back to the *postmortem* analysis of the brain of AD patients with varying degrees of the clinical manifestation of dementia, in which the authentic disease can be analyzed as a progressive process. We were able to describe that NFTs composed of either Asp^{421} or Glu^{391}-truncated tau were mutually exclusive in the brain of AD patients at any stage of AD progression, and that the advanced Glu^{391}-truncated variant of tau is a common feature of AD but not for other tauopathies (Basurto-Islas et al., 2008; Mondragon-Rodriguez et al., 2008). Interestingly we found that the initial Alz-50 conformational stage of tau protein residing in early NFTs is transiently transformed to the Tau-66 conformation, possibly caused by subtle truncation of the extreme C- terminus at the position Asp^{421} (Fig. 4 and Fig. 5). It is clearly seen that Alz-50 colocalizes with Tau-C3 in some of these structures (arrows in Fig. 4), but in others the Alz-50 conformation is lost coincidentally with the presence of truncation at the Asp^{421} residue (arrowheads in Fig. 4).

This result is intriguing because the major contributor for the Alz-50 folding is the N-terminus, completely opposite to the truncation site at the C-terminus. From these data, we have only inferred that the loss of these 20 amino acids may cause a rearrangement in the N-folding of the tau protein because it coincides with the increase of NFTs developing a new conformation now detected by the Tau-66 antibody (arrows in Fig. 5).

In relating cleavage and phosphorylation, abnormal phosphorylated sites in the tau protein, such as $Ser^{199, 202}$ Thr^{205}, $Ser^{396, 404}$, and Ser^{262}, were found coexisting in the Tau-C3 structures. Moreover and supporting those previous findings that come from AD brain tissue, chimeric NFTs composed of full-length tau and C-terminal-truncated tau at Asp^{421} were also found in this study (Guillozet-Bongaarts et al., 2005). Abnormal phosphorylation of tau protein has also been found in other tauopathies, such as Pick disease in which Asp^{421} cleavage of tau was colocalized into the characteristic Pick bodies (Mondragon-Rodriguez et al., 2008). These data suggest a close relationship of phosphorylation and cleavage for the tau processing (Guillozet-Bongaarts et al., 2007; Mondragon-Rodriguez et al., 2008).

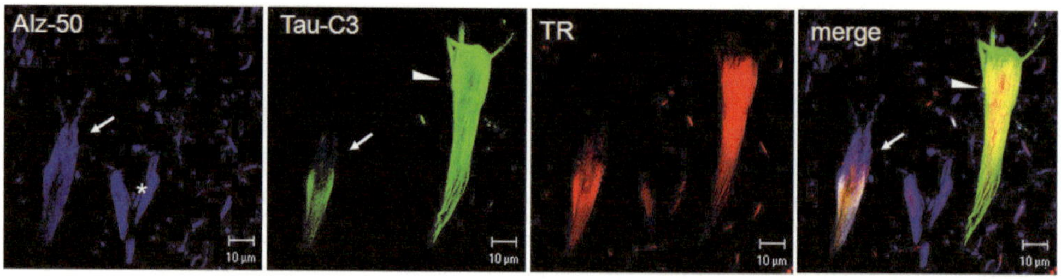

Fig. 4. Subtle truncation of the extreme C-terminus is occurring in tau protein adopting the Alz-50 conformation. In some intermediate-stage NFTs (arrows), the tau molecule adopting the Alz-50 conformation is subjected to proteolysis that cleaves the extreme C-terminus at the position Asp^{421} (Tau-C3 immunolabeling). In contrast, other NFTs have either the Alz-50 conformation (asterisk) or the truncation at the Asp^{421} (arrowhead). Images taken from the hippocampus.

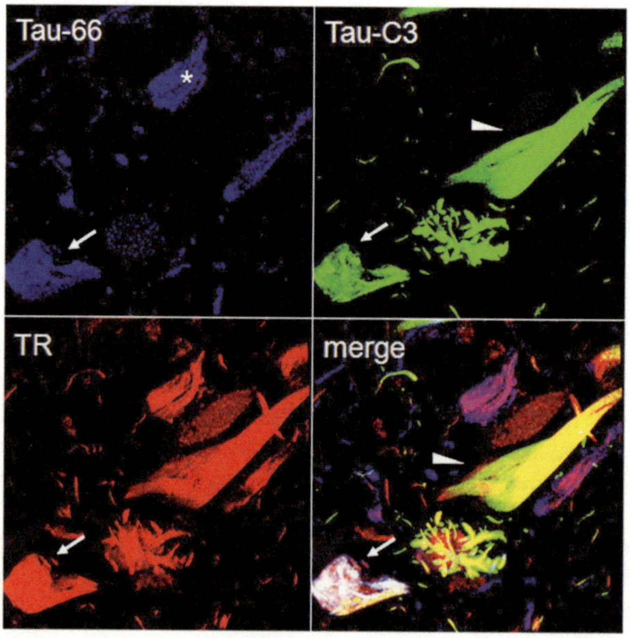

Fig. 5. Asp^{421}-truncation links a new conformation of tau protein in NFTs. From intermediate to advanced stages in AD, some NFTs are carrying tau molecules that have a new conformation recognized by the Tau-66 antibody and are also undergoing truncation at position Asp^{421} (arrows). In contrast other NFTs have either the Tau-66 conformation (asterisk) or the truncation at the Asp^{421} (arrowhead). Images taken from the hippocampus.

In contrast, phosphorylation of tau is able to prevent apoptosis in growing cells (Li et al., 2007) and the cleavage at the Asp^{421} residue is reduced *in vitro* by the pseudophosphorylation of the site Ser^{422} (Guillozet-Bongaarts et al., 2006). Similarly, dephosphorylation of the molecule is crucial for tau protein to undergo cleavage (Rametti et al., 2004). However, other experiments *in vitro* recapture the pathologic relationship between phosphorylation and the cleavage of tau protein. Alterations in the microtubule-binding properties were found in tau protein when the molecule was phosphorylated at specific sites, such as $Ser^{396, 404}$, and cleaved at the site Asp^{421} (Ding et al., 2006). It was also found that the combination of phosphorylated and truncated tau contributes to tau oligomerization (Cho & Johnson, 2004). Supporting the phosphorylation as a pathological event, upregulation of c-jun N-terminal kinase leading sequentially to tau phosphorylation and cleavage has also been reported (Sahara et al., 2008). Overall, and affirming the initial idea, it is clear that phosphorylation is highly related to the cleavage during tau processing, although the precise role still remains to be clarified.

As our data have shown, it is clear that a tau molecule truncated at Asp^{421} also attains a conformation recognized by Tau-66 (merged white tangle in Fig. 5), an event that can be the link between the Alz-50 and Tau-66 conformational stages. Different NFTs are not synchronized along the time-course of maturation and have either the truncation at the Asp^{421} of tau protein (arrowhead) (and probably are Alz-50 positive) but are negative to Tau-66 or have attained the Tau-66 conformation and are truncated at the C-terminus (asterisk in Fig. 5) (negative to Tau-C3). Putting these data together, we have concluded that the switching of conformations in the tau molecule in a polymeric state is a transient process occurring during the maturation of NFTs from early to intermediate stages of the disease. During this maturation, early NFTs will colonize new areas that follow the important perforant pathway of communication from the entorhinal cortex to the hippocampus, and later from this area to the isocortex via the subiculum and entorhinal cortex layer IV (Braak & Braak, 1991; Garcia-Sierra et al., 2001; Van Hoesen, Hyman & Damasio, 1991). The most mature structures and consequently the more proteolytically processed remain at the earlier invaded areas. From intermediate to advanced stages of AD, the Tau-66 conformation attained by tau protein after Asp^{421} truncation is altered by further truncation of the remaining C-terminus. This means the conformational folding and partial truncation of tau protein by caspases may cause rearrangements in the polymeric state of tau protein to expose occluded epitopes that in turn may be the target for other intracellular proteases, such as cathepsins, calpains, or more nonspecific carboxy-peptidases. Whatever the responsible enzyme is, the result is that tau protein is later truncated at the Glu^{391} site, which is still observed in NFTs carrying tau molecules having the Tau-66 conformation (arrows in Fig. 6). Frequently from the intermediate to the late stages of AD, Tau-66 and MN423 are observed to colocalize in both intracellular and extracellular NFTs, the latter commonly recognized by MN423 and having less intensity for TR staining (arrows in Fig. 6).

The Tau-66 conformation, even when present at late stages of AD, is finally lost when the NFTs are severely proteolyzed, leaving only a remainder PHF-core that is mostly composed of truncated tau at the Glu^{391} site (Mena et al., 1996; Novak et al., 1993). In the hippocampus of AD patients the maturation of NFTs is reported to be unsynchronized, therefore these structures have different stages of tau processing (Basurto-Islas et al., 2008). We found different populations of NFTs in the same hippocampal area that were mutually exclusive when they were composed of either Glu^{391}-truncation or Alz-50 conformation, but not colocalized at any single point during the maturation of the NFTs (Fig. 7).

Although phosphorylation of tau residues is believed to be reduced during the progression of the disease, NFTs recognized by the conformation-dependent antibody Tau-66 and tau truncated at Glu^{391} still preserve the phosphorylated residues $pSer^{199, 202}$ and $pSer^{396, 404}$ (arrows in Fig. 8), which is explained by the existence of chimeric NFTs composed of independent molecules of tau having different degrees of truncation. A clear example of how tau pathology is not synchronized in the hippocampal area is shown in Fig. 8, where somatic aggregation of advanced truncation of the tau protein (Glu^{391}) is observed in one NFT (asterisks), which is innervated by dystrophic neurites composed of phosphorylated tau ($pSer^{396, 404}$) (green channel), with the conformationally altered tau protein distributed only in the apical neurite (arrowheads in the blue channel).

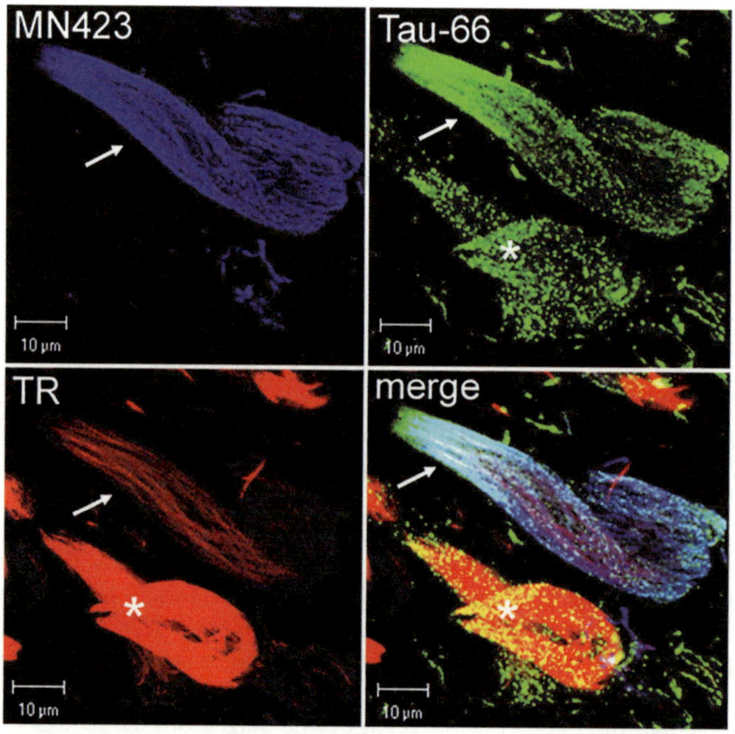

Fig. 6. Tau-66 conformation is strongly associated with truncation of tau protein at Glu^{391}. At intermediate and advanced stages of AD, significant numbers of NFTs acquire the conformational change detected by the Tau-66 antibody (channel green). In this conformation the tau molecule has lost both the N- and C- termini, and truncation of tau protein in some of these NFTs has reached the Glu^{391} position recognized by the MN423 antibody (arrows). In other NFTs, conformationally altered tau protein is expressed, but the Glu^{391} truncation is not yet reached (asterisks). Images taken from the hippocampus.

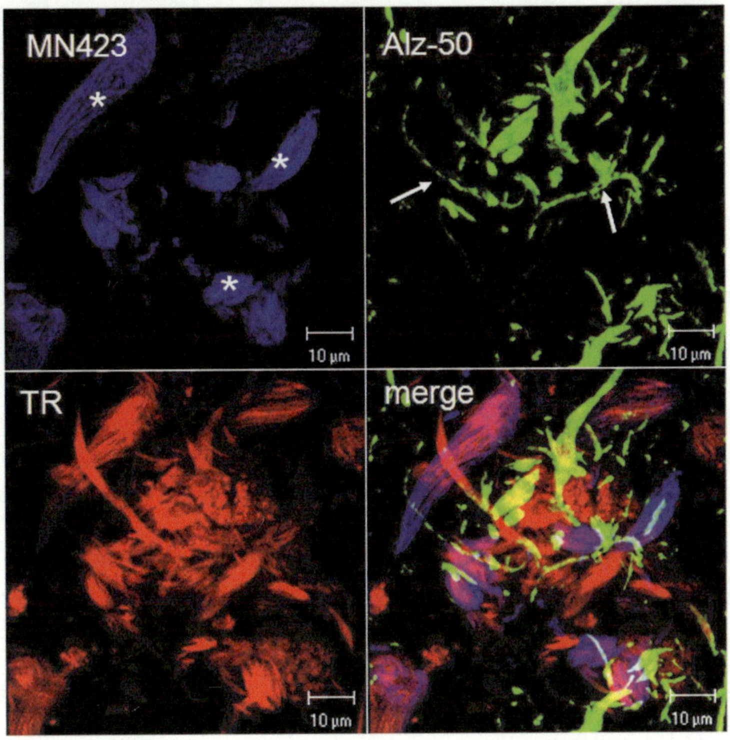

Fig. 7. Alz-50 conformation is not associated with truncation of tau at Glu[391]. As truncation of tau at Glu[391] was progressively occurring during the maturation of the NFTs, the conformational change recognized by Alz-50 was becoming lost. NFTs recognized by MN423 (to Glu[391]-truncated tau) (blue channel) were never detected with the Alz-50 antibody (green channel), which mostly detected dystrophic neurites. The picture corresponds to NFTs (asterisks) and neuritic components surrounding a β-amyloid plaque (see the red core of the β-amyloid in the merge channel) taken from the hippocampus.

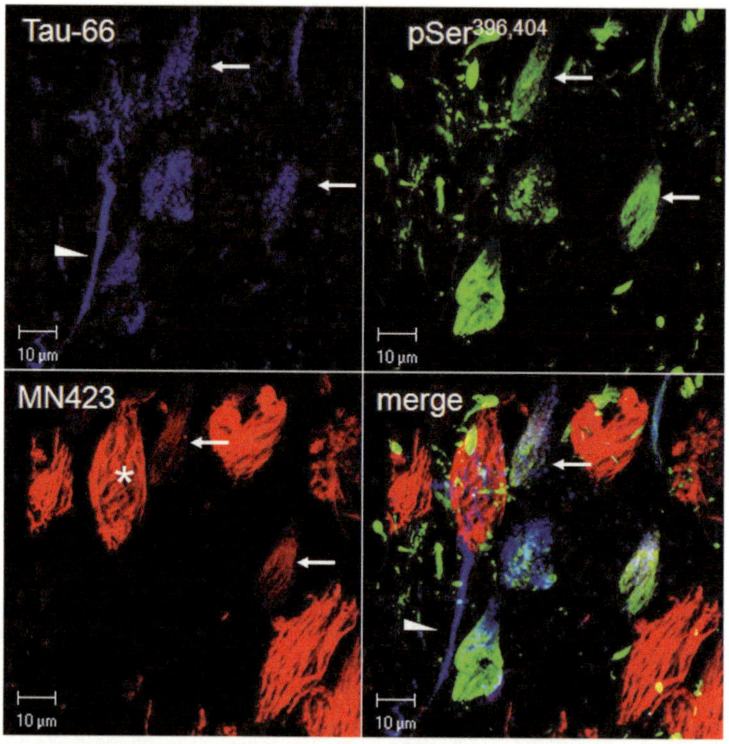

Fig. 8. Chimeric NFTs are composed of truncated and phosphorylated tau molecules. Some NFTs at advanced stages of AD show a chimeric profile (arrows) composed of truncated tau protein at Glu^{391} and more intact molecules phosphorylated at $Ser^{396,404}$. In another example, a well-defined extracellular NFT is composed of Glu^{391} truncated (asterisk) that is innervated by dystrophic neurites conformed by phosphorylated tau ($Ser^{396,404}$) (green channel) and the apical neurite filled with tau molecules displaying the Tau-66 conformational change (arrowhead in merge channel). Images taken from the hippocampus.

When we look at the entorhinal cortex at advanced stages of AD, the common scenario is the presence of extracellular NFTs formed inside multipolar neurons that are morphologically distinct from NFTs appearing in pyramidal neurons of the hippocampus. NFTs in the entorhinal cortex preserve the characteristic columnar arrangements shown by the islands of multipolar cells (Fig. 9). It is clearly seen how these NFTs strongly colocalize with TR, which indicates a well-synchronized processing mostly containing Glu^{391}-truncated tau (Fig. 9d-f). Interestingly, those NFTs mainly composed of Glu^{391}-truncated tau showed a distinct pattern around the hippocampal area (Fig. 9a-c), in which part of the whole population had only the Glu^{391} truncation of tau and the other is only recognized by TR, which suggests the presence of more intact tau protein in these structures. These data clearly show the unsynchronized, by time, processing of NFTs in the hippocampus and the late time processing of NFTs in the ERC-II area, emphasizing that this is the more vulnerable area for the onset of the AD neurofibrillary pathology. Regarding isocortical areas, which are the later affected regions in AD progression, most of the changes in tau protein that are seen in the NFTs, mostly correspond to increased phosphorylation (Thangavel et al., 2008). However along the progression of the disease, truncation of tau protein at Asp^{421} also has been described in some of NFTs proliferating in the temporal isocortex (Guillozet-Bongaarts et al., 2006). Moreover, at very advanced stages of the disease, some of these NFTs in the temporal isocortex also display tau molecules truncated at the Glu^{391} (Garcia-Sierra et al., 2001).

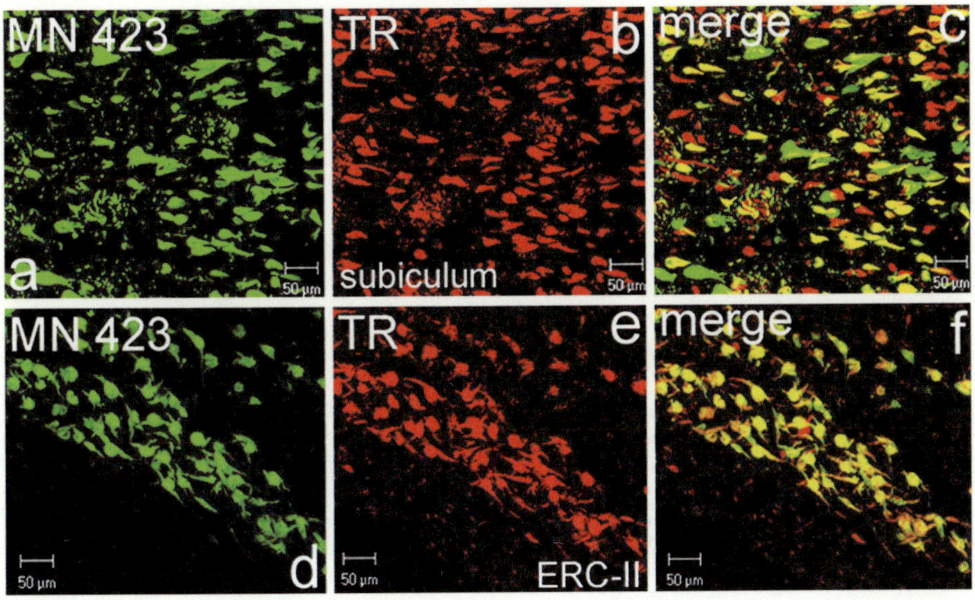

Fig. 9. Columnar arrangements of NFTs along the entorhinal cortex of AD patients. In the hippocampus of AD patients the neurofibrillary pathology is unsynchronized and selected populations of NFTs (a-c) have advanced truncation of tau protein at Glu^{391} (yellow NFTs in the merge channel). In contrast, in the layer II of the entorhinal cortex NFTs distributed along the columnar arrangements of neurons (d-f) are synchronically proteolyzed and have a uniform labeling with the MN423 antibody (note that most of the NFTs have a yellow pseudocolor in the merge channel).

8. Conclusion

We summarize that the chronological formation and maturation of NFTs in AD is made by a sequence of well-ordered events involving conformational changes in the tau molecule that may be driven by specific phosphorylations and sequential truncation of its C-terminus (Fig. 10). Early truncation at Asp^{421} is a pivotal modification that may produce more alterations on the tau structure, facilitating the exposure of different domains that can be lately proteolyzed by other non-apoptotic enzymes. *In situ*, we demonstrated a close association between Asp^{421}-truncated tau and several apoptotic markers. For diagnostic purposes, NFTs now can be classified according to their chimeric character that better predict the neuropathological evolution of AD. We currently are trying to reproduce this scenario by analyzing the polymerization properties of chimeric tau filaments assembled *in vitro*. Moreover we aim to evaluate the toxic effects of double expressed truncated and nontruncated tau variants in cultured neurons to validate the pathologic interaction of these proteins observed *in situ*.

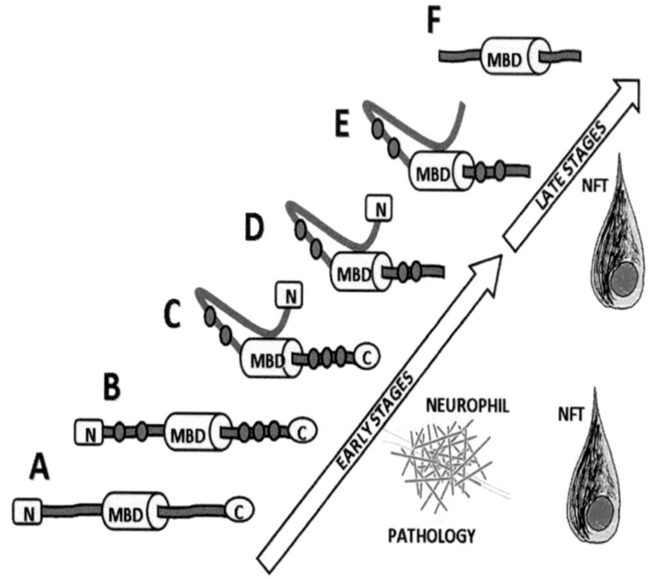

Fig. 10. Chronological formation and maturation of NFTs in AD. Formation and maturation of NFTs is based on conformational changes of tau protein (Alz-50) developed early by phosphorylation (p-p) of specific domains (A-C). These changes are modified at intermediate stages of the disease by early cleavage of tau protein at the Asp^{421} residue (D), leading to a new conformation (Tau-66) that is associated with further truncation of the molecule at the Glu^{391} (E-F). Advanced stages are characterized by the presence of the minimum PHF-core composed only of Glu^{391}-truncated tau protein (F). Tau protein in neuropil threads also undergoes a similar processing, however it is delayed in time and only reaches early conformational changes (Alz-50) and truncation at the Asp^{421} (A-D).

9. Acknowledgment

The authors thank Dr. Virginia Lee for the use of Tau-46.1 and PHF1 antibodies, Dr. Peter Davis for the use of Alz-50 and PHF1 antibodies, Michael Novak for the use of MN423 antibody. We also want to thank to Dr. Ellis Glazier who edited this English-language text. Financial support by CONACyT- México to FG-S grants 59651, 113772. RM was supported by CONACyT-México, grant 102278. Support from the Ministry of Health of the Czech Republic was for ZK and DR, project MZ0PCP2005.
HCC was supported by ICyT-México

10. References

Abraha, A., Ghoshal, N., Gamblin, T. C., Cryns, V., Berry, R. W., Kuret, J. & Binder, L. I. (2000). C-terminal inhibition of tau assembly *in vitro* and in Alzheimer's disease. *J Cell Sci* 113 Pt 21, 3737-45.

Alonso, A., Zaidi, T., Novak, M., Grundke-Iqbal, I. & Iqbal, K. (2001a). Hyperphosphorylation induces self-assembly of tau into tangles of paired helical filaments/straight filaments. *Proc Natl Acad Sci U S A* 98(12), 6923-8.

Alonso, A. D., Grundke-Iqbal, I., Barra, H. S. & Iqbal, K. (1997). Abnormal phosphorylation of tau and the mechanism of Alzheimer neurofibrillary degeneration: sequestration of microtubule-associated proteins 1 and 2 and the disassembly of microtubules by the abnormal tau. *Proc Natl Acad Sci U S A* 94(1), 298-303.

Arriagada, P. V., Marzloff, K. & Hyman, B. T. (1992). Distribution of Alzheimer-type pathologic changes in nondemented elderly individuals matches the pattern in Alzheimer's disease. *Neurology* 42(9), 1681-8.

Avila, J. (2008). Tau kinases and phosphatases. *Journal of cellular and molecular medicine* 12(1), 258-9.

Ballatore, C., Lee, V. M. & Trojanowski, J. Q. (2007). Tau-mediated neurodegeneration in Alzheimer's disease and related disorders. *Nature reviews* 8(9), 663-72.

Barghorn, S., Davies, P. & Mandelkow, E. (2004). Tau paired helical filaments from Alzheimer's disease brain and assembled *in vitro* are based on beta-structure in the core domain. *Biochemistry* 43(6), 1694-703.

Basurto-Islas, G., Luna-Munoz, J., Guillozet-Bongaarts, A. L., Binder, L. I., Mena, R. & Garcia-Sierra, F. (2008). Accumulation of aspartic acid421- and glutamic acid391-cleaved tau in neurofibrillary tangles correlates with progression in Alzheimer disease. *J Neuropathol Exp Neurol* 67(5), 470-83.

Berger, Z., Roder, H., Hanna, A., Carlson, A., Rangachari, V., Yue, M., Wszolek, Z., Ashe, K., Knight, J., Dickson, D., Andorfer, C., Rosenberry, T. L., Lewis, J., Hutton, M. & Janus, C. (2007). Accumulation of pathological tau species and memory loss in a conditional model of tauopathy. *J Neurosci* 27(14), 3650-62.

Bielska, A. A. & Zondlo, N. J. (2006). Hyperphosphorylation of tau induces local polyproline II helix. *Biochemistry* 45(17), 5527-37.

Biernat, J., Gustke, N., Drewes, G., Mandelkow, E. M. & Mandelkow, E. (1993). Phosphorylation of Ser262 strongly reduces binding of tau to microtubules: distinction between PHF-like immunoreactivity and microtubule binding. *Neuron* 11(1), 153-63.

Binder, L. I., Guillozet-Bongaarts, A. L., Garcia-Sierra, F. & Berry, R. W. (2005). Tau, tangles, and Alzheimer's disease. *Biochimica et biophysica acta* 1739(2-3), 216-23.

Braak, H. & Braak, E. (1991). Neuropathological stageing of Alzheimer-related changes. *Acta Neuropathol (Berl)* 82(4), 239-59.

Braak, H. & Braak, E. (1994). Morphological criteria for the recognition of Alzheimer's disease and the distribution pattern of cortical changes related to this disorder. *Neurobiol Aging* 15(3), 355-6; discussion 79-80.

Braak, H. & Braak, E. (1996). Evolution of the neuropathology of Alzheimer's disease. *Acta neurologica Scandinavica* 165, 3-12.

Braak, H. & Braak, E. (1997). Frequency of stages of Alzheimer-related lesions in different age categories. *Neurobiology of aging* 18(4), 351-7.

Braak, H., Braak, E. & Bohl, J. (1993). Staging of Alzheimer-related cortical destruction. *European neurology* 33(6), 403-8.

Brady, D. R. & Mufson, E. J. (1991). Alz-50 immunoreactive neuropil differentiates hippocampal complex subfields in Alzheimer's disease. *J Comp Neurol* 305(3), 489-507.

Bramblett, G. T., Goedert, M., Jakes, R., Merrick, S. E., Trojanowski, J. Q. & Lee, V. M. (1993). Abnormal tau phosphorylation at Ser396 in Alzheimer's disease recapitulates development and contributes to reduced microtubule binding. *Neuron* 10(6), 1089-99.

Brion, J. P., Hanger, D. P., Couck, A. M. & Anderton, B. H. (1991). A68 proteins in Alzheimer's disease are composed of several tau isoforms in a phosphorylated state which affects their electrophoretic mobilities. *Biochem J* 279 (Pt 3), 831-6.

Carmel, G., Mager, E. M., Binder, L. I. & Kuret, J. (1996). The structural basis of monoclonal antibody Alz50's selectivity for Alzheimer's disease pathology. *J Biol Chem* 271(51), 32789-95.

Carrell, R. W. & Gooptu, B. (1998). Conformational changes and disease--serpins, prions and Alzheimer's. *Curr Opin Struct Biol* 8(6), 799-809.

Congdon, E. E. & Duff, K. E. (2008). Is tau aggregation toxic or protective? *J Alzheimers Dis* 14(4), 453-7.

Cotman, C. W., Poon, W. W., Rissman, R. A. & Blurton-Jones, M. (2005). The role of caspase cleavage of tau in Alzheimer disease neuropathology. *J Neuropathol Exp Neurol* 64(2), 104-12.

Cho, J. H. & Johnson, G. V. (2004). Glycogen synthase kinase 3 beta induces caspase-cleaved tau aggregation *in situ*. *J Biol Chem* 279(52), 54716-23.

Chun, W. & Johnson, G. V. (2007). The role of tau phosphorylation and cleavage in neuronal cell death. *Front Biosci* 12, 733-56.

de la Monte, S. M., Spratt, R. A., Chong, J., Ghanbari H. A., Wands J. R. (1992). Immunohistochemical and histopathologic correlates of Alzheimer´s disease-associated Alz-50 immunoreactivity quantified in homogenates of cerebral tissue. American Journal of Pathology 141(6), 1459-69.

de la Monte, S. M., Sohn, Y. K. & Wands, J. R. (1997). Correlates of p53- and Fas (CD95)-mediated apoptosis in Alzheimer's disease. *Journal of the neurological sciences* 152(1), 73-83.

Delobel, P., Lavenir, I., Fraser, G., Ingram, E., Holzer, M., Ghetti, B., Spillantini, M. G., Crowther, R. A. & Goedert, M. (2008). Analysis of tau phosphorylation and truncation in a mouse model of human tauopathy. *Am J Pathol* 172(1), 123-31.

Dickson, D. W. (2004). Apoptotic mechanisms in Alzheimer neurofibrillary degeneration: cause or effect? *J Clin Invest* 114(1), 23-7.

Ding, H., Matthews, T. A. & Johnson, G. V. (2006). Site-specific phosphorylation and caspase cleavage differentially impact tau-microtubule interactions and tau aggregation. *J Biol Chem* 281(28), 19107-14.

Du, J. T., Yu, C. H., Zhou, L. X., Wu, W. H., Lei, P., Li, Y., Zhao, Y. F., Nakanishi, H. & Li, Y. M. (2007). Phosphorylation modulates the local conformation and self-aggregation ability of a peptide from the fourth tau microtubule-binding repeat. *Febs J* 274(19), 5012-20.

Fasulo, L., Ugolini, G., Visintin, M., Bradbury, A., Brancolini, C., Verzillo, V., Novak, M. & Cattaneo, A. (2000). The neuronal microtubule-associated protein tau is a substrate for caspase-3 and an effector of apoptosis. *Journal of neurochemistry* 75(2), 624-33.

Fox, N., Harvey, R. J. & Rossor, M. N. (1996). Protein folding, nucleation phenomena and delayed neurodegeneration in Alzheimer's disease. *Rev Neurosci* 7(1), 21-8.

Gamblin, T. C., Berry, R. W. & Binder, L. I. (2003a). Tau polymerization: role of the amino terminus. *Biochemistry* 42(7), 2252-7.

Gamblin, T. C., Chen, F., Zambrano, A., Abraha, A., Lagalwar, S., Guillozet, A. L., Lu, M., Fu, Y., Garcia-Sierra, F., LaPointe, N., Miller, R., Berry, R. W., Binder, L. I. & Cryns, V. L. (2003b). Caspase cleavage of tau: linking amyloid and neurofibrillary tangles in Alzheimer's disease. *Proc Natl Acad Sci U S A* 100(17), 10032-7.

Garcia-Sierra, F., Ghoshal, N., Quinn, B., Berry, R. W. & Binder, L. I. (2003). Conformational changes and truncation of tau protein during tangle evolution in Alzheimer's disease. *J. Alzheimers Dis.* 5(2), 65-77.

Garcia-Sierra, F., Hauw, J. J., Duyckaerts, C., Wischik, C. M., Luna-Munoz, J. & Mena, R. (2000). The extent of neurofibrillary pathology in perforant pathway neurons is the key determinant of dementia in the very old. *Acta Neuropathol (Berl)* 100(1), 29-35.

Garcia-Sierra, F., Mondragon-Rodriguez, S. & Basurto-Islas, G. (2008). Truncation of tau protein and its pathological significance in Alzheimer's disease. *J Alzheimers Dis* 14(4), 401-9.

Garcia-Sierra, F., Wischik, C. M., Harrington, C. R., Luna-Munoz, J. & Mena, R. (2001). Accumulation of C-terminally truncated tau protein associated with vulnerability of the perforant pathway in early stages of neurofibrillary pathology in Alzheimer's disease. *J Chem Neuroanat* 22(1-2), 65-77.

Ghoshal, N., Garcia-Sierra, F., Fu, Y., Beckett, L. A., Mufson, E. J., Kuret, J., Berry, R. W. & Binder, L. I. (2001). Tau-66: evidence for a novel tau conformation in Alzheimer's disease. *J Neurochem* 77(5), 1372-85.

Ghoshal, N., Garcia-Sierra, F., Wuu, J., Leurgans, S., Bennett, D. A., Berry, R. W. & Binder, L. I. (2002). Tau conformational changes correspond to impairments of episodic memory in mild cognitive impairment and Alzheimer's disease. *Exp Neurol* 177(2), 475-93.

Ghoshal, N., Smiley, J. F., DeMaggio, A. J., Hoekstra, M. F., Cochran, E. J., Binder, L. I. & Kuret, J. (1999). A new molecular link between the fibrillar and granulovacuolar lesions of Alzheimer's disease. *Am J Pathol* 155(4), 1163-72.

Gold, R., Schmied, M., Giegerich, G., Breitschopf, H., Hartung, H. P., Toyka, K. V. & Lassmann, H. (1994). Differentiation between cellular apoptosis and necrosis by the combined use of *in situ* tailing and nick translation techniques. *Laboratory investigation; a journal of technical methods and pathology* 71(2), 219-25.

Gomez-Isla, T., Hollister, R., West, H., Mui, S., Growdon, J. H., Petersen, R. C., Parisi, J. E. & Hyman, B. T. (1997). Neuronal loss correlates with but exceeds neurofibrillary tangles in Alzheimer's disease. *Annals of neurology* 41(1), 17-24.

Gotz, J., Ittner, L. M., Fandrich, M. & Schonrock, N. (2008). Is tau aggregation toxic or protective: a sensible question in the absence of sensitive methods? *J Alzheimers Dis* 14(4), 423-9.

Greenberg, S. G. & Davies, P. (1990). A preparation of Alzheimer paired helical filaments that displays distinct tau proteins by polyacrylamide gel electrophoresis. *Proc Natl Acad Sci U S A* 87(15), 5827-31.

Grundke-Iqbal, I., Iqbal, K., Quinlan, M., Tung, Y. C., Zaidi, M. S. & Wisniewski, H. M. (1986a). Microtubule-associated protein tau. A component of Alzheimer paired helical filaments. *J Biol Chem* 261(13), 6084-9.

Grundke-Iqbal, I., Iqbal, K., Tung, Y. C., Quinlan, M., Wisniewski, H. M. & Binder, L. I. (1986b). Abnormal phosphorylation of the microtubule-associated protein tau (tau) in Alzheimer cytoskeletal pathology. *Proc Natl Acad Sci U S A* 83(13), 4913-7.

Guillozet-Bongaarts, A. L., Cahill, M. E., Cryns, V. L., Reynolds, M. R., Berry, R. W. & Binder, L. I. (2006). Pseudophosphorylation of tau at serine 422 inhibits caspase cleavage: *in vitro* evidence and implications for tangle formation in vivo. *J Neurochem* 97(4), 1005-14.

Guillozet-Bongaarts, A. L., Garcia-Sierra, F., Reynolds, M. R., Horowitz, P. M., Fu, Y., Wang, T., Cahill, M. E., Bigio, E. H., Berry, R. W. & Binder, L. I. (2005). Tau truncation during neurofibrillary tangle evolution in Alzheimer's disease. *Neurobiology of aging* 26(7), 1015-22.

Guillozet-Bongaarts, A. L., Glajch, K. E., Libson, E. G., Cahill, M. E., Bigio, E., Berry, R. W. & Binder, L. I. (2007). Phosphorylation and cleavage of tau in non-AD tauopathies. *Acta Neuropathol (Berl)* 113(5), 513-20.

Guo, J. L. & Lee, V. M. (2011). Seeding of normal tau by pathological tau conformers drives pathogenesis of Alzheimer-like tangles. *The Journal of biological chemistry.*

Gustke, N., Steiner, B., Mandelkow, E. M., Biernat, J., Meyer, H. E., Goedert, M. & Mandelkow, E. (1992). The Alzheimer-like phosphorylation of tau protein reduces microtubule binding and involves Ser-Pro and Thr-Pro motifs. *FEBS Lett* 307(2), 199-205.

Honson, N. S. & Kuret, J. (2008). Tau aggregation and toxicity in tauopathic neurodegenerative diseases. *J Alzheimers Dis* 14(4), 417-22.

Hoozemans, J. J., van Haastert, E. S., Nijholt, D. A., Rozemuller, A. J., Eikelenboom, P. & Scheper, W. (2009). The unfolded protein response is activated in pretangle neurons in Alzheimer's disease hippocampus. *Am J Pathol* 174(4), 1241-51.

Horowitz, P. M., Patterson, K. R., Guillozet-Bongaarts, A. L., Reynolds, M. R., Carroll, C. A., Weintraub, S. T., Bennett, D. A., Cryns, V. L., Berry, R. W. & Binder, L. I. (2004). Early N-terminal changes and caspase-6 cleavage of tau in Alzheimer's disease. *J Neurosci* 24(36), 7895-902.

Hyman, B. T., Augustinack, J. C. & Ingelsson, M. (2005). Transcriptional and conformational changes of the tau molecule in Alzheimer's disease. *Biochim Biophys Acta* 1739(2-3), 150-7.

Hyman, B. T., Van Hoesen, G. W., Wolozin, B. L., Davies, P., Kromer, L. J. & Damasio, A. R. (1988). Alz-50 antibody recognizes Alzheimer-related neuronal changes. *Ann Neurol* 23(4), 371-9.

Iqbal, K., del, C. A. A. & Grundke-Iqbal, I. (2008). Cytosolic abnormally hyperphosphorylated tau but not paired helical filaments sequester normal MAPs and inhibit microtubule assembly. *J Alzheimers Dis* 14(4), 365-70.

Iqbal, K. & Grundke-Iqbal, I. (2008). Alzheimer neurofibrillary degeneration: significance, etiopathogenesis, therapeutics and prevention. *Journal of cellular and molecular medicine* 12(1), 38-55.

Iqbal, K., Wang, X., Blanchard, J., Liu, F., Gong, C. X. & Grundke-Iqbal, I. (2010). Alzheimer's disease neurofibrillary degeneration: pivotal and multifactorial. *Biochemical Society transactions* 38(4), 962-6.

Jeganathan, S., Hascher, A., Chinnathambi, S., Biernat, J., Mandelkow, E. M. & Mandelkow, E. (2008). Proline-directed pseudo-phosphorylation at AT8 and PHF1 epitopes induces a compaction of the paperclip folding of Tau and generates a pathological (MC-1) conformation. *J Biol Chem* 283(46), 32066-76.

Jicha, G. A., Bowser, R., Kazam, I. G. & Davies, P. (1997a). Alz-50 and MC-1, a new monoclonal antibody raised to paired helical filaments, recognize conformational epitopes on recombinant tau. *Journal of neuroscience research* 48(2), 128-32.

Jicha, G. A., Lane, E., Vincent, I., Otvos, L., Jr., Hoffmann, R. & Davies, P. (1997b). A conformation- and phosphorylation-dependent antibody recognizing the paired helical filaments of Alzheimer's disease. *J Neurochem* 69(5), 2087-95.

Kelly, J. W. (1996). Alternative conformations of amyloidogenic proteins govern their behavior. *Curr Opin Struct Biol* 6(1), 11-7.

Kidd, M. (2006). The history of the paired helical filaments. *J Alzheimers Dis* 9(3 Suppl), 71-5.

Kosik, K. S., Joachim, C. L. & Selkoe, D. J. (1986). Microtubule-associated protein tau (tau) is a major antigenic component of paired helical filaments in Alzheimer disease. *Proc Natl Acad Sci U S A* 83(11), 4044-8.

Kuhla, B., Haase, C., Flach, K., Luth, H. J., Arendt, T. & Munch, G. (2007). Effect of pseudophosphorylation and cross-linking by lipid peroxidation and advanced glycation end product precursors on tau aggregation and filament formation. *J Biol Chem* 282(10), 6984-91.

Lapointe, N. E., Morfini, G., Pigino, G., Gaisina, I. N., Kozikowski, A. P., Binder, L. I. & Brady, S. T. (2008). The amino terminus of tau inhibits kinesin-dependent axonal transport: Implications for filament toxicity. *J Neurosci Res.*

Latzer, J., Shen, T. & Wolynes, P. G. (2008). Conformational switching upon phosphorylation: a predictive framework based on energy landscape principles. *Biochemistry* 47(7), 2110-22.

Lee, H. G., Casadesus, G., Zhu, X., Takeda, A., Perry, G. & Smith, M. A. (2004). Challenging the amyloid cascade hypothesis: senile plaques and amyloid-beta as protective adaptations to Alzheimer disease. *Ann N Y Acad Sci* 1019, 1-4.

Lee, H. G., Castellani, R. J., Zhu, X., Perry, G. & Smith, M. A. (2005). Amyloid-beta in Alzheimer's disease: the horse or the cart? Pathogenic or protective? *Int J Exp Pathol* 86(3), 133-8.

Lee, V. M., Balin, B. J., Otvos, L., Jr. & Trojanowski, J. Q. (1991). A68: a major subunit of paired helical filaments and derivatized forms of normal Tau. *Science* 251(4994), 675-8.

Li, H. L., Wang, H. H., Liu, S. J., Deng, Y. Q., Zhang, Y. J., Tian, Q., Wang, X. C., Chen, X. Q., Yang, Y., Zhang, J. Y., Wang, Q., Xu, H., Liao, F. F. & Wang, J. Z. (2007). Phosphorylation of tau antagonizes apoptosis by stabilizing beta-catenin, a mechanism involved in Alzheimer's neurodegeneration. *Proc Natl Acad Sci U S A* 104(9), 3591-6.

Liu, F., Liang, Z. & Gong, C. X. (2006). Hyperphosphorylation of tau and protein phosphatases in Alzheimer disease. *Panminerva medica* 48(2), 97-108.

Lucassen, P. J., Chung, W. C., Kamphorst, W. & Swaab, D. F. (1997). DNA damage distribution in the human brain as shown by *in situ* end labeling; area-specific differences in aging and Alzheimer disease in the absence of apoptotic morphology. *Journal of neuropathology and experimental neurology* 56(8), 887-900.

Luna-Munoz, J., Chavez-Macias, L., Garcia-Sierra, F. & Mena, R. (2007). Earliest Stages of Tau Conformational Changes are Related to the Appearance of a Sequence of Specific Phospho-Dependent Tau Epitopes in Alzheimer's Disease. *J Alzheimers Dis* 12(4), 365-75.

Luna-Munoz, J., Garcia-Sierra, F., Falcon, V., Menendez, I., Chavez-Macias, L. & Mena, R. (2005). Regional conformational change involving phosphorylation of tau protein at the Thr231, precedes the structural change detected by Alz-50 antibody in Alzheimer's disease. *J Alzheimers Dis* 8(1), 29-41.

Maeda, S., Sahara, N., Saito, Y., Murayama, S., Ikai, A. & Takashima, A. (2006). Increased levels of granular tau oligomers: an early sign of brain aging and Alzheimer's disease. *Neuroscience research* 54(3), 197-201.

Mandelkow, E. M., Biernat, J., Drewes, G., Gustke, N., Trinczek, B. & Mandelkow, E. (1995). Tau domains, phosphorylation, and interactions with microtubules. *Neurobiology of aging* 16(3), 355-62; discussion 62-3.

Mandelkow, E. M., Drewes, G., Biernat, J., Gustke, N., Van Lint, J., Vandenheede, J. R. & Mandelkow, E. (1992). Glycogen synthase kinase-3 and the Alzheimer-like state of microtubule-associated protein tau. *FEBS Lett* 314(3), 315-21.

Mandelkow, E. M., Stamer, K., Vogel, R., Thies, E. & Mandelkow, E. (2003). Clogging of axons by tau, inhibition of axonal traffic and starvation of synapses. *Neurobiol Aging* 24(8), 1079-85.

Mena, R., Edwards, P., Perez-Olvera, O. & Wischik, C. M. (1995). Monitoring pathological assembly of tau and beta-amyloid proteins in Alzheimer's disease. *Acta Neuropathol (Berl)* 89(1), 50-6.

Mena, R., Edwards, P. C., Harrington, C. R., Mukaetova-Ladinska, E. B. & Wischik, C. M. (1996). Staging the pathological assembly of truncated tau protein into paired helical filaments in Alzheimer's disease. *Acta Neuropathol (Berl)* 91(6), 633-41.

Mondragon-Rodriguez, S., Basurto-Islas, G., Binder, L.I., & García-Sierra, F. (2009). Conformational changes and cleavage; are these responsible for the tau aggregation in Alzheimer's diasease?. *Future neurol* 4(1), 39-53.

Mondragon-Rodriguez, S., Mena, R., Binder, L. I., Smith, M. A., Perry, G. & Garcia-Sierra, F. (2008). Conformational changes and cleavage of tau in Pick bodies parallel the early processing of tau found in Alzheimer pathology. *Neuropathol Appl Neurobiol* 34(1), 62-75.

Murayama, S. & Saito, Y. (2004). Neuropathological diagnostic criteria for Alzheimer's disease. *Neuropathology* 24(3), 254-60.

Nagy, Z. S. & Esiri, M. M. (1997). Apoptosis-related protein expression in the hippocampus in Alzheimer's disease. *Neurobiology of aging* 18(6), 565-71.

Necula, M. & Kuret, J. (2004). Pseudophosphorylation and glycation of tau protein enhance but do not trigger fibrillization *in vitro*. *J Biol Chem* 279(48), 49694-703.

Newman, J., Rissman, R. A., Sarsoza, F., Kim, R. C., Dick, M., Bennett, D. A., Cotman, C. W., Rohn, T. T. & Head, E. (2005). Caspase-cleaved tau accumulation in neurodegenerative diseases associated with tau and alpha-synuclein pathology. *Acta Neuropathol* 110(2), 135-44.

Novak, M. (1994). Truncated tau protein as a new marker for Alzheimer's disease. *Acta Virol* 38(3), 173-89.

Novak, M., Jakes, R., Edwards, P. C., Milstein, C. & Wischik, C. M. (1991). Difference between the tau protein of Alzheimer paired helical filament core and normal tau revealed by epitope analysis of monoclonal antibodies 423 and 7.51. *Proceedings of the National Academy of Sciences of the United States of America* 88(13), 5837-41.

Novak, M., Kabat, J. & Wischik, C. M. (1993). Molecular characterization of the minimal protease resistant tau unit of the Alzheimer's disease paired helical filament. *Embo J* 12(1), 365-70.

Novak, M., Wischik, C. M., Edwards, P., Pannell, R. & Milstein, C. (1989). Characterisation of the first monoclonal antibody against the pronase resistant core of the Alzheimer PHF. *Prog Clin Biol Res* 317, 755-61.

Papasozomenos, S. C. & Binder, L. I. (1987). Phosphorylation determines two distinct species of Tau in the central nervous system. *Cell Motil Cytoskeleton* 8(3), 210-26.

Pritchard, S. M., Dolan, P. J., Vitkus, A. & Johnson, G. V. (2011). The Toxicity of Tau in Alzheimer Disease: Turnover, Targets and Potential Therapeutics. *Journal of cellular and molecular medicine.*

Rametti, A., Esclaire, F., Yardin, C. & Terro, F. (2004). Linking alterations in tau phosphorylation and cleavage during neuronal apoptosis. *J Biol Chem* 279(52), 54518-28.

Rissman, R. A., Poon, W. W., Blurton-Jones, M., Oddo, S., Torp, R., Vitek, M. P., LaFerla, F. M., Rohn, T. T. & Cotman, C. W. (2004). Caspase-cleavage of tau is an early event in Alzheimer disease tangle pathology. *J Clin Invest* 114(1), 121-30.

Rubinsztein, D. C. (2006). The roles of intracellular protein-degradation pathways in neurodegeneration. *Nature* 443(7113), 780-6.

Sadqi, M., Hernandez, F., Pan, U., Perez, M., Schaeberle, M. D., Avila, J. & Munoz, V. (2002). Alpha-helix structure in Alzheimer's disease aggregates of tau-protein. *Biochemistry* 41(22), 7150-5.

Sahara, N., Murayama, M., Lee, B., Park, J. M., Lagalwar, S., Binder, L. I. & Takashima, A. (2008). Active c-jun N-terminal kinase induces caspase cleavage of tau and additional phosphorylation by GSK-3beta is required for tau aggregation. *Eur J Neurosci* 27(11), 2897-906.

Salehi, A., Van de Nes, J. A., Hofman, M. A., Gonatas, N. K. & Swaab, D. F. (1995). Early cytoskeletal changes as shown by Alz-50 are not accompanied by decreased neuronal activity. *Brain Res* 678(1-2), 28-39.

Schaffer, B. A., Bertram, L., Miller, B. L., Mullin, K., Weintraub, S., Johnson, N., Bigio, E. H., Mesulam, M., Wiedau-Pazos, M., Jackson, G. R., Cummings, J. L., Cantor, R. M., Levey, A. I., Tanzi, R. E. & Geschwind, D. H. (2008). Association of GSK3B with Alzheimer disease and frontotemporal dementia. *Arch Neurol* 65(10), 1368-74.

Schneider, A., Biernat, J., von Bergen, M., Mandelkow, E. & Mandelkow, E. M. (1999). Phosphorylation that detaches tau protein from microtubules (Ser262, Ser214) also protects it against aggregation into Alzheimer paired helical filaments. *Biochemistry* 38(12), 3549-58.

Soto, C. (1999). Alzheimer's and prion disease as disorders of protein conformation: implications for the design of novel therapeutic approaches. *J Mol Med* 77(5), 412-8.

Stokin, G. B. & Goldstein, L. S. (2006). Axonal transport and Alzheimer's disease. *Annu Rev Biochem* 75, 607-27.

Thangavel, R., Sahu S. K., Van Hoesen, G. W., Zaheer, A. (2008). Modular and laminar pathology of Brosmann´s area 37 in Alzheimer´s disease. *Neuroscience* 152, 50-55.

Tourtellotte, W. G., Van Hoesen, G. W., Hyman, B. T., Tikoo, R. K. & Damasio, A. R. (1990). Alz-50 immunoreactivity in the thalamic reticular nucleus in Alzheimer's disease. *Brain Res* 515(1-2), 227-34.

Tseng, B. P., Kitazawa, M. & LaFerla, F. M. (2004). Amyloid beta-peptide: the inside story. *Curr Alzheimer Res* 1(4), 231-9.

van de Nes, J. A., Kamphorst, W., Ravid, R. & Swaab, D. F. (1998). Comparison of beta-protein/A4 deposits and Alz-50-stained cytoskeletal changes in the hypothalamus and adjoining areas of Alzheimer's disease patients: amorphic plaques and cytoskeletal changes occur independently. *Acta Neuropathol (Berl)* 96(2), 129-38.

Van Hoesen, G. W., Hyman, B. T. & Damasio, A. R. (1991). Entorhinal cortex pathology in Alzheimer's disease. *Hippocampus* 1(1), 1-8.

Vega, I. E., Cui, L., Propst, J. A., Hutton, M. L., Lee, G. & Yen, S. H. (2005). Increase in tau tyrosine phosphorylation correlates with the formation of tau aggregates. *Brain Res Mol Brain Res* 138(2), 135-44.

Vincent, I. J. & Davies, P. (1990). Phosphorylation characteristics of the A68 protein in Alzheimer's disease. *Brain Res* 531(1-2), 127-35.

Wang, J. Z., Grundke-Iqbal, I. & Iqbal, K. (1996). Restoration of biological activity of Alzheimer abnormally phosphorylated tau by dephosphorylation with protein phosphatase-2A, -2B and -1. *Brain Res Mol Brain Res* 38(2), 200-8.

Wang, J. Z., Wu, Q., Smith, A., Grundke-Iqbal, I. & Iqbal, K. (1998). Tau is phosphorylated by GSK-3 at several sites found in Alzheimer disease and its biological activity markedly inhibited only after it is prephosphorylated by A-kinase. *FEBS Lett* 436(1), 28-34.

Wang, Y., Martinez-Vicente, M., Kruger, U., Kaushik, S., Wong, E., Mandelkow, E. M., Cuervo, A. M. & Mandelkow, E. (2009). Tau fragmentation, aggregation and clearance: the dual role of lysosomal processing. *Human molecular genetics* 18(21), 4153-70.

Wischik, C. M., Edwards, P. C., Lai, R. Y., Gertz, H. N., Xuereb, J. H., Paykel, E. S., Brayne, C., Huppert, F. A., Mukaetova-Ladinska, E. B., Mena, R. & et al. (1995). Quantitative analysis of tau protein in paired helical filament preparations: implications for the role of tau protein phosphorylation in PHF assembly in Alzheimer's disease. *Neurobiol Aging* 16(3), 409-17; discussion 18-31.

Wischik, C. M., Novak, M., Edwards, P. C., Klug, A., Tichelaar, W. & Crowther, R. A. (1988a). Structural characterization of the core of the paired helical filament of Alzheimer disease. *Proceedings of the National Academy of Sciences of the United States of America* 85(13), 4884-8.

Wischik, C. M., Novak, M., Thogersen, H. C., Edwards, P. C., Runswick, M. J., Jakes, R., Walker, J. E., Milstein, C., Roth, M. & Klug, A. (1988b). Isolation of a fragment of tau derived from the core of the paired helical filament of Alzheimer disease. *Proceedings of the National Academy of Sciences of the United States of America* 85(12), 4506-10.

Wolozin, B. L., Pruchnicki, A., Dickson, D. W. & Davies, P. (1986). A neuronal antigen in the brains of Alzheimer patients. *Science* 232(4750), 648-50.

Yamamoto, H., Hiragami, Y., Murayama, M., Ishizuka, K., Kawahara, M. & Takashima, A. (2005). Phosphorylation of tau at serine 416 by Ca2+/calmodulin-dependent protein kinase II in neuronal soma in brain. *J Neurochem* 94(5), 1438-47.

Yang, L. S. & Ksiezak-Reding, H. (1995). Calpain-induced proteolysis of normal human tau and tau associated with paired helical filaments. *European journal of biochemistry / FEBS* 233(1), 9-17.

Yin, H. & Kuret, J. (2006). C-terminal truncation modulates both nucleation and extension phases of tau fibrillization. *FEBS Lett* 580(1), 211-5.

Zhu, X., Raina, A. K., Perry, G. & Smith, M. A. (2006). Apoptosis in Alzheimer disease: a mathematical improbability. *Curr Alzheimer Res* 3(4), 393-6.

8

Structure and Toxicity of the Prefibrillar Aggregation States of Beta Peptides in Alzheimer's Disease

Angelo Perico, Denise Galante and Cristina D'Arrigo
Institute for Macromolecular Studies (ISMAC, CNR)
Italy

1. Introduction

As in several neurodegenerative diseases, Alzheimer's disease (AD) arises when proteins fail to get their functional fold and aggregate in amyloid fibrils (Chiti & Dobson, 2006; Chiti et al., 2002). The Abeta peptides (Aβ), proteolytic products generated from beta-amyloid precursor protein (APP), are the subunits of amyloid fibrils that deposit in brain (Forloni et al., 2002; Selkoe, 1996, 2004). Aβ aggregates consist of a mixture of Aβ peptides around 40 aminoacids having different N- and C- termini (Russo et al., 2000). It is now largely accepted that the pathogenic species in AD are the toxic oligomeric aggregates of Aβ that assembly in the brain before the formation of amyloid fibrils (Chiti & Dobson, 2006; Kirkitadze et al., 2002; Walsh & Selkoe, 2007; Yankner & Lu, 2009). Oligomers extracted from AD brain potently impair synapse structure and function (Shankar et al, 2008). The structural characterization and neurotoxicity of these oligomeric aggregation states, even though very difficult to achieve due to the fast aggregation processes involved, to the heterogeneous peptide contents and transient organization, is of primary importance in the study of AD pathogenesis (Jahn et al., 2010).

Monomeric Aβ may assume in water a β-hairpin conformation stabilized by intramolecular H-bonds and antiparallel β-strands that lead to intermediate oligomeric states of Aβ subunits with intermolecular H-bonds and parallel β-strand organization (Campioni et al., 2010; Ono et al., 2009; Roychaudhuri et al., 2009; Sandbergh et al., 2010). More evidence of the structure of oligomers and protofibrils is required that may be obtained by TEM and AFM (Apetri et al., 2006; Pastor et al., 2008; Yoshiike et al., 2007). Recently, new AFM techniques enabled to image a dynamic of Aβ oligomer formation, consistent with the hairpin conformation hypothesis (Mastrangelo et al., 2006). Changing the peptide composition of these prefibrillar aggregates, significant differences in packing strength and solvent exposure are eventually achieved that may be strictly related to cell toxicity.

Between the different species of water-soluble β-peptides, found in abundance in the fibril brain deposits (full length Aβ1-42, Aβ1-40 and N-terminal truncated Aβs), Aβ*py*3-42, a peptide N-terminal truncated at residue 3 (Glu) and further modified by cyclization of Glu to pyroglutamic acid *py*Glu, (catalysed, both in vitro and in vivo, by glutamynil cyclase enzyme, upregulated in the cortices of AD individuals (Shilling et al., 2008)), may have an important role in the cooperative process leading to AD. The N termination at residue 3 in

Aβ*py*3-42 may change the attitude of the full length Aβ1-42 to aggregate gradually to a fibril organization, heading the β-peptide to a fast aggregation towards a relatively stable and toxic soluble oligomeric state.
Recently, the faster aggregation kinetics after incubation time of the N-terminal and pyro-modified peptides relative to the full length Aβ, were demonstrated together with significant morthological differences in the pure or mixed aggregation states (D'Arrigo et al., 2009; Shilling et al., 2006). Demuth and coll. gave indications that prevention of formation of pyroglutamate-modified N-terminally truncated Aβs, such as Aβ*py*3-42, by inhibition of glutaminyl cyclase, may represent a new therapeutic strategy for alleviating amyloidoses (Shilling et al., 2008). In general, N-terminal pyroglutamyl modifications increase the aggregation propensity and also enhances resistance to degradation by proteases (Shilling et al., 2004, 2006). Prevention of formation of pyroglutamate-modified N-terminally truncated Aβs may be beneficial for AD patients. The ratio of soluble Aβ species may dictate the role of these aggregates on the AD amyloidosis (He & Barrow, 1999): particularly the toxic effect of water-soluble Aβ on neurons seems to be related to the predominance of A*py*3-42 (Russo et al., 2002). This finding reinforces the idea that an adequate characterization of the oligomeric and prefibrillar states in terms of peptide content, structure and toxicity may be a promising appropriate strategy to design innovative therapies.
The intermedium water-soluble Aβ aggregation states and their assembly process, with a particular attention to the role of Aβ*py*3-42, will be the focus of the chapter.
In section 2., a review of the efforts to characterize the structure, organization and toxicity of the possible prefibrillar aggregation states is given. In section 3., the hypothesis of the possible role in AD of the N-truncated and pyromodified Aβ is described in comparison to full-length Aβ. In section 4., the inhibition of the most toxic prefibrillar aggregation states is discussed as a new therapeutic strategy in AD. In section 5., concluding remarks are reported on the possible new molecular therapeutic strategy in AD, based on the inhibition of the most toxic soluble Aβ oligomeric aggregation states.

2. Oligomeric aggregation states of beta amyloids in Alzheimer's disease

In this section we review recent advancements in the description and characterization of soluble oligomeric aggregates, their toxicity and possible role in Alzheimer pathogenesis (Campioni et al., 2010; Ono et al., 2009; Mastrangelo et al., 2006; Roychaudhuri et al., 2009; Sandbergh et al., 2010).
Soluble oligomers, as fractionated by size exclusion chromatography, are often classified as low molecular weight oligomers (< 10 monomers) and high molecular weight oligomers (in the range of 20-40 monomers) (Mastrangelo et al., 2006; Jahn et al., 2010; Walsh et al., 1999). Efforts to establish rigorous structure–toxicity correlations have been hindered by the complex, dynamic equilibria displayed by Aβ (Ono et al., 2009; Roychaudhuri et al., 2009) . To clarify this matter it is therefore preliminarly necessary to choose selected well-defined, stabilized oligomers for establishing rigorous structure activity correlations leading to knowledge-based therapeutic drug design (Ono et al., 2009). The technique of photo-induced cross-linking of unmodified proteins (PICUP) was used to stabilize oligomers of Aβ1-40 (Ono et al., 2009). The results are summarized quantitatively in Table1 where the oligomeric structure-toxicity characterization for uncross-linked, cross-linked, small oligomers and fibrils is reported from reference (Ono et al., 2009).
The data suggest that monomer/dimer transition involves the largest change in the conformation content, from random to β-sheet conformation, as observed by circular

dichroism (CD); while the three dimensional change in the dimensions (TEM and AFM) of the oligomers has its maximum in the dimer/trimer and trimer/tetramer transitions.

Sample	α-Helix*	β-Sheet*	SC*	Diameter†	Height‡	EC_{50}§
Uncross-linked	9.4	25.2	65.4	1.15 ± 0.17 (79)	0.14 ± 0.01 (135)	102.5 ± 5.6
Cross-linked	11.1	33.6	55.3	12.39 ± 2.13 (55)	2.93 ± 0.40 (56)	43.0 ± 2.7
Pure monomer	8.7	24.0	67.3	1.30 ± 0.13 (127)	0.24 ± 0.01 (178)	67.3 ± 8.7
Pure dimer	10.5	38.6	50.9	1.78 ± 0.23 (116)	0.53 ± 0.03 (165)	41.6 ± 3.9
Pure trimer	10.3	40.8	48.9	7.22 ± 1.12 (64)	0.94 ± 0.13 (67)	24.5 ± 1.9
Pure tetramer	12.7	44.9	42.4	11.00 ± 2.08 (39)	1.51 ± 0.30 (38)	20.5 ± 0.4
Fibrils	ND	57.0	43.0	ND	ND	57.6 ± 2.2

ND, not determined.
*CD data are expressed as percent of each secondary structure element.
†Mean diameter ± SE, in nm, is listed for (*n*) Aβ assemblies visualized by EM.
‡Mean height ± SE, in nm, is listed for (*n*) Aβ assemblies visualized by AFM.
§Effective concentration (EC_{50}) is the concentration of a particular Aβ assembly that produced a level of toxicity in MTT assays that was half maximal. EC_{50} [mean concentration (μM) ± SE] values were calculated after sigmoidal curve fitting of the data shown in Fig. S5, using GraphPad Prism software (version 4.0a).

Table 1. Characteristics of Aβ assemblies

Finally MTT analysis (last column in Table 1, represented as the concentration in μM of a particular assembly that produced a level of toxicity in MTT assays that was half maximal) says that both cross-linked oligomeric Aβ and fibrillar Aβ were significantly more toxic than unassembled Aβ (dimers three-fold and tetramers 13-fold more toxic than monomers). One of the main results is the confirmation that monomers have very low toxicity activity while only when Aβ self associate, toxicity rises substantially, even though it is impossible to establish a degree of increasing toxicity with the number of monomers in the given oligomer because of the decrease in occurrence frequency of higher order oligomers. The authors suggest as a possible therapeutic strategy in AD to target the low order oligomers to unstabilize the most toxic Aβ contributing to AD neurotoxicity (Ono et al., 2009).

Monomeric Aβ has the propensity to adopt in water solutions different conformations, including transient extended β-sheet conformations in the central and C-terminal regions, connected by turn between them, or β-hairpin (see Figure 1, panel A) (Hou et al., 2004; Mitternachet et al., 2010; Sandbergh et al., 2010).

When a synthetic or purified and denatured monomeric Aβ (say the full length peptide Aβ1-42 or the C-terminal truncated Aβ1-40 or the N-terminal truncated Aβ3-42 and modified Aβ*py*3-42,...) is incubated in a native buffer, peptide aggregates are formed showing oligomeric species increasing in molecular weight, initially found by CD in a disordered (random) conformation that may transiently convert into β-sheet oligomers that assemble further into protofibrils, following distinct pathways according to the original monomer peptide. Some of these transient oligomeric aggregation states may be built by subunits in the hairpin conformation after conversion of intramolecular Hbonds and antiparallel β-strands into intermolecular Hbonds and parallel β-sheets (Hoyer et al., 2008). By engineering a double cysteine mutant, in which the β-hairpin is stabilized by an intramolecular disulfide bond, Aβ1-40 and Aβ1-42 are transformed into Aβ40CC and Aβ42CC, becoming building block of toxic Aβ oligomers, unable to convert into amyloid fibrils (Sandbergh et al., 2010) (see figure 1).

In figure 1, panel A, the transient β-hairpin is first compared with the stabilized β-hairpin by the two disulfide bonds in the double cystein mutants, in panel B (ThT fluorescence assay) it is shown that Aβ40CC is unable to transform, after incubation, in fibrils being blocked in the oligomeric form (see relative TEM micrograpghs, panel C), evolution that is recovered after treatment of Aβ40CC with the reducing agent TCEP. The neurotoxicity of different AβCC aggregates was assayed by measuring their ability to induce apoptosis (level of caspase-3/7 activity in human neuroblastoma cell line, SH-SY5Y) (Sandbergh et al., 2010). Aβ42CC aggregates, pooled from SEC, all induce apoptosis 24 hr after addition to the cells, but β-sheet oligomer fractions are considerably more toxic than low molecular weight or high molecular weight fractions of Aβ42CC: the β-sheet oligomers (at 1μM) resulted 50 times more potent than wild-type Aβ42 monomer or fibril samples (see figure 2).

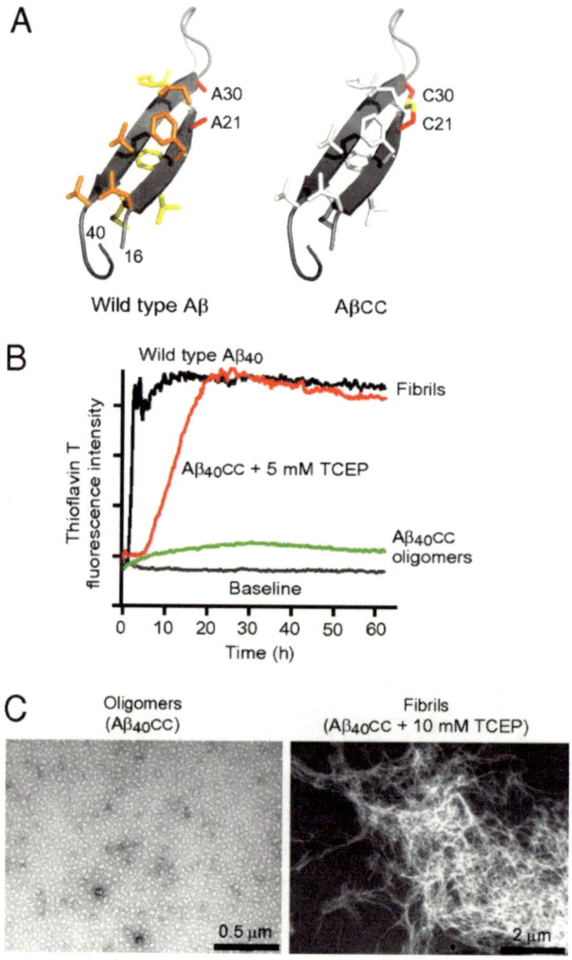

Fig. 1. Panel A. On the left, the β-hairpin conformation of $A\beta_{40}$ in complex with an Affibody binding protein [29]; the ALA21 and ALA30 methyls are located in close proximity on opposite β-strands. On the right, model of double-mutated Aβ A21C and A30C, AβCC, in which the β-hairpin conformation is locked by a disulfide bond. Panel B. ThT fluorescence assays of $A\beta_{40}CC$ aggregation in the absence or presence of reducing agent (TCEP), compared with wild-type $A\beta_{40}$ aggregation. Panel C. TEM micrographs of β-sheet oligomers of $A\beta_{40}CC$ (left) and of fibrils formed in presence of TCEP (right). Adapted from Figure 1 of reference (Sandbergh et al., 2010).

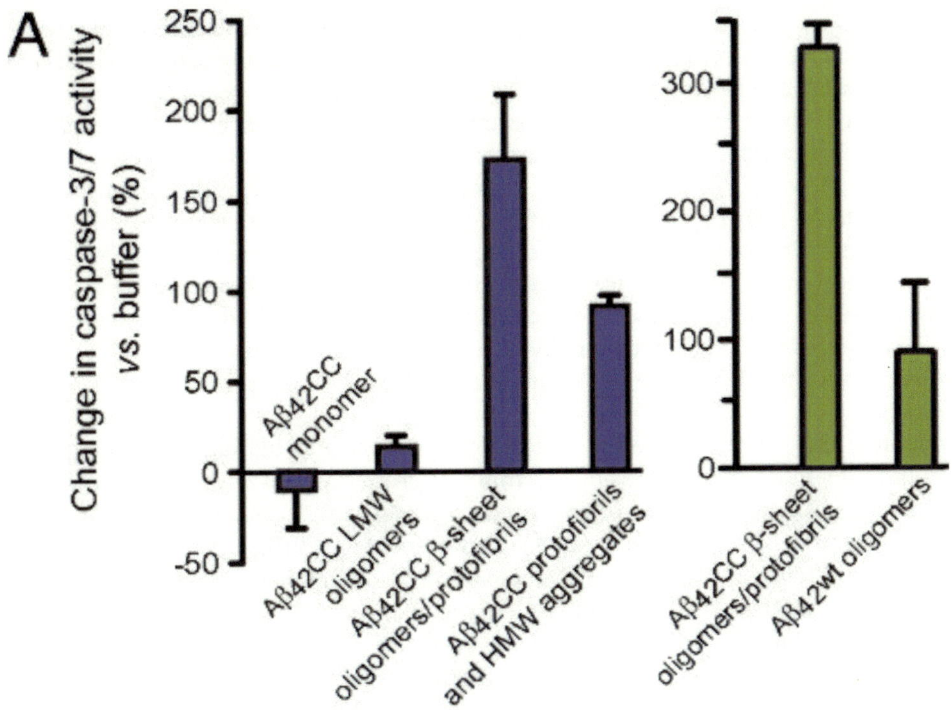

Fig. 2. Neutoxicity of AβCC to SH-SY5Y human neuroblastoma cells. Caspase-3/7 activity reporting on apoptosis was measured after 24 h of treatment with 10 μM of different $A\beta_{42}CC$ species (blue); $A\beta_{42}CC$ oligomers compared with wild-type $A\beta_{42}$ (green). Adapted from Figure 4 of reference (Sandbergh et al., 2010).

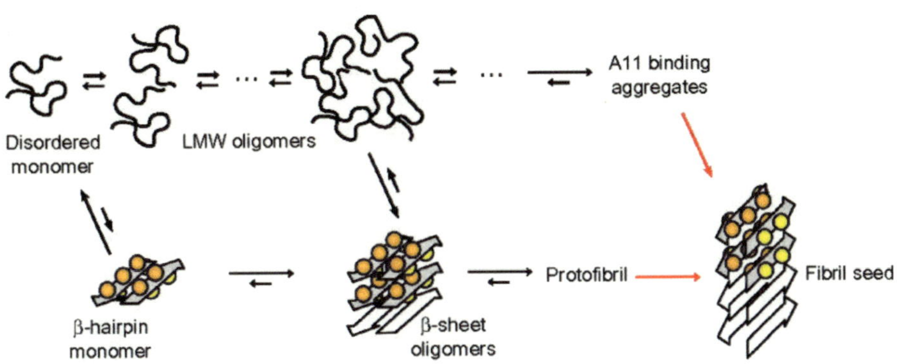

Fig. 3. Aβ aggregation via two pathways. Disordered pathway: upper; toxic β-sheet oligomers pathway: lower. Adapted from Figure 5 of reference (Sandbergh et al., 2010).

In conclusion an aggregation scheme was proposed as synthesized in figure 3 (Sandbergh et al., 2010). It is possible that the aggregation and kinetic plasticity of Aβ leads to different pathways for amyloid formation, having different impacts on AD pathogenesis (figure 3): one pathway involves disorganized oligomers and large non fibrillar aggregates (disordered less toxic pathway) and the other involves assembly in β-sheet oligomers which in turn may be the building blocks of protofibrils as the penultimate intermediate before fibril seeds formation (toxic β-sheet oligomers pathway). Aβ42CC more readily forms β-sheet oligomers than Aβ40CC, probably as a result of the presence of a kinetic barrier to oligomer formation that can only be overcome by Aβ40CC with the aid of heating and concentration (Sandbergh et al., 2010). It is possible that the stronger toxicity found for Aβ42 in respect to Aβ40 reflects different barriers to β-sheet oligomer formation. Accordingly, the former peptide may follow the toxic β-sheet oligomers pathway while the latter may follow the disordered pathway. This concept of kinetic partitioning of Aβ into two or more aggregation pathways may be important in AD progress, and at the same time the choice between the different pathways is very subtle because morphologically very similar oligomers may show different cell toxicity. A demonstration of this hyperfine behaviour was finely given by considering a protein model, the 91 residue N-terminal domain HypF-N of Escherichia coli (Campioni et al., 20 10).

This protein, prepared in different conditions, gives two stable oligomers HypF-N-A and HypF-N-B of similar morphological and tintorial properties but with the first one very toxic and the second one almost non toxic versus human neuroblastoma cells (SH-SY5Y), via MTT and Hend assays (figure 4, panel A) (Campioni et al., 2010).

To gain insight into the structural differences of the two oligomers HypF-N-A and HypF-N-B, 18 mutational variants of the protein were expressed, each carrying a single cysteine residue but located at different positions along the polypeptide chain, and labeled with a pyrene. Each labeled variant was allowed to aggregate separately, analysing the resulting fluorescence spectra with the eventual formation of pyrene excimers as a probe of the proximity (about 1 nm) of labelled pairs. It was shown that the structural hydrophobic core of the non-toxic HypF-N-B oligomers is more compact and less solved exposed (see figure 4, panel B) than the less tightly packed core of the toxic HypF-N-A oligomers. This demonstrates that the difference in cell membrane interaction and ability to cause cell dysfunction is due to the small differences in structural flexibility and solvent exposure of the core residues.

Toxicity is associated with the ability of the oligomeric species to form a more pronounced and disruptive interaction with cells, by exposure to the solvent of the surfaces of hydrophobic disorganized residues and thus leading to cell death. Thus, the protein model HypF-N has allowed oligomeric states, that would normally be metastable, to be trapped and therefore studied, with conclusions probably valid for the toxic properties of many oligomers in disease-related systems (Campioni et al., 2010).

Summarizing (Campioni et al., 2010; Sandbergh et al., 2010), to form amyloid-like structures is *generic* to polypeptide chains, but whether or not these species are pathogenic depends on their structural features, notably the extent to which hydrophobic residues are *flexible and exposed* on their surfaces within the environment of a living organism. Thus it seems that for therapeutic purposes the toxicity can be substantially reduced if the hydrophobic residues are incorporated to a greater extent within the interior of the oligomeric assemblies, even in the absence of an effective change in morphology: solvent-exposed structurally disorganized hydrophobic residues within small protein oligomers are at the origin of the pathogenesis of important human diseases.

Nevertheless the world of Aβ assembly still is too complex to be conclusive on the related biological activity in neurodegenerative diseases and fundamental questions remains to be clarified such as: is Aβ the main proximate etiologic agent of AD?; what is the structure of the proximate neurotoxic Aβ assembly? (Roychaudhuri et al., 2009).

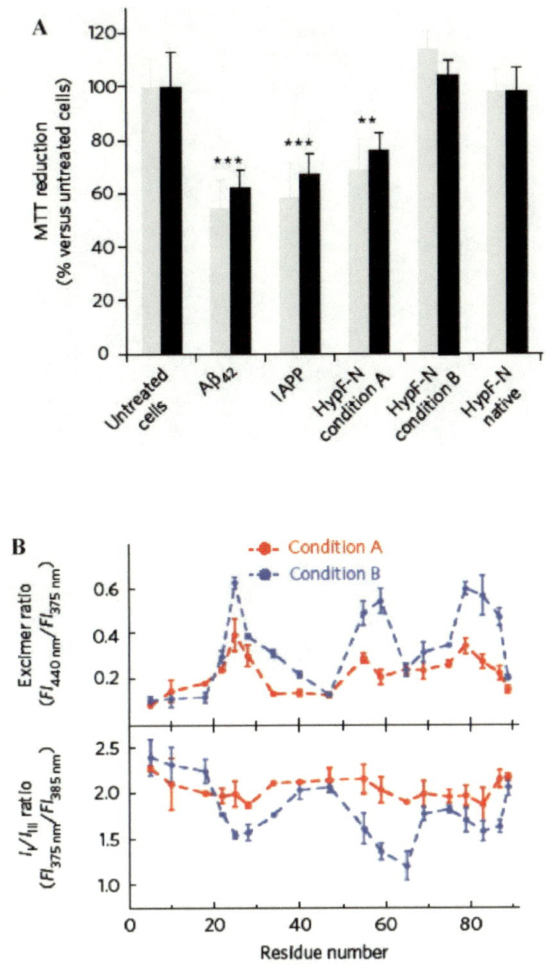

Fig. 4. Toxicity of HypF-N aggregates. Panel A. MTT reduction assay on SH-SY5Y (gray) and Hend (black) cells untreated (lane 1), or treated with Aβ1-42 oligomers (lane 2), control IAPP oligomers (lane 3), HypF-N aggregates under condition A (lane 4) and B (lane 5) and native HypF-N (lane 6). Panel B. Pyrene fluorescence emission spectra: excimer ratio profiles of HypF-N oligomers formed under condition A (red) and B(blue). Adapted from Figures 1 and 3 of reference (Campioni et al., 2010).

One of the main problems is to well characterize the structure of oligomeric states even when well followed: normally this is done by TEM and AFM with a lack of resolution to characterize such small and dynamic structures. Recently, a new approach in AFM was developed at LifeAFM , Port Jefferson (NY), that yields high-resolution images and allows to observe the structure of the smallest MW oligomers (Mastrangelo et al., 2006). The new AFM methodology, at difference with conventional tapping mode AFM, is based on a single low-force touch of the cantilever tip, enabling a non-destructive imaging of Aβ and observation of the small Mw oligomers. AFM of Aβ42 at early incubation time, give images of monomers, dimers, trimers, tetramers and other low Mw oligomers that are consistent with the hairpin structure, above described (Figure 5) (Mastrangelo et al., 2006).

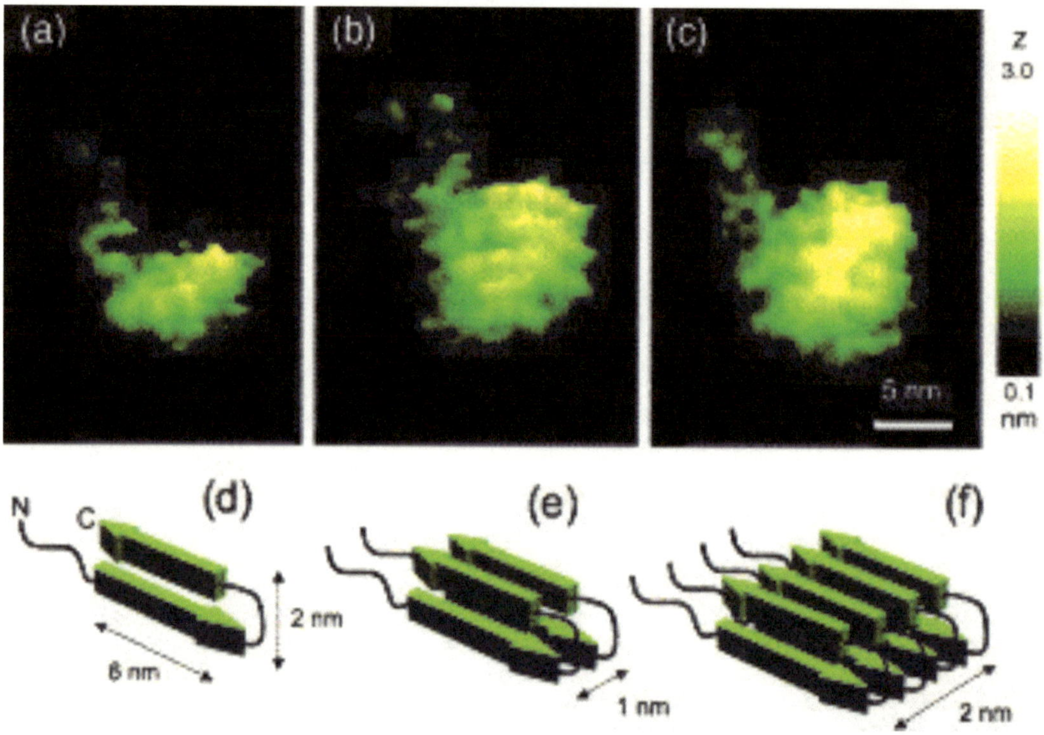

Fig. 5. High resolution AFM of Aβ1-42. AFM images are interpreted as panel A: a dimer; panel B and C: a tetramer. In each image the diffuse area to the left of the particle is interpreted as the disordered N-terminal region of the Aβ1-42 monomer. Adapted from Figure 4 of reference (Mastrangelo et al., 2006).

For the first time, images of such small oligomers were obtained, that may be interpreted as hairpin monomer, dimer and tetramer (see panels d, e and f). Note that the structures described above were found also in Alzheimer brains and should be present in the toxicity studies to clarify what structural features of the soluble oligomers are responsible of toxicity (Mastrangelo et al., 2006).

3. Comparison of N-truncated and pyromodified Aβ to full-length Aβ aggregation states: Transient aggregation states and kinetics

The N-terminal truncated and pyroglutamyl modified Aβ, as summarized in the introduction, accounts for the majority of the deposited peptides and of the most toxic effects on neurons. Recently, it was demonstrated that, in similar initial buffer conditions and using three different techniques (flow cytometry, ThT fluorescence and circular dichroism), these N-terminal modified peptides aggregate much faster than the full-length Aβ (D'Arrigo et al., 2009; Shilling et al., 2006). Altogether, the aggregation kinetics of Aβ*py*3-42 was found 20-250 by cytometry and ThT fluorescence (Shilling et al., 2006) and more than 30 times by CD (D'Arrigo et al., 2009) faster than that of Aβ1-42 respectively, depending upon the assay method. The oligomers that form β-structure rapidly are found to be more toxic (D'Arrigo et al., 2009; Mastrangelo et al., 2006; Shilling et al., 2006).

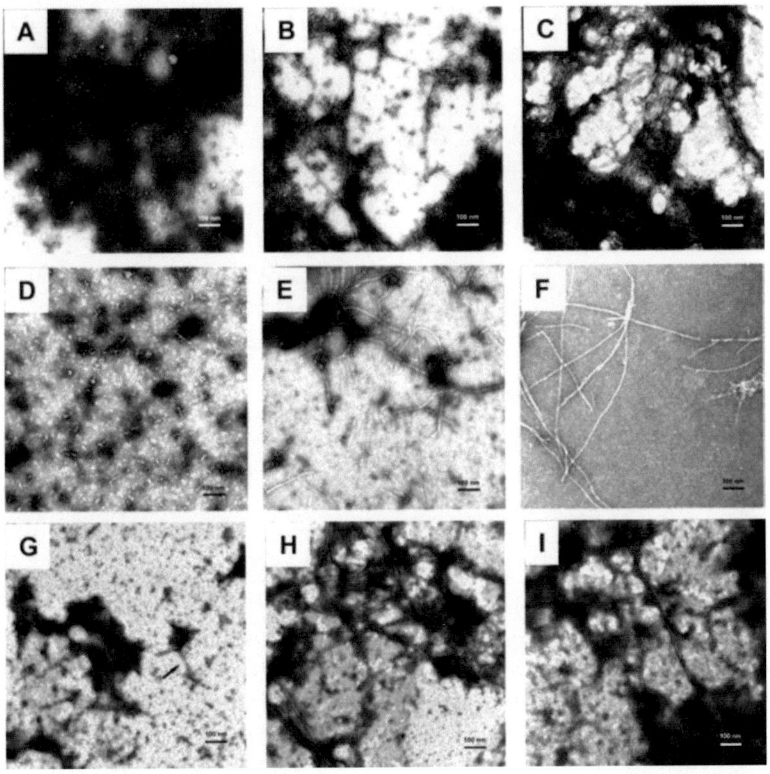

Fig. 6. The peptide TEM morphology after incubation in 20 mM phosphate buffer, pH 7.4 at 37 °C. Aβ1-42: panel A, at initial incubation time; panel B, after 1 day of incubation; panel C, after 2 days of incubation. Aβ*py*3-42: panel D, at initial incubation time; panel E, after 1 day of incubation; panel F, after 2 days of incubation. The 1:1 mixture Aβ1-42/Aβ*py*3-42: panel G, at initial incubation time (the arrow points to a protofibril); panel H, after 1 day incubation; panel I, after 2 days of incubation. Peptides concentrations: 50 μM. Adapted from Figures 6 and 7 of reference (D'Arrigo et al., 2009).

In addition the aggregation pathway of the two Aβ leads to more toxic dynamic oligomeric states for Aβ*py*3-42 and to fibril formation for Aβ1-42, see for instance (D'Arrigo et al., 2009) and (He & Barrow, 1999), while when the two are mixed (e.g. in a 1:1 ratio) Aβ*py*3-42 has an inhibitory effect on the fibrillogenesis of Aβ1-42, favouring prefibrillar aggregation states, that are more toxic for the cells (see Figure 6) (D'Arrigo et al., 2009).

These experiments confirm the strong role of Aβ*py*3-42 on the progression of Alzheimer pathogenesis (D'Arrigo et al., 2009; Jan et al., 2008).

The Aβ peptides display regions that are more affected by environmental conditions which may be responsible for conformational transitions and for different aggregation states and kinetics towards fibrillization (D'Arrigo et al., 2009). This has been confirmed experimentally, especially by NMR (Danielsson et al., 2006; Hou et al., 2004; Tomaselli et al., 2006), and it can be well illustrated by a simple model using the basic properties of the 20 aminoacids. In Figure 7 a model of the two Aβ peptides, Aβ1-42 and Aβ*py*3-42, is reported (D'Arrigo et al., 2009), as a string of pearls where each pearl represents one amino acid. Each aminoacid has one of 5 colours, each colour corresponding to the 5 generic standard classification of the 20 aminoacids: red, negatively charged residue; blue, positively charged residue; yellow, polar residue; black, hydrophobic residue; white, Gly residue. The C-terminals of the three peptides and the N-terminal of Aβ1-42 are represented by red and blue squares respectively.

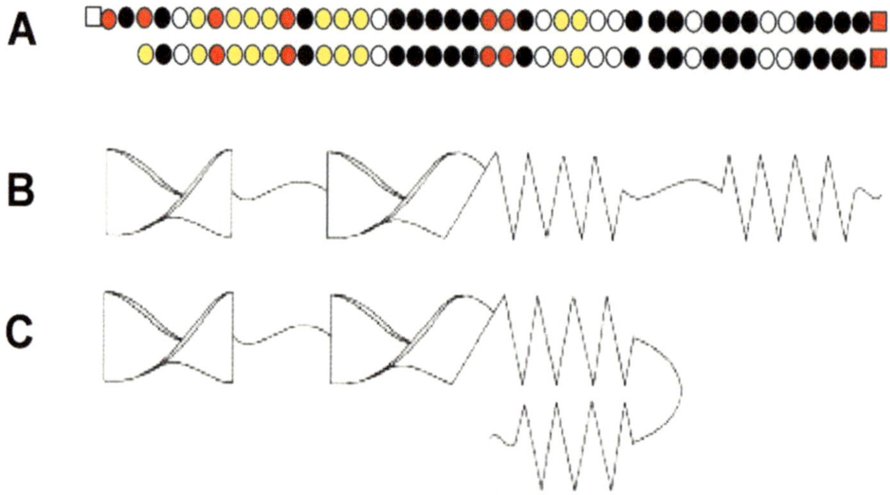

Fig. 7. Five colors representation pearl chain model of Aβ1-42 and Aβ*py*3-42 8 (panel A). Red pearl: negatively charged residue; Blue pearl: positively charged residue; Yellow pearl: polar residue; Black pearl: hydrophobic residue; White pearl: Gly residue. The C-terminals of the two peptides and the N-terminal of Aβ1-42 are represented by red and blue squares respectively. Conformation of Aβ1-40, according to NMR analysis (panel B) of ref. [32]. The proposed β-hairpin structure of toxic oligomers (panel C), see ref. [32]. Adapted from Figure 9 of reference (D'Arrigo et al., 2009) and Figure 6 of reference (Danielsson et al., 2006).

The central hydrophobic region 16-24 is crucial for the β-sheet forming oligomerization and subsequent fibril formation (Danielsson et al., 2006) and is well identified in the 5-colour representation. On the contrary the N-terminal region 1-16 has a large propensity, demonstrated by NMR, to be in an extended (especially at low temperature, where, accordingly, Aβ is found more soluble) PII-helix which is retained going from apolar to polar environments, or binding metal ions, or partially retained raising the temperature (Danielsson et al., 2006; Tomaselli et al., 2006). Again the NMR findings have a rough correspondence with the 1-16 sequence in the 5 colour representation of Aβ1-42, even though the correlation is less strong. Reducing or removing the helix propensity of the N-terminal region may favor a faster and different aggregation. One way to realize this enhancement of the aggregation process is just to destabilize the N-terminal region of Aβ1-42 by truncating the first two residues and by pyroglutamyl termination to Aβ*py*3-42. Going from Aβ1-42 to Aβ*py*3-42 the N-terminal portion of Aβ suffers important and indicative changes: the negative charges decrease from 7 to 5, the positive charges from 4 to 3, globally the terminal chain loosing 3 charges, while the hydrophobic residues decrease only by one in favour of an equal increase in polar residues. On this basis one may infer (D'Arrigo et al., 2009) that the helix propensity of the N-terminal is strongly reduced and the peptide, in which the central hydrophobic part did not make any change, is now more prone to the β conformational state and to aggregation, as observed by CD (D'Arrigo et al., 2009; He & Barrow, 1999).

Different Aβ peptides, full-length and truncated and modified, do have different attitude to develop the cross-β structure conformation with big consequences not only on fibrillization but also on the aggregation kinetics and on the formation of different prefibrillar aggregation states. So these N-terminal truncations and pyroglutamil modifications of Aβ1-42 have the consequences of accelerating the initial aggregation kinetics, directing it towards faster oligomerization. In addition, the *py*-Glu residue prevents degradation of the peptide by aminopeptidase (Shilling et al., 2004, 2006) and at the same time, as demonstrated by TEM, Aβ*py*3-42 inhibits the great propensity of the full-length peptide to aggregate in fibrils, favouring and stabilizing pre-fibrillar aggregation states that may be very toxic for the cells and for the progression of Alzheimer pathogenesis (D'Arrigo et al., 2009).

4. Inhibition of the most toxic prefibrillar aggregates as a new therapeutic strategy against Alzheimer pathogenesis

From sections 2 and 3 it comes out that a possible new therapeutic strategy against AD may be based on the inhibition of the highest toxic prefibrillar aggregates (Ono et al., 2009). As we have seen before, this means that attention should be directed to reduce the Aβ prefibrillar aggregations particularly of those more stable components which are organized in such a way to be greatly toxic to neuron cells. This logic suggests to target ordered oligomers and small ordered aggregates, destabilizing them in favour of disorder states. This is something that applies to all the forms of Aβ peptides, but it should be even of more importance to target special peptides such as the N-terminal truncated and pyroglutamyl modified peptides like Aβ*py*3-42. This strategy was strongly pursued by Demuth's group. In a remarkable 2008 paper on Nature Medicine (Shilling et al., 2008), Demuth and coll. Indicate, by experiments in vivo and in vitro, that inhibition of the level of glutaminyl cyclase (QC) in mammalian brains, where it is widely distributed, attenuates pyroglutamate Aβ and AD pathology.

To assess whether QC expression can be correlated with generation of Aβ*py*3-42 in AD, QC mRNA and protein concentrations in human neocortical brain samples post mortem were analysed (figure 8A). It was found that QC mRNA and protein were upregulated in samples from AD individuals, compared with samples from normal aging individuals; significantly larger concentrations of Aβ*py*3-42 were detected by ELISA analysis in the former individuals relative to the latter (figure 8B). This supports the role of QC in the generation of Aβ*py*3-42. In contrast high total Aβ*x*-42 concentrations in aged controls were found (figure 8B).

The protein APP and QC were co-expressed in HEK293 cells to study the correlations between QC expression and Aβ*py*3-42 generation (Shilling et al., 2008). When the first potent inhibitor for human QC, PDB150 (Buchholz et al., 2006), was added, the Aβ*py*3-42 formation was suppressed the most the highest the inhibitor dose, while the other non pyromodified peptides were not affected (figure 8C). This demonstrates the specific effect of the inhibitor on QC catalysis (figure 8C and 8D).

Subsequently PBD150 was orally applied to 4-month-old female Tg2576 mice for 6 months to study effects of QC inhibition on the Aβ*py*3-42 and on non pyromodified peptides in the insoluble Aβ pool (Shilling et al., 2008). Aβ*py*3-42 decreased by 23% and 65% according to the PBD150 dose as well as the non pyromodified peptides. Two are therefore the indications in vivo: Aβ*py*3-42 generation is mediated by QC and there is a correlation between Aβ*py*3-42 aggregation and total Aβ aggregation.

These interesting conlusions were confirmed by other experiments on the effects of QC inhibition on Tg256 mice and on TASD-41 mice (Shilling et al., 2008).

It seems to us that the conclusions of the authors of the above paper (Shilling et al., 2008), that prevention of pyroglutamate Aβ at the N-terminus by QC inhibition represents a new therapeutic strategy for alleviating amyloidoses caused by the seeding of amyloidogenic peptides, was well substantiated. This may represent an important step to get a first molecular strategy in AD therapy.

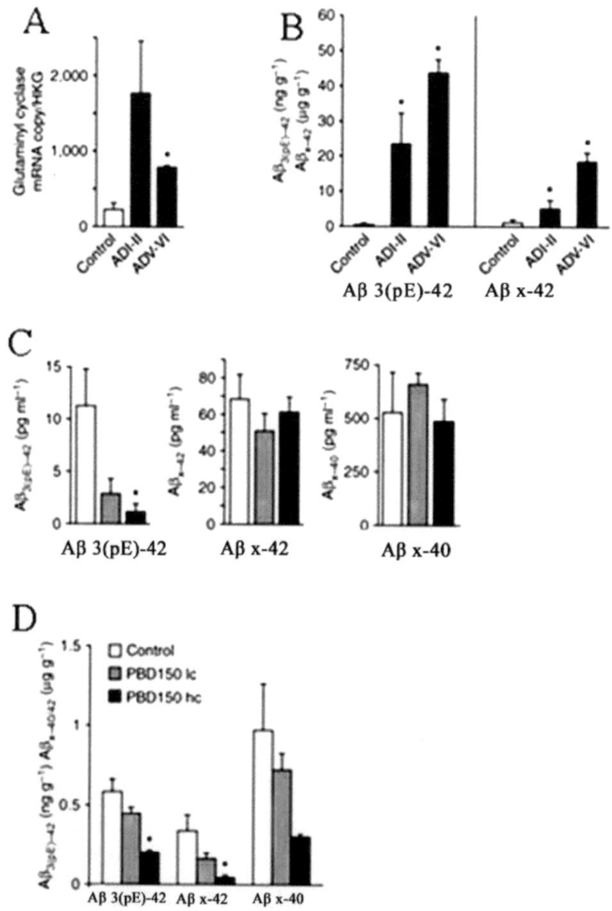

Fig. 8. Glutamynil cyclase (QC) expression and pyroglutamate-modified N-terminally truncated Aβ: prevention of Aβ*py* formation by glutamynil cyclase inhibition in vitro and in vivo. Panel A: quantitative analysis of QC transcript levels. Total RNA from human neocortical brain samples was isolated from aged controls and individuals with AD (the Roman numerals in ADI, ADII, ADV-VI refer to Braak stages). Panel B: Quantification of Aβ*py*3-42 and Aβ1-42 concentrations from the samples of Panel A by ELISA analysis. Panel C: quantification of Aβ concentrations in conditioned media of HEK293 cells, which were transiently transfected with an APPsw/l variant and human QC. PBD150 lc (low concentration) = 0.1μM; (high concentration) = 1 μM. Panel D: quantification of Aβ concentrations in the brains of 10-month old Tg2576 control mice and of age-matched littermates treated for 6 months with PBD150 at a concentration of 2.4 mg per g (PBD150lc) or 7.2 mg per g (PBD150lc) of food pellets. Only female mice were enrolled in the study. Adapted from Figure 1 of (Shilling et al., 2008).

5. Conclusion

We firstly introduced the prefibrillar aggregation states that are thought to be responsible of the progress of Alzheimer's pathogenesis, and then discussed the possible peptide conformation and assembly organization of them. These features has been correlated with their peptide content, particularly full-length Aβ1-42 and N-truncated and modified Aβ*py*3-42, their structure, kinetics and cell toxicity. We have reviewed the elements of a new therapeutic strategy generically based on opposing conformational diseases taking into account properly of the conformational and structural organization of most toxic oligomeric aggregates. One of the most toxic oligomeric aggregates is formed by Aβ*py*3-42: the new therapeutic strategy may be the prevention of pyroglutamyl termination by finding a well tolerated inhibitor of glutamynil cyclase, which is responsible of the catalysis in vivo of this termination. More difficult is to find conformational inhibitors of the more extended variety of amyloid peptides participating to the formation of the most toxic oligomeric aggregation states. If some steps in the new therapeutic strategy have been done, more work is required to determine more extensively the conformation and structure of the possible oligomeric states and their interaction with neuronal cells to clarify the mechanism of toxicity.
Finally, we have not treated here this topic, but evidence exists that metals are involved as well, in the pathogenesis of AD but the mechanism and role, although important it remains unclear.

6. Acknowledgement

Finantial support from Compagnia di San Paolo Foundation (Torino, Italy) in the framework of BASKO project is acknowledged.

7. References

Apetri, M. M.; Maiti, N.C.; Zagorski, M.G.; Carey, P.R; Anderson, V.E. (2006) Secondary structure of alpha-synuclein oligomers. Characterization by raman atomic force microscopy. *J. Mol. Biol. 355*, 63-71.

Buchholz, M., Heiser, U., Shilling S., Niestroj, A. J., Zunkel, K., Demuth, H. U. (2006). The first potent inhibitors for human glutaminyl cyclase: synthesis and structure-activity relationship *J. Med. Chem. 49*, 664-677.

Campioni, S., Mannini, B., Zampagni, M., Pensalfini, A., Parrini, C., Evangelisti, E., Relini, A., Stefani, M., Dobson C. M., Cecchi, C., Chiti, F. (2010). A causative link between the structure of aberrant protein oligomers and their toxicity. *Nature Chem. Biol. 6*, 140-147.

Chiti, F.; Taddei, N.; Baroni, F.; Capanni, C.; Stefani, M.; Ramponi, G.; Dobson, C. M. (2002).Kinetic partitioning of protein folding and aggregation. *Nature Structural Biology 9*, 137-143.

Chiti F., Dobson C. M. (2006). Protein misfolding, functional amyloid, and human disease. *Annu. Rev. Biochem. 75*, 333-366.

Danielsson, J.; Andersson, A.; Jarvet, J.; Graslund, A. (2006). ^{15}N relaxation study of theamyloid beta-peptide: struictural propensities and persistence length. *Magn. Reson. Chem. 44*, S114-S121.

D'Arrigo C., Tabaton, M., Perico, A. (2009). N-terminal truncated pyroglutamyl beta amyloid peptide Abeta*py*3-42 shows a faster aggregation kinetics than the full-length Abeta1-42 *Biopolymers 91*, 861-873.

Forloni, G.; Terreni, L.; Bertani, I.; Fogliarino, S.; Invernizzi, R.; Assini, A.; Ribizzi, G.; Negro, A.; Calabrese, E.; Volontè, M.A.; Mariani, C.; Franceschi, M.; Tabaton, M.; Bertoli, A. (2002). Protein misfolding in Alzheimer's and Parkinson's disease: genetics and molecular mechanisms.*Neurobiol. Aging, 23*, 957-976.

He, W.; Barrow, C. J. (1999). The Abeta 3-pyroglutamyl and 11-pyroglutamyl peptides foundin senile plaque have greater beta-sheet forming and aggregation propensities in vitro than full-length Abeta. *Biochemistry 38*, 10871-10877.

Hou L., Shao, H., Zhang, Y., Li, H., Menon, N. K., Neuhaus, E., B., Brewer, J. M., Byeon, I. L., Ray, D. G., Vitek, M. P., Iwashita, T., Makula, R. A., Przybyla, A. B., Zagorski, M. G. (2004). Solution NMR studies of the Abeta(1-40) and Abeta(1-42) peptides establish that the Met35 oxidation state affects the mechanism of amyloid formation. *J. Am. Chem. Soc. 126*, 1992-2005.

Hoyer V., Gronwall C., Jonsson A., Stahl S., Hard T. (2008). Stabilization of a beta-hairpin in monomeric Alzheimer's amyloid-beta peptide inhibits amyloid formation. *Proc. Natl. Acad. Sci. USA 105*, 5099-5104.

Jahn, A., Hartley, D. M., Lashuel, H. A. (2010). Preparation and characterization of toxic Abeta aggregates for structural and functional studies in Alzheimer's disease research. *Nature protocols 5*, 1186-1209.

Jan A., Gokce O., Luthi-Carter R., Lashuel H. A. (2008). The ratio of monomeric to aggregated forms of Abeta40 and Abeta42 is an important determinant of amyloid-beta aggregation, fibrillogenesis, and toxicity. *J. Biol. Chem. 283*, 28176-28189.

Kirkitadze M.D., Bitan G., Teplow D.B. (2002). Paradigm shifts in Alzheimer's disease and other neurodegenerative disorders: the emerging role of oligomeric assemblies. *J. Neurosci. Res. 69*, 567-577.

Mastrangelo, I. A., Ahmed, M., Sato, T., Liu, W., Wang, C., Hough, P., Smith, S. O. (2006). High-resolution atomic force microscopy of soluble Abeta42 oligomers. *J. Mol. Biol. 358*, 106-119.

Mitternacht S., Staneva I., Hard T., Irback A. (2010). Comparing the folding free-energy landscapes of Abeta42 variants wityh different aggregation properties. *Proteins 78*, 2600-2608.

Ono, K. Condron, M.M., Teplow, D. B. (2009). Structure-neurotoxicity relationships of amyloid beta-protein oligomers. *PNAS 106*, 14745-14750.

Pastor, M. T., Kummerer, N., Schubert, V., Esteras-Chopo, A., Dotti, FC. G., Lopez de la Paz, M., Serrano, L. (2008). Amyloid toxicity is independent of polypeptide sequence, length and chirality. *J. Mol. Biol. 375*, 695-707.

Roychaudhuri, R. Yang, M., Hoshi, M. M., Teplow, D. B. (2009). Amyloid beta-protein assembly and Alzheimer disease. *J. Biol. Chem. 284*, 4749-4753.

Russo, C.; Schettini, G.; Saido, T. C.; Hulette, C.; Lippa, C.; Lannfelt, L.; Ghetti, B.; Gambetti,P.; Tabaton, M.; Teller, J.K. (2000). Presenilin-1 mutations in Alzheimer's disease. *Nature 405*, 531-532.

Russo, C.; Violani, E.; Salis, F.; Venezia, V.; Dolcini, V.; Damonte, G.; Benatti, U.; D'Arrigo, C.; Patrone, E.; Carlo, P.; Schettini, G. (2002). Pyroglutamate-modified amyloid beta-peptides—AbetaN3(pE)—strongly affect cultured neuron and astrocyte survival. *J. Neurochem. 82*, 1480-1489.

Sandbergh, A., Luheshi, L. M., Sollvander, S., Pereira de Barros, T., Macao, B., Knowles, T. P. J., Biverstal, H., Lendel, C., Ekholm-Petterson, F., Dubnovitsky, A., Lannfelt, L., Dobson, C. M., Hard, T. (2010). Stabilization of neurotoxic Alzheimer amyloid-beta oligomers by protein engineering. *PNAS 107*, 15595-15600.

Selkoe D. J. (1996). Amyloid beta-protein and the genetics of Alzheimer's disease. *J.Biol. Chem. 271*, 18295-18298.

Selkoe D. J. (2004). Alzheimer disease: mechanistic understanding predicts novel therapies. *Ann. Intern. Med. 140*, 627-638.

Shankar G. M., Metha T. H., Garcia-Munoz, A., Shepardson, N. E., Smith, I., Brett, F. M., Farell, M. A., Rowan, M. J., Lemere, C. A., Regan, C. M., Walsh, D. M., Sabatini, B. L., Selkoe, D. J. (2008). Amyloid-beta protein dimmers isolated directly from Alzheimer's gbrains impair synaptic plasticity and memory. *Nat. Med. 14*, 837-842.

Schilling, S.; Hoffmann, T.; Manhart, S.; Hoffmann, M.; Demuth, H.U. (2004). Glutamynil cyclase unfold glutamyl cyclase activity under mild acid conditions. *FEBS Lett. 563*, 191-196.

Schilling, S., Lauber, T., Schaupp, M., manhart, S., Scheel, E., Bohm, G., Demuth H. U. (2006). On the seeding and oligomerization of pGlu-amyloid peptides. *Biochemistry 45*, 12393-12399.

Shilling S., Zeitschel, U., Hoffmann, T., Heiser, U., Francke, M., Kehlen, A., Holzer, M., Hutter-Paier, B., Prokesh, M., Windisch, M., Jagla, W., Schlenzig, D., Lindner, C., Rudolph, T., Reuter, G., Cynis, H., Montag, D., Demuth, H. U., Rossner, S. (2008). Glutaminyl cyclase inhibition attenuates pyroglutamate Abeta and Alzheimer's disease-like pathology. *Nature Medicine, Letters 14*, 1106.

Tomaselli, S.; Esposito, V.; Vangone, P.; van Nuland, N. A. J.; Bonvin, A.M.; Guerrini, R.; Tancredi, T.; Temussi, P.A.; Picone, D. (2006). The alfa-to-beta conformational transition of Alzheimer's Abeta(1-42) peptide in acqueous media is reversible: a step by step conformational analysis suggests the location of beta conformation seeding. *ChemBioChem 7*, 257-267.

Walsh, D. M., Hartley, D. M., Kusumoto, Y., Fezoui, Y., Condron M. M., Lomakin, A., Benedek, G. B., Selkoe, D. J., Teplow, D. B. (1999). Amyloid beta-protein fibrillogenesis. Structure and biological activity of protofibrillar intermediates. *J. Biol. Chem. 274*, 25945-25952.

Walsh D. M., Selkoe D.B. (2007). A beta oligomers-a decade of discovery. *J. Neurochem. 101*,1172-1184.

Yankner B. A., Lu T. (2009). Amyloid beta-protein toxicity and the pathogenesis of Alzheimer disease. *J. Biol. Chem. 284,* 4755-4759.

Yoshiike, Y., Akagi, T., Takashima, A. (2007). Surface structure of amyloid-beta fibrils contributes to cytotoxicity. *Biochemistry 46,* 9805-9812.

9

Structural and Toxic Properties of Protein Aggregates: Towards a Molecular Understanding of Alzheimer's Disease

Lei Wang and Silvia Campioni
Swiss Federal Institute of Technology (ETH) Zurich
Switzerland

1. Introduction

Alzheimer's disease (AD) is an age-related irreversible brain disorder that progresses over 10 to 20 years. AD gradually destroys human memory and thinking skills, leads to severe loss of mental function, and eventually causes death (Querfurth and LaFerla, 2010). Normally, AD symptoms first appear after age 65. It is estimated that AD affected 36 million people globally in 2009, and the number will be more than doubled by 2050. Currently, there is no cure for AD, except few medications that can relieve AD symptoms (Brunden et al., 2009; Citron, 2004).

AD is accompanied by a significant shrunk of brain tissue, which is a result of brain neuron degeneration. In the brains of AD patients, neurons are found to have lost their synaptic connections with other neurons and are unable to survive (Wenk, 2003). The synaptic failure is indeed the earliest event associated with the cognitive impairment caused by the disease (Selkoe, 2002). In addition, the brains of AD patients are characterized by the presence of two types of hystopathological hallmark lesions: amyloid plaques and neurofibrillary tangles (NFTs), which are composed of aggregated proteinaceous material (Tiraboschi et al., 2004). Although both amyloid plaques and NFTs are also present in brains of healthy individuals, the amount of these aggregates in the brains of AD patients is significantly higher. Early studies correlated neuron degeneration in AD with the formation of these insoluble protein aggregates. However, recent studies suggest that soluble protein aggregates of the same protein composition are more toxic to neurons (Rahimi et al., 2008). It has also been suggested that the insoluble aggregates actually play a beneficial role in that they sequester the toxic soluble aggregates into less toxic or non-toxic insoluble aggregates (Greenwald and Riek, 2010).

At current stage, we are still trying to understand how different protein aggregates in the brain mediate neuron degeneration and lead to AD. Like any other protein activity, the neurotoxicity of protein aggregates must be associated with their specific molecular structures. Therefore, investigating the high-resolution structures of amyloid plaques, NFTs and soluble aggregates would greatly facilitate the development of diagnostic and therapeutic strategies. Here, in this chapter, we review current knowledge about the structure and toxicity of the aggregates involved in AD.

2. Structure and toxicity of different protein aggregates involved in AD

2.1 Amyloid-β peptides, tau protein and their relation to AD

Amyloid plaques are extracellular deposits mainly composed of full length and truncated fragments of amyloid-β (Aβ) peptides. Aβ peptides are produced upon cleavage of the amyloid precursor protein (APP) by β- and γ- secretases (Hooper, 2005). APP is an integral membrane protein expressed in many tissues and concentrated in the neuronal synapses (Turner et al., 2003). The γ-secretase protease cleaves APP at different positions, thus producing different Aβ fragments composed by 36 to 43 amino-acid-residues (Kang et al., 1987; Masters et al., 1985). Among those, the Aβ fragments having 40 ($A\beta_{40}$) or 42 ($A\beta_{42}$) amino-acid-residues are the most common (Hartmann et al., 1997). The amino-acid sequences of $A\beta_{40}$ and $A\beta_{42}$ are:

$A\beta_{40}$: DAEFRHDSGYEVHHQKLVFFAEDVGSNKGAIIGLMVGGVV

$A\beta_{42}$: DAEFRHDSGYEVHHQKLVFFAEDVGSNKGAIIGLMVGGVVIA

In the amyloid plaques, Aβ peptides form highly-ordered insoluble fibrillar aggregates, termed amyloid fibrils (Ohnishi and Takano, 2004). Besides, in the brain of AD patients, Aβ peptides can also form different types of soluble aggregates, such as small spherical aggregates, large spherical aggregates and small curved fibrils that are different from mature amyloid fibrils found in amyloid plaques (Dahlgren et al., 2002). An important role for of Aβ peptides in AD pathogenesis is also suggested by the fact that many mutations related to early-onset familial forms of AD increase total Aβ peptides levels and/or the relative concentration of $A\beta_{40}$ and $A\beta_{42}$, which is an important factor for AD since the latter peptide is more hydrophobic and hince aggregation prone (Borchelt et al., 1996; Eckman et al., 1997).

Neurofibrillary tangles (NFTs) are intracellular deposits mainly composed of the tau protein. Normally, tau interacts with tubulins and facilitates their assembly into microtubules, which act as cell skeleton and are important for cell health (Hernandez and Avila, 2007). Tau sequence can be divided into two major domains: a projection domain and a C-terminal microtubules binding domain. The latter contains similar but not identical repeats of 31-32 residues responsible for tubulin binding (Kosik, 1990). Six isoforms of tau are present in the brain, with 352 to 441 amino-acid-residues (Goedert et al., 1992). They differ from each other in the number of tubulin binding domains. Tau can undergo multiple types of post-translational modification. Its most important modification in AD is phosphorylation. When tau is hyperphosphorylated, it looses binding affinity to the microtubules, and starts to self-assemble into paired helical filaments (PHFs), which in turn deposit into NFTs (Alonso et al., 2001). Tau deposition as NFTs is also a characteristics of a subset of frontotemporal dementia. The fact that mutations in the gene encoding for tau are related to familial forms of frontotemporal dementia indicate an important role for tau in neurodegeneration (Heutink, 2000).

In early reports, spreading of NFTs in the brain had been observed to correlate with the progression of AD, suggesting a central role for tau in AD, but later studies rather led to the dominant idea that the aggregation of Aβ peptides in the brain is the primary event in AD and occurs before tau aggregation (Hardy and Selkoe, 2002). The amyloid cascade hypothesis for AD proposes that the imbalance between the production and clearance of Aβ peptides leads to Aβ aggregation and plaques formation, initiating a complex cascade of events, such as synaptic failure, tau hyperphosphorylation and inflammation, that finally lead to AD (Tanzi and Bertram, 2005). So far, the correlation between Aβ amyloid fibrils and AD onset remains weak (Schmitz et al., 2004), wheareas soluble Aβ aggregates are believed to play the most important role in AD (Rahimi et al., 2008).

Despite the primary role of Aβ aggregates in AD, Aβ and tau have been demonstrated to interact with each other and most likely they cause AD through synergic effects. Indeed, the presence of Aβ peptides in transgenic mice influences the aggregation of tau into NFTs and, on the other hand, tau protein mediates Aβ toxicity (Lewis et al., 2001; Rapoport et al., 2002). Recently, a novel hypothesis linking Aβ and tau has been proposed on the basis of the observation that tau can also have a dendritic localization under physiological conditions and that tau-mediated postsynaptic targeting of the tyrosine protein kinase FYN confers Aβ toxicity (Ittner et al., 2010).

2.2 Structure of $A\beta_{42}$ amyloid fibrils

$A\beta_{42}$ amyloid fibrils are the most abundant aggregates in amyloid plaques (Roher et al., 1993). Under electron microscope, they look like unbranched filaments with a diameter of ~ 10 nm, and their length can reach up to several micrometer (Antzutkin et al., 2002) (Figure 1A). The X-ray diffraction pattern of aligned $A\beta_{42}$ amyloid fibrils shows two characteristic bands: one sharp band at ~ 4.7 Å position, and another diffused orthogonal band at ~ 10 Å (Kirschner et al., 1986) (Figure 1B).

Two structural models of $A\beta_{42}$ amyloid fibrils are available. In the first model, the structural information was obtained by using solid-state nuclear magnetic resonance (ssNMR) and solution NMR combined with the hydrogen/deuterium exchange (H/D-exchange) method. The ssNMR techinque provides distance restraints within amyloid fibrils while H/D-exchange monitored with solution NMR allows the identification of the regions of the protein sequence involved in the core structure of amyloid fibrils (Hoshino et al., 2002; Wang et al., 2008; Wang et al., 2010). The obtained model shows that: (a) in amyloid fibrils, amino-acid-residues 1-10 of $A\beta_{42}$ are unstructured, residues 11-22 and 31-42 form two β-strands (β1 and β2), and residues 23-30 form a bend (Figure 1C) (Ahmed et al., 2010; Olofsson et al., 2006); (b) through backbone hydrogen bonds, β1- and β2-strands interact with β1- and β2-strands in other $A\beta_{42}$ molecules and form two parallel β-sheets. All β-strands are perpendicular to the fibril axis, and both β-sheets are parallel to the fibril axis. This structure is called the cross-β-sheet structure (Figure 1E) (Balbach et al., 2002; Kirschner et al., 1986; Tycko, 2004); (c) the two β-sheets are connected by the intramolecular side chain interaction between Phe19 and Leu34, the salt bridge between Asp23 and Lys28, and the intermolecular side chain interaction between Gln15 and Gly37 (Figure 1C & 1F) (Ahmed et al., 2010). The distance between two adjacent β-strands is ~ 4.7 Å, and the distance between two β-sheets is ~ 10 Å, corresponding to the two characteristic bands observed in X-ray diffraction of amyloid fibrils.

In the second model, $^{35Mox}A\beta_{42}$ was used to produce amyloid fibrils. $^{35Mox}A\beta_{42}$ contains a methionine sulfoxide at position 35. This structural model was obtained by using solution NMR combined with H/D-exchange method and pairwise mutagenesis experiments. The resulting structure shows that: (a) in the fibrils, amino-acid-residues 1-17 of $^{35Mox}A\beta_{42}$ are unstructured, residues 18-26 and 31-42 form two β-strands (β1 and β2), and residues 27-30 form a bend (Figure 1D) (Luhrs et al., 2005); (b) β1- and β2-strands in different

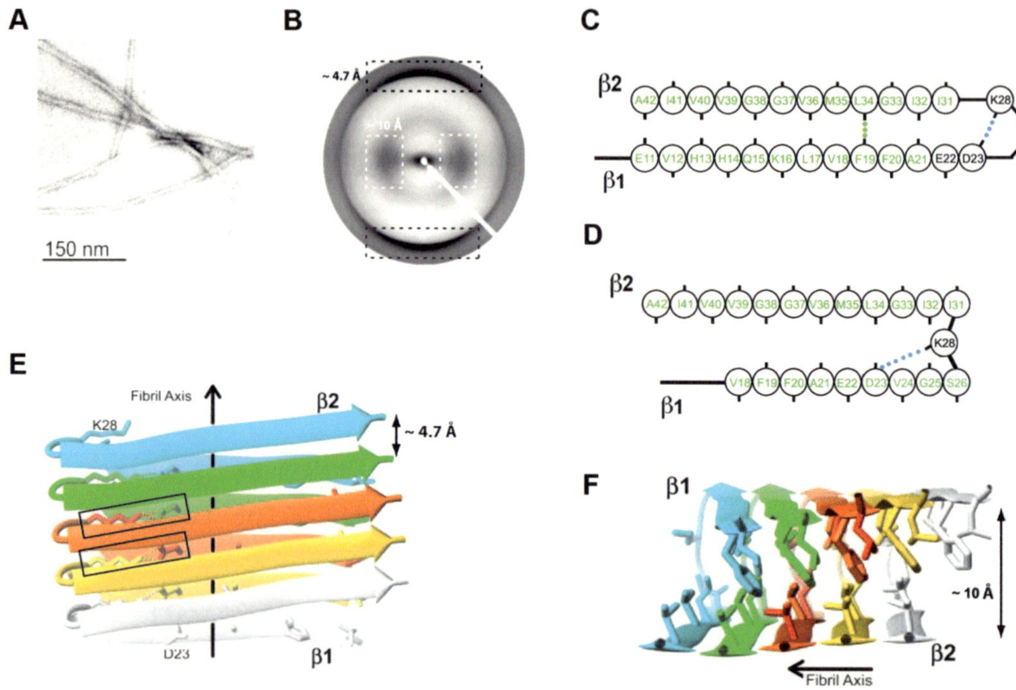

Fig. 1. Structural model of $A\beta_{42}$ amyloid fibrils. (A)Electron microscope image of $A\beta_{42}$ amyloid fibrils. (B) X-ray diffraction pattern of amyloid fibrils. (C) Illustration of $A\beta_{42}$ in amyloid fibrils. (D) Illustration of ${}^{Mox}A\beta_{42}$ in amyloid fibrils. (E) The cross-β-sheet structure of amyloid fibrils. (F) The side chain arrangement in amyloid fibrils. This figure is adapted from Fig 4 (Antzutkin et al., 2002), Fig 1 (Ahmed et al., 2010) and Fig 4 (Luhrs et al., 2005).

${}^{35Mox}A\beta_{42}$ molecules interconnect and form the cross-β-sheet structure (Figure 1E); (c) the two β-sheets are connected by the intermolecular side chain interactions between Phe19 and Gly38, Ala21 and Val36, and the salt bridge between Asp23 and Lys28 (Figure 1D & 1F) (Luhrs et al., 2005). Compared to the structure of $A\beta_{42}$ amyloid fibrils, the structural difference of ${}^{35Mox}A\beta_{42}$ amyloid fibrils may reflect the effect of Met35 modification, or, it may reflect the a structural polymorphism of $A\beta_{42}$ amyloid fibrils.

2.3 Structure of $A\beta_{40}$ amyloid fibrils

$A\beta_{40}$ can form at least three types of amyloid fibrils with distinct morphology, which include striated-ribbon fibrils (Figure 2A), twisted-pair fibrils (Figure 2B) and brain-seeded fibrils (Figure 2C) (Paravastu et al., 2009; Petkova et al., 2005). The polymorphism of the fibrils is induced by the different conditions used to form them. In particular, incubation of $A\beta_{40}$ under agitation leads to the formation of straight-rod shaped protofilaments with a width of 6 nm, and these protofilaments associate laterally to form striated-ribbon fibrils. Quiescent growth rather leads to the formation of twisted-pair fibrils that are composed of single protofilaments (Petkova et al., 2005). Seeding $A\beta_{40}$ aggregation with purified fibrils from brain tissue of AD patients leads to the formation of curved and untwisted fibrils (Paravastu et al., 2009). All three $A\beta_{40}$ fibrils have different underlying molecular structures.

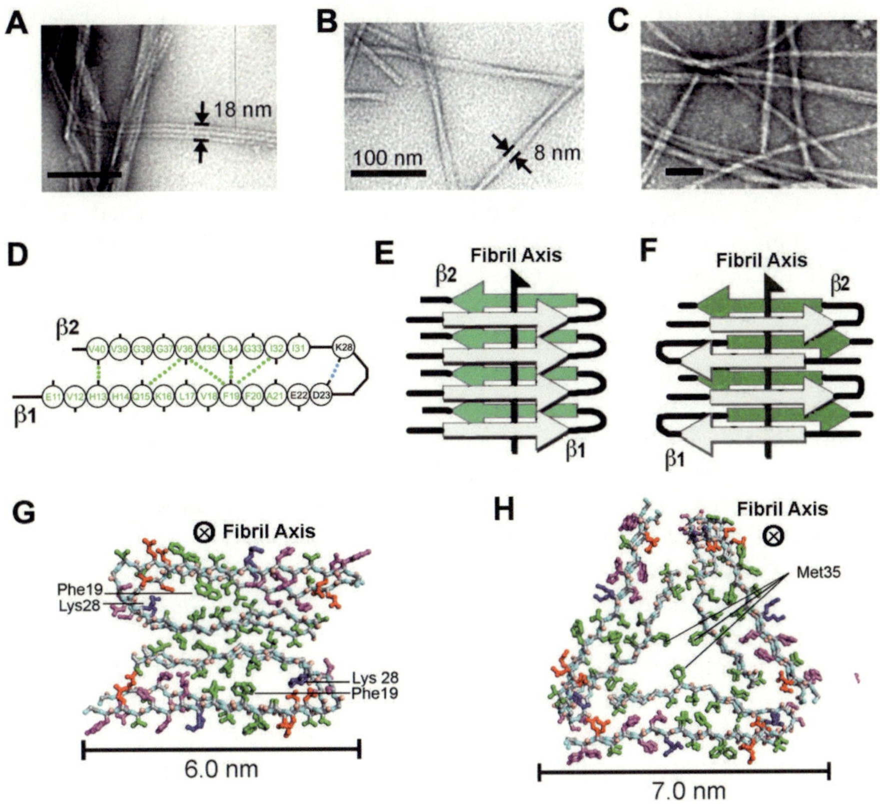

Fig. 2. Structural model of $A\beta_{40}$ amyloid fibrils. (A-C) Electron microscope images of striated-ribbon fibrils (A), twisted-pair fibrils (B) and brain-seeded (C) amyloid fibrils of $A\beta_{40}$. Scale bar = 100 nm. (D) Illustration of $A\beta_{40}$ in amyloid fibrils. (E) The parallel cross-β-sheet structure of $A\beta_{40}$ amyloid fibrils. (F) The antiparallel cross-β-sheet structure of $A\beta_{40}$–D23N amyloid fibrils. (G) One protofilament in the striated-ribbon fibrils is composed of two cross-β-sheet units. (H) One protofilament in the twisted-pair fibrils is composed of three cross-β-sheet units. This figure is adapted from Fig 4 (Paravastu et al., 2008), Fig 1 (Paravastu et al., 2009), and Fig 4 (Sawaya et al., 2007).

A structural model for striated-ribbon fibrils of $A\beta_{40}$ was obtained using solid-state NMR spectroscopy and electron microscopy. It shows that: (a) in amyloid fibrils, amino-acid-residues 1-9 of $A\beta_{40}$ are unstructured, residues 10-22 and 30-40 form two β-strands (β1 and β2), and residues 23-29 form a bend (Figure 2D) (Petkova et al., 2006); (b) through backbone hydrogen bonds, β1- and β2-strands interact with β1- and β2-strands in other $A\beta_{40}$ molecules and form two parallel β-sheets. All β-strands are perpendicular to the fibril axis, and both β-sheets are parallel to the fibril axis. This structure is considered as one cross-β-sheet unit (Figure 2E); (c) the two β-sheets are connected by side chain interactions, including the intermolecular interaction between Phe19 in one molecule and Leu34 in the neighboring molecule, and the intramolecular salt bridge between Asp23 and Lys28 (Petkova et al., 2006) (Figure 2D); (d) the individual protofilament in the striated-ribbon fibrils is composed of two cross-β-sheet units, which are two-fold rotationally symmetric to each other along the fibril axis (Sciarretta et al., 2005; Tycko, 2010) (Figure 2G).

The structural model for twisted-pair fibrils of $A\beta_{40}$ contains similar cross-β-sheet unit as in striated-ribbon fibrils (Petkova et al., 2006) (Figure 2D & 2E). But the individual protofilament in the twisted-pair fibrils is composed of three cross-β-sheet units, which are three-fold rotationally symmetric to each other along the fibril axis (Sciarretta et al., 2005) (Figure 2H). This is the biggest difference from the protofilament composed of two cross-β-sheet units obtained for striated-ribbon fibrils. Other structural differences in twisted-pair fibrils include the absence of the salt bridge between Asp23 and Lys28, and different side chain interactions among cross-β-sheet units.

Brain-seeded fibrils have been produced to mimic amyloid fibrils of $A\beta_{40}$ formed *in vivo*. Due to experimental limit, currently it is not possible to measure the structure of fibrils directly from human tissue. As an alternative, fibrils extracted from the brain tissue of AD patients were used as seeds to produce large amount of isotopically labeled brain-seeded fibrils for structural study (Paravastu et al., 2009). These fibrils are thus likely to represent the amyloid fibrils formed *in vivo*. It has been shown that the ssNMR spectra of the brain-seeded fibrils are different from that of the striated-ribbon or twisted-pair fibrils, suggesting that brain-seeded fibrils have a different structure than previous identified structures of $A\beta_{40}$ fibrils (Tycko, 2010). However, a detailed structural model for brain-seeded fibrils is not yet available.

Disease-related mutants of $A\beta_{40}$ also form amyloid fibrils. The structure of the amyloid fibrils formed by the Iowa mutant ($A\beta_{40}$-D23N), associated with early-onset familial AD, is composed of a different cross-β-sheet unit, in which β1- and β2-strands of $A\beta_{40}$-D23N molecules are interconnected and form two antiparallel β-sheets (Tycko et al., 2009) (Figure 2F).

2.4 Structure of paired helical filaments of tau

As mentioned before, neurofibrillary tangles (NFTs) deposits are composed of paired helical filaments (PHFs) of tau protein (Wischik et al., 1988) (Figure 3A). Although the high-resolution structure of tau PHFs has not been solved yet, several structural models are available based on various experimental data. Fourier transform infrared (FT-IR) spectroscopy experiments show that tau PHFs are composed of a large amount of random coil structure together with some α-helical and β-sheet structure (Sadqi et al., 2002). It has also been found that the residues 265-338 in PHFs (PHF43) are protected against proteases digestion, and PHF43 alone can also form amyloid fibrils (von Bergen et al., 2000). Further investigation shows that the amino-acid-residues 306-311 (sequence: VQIVYK) (PHF6) within PHF43 are responsible for PHF43 amyloid fibrils formation. PHF6 alone forms amyloid fibrils that resemble tau PHFs (von Bergen et al., 2005; von Bergen et al., 2000). X-ray microcrystallography data show that PHF6 forms parallel β-sheets in amyloid fibrils, and the β-sheets are connected by side chains that form steric zippers (Sawaya et al., 2007) (Figure 3B & 3C).

One structural model of tau PHFs suggests that they contain one cross-β sheet composed of PHF6 while the rest of the sequence is structurally disordered or contains some α-helical structure (von Bergen et al., 2005) (Figure 3D). Another structural model suggests that PHFs may contain an additional cross-β sheet, which is composed of amino-acid-residues 272-289 (S2) (Figure 3E). This model is based on the finding that isolated S2 can also form amyloid fibrils under certain conditions (Margittai and Langen, 2006).

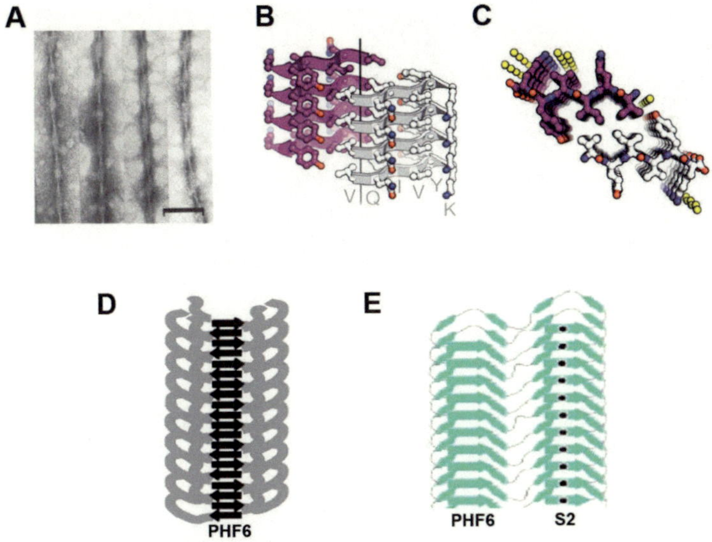

Fig. 3. Structural model of paired helical filaments (PHFs) of tau. (A) Electron microscope image of tau PHFs. Scale bar = 100 nm. (B-C) The side and top view of the cross-β-sheet structure of PHF6 amyloid fibrils. (D) The proposed structural model for tau PHFs, in which PHF6 form the cross-β-sheet structure, and the rest of tau PHFs is not/least structured. (E) Another proposed structural model for tau PHFs, in which PHF6 and S2 form two cross-β-sheet structures. This figure is adapted from Fig 1B (Wischik et al., 1988), Fig 2 & 3 (Sawaya et al., 2007), Fig 6 (von Bergen et al., 2005) and Fig 4A (Margittai and Langen, 2006).

2.5 Soluble Aβ aggregates: Mechanism of toxicity and structure

Increasing evidence suggest that the pathogenic agents in amyloid-related diseases are the transient, pre-fibrillar Aβ assemblies preceding the formation of mature fibrils, whereas amyloid fibrils rather represent the protective end state of the protein misfolding event (Sakono and Zako, 2010; Rahimi et al., 2008; Chiti and Dobson, 2006). This is particularly valid in the case of AD, where a weak correlation exists between cognitive impairment and amyloid plaques formation (Terry et al., 1991) and, in transgenic mouse lines used to model AD, synaptotoxicity is observed before and/or independently of amyloid plaque formation (Mucke et al., 2000). Instead, the levels of soluble Aβ oligomers in AD patients correlate much better with the onset of neurodegeneration (for a review on the oligomer-toxicity hypothesis see Klein et al., 2001). Remarkably, a mutated form of Aβ showing enhanced oligomerization but no fibrillation was identified in a Japanese pedigree of AD patients with little deposition of fibrillar amyloid (Tomiyama et al., 2008).
Despite their relevance to disease, a detailed structural and functional characterization of amyloid pre-fibrillar species is considerably hampered by their transient and heterogeneous nature. In addition, in the case of Aβ pre-fibrillar species, further complications arise due to the various methods used to produce the synthetic peptide/s used in the experiments and the fact that the $A\beta_{40}$ and $A\beta_{42}$ are more aggregation prone than other amyloidogenic peptides and protein and form ensembles of oligomeric species already upon dissolution of the lyophilized peptides in aqueous buffer (Teplow, 2006). Describing in detail all types of Aβ oligomers reported in the literature up to date would be beyond the scopes of this book chapter; we will

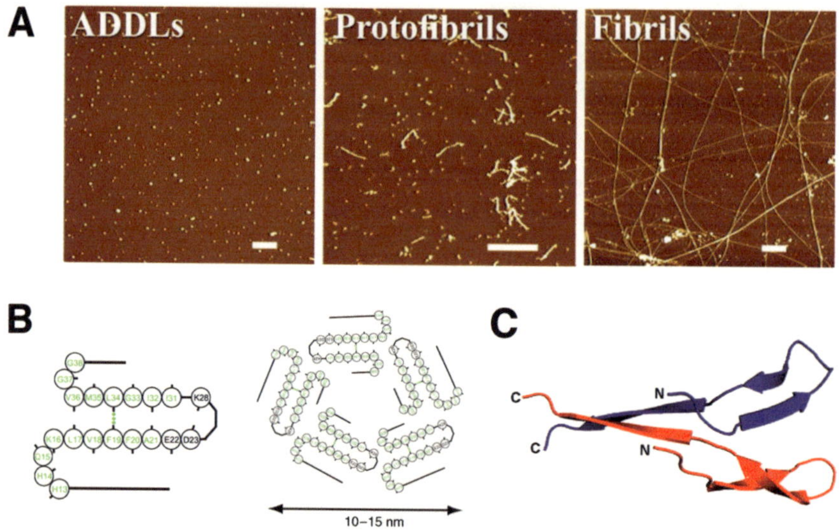

Fig. 4. Morphology and conformation of different aggregates formed by $A\beta_{42}$ under different incubation conditions. (A) Atomic force microscopy images of ADDLs (left), protofibrils (middle) and mature fibrils (right). (B) Schematic model of $A\beta_{42}$ monomer within a spherical pentameric aggregated from solid-state magic angle spinning data. Light blue squares connect Phe19 and Leu34. The areas showing little protection from hydrogen-deuterium exchange are coloured in green. (C) Model for the structure of $A\beta_{42}$ preglobulomers obtained from solution state NMR. According to this model, preglobulomers are formed by dimer units adopting mixed parallel and antiparallel structure. This figure is adapted from Fig 2 & 4 (Klein et al., 2001), and Fig 3 (Yu et al., 2009).

thus limit our description to a summary of the most consolidated and recent information on the species thought to play an important role in AD disease. Although all these species are generally referred to as "Aβ oligomers", the readers should keep in mind that they may differ in structure, pathway of formation and mechanism of toxicity as well.

2.5.1 Aβ pre-fibrillar aggregates formed in vitro

In studies performed *in vitro,* Aβ peptides have been found to form various types of aggregates having spherical morphology. Cross-linking experiments show that $A\beta_{40}$ and $A\beta_{42}$ preparations differ in their oligomers distributions, with the former peptide forming roughly equimolar mixtures of aggregates ranging from dimers to tetramers, whereas the latter preferentially forms pentamers/hexamers (termed paranuclei), which self-associate into dodecamers and octadecamers (Bitan et al., 2001; Bitan et al., 2003). These larger species appear not to be artifacts of the cross-linking technique since $A\beta_{42}$ stable dodecamers formed by stacked hexamer units have been detected also in the absence of any cross-linking (Bernstein et al., 2009). Here we will summarize present information on the toxic effect and the conformational properties of the most investigated oligomeric species.

Aβ-derived diffusible ligands (ADDLs) are slowly sedimenting aggregates observed only in preparations of synthetic $A\beta_{42}$ peptides; they appear as globular species with 3-8 nm height (Figure 4A) and they are believed to be composed of 3-24 monomers (Oda et al., 1995;

Lambert et al., 1998; Klein et al., 2002; Chromy et al., 2003). Their pathological relevance is supported by the detection of aggregates (in particular dodecamers) immunoreactive to anti-ADDLs antibodies in the brain and cerebrospinal fluid of AD patients (Gong et al., 2003; Georganopoulou et al., 2005). ADDLs are potent neurotoxins: they induce the death of principal neurons of the hippocampus and, in rat hippocampal brain slices, they inhibit long-term potentiation (LTP) but not long-term depression (LTD), two forms of synaptic plasticity implicated in learning and memory (Lambert et al., 1998; Wang et al., 2002). Binding of ADDLs to hippocampal neurons appears to occur at the postsynaptic termini of excitatory synapses and stimulates aberrant expression of the activity-regulated cytoskeletal-associated (Arc) protein (implicated in long-term memory formation), tau hyperphosphorylation, synapses deterioration and loss, and enhanced formation of reactive oxygen species (ROS) thought to play a major role in the pathogenesis of AD (Lacor et al., 2004; Guzowski 2002; Hsieh et al., 2006; De Felice et al., 2007a; De Felice et al., 2007b; Lacor et al., 2007; Shankar et al., 2007). Monoclonal antibodies targeting ADDLs can prevent their aberrant binding and synaptotoxicity (Lambert et al., 2007). *In vivo*, insulin signaling and the cellular prion protein (PrP^C) have been suggested to mediate the toxicity of ADDLs, even if in the latter case an effective involvement in AD is currently under debate (De Felice et al., 2009; Laurén et al., 2009; Gimbel et al., 2010; Calella et al., 2010; Caetano et al., 2011). Despite the large amount of data on the toxic effect of ADDLs, still little is known about their structure; mainly because they are heterogeneous mixtures of oligomers of different sizes. The structure of neurotoxic $A\beta_{42}$ pentamers has been recently investigated (Figure 4B). Hydrogen-deuterium exchange measurements indicate that the first nine residues are solvent exposed, as well as residues 13-15, 25-29 and 37-38 that presumably form solvent-accessible turns (Ahmed et al., 2010). Solid-state magic angle spinning measurements show the lack of parallel, in-register β-sheets, but the C-terminal regions of the constituting monomers are packed together and adopt a conformation similar to that observed in the mature fibrils (U-shaped hairpin structure), with Phe19 in contact with Leu34 (Ahmed et al., 2010).

Globular oligomers having a size of 4-5 nm, composed of twelve monomeric units and forming independently from fibril formation have been obtained from $A\beta_{42}$ samples incubated at high concentration (400 μM) in the presence of sodium dodecyl sulfate (SDS) or fatty acids; such species are known as Aβ globulomers (Barghorn et al., 2005; Gellermann et al., 2008; Yu et al., 2009). Similarly to ADDLs, globulomers selectively bind to neuronal cells, inhibit LTP in hippocampal brain slices and their toxicity can be rescued with a globulomer-specific antibody (Barghorn et al., 2005; Hillen et al., 2010). Moreover, antibodies against globulomers detect immunoreactive species in tissue sections from the brains of AD patients and human APP transgenic mice (Barghorn et al., 2005). In contrast to ADDLs preparations, globulomer samples are stable and homogeneous; thus can be used for structural studies. Protease digestion, cross-linking and antibody binding data suggest that residues 1-20 of $A\beta_{42}$ are accessible to the solvent while the rest of the sequence forms the core of the aggregates. Solution NMR data on smaller pre-globulomeric species (tetramers) indicate that they are composed of dimer repeating units (Figure 4C) with residues 18-23 and 28-40 forming β-structure in mixed parallel and antiparallel β-sheets (Yu et al., 2009). Finally, hydrogen-deuterium exchange measurements indicate that globulomers and pre-globulomers have similar secondary structures and that the former species result from association of pre-globulomeric units.

$A\beta_{40}$ and $A\beta_{42}$ can also form, off-pathway from fibril formation, large globular aggregates with little or no cross-β structure (they do not bind the amyloid-specific dye thioflavin T) termed amylospheroids (ASPDs) (Hoschi et al., 2003; Matsumura et al., 2011). ASPDs of 10-15 nm diameter are potent neurotoxins to primary cultures from rat septum regions; the most toxic species being 32-mers (Hoschi et al., 2003; Matsumura et al., 2011). Antibodies generated to recognize ASPDs stain AD brains and have been used to immunoisolate ASPDs directly from AD and dementia with Lewy bodies brains (Noguchi et al., 2009). Levels of ASPDs in AD patients correlate with the severity of disease and the immunoprecipitated species induce degeneration on neurons *in vitro* (Noguchi et al., 2009). Chimon et al. investigated the structure of globular $A\beta_{40}$ aggregates formed by at least 150 monomers that impair the viability of cultured PC-12 cells and have a diameter similar to that of ASPDs, but, in contrast to ASPDs, they are rich in β-sheet structure and are on-pathway intermediates of fibril formation (Chimon and Ishii, 2005; Chimon et al., 2007). Solid-state NMR spectra show that these assemblies have ordered parallel, in regisister, β-stucture, extremely similar to that of mature $A\beta_{40}$ fibrils, particularly in the hydrophobic core and C-terminal regions (Chimon and Ishii, 2005; Chimon et al., 2007).

Aβ protofibrils (Figure 4A) also belong to the wide range of possible Aβ pre-fibrillar aggregates. These are soluble aggregates formed by both $A\beta_{40}$ and $A\beta_{42}$ *via* association of smaller globular units, with an apparent mass higher than 100 kDa and appearing as curved fibril-like structures of 3-8 nm diameter and less than 200 nm length (Harper et al., 1997; Walsh et al., 1997; Walsh et al., 1999; Harper et al., 1999). PFs formed *in vitro* alter the viability of cultured rat primary cortical neurons and induce neuronal injury, impaired electrophysiological activities and neuronal loss (Walsh et al., 1999; Hartley et al., 1999). The fact that the early-onset AD-related Arctic mutation enhances PF formation suggests that these species might be relevant for the disease (Nilsberth et al., 2001). Moreover, 4-hydroxy-2-nonenal (HNE), a metabolite of oxidative stress found to exist at increased concentrations in AD patients and to co-localize with Aβ deposits, causes *in vitro* accumulation of $A\beta_{40}$ PFs and prevents their conversion into mature fibrils, thus leading to sustained neurotoxicity to cultured cells (Sayre et al., 1997; Siegel et al., 2007; Johansson et al., 2007). PFs appear transiently and are considered to be the direct precursors of long and rigid amyloid fibrils (Harper et al., 1997; Walsh et al., 1997). Indeed, they already possess a high content of β-sheet structure and the capability to bind the WO1 amyloid fibrils-specific antibody (Williams et al., 2005). Nonetheless, they are still metastable and can dissociate into low molecular weight oligomers (Walsh et al., 1999; Harper et al., 1999). $A\beta_{40}$ PFs possess a stable structural core (Kheterpal et al., 2003). Proline substitution and hydrogen-deuterium exchange experiments on $A\beta_{40}$ PFs stabilized by a small molecule show that the first N-terminal 14-19 residues and the C-terminal 3-5 residues are not involved in the formation of their structural core and that, in comparison to mature fibrils, PFs are less structured in the fragment spanning residues 20-34 (Williams et al., 2005; Kheterpal et al., 2006).

Protofibrillar aggregates formed by the E22G (Arctic mutation) mutant of $A\beta_{40}$ can also adopt annular structures (Lashuel et al., 2002). These species have a pore-like appearance with an outer diameter of 7-10 nm and an inner diameter of 1.5-2.0 nm, and appear to be composed of 40-60 peptide molecules (Lashuel et al., 2002). Structures similar to annular PFs have been observed upon incorporation of different Aβ peptides into artificial and natural membranes and have been hypothesized to serve as calcium channels that mediate Aβ-induced toxicity in AD (Arispe et al., 2007). However, the formation of Aβ pores is still debated since spherical Aβ aggregates can increase membrane permeability and intracellular calcium levels without any evidence of discrete channel of pore formation (Kayed et al., 2004; Demuro et al., 2005). Antibodies specific for annular protofibrils, but not spherical oligomers and fibrils, also recognize heptameric alpha-hemolysin pores, suggesting that the antibody recognizes an epitope that is specific for a β barrel structural motif (Kayed et al., 2009).

2.5.2 Cell-derived pre-fibrillar aggregates

Oligomerization studies performed *in vitro* with synthetic peptides have various limitations: 1) the usually employed peptide concentrations are in the micromolar range, whereas Aβ concentration *in vivo* is rather in the nanomolar or even subnanomolar range (Seubert et al., 1992; Suzuki et al., 1994; Tabaton et al., 1994); 2) *in vitro*, peptides of specified lengths are used, whereas numerous Aβ species, with extensive amino and carboxyl terminal heterogeneity, are usually present *in vivo* (reviewed in Golde and Younkin, 1996); 3) aggregation is usually examined under non-physiological conditions, with the peptides solubilized in organic solvents and then diluted in water or aqueous buffers free of other proteins, macromolecules or small molecules. These limitations imply that pathologically relevant aggregates may differ substantially from those produced *in vitro*. Thus, considerable effort has been recently spent in isolating and characterizing Aβ oligomers formed *in vivo*. Detailed structural characterization of cell-derived oligomers is lacking due to their low concentration, but their ability to cause toxicity and cognitive impairment has been deeply investigated.

Small SDS-stable oligomers have been isolated at nanomolar concentration from the medium of caltured cells, human cerebrospinal fluid, APP transgenic mouse brain and human brain (reviewed in Selkoe 2008; Rahimi et al., 2008). Aβ dimers have been detected and proved to form intracellularly in primary human neurons and in both neuronal and non-neural cell lines (Walsh et al., 2000). Stable dimers and trimers of Aβ isolated from the neuritic plaques of AD patients and leptomeningeal vessels compromise the viability of cultured rat hippocampal neuron glia cells through a microglia-dependent mechanism and Aβ dimers from the cerebral cortex of AD patients can also impair synaptic plasticity and memory in rats (Roher et al., 1996; Shankar et al., 2008). Synaptic dysfunction is also caused by dimers from *ex vivo* human cerebrospinal fluid (Klyubin et al., 2008).

Oligomers (in particular trimers) secreted in the medium of Chinese Hamster Ovary cells over-expressing the β-amyloid precursor protein inhibit hippocampal LTP, decrease the density of dendritic spines, impair cognitive function in rats and inhibit the remodeling of synapses, a prerequisite for memory consolidation (Walsh et al., 2002; Cleary et al., 2005; Townsend et al., 2006; Shankar et al., 2007; Poling et al., 2008; Freir et al., 2010). Compounds that inhibit oligomers formation or antibodies that bind to the oligomers rescue their toxic effects (Walsh et al., 2005a; Walsh et al., 2005b).

A soluble, SDS-stable dodecamer termed Aβ*56 was found in the brain of middle-aged APP transgenic mice carrying a familial AD-linked double mutation (Lesné et al., 2006). Levels of Aβ*56 dodecamers in middle-aged APP transgenic mice correlate with cognitive deficits and administration of purified Aβ*56 to young rats disrupts their memory (Lesné et al., 2006). In a recent study, synthetic $A\beta_{42}$-derived oligomers, cell- and brain-derived low molecular weight oligomers, and Aβ*56 have been compared for their ability to produce deficits in learned behavior of rats, finding that dimers derived from the culture medium of APP transgenic cells are the most potent neurotoxins (Reed et al., 2009).

Oligomers of modified forms of N-terminally truncated Aβ peptides having pyroglutamate as first residue in the sequence (pE-Aβ) have also been detected in the cerebral cortex of AD patients (Piccini et al., 2005). pE-Aβ peptides are believed to play an important role in the pathogenesis of AD because they are highly abundant in the brains of AD patients and they are major constituents of the amyloid plaques (for a recent review, see Gunn et al., 2010). *In vitro* studies indicate that pE-Aβ peptides are more aggregation prone and neurotoxic than full length Aβ (Harigaya et al., 2000; Russo et al., 2002). When a novel mouse monoclonal antibody specifically targeting low molecular weights oligomers of pE-Aβ is used to passively immunize transgenic mice, plaque load and Aβ levels are reduced and behavioral deficits are normalized, suggesting that pE-Aβ oligomers are valuable targets for AD diagnosis and therapeutic intervention (Wirths et al., 2010).

3. Conclusion

In this chapter, we reviewed current knowledge of the structure and toxicity of different protein aggregates that are involved in Alzheimer's disease (AD). Currently, two structural models are available for $A\beta_{42}$ amyloid fibrils. Both models show a parallel cross-β-sheet structure. But in the first model, amino-acid-residues 11-22 and 31-42 adopt β-strand conformation ($A\beta_{42}$); wheareas in the second model, residues 18-26 and 31-42 adopt β-strand conformation ($^{35Mox}A\beta_{42}$). For $A\beta_{40}$ amyloid fibrils, structural polymorphism has been observed. The striated-ribbon fibrils, twisted-pair fibrils and brain-seeded fibrils of $A\beta_{40}$ all have different morphology and molecular structure. Tau PHFs also contain a cross-β-sheet structure, in which amino-acid-residues 306-311 and possibly 272-289 adopt the β-strand conformation. The rest of tau is either disordered or contains small amount of α-helical structure.

Recent studies suggest that the soluble Aβ aggregates (pre-fibrillar aggregates), instead of Aβ amyloid fibrils and tau PHFs, correlate more closelly with neuron degeneration in AD. Several types of Aβ pre-fibrillar aggregates have been described. Their common toxicity may be due to multiple reasons such as the heterogeneity of Aβ aggregates preparations, most likely containing different amounts of monomeric, oligomeric and fibrillar Aβ rather than single species, and the fact that all these species may share a "misfolded" nature, meaning that they most likely expose on their surfaces repetitive clusters and/or arrays of groups that enable their interaction with different targets. It has been recently suggested that it's the ongoing Aβ polymerization process involving the elongation and growth of pre-fibrillar aggregates such as protofibrils, rather than the formation of a specific toxic oligomeric species to be responsible for Aβ toxicity in AD (Jan et al., 2011). Similarly to what has been proposed for another amyloid forming peptide, the cooperative binding of Aβ peptides to cell membranes, and the growth and elongation of Aβ aggregates at the level of the membrane could result in changes in membrane curvature and weakened lipid packing, leading to membrane permeabilization and toxicity (Engel et al., 2008; Friedman et al., 2009). Further studies are therefore necessary to clearly elucidate the structural properties and mechanism of toxicity of Aβ aggregates in order to develop efficient therapeutic strategies for AD.

4. Acknowledgment

We would like to thank Prof. Roland Riek for his helpful comments and suggestions.

5. References

Ahmed, M., Davis, J., Aucoin, D., Sato, T., Ahuja, S., Aimoto, S., Elliott, J.I., Van Nostrand, W.E., & Smith, S.O. (2010). Structural conversion of neurotoxic amyloid-β_{1-42} oligomers to fibrils. *Nat Struct Mol Biol.*, 17, 561-567.

Alonso, A., Zaidi, T., Novak, M., Grundke-Iqbal, I., & Iqbal, K. (2001). Hyperphosphorylation induces self-assembly of tau into tangles of paired helical filaments/straight filaments. *Proc Natl Acad Sci U S A*, 98, 6923-6928.

Antzutkin, O.N., Leapman, R.D., Balbach, J.J., & Tycko, R. (2002). Supramolecular structural constraints on Alzheimer's beta-amyloid fibrils from electron microscopy and solid-state nuclear magnetic resonance. *Biochemistry*, 41, 15436-15450.

Arispe, N., Diaz, J.C., & Simakova, O. (2007). Abeta ion channels. Prospects for treating Alzheimer's disease with Abeta channel blockers. *Biochim Biophys Acta.*, 1768, 1952-1965.

Balbach, J.J., Petkova, A.T., Oyler, N.A., Antzutkin, O.N., Gordon, D.J., Meredith, S.C., & Tycko, R. (2002). Supramolecular structure in full-length Alzheimer's beta-amyloid fibrils: evidence for a parallel beta-sheet organization from solid-state nuclear magnetic resonance. *Biophys J.*, 83, 1205-1216.

Barghorn, S., Nimmrich, V., Striebinger, A., Krantz, C., Keller, P., Janson, B., Bahr, M., Schmidt, M., Bitner, R.S., Harlan, J., Barlow, E., Ebert, U., & Hillen, H. (2005). Globular amyloid beta-peptide oligomer – a homogeneous and stable neuropathological protein in Alzheimer's disease. *J Neurochem.*, 95, 834-847.

Bernstein, S.L., Dupuis, N.F., Lazo, N.D., Wyttenbach, T., Condron, M.M., Bitan, G., Teplow, D.B., Shea, J.E., Ruotolo, B.T., Robinson, C.V., & Bowers, M.T. (2009). Amyloid-β protein oligomerization and the importance of tetramers and dodecamers in the aetiology of Alzheimer's disease. *Nat Chem.*, 1, 326-331.

Bitan, G., Lomakin, A., & Teplow, D.B. (2001). Amyloid beta-protein oligomerization: prenucleation interactions revealed by photo-induced cross-linking of unmodified proteins. *J Biol Chem.*, 276, 35176-35184.

Bitan, G., Kirkitadze, M.D., Lomakin, A., Vollers, S.S., Benedek, G.B., & Teplow, D.B. (2003). Amyloid beta -protein (Abeta) assembly: Abeta 40 and Abeta 42 oligomerize through distinct pathways. *Proc Natl Acad Sci USA*, 100, 330-335.

Borchelt, D.R., Thinakaran, G., Eckman, C.B., Lee, M.K., Davenport, F., Ratovitsky, T., Prada, C.M., Kim, G., Seekins, S., Yager, D., Slunt, H.H., Wang, R., Seeger, M., Levey, A.I., Gandy, S.E., Copeland, N.G., Jenkins, N.A., Price, D.L., Younkin, S.G., & Sisodia, S.S. (1996). Familial Alzheimer's disease-linked presenilin 1 variants elevate Abeta1-42/1-40 ratio in vitro and in vivo. *Neuron*, 17, 1005-1013.

Braak, H., & Braak, E. (1995) Staging of Alzheimer's disease-related neurofibrillary changes. *Neurobiol Aging*, 16, 271–278.

Brunden, K.R., Trojanowski, J.Q., & Lee, V.M. (2009). Advances in tau-focused drug discovery for Alzheimer's disease and related tauopathies. *Nat Rev Drug Discov*, 8, 783-793.

Caetano, F.A., Beraldo, F.H., Hajj, G.N., Guimaraes, A.L., Jürgensen, S., Wasilewska-Sampaio, A.P., Hirata, P.H., Souza, I., Machado, C.F., Wong, D.Y., De Felice, F.G., Ferreira, S.T., Prado, V.F., Rylett, R.J., Martins, V.R., & Prado, M.A. (2011). Amyloid-beta oligomers increase the localization of prion protein at the cell surface. *J Neurosci.*, 117, 538-553.

Calella, A.M., Farinelli, M., Nuvolone, M., Mirante, O., Moos, R., Falsig, J., Mansuy, I.M., & Aguzzi, A. (2010). Prion protein and Abeta-related synaptic toxicity impairment. *EMBO Mol Med.*, 2, 306-314.

Chimon, S., & Ishii, Y. (2005). Capturing intermediate structures of Alzheimer's b-amyloid, Abeta (1-40), by solid-state NMR spectroscopy. *J Am Chem Soc.*, 127, 13472-13473.

Chimon, S., Shaibat, M.A., Jones, C.R., Calero, D.C., Aizezi, B., & Ishii, Y. (2007). Evidence of fibril-like beta-sheet structures in a neurotoxic amyloid intermediate of Alzheimer's beta-amyloid. *Nat Struct Mol Biol.*, 14, 1157-1164.

Chiti, F., & Dobson, C.M. (2006). Protein misfolding, functional amyloid, and human disease. *Annu Rev Biochem.*, 75, 333-366.

Chromy, B.A., Nowak, R.J., Lambert, M.P., Viola, K.L., Chang, L., Velasco, P.T., Jones, B.W., Fernandez, S.J., Lacor, P.N., Horowitz, P., Finch, C.E., Krafft, G.A., & Klein, W.L. (2003). Self-assembly of Abeta(1-42) into globular neurotoxins. *Biochemistry*, 42, 12749-12760.

Cleary, J.P., Walsh, D.M., Hofmeister, J.J., Shankar, G.M., Kuskowski, M.A., Selkoe, D.J., Ashe, K.H. (2005). Natural oligomers of the amyloid-beta protein specifically disrupt cognitive function. *Nat Neurosci.*, 8, 79-84.

Citron, M. (2004). Strategies for disease modification in Alzheimer's disease. *Nat Rev Neurosci* 5, 677-685.

Dahlgren, K.N., Manelli, A.M., Stine, W.B., Jr., Baker, L.K., Krafft, G.A., & LaDu, M.J. (2002). Oligomeric and fibrillar species of amyloid-beta peptides differentially affect neuronal viability. *J Biol Chem.*, 277, 32046-32053.

De Felice, F.G., Velasco, P.Y., Lambert, M.P., Viola, K., Fernandez, S.J., Ferreira, S.T., & Klein, W.L. (2007a) Abeta oligomers induce neuronal oxidative stress through an N-methyl-D-aspartate receptor-dependent mechanism that is blocked by the Alzheimer drug memantine. *J Biol Chem.*, 282, 11590-11601.

De Felice, F.G., Wu, D., Lambert, M.P., Fernandez, S.J., Velasco, P.T., Lacor, P.N., Bigio, E.H., Jerecic, J., Acton, P.J., Shughrue, P.J., Chen-Dodson, E., Kinney, G.G., & Klein, W.L. (2007b) Alzheimer's disease-type neuronal tau hyperphosphorylation induced by Abeta oligomers. *Neurobiol Aging.*, 29, 1334-1347.

De Felice, F.G., Vieira, M.N.N., Bomfim, T.R., Decker, H., Velasco, P.T., Lambert, M.P., Viola, K.L., Zhao, W.Q., Ferreira, S.T., Klein, W.L. (2009) Protection of synapses against Alzheimer's-linked toxins: insulin signaling prevents the pathogenic binding of Abeta oligomers. *Proc Natl Acad Sci U S A*, 106, 1971-1976.

Demuro, A., Mina, E., Kayed, R., Milton, S.C., Parker, I., & Glabe, C.G. (2005). Calcium dysregulation and membrane disruption as a ubiquitous neurotoxic mechanism of soluble amyloid oligomers. *J Biol Chem.*, 280, 17294-17300.

Dovey, H.F., Suomonsaari-Chrysler, S., Lieberburg, I., Sinha, S., & Keim, P.S. (1993). Cells with a familial Alzheimer's disease mutation produce authentic beta-peptide. *Neuroreport.*, 4, 1039-1042.

Eckman, C.B., Mehta, N.D., Crook, R., Perez-tur, J., Prihar, G., Pfeiffer, E., Graff-Radford, N., Hinder, P., Yager, D., Zenk, B., Refolo, L.M., Prada, C.M., Younkin, S.G., Hutton, M., Hardy, J. (1997). A new pathogenic mutation in the APP gene (I716V) increases the relative proportion of A beta 42(43). *Hum Mol Genet.*, 6, 2087-2089.

Engel, M.F.M., Khemtemourian, L., Kleijer, C., Meeldijk, H.J.D., Jacobs, J., Verkleij, A.J., de Kruijff, B., Killian, J.A., & Höppener, J.W. (2008). Membrane damage by human islet amyloid polypeptide through fibril growth at the membrane. *Proc Natl Acad Sci U S A*, 105, 6033-6038.

Freir, D.B., Fedriani, R., Scully, D., Smith, I.M., Selkoe D.J., Walsh, D.M., & Regan, C.M. (2010) Abeta oligomers inhibit synapse remodeling necessary for memory consolidation. *Neurobiol Aging*. Epub ahead of print.

Friedman, R., Pellarin, R., & Caflisch, A. (2009) Amyloid aggregation on lipid bilayers and its impact on membrane permeability. *J Mol Biol.*, 387, 407-415.

Gellermann, G.P., Byrnes, H., Striebinger, A., Ullrich, K., Mueller, R., Hillen, H., & Barghorn, S. (2008). Abeta-globulomers are formed independently of the fibril pathway. Neurobiol Dis., 30, 212-220.

Georganopoulou, D.G., Chang, L., Nam, J-M., Thaxton, C.S., Mufson, E.J., Klein, W.L., & Mirkin, C.A. (2005). Nanoparticle-based detection in cerebral spinal fluid of a soluble pathogenic biomarker for Alzheimer's disease. *Proc Natl Acad Sci U S A*, 102, 2273-2276.

Gimbel, D.A., Nygaard, H.B., Coffey, E.E., Gunther, E.C., Laurén, J., Gimbel, Z.A., & Strittmatter, S.M. (2010). Memory impairment in transgenic Alzheimer mice requires cellular prion protein. *J Neurosci.*, 30, 6367-6374.

Golde, T.E., & Younkin, S.G. (1996) in *Pathology of Alzheimer's Disease*, Goate A. (Ed.), p. 113, Academic press, New York.

Gong, Y., Chang, L., Viola, K.L., Lacor, P.N., Lambert, M.P., Finch, C.E., Krafft, G.A., & Klein, W.L. (2003). Alzheimer's disease-affected brain: presence of oligomeric Abeta ligands (ADDLs) suggests a molecular basis for reversible memory loss. *Proc Natl Acad Sci U S A*, 100, 10417-10422.

Gunn, A.P., Masters, C.L., & Cherny, R.A. (2010) Pyroglutamate-Aβ: Role in the natural history of Alzheimer's disease. *Int J Biochem Cell Biol.*, 42, 1915-1918.

Guzowski, J.F. (2002). Insights into immediate-early gene function in hippocampal memory consolidation using antisense oligonucleotide and fluorescent imaging approaches. *Hippocampus*, 12, 86-104.

Goedert, M., Spillantini, M.G., Cairns, N.J., & Crowther, R.A. (1992). Tau proteins of Alzheimer paired helical filaments: abnormal phosphorylation of all six brain isoforms. *Neuron*, 8, 159-168.

Greenwald, J., & Riek, R. (2010). Biology of amyloid: structure, function, and regulation. *Structure*, 18, 1244-1260.

Hardy, J., & Selkoe, D.J. (2002). The amyloid hypothesis of Alzheimer's disease: progress and problems on the road to therapeutics. *Science*, 297, 353-356.

Hartmann, T., Bieger, S.C., Bruhl, B., Tienari, P.J., Ida, N., Allsop, D., Roberts, G.W., Masters, C.L., Dotti, C.G., Unsicker, K., & Beyreuther, K. (1997). Distinct sites of intracellular production for Alzheimer's disease A beta40/42 amyloid peptides. *Nat Med.*, 3, 1016-1020.

Hernandez, F., & Avila, J. (2007). Tauopathies. *Cell Mol Life Sci.*, 64, 2219-2233.

Heutink, P. (2000). Untangling tau-related dementia. *Hum Mol Genet.*, 9, 979-986.

Hooper, N.M. (2005). Roles of proteolysis and lipid rafts in the processing of the amyloid precursor protein and prion protein. *Biochem Soc Trans.*, 33, 335-338.

Hoshino, M., Katou, H., Hagihara, Y., Hasegawa, K., Naiki, H., & Goto, Y. (2002). Mapping the core of the beta(2)-microglobulin amyloid fibril by H/D exchange. *Nat Struct Biol.*, 9, 332-336.

Haass, C., Schlossmacher, M.G., Hung, A.Y., Vigo-Pelfrey, C., Mellon, A., Ostaszewski, B.L., Lieberburg, I., Koo, E.H., Schenk, D., Teplow, D.B. et al. (1992). Amyloid beta-peptide is produced by cultured cells during normal metabolism. *Nature*, 359, 322-325.

Hardy, J., & Selkoe, D.J. (2002). The amyloid hypothesis of Alzheimer's disease: progress and problems on the road to therapeutics. *Science*, 297, 353-356.

Harigaya, Y., Saido, T.C., Eckman, C.B., Prada, C.M., Shoji, M., & Younkin, S.G. (2000). Amyloid beta protein starting pyroglutamate at position 3 is a major component of the amyloid deposits in the Alzheimer's disease brain. *Biochem Biophys Res Commun.*, 276, 422-427.

Harper, J.D., Wong, S.S., Lieber, C.M., & Lansbury, P.T. (1997) Observation of metastable Aβ amyloid protofibrils by atomic force microscopy. *Chem Biol.*, 4, 119-125.

Harper, J.D., Wong, S.S., Lieber, C.M., & Lansbury, P.T. (1999) Assembly of Abeta amyloid protofibrils: an *in vitro* model for a possible early event in Alzheimer's disease. *Biochemistry*, 38, 8972-8980.

Hartley, D.M., Walsh, D.M., Ye, C.P., Diehl, T., Vasquez, S., Vassilev, P.M., Teplow, D.B., & Selkoe, D.J. (1999). Protofibrillar intermediates of amyloid β-protein induce acute electrophysiological changes and progressive neurotoxicity in onrtical neurons. *J Neurosci.*, 19, 8876-8884.

Hillen, H., Barghorn, S., Striebinger, A., Labkovsky, B., Müller, R., Nimmrich, V., Nolte, M.W., Perez-Cruz, C., van der Auwera, I., van Leuven, F., van Gaalen, M., Bespalov, A.Y., Schoemaker, H., Sullivan, J.P., & Ebert, U. (2010). Generation and therapeutic efficacy of highly oligomer-specific beta-amyloid antibodies. *J Neurosci.*, 30, 10369-10379.

Hoshi, M., Sato, M., Matsumoto, S., Noguchi, A., Yasutake, K., Yoshida, N., & Sato, K. (2003). Spherical aggregates of beta-amyloid (amylospheroid) show high neurotoxicity and activate tau protein kinase I/glycogen synthase kinase-3b. *Proc Natl Acad Sci U S A*, 100, 6370-6375.

Hsieh, H., Boehm, J., Sato, C., Iwatsubo, T., Tomita, T., Sisodia, S., & Malinow, R. (2006). AMPAR removal underlies Abeta-induced synaptic depression and dendritic spine loss. *Neuron*, 52, 831-43.

Ittner, L.M., Ke, Y.D., Delerue, F., Bi, M., Gladbach, A., van Eersel, J., Wolfing, H., Chieng, B.C., Christie, M.J., Napier, I.A., Eckert, A., Staufenbiel, M., Hardeman, E., & Götz, J. (2010). Dendritic function of tau mediates amyloid-beta toxicity in Alzheimer's disease mouse models. *Cell*, 142, 387-397.

Johansson, A.S., Garlind, A., Berlind-Dehlin, F., Karlsson, G., Edwards, K., Gellerfors, P., Ekholm-Pettersson, F., Palmblad, J., & Lannfelt, L. (2007). Docosahexaenoic acid stabilizes soluble amyloid-beta protofibrils and sustains amyloid-β-induced neurotoxicity in vitro. *FEBS J.*, 274, 990-1000.

Kayed, R., Head, E., Thompson, J.L., McIntire, T.M., Milton, S.C., Cotman, C.W., & Glabe, C.G. (2003). Common structure of soluble amyloid oligomers implies common mechanism of pathogenesis. *Science*, 300, 486-489.

Kayed, R., Sokolov, Y., Edmonds, B., McIntire, T.M., Milton, S.C., Hall, J.E., & Glabe, C.G. (2004). Permeabilization of lipid bilayers is a common conformation-dependent activity of soluble amyloid oligomers in protein misfolding diseases. J Biol Chem., 279, 46363-46366.

Kayed, R., Pensalfini, A., Margol, L., Sokolov, Y., Sarsoza, F., Head, E., Hall, J., & Glabe, C. (2009). Annular protofibrils are a structurally and functionally distinct type of amyloid oligomer. *J Biol Chem.*, 284, 4230-4237.

Kheterpal, I., Lashuel, H.A., Hartley, D.M., Walz, T., Lansbury, P.T.Jr., & Wetzel, R. (2003). Abeta protofibrils possess a stable core structure resistant to exchange. *Biochemistry*, 42, 4092-4098.

Kheterpal, I., Chen, M., Cook, K.D., & Wetzel, R. (2006). Structural differences in Aβ amyloid protofibrils and fibrils mapped by hydrogen exchange--mass spectrometry with on-line proteolytic fragmentation. *J Mol Biol.*, 361, 785-795.

Klein, W.L., Krafft, G.A., & Finch, C.E. (2001). Targeting small Abeta oligomers: the solution to an Alzheimer's disease conundrum? *Trends Neurosci.*, 24, 219-224.

Klein, W.L. (2002) Abeta toxicity in Alzheimer's disease: globular oligomers (ADDLs) as new vaccine and drug targets. *Neurochem Int.*, 41, 345-352.

Klyubin, I., Betts, V., Wetzel, A.T., Blennow, K., Zetterberg, H., Wallin, A., Lemere, C.A., Cullen, W.K., Peng, Y., Wisniewski, T., Selkoe, D.J., Anwyl, R., Walsh, D.M., & Rowan, M.J. (2008). Amyloid beta protein dimer-containing human CSF disrupts synaptic plasticity: prevention by systemic passive immunization. *J Neurosci.*, 28, 4231-4237.

Kang, J., Lemaire, H.G., Unterbeck, A., Salbaum, J.M., Masters, C.L., Grzeschik, K.H., Multhaup, G., Beyreuther, K., & Muller-Hill, B. (1987). The precursor of Alzheimer's disease amyloid A4 protein resembles a cell-surface receptor. *Nature*, 325, 733-736.

Kosik, K.S. (1990). Tau protein and Alzheimer's disease. *Curr Opin Cell Biol.*, 2, 101-104.

Kirschner, D.A., Abraham, C., & Selkoe, D.J. (1986). X-ray diffraction from intraneuronal paired helical filaments and extraneuronal amyloid fibers in Alzheimer disease indicates cross-beta conformation. *Proc Natl Acad Sci U S A*, 83, 503-507.

Lewis, J., Dickson, D.W., Lin, W.L., Chisholm, L., Corral, A., Jones, G., Yen, S.H., Sahara, N., Skipper, L., Yager, D., Eckman, C., Hardy, J., Hutton, M., & McGowan, E. (2001). Enhanced neurofibrillary degeneration in transgenic mice expressing mutant tau and APP. *Science*, 293, 1487-1491.

Luhrs, T., Ritter, C., Adrian, M., Riek-Loher, D., Bohrmann, B., Dobeli, H., Schubert, D., & Riek, R. (2005). 3D structure of Alzheimer's amyloid-beta(1-42) fibrils. *Proc Natl Acad Sci U S A*, 102, 17342-17347.

Lacor, P.N, Buniel, M.C, Chang, L., Fernandez, S.J., Gong, Y., Viola, K.L., Lambert, M.P., Velasco, P.T., Bigio, E.H., Finch, C.E., Krafft, G.A., & Klein, W.L. (2004) Synaptic targeting by Alzheimer's-related amyloid b oligomers. J Neurosci., 24, 10191-10200.

Lacor, P.N., Buniel, M.C., Furlow, P.W., Clemente, A.S., Velasco, P.T., Wood, M., Viola, K.L., & Klein, W.L. (2007) Abeta oligomer-induced aberrations in synapse composition, shape, and density provide a molecular basis for loss of connectivity in Alzheimer's disease. *J Neurosci.*, 27, 796-807.

Lambert, M.P., Barlow, A.K., Chomy, B.A., Edwards, C, Freed, R., Liosatos, M., Morgan, T.E., Rozovsky, I., Trommer, B., Viola, K.L., Wals, P., Zhang, C., Finch, C.E., Krafft, G.A., & Klein, W.L. (1998) Diffusible, nonfibrillar ligands derived from $A\beta_{1\text{-}42}$ are potent central nervous system neurotoxins. *Proc Natl Acad Sci U S A*, 95, 6448-6453.

Lambert, M.P., Velasco, P.T., Chang, L., Viola, K.L., Fernandez, S., Lacor, P.N., Khuon, D., Gong, Y., Bigio, E.H., Shaw, P., De felice, F.G., Krafft, G.A., & Klein, W.L. (2007) Monoclonal antibodies that target pathological assemblies of Abeta. *J Neurochem.*, 199, 23-35.

Lashuel, H.A., Hartley, D., Petre, B.M., Walz, T., & Lansbury, P.T.Jr. (2002) Neurodegenerative disease: amyloid pores from pathogenic mutations. *Nature*, 418, 291.

Laurén, J., Gimbel, D.A., Nygaard, H.B., Gilbert, J.W., & Strittmatter, S.M. (2009) Cellular prion protein mediates impairment of synaptic plasticity by amyloid-beta oligomers. *Nature*, 457, 1128-1132.

Lesné, S., Koh, M.T., Kotilinek, L., Kayed, R., Glabe, C.G., Yang, A., Gallagher, M., & Ashe, K.H. (2006) A specific amyloid-beta protein assembly in the brain impairs memory. *Nature*, 440, 352-357.

Lewis, J., Dickson, D.W., Lin, W.L., Chisholm, L., Corral, A., Jones, G., Yen, S.H., Sahara, N., Skipper, L., Yager, D., Eckman, C., Hardy, J., Hutton, M., & McGowan, E. (2001). Enhanced neurofibrillary degeneration in transgenic mice expressing mutant tau and APP. *Science*, 293, 1487-1491.

Margittai, M., & Langen, R. (2006). Side chain-dependent stacking modulates tau filament structure. *J Biol Chem.*, 281, 37820-37827.

Masters, C.L., Simms, G., Weinman, N.A., Multhaup, G., McDonald, B.L., & Beyreuther, K. (1985). Amyloid plaque core protein in Alzheimer disease and Down syndrome. *Proc Natl Acad Sci U S A*, 82, 4245-4249.

Matsumura, S., Shinoda, K., Yamada, M., Yokojima, S., Inoue, M., Ohnishi, T., Shimada, T., Kikuchi, K., Masui, D., Hashimoto, S., Sato, M., Ito, A., Akioka, M., Takagi, S., Nakamura, Y., Nemoto, K., Hasegawa, Y., Takamoto, H., Inoue, H., Nakamura, S., Nabeshima, Y., Teplow, D.B., Kinjo, M., & Hoshi, M. (2011). Two distinct amyloid beta-protein (Abeta) assembly pathways leading to oligomers and fibrils identified by combined fluorescence correlation spectroscopy, morphology and toxicity analyses. *J Biol Chem.*, 286, 11555-11562.

Mori, H., Takio, K., Ogawara, M., & Selkoe, D.J. (1992). Mass spectrometry of purified amyloid beta protein in Alzheimer's disease. *J Biol Chem.*, 267, 17082-17086.

Nilsberth, C., Westlind-Danielsson, A., Eckman, C.B., Condron, M.M., Axelman, K., Forsell, C., Stenh, C., Luthman, J., Teplow, D.B., Younkin, S.G., Naslund, J., & Lannfelt, L. (2001). The 'Arctic' APP mutation (E693G) causes Alzheimer's disease by enhanced Ab protofibril formation. *Nat Neurosci.*, 4, 887-893.

Noguchi, A., Matsumura, S., Dezawa, M., Tada, M., Yanazawa, M., Ito, A., Akloka, M., Kikuchi, S., Sato, M., Ideno, S., Noda, M., Fukunari, A., Maramatsu, S., Itokazu, Y., Sato, K., Takahashi, H., Teplow, D.B., Nabeshima, Y., Kakita, A., Imahori, K., & Hoshi, M. (2009). Isolation and characterization of patient-derived, toxic, high mass amyloid beta-protein (Abeta) assembly from Alzheimer disease brains. *J Biol Chem.*, 284, 32895-32905.

Oda, T., Wals, P., Osterburg, H.H., Johnson, S.A., Pasinetti, G.M., Morgan, T.E., Rozovsky, I., Stine, W.B., Snyder, S.W., Holzman, T.F. *et al.* (1995). Clusterin (apoJ) alters the aggregation of amyloid beta-peptide (A beta 1-42) and forms slowly sedimenting A beta complexes that cause oxidative stress. *Exp Neurol.*, 136, 22-31.

Ohnishi, S., & Takano, K. (2004). Amyloid fibrils from the viewpoint of protein folding. *Cell Mol Life Sci.*, 61, 511-524.

Olofsson, A., Sauer-Eriksson, A.E., & Ohman, A. (2006). The solvent protection of alzheimer amyloid-beta-(1-42) fibrils as determined by solution NMR spectroscopy. *J Biol Chem.*, 281, 477-483.

Paravastu, A.K., Qahwash, I., Leapman, R.D., Meredith, S.C., & Tycko, R. (2009). Seeded growth of beta-amyloid fibrils from Alzheimer's brain-derived fibrils produces a distinct fibril structure. *Proc Natl Acad Sci U S A*, 106, 7443-7448.

Paravastu, A.K., Leapman, R.D., Yau, W.M., & Tycko, R. (2008). Molecular structural basis for polymorphism in Alzheimer's beta-amyloid fibrils. *Proc Natl Acad Sci U S A*, 105, 18349-18354.

Petkova, A.T., Leapman, R.D., Guo, Z., Yau, W.M., Mattson, M.P., & Tycko, R. (2005). Self-propagating, molecular-level polymorphism in Alzheimer's beta-amyloid fibrils. *Science*, 307, 262-265.

Petkova, A.T., Yau, W.M., & Tycko, R. (2006). Experimental constraints on quaternary structure in Alzheimer's beta-amyloid fibrils. *Biochemistry*, 45, 498-512.

Piccini, A., Russo, C., Gliozzi, A., Relini, A.,Vitali, A., Borghi, R., Giliberto, L., Armirotti, A., D'Arrigo, C., Bachi, A., Cattaneo, A., Canale, C., Torrassa, S., Saldo, T.C., Markesbery, W., Gambetti, P., & Tabaton, M. (2005). beta-Amyloid is different in normal aging and in Alzheimer disease. *J Biol Chem.*, 280, 34186-34192.

Poling, A., Morgan-Paisley, K., Panos, J.J., Kim, E.M., O'Hare, E., Cleary, J.P., Lesné, S., Ashe, K.H., Porritt, M., & Baker, L.E. (2008). Oligomers of the amyloid-beta protein disrupt working memory: confirmation with two behavioral procedures. *Behav Brain Res.*, 193, 230-234.

Portelius, E., Bogdanovic, N., Gustavsson, M.K., Volkmann, I., Brinkmalm, G., Zetterberg, H., Winblad, B., & Blennow, K. (2010). Mass spectrometric characterization of brain amyloid beta isoform signatures in familial and sporadic Alzheimer's disease. *Acta Neuropathol.*, 120, 185-193.

Querfurth, H.W., & LaFerla, F.M. (2010). Alzheimer's disease. *N Engl J Med.*, 362, 329-344.

Rahimi, F., Shanmugam, A., & Bitan, G. (2008). Structure-function relationships of pre-fibrillar protein assemblies in Alzheimer's disease and related disorders. *Curr Alzheimer Res.*, 5, 319-341.

Rapoport, M., Dawson, H.N., Binder, L.I., Vitek, M.P., & Ferreira, A. (2002). Tau is essential to beta -amyloid-induced neurotoxicity. *Proc Natl Acad Sci U S A*, 99, 6364-6369.

Roher, A.E., Lowenson, J.D., Clarke, S., Woods, A.S., Cotter, R.J., Gowing, E., & Ball, M.J. (1993). beta-Amyloid-(1-42) is a major component of cerebrovascular amyloid deposits: implications for the pathology of Alzheimer disease. *Proc Natl Acad Sci U S A*, 90, 10836-10840.

Reed, M.N., Hofmeister, J.J., Jungbauer, L., Welzel, A.T., Yu, C., Sherman, M.A., Lesné, S., Ladu, M.J., Walsh, D.M., Ashe, K.H., & Cleary, J.P. (2009). Cognitive effects of cell-derived and synthetically derived Abeta oligomers. Neurobiol Aging., Ebup ahead of print.

Roher, A.E., Chaney, M.O., Kuo, Y.M., Webster, S.D., Stine, W.B., Haverkamp, L.J., Woods, A.S., Cotter, R.J., Tuohy, J.M., Krafft, G.A., Bonnell, B.S., & Emmerling, M.R. (1996). Morphology and toxicity of Abeta-(1-42) dimer derived from neuritic and vascular amyloid deposits of Alzheimer's disease. *J Biol Chem.*, 271, 20631-20635.

Russo, C., Violani, E., Salis, S., Venezia, V., Dolcini, V., Damonte, G., Benatti, U., D'Arrigo, C., Patrone, E., Carlo, P., & Schettini, G. (2002). Pyroglutamate-modified amyloid beta-peptides - AbetaN3(pE) - strongly affects cultured neuron and astrocyte survival. *J Neurochem.*, 82, 1480-1489.

Sakono, M., & Zako, T. (2010). Amyloid oligomers: formation and toxicity of Abeta oligomers. *FEBS J.*, 277, 1348-1358.

Saido, T.C., Iwatsubo, T., Mann, D.M., Shimada, H., Ihara, Y., & Kawashima, S. (1995). Dominant and differential deposition of distinct beta-amyloid peptide species, A beta N3(pE), in senile plaques. *Neuron*, 14, 457-466.

Sayre, L.M., Zelasko, D.A., Harris, P.L., Perry, G., Salomon, R.G., & Smith, M.A. (1997). 4-Hydroxynonenal-derived advanced lipid peroxidation end products are increased in Alzheimer's disease. J Neurochem., 68, 2092-2097.

Selkoe, D.J. (2008). Soluble oligomers of the amyloid beta-protein impair synaptic plasticity and behavior. *Behav Brain Res.*, 192, 106-113.

Seubert, P., Vigo-Pelfrey, C., Esch, F., Lee, M., Dovey, H., Davis, D., Sinha, S., Schlossmacher, M., Whaley, J., Swindlehurst, C. et al. (1992). Isolation and quantification of soluble Alzheimer's beta-peptide from biological fluids. *Nature,* 359, 325-327.

Shankar, G.M., Bloodgood, B.L., Townsend, M., Walsh, D.M., Selkoe, D.J., & Sabatini, B.L. (2007). Natural oligomers of the Alzheimer amyloid-beta peptide induce reversible synapse loss by modulating an NMDA-type glutamate receptor-dependent signaling pathway. *J Neurosci.,* 27, 2866-2875.

Shankar G.M., Li S., Mehta T.H., Garcia-Munoz A., Shepardson N.E., Smith, I., Brett, F.M., Farrell, M.A., Rowan, M.J., Lemere, C.A., Regan, C.M., Walsh, D.M., Sabatini, B.L., & Selkoe, D.J. (2008). Amyloid-beta protein dimers isolated directly from Alzheimer's brains impair synaptic plasticity and memory. *Nat Med.,* 14, 837-842.

Siegel, S.J., Bieschke, J., Powers, E.T., & Kelly, J.W. (2007). The oxidative stress metabolite 4-hydroxynonenal promotes Alzheimer protofibril formation. *Biochemistry,* 46, 1503-1510.

Suzuki, N., Cheung, T.T., Cai, X.D., Odaka, A., Otvos, L.Jr., Eckman, C., Golde, T.E., & Younkin, S.G. (1994). An increased percentage of long amyloid beta protein secreted by familial amyloid beta protein precursor (beta APP717) mutants. *Science,* 264, 1336-1340.

Sadqi, M., Hernandez, F., Pan, U., Perez, M., Schaeberle, M.D., Avila, J., & Munoz, V. (2002). Alpha-helix structure in Alzheimer's disease aggregates of tau-protein. *Biochemistry,* 41, 7150-7155.

Sawaya, M.R., Sambashivan, S., Nelson, R., Ivanova, M.I., Sievers, S.A., Apostol, M.I., Thompson, M.J., Balbirnie, M., Wiltzius, J.J., McFarlane, H.T., *et al.* (2007). Atomic structures of amyloid cross-beta spines reveal varied steric zippers. *Nature,* 447, 453-457.

Schmitz, C., Rutten, B.P., Pielen, A., Schafer, S., Wirths, O., Tremp, G., Czech, C., Blanchard, V., Multhaup, G., Rezaie, P., *et al.* (2004). Hippocampal neuron loss exceeds amyloid plaque load in a transgenic mouse model of Alzheimer's disease. *Am J Pathol.,* 164, 1495-1502.

Sciarretta, K.L., Gordon, D.J., Petkova, A.T., Tycko, R., & Meredith, S.C. (2005). Abeta40-Lactam(D23/K28) models a conformation highly favorable for nucleation of amyloid. *Biochemistry,* 44, 6003-6014.

Selkoe, D.J. (2002). Alzheimer's disease is a synaptic failure. *Science,* 298, 789-791.

Tanzi, R.E., & Bertram, L. (2005). Twenty years of the Alzheimer's disease amyloid hypothesis: a genetic perspective. *Cell,* 120, 545-555.

Tiraboschi, P., Hansen, L.A., Thal, L.J., & Corey-Bloom, J. (2004). The importance of neuritic plaques and tangles to the development and evolution of AD. *Neurology,* 62, 1984-1989.

Turner, P.R., O'Connor, K., Tate, W.P., & Abraham, W.C. (2003). Roles of amyloid precursor protein and its fragments in regulating neural activity, plasticity and memory. *Prog Neurobiol.,* 70, 1-32.

Tycko, R. (2004). Progress towards a molecular-level structural understanding of amyloid fibrils. *Curr Opin Struct Biol.,* 14, 96-103.

Tycko, R. (2010). Solid-State NMR Studies of Amyloid Fibril Structure. Annu Rev Phys Chem.

Tycko, R., Sciarretta, K.L., Orgel, J.P., & Meredith, S.C. (2009). Evidence for novel beta-sheet structures in Iowa mutant beta-amyloid fibrils. *Biochemistry,* 48, 6072-6084.

Tabaton, M., Nunzi, M.G., Xue, R., Usiak, M., Autilio-Gambetti, L., & Gambetti, P. (1994). Soluble amyloid beta-protein is a marker of Alzheimer amyloid in brain but not in cerebrospinal fluid. *Biochem Biophys Res Commun.,* 200, 1598-1603.

Teplow, D.B. (2006). Preparation of amyloid beta-protein for structural and functional studies. *Methods Enzymol.*, 413, 20-33.

Terry, R.D., Masliah, E., Salmon, D.P., Butters, N., De Teresa, R., Hill, R., Hansen, L.A., & Katzman, R. (1991). Physical basis of cognitive alterations in Alzheimer's disease: synapse loss is the major correlate of cognitive impairment. *Ann Neurol.*, 30, 572-580.

Tomiyama, T., Nagata, T., Shimada, H., Teraoka, R., Fukushima, A., Kanemitsu, H., Takuma, H., Kuwano, R., Imagawa, M., Ataka, S., Wada, Y., Yoshioka, E., Nishizaki, T., Watanabe, Y., & Mori, H. (2008). A new amyloid beta variant favoring oligomerization in Alzheimer's-type dementia. *Ann. Neurol.*, 63, 377-387.

Townsend, M., Shankar, G.M., Mehta, T., Walsh, D.M., & Selkoe, D.J. (2006). Effects of secreted oligomers of amyloid beta-protein on hyppocampal synaptic plasticity: a potent role for trimers. *J Physiol.*, 572, 477-492.

Vigo-Pelfrey, C., Lee, D., Keim, P., Lieberburg, I., & Schenk, D.B. (1993). Characterization of beta-amyloid peptide from human cerebrospinal fluid. *J Neurochem.*, 61, 1965-1968.

von Bergen, M., Barghorn, S., Biernat, J., Mandelkow, E.M., & Mandelkow, E. (2005). Tau aggregation is driven by a transition from random coil to beta sheet structure. *Biochim Biophys Acta*, 1739, 158-166.

von Bergen, M., Friedhoff, P., Biernat, J., Heberle, J., Mandelkow, E.M., & Mandelkow, E. (2000). Assembly of tau protein into Alzheimer paired helical filaments depends on a local sequence motif ((306)VQIVYK(311)) forming beta structure. *Proc Natl Acad Sci U S A*, 97, 5129-5134.

Walsh, D.M., Lomakin, A., Benedeck, G.B., Condron, M.M., & Teplow, D.B. (1997). Amyloid-beta protein fibrillogenesis. Detection of a protofibrillar intermediate. *J Biol Chem.*, 292, 22364-22372.

Walsh, D.M., Hartley, D.M., Kusumoto, Y., Fezoui, Y., Condron, M.M., Lomakin, A., Benedek, G.B., Selkoe, D.J., & Teplow, D.B. (1999). Amyloid-beta protein fibrillogenesis. Structure and biological activity of protofibrillar intermediates. *J Biol Chem.*, 274, 25945-25952.

Walsh, D.M., Tseng, B.P., Rydel, R.E., Podlisny, M.B., & Slekoe, D.J. (2000). The oligomerization of amyloid beta-protein begins intracellularly in cells derived from human brain. *Biochemistry*, 39, 10831-10839.

Walsh, D.M., Klyubin, I., Fadeeva, J., Cullen, W.K., Anwyl, R., Wolfe, M.S., Rowan, M.J., & Selkoe, D.J. (2002). Naturally secreted oligomers if the Alzheimer amiloid beta-protein potently inhibit hippocampal long-term potentiation in vivo. *Nature*, 416, 535-539.

Walsh, D.M., Townsend, M., Podlisny, M.B., Shankar, G.M. Fadeeva, J.V., El Agnaf, O., Hartley, D.M., & Selkoe, D.J. (2005a). Certain inhibitors of synthetic amyloid beta-peptide (Abeta) fibrillogenesis block oligomerization of natural Abeta and thereby rescue long-term potentiation. *J Neurosci.*, 25, 2455-2462.

Walsh, D.M., Klyubin, I., Shankar, G.M., Townsend, M., Fadeeva, J.V., Betts, V., Podlisny, M.B., Cleary, J.P., Ashe, K.H., Rowan, M.J., & Selkoe, D.J. (2005b). The role of cell-derived oligomers of Abeta in Alzheimer's disease and avenues for therapeutic intervention. *Biochem Soc Trans.*, 33, 1087-1090.

Wang, H.W., Pasternak, J.F., Kuo, H., Ristic, H., Lambert, M.P., Chromy, B., Viola, K.L., Klein, W.L., Stine, W.B., Krafft, G.A., & Trommer, B.L. (2002). Soluble oligomers of beta amyloid (1-42) inhibit long-term potentiation but not long-term depression in rat dentate gyratus. *Brain Res.*, 924, 133-140.

Wang, L., Maji, S.K., Sawaya, M.R., Eisenberg, D., & Riek, R. (2008). Bacterial inclusion bodies contain amyloid-like structure. *PLoS Biol.*, 6, e195.

Wang, L., Schubert, D., Sawaya, M.R., Eisenberg, D., & Riek, R. (2010). Multidimensional structure-activity relationship of a protein in its aggregated states. *Angew Chem Int Ed Engl.*, 49, 3904-3908.

Westlind-Danielsson, A., & Arnerup, G. (2001). Spontaneous in vitro formation of supramolecula b-amyloid structures, "betaamy balls", by beta-amyloid 1-40 peptide. *Biochemistry*, 40, 14736-14743.

Wenk, G.L. (2003). Neuropathologic changes in Alzheimer's disease. *J Clin Psychiatry*, 64 Suppl 9, 7-10.

Wischik, C.M., Novak, M., Edwards, P.C., Klug, A., Tichelaar, W., & Crowther, R.A. (1988). Structural characterization of the core of the paired helical filament of Alzheimer disease. *Proc Natl Acad Sci U S A*, 85, 4884-4888.

Williams, A.D., Sega, M., Chen, M., Kheterpal, I., Geva, M., Berthelier, V., Kaleta, D.T., Cook, K.D., & Wetzel, R. (2005). Structural properties of Abeta protofibrils stabilized by a small molecule. *Proc Natl Acad Sci U S A*, 102, 7115-7120.

Wirths, O., Erck, C., Martens, H., Harmeier, A., Geumann, C., Jawhar, S., Kumar, S., Multhauo, G., Walter, J., Ingelsson, M., Degerman-Gunnarsson, M. *et al.* (2010). Identification of low molecular weight pyroglutamate Abeta oligomers in Alzheimer disease: a novel tool for therapy and diagnosis. *J Biol Chem.*, 285, 41517-41524.

Yu, L., Edalji, R., Harlan, J.E., Holzman, T.F., Lopez, A.P., Labkovsky, B., Hillen, H., Barghorn, S., Ebert, U., Richardson, P.L. *et al.* (2009). Structural characterization of a soluble amyloid b-peptide oligomer. *Biochemistry*, 48, 1870-1877.

Part 3

Abnormalities in Signal Trandusction, Neurotransmission, and Gene Regulation

10

The Role of Glycogen Synthase Kinase-3 (GSK-3) in Alzheimer's Disease

Miguel Medina[1] and Jesús Avila[2]
[1]*Noscira S.A., Tres Cantos*
[2]*Centro de Biología Molecular "Severo Ochoa" CSIC-UAM, Cantoblanco*
Spain

1. Introduction

Despite its initial discovery as one of five protein kinases activities found to phosphorylate glycogen synthase (GS) in fractioned extracts of rabbit skeletal muscle (Embi et al., 1980; Hemmings et al., 1981), Glycogen Synthase Kinase 3 (GSK-3) is by no means restricted to a role in glycogen metabolism. Indeed, the enzyme targets a wide variety of proteins involved in signalling, metabolism, structural proteins and a remarkable number of transcription factors and plays a far more pleiotropic role than first imagined (Woodgett, 2006). Genetic analyses and the use of selective inhibitors have shown that GSK-3 plays critical roles in development, metabolic homeostasis, neuronal growth and differentiation (Hur & Zhon, 2010), cell polarity, cell fate and apoptosis. Its unique position in modulating the function of a diverse series of proteins in combination with its association with a wide variety of human disorders, from neurodegenerative diseases, stroke, bipolar disorder to diabetes and cancer, has attracted significant attention to the protein both as a therapeutic target and as a means to understand the molecular basis of these disorders.

In particular, the involvement of GSK-3 in several key pathophyisiological pathways leading to Alzheimer's disease (AD) and neurodegenerative diseases has placed this enzyme in a central position in this disorder. Thus, GSK-3 has recently been proposed as a link between the two major pathological pathways in AD, amyloid and tau (Hernández et al., 2010; Muyllaert et al., 2008) and even a "GSK-3 hypothesis of AD", suggesting that GSK-3 might be a casual mediator of the disease, has been put forward (Hooper et al., 2008). This review will focus on describing the key role that GSK-3 plays in AD pathobiology and the use of GSK-3 inhibition as a potential therapeutic approach to treat this disease.

2. GSK-3 structure and regulation

GSK-3 is a highly conserved protein kinase belonging to the CMGC family of serine/threonine protein kinases, as genes encoding the enzyme have been identified in every eukaryotic genome that has been investigated, such as *Dictyostelium discoideum* (Kim et al., 1999), *Xenopus laevis* (Itoh et al., 1995), *Drosophila melanogaster* (Ruel et al., 1993) or parasites such like *Plasmodium falciparum, Trypanosoma brucei* or *Leishmania donovani* (Osolodkin et al., 2011). Mammalian GSK-3 is encoded by two genes, *gsk-3α* and *gsk-3β*

(Frame & Cohen, 2001; Grimes & Jope, 2001), that encode proteins of 51 and 47 kDa, respectively and which display 84% overall identity (98% within their catalytic domains), with the main difference being an extra Gly-rich stretch in the N-terminal domain of GSK-3α (Woodgett, 1990). Mammalian GSK-3α and β are each widely expressed although some tissues show preferential levels of some of the two proteins. Furthermore, an alternatively splicing event between exons 8 and 9 of GSK-3β gives rise in neurons to a splice variant (GSK-3β2) containing a 13 amino acids insertion within the kinase domain near to the substrate binding pocket (Mukai et al., 2002). How this insertion affects kinase activity or regulation remains unclear, although some differences between GSK-3β1 and GSK-3β2 isoforms have already been described (see below).

Crystallographic studies have revealed the three-dimensional structure of GSK-3β (Dajani et al., 2001; ter Haar et al., 2001), having the overall shape common to most kinases, with a small N-terminal lobe mostly consisting of β-sheets and a large C-terminal lobe essentially formed of α-helices (Noble et al., 2005). The ATP binding pocket is located between the two lobes and it is well conserved among kinases (Bain et al., 2007). Very recently, a comparison of the human and parasite GSK-3 ATP binding sites has opened the possibility of developing selective drugs specifically affecting parasite GSK-3 (Osolodkin et al., 2011).

Some GSK-3 substrates do not require a very specific sequence but rather a previous (*primed*) phosphorylation by a *priming* kinase on a Ser or Thr residue located four amino acids C-terminal to the Ser or Thr residue to be modified by GSK-3 (see below for regulation through primed phosphorylation). The crystal structure of human GSK-3β has also provided a model for the binding of pre-phosphorylated substrates to the kinase. According to it, primed Ser/Thr is recognized by a positively charged binding pocket formed by residues Arg96, Arg180 and Lys205 that facilitates the binding of the phosphate group of primed substrates. GSK-3β uses the phosphorylated serine or threonine at position +4 of the substrate to align the two domains for optimal catalytic activity (Dajani et al., 2001; ter Haar et al., 2001).

Furthermore, crystal structures of GSK-3β complexes with interacting proteins FRAT/GBP and axin have allowed defining the molecular basis for those interactions, which play critical roles in some signalling pathways (see below for regulation through protein complex formation). These studies confirm the partial overlap of the binding sites of axin and FRAT1/GBP predicted from genetic and biochemical studies (Ferkey & Kimelman, 2002; Fraser et al., 2002) but reveal significant differences in the detailed interactions, and identify key residues mediating the differential interaction with both proteins. This ability of GSK-3β to bind two different proteins with high specificity *via* the same binding site is mediated by the conformational plasticity of the 285-299 loop, while some residues in this versatile binding site are involved in interactions with both axin and FRAT, others are involved uniquely with one or the other (Dajani et al., 2003).

GSK-3 is ubiquitously expressed and, unlike most kinases, has a relatively high activity in resting, unstimulated cells while it is normally reduced in response to a variety of extracellular stimuli (Frame & Cohen, 2001). In mammals, GSK-3α and β are each expressed widely at both the RNA and protein levels, although some tissues show preferential levels of some of the two proteins as for instance, both isoforms are highly expressed in neural tissue. Neither gene appears to be acutely regulated at the transcriptional level whereas the proteins are controlled post-translationally, largely through protein-protein interactions or by post-translational regulation.

Given that chemical inhibitors of GSK-3 are unable to discriminate between the various GSK-3 isoforms, evaluation of isoform-specific functions it is not possible by using these compounds. However, evidence for isoform-specific roles has now emerged from mouse models (see below). For instance, some recent findings suggest that there are tissue- and isoform-specific roles in regulation of glucose metabolism (Patel et al., 2008; Mol Cell Biol), as GSK-3α seems to be the predominant regulator of GS and glycogen synthesis in liver whereas GSK-3β has a more prevalent role within skeletal muscle and pancreas. Also, although the effect of the inserted sequence on kinase activity, substrate specificity or requirement for priming of substrates remains unclear, the neuron-specific alternatively spliced GSK-3β2 isoform appears to phosphorylate unprimed residues on tau and MAP1B to a lesser extent than GSK-3β1 (Mukai et al. 2002, Wood-Kaczmar *et al.* 2009).

Three decades after its discovery as a protein kinase involved in glycogen metabolism, GSK-3 has revealed as a key enzyme in regulating many critical cellular processes, providing a link between many different substrates and various signalling pathways as well as gene expression. Modulation of its activity has also turned out to be much more complex than originally thought. As already mentioned above, one of the main characteristics of GSK-3 is that its activity is high in resting, unstimulated cells while regulated by extracellular signals that typically induce a rapid and reversible decrease in enzymatic activity. Control of GSK-3 activity occurs by complex mechanisms that are each dependent upon specific signalling pathways (for a recent review see Medina & Wandosell, 2011).

Early on, GSK-3 was proved to be a dual specificity kinase differentially regulated by tyrosine and serine/threonine phosphorylation (Wang et al., 1994). The first regulatory mechanism described of GSK-3 activity involved the phosphorylation of specific residues of GSK-3 by other kinases; and more recently through auto-phosphorylation (Frame & Cohen, 2001; Harwood, 2001). Thus, four different regions and residues have been described in the GSK-3 molecule. First, it has been clearly established that phosphorylation of serine residue at positions 21 in GSK-3α and 9 in GSK-3β, correlates with the inhibition of its kinase activity (Frame et al., 2001; Stambolic et al., 1994; Sutherland et al., 1993). Many protein kinases are capable of phosphorylating GSK-3 at this residue, such as Akt, ILK, PKA, p90Rsk (Delcommenne et al., 1998; Fang et al., 2000), and many physiological situations of inhibition of GSK-3 correlate with serine phosphorylation, such as Insulin/IGF1, NGF, or Estradiol treatments, not only in neurons but also in other cell types (Cardona-Gomez et al., 2004). In addition, phosphorylation at threonine 43, present only in the isoform GSK-3β, by ERK also correlates with GSK-3 inhibition (Ding et al., 2005), whereas residues serine 389 and threonine 390 present in GSK-3β have been shown to be phosphorylated by p38 MAPK (Thornton et al., 2008), increasing the capacity of Ser-9 to be phosphorylated rather than promoting a direct inhibition.

In contrast, tyrosine phosphorylation present in positions 279 in GSK-3α or 216 in GSK-3β, correlates with an increase of its kinase activity (Hughes et al., 1993). Different candidate kinases such as Pyk-2 and Fyn have been reported to be able to phosphorylate GSK-3 on this residue *in vitro*, as MEK1/2 has been shown to do it in mammalian fibroblasts (Hartigan et al., 2001; Lesort et al., 1999) or ZAK1 in *Dictyostelium discoideum* (Kim et al., 1999; 2002), although no homologue of this latter kinase has been found in mammals. More recently, it has been suggested that phosphotyrosine in GSK-3 in mammalian systems might arise from a chaperone-dependent intra-molecular autophosphorylation event perhaps regulated by Hsp90 (Cole et al., 2004 Biochem J; Lockhead et al., 2006; Wang et al., 1994). Molecular dynamics and crystallographic studies clearly suggest that pTyr216 renders the kinase active through interactions with Arg220 and Arg223, stabilizing the activation loop and allowing full substrate accessibility (Buch et al., 2010; Cohen & Goedert, 2004). Very recently, it has been also shown that the extent of phosphorylation at both Ser9 and Tyr216 residues is very similar in both GSK-3β splice variants, β1 and β2 (Soutar et al., 2010).

On the other hand, tyrosine phosphorylation of residue 216 or 279 increased in neuronal cells following exposure to LPA (Sayas et al., 1999) and also upon exposure of neurons to β-amyloid or PrP (Muñoz-Montaño et al., 1997; Perez et al., 2003; Takashima et al., 1998) in a clear correlation with an increase on GSK-3 activity. In addition, in many neuronal cells the pharmacological inhibition of tyrosine phosphatases with *ortho*-vanadate increases the basal level of GSK-3-pTyr (Simon et al., 2008). Thus, taken all together, in addition to the reported tyrosine 216/279 autophosphorylation mechanism proposed, some as-yet-unidentified tyrosine kinases and/or phosphatases may also regulate GSK-3 activity by phosphorylation of this particular residue.

Another mechanism of GSK-3 regulation through post-translational modification involves the removal by calpain of a fragment from the N-terminal region of GSK-3, including the regulatory serines 9/21. After removal of that fragment GSK-3 becomes activated (Goñi-Oliver et al., 2007). The same study showed that both isoforms α and β are cleaved by calpain, although with different susceptibility. Moreover, GSK-3 truncation has been observed in human and mouse post-mortem brain tissue (Goñi-Oliver et al., 2009a). It is noteworthy to consider that a similar mechanism has been described for β-catenin in hippocampal neurons, where after NMDA-receptor-dependent activation; calpain induces the cleavage of β-catenin at the N-terminus, generating stable and truncated forms which maintain its transcriptional capacity (Abe & Takeichi, 2007). Likewise, GSK-3 truncation is mediated by extracellular calcium and can be inhibited by memantine (Goñi-Oliver et al., 2009b), a NMDA antagonist used for the treatment of Alzheimer's disease. Interestingly, GSK-3β has also been recently shown to be cleaved at the N-terminus (and subsequently activated) by matrix metallo-proteinase 2 (MMP-2) in cardiomyoblasts (Kanadasamy & Schulz, 2009).

Besides post-translational modifications, GSK-3 activity can also be regulated by protein complex association, for instance through its interaction with structural (scaffold) proteins. It is well known that GSK-3 contributes to Wnt signalling by participating in a multiprotein complex formed by axin, β-catenin and adenomatous polyposis coli (APC), among others (for review see, i.e. Moon et al., 2004). Indeed, in the absence of the Wnt ligand, GSK-3 it is able to phosphorylate β-catenin and targeting it for proteasome degradation (Aberle et al., 1997) whereas in its presence GSK-3 is unable to do that, increasing β-catenin cytosolic levels and eventually mediating TCF/LEF-mediated transcription at the nucleus. Recent data suggest that this complex may be specific for the GSK-3β2 splice isoform (Castaño et al., 2010). Recent evidence also supports a neuroprotective role for *Wnt* signaling in neurodegenerative disorders such as AD (Inestrosa & Toledo, 2008).

Moreover, another GSK-3-binding protein (GBP or FRAT) has been reported to regulate GSK-3 enzymatic activity (Itoh et al., 1995; Li et al., 1999). From the three different FRATs that have been cloned and characterized, FRAT1 appears to act as an inhibitory system (Yost et al., 1998) whereas FRAT2 appears to preferentially increase GSK-3-mediated phosphorylation in some residues (Stoothoff et al., 2005). Surprisingly, the triple FRAT-knockout mouse lacks any major defect in brain development (van Amerongen et al., 2005), which underlines the need to better define the precise role of FRAT in GSK-3 regulation and brain physiology. Furthermore, using the binding site on GSK-3 for FRAT/GBP, a GSK-3-interacting protein (GSKIP) has been identified that can block phosphorylation of different substrates and functions as a negative regulator of GSK-3β (Chou et al., 2006). Other proteins have also been proposed to further contribute to GSK-3 regulation through physical interaction with it. Thus, DISC-1 (Disrupted In Schizophrenia-1) regulates neural progenitor proliferation via the β-catenin/GSK-3β pathway, whereby DISC-1 stabilizes β-catenin by inhibiting GSK-3β activity through a direct binding (Mao et al., 2009). Finally, the dimeric scaffold protein 14-3-3 has been shown to co-elute from brain microtubules together with tau and GSK-3β and this interaction has been proposed to facilitate the interaction of the kinase with some of its substrates (Agarwal-Mawal et al., 2003).

As already mentioned, an unusual property of GSK3 is that most of its substrates require prior phosphorylation (priming) at a residue 4 or 5 amino acids C-terminal to the target residue (Frame & Cohen 2001), thus providing another mechanism of regulation of the GSK-3 activity. Some priming kinases have been identified, such as cdk5 (Alonso et al., 2006; Noble et al., 2003; Sengupta et al., 1997), PAR-1 (Nishimura et al., 2004), casein kinase I (Amit et al. 2002), PKC (Liu et al., 2003) or PKA (Sengupta et al., 1997). That said, there are examples of unprimed substrates reported, although is not entirely clear as yet whether this second set of unprimed substrates may define a different group of functions (Twomey & McCArthy, 2006).

3. GSK-3 activity in AD brain

Compared to age-matched control samples, increased levels of GSK-3 have been found in post-mortem analysis of brains from AD patients (Pei et al., 1997) while a spatial and temporal pattern of increased active GSK-3β expression correlating with the progression of neurofibrillary tangles (NFT) and neurodegeneration has also been shown (Leroy et al., 2002). Thus, GSK-3 has been shown to localize to pre-tangle neurons, dystrophic neurites and NFTs in AD brain (Pei et al., 1997). Neurons actively undergoing granulovacuolar degeneration are also immunopositive for active GSK3β (Leroy et al., 2002). Taken all together, although direct evidence might be lacking, all these studies strongly suggest that GSK-3β activity is increased in the brains of patients suffering from AD.

GSK-3β is the major kinase to phosphorylate tau protein both *in vitro* and *in vivo*. Furthermore, GSK-3β has been proposed as the link between the two major histopathological hallmarks of AD, the extracellular amyloid plaques and the intracellular NFT (Hernández et al., 2010; Ittner and Götz, 2011; Muyllaert et al., 2008). Exposure of primary neuronal cultures to Aβ induces activation of GSK-3β, tau phosphorylation and cell death, whereas blockade of GSK-3 expression by antisense oligonucleotides or its activity by lithium inhibits Aβ-induced toxicity (Alvarez et al., 1999; Hoshi et al., 2003; Wei et al., 2000). GSK-3β-deficient mice die during embryonic development (Hoeflich *et al.* 2000, Liu *et al.* 2007) whereas GSK-3β heterozygous (+/-) mice are viable, although they show some neurological abnormalities, including reduced aggression, increased anxiety, reduced exploratory activity, poor memory consolidation and reduced responsiveness to amphetamine (O'Brien *et al.* 2004, Kimura *et al.* 2008, Beaulieu *et al.* 2008). Conversely, transgenic mice over-expressing GSK-3β result in behavioural changes that appear to recapitulate hyperactivity observed in the manic phase of bipolar disorder (Prickaerts *et al.* 2006).

On the other hand, mice lacking GSK-3α are viable and develop normally (MacAulay *et al.* 2007), but display enhanced glucose tolerance and insulin sensitivity accompanied by reduced fat mass. Interestingly, GSK-3α knock-out mice show reduced exploratory activity and aggression, similar to the GSK-3β heterozygotes, but in addition have decreased locomotion, impaired co-ordination and a deficit in fear conditioning (Kaidanovich-Beilin *et al.* 2009). These different in phenotypes in mice lacking one isoform or the other suggest non-redundant functions of the GSK-3 genes in the brain, while the overlapping behavioural problems between GSK-3α knockout (KO) and GSK-3β heterozygous (+/-) mice suggest some common substrates.

Furthermore, loss of both GSK-3 isoforms specifically in the brain results in increased self-renewal of neuronal progenitor cells, but reduced neurogenesis (Kim *et al.* 2009), while double GSK3α/β knock-in mice in which endogenous isoforms are replaced by mutant proteins where Ser21/9 have been mutated to Ala21/9 respectively, thus preventing repression by growth factor signalling, exhibit impaired neuronal precursor cell proliferation (Eom & Jope 2009). These data underscore the critical role that proper regulation of expression and activity of GSK-3 play in the maturation of these cells during mammalian brain development.

However, we must be careful when interpreting data from transgenic or KO animals since some strain specificity has been recently observed, at least in the case of improved insulin sensitivity and hepatic glucose homeostasis phenotype observed upon global inactivation of GSK-3α (Patel et al., 2011).

All these observations and the ones described below strongly suggest a central role of GSK-3 in AD pathogenesis and have also led to several efforts trying to identify sequence variations in the *gsk-3* gene and its promoter. Despite early reports of a lack of genetic association between the *gsk-3* coding sequence or its promoter with AD (Russ et al., 2001), several groups have now reported this association. Thus, a polymorphism in the promoter region (-50) of the *gsk-3β* gene appears associated with a two-fold increased risk for sporadic AD when analysing 333 sporadic AD patients and 307 control subjects from Spain (Mateo et al., 2006). More recently, a case-control study has found a rare intronic polymorphism in *gsk-3β* that occurred twice more frequently in AD patients than in aged healthy controls (Schaffer et al., 2010), strongly supporting the notion of a genetic association of the *gsk-3β* gene with AD. Furthermore, two additional independent studies have reported synergistic effects (epistasis) between the *gsk-3β* and either the *MAPT* (tau) genes (Kwok et al., 2008) or the p35 subunit of cdk5 (Mateo et al., 2009) in late-onset AD, further supporting a genetic association between *gsk-3β* and AD. Interestingly, a genetic polymorphism that increases the ratio of GSK-3β1 to GSK-3β2 interacts with tau haplotypes and modifies risk in Parkinson's and Alzheimer's disease (Kwok et al. 2005, 2008).

4. The role of GSK-3 in tau phosphorylation

Tau protein is a microtubule-associated protein (MAP) that in normal physiological conditions binds to microtubules (MT), regulating their assembly, dynamic behaviour, and spatial organization (Drechsel et al., 1992; LoPresti et al., 1995). Later on, tau has also been shown to regulate the axonal transport of organelles, including mitochondria (Ebneth et al., 1998). Tau is primarily, though not exclusively, a neuronal protein encoded by a single gene but with six major isoforms derived by alternative splicing (Goedert et al., 1989; Himmler et al., 1989). The interaction between tau and tubulin is mediated by four imperfect repeat domains (31-32 residues) encoded by exons 9-12 (Lee et al., 1989). Alternative splicing of exon 10 gives rise to isoforms with 3 or 4 binding domains (3R and 4R tau) (Goedert et al., 1989). Adult human brain shows a 1:1 ratio of 3R and 4R isoforms whereas foetal brain, however, only expresses 3R tau, demonstrating developmental regulation of exon 10 splicing. Different brain regions also differ in the relative levels of 3R and 4R isoforms with granule cells in the hippocampal formation reported to have only 3R tau (Goedert et al., 1989). Disturbances in this ratio are a common feature in most neurodegenerative tauopathies, including AD.

Within neurons, tau is predominantly found in axons as a highly soluble phosphoprotein. As mentioned in the case of alternative splicing, phosphorylation is also developmentally regulated, with a high tau phosphorylation level during embryogenesis and early development, when only the shortest of the isoforms is being expressed. By contrast, adult brain expresses all six isoforms with relatively reduced phosphorylation levels compared with the foetal one (see [Hanger et al., 2009] for a review).

Upon abnormal phosphorylation, the microtubule-associated protein tau reduces its affinity for and dissociates from microtubules. In AD brains tau accumulates in the neuronal perikarya and processes as paired helical filaments (PHF). It has been suggested that at the single-cell level the defects start with a modification of tau by phosphorylation, resulting in a destabilization of microtubules giving rise to a "pre-tangle" stage. After this stage, the destabilization of microtubules leads to loss of dendritic microtubules and synapses, plasma membrane degeneration, and eventually cell death (Iqbal et al., 2009).

The knowledge accumulated in the last years strongly suggest that tau-induced neurodegeneration is most likely a consequence of a combination of loss of (tau) function as well as gain of (toxic) function. On one hand, tau detachment from microtubules after hyperphosphorylation (or mutations) causes impaired microtubule function and axonal transport and eventually synaptic dysfunction and neurodegeneration (Jaworski et al., 2010). On the other hand, hyperphosphorylated tau molecules tend to self-assemble into filaments such as PHF or straight filaments (SF) that form the NFT. But hyperphosphorylated tau seems to also have the capacity of sequestering normal tau molecules (and perhaps other microtubule-associated proteins) into the aggregates, which will also have a negative impact on the normal microtubule function. At some point after detaching from microtubules and getting into the aggregation process, tau molecules also suffer other post-translational modifications such as truncation (Delobel et al., 2008; Gamblin et al., 2003; Nvak et al., 1993), glycosylation (Wang et al., 1996), O-GlcNAcylation (Arnold et al., 1996; Hart et al., 1996), and ubiquitination (Bancher et al., 1991; Mori et al., 1987), which could also contribute to the pathology. For a recent review on the molecular mechanisms by which tau induces neurodegeneration please refer to (Brunden et al., 2009; Iqbal et al., 2009).

Interestingly, recent data strongly indicates that some soluble, oligomeric (pre-filament, immature filaments) tau species, rather than the tangles, are indeed the pathogenic ones (Bretteville & Planel, 2008, Congdon & Duff, 2008), reminiscent of what has happened in recent years in the amyloid field regarding plaques and intermediate Aβ oligomers (Haass & Selkoe, 2007; Walsh & Selkoe, 2007). For a very long time, tangles or fibrils have been considered to be the pathological species, but it has become clear now that, much like amyloid plaques, NFT are the final stages of a pathological process, but the real damage might actually be done by some intermediate hyperphosphorylated, most likely soluble tau species (Brunden et al., 2009; Iqbal et al., 2009; Jaworski et al., 2010). In fact, there is some evidence suggesting that NFT might be protective indeed, as tangle-bearing neurons seem to survive for long periods of time (Andorfer et al., 2005; de Calignon et al., 2009; Morsch et al., 1999). More recently, some novel mechanisms of propagation of tau protein misfolding from the extracellular to the intracellular space, both *in vitro* (Frost et al., 2009) and *in vivo* (Clavaguera et al., 2010) have been described. The demonstration of a link between tau oligomers and brain pathology in animal models has lately sparked the interest of tau immunotherapies (Boutajangout et al., 2010; Kayed & Jackson, 2009; Medina, 2011; Sigurdsson, 2008).

GSK-3 induces tau phosporylation in several primed and unprimed PHF phosphoepitopes, both *in vitro* and in cell cultures. Activation of the insulin or Wnt signalling pathways increase tau phosphorylation mediated by GSK-3 (Caricasole et al., 2004; Lesort et al., 1999). Furthermore, some genetic studies show an association of Wnt signalling with AD through the low-density lipoprotein receptor-related protein 6 (LRP6), a co-receptor for Wnt signalling, which has been identified as a genetic risk for a subpopulation of late onset AD (De Ferrari et al., 2007). In addition, epidemiological and genetic studies also associate diabetes and insulin resistance with AD (Biessels & Kappelle, 2005; Hamilton et al., 2007; Reiman et al., 2007).

Persistent tau phosphorylation might results in neuritic dystrophy. Lipophosphatidic acid treated neurons result in GSK-3-dependent persistent tau phosphorylation followed by neurite retraction and growth cone collapse (Sayas et al., 2002). Several animal models, which exhibit persistent tau phosphorylation, also display neuritic dystrophy. For instance mice lacking either Reelin, mammalian disabled (mDab1), or VLDLR2 and ApoER2 exhibit persistent tau phosphorylation and have neuritic dystrophy and cytoskeletal abnormalities associated with them (Hiesberger et al., 1999; Sheldon et al., 1997). It is conceivable that persistent phosphorylation by GSK-3 results in neuritic dystrophy and subsequent cytoskeletal breakdown. In *Drosophila,* tau overexpression in combination with phosphorylation by the *Drosophila* GSK-3 homolog *Shaggy,* exacerbated neurodegeneration induced by tau overexpression alone, leading to neurofibrillary pathology (Jackson et al., 2002).

Recent evidence points out to GSK-3 linking tau and neuronal polarity through a protein called CRMP-2 (collapsing response mediator protein-2) which is essential for regulating axon growth and promotes assembly of microtubules (Cole et al., 2004). GSK-3 not only phosphorylates tau but also several CRMPs (Cole et al., 2006), including CRMP-2 (Yoshimura et al., 2005) at Thr514, a residue crucial for controlling its activity. Low levels of phosphorylated CRMP-2 at that residue are present in the growth cone and are associated with axon growth, which is consistent with previous data demonstrating that inhibition of GSK-3 results in enhanced neurite outgrowth (Muñoz-Montaño et al., 1999). These data were substantially backed up by a different group (Jiang et al., 2005) that also found that GSK-3 is spatially regulated, with the ratio of inactive (phosphorylated at S9) versus active (unphosphorylated) being highest in the axon tips, consistent with the fact that higher levels of unphosphorylated CRMP-2 drive axon development, and hence, neural polarity.

5. The role of GSK-3 in Aβ formation and neurotoxicity

While not universally accepted, the so-called amyloid hypothesis of AD has provided the main conceptual framework for studying the causes of the diseases and developing new therapeutic interventions during the last quarter of century. According to it, the gradual cerebral accumulation of soluble and insoluble assemblies of the amyloid Aβ peptide triggers a cascade of biochemical and cellular alterations that produce the clinical phenotype of AD (Hardy & Higgins, 1992; Hardy & Selkoe, 2002; Selkoe, 1991). The reasons for elevated Aβ levels in most patients with sporadic, late-onset AD are unknown, but recent evidence suggest that these could turn out to include increased neuronal release of Aβ during some kind of synaptic activity (Selkoe, 2002; 2008).

GSK-3 inhibition *per se* decreases Aβ production in cells and in an animal model of amyloidosis, as shown using non-isoform selective pharmacological inhibitors such as lithium, kenpaullone as well as small interfering RNA against the α isoform of GSK-3 (Phiel et al., 2003; Su et al., 2004; Sun et al., 2002). The exact mechanism by which this occurs remains unclear and in fact the isoform specificity of the effect on Aβ production is still highly controversial. However, the observation that amyloid precursor protein (APP) C-terminal fragments accumulate in the presence of these inhibitors suggests that GSK-3 may influence γ-secretase activity. γ-secretase activity is a multiprotein complex that is necessary for the terminal cleavage of APP to generate the Aβ fragment. Interestingly, inhibition of GSK-3 failed to demonstrate accumulation of C-terminal fragments of the Notch protein, which is also a substrate for γ-secretase (Phiel et al., 2003). Actually, GSK-3 has been shown to bind and phosphorylate presenilin 1 (PS1), the catalytic component of the γ-secretase complex, acting perhaps as a docking protein and regulating phosphorylation of some GSK-3 substrates such as tau and β-catenin (Palacino et al., 2001; Su et al., 2004; Takashima et al., 1998; Tesco & Tanzi, 2002; Twomey & McCarthy, 2006). PS1 has been shown to inactivate GSK-3 through PI3K/Akt signalling, preventing tau phosphorylation and apoptosis. Interestingly, PS1 FAD mutations inhibit PS1-dependent PI3K/Akt signalling, facilitating GSK-3 and thus tau phosphorylation (Baki et al., 2004). Furthermore, APP has also been shown to be a substrate for GSK-3 *in vitro* (Aplin et al., 1996) and *in vivo* (Rockenstein et al., 2007), suggesting a role of GSK-3 in APP transport and maturation (da Cruz e Silva & da Cruz e Silva, 2003; Lee et al., 2003) from the early secretory pathway through the axon terminals, perhaps controlling APP processing. Finally, modulation of the GSK-3 signalling pathway by chronic lithium treatment of transgenic animals has been shown to have neuroprotective effects by regulating APP maturation and processing (Rockenstein et al., 2007).

A substantial body of evidence has established the toxic properties of extracellular Aβ peptides on neuronal cells (Selkoe, 2008). Non-neuronal cells however are generally resistant to Aβ treatment, with some exceptions such as endothelial cells and smooth muscle cells (Suhara et al., 2003). On the other hand, oligomers of the Aβ peptide have been reported to act as antagonists for insulin (Towsend et al. 2007) or Wnt (Magdesian et al. 2008) receptors, resulting in an increase in GSK-3 activity. Also, a PS1 lack of function by mutations such as those present in some familial AD patients has been suggested to result in an increase of GSK-3 activity (Baki et al., 2004).

As mentioned, the aggregation of Aβ peptide into soluble oligomers is considered an early event in Alzheimer's disease and the presence of these aggregates seems to lead to neurodegeneration in the context of this disease. However, the mechanisms underlying Aβ-induced neurotoxicity are not completely understood. Although previous studies in mice have suggested that GSK-3 alters Aβ levels via modulation of APP processing (Phiel et al., 2003; Rockenstein et al., 2007), the direct effects of the enzyme on Aβ toxicity, and in the adult nervous system, have not been examined in depth. A recent study has tackled this particular issue of the specific role of GSK-3 in regulating Aβ42 toxicity in adult neurons *in vivo*, by modulating its activity in an adult-onset *Drosophila* model of Alzheimer's disease (Sofola et al., 2010). This study shows that GSK-3 inhibition ameliorates Aβ42 toxicity in adult flies, and also highlights a novel mechanism of protection by which GSK-3 directly regulates Aβ42 levels in the absence of any effects on APP processing.

6. The role of GSK-3 in synaptic plasticity, learning and memory

GSK-3 has also been shown to phosphorylate and inhibit kinesin-mediated motility. Fast axonal transport misregulation has been hypothesized to play a role in Alzheimer's disease pathogenesis (Morfini et al., 2002). Fibrillar Aβ binds to and induces the clustering of the integrin receptors, leading to the activation of paxillin and focal adhesion kinases. Interestingly, active GSK-3 associates with focal adhesion proteins suggesting the possibility that GSK-3 might mediate neuritic dystrophy via these interactions (Grace & Busciglio, 2003). Abnormal increase in GSK-3 activity has been shown to cause neurodegeneration and interfere with synaptic plasticity (for review see Bhat & Budd, 2002; Bhat & Froelich-Fabre, 2004).

Another important aspect of GSK-3 function is its role in the assembly and disassembly of synapses determining synaptic plasticity. Regarding memory, some states of synaptic plasticity may be considered as a balance between long-term potentiation (LTP) and long-term depression (LTD), with the former strengthening synaptic connections and the latter weakening them. Interestingly, GSK-3 appears to be a key factor in swaying that balance (Hooper et al., 2007; Peineau et al., 2007) since after LTP induction, GSK-3 becomes temporarily inactivated, support for LTD is lost and LTP comes out on top. This is relevant from the drug discovery point of view, since it implies that inhibition of GSK-3 might boost LTP and depress LTD, in principle a good thing for learning and memory. The precise molecular mechanism by which GSK-3 influences these processes remains to be elucidated, although some preliminary data seems to suggest that installation or maintenance of AMPA receptors might play a role (Peinau et al., 2007). Several GSK-3 downstream substrates such as CRMP-2 or the cAMP responsive element-binding protein (CREB) are also involved in synaptic remodelling, a key process required for memory formation. All this evidence has led to propose that GSK-3 acts as a gate through which LTP and memory are established (Hooper et al., 2008) and that memory failure in AD may be due to the inhibition of LTP by GSK-3 overactivity, with neuronal loss ensuing during disease progression.

It is well established that Aβ oligomers inhibit LTP and enhance LTD (Shieh et al., 2003; Walsh et al., 2002; Selkoe, 2008), although the precise mechanisms by which Aβ interferes with long-term plasticity have remained largely unknown. Very recently, GSK-3 has revealed as a key enzyme in mediating Aβ-induced LTP inhibition (Jo et al., 2011). In this study, treatment of rat hippocampal slices with Aβ oligomers induced caspase 3-mediated cleavage of Akt-1, resulting in GSK-3 activation. Consistent with it, treatment with a GSK-3 inhibitor completely prevented Aβ oligomers from inhibiting LTP.

7. Lithium as a GSK-3 inhibitor

The finding that the mood stabilizing drug lithium directly inhibited GSK-3 initially sparked the interest for this enzyme as a potential target for mood disorders. Lithium and valproic acid are mood stabilizers widely used in the chronic treatment of bipolar disorders. Lithium ions directly inhibit GSK-3 (Klein & Melton, 1996), most likely by competing with magnesium, while valproic acid inhibits GSK-3 activity in relevant therapeutic concentrations in human neuroblastoma cells (Chen et al., 1999), most likely through an indirect mechanism (Rosenberg, 2007).

The mechanism of action by which lithium exerts its therapeutic effects is not known but it is conceivable that the acute effects on GSK-3 results in changes in gene regulation and cellular changes which could affect the neuronal plasticity over time (Gould & Manji, 2002; Jope, 1999; Lennox & Hahn, 2000). Lithium also inhibits at least four phosphomonoesterases (including inositol monophosphatase) (York et al., 1995), and phosphoglucomutase (Ray & Szymanki, 1978; Stambolic & Woodgett, 1994), apart from GSK-3 (Klein & Melton, 1996; Li-Smerin et al., 2001). That said, GSK-3 is significantly inhibited at therapeutic lithium concentrations (Gould & Manji, 2002; Phiel et al., 2003; Shaldubina et al., 2001). Thus, if a significant proportion of lithium's therapeutic actions in bipolar disorder results from the inhibition of GSK-3, then this enzyme would be an important target for bipolar disorder (Li et al., 2002; Rowe et al., 2007).

In spite of these attributes, lithium has a narrow therapeutic window (blood serum levels 0.6 to 1.2 mM) above which side effects are intolerable. Overdose can lead to severe neurological dysfunction and in some cases death. Non-CNS side effects of lithium (not uncommonly within therapeutic levels) include tremor, polyuria, polydipsia, nausea, and weight gain. Lithium can have adverse reactions with other drug classes including diuretics, NSAIDS, and other drugs that alter kidney function (see Gould & Manji, 2006 for a review).

There are only a few observational studies that have attempted to address the clinical effect of lithium in patients with AD. A retrospective study with a large sample of patients with dementia resulted in an increased risk of AD in patients who had been treated with lithium within 4 years prior to diagnosis (Ayuso-Mateo et al., 2001), although it is possible that this is partially accounted for by the increased occurrence of depression associated with AD. Moreover, a single case study reported in dementia patient showed that lithium treatment alleviated symptoms of aggression and agitation, while cognition persisted after 1.5 years of treatment (Havens et al., 1982). Furthermore, a significantly increased global cognitive ability as measured by MMSE in non-demented patients appears associated with lithium intake (Terao et al., 2006). The study design and low sample size precludes however to draw any causative conclusion from those studies.

Some pilot studies have been carried out to directly address the effect of lithium treatment in AD patients. An open label feasibility and tolerability study on a small cohort of 22 subjects patients receiving a low dose of lithium was carried out in UK, reported a high discontinuation rate despite few, relatively mild and reversible side effects (MacDonald et al., 2008). A second randomized, single-blind, placebo-controlled, parallel group, multicentre 10-week study was carried out in Germany as a proof-of-principle (Hampel et al., 2009). A total of 71 patients with mild AD (MMSE scores between 21 and 26) were treated with lithium or placebo for 10 weeks after which neuropsychological and neuropsychiatric assessment was performed together with some biomarkers determinations in plasma (Aβ1-42), lymphocytes (GSK-3 activity) and CSF (total tau, phospho-tau, and Aβ1-42). In spite of the fact that lithium plasma levels were within the therapeutic range, no treatment effect was observed in any the cognition assessment scales used or the selected biomarkers. Given the short time of treatment of this study, the possibility that lithium has long-term effects on cognition or any other biomarker in AD remains to be tested.

8. Development of GSK-3 inhibitors and their therapeutic potential

The unique position of GSK-3 as a pivotal and central player in the pathogenesis of both sporadic and familial forms of AD has attracted significant attention to this enzyme as a therapeutic target and also as a means to understand the molecular basis underlying AD and related disorders. This has led to the synthesis of a high number of GSK-3 inhibitors, some of which are currently being tested in phase II proof-of-concept clinical trials (Mangialasche et al., 2010; Medina & Avila, 2010). Inhibition of GSK-3 with small molecules would be expected to slow down progression of neurodegeneration in AD and perhaps other tauopathies as well.

A number of novel potent and fairly selective small-molecule inhibitors of GSK-3 activity from different chemical families have recently been described, including hymenialdisine, indirubins, paullones, maleimides, amino pyrazoles, thiazoles, and 2,4-disubstituted thiadiazolidinones (TDZD) (reviewed in Medina & Castro, 2008). Most of them are ATP-competitive inhibitors, although more recently new small molecule derivatives that exhibit substrate competitive inhibition activity toward GSK-3 have been reported. Since the different GSK-3 isoforms display a high degree of homology within the ATP binding site, inhibitors are unable to exhibit isoform selectivity, as they all show similar potencies towards purified GSK-3α and GSK-3β.

Although the ATP-competitive inhibitors occupy the general area of the highly conserved ATP-binding site, they do explore other available space nearby depending upon their structure and it is possible to obtain selective inhibitors by taking advantage of the small differences that exist between the different kinases. Crystal structures of GSK-3β complexed with a variety of ligands, together with molecular modelling approaches, provide the necessary clues for enhancing selectivity towards GSK-3 (Patel et al., 2007; ter Haar et al., 2001). All ATP-binding site inhibitors make hydrogen bonds with backbone atoms of the kinase domain hinge (residues Asp 133 to Thr 138). The hydrogen bonds are the same as observed with ATP although different inhibitors make different combinations of hydrogen bonds. For instance, the two indirubin complexes (PDB 1UV5 and 1Q41) have four hydrogen bonds. In contrast, the Alsterpaullone complex (PDB 1Q3W) only has three hydrogen bonds (with the two backbone atoms of Val 135).

Some GSK-3 inhibitors also target other areas of the ATP pocket. For instance the nitro-group of the Alsterpaullone (PDB 1Q3W) and the chlorine of I-5 (3-anilino-4-arylmaleimide) interact with the conserved catalytic lysine, Lys 85. The bromine atom of 6-bromoindirubin (PDB 1UV5) is buried in the hydrophobic pocket of GSK-3β between residues Leu 132, Leu 130 and Met 101. This is a pocket that is often targeted to increase the selectivity of the inhibitor since it is one of the most diverse areas in the ATP-binding site of kinases and has been successfully used for instance to increase the selectivity in favour of p38α over ERK2. The GSK-3β ATP-binding site inhibitors do not cover the γ-phosphate transfer area. Targeting this part of the ATP-binding site does not appear to improve the selectivity of the inhibitor, although it may improve the potency as additional contacts between the inhibitor and the protein are established (ter Haar et al., 2006).

Some physiological peptides act as GSK-3 inhibitors, including GBP, a maternal *Xenopus* GSK-3 binding protein homologous to a mammalian T cell proto-oncogene (Yost et al., 1998) and p24, a heat resistant GSK-3 binding protein (Martín et al., 2002). That finding led to a synthetic strategy to develop new inhibitors, such as L803-mts, a peptidic inhibitor that binds to the substrate site (Plotkin et al., 2003). L803-mts has been more recently used to examine the impact of long-term *in vivo* inhibition of GSK-3 and its effects in specific tissues (Kaidanocih-Beilin & Eldar-Finkelman, 2006).

One classical approach for identifying GSK-3 inhibitors has exploited screening programs specifically aimed at finding new hits among compounds that exhibit other pharmacological profiles. However, the availability of X-ray crystallographic data of GSK-3β and several of its complexes with different inhibitors (ter Haar, 2006) in recent years has enabled the application of rational drug optimisation programs to discover new lead compounds. Molecular docking studies on the inhibitors of GSK-3 kinase in the enzyme binding sites of the X-ray complexes studies provide valuable insights into computational strategies useful for the identification of potential GSK-3 inhibitors (Gadakar et al., 2007). As a result of the great amount of information concerning current GSK-3 inhibitors, there are a huge number of reported empirical structure-activity relationships (SAR) that may guide a rational design of more potent and selective inhibitors. However, only a few studies based on Quantitative Structure-Activity Relationships (QSAR) are available for predicting the inhibitor potency against this specific kinase, and they involve mainly molecular modelling and 3D-QSAR (Medina & Castro, 2008).

The last few years have seen the synthesis of quite a number of fairly selective, potent GSK-3 inhibitors which have started to show *in vivo* efficacy in a diverse array of animal models of human diseases, including Alzheimer's disease. Despite the challenges faced by this approach with respect to safety and specificity, a number of efforts are underway to develop kinase inhibitors and in fact, Noscira's tideglusib (NP12), is already in phase II clinical trials for the treatment of both Alzheimer's disease and progressive supranuclear palsy (PSP), a tauopathy (Medina & Castro, 2008; Medina & Avila, 2010).

9. Conclusion

Three decades after its discovery as a protein kinase involved in glycogen metabolism, GSK-3 has revealed as a cellular nexus, integrating several signalling systems, including several second messengers and a wide selection of cellular stimulants. Modulation of its activity has also turned out to be much more complex than originally thought as control of GSK-3 activity occurs by complex mechanisms that are each dependent upon specific signalling pathways, including post-translational modifications, protein complex formation and subcellular localization. Although there seems to be a good degree of functional overlapping between the different isoforms, some tissue- and isoform-specific functions and substrates are starting to emerge and more will most likely be discovered within the next few years and will open the possibility to design better, more specific inhibitors.

Deregulation or abnormal GSK-3 activity appears to be associated with various relevant pathologies, including Alzheimer's disease, as the enzyme is uniquely positioned as a key, central player in AD pathogenesis, having a critical role in key events such as tau phosphorylation, Aβ formation and neurotoxicity, microtubule dynamics, synaptic plasticity, neuritic dystrophy, cognition, neuronal survival, and neurodegeneration. Furthermore, recent reports point out to a genetic association of the *gsk-3* gene with the risk of AD either by itself or synergistically with tau or cdk5 genes.

Drug discovery and development efforts for AD in the last two decades have primarily focused on targets defined by the amyloid cascade hypothesis, so far with disappointing results, underscoring the need of novel therapeutic approaches and targets. A significant effort has being made in the last few years to synthesize a high number of fairly selective, potent GSK-3 inhibitors, while some of them have shown *in vivo* efficacy in various animal models of AD. Some of the known drug discovery and development challenges will be faced: lack of good predictive animal models, lack of good validated biomarkers of disease progression, clinical trial design, early diagnosis and treatment, definition of target population, difficulties in demonstrating disease modifying effects, etc. Despite the challenges faced by this approach with respect to safety and specificity, a number of efforts are underway to develop GSK-3 inhibitors as useful drugs for the treatment of AD as some compounds have already reached phase II clinical trials and some proof-of-concept studies are currently ongoing or planned.

10. Acknowledgments

MM acknowledges grant support from EU-FP7 (Neuro.GSK3, project # 223276) and from CDTI's CENIT program (DENDRIA, project # CEN-20101023).

11. References

Abe K, and Takeichi M (2007) NMDA-receptor activation induces calpain-mediated beta-catenin cleavages for triggering gene expression. *Neuron* 53: 387-97.

Aberle H, Bauer A, Stappert J, Kispert A, Kemler R (1997) Beta-catenin is a target for the ubiquitin-proteasome pathway. *EMBO J* 16(13): 3797-804.

Agarwal-Mawal A, Qureshi HY, Cafferty PW, Yuan Z, Han D, Lin R, and Paudel HK (2003) 14-3-3 connects glycogen synthase kinase-3 beta to tau within a brain microtubule-associated tau phosphorylation complex. *J Biol Chem* 278 (15): 12722-8.

Alonso A del C, Li B, Grundke-Iqbal I, and Iqbal K (2006) Polymerization of hyperphosphorylated tau into filaments eliminates its inhibitory activity. *Proc Natl Acad Sci U S A* 103: 8864-9

Alvarez G, Muñoz-Montaño JR, Satrústegui J, Avila J, Bogónez E, Díaz-Nido J. (1999) Lithium protects cultured neurons against beta-amyloid-induced neurodegeneration. *FEBS Lett* 453(3): 260-4.

Amit S, Hatzubai A, Birman Y, Andersen JS, Ben-Shushan E, Mann M, Ben-Neriah Y, and Alkalay I (2002) Axin-mediated CKI phosphorylation of beta-catenin at Ser 45: a molecular switch for the Wnt pathway. *Genes Dev* 16: 1066-76

Andorfer C, Acker CM, Kress Y, Hof PR, Duff K, Davies P (2005) Cell-cycle reentry and cell death in transgenic mice expressing nonmutant human tau isoforms. *J Neurosci* 25(22): 5446-54.

Aplin AE, Gibb GM, Jacobsen JS, Gallo JM, Anderton BH. (1996) In vitro phosphorylation of the cytoplasmic domain of the amyloid precursor protein by glycogen synthase kinase-3b. *J. Neurochem.* 67(2):699-707

Arnold CS, Johnson GV, Cole RN, Dong DL, Lee M, Hart GW (1996) The microtubule-associated protein tau is extensively modified with O-linked N- acetylglucosamine. *J Biol Chem* 271(46): 28741-4.

Ayuso-Mateos JL, Vázquez-Barquero JL, Dowrick C, Lehtinen V, Dalgard OS, Casey P, Wilkinson C, Lasa L, Page H, Dunn G, Wilkinson G; ODIN Group (2001) Depressive disorders in Europe: prevalence figures from the ODIN study. *Br J Psychiatry* 179: 308-16.

Bain J, Plater L, Elliott M, Shpiro N, Hastie CJ, McLauchlan H, Klevernic I, Arthur JS, Alessi DR, and Cohen P (2007) The selectivity of protein kinase inhibitors: a further update. *Biochem J* 408: 297-315.

Baki L, Shioi J, Wen P, Shao Z, Schwarzman A, Gama-Sosa M, Neve R and Robakis NK (2004) PS1 activates PI3K thus inhibiting GSK-3 activity and tau overphosphorylation: effects of FAD mutations. *EMBO J* 23: 2586-96.

Baki, L., Shioi, J., Wen, P., Shao, Z., Schwarzman, A., Gama-Sosa, M., Neve, R. and Robakis, N.K. (2004) PS1 activates PI3K thus inhibiting GSK-3 activity and tau overphosphorylation: effects of FAD mutations. EMBO J. 23, 2586-96.

Bancher C, Grundke-Iqbal I, Iqbal K, Fried VA, Smith HT, Wisniewski HM (1991) Abnormal phosphorylation of tau precedes ubiquitination in neurofibrillary pathology of Alzheimer disease. *Brain Res* 539(1): 11-8.

Beaulieu JM, Zhang X, Rodriguez RM, Sotnikova TD, Cools MJ, Wetsel WC, Gainetdinov RR and Caron MG (2008) Role of GSK3 beta in behavioralabnormalities induced by serotonin deficiency. *Proc Natl Acad Sci USA* 105: 1333-1338.

Bhat R.V. and Froelich-Fabre S. (2004) Mechanisms of Tauopathies. *Drug Disc. Today Drug Disc.: Dis. Mech.*, 1, 391-8.

Bhat R.V., and Budd S. (2002) GSK3□ signaling: casting a wide net in Alzheimer´s Disease. *Neurosignals*, 11, 251-61.

Biessels GJ and Kappelle LJ (2005) Increased risk of Alzheime's disease in Type II diabetes: insulin resistance of the brain or insulin-induced amyloid pathology? *Biochem. Soc. Trans.* 33, 1041-4.

Boutajangout A, Quartermain D, Sigurdsson EM. (2010) Immunotherapy targeting pathological tau prevents cognitive decline in a new tangle mouse model. *J Neurosci* 30(49): 16559-66.

Bretteville A, Planel E (2008) Tau aggregates: toxic, inert, or protective species? *J Alzheimers Dis* 14(4): 431-6

Brunden KR, Trojanowski JQ, Lee VM (2009) Advances in tau-focused drug discovery for Alzheimer's disease and related tauopathies. *Nat Rev Drug Discov* 8(10): 783-93.

Buch I, Fishelovitch D, London N, Raveh B, Wolfson HJ, and Nussinov R (2010). Allosteric regulation of glycogen synthase kinase 3beta: a theoretical study. *Biochemistry* 49: 10890-901.

Cardona-Gomez P, Perez M, Avila J, Garcia-Segura LM, and Wandosell F (2004) Estradiol inhibits GSK3 and regulates interaction of estrogen receptors, GSK3, and beta-catenin in the hippocampus. *Mol Cell Neurosci* 25: 363-73.

Caricasole A, Copani A, Caraci F, Aronica E, Rozemuller AJ, Caruso A, Storto M, gaviraghi G, Terstappen GC and Nicoletti F (2004) Induction of Dikkopft-1, a negative modulator of the Wnt pathway, is associated with neuronal degeneration in Alzheimer's brain. *J. Neurosci*. 24, 6021-27.

Castano Z, Gordon-Weeks PR and Kypta RM (2010) The neuron-specific isoform of glycogen synthase kinase-3beta is required for axon growth. *J Neurochem* 113: 117-130.

Chen G, Huang LD, Jiang YM, Manji HK (1999) The mood-stabilizing agent valproate inhibits the activity of glycogen synthase kinase-3. *J Neurochem* 72(3): 1327-30.

Chou HY, Howng SL, Cheng TS, Hsiao YL, Lieu AS, Loh JK, Hwang SL, Lin CC, Hsu CM, Wang C, Lee CI, Lu PJ, Chou CK, Huang CY, and Hong YR (2006) GSKIP is homologous to the Axin GSK3beta interaction domain and functions as a negative regulator of GSK3beta. *Biochemistry* 45: 11379-89.

Clavaguera F, Bolmont T, Crowther RA, Abramowski D, Frank S, Probst A, Fraser G, *et al.* (2010) Transmission and spreading of tauopathy in transgenic mouse brain. *Nat Cell Biol* 11(7): 909-13.

Cohen P, and Goedert M (2004) GSK3 inhibitors: development and therapeutic potential. *Nat Rev Drug Discov* 3: 479-87.

Cole A, Frame S, and Cohen P (2004) Further evidence that the tyrosine phosphorylation of glycogen synthase kinase-3 (GSK3) in mammalian cells is an autophosphorylation event. *Biochem J* 377: 249-55.

Cole AR, Causeret F, Yadirgi G, Hastie CJ, McLauchlan H, McManus EJ, Hernández F, Eickholt BJ, Nikolic M, and Sutherland C (2006) "Distinct priming kinases contribute to differential regulation of collapsin response mediator proteins by glycogen synthase kinase-3 in vivo" *J. Biol. Chem.* 281(24):16591-8.

Congdon EE, Duff KE (2008) Is tau aggregation toxic or protective? *J Alzheimers Dis* 14(4): 453-7.

da Cruz e Silva EF and da Cruz e Silva OA. (2003) Protein phosphorylation and APP metabolism. *Neurochem. Res.* 28(10): 1553-61.

Dajani R, Fraser E, Roe SM, Yeo M, Good VM, Thompson V, Dale TC, and Pearl LH (2003) Structural basis for recruitment of glycogen synthase kinase 3beta to the axin-APC scaffold complex. *EMBO J* 22: 494-501.

Dajani R, Fraser E, Roe SM, Young N, Good V, Dale TC, and Pearl LH (2001) Crystal structure of glycogen synthase kinase 3 beta: structural basis for phosphate-primed substrate specificity and autoinhibition. *Cell* 105: 721-32.

de Calignon A, Spires-Jones TL, Pitstick R, Carlson GA, Hyman BT (2009) Tangle-bearing neurons survive despite disruption of membrane integrity in a mouse model of tauopathy. *J Neuropathol Exp Neurol* 68(7): 757-61.

De Ferrari G.V., Papassotiropoulos A, Biechele T, Wavrant De-Vrieze F, Avila ME, Major MB, Myers A, Sáez K, Henríquez JP, Zhao A, Wollmer MA, Nitsch RM, Hock C, Morris CM, Hardy J, Moon RT. (2007) Common genetic variation within the low-density lipoprotein receptor-related protein 6 and late-onset Alzheimer's disease. *Proc. Natl. Acad. Sci.* 104, 9434-39.

Delcommenne M, Tan C, Gray V, Rue L, Woodgett J, and Dedhar S (1998) Phosphoinositide-3-OH kinase-dependent regulation of glycogen synthase kinase 3 and protein kinase B/AKT by the integrin-linked kinase. *Proc Natl Acad Sci U S A* 95: 11211-6.

Delobel P, Lavenir I, Fraser G, Ingram E, Holzer M, Ghetti B, Spillantini MG, Crowther RA, Goedert M. (2008) Analysis of tau phosphorylation and truncation in a mouse model of human tauopathy. *Am J Pathol* 172(1): 123-31.

Ding Q, Xia W, Liu JC, Yang JY, Lee DF, Xia J, Bartholomeusz G, Li Y, Pan Y, Li Z, Bargou RC, Qin J, Lai CC, Tsai FJ, Tsai CH, and Hung MC (2005) Erk associates with and primes GSK-3beta for its inactivation resulting in upregulation of beta-catenin. *Mol Cell* 19: 159-70.

Drechsel DN, Hyman AA, Cobb MH, Kirschner MW (1992) Modulation of the dynamic instability of tubulin assembly by the microtubule-associated protein tau. *Mol Biol Cell* 3(10): 1141-54.

Ebneth A, Godemann R, Stamer K, Illenberger S, Trinczek B, Mandelkow E (1998) Overexpression of tau protein inhibits kinesin-dependent trafficking of vesicles, mitochondria, and endoplasmic reticulum: Implications for Alzheimer's disease. *J Cell Biol* 143(3): 777-94.

Embi N, Rylatt DB, and Cohen P (1980) Glycogen synthase kinase-3 from rabbit skeletal muscle. Separation from cyclic-AMP-dependent protein kinase and phosphorylase kinase. *Eur. J. Biochem.* 107(2):519-27.

Eom TY and Jope RS (2009) Blocked inhibitory serine-phosphorylation of glycogen synthase kinase-3alpha/beta impairs in vivo neural precursor cell proliferation. *Biol Psychiatry* 66: 494-502.

Fang X, Yu SX, Lu Y, Bast RC Jr., Woodgett JR, and Mills GB (2000) Phosphorylation and inactivation of glycogen synthase kinase 3 by protein kinase A. *Proc Natl Acad Sci U S A* 97: 11960-5.

Ferkey DM & Kimelman D (2002) Glycogen synthase kinase-3 beta mutagenesis identifies a common binding domain for GBP and Axin. *J Biol Chem* 277: 16147-52.

Frame S and Cohen P (2001) GSK3 takes centre stage more than 20 years after its discovery. *Biochem J* 359: 1-16.

Frame S, Cohen P, and Biondi RM (2001) A common phosphate binding site explains the unique substrate specificity of GSK3 and its inactivation by phosphorylation. *Mol Cell* 7: 1321-7.

Fraser E, Young N, Dajani R, Franca-Koh J, Ryves J, Williams RS, Yeo M, Webster MT, Richardson C, Smalley CM, Pearl LH, Harwood A, and Dale TC (2002) Identification of the Axin and Frat binding region of glycogen synthase kinase-3. *J Biol Chem* 277: 2176-85.

Frost B, Jacks RL, Diamond MI. Propagation of tau misfolding from the outside to the inside of a cell (2009) *J Biol Chem* 284(19): 12845-52.

Gadakar PK, Phukan S, Dattatreya P, Balaji VN (2007) Pose prediction accuracy in docking studies and enrichment of actives in the active site of GSK-3beta. *J Chem Inf Model* 47(4):446-59.

Gamblin TC, Chen F, Zambrano A, Abraha A, Lagalwar S, Guillozet AL, Lu M, Fu Y, Garcia-Sierra F, LaPointe N, Miller R, Berry RW, Binder LI, Cryns VL (2993) Caspase cleavage of tau: linking amyloid and neurofibrillary tangles in Alzheimer's disease. *Proc Natl Acad Sci USA* 100(17): 10032-7

Goedert M, Spillantini MG, Potier MC, Ulrich J, Crowther RA (1989) Cloning and sequencing of the cDNA encoding an isoform of microtubule-associated protein tau containing four tandem repeats: differential expression of tau protein mRNAs in human brain. *EMBO J* 8(2): 393-9.

Goñi-Oliver P, Avila J, and Hernández F (2009a) Calpain-mediated truncation of GSK-3 in post-mortem brain samples. *J Neurosci Res* 87: 1156-61.

Goñi-Oliver P, Avila J, and Hernández F (2009b) Memantine inhibits calpain-mediated truncation of GSK-3 induced by NMDA: implications in Alzheimer's disease. *J Alzheimers Dis.* 18(4): 843-8.

Goñi-Oliver P, Lucas JJ, Avila J, and Hernández F (2007) N-terminal cleavage of GSK-3 by calpain: a new form of GSK-3 regulation. *J Biol Chem* 282: 22406-13.

Gould TD and Manji HK (2006) Glycogen synthase kinase 3: a target for novel mood disorder treatments. In: *Glycogen Synthase Kinase 3 (GSK-3) and Its Inhibitors-Drug discovery and Development.* Wang B (Ed), Ch 7, pp. 125-154. Wiley Series in Drug Discovery and Development. New Jersey, USA..

Gould TD, Manji HK (1995) The Wnt signaling pathway in bipolar disorder. *Neuroscientist* 8(5): 497-511.

Grace EA and Busciglio J (2003) Aberrant activation of focal adhesion proteins mediates fibrillar amyloid β-induced neuronal dystrophy. *J. Neurosci.* 23, 493-502.

Grimes CA, and Jope RS (2001) The multifaceted roles of glycogen synthase kinase 3beta in cellular signaling. *Prog Neurobiol* 65: 391-426.

Haass C, Selkoe DJ (2007) protein oligomers in neurodegeneration: Lessons from the Alzheimer's amyloid beta-peptide. *Nat Rev Mol Cell Biol* 8(2): 101-12.

Hamilton G, Proitsi P, Jehu L, Morgan A, Williams J, O'Donovan M, Owen MJ, Powell JF and Lovestone S (2007) Candidate gene association study of insulin signalling genes and Alzheimer's disease: evidence for SOS2, PCK1, and PPARgamma as susceptibility loci. *Am. J. Med. Genet. B Neuropsychiatr. Genet.* 144, 508-16.

Hampel H, Ewers M, Bürger K, Annas P, Mörtberg A, Bogstedt A, Frölich L, Schröder J, Schönknecht P, Riepe MW, Kraft I, Gasser T, Leyhe T, Möller HJ, Kurz A, Basun H (2009) Lithium trial in Alzheimer's disease: a randomized, single-blind, placebo-controlled, multicenter 10-week study. *J Clin Psychiatry* 70(6): 922-31.

Hanger DP, Anderton BH, Noble W (2009) Tau phosphorylation: The therapeutic challenge for neurodegenerative disease. *Trends Mol Med* 15(3): 112-9.

Hardy J, Selkoe DJ (2002) The amyloid hypothesis of Alzheimer's disease: progress and problems on the road to therapeutics. Science 297: 353–356.

Hardy JA, Higgins GA (1992) Alzheimer's disease: the amyloid cascade hypothesis. *Science* 256: 184–185.

Hart GW, Kreppel LK, Comer FI, Arnold CS, Snow DM, Ye Z, Cheng X, DellaManna D, Caine DS, Earles BJ, Akimoto Y, Cole RN, Hayes BK (1996) O-GlcNAcylation of key nuclear and cytoskeletal proteins: reciprocity with O-phosphorylation and putative roles in protein multimerization. *Glycobiology* 6(7): 711-6.

Hartigan JA, Xiong WC, and Johnson GV (2001) Glycogen synthase kinase 3beta is tyrosine phosphorylated by PYK2. *Biochem Biophys Res Commun* 284: 485-9.

Harwood AJ (2001) Regulation of GSK-3: a cellular multiprocessor. *Cell* 105: 821-4.

Havens WW 2nd, Cole J (1982) Successful treatment of dementia with lithium. *J Clin Psychopharmacol* 2(1): 71-2.

Hemmings BA, Yellowlees D, Kernohan JC, and Cohen P (1981) Purification of glycogen synthase kinase 3 from rabbit skeletal muscle. Copurification with the activating factor (FA) of the (Mg-ATP) dependent protein phosphatase. *Eur. J. Biochem.* 119(3):443-51.

Hernández F, Gómez de Barreda E, Fuster-Matanzo A, Lucas JJ, Avila J (2010) GSK3: a possible link between beta amyloid peptide and tau protein. *Exp Neurol.* 223(2): 322-5.

Hiesberger T., Trommsdorff M., Howell B. W., Goffinet A., Mumby M. C., Cooper J. A. and Herz J. (1999) Direct binding of Reelin to VLDL receptor and ApoE receptor 2 induces tyrosine phosphorylation of disabled-1 and modulates tau phosphorylation. *Neuron* 24, 481-9.

Himmler A, Drechsel D, Kirschner MW, Martin DW Jr (1989) Tau consists of a set of proteins with repeated C-terminal microtubule-binding domains and variable N-terminal domains. *Mol Cell Biol* 9(4): 1381-8.

Hoeflich KP, Luo J, Rubie EA, Tsao M-S, Jin O and Woodgett JR (2000) Requirement for GSK3beta in cell surival and NFkB activation. *Nature* 406: 86-90.

Hooper C, Killick R, and Lovestone S (2008) The GSK3 hypothesis of Alzheimer's disease. *J. Neurochem.* 104: 1433-9.

Hooper C, Markevich V, Plattner F, Killick R, Schofield E, Engel T, Hernandez F, Anderton B, Rosenblum K, Bliss T, Cooke SF, Avila J, Lucas JJ, Giese KP, Stephenson J, and Lovestone S (2007) Glycogen synthase kinase-3 inhibition is integral to long-term potentiation. Eur. J. Neurosci. 25(1): 81-6.

Hoshi M, Sato M, Matsumoto S, Noguchi A, Yasutake K, Yoshida N, Sato K (2003) Spherical aggregates of beta-amyloid (amylospheroid) show high neurotoxicity and activate tau protein kinase I/glycogen synthase kinase-3beta. *Proc Natl Acad Sci U S A* 100(11): 6370-6375.

Hsieh H, Boehm J, Sato C, Iwatsubo T, Tomita T, Sisodia S, Malinow R (2006) AMPAR removal underlies Abeta-induced synaptic depression and dendritic spine loss. Neuron 52(5): 831-43.

Hughes K, Nikolakaki E, Plyte SE, Totty NF, Woodgett JR (1993) Modulation of the glycogen synthase kinase-3 family by tyrosine phosphorylation. *EMBO J* 12(2): 803-8.

Hur EM and Zhon FP (2010) GSK3 signalling in neural development. *Nat Rev Neurosci* 11: 539-51.

Inestrosa NC, Toledo EM (2008) The role of Wnt signaling in neuronal dysfunction in Alzheimer's Disease. *Mol Neurodegener* 24: 3-9.

Iqbal K, Liu F, Gong CX, Alonso Adel C, Grundke-Iqbal I (2009) Mechanisms of tau-induced neurdegeneration. *Acta Neuropathol* 118(1): 53-69.

Itoh K, Tang TL, Neel BG, and Sokol SY (1995) Specific modulation of ectodermal cell fates in Xenopus embryos by glycogen synthase kinase. *Development* 121, 3979-88.

Ittner LM, Götz J (2011) Amyloid-β and tau--a toxic pas de deux in Alzheimer's disease. *Nat Rev Neurosci* 12(2): 65-72.

Jackson G. R., Wiedau-Pazos M., Sang T. K., Wagle N., Brown C. A., Massachi S. and Geschwind D. H. (2002) Human wild-type tau interacts with wingless pathway components and produces neurofibrillary pathology in Drosophila. *Neuron* 34, 509-19

Jaworski T, Kügler S, Van Leuven F (2010) Modeling of tau-mediated synaptic and neuronal degeneration in Alzheimer's disease. *Int J Alzheimers Dis.* pii: 573138.

Jiang H, Guo W, Liang X, Rao Y. (2005) Both the establishment and the maintenance of neuronal polarity require active mechanisms: critical roles of GSK-3β and its upstream regulators. Cell. 120:123-35.

Jo J, Whitcomb DJ, Olsen KM, Kerrigan TL, Lo SC, Bru-Mercier G, Dickinson B, Scullion S, Sheng M, Collingridge G, Cho K (2011) Aβ(1-42) inhibition of LTP is mediated by a signaling pathway involving caspase-3, Akt1 and GSK-3β. Nat Neurosci [Epub ahead of print]. PMID: 21441921.

Jope RS (1999) Anti-bipolar therapy: mechanism of action of lithium. *Mol Psychiatry* 4(2): 117-28.

Kaidanovich-Beilin O, Eldar-Finkelman H (2006) Long-term treatment with novel glycogen synthase kinase-3 inhibitor improves glucose homeostasis in ob/ob mice: molecular characterization in liver and muscle. *J Pharmacol Exp Ther* 316(1): 17-24.

Kaidanovich-Beilin O, Lipina TV, Takao K van Eede M, Hattori S, Laliberté C, Khan M, Okamoto K, Chambers JW, Fletcher PJ, MacAulay K, Doble BW, Henkelman M, Miyakawa T, Roder J, Woodgett JR. (2009) Abnormalities in brain structure and behavior in GSK-3alpha mutant mice. *Mol Brain* 2: 35.

Kandasamy AD, and Schulz R (2009) Glycogen synthase kinase-3beta is activated by matrix metalloproteinase-2 mediated proteolysis in cardiomyoblasts. *Cardiovasc Res* 83: 698-706.

Kayed R, Jackson GR. Prefilament tau species as potential targets for immunotherapy for Alzheimer disease and related disorders (2009) *Curr Opin Immunol* 21(3): 359-63.

Kim L, Harwood A, and Kimmel AR (2002) Receptor-dependent and tyrosine phosphatase-mediated inhibition of GSK3 regulates cell fate choice. *Dev Cell* 3: 23-32.

Kim L, Liu J, and Kimmel AR (1999).The novel tyrosine kinase ZAK1 activates GSK3 to direct cell fate specification. *Cell* 99: 399-408.

Kim WY, Wang X, Wu Y, Doble BW, Patel S, Woodgett JR and Snider WD (2009) GSK-3 is a master regulator of neural progenitor homeostasis. *Nat Neurosci* 12: 1390-1397.

Kimura T, Yamashita S, Nakao S, Park JM, Murayama M, Mizoroki T, Yoshiike Y, Sahara N and Takashima A (2008) GSK-3beta is required for memory reconsolidation in adult brain. *PLoS One,* 3(10): e3540.

Klein PS, Melton DA (1996) A molecular mechanism for the effect of lithium on development. *Proc Natl Acad Sci USA* 93(16): 8455-9.

Kwok JB, Hallupp M, Loy CT, Chan DK, Woo J, Mellick GD, Buchanan DD, Silburn PA, Halliday GM, Schofield PR (2005) GSK3B polymorphisms alter transcription and splicing in Parkinson's disease. *Ann Neurol* 58(6): 829-39.

Kwok JB, Loy CT, Hamilton G, Lau E, Hallupp M, Williams J, Owen MJ, Broe GA, Tang N, Lam L, Powell JF, Lovestone S, Schofield PR (2008) Glycogen synthase kinase-3beta and tau genes interact in Alzheimer's disease. *Ann Neurol* 64(4): 446-54.

Lee G, Neve RL, Kosik KS (1989) The microtubule binding domain of tau protein. *Neuron* 2(6): 1615-24.

Lee JH, Lau KF, Perkinton MS, Standen CL, Shemilt SJ, Mercken L, Cooper JD, McLoughlin DM, Miller CC. (2003) The neuronal adaptor protein X11a reduces Aβ levels in the brains of Alzheimer's APPswe Tg2576 transgenic mice. *J Biol Chem.* 278(47): 47025-9.

Lenox RH, Hahn CG (2000) Overview of the mechanism of action of lithium in the brain: fifty-year update. *J Clin Psychiatry* 61(Suppl 9): 5-15.

Leroy K, Boutajangout A, Authelet M, Woodgett JR, Anderton BH, and Brion JP (2002) The active form of glycogen synthase kinase-3b is associated with granulovacuolar degeneration in neurons in Alzheimer's disease. *Acta Neuropathol.* 103(2):91-9.

Lesort M, Jope RS, and Johnson GV (1999) Insulin transiently increases tau phosphorylation: involvement of glycogen synthase kinase-3beta and Fyn tyrosine kinase. *J Neurochem* 72: 576-84.

Li L, Yuan H, Weaver CD, Mao J, Farr GH 3rd, Sussman DJ, Jonkers J, Kimelman D, and Wu D (1999) Axin and Frat1 interact with dvl and GSK, bridging Dvl to GSK in Wnt-mediated regulation of LEF-1. *EMBO J* 18: 4233-40.

Li X, Bijur GN, Jope RS (2002) Glycogen synthase kinase-3beta, mood stabilizers, and neuroprotection. *Bipolar Disord* 4(2): 137-44.

Li-Smerin, Y, Levitan ES and Johnson JW (2001) Free intracellular Mg(2+) concentration and inhibition of NMDA responses in cultured rat neurons. *J Physiol* 533: 729-43.

Liu KJ, Arron JR, Stankunas K, Crabtree GR and Longaker MT (2007) Chemical rescue of cleft palate and midline defects in conditional GSK3b mice. *Nature* 446: 79-82.

Liu SJ, AH Zhang, Li HL, Wang Q, Deng HM, Netzer WJ, Xu H, and Wang JZ (2003) Overactivation of glycogen synthase kinase-3 by inhibition of phosphoinositol-3 kinase and protein kinase C leads to hyperphosphorylation of tau and impairment of spatial memory. *J Neurochem* 87: 1333-44.

Lochhead PA, Kinstrie R, Sibbet G, Rawjee T, Morrice N and Cleghon V (2006) A chaperone-dependent GSK3beta transitional intermediate mediates activation-loop autophosphorylation. *Mol Cell* 24: 627-633.

LoPresti P, Szuchet S, Papasozomenos SC, Zinkowski RP, Binder LI (1995) Functional implications for the microtubule-associated protein tau: Localization in oligodendrocytes. *Proc Natl Acad Sci USA* 92(22): 10369-73.

MacAulay K, Doble BW, Patel S, Hansotia T, Sinclair EM, Drucker DJ, Nagy A and Woodgett JR (2007) Glycogen synthase kinase 3alpha-specific regulation of murine hepatic glycogen metabolism. *Cell Metab* 6: 329-337.

Macdonald A, Briggs K, Poppe M, Higgins A, Velayudhan L, Lovestone S (2008) A feasibility and tolerability study of lithium in Alzheimer's disease. *Int J Geriatr Psychiatry* 23(7): 704-11.

Magdesian MH, Carvalho MM, Mendes FA, Saraiva LM, Juliano MA, Juliano L, Garcia-Abreu J, and Ferreira ST (2008) Amyloid-beta binds to the extracellular cysteine-rich domain of Frizzled and inhibits Wnt/beta-catenin signaling. *J Biol Chem.* 283(14): 9359-68

Mangialasche F, Solomon A, Winblad B, Mecocci P, Kivipelto M (2010) Alzheimer's disease: clinical trials and drug development. *Lancet Neurol* 9(7): 702-16.

Mao Y, Ge X, Frank CL, Madison JM, Koehler AN, Doud MK, Tassa C, Berry EM, Soda T, Singh KK, Biechele T, Petryshen TL, Moon RT, Haggarty SJ, and Tsai LH (2009) Disrupted in schizophrenia 1 regulates neuronal progenitor proliferation via modulation of GSK3beta/beta-catenin signaling. *Cell* 136 (6), 1017-31.

Martín CP, Vázquez J, Avila J, Moreno FJ (2002) P24, a glycogen synthase kinase 3 (GSK 3) inhibitor. Biochim Biophys Acta. 2002 Jan 2;1586(1):113-22.

Mateo I, Infante J, Llorca J, Rodríguez E, Berciano J, Combarros O (2006) Association between glycogen synthase kinase-3beta genetic polymorphism and late-onset Alzheimer's disease. *Dement Geriatr Cogn Disord* 21(4): 228-32.

Mateo I, Vázquez-Higuera JL, Sánchez-Juan P, Rodríguez-Rodríguez E, Infante J, García-Gorostiaga I, Berciano J, Combarros O (2009) Epistasis between tau phosphorylation regulating genes (CDK5R1 and GSK-3beta) and Alzheimer's disease risk. *Acta Neurol Scand* 120(2): 130-3.

Medina M & Wandosell F (2011) Deconstructing GSK-3: the fine regulation of its activity) *Int J Alz Dis* (in press).

Medina M (2011) Recent developments in tau-based therapeutics for neurodegenerative diseases. *Recent Pat CNS Drug Discov* 6(1): 20-30

Medina M, Avila J (2010) Glycogen synthase kinase-3 (GSK-3) inhibitors for the treatment of Alzheimer's disease. *Curr Pharm Des* 16(25): 2790-8.

Medina M, Castro A (2008) Glycogen synthase kinase-3 (GSK-3) inhibitors reach the clinic. *Curr Opin Drug Discov Devel* 11(4): 533-43.

Moon RT, Kohn AD, De Ferrari GV, and Kaykas A (2004) Wnt and beta-catenin signalling: diseases and therapies. *Nat Rev Genet* 5: 691-701.

Morfini G., Pigino G., Beffert U., Busciglio J. and Brady S. T. (2002) Fast axonal transport misregulation and Alzheimer's disease. *Neuromol. Med.* 2, 89-99.

Mori H, Kondo J, Ihara Y. (1987) Ubiquitin is a component of paired helical filaments in Alzheimer's disease. *Science* 235(4796): 1641-4.

Morsch R, Simon W, Coleman PD (1999) Neurons may live for decades with neurofibrillary tangles. *J Neuropathol Exp Neurol* 58(2): 188-97.

Mukai F, Ishiguro K, Sano Y, Fujita SC (2002) Alternative splicing isoform of tau protein kinase I/glycogen synthase kinase 3 beta. *J Neurochem.* 81(5):1073-83.

Muñoz-Montaño JR, Lim F, Moreno FJ, Avila J, and Díaz-Nido J. (1999) Glycogen Synthase Kinase-3 Modulates Neurite Outgrowth in Cultured Neurons: Possible Implications for Neurite Pathology in Alzheimer's Disease. *J. Alzheimers Dis.* 1(6):361-78.

Munoz-Montano JR, Moreno FJ, Avila J, and Diaz-Nido J (1997) Lithium inhibits Alzheimer's disease-like tau protein phosphorylation in neurons. *FEBS Lett* 411: 183-8.

Muyllaert D, Kremer A, Jaworski T, Borghgraef P, Devijver H, Croes S, Dewatcher I, and Van Leuven F. (2008) Glycogen synthase kinase-3beta, or a link between amyloid and tau pathology? *Genes Brain Behav.* 7 (suppl. 1): 57-66.

Nishimura I, Yang Y, and Lu B (2004) PAR-1 kinase plays an initiator role in a temporally ordered phosphorylation process that confers tau toxicity in Drosophila. *Cell* 116: 671-82.

Noble W, Olm V, Takata K, Casey E, Mary O, Meyerson J, Gaynor K, LaFrancois J, Wang L, Kondo T, Davies P, Burns M, Veeranna, Nixon R, Dickson D, Matsuoka Y, Ahlijanian M, Lau LF, and Duff K (2003) Cdk5 is a key factor in tau aggregation and tangle formation in vivo. *Neuron* 38: 555-65.

Noble W, Planel E, Zehr C, Olm V, Meyerson J, Suleman F, Gaynor K, Wang L, LaFrancois J, Feinstein B, Burns M, Krishnamurthy P, Wen Y, Bhat R, Lewis J, Dickson D, and Duff K (2005) Inhibition of glycogen synthase kinase-3 by lithium correlates with reduced tauopathy and degeneration in vivo. *Proc Natl Acad Sci U S A* 102: 6990-5.

O'Brien WT, Harper AD, Jove F, Woodgett JR, Maretto S, Piccolo S and Klein PS (2004) Glycogen synthase kinase-3beta haploinsufficiency mimics the behavioral and molecular effects of lithium. *J Neurosci* 24: 6791-6798.

Osolodkin DI, Zakharevich NV, Palyulin VA, Danilenko VN, and Zefirov NS (2011) Bioinformatic analysis of glycogen synthase kinase 3: human versus parasite kinases.*Parasitology* Feb 24: 1-11.

Palacino J.J., Murphy M.P., Murayama O., Iwasaki K., Fujiwara M., Takashima A., Golde T.E., and Wolozin B. (2001) Presenilin 1 regulates β-catenin-mediated transcription in a glycogen synthase kinase-3-independent fashion. *J. Biol. Chem.* 276(42):38563-9.

Patel DS, Dessalew N, Iqbal P, Bharatam PV (2007) Structure-based approaches in the design of GSK-3 selective inhibitors. *Curr Protein Pept Sci* 8(4):352-64.

Patel S, Doble BW, MacAulay K, Sinclair EM, Drucker DJ, Woodgett JR (2008) Tissue-specific role of glycogen synthase kinase 3beta in glucose homeostasis and insulin action. *Mol Cell Biol* 28(20): 6314-28.

Patel S, Macaulay K, Woodgett JR (2011) Tissue-specific analysis of glycogen synthase kinase-3α (GSK-3α) in glucose metabolism: effect of strain variation. *PLoS One* 6(1): e15845.

Pei JJ, Tanaka T, Tung YC, Braak E, Iqbal K, and Grundke-Iqbal I (1997) Distribution, levels, and activity of glycogen synthase kinase-3 in the Alzheimer disease brain. J *Neuropathol Exp Neurol*. 56(1):70-8.

Peineau S, Taghibiglou C, Bradley C, Wong TP, Liu L, Lu J, Lo E, Wu D, Saule E, Bouschet T, Matthews P, Isaac JT, Bortolotto ZA, Wang YT, and Collingridge GL (2007) LTP inhibits LTD in the hippocampus via regulation of GSK-3ba. *Neuron*. 53(5):703-17.

Perez M, Rojo AI, Wandosell F, Diaz-Nido J, and Avila J (2003) Prion peptide induces neuronal cell death through a pathway involving glycogen synthase kinase 3. *Biochem J* 372: 129-36.

Phiel CJ, Wilson CA, Lee VM, and Klein PS (2003) GSK-3alpha regulates production of Alzheimer's disease amyloid-b peptides *Nature*. 423(6938):435-9.

Plotkin B, Kaidanovich O, Talior I, Eldar-Finkelman H (2003) Insulin mimetic action of synthetic phosphorylated peptide inhibitors of glycogen synthase kinase-3. J Pharmacol Exp Ther 305(3): 974-80.

Prickaerts J, Moechars D, Cryns K, Lenaerts I, van Craenendonck H, Goris I, Daneels G, Bouwknecht JA and Steckler T (2006) Transgenic mice overexpressing glycogen synthase kinase 3beta: a putative model of hyperactivity and mania. *J Neurosci* 26: 9022-9029.

Ray WJ Jr, Szymanki ES, Ng L (1978) The binding of lithium and of anionic metabolites to phosphoglucomutase. *Biochim Biophys Acta* 522(2): 434-42.

Reiman EM, Webster JA, Myers AL, Hardy J, Dunckley T, Zismann VL, Joshipura KD, Pearson JV, Hu-Lince D, Huentelman MJ, Craig DW, Coon KD, Liang WS, Herbert RH, Beach T, Rohrer KC, Zhao AS, Leung D, Bryden L, Marlowe L, Kaleem M, Mastroeni D, Grover A, Heward CB, Ravid R, Rogers J, Hutton ML, Melquist S, Petersen RC, Alexander GE, Caselli RJ, Kukull W, Papassotiropoulos A, Stephan DA. (2007) GAB2 alleles modify Alzheimer's risk in ApoE4 carriers. *Neuron* 54, 713-20.

Rockenstein E, Torrance M, Adame A, Mante M, Bar-on P, Rose JB, Crews L, and Masliah E. (2007) Neuroprotective effects of regulators of the glycogen synthase kinase-3b signaling pathway in a transgenic model of Alzheimer's disease are associated with reduced amyloid precursor protein phosphorylation. *J. Neurosci*. 27(8):1981-91.

Rosenberg (2007) The mechanisms of action of valproate in neuropsychiatric disorders: can we see the forest for the trees? *Cell Mol Life Sci* 64(16): 2090-103.

Ruel L, Bourouis M, Heitzler P, Pantesco V, and Simpson P (1993) Drosophila shaggy kinase and rat glycogen synthase kinase-3 have conserved activities and act downstream of Notch. *Nature* 362 57-60.

Russ C, Lovestone S, Powell JF (2001) Identification of sequence variants and analysis of the role of the glycogen synthase kinase 3 beta gene and promoter in late onset Alzheimer's disease. *Mol Psychiatry* 6(3): 320-4

Sayas C. L., Avila J. and Wandosell F. (2002) Regulation of neuronal cytoskeleton by lysophosphatidic acid: role of GSK-3. *Biochim. Biophys. Acta* 1582, 144-53.

Sayas CL, Moreno-Flores MT, Avila J, Wandosell F (1999) The neurite retraction induced by lysophosphatidic acid increases Alzheimer's disease-like Tau phosphorylation. *J Biol Chem* 274(52): 37046-52.

Schaffer BA, Bertram L, Miller BL, Mullin K, Weintraub S, Johnson N, Bigio EH, Mesulam M, Wiedau-Pazos M, Jackson GR, Cummings JL, Cantor RM, Levey AI, Tanzi RE, Geschwind DH (2008) Association of GSK3B with Alzheimer disease and frontotemporal dementia. *Arch Neurol* 65(10): 1368-74.

Selkoe DJ (1991) The molecular pathology of Alzheimer's disease. *Neuron* 6: 487–498.

Selkoe DJ (2002) Alzheimer's disease is a synaptic failure. *Science* 298: 789–791.

Selkoe DJ (2008) Soluble oligomers of the amyloid β-protein impair synaptic plasticity and behaviour. *Behav Brain Res* 192(1): 106-13.

Sengupta A, Wu Q, Grundke-Iqbal I, Iqbal K, and Singh TJ (1997) Potentiation of GSK-3-catalyzed Alzheimer-like phosphorylation of human tau by cdk5. *Mol Cell Biochem* 167: 99-105.

Shaldubina A, Agam G, Belmaker RH (2001) The mechanism of lithium action: state of the art, ten years later. *Prog Neuropsychopharmacol Biol Psychiatry* 25(4): 855-66.

Sheldon M., Rice D. S., D'Arcangelo G., Yoneshima H., Nakajima K., Mikoshiba K., Howell B. W., Cooper J. A., Goldowitz D., and Curran T. (1997) Scrambler and yotari disrupt the disabled gene and produce a reeler-like phenotype in mice. *Nature* 389, 730-3.

Sigurdsson EM (2008). Immunotherapy targeting pathological tau protein in Alzheimer's disease and related tauopathies *J Alzheimers Dis* 15(2): 157-68.

Simon D, Benitez MJ, Gimenez-Cassina A, Garrido JJ, Bhat RV, Diaz-Nido J, and Wandosell F (2008) Pharmacological inhibition of GSK-3 is not strictly correlated with a decrease in tyrosine phosphorylation of residues 216/279. *J Neurosci Res* 86: 668-74.

Sofola O, Kerr F, Rogers I, Killick R, Augustin H, Gandy C, Allen MJ, Hardy J, Lovestone S, Partridge L (2010) Inhibition of GSK-3 ameliorates Abeta pathology in an adult-onset Drosophila model of Alzheimer's disease. *PLoS Genet* 6(9). pii: e1001087.

Soutar MP, Kim WY, Williamson R, Peggie M, Hastie CJ, McLauchlan H, Snider WD, Gordon-Weeks PR, and Sutherland C (2010) Evidence that glycogen synthase kinase-3 isoforms have distinct substrate preference in the brain. *J Neurochem* 115: 974-83.

Stambolic V, and Woodgett JR (1994) Mitogen inactivation of glycogen synthase kinase-3 beta in intact cells via serine 9 phosphorylation. *Biochem J* 303 (3): 701-4.

Stambolic V, Ruel L, Woodgett JR (1997) Lithium inhibits glycogen synthase kinase-3 activity and mimics wingless signalling in intact cells. *Curr Biol* 6(12): 1664-8.

Stoothoff WH, Cho JH, McDonald RP, and Johnson GV (2005) FRAT-2 preferentially increases glycogen synthase kinase 3 beta-mediated phosphorylation of primed sites, which results in enhanced tau phosphorylation. *J Biol Chem* 280: 270-6.

Su Y Ryder J., Li B., Wu X., Fox N., Solenberg, P., Brune K., Paul S., Zhou Y., Liu F., and Ni B. (2004) Lithium, a common drug for bipolar disorder treatment, regulates amyloid-β precursor protein processing. *Biochemistry* 43(22):6899-908.

Suhara T, Magrané J, Rosen K, Christensen R, Kim HS, Zheng B, McPhie DL, Walsh K, Querfurth H (2003) Abeta42 generation is toxic to endothelial cells and inhibits eNOS function through an Akt/GSK-3beta signaling-dependent mechanism. *Neurobiol Aging* 24(3): 437-51.

Sun X., Sato S., Murayama O., Murayama M., Park J.M., Yamaguchi H., and Takashima A. (2002) Lithium inhibits amyloid secretion in COS7 cells transfected with amyloid precursor protein C100. *Neurosci. Lett.* 321(1-2):61-4.

Sutherland C, Leighton IA, and Cohen P (1993) Inactivation of glycogen synthase kinase-3 beta by phosphorylation: new kinase connections in insulin and growth-factor signalling. *Biochem J* 296: 15-9.

Takashima A, Honda T, Yasutake K, Michel G, Murayama O, Murayama M, Ishiguro K, and Yamaguchi H (1998a) Activation of tau protein kinase I/glycogen synthase kinase-3beta by amyloid beta peptide (25-35) enhances phosphorylation of tau in hippocampal neurons. *Neurosci Res* 31: 317-23.

Takashima A., Murayama O., Kohno T., Honda T., Yasutake K., Nihonmatsu N., Mercken M., Yamaguchi H., Sugihara S., and Wolozin B. (1998b) Presenilin 1 associates with glycogen synthase kinase-3β and its substrate tau. *Proc. Natl. Acad. Sci. U S A.* 95(16):9637-41.

ter Haar E (2006) The crystal structure of glycogen synthase kinase 3. In: *Glycogen Synthase Kinase 3 (GSK-3) and Its Inhibitors-Drug discovery and Development.* Wang B (Ed), Ch 5, pp. 61-82. Wiley Series in Drug Discovery and Development. New Jersey, USA..

ter Haar E, Coll JT, Austen DA, Hsiao HM, Swenson L, and Jain J (2001) Structure of GSK3beta reveals a primed phosphorylation mechanism. *Nat Struct Biol* 8: 593-6.

Terao T, Nakano H, Inoue Y, Okamoto T, Nakamura J, Iwata N (2006) Lithium and dementia: a preliminary study. *Prog Neuropsychopharmacol Biol Psychiatry*30(6): 1125-8.

Tesco G. and Tanzi R.E. (2000) GSK-3β forms a tetrameric complex with endogenous PS1-CTF/NTF and β-catenin. Effects of the D257/D385A and FAD-linked mutations. *Ann. NY Acad. Sci.* 920:227-32.

Thornton TM, Pedraza-Alva G, Deng B, Wood CD, Aronshtam A, Clements JL, Sabio G, Davis RJ, Matthews DE, Doble B, and Rincon M (2008) Phosphorylation by p38 MAPK as an alternative pathway for GSK3beta inactivation. *Science* 320: 667-70.

Townsend M, Mehta T, and Selkoe DJ (2007) Soluble Abeta inhibits specific signal transduction cascades common to the insulin receptor pathway. *J Biol Chem* 282 (46): 33305-12.

Twomey C and McCarthy JV (2006) Presenilin-1 is an unprimed glycogen synthase kinase-3beta substrate. *FEBS Lett* 580: 4015-20.

van Amerongen R, Nawijn M, Franca-Koh J, Zevenhoven J, van der Gulden H, Jonkers J, and Berns A (2005) Frat is dispensable for canonical Wnt signaling in mammals. *Genes Dev* 19: 425-30.

Walsh DM, Klyubin I, Fadeeva JV, Cullen WK, Anwyl R, Wolfe MS, Rowan MJ, Selkoe DJ (2002) Naturally secreted oligomers of amyloid beta protein potently inhibit hippocampal long-term potentiation in vivo. Nature 416(6880): 535-9.

Walsh DM, Selkoe DJ (2007) A beta oligomers - a decade of discovery. *J Neurochem* 101(5): 1172-84

Wang JZ, Grundke-Iqbal I, Iqbal K (1996) Glycosylation of microtubule-associated protein tau: an abnormal posttranslational modification in Alzheimer's disease. *Nat Med* 2(8): 871-5.

Wang QM, Fiol CJ, DePaoli-Roach AA, and Roach PJ (1994) Glycogen synthase kinase-3 beta is a dual specificity kinase differentially regulated by tyrosine and serine/threonine phosphorylation. *J Biol Chem* 269: 14566-74.

Wei H, Leeds PR, Qian Y, Wei W, Chen R, Chuang D (2000) Beta-amyloid peptide-induced death of PC 12 cells and cerebellar granule cell neurons is inhibited by long-term lithium treatment. *Eur J Pharmacol* 392(3): 117-23.

Woodgett JR (2006) Glycogen synthase Kinase 3: an introductory synopsis. In: *Glycogen Synthase Kinase 3 (GSK-3) and Its Inhibitors-Drug discovery and Development.* Wang B (Ed), Ch 1, pp. 3-24. Wiley Series in Drug Discovery and Development. New Jersey, USA..

Woodgett JR: Molecular cloning and expression of glycogen synthase kinase-3/factor A. *EMBO J.* (1990) 9(8):2431-8.

Wood-Kaczmar A, Kraus M, Ishiguro K, Philpott KL and Gordon-Weeks PR (2009) An alternatively spliced form of glycogen synthase kinase-3beta is targeted to growing neurites and growth cones. *Mol Cell Neurosci* 42: 184-194.

York JD, Ponder JW, Majerus PW (1995) Definition of a metal-dependent/Li(+)-inhibited phosphomonoesterase protein family based upon a conserved three-dimensional core structure. *Proc Natl Acad Sci USA* 92(11): 5149-53.

Yoshimura T, Kawano Y, Arimura N, Kawabata S, Kikuchi A, Kaibuchi K. (2005) GSK-3β regulates phosphorylation of CRMP-2 and neuronal polarity. Cell 120:137-49.

Yost C, Farr GH 3rd, Pierce SB, Ferkey DM, Chen MM, and Kimelman D (1998)GBP, an inhibitor of GSK-3, is implicated in Xenopus development and oncogenesis. *Cell* 93: 1031-41.

11

Pin1: A New Enzyme Pivotal for Protecting Against Alzheimer's Disease

Kazuhiro Nakamura, Suk Ling Ma and Kun Ping Lu
Department of Medicine, Beth Israel Deaconess Medical Center
Harvard Medical School, Boston
USA

1. Introduction

Alzheimer's disease (AD) affects more than 35 million people worldwide, and the prevalence of AD increases with age and doubles every 5 years after the age of 65 (Evans et al., 1989). AD is characterized by intracellular neurofibrillary tangles (NFTs) and extracellular amyloid fibrils composed of amyloid beta peptides (Aβ). Accordingly, both tau and amyloid have been the targets for development of treatment for AD.

Tau-mediated neurodegeneration may result from the combination of toxic gains-of-function acquired by the aggregates or their precursors and the detrimental effects that arise from the loss of the normal function(s) of tau in the disease state (Ballatore et al., 2007). The toxic gains-of-function includes sequestration of normal tau function by NFTs made of hyperphosphorylated tau. NFTs also become physical obstacles to the transport of vesicles and other cargos (Ballatore et al., 2007). The loss of the normal function of tau includes detachment of tau from microtubules that causes loss of microtubule-stabilizing function (Stoothoff & Johnson, 2005). Although dynamic tau phosphorylation occurs during embryonic development (Mawal-Dewan et al., 1994), aberrant tau phosphorylation in mature neurons is harmful to the neuron (Matsuo et al., 1994). Tau hyperphosphorylation is a key regulatory mechanism that leads to both such toxic gains-of-function and the loss of the normal function(s) of tau (Ballatore et al., 2007).

Upregulation of aberrant activation of tau kinases and downregulation of phosphatases are major mechanisms possibly involved in tau hyperphosphorylation (Ballatore et al., 2007). Consistently, tau phosphorylation on Ser/Thr-Pro by Pro-directed kinases (Illenberger et al., 1998; Pelech, 1995) or phosphatases such as phosphatase2A (PP2A) (Goedert et al., 2000; Sontag et al., 1996) play pivotal roles in tauopathy. Indeed, overexpression of glycogen synthase kinase-3β (GSK3β) or cyclin-dependent protein kinases (CDK5) and its activator p25 or inhibition of PP2A enhances or induces tau-related phenotypes in mice (Ahlijanian et al., 2000; Augustinack et al., 2002; Cruz et al., 2003; Kins et al., 2001; Noble et al., 2003). In addition, tau phosphorylation has been shown to promote tau degradation via chaperone-interacting protein/Hsp70 (Dickey et al., 2007; Kosik & Shimura, 2005; Petrucelli et al., 2004). These results indicate that kinases and phosphatases that increase and decrease phosphorylated tau, respectively, are crucial targets for treatment of AD. Design of inhibitors for these kinases is undertaken as potential drug targets (reviewed in (Mazanetz and Fischer, 2007).

Regarding amyloid, Aβ varies from 39 to 43 amino acids and arises from sequential β- and γ-secretases processing of the amyloid precursor protein (APP). Presenilin 1 (PS1) is a catalytic subunit of γ-secretase. Several active and passive immunotherapy approaches such as acceleration of clearance of Aβ from the brain of the AD patients using brain penetrant inhibitors of Aβ aggregation and anti-Aβ monoclonal antibodies are undertaken (Frisardi et al.). Inhibitors of proteases such as β- and γ-secretase regulating Aβ formation from APP and compounds that stimulate α-secretase, the enzyme responsible for the non-amyloidogenic metabolism of APP are also investigated (reviewed in Frisardi et al.).

In addition to inhibition of tau phosphorylation and clearance of Aβ, an approach that targets protein conformations of tau and APP has been proposed as a new therapeutic target treating AD. Phosphorylation of serine and threonine residues preceding proline (pSer/Thr–Pro) mediated by a large number of so-called Pro-directed protein kinases is a major signaling mechanism (Hunter, 1995; Lu, 2004; Lu et al., 2002). Specific pSer/Thr-Pro motifs in certain proteins such as tau can exist in 2 distinct *cis* and *trans* conformations, whose conversion can be greatly accelerated by Pin1 (protein interacting with NIMA 1), a unique prolyl *cis-trans* isomerase (Lu et al., 1996; Lu et al., 1999b; Yaffe et al., 1997; Zhou et al., 1999). Such Pin1-catalyzed conformational changes, which can now be visualized by nuclear magnetic resonance (NMR) (Pastorino et al., 2006), have a profound impact on phosphorylation signaling, achieved by regulating a spectrum of target activities (Lu, 2004; Lu & Zhou, 2007; Wulf et al., 2005). Pin1 is tightly regulated and its deregulation contributes to pathological conditions, notably AD and cancer (Butterfield et al., 2006; Lu, 2004; Lu & Zhou, 2007; Pastorino et al., 2006; Shen et al., 2005; Suizu et al., 2006; Wulf et al., 2005). Remarkably, deletion of Pin1 in mice causes progressive age-dependent tauopathy (Liou et al., 2003). The observation that deprivation of a single molecule causes tauopathy verifies the importance of Pin1 on tauopathy. Conversely, neuronal Pin1 overexpression decreases the stability of tau, and greatly inhibits the tauopathy phenotype in wild-type tau transgenic mice (Lim et al., 2008). In AD, Pin1 binds to and isomerizes the pThr231-Pro motif in tau to restore its ability to bind to microtubules and to promote their assembly (Lu et al., 1999a) by facilitating tau dephosphorylation by PP2A (Liou et al., 2003; Zhou et al., 2000). Moreover, Pin1 binds to the pThr668-Pro motif of APP in the *cis* and *trans* conformations, accelerates the isomerization rate (Pastorino et al., 2006) and promotes nonamyloidogenic APP processing, thereby producing neurotrophic αAPPs and reducing neurotoxic Aβ peptides (Pastorino et al., 2006).

Because such neurodegeneration-protecting effects by Pin1 are generally believed to be ascribable to *cis trans* conformational changes by Pin1, regulation of the conformations of tau and APP after phosphorylation likely serves as potential therapeutic target for AD.

In this chapter, we summarize the current understanding of the mechanisms on how Pin1 acts as a protecting molecule against neurodegeneration in AD mouse models, followed by evidences of the pivotal roles of Pin1 in human AD.

2. Contribution of *cis-trans* isomerization to neural functions

The unique stereochemistry of Pro means that it can adopt two completely different conformational states (*trans* and *cis*). The significance of this with respect to the fact that Pro is often found next to phosphorylated Ser/Thr residues was not appreciated for a long time (Lu, 2004; Wulf et al., 2005). A breakthrough in understanding the conformational importance of Pro-directed phosphorylation motifs was the discovery of a unique and conserved peptidyl-prolyl *cis/trans* isomerase (PPIase), Pin1 (Lu, 2004; Lu et al., 1996; Ranganathan et al., 1997; Yaffe et al., 1997). Although Pin1 belongs to the parvulin subfamily of PPIases, it is the only PPIase that specifically recognizes pSer/Thr-Pro peptide sequences (Lu, 2004; Lu et al., 1996; Ranganathan et al., 1997; Yaffe et al., 1997), which is especially important because Pro-directed kinases and phosphatases are conformation-specific and act only on the *trans* conformation (Brown et al., 1999; Weiwad et al., 2000; Zhou et al., 2000). The identification of Pin1 as a phosphorylation-specific PPIase led to a new concept that Pin1 catalytically regulates the conformation of substrates after their phosphorylation to further control protein function (Lu et al., 1999b; Ranganathan et al., 1997; Yaffe et al., 1997; Zhou et al., 1999).

Phosphorylation dramatically slows down the already slow rate of isomerization of Ser/Thr-Pro bonds and renders the phosphopeptide bond resistant to the catalytic action of conventional PPIases (Yaffe et al., 1997). Pro-directed phosphorylation also induces local structural changes that make it accessible to further modifications (Kipping et al., 2001). The striking substrate specificity of Pin1 towards certain pSer/Thr–Pro bonds results from its unique two domain structure consisting of an N-terminal WW domain and a C-terminal PPIase domain, which form a "double-check" mechanism (Ranganathan et al., 1997; Yaffe et al., 1997; Zhou et al., 2000). The WW domain of Pin1 binds only to specific pSer/Thr–Pro motifs, which are often critical regulatory phosphorylation sites in Pin1 substrates (Shen et al. 1998; Lu et al. 1999; Lu et al. 1999; Zhou et al. 2000; Ryo et al. 2001; Wulf et al. 2001; Lu et al. 2002). This WW domain binding targets the Pin1 catalytic domain close to its substrates, where the PPIase domain isomerizes specific pSer/Thr–Pro motifs and catalytically induces conformational changes in proteins (Lu et al., 1999b; Zhou et al., 2000). It remains to be solved why Pin1 binds only to specific pSer/Thr-Pro motifs in certain proteins but it may be due to combined primary (and other) structural determinants. Furthermore, the WW domain can increase or inhibit Pin1 isomerase activity depending on whether a peptide substrate is phosphorylated on a single site or on multiple sites *in vitro* (Smet et al., 2005), although the biological significance of these findings is unclear. The findings that many substrates contain a single phosphorylation target site for Pin1 suggest that when it is targeted to the substrate by the WW domain, the PPIase domain would have to act on the same pSer/Thr-Pro motif to accelerate its isomerization. Another possibility is that the WW domain and PPIase domain might act on different pSer/Thr-Pro motifs in the same protein or in different ones when a Pin1 substrate is multiphosphorylated or in a multiprotein complex. In contrast to most other constitutively active PPIases (Fischer & Aumuller, 2003), Pin1 function is tightly regulated at multiple levels under physiological conditions, as expected given the tight regulation of Pro-directed phosphorylation signalling. For example, in neurons, Pin1 expression is induced upon neuronal differentiation (Hamdane et al., 2006; Liou et al., 2003; Lu et al., 1999a). This observation raises the link between prolyl *cis-trans* isomerization and neural functions.

Indeed, prolyl *cis-trans* isomerization has been shown to control neural functions. The study that took an initiative in this field is *cis* and *trans* specific functions on the opening of a neurotransmitter-gated ion channel *in vitro* (Lummis et al., 2005). Serotonin (5-hydroxytryptamine type 3, 5-HT3) receptors are members of the cysteine-loop receptor superfamily (Lester et al., 2004). Neurotransmitter binding in these proteins triggers the opening of an ion channel by inducing *cis-trans* conformational change (Lummis et al., 2005).

5-HT3 receptors have a specific proline (P*8) located at the apex of the loop between the second and third transmembrane helices (M2 and M3). When P*8 is replaced with analogs that favor the *trans* conformation, closed channels are observed. Conversely, unnatural amino acids that have high *cis* preference resulted in irreversible open channels. These results suggest that neurotransmitter binding may trigger a conformational change that isomerizes P*8 from *trans* to *cis* (Lummis et al., 2005). Interestingly, proline is often found in the transmembrane regions of ion channels and transporters (Sansom & Weinstein, 2000), which suggests an important role for the conformational changes in regulating the gating of 5HT3 receptor channel. These results clearly show that prolyl *cis-trans* isomerization controls physiological neural functions *in vitro*. A finding that Pin1, a PPIase, enhances the ability of gephyrin to bind the β-subunit of glycine receptors, which is important for maintaining a high concentration of inhibitory glycine receptors juxtaposed to presynaptic releasing sites (Zita et al., 2007), further suggests an intriguing hypothesis that PPIases might be involved in neural functions, especially pathological neural functions.

Exploration of the contributions of Pin1, a PPIase, to pathological neural functions gave an answer for the hypothesis. Pin1 protects against spinal cord injury by preventing JNK3-induced MCL1 degradation, cytochrome *c* release and apoptosis *in vitro* and *in vivo* (Li et al., 2007), which are opposite to the *in vitro* findings that Pin1 acts on bimEL (also known as B-cell lymphoma protein-2 (bcl2)-like-11) to induce apoptosis (Becker & Bonni, 2006). Furthermore, evidences for Pin1's protection against neurodegeneration through tau and APP *in vitro* and *in vivo* as shown in the next section confirmed the pivotal role of the PPIase in pathological neural conditions.

3. Pin1 restores tauopathy phenotype in mice

3.1 Pin1 recognizes phosphorylated Thr231 in tau

Various isoforms of tau appear to be differentially expressed during development, however, the tau isoforms with 3 and 4 tubulin-binding repeats are expressed in a one-to-one ratio in most regions of the adult brain (Ballatore et al., 2007). The primary function of tau is to stabilize microtubules. Tau proteins promote tubulin polymerization and stabilize microtubule structure *in vivo* (Lindwall & Cole, 1984; Weingarten et al., 1975). Tau deletion also potentiates the phenotypes of axon tracts and neuronal layers in mice lacking MAP1B, another major MT-associated protein (Takei et al., 2000). In AD brains, neuronal cytoskeleton is progressively disrupted and replaced by NFTs (Alonso et al., 1996). NFTs in AD are composed of hyperphosphorylated tau in two forms (paired helical filaments (PHF) and straight filaments (SF)). Tau hyperphosphorylation appears to precede tangle formation and neurodegeneration in AD. Hyperphosphorylated tau shows defective microtubule binding, fails to promote microtubule assembly, and self-assembles into NFTs *in vitro* (Mandelkow, 1999). In contrast, dephosphorylation *in vitro* can restore the microtubule-binding function and abolish the aggregation of AD phospho-tau (ptau) (Alonso et al., 1996). Taken together, these results indicate that increased tau phosphorylation is a key and an early event in the pathogenesis of human tauopathies, and therefore, dephosphorylation of hyperphosphorylated tau could be an attractive way to restore physiological tau function.

Ser/Thr-Pro sites are major regulatory phosphorylation motif in cells (Blume-Jensen & Hunter, 2001; Lee & Tsai, 2003; Lu, 2004; Lu et al., 2003; Nigg, 2001). Enzymes that are responsible for such phosphorylation belong to a large superfamily of Pro-directed protein kinases, which include extracellular signal-regulated kinases (ERKs), stress-activated protein kinases/c-Jun-N-

terminal kinases (SAPKs/JNKs), p38 kinases and Polo-like kinases (PLKs) in addition to CDKs and GSKs. These kinases have a crucial role in diverse cellular processes such as cell growth regulation, stress responses and neuronal survival, as well as in human diseases such as cancer and AD (Blume-Jensen & Hunter, 2001; Lee & Tsai, 2003; Lu, 2004; Lu et al., 2003; Nigg, 2001).
Pin1 binds to tau in a phosphorylation-dependent manner and the binding site was mapped to pThr231 of tau *in vitro* (Lu et al., 1999a). This phospho-epitope has been proposed to be diagnostic for AD because its levels in the cerebrospinal fluid correlate with the progression of the disease (Hampel et al., 2001; Kohnken et al., 2000). In addition, the mobility shifted ptau was positively probed by both CP9, an antibody specific for pThr231, and TG3, an antibody detecting Alzheimer-specific conformation of pThr231. In AD brain sections, exogenous Pin1 specifically bound to NFTs and neurites, which were also reactive to Pin1 antibody and TG3, indicating endogenous Pin1 is also localized to the pThr231 site. Biochemically, Pin1 was co-purified with PHF. Thus, the Pin1 interaction with ptau has been established.

3.2 Pin1 restores normal tau function through dephosphorylation of pThr231 of tau in vitro

Tau phosphorylated by Cdc2 showed a marked decrease in microtubule binding compared to unphosphorylated tau in tau biochemical assay *in vitro* (Lu et al., 1999a). Pin1-directed restoration of tau's ability to bind to microtubule was revealed by several observations. The loss of ptau's affinity to microtubules could be dramatically rescued by the sole presence of Pin1. The functional consequence of application of Pin1 was derived when microtubule assembly from tubulin was measured based on turbidity changes detected by spectrophotometer. The ability of tau to promote tubulin polymerization was abolished after tau was phosphorylated by Cdc2. Wild-type Pin1, but not the binding of defective point mutant, restored the function.
The involvement of dephosphorylation in the restoration by Pin1 was led by the observations that many of phosphoproteins Pin1 binds to are also recognized by the mitosis- and phosphorylation-specific antibody (mAb) MPM-2, and induction of MPM-2 epitopes is a prominent common feature shared by AD, frontotemporal dementia and parkinsonism linked to chromosome 17 (FTDP-17), Down Syndrome, corticobasal degeneration, progressive supranuclear palsy and Pick's disease. Furthermore, various studies have shown that mitotic events, including Cdc2 kinase, are aberrantly activated in the AD brain (Vincent et al., 1997; Vincent et al., 1996) and the phosphorylation pattern of tau in mitotic cells is strikingly similar to that in the AD brain (Kondratick et al. 1996; Vincent et al. 1996; Vincent et al. 1997; Illenberger et al. 1998; Preuss et al. 1998; Vincent et al. 1998). Indeed, both mitotic and AD tau proteins are recognized by mitosis-specific or AD-specific mAbs that are phosphorylation-dependent. Pin1 binds to pSer/Thr–Pro sites of many MPM-2 antigens, including tau. The phosphorylation dependent *cis/trans*-isomerization of pSer/Thr–Pro of many MPM-2 antigens is important for cell cycle control (Ding et al., 2000; Lane & Nigg, 1996; Wells et al., 1999; Winkler et al., 2000). On the other hand, dephosphorylation of the MPM-2 epitopes by phosphatases, notably PP2A, also plays an essential role in the regulation of Cdc2 activation and mitosis (Evans & Stark, 1997; Kawabe et al., 1997; Kinoshita et al., 1990; Lee, 1995; Lin & Arndt, 1995; Sontag et al., 1995). Interestingly, using metabolically active rat brain slices as a model, Gong *et al.* (Gong et al., 2000) showed that down-regulation of PP2A by okadaic acid induced Alzheimer-like hyperphosphorylation of tau. In contrast, the inhibition of PP2B by cyclosporin A in the same system did not significantly affect tau phosphorylation.

The pure *cis* isomer of tau peptide can be obtained using *trans*-specific α-chymotrypsin to eliminate the *trans* isomer (Zhou et al., 2000). In the absence of any PPIases, it took about 2.5 h to convert the pure *cis* peptide to equilibrium state, which is about 15% *cis*. Importantly, the pure *cis* peptides cannot be dephosphorylated by PP2A (Zhou et al., 2000). The pThr–Pro peptides were dephosphorylated by PP2A with a rate almost identical to that of *trans* isomer appearance. The *trans* isomer-dependent dephosphorylation was neither observed with alkaline phosphatase nor with a non-Pro-containing peptide. These experiments indicated that PP2A is a *trans* conformation-specific phosphatase. Indeed, the presence of Pin1 accelerated the dephosphorylation of tau by PP2A. However, the effect of Pin1 on PP2A dephosphorylation was not observed in tau Thr231Ala mutant. Taken together, Pin1 facilitates the dephosphorylation of pThr231-Pro site in tau through PP2A likely leads to the restoration of tau-mediated microtubule function.

3.3 Pin1 degrades hyperphosphorylated tau

Another effective way to treat tauopathy might be the elimination of hyperphosphorylated tau. It has been shown that tau phosphorylation regulates its degradation (Dickey et al., 2007; Kosik & Shimura, 2005; Petrucelli et al., 2004; Poppek et al., 2006) and that protein degradation is modulated by Pin1 (Lu & Zhou, 2007). These results suggest that Pin1 might act on the pThr231-Pro motif in tau to regulate the protein stability. Pin1 knockdown caused tau to become highly stable in neuron-like SH-SY5Y cells under cycloheximide experiment (Lim et al., 2008). Importantly, the effect of Pin1 knockdown on tau protein stability was completely abolished in the presence of the proteosome inhibitor MG132, demonstrating that the effect of Pin1 knockdown depends on functional proteosome, as shown for other Pin1 substrates (Lu & Zhou, 2007). The result was replicated in neurons isolated from mice. Transfected tau protein in primary cultured neurons and tau protein in brain slices from tau transgenic mouse were significantly more stable in Pin1-knockout background (Lu & Zhou, 2007). Further examination was carried out under Pin1 transgenic background in mice in which Pin1 transgene is expressed under Thy1.2 promoter that is active in neurons approximately 10 days after birth (Caroni, 1997). In the double transgenic mice having both tau transgene and Pin1 transgene, tau phosphorylation on Thr231 was reduced compared to tau transgene alone.

Tau phosphorylation has been shown to promote tau degradation via chaperone-interacting protein/Hsp70 (Dickey et al., 2007; Kosik & Shimura, 2005; Petrucelli et al., 2004) or inhibit tau degradation (Poppek et al., 2006). Interestingly, F-box proteins, which target phosphorylated proteins to ubiquitin-mediated proteolysis, bind to pSer/Thr-Pro motifs only in *trans*, but not *cis* (Orlicky et al., 2003). One model is that proteins targeting phosphorylated tau for degradation might bind to certain pSer/Thr-Pro motif(s) in tau only in *trans* conformation that would promote this interaction to promote degradation of tau. In this model, although tau is probably phosphorylated on certain Ser/Thr-Pro motifs such as the Thr231-Pro motif in *trans* due to the conformation specificity of kinases (Lu & Zhou, 2007), the pThr231-Pro motif in tau might have a tendency to be in the *cis* conformation due to local structural constraints after phosphorylation, as shown for APP (Ramelot & Nicholson, 2001). Therefore, in the nonequilibrium cellular environment, Pin1 overexpression might greatly accelerate the *cis* to *trans* isomerization to promote tau degradation, whereas Pin1 inhibition might allow a higher concentration of *cis* pThr231-Pro motif to be present for a longer time, which might inhibit tau degradation (Figure 1).

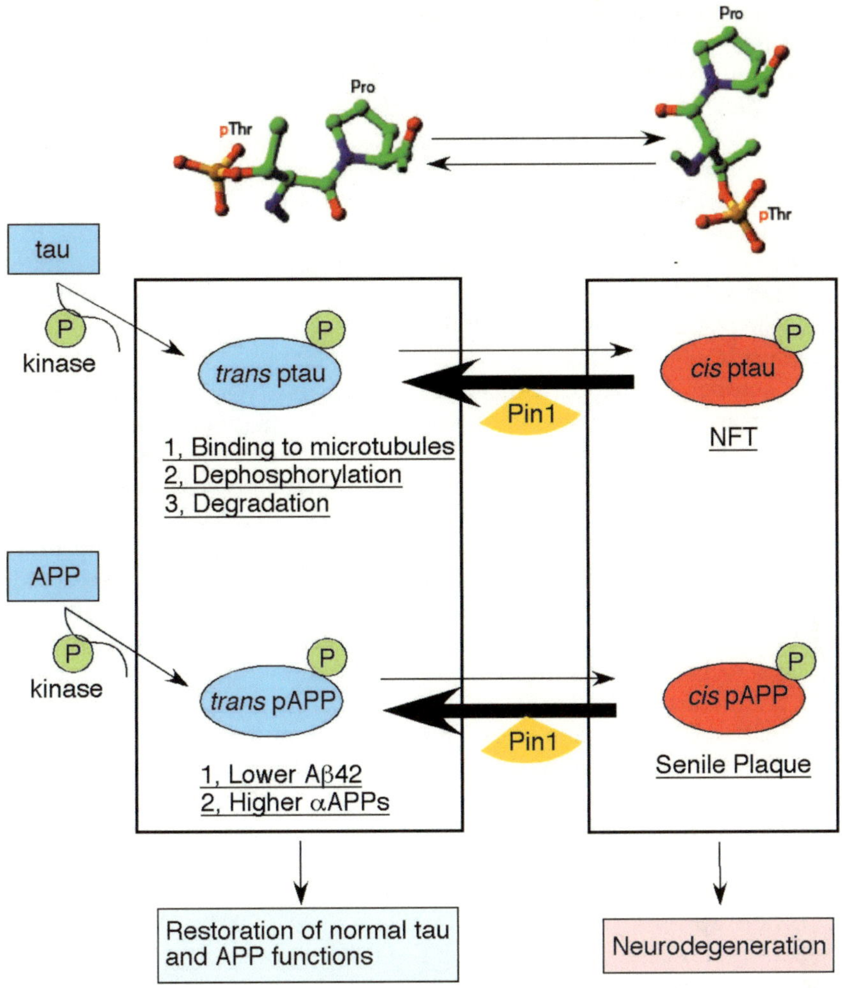

Tau and APP may be phosphorylated by protein kinases as part of their normal functions. *Cis*-ptau is resistant to binding to microtubules, protein phosphatases and degradation. By catalysing isomerization of the *cis* to *trans* conformation, Pin1 facilitates binding to microtubules and restores normal tau function. Pin1 also promotes tau dephosphorylation by phosphatases that contributes to the binding to microtubules. The *cis* to *trans* transition by Pin1 also facilitates degradation of phosphorylated tau. Regarding APP, *cis*-pAPP represents amyloidogenic APP processing. Pin1 catalyses isomerization of the *cis* to *trans* conformation, thereby, inducing decreased Aβ42 and increased αAPPs. The *trans*-conformations of ptau and pAPP may represent the physiological conformations that promote their normal functions.

Fig. 1. Restoration of tau and APP functions by Pin1.

Importantly, in 18-month-old tau transgenic mice, neuropathological changes, as demonstrated by the presence of some silver-positive neurons in the ventral horn of spinal cord and several degenerating or demyelinated axons within the sciatic nerves were found. However, neither silver-positive neurons in the spinal cord nor degenerated neurons within the sciatic nerve was observed in double transgenic mice having both Pin1 transgene and wild-type tau transgene (Lim et al., 2008). This result indicates that Pin1 overexpression effectively inhibits spinal and peripheral neuropathies induced by tau overexpression.

3.4 Deletion of Pin1 causes tauopathy in mice

Pin1 knockout mice (Liou et al., 2003) serves as a good tool to investigate the effect of Pin1 on endogenous tau *in vivo*. Pin1-deficient mice showed progressive age-dependent motor and behavioral deficits including abnormal limb-clasping reflexes, hunched postures and reduced mobility (Liou et al., 2003) similar to tau transgenic mice (Allen et al., 2002; Lewis et al., 2000). These phenotypes in Pin1 mutant mice are significant because the total level of NFTs correlates with the degree of cognitive impairment (Arriagada et al., 1992a; Arriagada et al., 1992b). Pioneering studies that used immunohistochemical techniques to determine the level of both NFTs and senile plaques in different brain regions of AD patients, as well as non-demented elderly individuals, demonstrated that the number of NFTs, but not the numbers of senile plaques, correlates with the degree of cognitive impairment (Arriagada et al., 1992a; Arriagada et al., 1992b).

Since neuron number in the parietal cortex of old, but not young mutant mice were significantly decreased, these phenotypes were caused by neuronal loss. A similar neuronal degeneration was found in spinal cords of the knockout mice (Liou et al., 2003). Tau hyperphosphorylation has been observed in aged mutant mice, with a dramatic mobility shift that is reversed by phosphatase treatment (Liou et al., 2003). The retarded forms of ptau in the mutant mice were also detected by various phospho-specific or Alzheimer-conformation-specific antibodies, such as AT180 and TG3. The phosphatase activity specific to pThr231 peptide motif was significantly reduced in the mutant mice, which is in agreement with Pin1's role in facilitating PP2A phosphatase activity. In aged Pin1-deficient mice, immunohistochemical staining of the hippocampus, cortex and spinal cord with specific ptau antibodies showed distinct somatodendritic signals, indicating pathological localization of tau. In Pin1-deficient mice, immunoelectronmicroscopic analysis showed that NFT-like tau filaments decorated by AT180 gold label were isolated from sarkosyl insoluble fractions (Liou et al., 2003). The tau filaments isolated resembled some of the human FTDP-17 mutants (Allen et al., 2002; Gotz et al., 2001; Lewis et al., 2000; Lim et al., 2001; Tanemura et al., 2002). Gallyas and thioflavin-staining, two established methods detecting NFTs in AD brains, were immense in entorhinal cortex and hippocampus, brain regions where impaired neuronal function appears initially in AD (Liou et al., 2003). These phenotypes are noteworthy because no gene deletion model has been reported to spontaneously cause tau pathology, thus no endogenous protective mechanism has been proposed.

4. Pin1 reduces Ab in mice

Tau and APP are two major molecules for AD. A growing body of evidence indicates some common features between the normal cell cycle and degenerated AD neurons, especially mitotic phosphorylation on certain Ser/Thr-Pro motifs (Lu et al., 2003; Yang & Herrup, 2007). Phosphorylation of APP on the Thr668-Pro motif, which occurs in mitotic cells (Suzuki et al., 1994), is also increased in AD brains and can elevate Aβ secretion *in vitro* (Lee et al., 2003).

Nuclear magnetic resonance (NMR) analysis of the action of Pin1 on APP has revealed the dynamic regulation of the intracellular domain of APP between the two completely distinct structures (Pastorino et al., 2006). APP possesses a Thr668-Pro motif that exists in *trans* before phosphorylation. The *cis* conformation appears only after phosphorylation due to local structural constraints, with ~10% of the phosphorylated motifs existing in the *cis* conformation (Ramelot & Nicholson, 2001). Pin1 binds to the pThr668-Pro motif in the *cis* and *trans* conformations and also accelerates the isomerization rate >1000-fold (in the millisecond timescale) compared with the typical uncatalysed reaction (which is in the minute timescale), with the catalysed *cis* to *trans* rate being 10-fold faster than the reverse rate (Pastorino et al., 2006), in contrast to a recent report that Pin1 does not act on full-length protein (Akiyama et al., 2005). Therefore, Pin1 would rapidly re-establish *cis/trans* equilibrium if either population was suddenly depleted in the cell.

APP processing is determined by APP subcellular localization and occurs through non-amyloidogenic processing at the plasma membrane by α-secretases or amyloidogenic processing at endosomes by β-secretase (De Strooper & Annaert, 2000; Esler & Wolfe, 2001; Hardy & Selkoe, 2002; Mattson, 2004; Selkoe et al., 1996). There is observation Pin1 co-localizes with APP at plasma membrane but not at endosomes, suggesting Pin1 affects APP intracellular localization and therefore affect APP processing and Aβ production (Pastorino et al., 2006). In addition, in Pin1 knockout mice, a significant increase in Aβ42 level in brain is observed (Pastorino et al., 2006).

Importantly, functional consequence of Pin1 deregulation revealed that the *cis* pThr668-Pro motif has a longer lifetime and its population relative to *trans* can be shifted far from its equilibrium depending on isomer-specific interactions, which might favor more amyloidogenic APP processing and Aβ production without proper Pin1 function (Figure 1). Therefore, in collaboration with other Alzheimer's disease factors, Pin1 deregulation might promote amyloidogenic APP processing and Aβ production and thus contribute to the pathology of AD (Pastorino et al., 2006).

5. Involvement of Pin1 in human AD

Positional cloning led to the identification of rare, disease-causing mutations in APP, PSEN1, and PSEN2 causing early-onset familial AD, followed by the discovery of ApoE as the only widely accepted and replicated risk factor for late-onset AD. In addition, recent genome-wide association approaches have delivered several additional AD susceptibility loci that are common in the general population (reviewed in Bertram & Tanzi, 2009).

Pin1 is mapped to 19p13.2, which has been identified as a novel locus for late onset AD that is independent of the effect of ApoE4 (Butler et al., 2009; Wijsman et al., 2004). Several common polymorphisms have been identified in the coding and promoter regions of Pin1. The relationship between Pin1 level and AD is of particular interest because Pin1 is downregulated and/or inhibited by oxidative modifications in AD (Liou et al., 2003; Sultana et al., 2006). Previous studies showed that Pin1 promoter single nucleotide polymorphism (SNP) (842G>C) is associated with reduced level of Pin1 in blood cells and increased risk for AD in an Italian cohort (Segat et al., 2007), although not in other cohorts (Lambert et al., 2009; Nowotny et al., 2007). Further studies have confirmed that this SNP abolishes Pin1 promoter activity and is associated with reduced risk for multiple cancers(Han et al., 2010). It is possible that the undetected population structure in studies with heterogeneous populations of subjects can lead to false positive results or failures in detecting the association with disease (Marchini et al., 2004) and this effect increased with samples size which might explain the conflicting results among the studies on Pin1 promoter polymorphisms. It has been shown that Chinese and Japanese subpopulations are more homogeneous and have a lower degree of population admixture (Marchini et al., 2004). Using Chinese subjects, we recently studied the onset of AD and Pin1 polymorphism. A functional polymorphism in the Pin1 promoter (rs2287839) was identified and this polymorphism was significantly associated with a 3-year delay in the onset of AD (Ma et al.). The base change of the SNP abolished the binding site of AP4 and increased the expression level of Pin1 in AD (Ma et al.). AP4 belongs to the basic helix-loop-helix leucine-zipper (bHLH-LZ) subgroup of bHLH proteins and recognizes the symmetrical DNA core sequence CAGCTG (Hu et al., 1990). Our result on AP4 RNAi and AP4 overexpression in H4 cells showed AP4 was able to repress the expression of Pin1 through the AP4 binding site in the promoter region of Pin1.

The above result is confirmed by biochemical and histochemical approaches using AD brain. Pin1 translocation from the soluble fractions to the insoluble fractions was reported in AD brains, while it was mainly present in the soluble fraction in age matched normal brain samples (Lu et al., 1999a). Further histological studies clarified Pin1's impact on AD. In the hippocampus and neocortex, the neurons in specific subregions are more prone to neurofibrillary degeneration than the neighboring subregions, indicating stereotypical patterns of neurodegeneration in AD. In the hippocampus, expression of Pin1 was relatively higher in CA4, CA3, CA2 and presubiculum, and lower in CA1 and subiculum. In the parietal cortex, expression of Pin1 was relatively higher in layer IIIb-c neurons, and lower in layer V neurons. The subregions with low expression of Pin1 coincide with the subregions that are more susceptible to neurofibrillary degeneration in AD, whereas those containing high Pin1 expression are not, showing an inverse correlation between Pin1 expression and predicted vulnerability (Liou et al., 2003). In AD brains, tangle-bearing neurons were enriched in CA1 and subiculum of the hippocampus and in layer V of the parietal cortex (Arriagada et al., 1992b; Davies et al., 1992; Hof & Morrison, 1991; Pearson et al., 1985). Overall, Pin1 level is generally low in these regions (Liou et al., 2003).

Because Pin1 is important in modulating APP processing in mice and has an inverse relationship with tau accumulation in human AD, increased Pin1 expression resulting from the base substitution of the SNP might delay the pathological process of AD, thus delaying the age of onset of AD (Figure 2). This result is significant because an intervention that could delay the average age of onset of AD by only 2 years has been predicted to reduce the expected prevalence by 23% by 2050 (Brookmeyer et al., 1998).

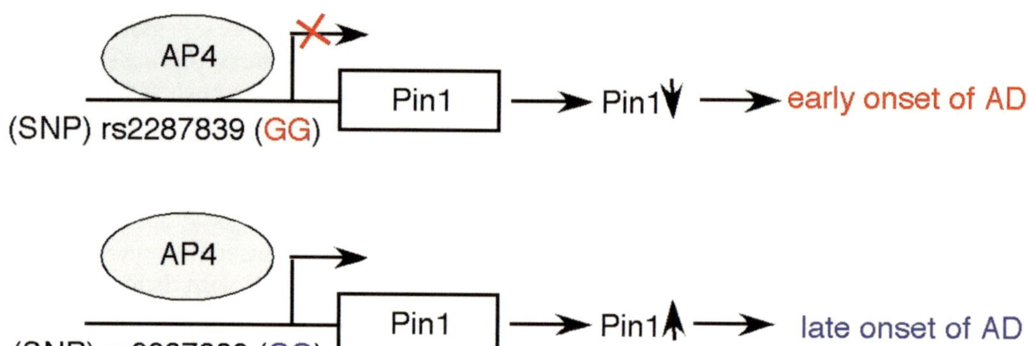

A transcription factor AP4 binds to wild type GG genotype in the Pin1 promoter (rs2287839) and represses its transcription. The polymorphism (CG) abolishes the binding site of AP4 and disinhibits the repression, thereby increases Pin1 expression level in AD. The polymorphism results in 3-year delay of the onset of AD.

Fig. 2. A Pin1 polymorphism associates with delayed onset of AD.

6. Conclusions

Tau and APP, two major causative molecules for AD, are reasonable and attractive therapeutic targets. The links between tau malfunctions and an overall imbalance in the activity levels or regulation of tau kinases and phosphatases have been established (Churcher, 2006; Mazanetz & Fischer, 2007). Although, attempts to identify AD-specific phosphorylation sites on tau have yet to yield conclusive results (Gordon-Krajcer et al., 2000; Schneider et al., 1999), the most probable candidates are Ser262 and the region around Thr231 and Ser235 (Hasegawa et al., 1992; Kohnken et al., 2000). Among these sites, Ser262 is identified as a Lys-Xaa-Gly-Ser motif recognized by Par1 kinase (microtubule associated regulating kinase) (Doerflinger et al., 2003; Drewes et al., 1995; Nishimura et al., 2004), whereas pSer/Thr–Pro sites of Thr231 and Ser235 are phosphorylated by CDKs, MAPKs, and/or GSKs (Ishiguro et al. 1993; Sperber et al. 1995; Zheng-Fischhofer et al. 1998; Ahlijanian et al. 2000; Reynolds et al. 2000; Takashima et al. 2001). These pro-directed kinases also target other pSer/Thr–Pro sites of tau. A hierarchy of phosphorylation regulation by different kinases has been implicated in the cascade of hyperphosphorylation and certain sites may play an initiative role (Jicha et al., 1999; Zheng-Fischhofer et al., 1998). GSK3β or CDK5 has been suggested to induce pre-tangle or NFT phenotypes, respectively (Lucas et al., 2001; Noble et al., 2003; Phiel et al., 2003). Thus, these tau kinases have received particular attention as targets for disease-modifying therapies using inhibitory compounds. Clearance of Aβ is also a logical therapeutic approach. If these inhibitor drugs can reach the brain efficiently from systemic circulation by crossing the blood–brain barrier, those might be attractive therapeutic approaches.

The discovery of the phosphorylation-specific PPIase Pin1 has established conformational regulation after phosphorylation as a new signaling mechanism. Pin1 could restore both tau and APP processing through their conformational changes. Thus, Pin1 might provide the opportunity for exploring more efficient therapy for AD than that targeting either tau or APP. A major challenge for the future will be to stably express Pin1 in the AD brain to normalize tau and APP processing.

7. References

Ahlijanian, M.K., Barrezueta, N.X., Williams, R.D., Jakowski, A., Kowsz, K.P., McCarthy, S., Coskran, T., Carlo, A., Seymour, P.A., Burkhardt, J.E., Nelson, R.B. & McNeish, J.D. (2000). Hyperphosphorylated tau and neurofilament and cytoskeletal disruptions in mice overexpressing human p25, an activator of cdk5. *Proceedings of the National Academy of Sciences USA*, Vol. 97, No. 6, pp. 2910-2915, ISSN 0027-8424

Akiyama, H., Shin, R.W., Uchida, C., Kitamoto, T. & Uchida, T. (2005). Pin1 promotes production of Alzheimer's amyloid beta from beta-cleaved amyloid precursor protein. *Biochemical and Biophysical Research Communications*, Vol. 336, No. 2, pp. 521-529, ISSN 0006-291X

Allen, B., Ingram, E., Takao, M., Smith, M.J., Jakes, R., Virdee, K., Yoshida, H., Holzer, M., Craxton, M., Emson, P.C., Atzori, C., Migheli, A., Crowther, R.A., Ghetti, B., Spillantini, M.G. & Goedert, M. (2002). Abundant tau filaments and nonapoptotic neurodegeneration in transgenic mice expressing human P301S tau protein. *Journal of Neuroscience*, Vol. 22, No. 21, pp. 9340-9351, ISSN 0270-6474

Alonso, A.C., Grundke-Iqbal, I. & Iqbal, K. (1996). Alzheimer's disease hyperphosphorylated tau sequesters normal tau into tangles of filaments and disassembles microtubules. *Nature Medicine*, Vol. 2, No. 7, pp. 783-787, ISSN 1078-8956

Arriagada, P.V., Growdon, J.H., Hedley-Whyte, E.T. & Hyman, B.T. (1992a). Neurofibrillary tangles but not senile plaques parallel duration and severity of Alzheimer's disease. *Neurology*, Vol. 42, No. 3 Pt 1, pp. 631-639, ISSN 0028-3878

Arriagada, P.V., Marzloff, K. & Hyman, B.T. (1992b). Distribution of Alzheimer-type pathologic changes in nondemented elderly individuals matches the pattern in Alzheimer's disease. *Neurology*, Vol. 42, No. 9, pp. 1681-1688, ISSN 0028-3878

Augustinack, J.C., Schneider, A., Mandelkow, E.M. & Hyman, B.T. (2002). Specific tau phosphorylation sites correlate with severity of neuronal cytopathology in Alzheimer's disease. *Acta Neuropathologica*, Vol. 103, No. 1, pp. 26-35, ISSN 0001-6322

Ballatore, C., Lee, V.M. & Trojanowski, J.Q. (2007). Tau-mediated neurodegeneration in Alzheimer's disease and related disorders. *Nature Reviews Neuroscience*, Vol. 8, No. 9, pp. 663-672, ISSN 1471-0048

Becker, E.B. & Bonni, A. (2006). Pin1 mediates neural-specific activation of the mitochondrial apoptotic machinery. *Neuron*, Vol. 49, No. 5, pp. 655-662, ISSN 0896-6273

Bertram, L. & Tanzi, R.E. (2009). Genome-wide association studies in Alzheimer's disease. *Human Molecular Genetics*, Vol. 18 (R2), pp. R137-145, ISSN 0964-6906

Blume-Jensen, P. & Hunter, T. (2001). Oncogenic kinase signalling. *Nature*, Vol. 411, No. 6835, pp. 355-365, ISSN 0028-0836

Brookmeyer, R., Gray, S. & Kawas, C. (1998). Projections of Alzheimer's disease in the United States and the public health impact of delaying disease onset. *American Journal of Public Health*, Vol. 88, No. 9, pp. 1337-1342, ISSN 0090-0036

Brown, N.R., Noble, M.E., Endicott, J.A. & Johnson, L.N. (1999). The structural basis for specificity of substrate and recruitment peptides for cyclin-dependent kinases. *Nature Cell Biology*, Vol. 1, No.7, pp. 438-443, ISSN 1097-6256

Butler, A.W., Ng, M.Y., Hamshere, M.L., Forabosco, P., Wroe, R., Al-Chalabi, A., Lewis, C.M. & Powell, J.F. (2009). Meta-analysis of linkage studies for Alzheimer's disease--a web resource. *Neurobiology of Aging*, Vol. 30, No. 7, pp. 1037-1047, ISSN 0197-4580

Butterfield, D.A., Abdul, H.M., Opii, W., Newman, S.F., Joshi, G., Ansari, M.A. & Sultana, R. (2006). Pin1 in Alzheimer's disease. *Journal of Neurochemistry*, Vol. 98, No. 6, pp. 1697-1706, ISSN 0022-3042

Caroni, P. (1997). Overexpression of growth-associated proteins in the neurons of adult transgenic mice. *Journal of Neuroscience Methods*, Vol. 71, No. 1, pp. 3-9, ISSN 0165-0270

Churcher, I. (2006). Tau therapeutic strategies for the treatment of Alzheimer's disease. *Current Topics in Medicinal Chemistry*, Vol. 6, No. 6, pp. 579-595, ISSN 1568-0266

Cruz, J.C., Tseng, H.C., Goldman, J.A., Shih, H. & Tsai, L.H. (2003). Aberrant Cdk5 activation by p25 triggers pathological events leading to neurodegeneration and neurofibrillary tangles. *Neuron*, Vol. 40, No. 3, pp. 471-483, ISSN 0896-6273

Davies, D.C., Horwood, N., Isaacs, S.L. & Mann, D.M. (1992). The effect of age and Alzheimer's disease on pyramidal neuron density in the individual fields of the hippocampal formation. *Acta Neuropathologica*, Vol. 83, No. 5, pp. 510-517, ISSN 0001-6322

De Strooper, B. & Annaert, W. (2000). Proteolytic processing and cell biological functions of the amyloid precursor protein. *Journal of Cell Science*, Vol. 113 (Pt 11), pp. 1857-1870, ISSN 0021-9533

Dickey, C.A., Kamal, A., Lundgren, K., Klosak, N., Bailey, R.M., Dunmore, J., Ash, P., Shoraka, S., Zlatkovic, J., Eckman, C.B., Patterson, C., Dickson, D.W., Nahman, N.S., Jr., Hutton, M., Burrows, F. & Petrucelli, L. (2007). The high-affinity HSP90-CHIP complex recognizes and selectively degrades phosphorylated tau client proteins. *Journal of Clinical Investigation*, Vol. 117, No. 3, pp. 648-658, ISSN 0021-9738

Ding, X.L., Husseman, J., Tomashevski, A., Nochlin, D., Jin, L.W. & Vincent, I. (2000). The cell cycle Cdc25A tyrosine phosphatase is activated in degenerating postmitotic neurons in Alzheimer's disease. *American Journal of Pathology*, Vol. 157, No. 6, pp. 1983-1990, ISSN 1525-2191

Doerflinger, H., Benton, R., Shulman, J.M. & St Johnston, D. (2003). The role of PAR-1 in regulating the polarised microtubule cytoskeleton in the Drosophila follicular epithelium. *Development*, Vol. 130, No. 17, pp. 3965-3975, ISSN 0950-1991

Drewes, G., Trinczek, B., Illenberger, S., Biernat, J., Schmitt-Ulms, G., Meyer, H.E., Mandelkow, E.M. & Mandelkow, E. (1995). Microtubule-associated protein/microtubule affinity-regulating kinase (p110mark). A novel protein kinase that regulates tau-microtubule interactions and dynamic instability by phosphorylation at the Alzheimer-specific site serine 262. *Journal of Biological Chemistry*, Vol. 270, No. 13, pp 7679-7688, ISSN 0021-9258

Esler, W.P. & Wolfe, M.S. (2001). A portrait of Alzheimer secretases--new features and familiar faces. *Science*, Vol. 293, No. 5534, pp 1449-1454, ISSN 0036-8075

Evans, D.A., Funkenstein, H.H., Albert, M.S., Scherr, P.A., Cook, N.R., Chown, M.J., Hebert, L.E., Hennekens, C.H. & Taylor, J.O. (1989). Prevalence of Alzheimer's disease in a community population of older persons. Higher than previously reported. *JAMA*, Vol. 262, No. 18, pp. 2551-2556, ISSN 0002-9955

Evans, D.R. & Stark, M.J. (1997). Mutations in the Saccharomyces cerevisiae type 2A protein phosphatase catalytic subunit reveal roles in cell wall integrity, actin cytoskeleton organization and mitosis. *Genetics*, Vol. 145, No. 2, pp. 227-241, ISSN 0016-6731

Fischer, G. & Aumuller, T. (2003). Regulation of peptide bond cis/trans isomerization by enzyme catalysis and its implication in physiological processes. *Reviews of Physiology, Biochemistry & Pharmacology*, Vol. 148, pp. 105-150, ISSN 0303-4240

Frisardi, V., Solfrizzi, V., Imbimbo, P.B., Capurso, C., D'Introno, A., Colacicco, A.M., Vendemiale, G., Seripa, D., Pilotto, A., Capurso, A. & Panza, F. (2010). Towards disease-modifying treatment of Alzheimer's disease: drugs targeting beta-amyloid. *Current Alzheimer Research*, Vol. 7, No. 1, pp. 40-55, ISSN 1567-2050

Goedert, M., Satumtira, S., Jakes, R., Smith, M.J., Kamibayashi, C., White, C.L., 3rd & Sontag, E. (2000). Reduced binding of protein phosphatase 2A to tau protein with frontotemporal dementia and parkinsonism linked to chromosome 17 mutations. *Journal of Neurochemistry*, Vol. 75, No. 5, pp. 2155-2162, ISSN 0022-3042

Gong, C.X., Lidsky, T., Wegiel, J., Zuck, L., Grundke-Iqbal, I. & Iqbal, K. (2000). Phosphorylation of microtubule-associated protein tau is regulated by protein phosphatase 2A in mammalian brain. Implications for neurofibrillary degeneration in Alzheimer's disease. *Journal of Biological Chemistry*, Vol. 275, No. 8, pp. 5535-5544, ISSN 0021-9258

Gordon-Krajcer, W., Yang, L. & Ksiezak-Reding, H. (2000). Conformation of paired helical filaments blocks dephosphorylation of epitopes shared with fetal tau except

Ser199/202 and Ser202/Thr205. *Brain Research*, Vol. 856, No. 1-2, pp. 163-175, ISSN 0006-8993

Gotz, J., Chen, F., Barmettler, R. & Nitsch, R.M. (2001). Tau filament formation in transgenic mice expressing P301L tau. *Journal of Biological Chemistry*, Vol. 276, No. 1, pp. 529-534, ISSN 0021-9258

Hamdane, M., Dourlen, P., Bretteville, A., Sambo, A.V., Ferreira, S., Ando, K., Kerdraon, O., Begard, S., Geay, L., Lippens, G., Sergeant, N., Delacourte, A., Maurage, C.A., Galas, M.C. & Buee, L. (2006). Pin1 allows for differential Tau dephosphorylation in neuronal cells. *Molecular and Cellular Neurosciences*, Vol. 32, No. 1-2, pp. 155-160, ISSN 1044-7431

Hampel, H., Buerger, K., Kohnken, R., Teipel, S.J., Zinkowski, R., Moeller, H.J., Rapoport, S.I. & Davies, P. (2001). Tracking of Alzheimer's disease progression with cerebrospinal fluid tau protein phosphorylated at threonine 231. *Annals of Neurology*, Vol. 49, No. 4, pp. 545-546, ISSN 0364-5134

Han, C.H., Lu, J., Wei, Q., Bondy, M.L., Brewster, A.M., Yu, T.K., Buchholz, T.A., Arun, B.K. & Wang, L.E. (2010). The functional promoter polymorphism (-842G>C) in the PIN1 gene is associated with decreased risk of breast cancer in non-Hispanic white women 55 years and younger. *Breast cancer research and treatment*, Vol. 122, No. 1, pp. 243-249, ISSN 0167-6806

Hardy, J. & Selkoe, D.J. (2002). The amyloid hypothesis of Alzheimer's disease: progress and problems on the road to therapeutics. *Science*, Vol. 297, No. 5580, pp. 353-356, ISSN 0036-8075

Hasegawa, M., Morishima-Kawashima, M., Takio, K., Suzuki, M., Titani, K. & Ihara, Y. (1992). Protein sequence and mass spectrometric analyses of tau in the Alzheimer's disease brain. *Journal of Biological Chemistry*, Vol. 267, No. 24, pp. 17047-17054, ISSN 0021-9258

Hof, P.R. & Morrison, J.H. (1991). Neocortical neuronal subpopulations labeled by a monoclonal antibody to calbindin exhibit differential vulnerability in Alzheimer's disease. *Experimantal Neurology*, Vol. 111, No. 3, pp. 293-301, ISSN 0014-4886

Hu, Y.F., Luscher, B., Admon, A., Mermod, N. & Tjian, R. (1990). Transcription factor AP-4 contains multiple dimerization domains that regulate dimer specificity. *Genes & Development*, Vol. 4, No. 10, pp. 1741-1752, ISSN 0890-9369

Hunter, T. (1995). Protein kinases and phosphatases: the yin and yang of protein phosphorylation and signaling. *Cell*, Vol. 80, No. 2, pp. 225-236, ISSN 0092-8674

Illenberger, S., Zheng-Fischhofer, Q., Preuss, U., Stamer, K., Baumann, K., Trinczek, B., Biernat, J., Godemann, R., Mandelkow, E.M. & Mandelkow, E. (1998). The endogenous and cell cycle-dependent phosphorylation of tau protein in living cells: implications for Alzheimer's disease. *Molecular Biology of the Cell*, Vol. 9, No. 6, pp. 1495-1512, ISSN 1059-1524

Jicha, G.A., O'Donnell, A., Weaver, C., Angeletti, R. & Davies, P. (1999). Hierarchical phosphorylation of recombinant tau by the paired-helical filament-associated protein kinase is dependent on cyclic AMP-dependent protein kinase. *Journal of Neurochemistry*, Vol. 72, No. 1, pp. 214-224, ISSN 0022-3042

Kawabe, T., Muslin, A.J. & Korsmeyer, S.J. (1997). HOX11 interacts with protein phosphatases PP2A and PP1 and disrupts a G2/M cell-cycle checkpoint. *Nature*, Vol. 385, No. 6615, pp. 454-458, ISSN 0028-0836

Kinoshita, N., Ohkura, H. & Yanagida, M. (1990). Distinct, essential roles of type 1 and 2A protein phosphatases in the control of the fission yeast cell division cycle. *Cell*, Vol. 63, No. 2, pp. 405-415, ISSN 0092-8674

Kins, S., Crameri, A., Evans, D.R., Hemmings, B.A., Nitsch, R.M. & Gotz, J. (2001). Reduced protein phosphatase 2A activity induces hyperphosphorylation and altered compartmentalization of tau in transgenic mice. *Journal of Biological Chemistry*, Vol. 276, No. 41, pp. 38193-38200, ISSN 0021-9258

Kipping, M., Zarnt, T., Kiessig, S., Reimer, U., Fischer, G. & Bayer, P. (2001). Increased backbone flexibility in threonine45-phosphorylated hirudin upon pH change. *Biochemistry*, Vol. 40, No. 27, pp. 7957-7963, ISSN 0006-2960

Kohnken, R., Buerger, K., Zinkowski, R., Miller, C., Kerkman, D., DeBernardis, J., Shen, J., Moller, H.J., Davies, P. & Hampel, H. (2000). Detection of tau phosphorylated at threonine 231 in cerebrospinal fluid of Alzheimer's disease patients. *Neuroscience Letters*, Vol. 287, No. 3, pp. 187-190, ISSN 0304-3940

Kosik, K.S. & Shimura, H. (2005). Phosphorylated tau and the neurodegenerative foldopathies. *Biochimica et Biophysica Acta*, Vol. 1739, No. 2-3, pp. 298-310, ISSN 0006-3002

Lambert, J.C., Heath, S., Even, G., Campion, D., Sleegers, K., Hiltunen, M., Combarros, O., Zelenika, D., Bullido, M.J., Tavernier, B., Letenneur, L., Bettens, K., Berr, C., Pasquier, F., Fievet, N., Barberger-Gateau, P., Engelborghs, S., De Deyn, P., Mateo, I., Franck, A., Helisalmi, S., Porcellini, E., Hanon, O., de Pancorbo, M.M., Lendon, C., Dufouil, C., Jaillard, C., Leveillard, T., Alvarez, V., Bosco, P., Mancuso, M., Panza, F., Nacmias, B., Bossu, P., Piccardi, P., Annoni, G., Seripa, D., Galimberti, D., Hannequin, D., Licastro, F., Soininen, H., Ritchie, K., Blanche, H., Dartigues, J.F., Tzourio, C., Gut, I., Van Broeckhoven, C., Alperovitch, A., Lathrop, M. & Amouyel, P. (2009). Genome-wide association study identifies variants at CLU and CR1 associated with Alzheimer's disease. *Nature Genetics*, Vol. 41, No. 10, pp. 1094-1099, ISSN 1061-4036

Lane, H.A. & Nigg, E.A. (1996). Antibody microinjection reveals an essential role for human polo-like kinase 1 (Plk1) in the functional maturation of mitotic centrosomes. *Journal of Cell Biology*, Vol. 135, No. 6 Pt 2, pp. 1701-1713, ISSN 0021-9525

Lee, M.S., Kao, S.C., Lemere, C.A., Xia, W., Tseng, H.C., Zhou, Y., Neve, R., Ahlijanian, M.K. & Tsai, L.H. (2003). APP processing is regulated by cytoplasmic phosphorylation. *Journal of Cell Biology*, Vol. 163, No. 1, pp. 83-95, ISSN 0021-9525

Lee, M.S. & Tsai, L.H. (2003). Cdk5: one of the links between senile plaques and neurofibrillary tangles? *Journal of Alzheimer's Disease*, Vol. 5, No. 2, pp. 127-137, ISSN 1387-2877

Lee, T.H. (1995). The role of protein phosphatase type-2A in the Xenopus cell cycle: initiation of the G2/M transition. *Seminars in Cancer Biology*, Vol. 6, No. 4, pp. 203-209, ISSN 1044-579X

Lester, H.A., Dibas, M.I., Dahan, D.S., Leite, J.F. & Dougherty, D.A. (2004). Cys-loop receptors: new twists and turns. *Trends in Neurosciences*, Vol. 27, No. 6, pp. 329-336, ISSN 0166-2236

Lewis, J., McGowan, E., Rockwood, J., Melrose, H., Nacharaju, P., Van Slegtenhorst, M., Gwinn-Hardy, K., Paul Murphy, M., Baker, M., Yu, X., Duff, K., Hardy, J., Corral, A., Lin, W.L., Yen, S.H., Dickson, D.W., Davies, P. & Hutton, M. (2000). Neurofibrillary tangles, amyotrophy and progressive motor disturbance in mice expressing mutant (P301L) tau protein. *Nature Genetics*, Vol. 25, No. 4, pp. 402-405, ISSN 1061-4036

Li, Q.M., Tep, C., Yune, T.Y., Zhou, X.Z., Uchida, T., Lu, K.P. & Yoon, S.O. (2007). Opposite regulation of oligodendrocyte apoptosis by JNK3 and Pin1 after spinal cord injury. *Journal of Neuroscience*, Vol. 27, No. 31, pp. 8395-8404, ISSN 0270-6474

Lim, F., Hernandez, F., Lucas, J.J., Gomez-Ramos, P., Moran, M.A. & Avila, J. (2001). FTDP-17 mutations in tau transgenic mice provoke lysosomal abnormalities and Tau filaments in forebrain. *Molecular and Cellular Neurosciences*, Vol. 18, No. 6, pp. 702-714, ISSN 1044-7431

Lim, J., Balastik, M., Lee, T.H., Nakamura, K., Liou, Y.C., Sun, A., Finn, G., Pastorino, L., Lee, V.M. & Lu, K.P. (2008). Pin1 has opposite effects on wild-type and P301L tau stability and tauopathy. *Journal of Clinical Investigation*, Vol. 118, No. 5, pp. 1877-1889, ISSN 0021-9738

Lin, F.C. & Arndt, K.T. (1995). The role of Saccharomyces cerevisiae type 2A phosphatase in the actin cytoskeleton and in entry into mitosis. *EMBO Journal*, Vol. 14, No. 12, pp. 2745-2759, ISSN 0261-4189

Lindwall, G. & Cole, R.D. (1984). Phosphorylation affects the ability of tau protein to promote microtubule assembly. *The Journal of Biological Chemistry*, Vol. 259, No. 8, pp. 5301-5305, ISSN 0021-9258

Liou, Y.C., Sun, A., Ryo, A., Zhou, X.Z., Yu, Z.X., Huang, H.K., Uchida, T., Bronson, R., Bing, G., Li, X., Hunter, T. & Lu, K.P. (2003). Role of the prolyl isomerase Pin1 in protecting against age-dependent neurodegeneration. *Nature*, Vol. 424, No. 6948, pp. 556-561, ISSN 0028-0836

Lu, K.P. (2004). Pinning down cell signaling, cancer and Alzheimer's disease. *Trends in Biochemical Sciences*, Vol. 29, No. 4, pp. 200-209, ISSN 0968-0004

Lu, K.P., Hanes, S.D. & Hunter, T. (1996). A human peptidyl-prolyl isomerase essential for regulation of mitosis. *Nature*, Vol. 380, No. 6574, pp. 544-547, ISSN 0028-0836

Lu, K.P., Liou, Y.C. & Vincent, I. (2003). Proline-directed phosphorylation and isomerization in mitotic regulation and in Alzheimer's Disease. *Bioessays*, Vol. 25, No. 2, pp. 174-181, ISSN 0265-9247

Lu, K.P., Liou, Y.C. & Zhou, X.Z. (2002). Pinning down proline-directed phosphorylation signaling. *Trends in Cell Biology*, Vol. 12, No. 4, pp. 164-172, ISSN 0962-8924

Lu, K.P. & Zhou, X.Z. (2007). The prolyl isomerase PIN1: a pivotal new twist in phosphorylation signalling and disease. *Nature Reviews Molecular Cell Biology*, Vol. 8, No. 11, pp. 904-916, ISSN 1471-0072

Lu, P.J., Wulf, G., Zhou, X.Z., Davies, P. & Lu, K.P. (1999a). The prolyl isomerase Pin1 restores the function of Alzheimer-associated phosphorylated tau protein. *Nature*, Vol. 399, No. 6738, pp. 784-788, ISSN 0028-0836

Lu, P.J., Zhou, X.Z., Shen, M. & Lu, K.P. (1999b). Function of WW domains as phosphoserine- or phosphothreonine-binding modules. *Science*, Vol. 283, No. 5406, pp. 1325-1328, ISSN 0036-8075

Lucas, J.J., Hernandez, F., Gomez-Ramos, P., Moran, M.A., Hen, R. & Avila, J. (2001). Decreased nuclear beta-catenin, tau hyperphosphorylation and neurodegeneration in GSK-3beta conditional transgenic mice. *EMBO Journal*, Vol. 20, No. 1-2, pp. 27-39, ISSN 0261-4189

Lummis, S.C., Beene, D.L., Lee, L.W., Lester, H.A., Broadhurst, R.W. & Dougherty, D.A. (2005). Cis-trans isomerization at a proline opens the pore of a neurotransmitter-gated ion channel. *Nature*, Vol. 438, No. 7065, pp. 248-252, ISSN 0028-0836

Ma, S.L., Tang, N.L., Tam, C.W., Cheong Lui, V.W., Lam, L.C., Chiu, H.F., Driver, J.A., Pastorino, L. & Lu, K.P. (2010) A PIN1 polymorphism that prevents its suppression by AP4 associates with delayed onset of Alzheimer's disease. *Neurobiology of Aging*, ISSN 0197-4580

Mandelkow, E. (1999). Alzheimer's disease. The tangled tale of tau. *Nature*, Vol. 402, No. 6762, pp. 588-589, ISSN 0028-0836

Marchini, J., Cardon, L.R., Phillips, M.S. & Donnelly, P. (2004). The effects of human population structure on large genetic association studies. *Nature Genetics*, Vol. 36, No. 5, pp. 512-517, ISSN 1061-4036

Matsuo, E.S., Shin, R.W., Billingsley, M.L., Van deVoorde, A., O'Connor, M., Trojanowski, J.Q. & Lee, V.M. (1994). Biopsy-derived adult human brain tau is phosphorylated at many of the same sites as Alzheimer's disease paired helical filament tau. *Neuron*, Vol. 13, No. 4, pp. 989-1002, ISSN 0896-6273

Mattson, M.P. (2004). Pathways towards and away from Alzheimer's disease. *Nature*, Vol. 430, No. 7000, pp. 631-639, ISSN 0028-0836

Mawal-Dewan, M., Henley, J., Van de Voorde, A., Trojanowski, J.Q. & Lee, V.M. (1994). The phosphorylation state of tau in the developing rat brain is regulated by phosphoprotein phosphatases. *The Journal of Biological Chemistry*, Vol. 269, No. 49, pp. 30981-30987, ISSN 0021-9258

Mazanetz, M.P. & Fischer, P.M. (2007). Untangling tau hyperphosphorylation in drug design for neurodegenerative diseases. *Nature Reviews Drug Discovery*, Vol. 6, No. 6, pp. 464-479, ISSN 1474-1776

Nigg, E.A. (2001). Mitotic kinases as regulators of cell division and its checkpoints. *Nature Reviews Molecular Cell Biology*, Vol. 2, No. 1, pp. 21-32, ISSN 1471-0072

Nishimura, I., Yang, Y. & Lu, B. (2004). PAR-1 kinase plays an initiator role in a temporally ordered phosphorylation process that confers tau toxicity in Drosophila. *Cell*, Vol. 116, No. 5, pp. 671-682, ISSN 0092-8674

Noble, W., Olm, V., Takata, K., Casey, E., Mary, O., Meyerson, J., Gaynor, K., LaFrancois, J., Wang, L., Kondo, T., Davies, P., Burns, M., Veeranna, Nixon, R., Dickson, D., Matsuoka, Y., Ahlijanian, M., Lau, L.F. & Duff, K. (2003). Cdk5 is a key factor in tau aggregation and tangle formation in vivo. *Neuron*, Vol. 38, No. 4, pp. 555-565, ISSN 0896-6273

Nowotny, P., Bertelsen, S., Hinrichs, A.L., Kauwe, J.S., Mayo, K., Jacquart, S., Morris, J.C. & Goate, A. (2007). Association studies between common variants in prolyl isomerase Pin1 and the risk for late-onset Alzheimer's disease. *Neuroscience Letters*, Vol. 419, No. 1, pp. 15-17, ISSN 0304-3940

Orlicky, S., Tang, X., Willems, A., Tyers, M. & Sicheri, F. (2003). Structural basis for phosphodependent substrate selection and orientation by the SCFCdc4 ubiquitin ligase. *Cell*, Vol. 112, No. 2, pp. 243-256, ISSN 0092-8674

Pastorino, L., Sun, A., Lu, P.J., Zhou, X.Z., Balastik, M., Finn, G., Wulf, G., Lim, J., Li, S.H., Li, X., Xia, W., Nicholson, L.K. & Lu, K.P. (2006). The prolyl isomerase Pin1 regulates amyloid precursor protein processing and amyloid-beta production. *Nature*, Vol. 440, No. 7083, pp. 528-534, ISSN 0028-0836

Pearson, R.C., Esiri, M.M., Hiorns, R.W., Wilcock, G.K. & Powell, T.P. (1985). Anatomical correlates of the distribution of the pathological changes in the neocortex in Alzheimer disease. *Proceedings of the National Academy of Sciences USA*, Vol. 82, No. 13, pp. 4531-4534, ISSN 0027-8424

Pelech, S.L. (1995). Networking with proline-directed protein kinases implicated in tau phosphorylation. *Neurobiology of Aging*, Vol. 16, No. 3, pp. 247-256; discussion pp. 257-261, ISSN 0197-4580

Petrucelli, L., Dickson, D., Kehoe, K., Taylor, J., Snyder, H., Grover, A., De Lucia, M., McGowan, E., Lewis, J., Prihar, G., Kim, J., Dillmann, W.H., Browne, S.E., Hall, A., Voellmy, R., Tsuboi, Y., Dawson, T.M., Wolozin, B., Hardy, J. & Hutton, M. (2004). CHIP and Hsp70 regulate tau ubiquitination, degradation and aggregation. *Human Molecular Genetics*, Vol. 13, No. 7, pp. 703-714, ISSN 0964-6906

Phiel, C.J., Wilson, C.A., Lee, V.M. & Klein, P.S. (2003). GSK-3alpha regulates production of Alzheimer's disease amyloid-beta peptides. *Nature*, Vol. 423, No. 6938, pp. 435-439, ISSN 0028-0836

Poppek, D., Keck, S., Ermak, G., Jung, T., Stolzing, A., Ullrich, O., Davies, K.J. & Grune, T. (2006). Phosphorylation inhibits turnover of the tau protein by the proteasome: influence of RCAN1 and oxidative stress. *Biochemical Journal*, Vol. 400, No. 3, pp. 511-520, ISSN 0264-6021

Ramelot, T.A. & Nicholson, L.K. (2001). Phosphorylation-induced structural changes in the amyloid precursor protein cytoplasmic tail detected by NMR. *Journal of Molecular Biology*, Vol. 307, No. 3, pp. 871-884, ISSN 0022-2836

Ranganathan, R., Lu, K.P., Hunter, T. & Noel, J.P. (1997). Structural and functional analysis of the mitotic rotamase Pin1 suggests substrate recognition is phosphorylation dependent. *Cell*, Vol. 89, No. 6, pp. 875-886, ISSN 0092-8674

Sansom, M.S. & Weinstein, H. (2000). Hinges, swivels and switches: the role of prolines in signalling via transmembrane alpha-helices. *Trends in Pharmacological Sciences*, Vol. 21, No. 11, pp. 445-451, ISSN 0165-6147

Schneider, A., Biernat, J., von Bergen, M., Mandelkow, E. & Mandelkow, E.M. (1999). Phosphorylation that detaches tau protein from microtubules (Ser262, Ser214) also protects it against aggregation into Alzheimer paired helical filaments. *Biochemistry*, Vol. 38, No. 12, pp. 3549-3558, ISSN 0006-2960

Segat, L., Pontillo, A., Annoni, G., Trabattoni, D., Vergani, C., Clerici, M., Arosio, B. & Crovella, S. (2007). PIN1 promoter polymorphisms are associated with Alzheimer's disease. *Neurobiology of Aging*, Vol. 28, No. 1, pp. 69-74, ISSN 0197-4580

Selkoe, D.J., Yamazaki, T., Citron, M., Podlisny, M.B., Koo, E.H., Teplow, D.B. & Haass, C. (1996). The role of APP processing and trafficking pathways in the formation of amyloid beta-protein. *Annals of the New York Academy of Sciences*, Vol. 777, pp. 57-64, ISSN 1749-6632

Shen, Z.J., Esnault, S. & Malter, J.S. (2005). The peptidyl-prolyl isomerase Pin1 regulates the stability of granulocyte-macrophage colony-stimulating factor mRNA in activated eosinophils. *Nature Immunology*, Vol. 6, No. 12, pp. 1280-1287, ISSN 1529-2908

Smet, C., Wieruszeski, J.M., Buee, L., Landrieu, I. & Lippens, G. (2005). Regulation of Pin1 peptidyl-prolyl cis/trans isomerase activity by its WW binding module on a multi-phosphorylated peptide of Tau protein. *FEBS Letters*, Vol. 579, No. 19, pp. 4159-4164, ISSN 0014-5793.

Sontag, E., Nunbhakdi-Craig, V., Bloom, G.S. & Mumby, M.C. (1995). A novel pool of protein phosphatase 2A is associated with microtubules and is regulated during the cell cycle. *Journal of Cell Biology*, Vol. 128, No. 6, pp. 1131-1144, ISSN 0021-9525

Sontag, E., Nunbhakdi-Craig, V., Lee, G., Bloom, G.S. & Mumby, M.C. (1996). Regulation of the phosphorylation state and microtubule-binding activity of Tau by protein phosphatase 2A. *Neuron*, Vol. 17, No. 6, pp. 1201-1207, ISSN 0896-6273

Stoothoff, W.H. & Johnson, G.V. (2005). Tau phosphorylation: physiological and pathological consequences. *Biochimica et Biophysica Acta*, Vol. 1739, No. 2-3, pp. 280-297, ISSN 0006-3002

Suizu, F., Ryo, A., Wulf, G., Lim, J. & Lu, K.P. (2006). Pin1 regulates centrosome duplication, and its overexpression induces centrosome amplification, chromosome instability, and oncogenesis. *Molecular and Cellular Biology*, Vol. 26, No. 4, pp. 1463-1479, ISSN 0270-7306

Sultana, R., Boyd-Kimball, D., Poon, H.F., Cai, J., Pierce, W.M., Klein, J.B., Markesbery, W.R., Zhou, X.Z., Lu, K.P. & Butterfield, D.A. (2006). Oxidative modification and down-regulation of Pin1 in Alzheimer's disease hippocampus: A redox proteomics analysis. *Neurobiology of Aging*, Vol. 27, No. 7, pp. 918-925, ISSN 0197- 4580

Suzuki, T., Oishi, M., Marshak, D.R., Czernik, A.J., Nairn, A.C. & Greengard, P. (1994). Cell cycle-dependent regulation of the phosphorylation and metabolism of the Alzheimer amyloid precursor protein. *EMBO Journal*, Vol. 13, No. 5, pp. 1114-1122, ISSN 0261-4189

Takei, Y., Teng, J., Harada, A. & Hirokawa, N. (2000). Defects in axonal elongation and neuronal migration in mice with disrupted tau and map1b genes. *Journal of Cell Biology*, Vol. 150, No. 5, pp. 989-1000, ISSN 0021-9525

Tanemura, K., Murayama, M., Akagi, T., Hashikawa, T., Tominaga, T., Ichikawa, M., Yamaguchi, H. & Takashima, A. (2002). Neurodegeneration with tau accumulation in a transgenic mouse expressing V337M human tau. *Journal of Neuroscience*, Vol. 22, No. 1, pp. 133-141, ISSN 0270-6474

Vincent, I., Jicha, G., Rosado, M. & Dickson, D.W. (1997). Aberrant expression of mitotic cdc2/cyclin B1 kinase in degenerating neurons of Alzheimer's disease brain. *Journal of Neuroscience*, Vol. 17, No. 10, pp. 3588-3598, ISSN 0270-6474

Vincent, I., Rosado, M. & Davies, P. (1996). Mitotic mechanisms in Alzheimer's disease? *Journal of Cell Biology*, Vol. 132, No. 3, pp. 413-425, ISSN 0021-9525

Weingarten, M.D., Lockwood, A.H., Hwo, S.Y. & Kirschner, M.W. (1975). A protein factor essential for microtubule assembly. *Proceedings of the National Academy of Sciences USA*, Vol. 72, No. 5, pp. 1858-1862, ISSN 0027-8424

Weiwad, M., Kullertz, G., Schutkowski, M. & Fischer, G. (2000). Evidence that the substrate backbone conformation is critical to phosphorylation by p42 MAP kinase. *FEBS Letters*, Vol. 478, No. 1-2, pp. 39-42, ISSN 0014-5793

Wells, N.J., Watanabe, N., Tokusumi, T., Jiang, W., Verdecia, M.A. & Hunter, T. (1999). The C-terminal domain of the Cdc2 inhibitory kinase Myt1 interacts with Cdc2 complexes and is required for inhibition of G(2)/M progression. *Journal of Cell Science*, Vol. 112 (Pt 19), pp. 3361-3371, ISSN 0021-9533

Wijsman, E.M., Daw, E.W., Yu, C.E., Payami, H., Steinbart, E.J., Nochlin, D., Conlon, E.M., Bird, T.D. & Schellenberg, G.D. (2004). Evidence for a novel late-onset Alzheimer disease locus on chromosome 19p13.2. *Amwrican Journal of Human Genetics*, Vol. 75, No. 3, pp. 398-409, ISSN 0002-9297

Winkler, K.E., Swenson, K.I., Kornbluth, S. & Means, A.R. (2000). Requirement of the prolyl isomerase Pin1 for the replication checkpoint. *Science*, Vol. 287, No. 5458, pp. 1644-1647, ISSN 0036-8075

Wulf, G., Finn, G., Suizu, F. & Lu, K.P. (2005). Phosphorylation-specific prolyl isomerization: is there an underlying theme? *Nature Cell Biology*, Vol. 7, No. 5, pp. 435-441, ISSN 1097-6256

Yaffe, M.B., Schutkowski, M., Shen, M., Zhou, X.Z., Stukenberg, P.T., Rahfeld, J.U., Xu, J., Kuang, J., Kirschner, M.W., Fischer, G., Cantley, L.C. & Lu, K.P. (1997). Sequence-specific and phosphorylation-dependent proline isomerization: a potential mitotic regulatory mechanism. *Science*, Vol. 278, No. 5345, pp. 1957-1960, ISSN 0036-8075

Yang, Y. & Herrup, K. (2007). Cell division in the CNS: protective response or lethal event in post-mitotic neurons? *Biochimica et Biophysica Acta*, Vol. 1772, No. 4, pp. 457-466, ISSN 0006-3002

Zheng-Fischhofer, Q., Biernat, J., Mandelkow, E.M., Illenberger, S., Godemann, R. & Mandelkow, E. (1998). Sequential phosphorylation of Tau by glycogen synthase kinase-3beta and protein kinase A at Thr212 and Ser214 generates the Alzheimer-specific epitope of antibody AT100 and requires a paired-helical-filament-like conformation. *European Journal of Biochemistry*, Vol. 252, No. 3, pp. 542-552, ISSN 0014-2956

Zhou, X.Z., Kops, O., Werner, A., Lu, P.J., Shen, M., Stoller, G., Kullertz, G., Stark, M., Fischer, G. & Lu, K.P. (2000). Pin1-dependent prolyl isomerization regulates dephosphorylation of Cdc25C and tau proteins. Molecular *Cell*, Vol. 6, No. 4, pp. 873-883, ISSN 1097-2765

Zhou, X.Z., Lu, P.J., Wulf, G. & Lu, K.P. (1999). Phosphorylation-dependent prolyl isomerization: a novel signaling regulatory mechanism. *Cellular and Molecular Life Sciences*, Vol. 56, No. 9-10, pp. 788-806, ISSN 1420-682X

Zita, M.M., Marchionni, I., Bottos, E., Righi, M., Del Sal, G., Cherubini, E. & Zacchi, P. (2007). Post-phosphorylation prolyl isomerisation of gephyrin represents a mechanism to modulate glycine receptors function. *EMBO Journal*, Vol. 26, No. 7, pp. 1761-1771, ISSN 0261-4189

12

Selectivity of Cell Signaling in the Neuronal Response Based on NGF Mutations and Peptidomimetics in the Treatment of Alzheimers Disease

Kenneth E. Neet[1], Sidharth Mahapatra[2], Hrishikesh M. Mehta[3]
[1]*Department of Biochemistry and Molecular Biology, The Chicago Medical School, Rosalind Franklin University of Medicine and Science, North Chicago*
[2]*Department of Pediatrics, School of Medicine, Stanford University, Palo Alto*
[3]*Department of Pediatrics, Division of Hematology/Oncology/Stem Cell Transplantation Children's Memorial Hospital, Northwestern Feinberg School of Medicine, Lurie Comprehensive Cancer Center, Chicago Northwestern University, Chicago USA*

1. Introduction

Neurotrophins are maintained at low concentrations by target tissues. They form highly selective interactions with their respective cognate receptors and maintain the viability of neurons in the central and peripheral nervous systems. Overlap in receptor specificities for neurotrophins, in the tissue distribution of the specific receptors, and in the expression of the high affinity receptors enable growth- and survival-enhancing signals to be transduced with great efficiency and specificity over a wide variety of neuronal cells. Early studies suggested that alterations in neurotrophin levels might underlie the pathogenesis of Alzheimer's disease (AD), Parkinson's disease (PD), Huntington's disease (HD) and other neurodegenerative disorders (Apfel et al., 1991; Emilien et al., 2000; Hefti, 1983) [reviewed in (Lad et al., 2003a)]. Today, a strong link between such a neurodegenerative condition and an imbalance in neurotrophin and/or receptor levels has been supported with nerve growth factor (NGF) and AD. A disruption or reduction in critical neurotrophin levels thus leads to widespread neurodegeneration. Conversely, administration of NGF and/or its related family of neurotrophins can potentially play a role in treatment of AD or other degenerative neurological disorders. NGF and its peptidomimetics have been proposed and tested in animal studies and clinical trials for AD with complex responses observed in some patients. Intracellular signaling from the NGF receptors is complex, giving rise to neuronal responses that include differentiation, survival, and apoptosis. This review will focus on novel approaches to eliciting selectivity of a cellular response, based on alterations in the NGF molecule or in the peptidomimetic, that may lead to more effective treatments of AD with NGF-related therapeutics. A conceptual comparison to selectivity in other growth factor receptor systems, such as epidermal growth factor (EGF) and insulin, will also be made.

2. Neurotrophins, their receptors, and neurodegenerative disease

2.1 Neurotrophin receptor interactions

Neurotrophins (NTs) are a family of closely related proteins that have diverse functions ranging from neuronal development, differentiation, and survival to regulation of axonal and dendritic outgrowth, activity-dependent synaptic formation and regulation, cell migration, and cellular proliferation (Diamond et al., 1992; Katz et al., 1990; Levi-Montalcini, 1987; Lindsay, 1988; Segal, 2003). The family of neurotrophins includes nerve growth factor (NGF), brain-derived neurotrophic factor (BDNF), neurotrophin 3 (NT-3), and neurotrophin 4 (NT-4) (Ibanez, 1994; Lad et al., 2003a) . They possess high sequence homology (ca. ~50%) and adopt similar tertiary structures (Fig. 1A) (Bibel & Barde, 2000; Korsching, 1993). The same neurotrophin can affect a variety of neuronal populations and, conversely, the same tissue is capable of receiving stimulatory inputs from multiple neurotrophins. For example, cholinergic basal forebrain (CBF) neurons are attuned to NGF for their maintenance but have been shown to respond to BDNF and NT-3 (Bibel & Barde, 2000; Korsching, 1993; Lad et al., 2003a). The viability of dopaminergic neurons of the substantia nigra has been linked to the actions of BDNF and NT-4 (Hyman et al., 1991; Lad et al., 2003a; Parain et al., 1999). Also, BDNF can act on the entorhinal cortex, the substantia nigra, and the striatum to affect AD, PD, and PD/HD, respectively (Nagahara & Tuszynski, 2011). Each of these neurotrophins binds selectively to a 140-kDa tropomyosin-receptor-kinase, i.e. NGF to TrkA, BDNF and NT-4 to TrkB, and NT-3 to TrkC (Cordon-Cardo et al., 1991; Kaplan et al., 1991; Soppet et al., 1991). Binding to Trk enables the transduction of positive signals, i.e. survival and differentiation through its intracellullar tyrosine kinase domain. In contrast, all neurotrophins can bind a 75-kDa common neurotrophin receptor, p75 (or $p75^{NTR}$), involved in the transduction of negative signals, i.e. growth arrest or apoptosis, when expressed exclusively, or positive signals when co-expressed with Trk receptors (Lad et al., 2003a). The central and peripheral nervous systems possess multiple neurotrophin-dependent cells and tissues that demonstrate co-expression of TrkA and p75.

2.2 Importance of neurotrophins in neurodegenerative disorders

Numerous studies have now demonstrated an imbalance between neurotrophins and their receptors in AD, appearing even in early cognitive defects (Mufson et al., 2007; 2008; Lad, et al., 2003a). In cholinergic basal forebrain (CBF) neurons in AD, TrkA and p75 are decreased at both the mRNA and proteins levels and NGF mRNA is not changed (Mufson et al., 1995; Salehi et al., 2000; S. A. Scott et al., 1995). NGF protein is down in CBF neurons with accumulation of NGF in the cortex, suggesting that retrograde transport to provide the neurotrophic factor to the basal forebrain is impaired (Schindowski et al., 2008). These changes begin to appear in early, pre-clinical stages of cognitive impairment (Ginsberg et al., 2006; Mufson et al., 1995; Mufson et al., 2000; Mufson et al., 2002; Schulte-Herbruggen et al., 2008). In addition, the pro-apoptotic proNGF is elevated, suggesting destruction of neurons containing p75 (Cuello et al., 2010; Fahnestock et al., 2001). A relationship of neurotrophins and their receptors to Aβ toxicity and/or deposition is also becoming apparent (Calissano et al., 2010a; Peng et al., 2004). Finally, BDNF, and possibly its precursor form, is implicated in neuronal survival imbalance in AD (Garzon & Fahnestock, 2007; Peng et al., 2005), particularly in the entorhinal cortex region of the brain (Nagahara & Tuszynski, 2011). Consequently, various treatment strategies have been suggested to slow or reverse cognitive symptoms, utilizing administration of neurotrophins (Mufson et al., 2008; Nagahara & Tuszynski, 2011; Nilsson et al., 2010; Schulte-Herbruggen et al., 2008).

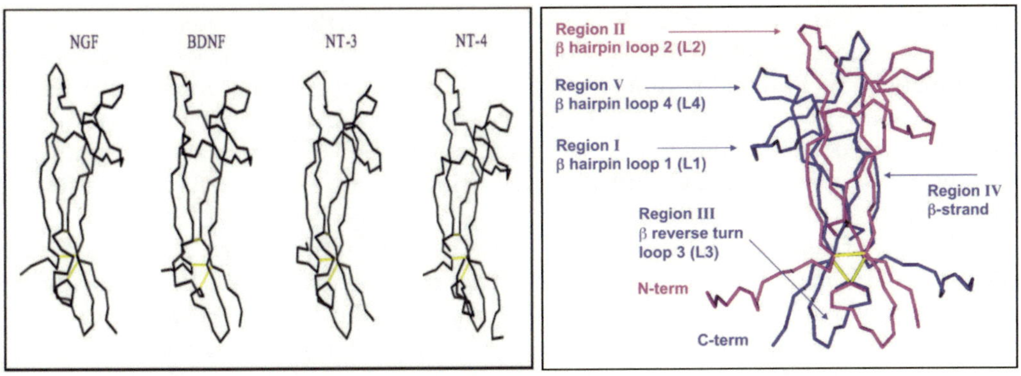

Fig. 1. A (left). Folding of the protomer of the four neurotrophins. B (right). Structure of dimeric NGF showing the loop regions that interact with the receptors. The yellow bonds represent the cystine knot motif. From PDB 1WWW. Note: the variable regions I, II and V defined by sequence homology (Ibanez et al., 1991; Ibanez et al., 1993; Ilag et al., 1994) are equivalent to loops 1, 2, and 4 (L1, L2, L4) defined in the structure (Wiesmann et al., 1999).

2.3 Alzheimer's disease – Treatment strategies

The pathogenesis of Alzheimer's disease is related to loss of NGF-mediated survival signals, receptor imbalances at the cell surface, and a shift to proprotein forms capable of inducing apoptosis. Without these positive signals, the progression of intracellular events that ultimately lead to deposition of tangles and plaques occurs uninterrupted. As a result, neurodegeneration in the cholinergic basal forebrain leads to cognitive and memory deficits demonstrable in AD patients. In the current treatment of Alzheimer's disease, the use of cholinesterase therapies to re-establish critical levels of acetylcholine in the inflicted areas are unable to deter the loss of neuronal populations from the CBF and hence to slow the progression of the disease (Bierer et al., 1995; Lad et al., 2003a). Based on these findings, an appropriate way to reduce or prevent neurodegeneration and maintain viability in Alzheimer's disease is to re-establish NGF signaling within the CBF. Additionally, the administered protein must be well-tolerated and stably released over a long period of time to achieve its trophic effects (Apfel, 2002). However, the direct administration of NGF to the CNS via the circulation is precluded by its inability to cross the blood brain barrier (BBB) (Lad et al., 2003a). Furthermore, subcutaneous delivery of NGF elicits acutely painful phenomena due to the presence of TrkA receptors at free nerve endings of pain fibers (Apfel et al., 1998; Lad et al., 2003a). Finally, gastric secretions would rapidly degrade the protein, making oral preparations ineffective.

Other methods have been considered for delivery of growth factors or protein drugs to the brain [for a broad review see references (Alam et al., 2010; Cattaneo et al., 2008)]. Intranasal inhalation has been demonstrated to be a promising mode of non-invasive, facile delivery of biologics to the brain (Benedict et al., 2011). Monocytes can be loaded to secrete NGF and, in proof of principle, shown to migrate across an *in vitro* BBB model consisting of a brain capillary endothelial cell system (Bottger et al., 2010). Encapsulated cell biodelivery is a modified gene therapy approach which encapsulates cells in a immunoprotective semi-permeable hollow fiber synthetic membrane to secrete the protein factor of interest into the desired region of the brain (Fjord-Larsen et al., 2010); NGF and glial derived neurotrophic factor (GDNF) are currently undergoing clinical trials with this method in Sweden. Transcranial focused ultrasound (FUS) has been shown to transiently-enhance the permeability of the BBB and permit antibodies, and probably other macromolecules into the intrathecal space (Jordão et al., 2010). Early interest in conjugation of NGF to transferrin or transferrin antibodies as a means of transport across the BBB (Friden et al., 1993; Liao et al., 2001) seems to have waned and shifted toward using this means of cellular uptake for anti-cancer or diabetic drugs.

Gene therapy presents the most-advanced, current means of delivering NGF in a cerebral region-specific manner (Lad et al., 2003a; Nagahara & Tuszynski, 2011). The two main forms of gene therapy that have been used in the delivery of NGF include an *in vivo* approach and an *ex vivo* approach. The former requires the injection of a viral vector containing the gene of interest directly into the region of interest. The latter can be done by transfecting cells with the gene of interest *in vitro* and subsequently transplanting the transfected cells into the region of interest. These techniques overcome the problems initially encountered with NGF delivery by circumventing the BBB, but require surgical manipulation. Additionally, by using viral vectors as the mode of NGF gene delivery into a specific target within the brain, these methods provide a stable, renewable system of NGF synthesis, which can help re-establish receptor levels and counter apoptosis driven by proNGF. However, these forms of therapy provide the greatest benefit during early stages of AD before cholinergic deficits set in.

Initial positive results in rat and primate animal models supported studies of NGF in clinical trials of AD (Bishop et al., 2008; Eriksdotter Jonhagen et al., 1998; Tuszynski et al., 2005). The early clinical trials met with a lack of success due to lack of efficacy, toxicity or both. Common problems in these clinical studies, as well as corresponding animal studies, include undesirable side effects (e.g. hyperinnervation, sprouting, sympathetic stimulation, cachexia, hyperalgesia) (Apfel, 2002; Thoenen & Sendtner, 2002; Winkler et al., 1997) [reviewed in (Nagahara & Tuszynski, 2011)]. Intriguingly, a phase I trial of *ex vivo* NGF gene delivery in mild Alzheimer's disease has shown some promise (Tuszynski et al., 2005). Briefly, eight individuals with early-stage, probable AD were administered primary autologous fibroblasts, which had been genetically modified to synthesize and secrete NGF, via stereotaxic injections to the CBF. This approach was shown to survive grafting into the brain and provided stable NGF secretion for up to 18 months in animal studies with improvement of cholinergic function and memory (Emerich et al., 1994; Tuszynski et al., 2002; Tuszynski et al., 2005). At 22 months of follow up, no adverse side effects were reported in the clinical trial. Mini-Mental State Exam scores demonstrated a reduction in the rate of cognitive decline and 18-fluorodeoxyglucose PET scans demonstrated significantly greater cortical glucose uptake (Tuszynski et al., 2005). Although these observations were encouraging, results must be considered with caution because of the small data set used and the absence of placebo groups. Additionally, NGF demonstrated a large trophic response in the CBF of some of these patients. While this response is necessary for target innervation during development of the nervous system, an adult brain where the axonal infrastructure is well-established might suffer from new and incomplete neuritogenesis in an area receiving dense axonal support. Hence, the generation of a more refined therapeutic molecule is desirable. Since this *ex vivo* trial, the focus of the scientific community has largely shifted to *in vivo* delivery with adeno-associated virus (AAV) (Table 1 and (Nagahara & Tuszynski, 2011; Nilsson et al., 2010).

Interestingly, monoclonal antibodies to NGF were so effective that a Phase III clinical trial for treatment of osteoarthritis of the knee was discontinued because of joint failure due to excessive wear and tear in the absence of the pain sensation (Lane et al., 2010; Wood, 2010).

Disorder	Phase	#	Delivery*	Status	Sponsor
AD	I	8	ex vivo NGF	end 2005 some cognitive improvement (see text)	UCSD
AD	II	50	ICV AAV-NGF Cere-110	Ongoing Recruiting	Ceregene
AD	Ib	6	Encapsulated cell biodelivery NGF	Ongoing	NsGene (Sweden)
HIV associated sensory neuropathy	II	270	SQ NGF	end 2005	NIAID
Osteo-arthritis of knee	III	(a)697 (b)848	IV mAb to NGF	Completed Discontinued (see text)	Pfizer

Table 1. Selected clinical trials of NGF for AD or pain. From clinicaltrials.gov, April 2011. *Abbreviations: #, number of patients; ICV, intracerebroventricular; AAV, adeno-associated virus; SQ, subcutaneous; IV, intravenous.

3. Signal transduction by neurotrophins

3.1 TrkA signaling

Neurotrophin-mediated signal transduction via the Trk receptors leads to an activation of downstream signaling pathways for survival and differentiation (Bibel & Barde, 2000; Ibanez, 1994; Kaplan & Miller, 2000; Levi-Montalcini, 1987). NGF binding induces TrkA receptor dimerization, transautophosphorylation, and tyrosine kinase ICD activation (Bibel & Barde, 2000; Cunningham & Greene, 1998; Cunningham et al., 1997; Friedman & Greene, 1999). The three major signaling pathways are the phosphotidylinositol-3-kinase (PI3 kinase)/Akt pathway, the Ras/mitogen-activated protein kinase (MAPK) pathway, and the phospholipase C gamma (PLCγ) pathway (Bibel & Barde, 2000; Kaplan & Miller, 2000; Lad et al., 2003a) (See Fig. 2). The PI3 kinase pathway through Akt mediates survival via the suppression of apoptotic proteins and accounts for over 80% of neurotrophin-mediated survival in neurons (Bartlett et al., 1997; Crowder & Freeman, 1998; Kaplan & Miller, 2000). The MAPK pathway, has been implicated in both survival and differentiation, although it has also been implicated in such diverse functions as synaptic plasticity and long-term potentiation (Kaplan & Miller, 2000; Lad et al., 2003a). Depending on the upstream activators and downstream effectors of MAPK, survival, differentiation or both signals can be transduced. For the specific induction of differentiation, a sustained MAPK activation is necessary. The third signal transduction pathway is the PLCγ pathway, involved primarily in Ca2+ regulation of calcium regulated enzymes, neurotrophin secretion, and synaptic plasticity (Bibel & Barde, 2000; Canossa et al., 1997). These conclusions about distinct pathways have been reached by mutagenesis of the Tyr residues of the Trk-ICD and demonstrate that these signaling pathways can be individually dissected by manipulation of the intracellular initiation of each pathway. TrkB and TrkC have similar signaling pathways but with some individual differences because of the different neuronal environment of these receptors. The division of TrkA signaling into three discrete, but overlapping signal pathways, suggests that pharmaceutical approaches for design of signal selective neurotrophic therapeutics (see Section 5.2) may be able to discriminate among selected paths toward cellular outcomes.

TrkA	**Outcome**
p-Y490→Ras→PI3K→Akt→	***survival*[1]**
p-Y490→Shc→MAPK→pMEK→Bcl2→	***survival*[2]**
p-Y490→FRS2→MAPK→p-Elk1, pCREB→	***differentiation*[2]**
p-Y785*→PLCγ→PI→DAG, IP3→Ca^{++}→	***synaptic plasticity*[3]**

Fig. 2. Signaling pathways, PI3K, MAPK, PLCγ , from TrkA phospho-tyrosines to cell outcomes. *Phosphorylation of Y785 is dependent on phosphorylaton of Y670, Y674, Y675. [1]Bartlett et al., 1997; Crowder & Freeman, 1998; Rodriguez-Viciana et al., 1994; Holgado-Madruga et al., 1997. [2]Kao et al., 2001; Loeb et al., 1994; Gomez & Cohen, 1991; Qian et al., 1998; [3]Loeb et al., 1994; Canossa et al., 1997; Cunningham et al., 1997.

Phosphorylation of a specific set of tyrosines ensues within the activation loop of the kinase domain. These include two tyrosines located in the juxtamembrane domain (Y490) and C-terminus (Y785) of Trk that serve as docking sites for adaptor proteins and three tyrosines (Y670, Y674, and Y675) within the activation loop that interact with nearby basic residues to stabilize a fully functional, active catalytic core and potentiate transduction of downstream signals (Bibel & Barde, 2000; Cunningham & Greene, 1998; Friedman & Greene, 1999; Grewal et al., 1999; Huang & Reichardt, 2003; Kaplan & Miller, 2000; Lad et al., 2003a).

3.2 p75 signaling

Classically, p75 has been thought to be involved in the induction of negative signals like apoptosis and growth arrest in oligodendrocytes, Schwann cells, sympathetic neurons, motor neurons, and sensory neurons (Bamji et al., 1998; Barrett & Bartlett, 1994; Casaccia-Bonnefil et al., 1996; Kaplan & Miller, 2000) in a Trk-independent fashion, (Davey & Davies, 1998; Kaplan & Miller, 2000; Soilu-Hanninen et al., 1999). The co-presence of Trk on a neuron silences pro-apoptotic pathways by activation of the pro-survival transcription factor, NF-κB, which subsequently activates Akt (Bibel & Barde, 2000; Kaplan & Miller, 2000; Khursigara et al., 1999). Sympathetic neurons and basal forebrain neurons that were p75-deficient in p75-/- mice underwent robust axonal sprouting, hypertrophy, or target innervation with naturally-occurring developmental apoptosis being significantly delayed (Kaplan & Miller, 2000; Walsh et al., 1999; Yeo et al., 1997; Bamji et al., 1998). Without intrinsic catalytic activity, the p75 ICD appears to rely on docking of adaptor proteins. The complexities of the p75 signaling are outlined by representative examples shown in Fig. 3.

p75	**Outcome**
Traf6 → JNK → Bax, p53, & caspases NRAGE → JNK → caspases Ceramide → inhibition of Raf-1 & Akt NRIF → nucleus	*Pro-apoptosis*[1]
SC-1	*Growth arrest*[2]
Lingo-1-p75-NgR → p75-ICD → RhoA	*Inhibit neurite outgrowth*[3]
TRAF-6 → NF-kB SHC → PI3K to Akt	*Pro-survival*[4]
MAPK	*Pro-survival or pro-apoptosis*[5]

Fig. 3. Some signaling pathways from p75 to cell outcomes. Adaptor proteins interact with p75 to generate most cellular effects of a diverse nature. Uncommon abbrevations: NRAGE, Neurotrophin receptor-interacting MAGE homolog; NRIF, neurotrophin receptor interacting factor, Zn finger transcriptional factor; SC-1, Schwann cell factor 1; NgR, Nogo receptor. RhoA, Ras homolog A. (For reviews see Kaplan & Miller, 2000; Bibel & Barde, 2000; Schecterson & Bothwell, 2010). [1]Aloyz et al., 1998; Salehi, et al., 2002; Muller, et al., 1998; de Chaves et al., 1997; Casademunt, et al., 1999; [2]Chittka & Chao, 1999; [3]Domeniconi et al., 2005; [4]Khursigara et al., 1999; [5]Susen, et al., 1999; Lad & Neet, 2003.

The self-interaction of p75 also influences cellular outcome. Biophysical and biochemical methods have suggested that homomeric p75 plays a pro-apoptotic role while formation of oligomers abolishes this effect and may even serve an anti-apoptotic role (Kaplan & Miller, 2000; Lad et al., 2003a; Wang et al., 2000). Recently, evidence has been provided to support a model in which the formation of an inter-protomer disulfide bond in p75 allows a scissoring (or snail-tong) action upon NGF binding that promotes binding of intracellular adaptor proteins (Simi & Ibanez, 2010; Vilar et al., 2009).

As mentioned above (Section 2.2), proneurotrophins may play significant role in AD, due to their ability to stimulate p75 in the absence of positive Trk signals thereby promoting apoptosis and death of neurons or glia (Cuello et al., 2010; Fahnestock et al., 2001; Teng, et al. 2010). These effects are thought to be mediated by the same pathways (Fig. 3) as presented for mature NGF (or other neurotrophins). In addition, soluble oligomers of β-amyloid may also interact with p75 to cause apoptotic signals in neuronal tissue of AD or pre-AD patients (Dechant & Barde, 2002; Diarra et al. 2009; Coulson, et al., 2009; Calissano, et al. 2010a; 2010b; Peng, et al., 2004; Susen & Blochl, 2005).

These studies demonstrate that the interaction of neurotrophins or proneurotrophins with p75 can lead to diverse effects that are determined by the developmental state of the organism, the particular cell type within which it is expressed, the additional expression of co-receptors, receptor oligomerization states, and the binding of intracellular adaptors or effectors. The complexity of the p75 pathways suggests that developing signal selective muteins for this receptor would be much more difficult than those outlined for the Trk receptor (Section 5.2) with its more clearly initiated signaling. Since the response of cells is, basically, apoptosis or not, then there would be less advantage at this point in time in generating such reagents for p75.

4. Molecular analysis of neurotrophin structure and rationale of mutations

4.1 Conserved and variable regions defined from sequence and 3-D crystallographic structures

Functional data gathered from systematic mutagenesis studies and through the construction of inter-neurotrophin chimeras coupled with structural data from crystallographic studies have implicated several spatially distinct patches of residues in bestowing receptor specificity to each neurotrophin (Casademunt et al., 1999; de Chaves et al., 1997; Grimes et al., 1997; Ilag et al., 1994; Lad et al., 2003a; Ninkina et al., 1997; Rabizadeh et al., 1993; J. Scott et al., 1983; Walsh et al., 1999; Wiesmann et al., 1999; Yeo et al., 1997) . Sequence alignments of NGF, BDNF, and NT-3 (Ibanez et al., 1992; Ibanez et al., 1991; Ibanez et al., 1993; Ilag et al., 1994; Kullander & Ebendal, 1994; Kullander et al., 1997) demonstrate that each neurotrophin possesses seven variable regions that include the same residue positions. These are the N-terminus (residues 1-9), variable region I (β-hairpin loop 1, residues 23-35), variable region II (β-hairpin loop 2, residues 40-49), variable region III (β-reverse turn loop 3, residues 59-66), variable region IV (β-strand, residues 79-88), variable region V (β-hairpin loop 4, residues 95-99), and the C-terminus (residues 111-118) (Fig. 1B). This homology in clustering translates structurally to variable regions occupying complementary sites on each neurotrophin molecule, which are surface-exposed, enabling these regions to function as sites of receptor contacts (Fig. 4). These regions also define amino acid residues to target for redesign of molecules to alter signaling (see Section 5.2).

4.1.1 The specificity patch

Chimeric molecules retaining the amino terminus, carboxyl terminus, and variable region II of NGF possessed the ability to differentiate sympathetic neurons and activate the TrkA receptor (Ibanez et al., 1991). However, a chimeric molecule that additionally replaced residues 3-9 of the N-terminus reduced TrkA binding, activation, and biological activity to <1% (Ibanez et al., 1993). Other substitution and deletion studies confirmed the importance of the N-terminus in specificity (Kullander et al., 1997; Woo et al., 1995; Kahle et al., 1992; Shih et al., 1994). Data from the crystal structure of human recombinant NGF complexed with the TrkA-d5 domains showed that the amino terminal residues 6-9, which were not well-defined in the original NGF crystal structure, adopted a helical conformation upon complex formation with their side chains almost completely buried in the interface (McDonald et al., 1991; Wiesmann et al., 1999) (Fig. 4). Within the same region, H4, I6, and E11 participated in strong interactions with residues in the ABED TrkA β-sheet. The authors labeled this region the specificity patch suggesting that the most important Trk receptor-binding determinants lie within the amino terminus (Wiesmann et al., 1999). Residues spanning the specificity patch, i.e. H4, P5, I6, F7, E11, and F12, are clearly important for neurotrophin-Trk interactions and activation.

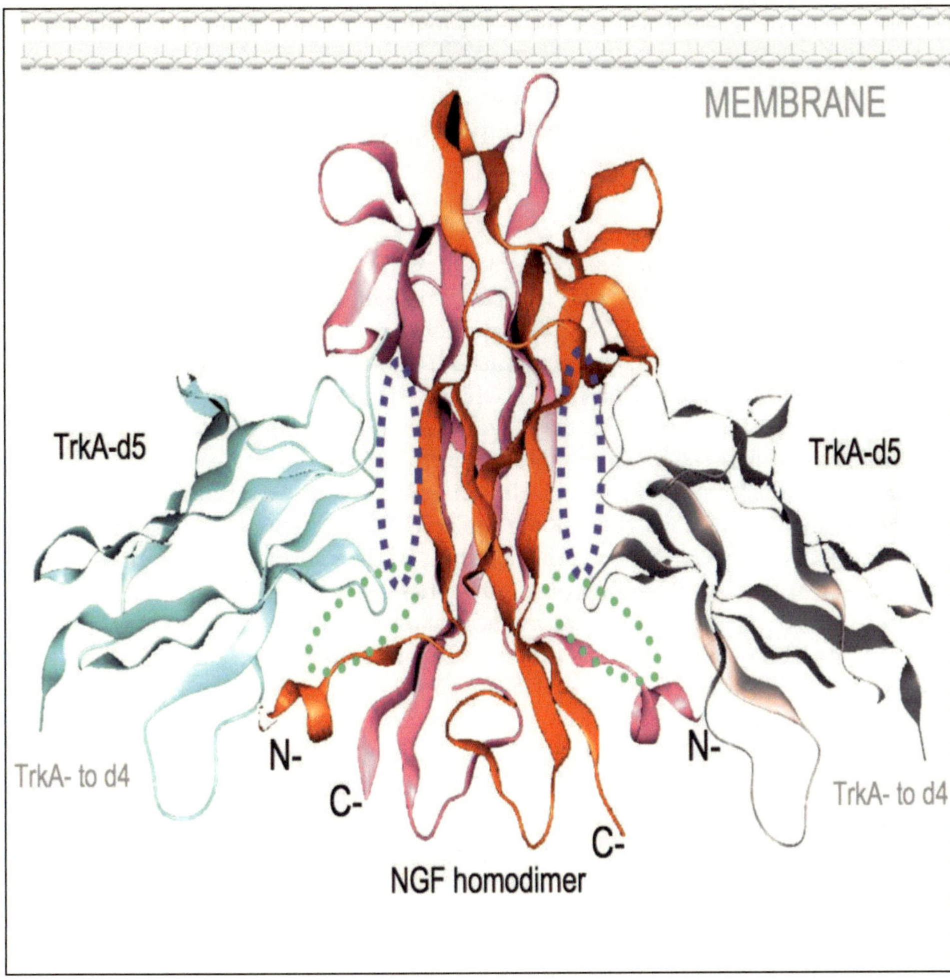

Fig. 4. Schematic representation of dimeric nerve growth factor complexed with two TrkA-d5 domains. NGF and TrkA (PDB 1WWW) form highly specific interactions at the specificity (green dotted oval) and the conserved patch (blue dotted oval). Additional contacts are provided by variable loops I, II, and V (loop 4) that form a continuous surface of binding. Each TrkA-d5 binding site is derived from contributions from loops in both protomers in the NGF dimer. NGF protomers, pink and orange. 1st TrkA-d5; cyan: 2nd TrkA-d5; grey.

4.1.2 The variable regions

The variable regions (Fig. 1B), in general, correspond to loops and surface residues in NGF and the other neurotrophins. Generation of NGF-BDNF chimeras identified variable region II as holding important receptor binding determinants (Ibanez et al., 1991; Ibanez et al., 1993; Ilag et al., 1994; Kullander & Ebendal, 1994; Kullander et al., 1997). The variable region was further dissected into IIa (residues 40-44) and IIb (residues 45-49) (Ibanez et al., 1993). Region IIb was shown to play a more pivotal role than IIa when replacement of only the latter led to a dramatic reduction in receptor activation and biological activity (Ibanez et al., 1993). The variable region II, with help from variable region V (loop 4), was also shown to confer specificity between NT-3 and NGF (Ilag et al., 1994; Kullander & Ebendal, 1994; Kullander et al., 1997). The C-terminal linker region of TrkA could serve as a possible binding partner of this region (Wiesmann et al., 1999) (Fig. 4). Therefore, residues within variable regions IIa and IIb are considered important for neurotrophin activity, i.e. E41, N43, I44, N45, V48, and F49.

4.1.3 The conserved patch

Crystallographic data of dimeric NGF complexed with TrkA-d5 demonstrated that 5 of 10 residues in variable region IV (Y79, T81, T83, H84, and F86) actually form part of the conserved patch that interacts intimately with the TrkA-d5 domains (Wiesmann & de Vos, 2001) (Fig. 4). This 'conserved' patch was so named because 14 of 23 NGF residues are occupied by homologous amino acids in BDNF and NT-3, while 8 of 15 TrkA residues are conserved in TrkB and TrkC (Wiesmann et al., 1999). The conserved patch forms a continuous binding surface for TrkA-d5 and retains high sequence homology across species (Wiesmann et al., 1999) (Fig. 4). Variable region IV, a β-strand, was specifically shown to retain ~90% homology across species. Within this region, T81 and H84 of NGF are replaced by non-homologous amino acids in the other neurotrophins, suggesting that variable region IV does form specific contacts with TrkA (Ibanez et al., 1993) (Fig. 4). Alanine point mutagenesis of H84 and H75 indicated that these residues participated in receptor binding and activation based on a decline in neuritogenesis in PC12 cells and the ability to compete for binding sites with radioactively-labeled wild-type NGF (Woo & Neet, 1996). Similarly, R100 and R103 showed trends akin to H84 with respect to sequence alignment analysis, mutagenesis studies, and crystallographic data. R100 and R103 are not only strictly conserved across species but also within the family of neurotrophins. Crystallographic data suggested that R103 was the most important binding determinant in the conserved patch (Wiesmann et al., 1999) (Fig. 4). [Also see Section 5.1.] Residues V22, I31, F53, and F54 within the conserved patch are also highly conserved across species and between neurotrophin family members. Alanine substitution of these four residues significantly affect TrkA binding by competition assays, intracellular receptor phosphorylation studies, and biological activity in PC12 cells (Ibanez et al., 1990; Ibanez et al., 1992; Ibanez et al., 1993; Guo et al., 1996). Hence, the conserved patch represents a binding epitope wherein residues help form critical interactions between neurotrophins and Trk receptors.

4.1.4 Summary of important regions and residues of the neurotrophin family

Sixteen residues of NGF may be identified as most important for function (Table 2) and can be designated as the specificity patch (H4, P5, I6, F7, E11, and F12), the variable loops (I31, E41, N43, I44, N45, V48, and F49), or the conserved patch (I31, F54, H84, and R103). Additional residues, V22, F53, H75, and R100, may not occupy the conserved patch, *per se*, but are as highly conserved as residues residing within or near the patch. Similar considerations have been made for BDNF and NT-3 (Ibanez et al., 1992; Ibanez et al., 1991; Ibanez et al., 1993; Ilag et al., 1994; Kullander & Ebendal, 1994; Kullander et al., 1997; Suter et al., 1992; Urfer et al., 1997). These regions of the NGF molecule were targeted to obtain the signal selective muteins discussed in Section 5.2.

Specificity Patch - induced N-terminal α-helix; mainly hydrophobic and some H-bond interactions to β-strands ABED of TrkA-d5.	**NGF:** H4, P5, I6, F7, E11, F12 **BDNF:** S4, D5, P6, A7, E11, L12
Conserved Patch - part of hydrophobic core of NGF; interacts with loop EF and C-terminus of TrkA-d5	**NGF:** V22, I31*, F53, F54, H75, H84*, R103 **BDNF:** V22, M31, F53, Y54, H75, Q84, R103
Specificity for NGF vs NT-3: **Loop II-**	**NGF:** E41, N43, I44, N45, V48, F49 **BDNF:** K41, P43, V44, S45 - - **NT-3:** E41, K43, T44, G45, P48, V49
N-terminus-	**NGF:** P5, F7 **NT-3:** H5, S7

Table 2. Important regions of Trk receptor interaction in human NGF and BDNF. Based on crystal structure and mutagenesis analysis of NGF (Mahapatra, 2008; Ibanez et al., 1992; Ibanez et al., 1991; Ibanez et al., 1993; Ilag et al., 1994; Kullander & Ebendal, 1994; Kullander et al., 1997; Wiesmann & de Vos, 2001) and the corresponding regions in BDNF and NT-3. Note: I31 and H84 (with *) also participate in Loop 1 and Loop 4, respectively, as well as the conserved patch.

5. Development of neurotrophin muteins that have potentially improved therapeutic properties

5.1 Receptor selective muteins

Two interesting, complementary, and useful muteins have helped elucidate the role of the two receptors in neurotrophin action. The first discovery was that mutations in the 32-35, loop I area would greatly reduce or eliminate binding to the p75 receptor and leave TrkA binding unimpaired (Ibanez et al 1992; 1993). The triNGF (or KKE) mutein contained the three mutations, K32A/K34A/E35A, and was used to demonstrate the functional interaction between p75 and TrkA in the developing embryo (Ryden, et al., 1997). The mutations in the N-terminus of NGF were shown to be important for TrkA binding in several laboratories (Section 4.1.1). One noteable mutein was the Δ9/13 mutein that bound p75 but not TrkA (Woo et al., 1995), and helped distinguish between differentiation, cell cycle regulation, and apoptosis in PC12 cells (Hughes et al., 2001). Utilization of this Δ9/13 mutein also later indicated a unique role for the 'high affinity' binding complex of p75 and TrkA in PC12 cells (Lad, et al., 2003b). Indeed, the combination of these two receptor muteins, KKE/Δ9/13 has been studied, briefly, and shown to have no observable activity, as expected (Mahapatra, et al., 2009). Both muteins, KKE and Δ9/13, have been used in a rat glaucoma model to interpret the roles of TrkA (neuroprotective) and p75 (neurotoxic) in retinal degeneration (Bai, et al., 2010). KKE, but not wild type NGF, has recently been reported to partially improve learning in a transgenic APP mouse model (overexpression of Swedish and Indiana mutations) with a reduction of soluble cortical β-amyloid levels, but with no improvement in long-term memory (Aboulkassim, et al., 2011). These two receptor selective muteins have potential as an improved therapeutic for disorders in which either TrkA or p75 can be expected, with improved targeting in that case.

In the opposite direction, a neurotrophin mutein has been made that is less restrictive, rather than more restrictive, in binding to Trk receptors. The pan-neurotrophin, PNT, incorporated elements of variable and conserved regions to produce a mutein that binds to all three receptors, TrkA, TrkB, TrkC (Ibanez, et al., 1993; Ilag, et al., 1995). To the authors' knowledge, a pan-neurotrophin has not been made that was promiscuous for Trk receptors but restricted so as to not bind p75. Such pan-neurotrophins might have utility in the treatment of some neurodegenerative disorders in which multiple receptors indiscriminately needed extra support (Funakoshi, et al., 1998).

The observation of a mutation in NGF that affects the pain response suggests that changes in signaling from mutations in the ligand have already occurred in nature. A nociceptive response is mediated by NGF (Pezet & McMahon, 2006), partly through the TrkA receptor and partly through p75 (Einarsdottir et al., 2004; Indo, 2002; Nicol & Vasko, 2007). In a large family from northern Sweden, an R100W mutation was uncovered within the coding region of NGF. Individuals from this family suffered from insensitivity to both temperature and deep pain perception, while retaining normal mental abilities, a disorder termed hereditary sensory and autonomic neuropathy type V (HSANV) (Einarsdottir et al., 2004). The R100W mutation selectively disrupts binding of NGF to the p75 receptor, while the affinity for TrkA receptor is less affected (Covaceuszach et al., 2010). Also, the consequence of the R100W mutation on p75 receptor binding is greater for mature NGF rather than proNGF. Signaling pathways reflect this selectivity (Capsoni et al., 2011), suggesting that these findings might lead to a 'painless' NGF protein with therapeutic potential. This NGF mutation is an example of a naturally-occurring, receptor-selective change in the neurotrophin.

5.2 Development of signal selective muteins

To alleviate the potentially undesirable effects of inappropriate over extension of neurites during clinical trials (Section 2.3), designer neurotrophins have been developed (Mahapatra et al., 2009). Two survival-specific (or signal-selective, SS) recombinant NGF muteins with decreased differentiation potential were designed from a set of rationally selected mutations within the specificity, conserved, and variable regions of NGF that may play a discriminatory role in signal transduction. One of these muteins is the F7A/H84A/R103A NGF triple mutein, also called SS-1 or 7-84-103 for short. The other signal-selective hextuple mutein is the K32A/K34A/E35A/F7A/H84A/R103A NGF mutein, or called SS-2 or KKE/7-84-103 (Mahapatra et al., 2009). The main difference between the two SS muteins is that the KKE addition to the F7A/H84A/R103A mutation simply makes the hextuple mutein, SS2, incapable of binding p75 (see Section 5.1).

Survival in several cell lines and differentiation in PC12 cells were studied with these recombinant NGF triple and hextuple muteins and compared to wild type NGF. Each of these two muteins induced slightly lower levels of survival in MG139 and PC12 cells with greatly reduced neuritogenesis in PC12 cells. Neuritogenesis data indicated that residues Phe7, His84, and Arg103 played a critical role in biological activity, in agreement with earlier data in the literature (see Section 4). The observed neuritogenic potential of each recombinant triple mutein suggested that His84 (conserved patch) played a discriminatory role in neurite outgrowth. When His84 was mutated to alanine, to make 7-84-103 and KKE/7-84-103, the maximum neuritic response was almost 40% lower than when His84 was left unaltered. With 7-84-103 and KKE/7-84-103, a synergistic effect also occurred when combining mutations to these three residues. These data suggested that mutations within the specificity and conserved patches were more than additive and led to a reduction of neuritogenesis. In 7-84-103 and KKE/7-84-103, the two point mutations were made in close proximity within the same spatial region, *i.e.* His84 and Arg103, within the conserved patch. Combining mutations in close proximity may have a cumulative effect on ligand-receptor interactions and ultimately reduce the efficiency of some aspects of intracellular signaling. When independent single mutations were incorporated in close proximity within critical regions at the ligand-receptor interface, survival and differentiation were both affected, with a more pronounced effect on neuritogenesis. The greater decrease in differentiation suggests the possibility of multiple binding epitopes for the mediation of survival, while suggesting more limited patches needed for the induction of differentiation. Comparison with binding to immobilized TrkA by surface plasmon resonance suggested that differentiation more closely follows affinity than does survival. Furthermore, similarity in measurements between the recombinant NGF triple mutein and its KKE hextuple counterpart suggested that p75 binding was inconsequential to the induction of survival or differentiation in these cell lines. Studies with ectopically expressed receptors in fibroblast cell lines, MG139 (TrkA+, p75-) and PCNA (TrkA-, p75+), also supported the interpretation that the distinction in signaling properties was due to signaling from the TrkA tyrosine kinase receptor.

The 7-84-103 mutein supported better activation of the PI 3-kinase/Akt survival pathway than the Ras/MAPK pathway, from which differentiation results. These differences in signaling pathways (Akt vs MAPK, see Section 3) indicate that qualitative differences result from a different mode of binding to the receptor, or re-orientation of the receptor upon binding (see Section 6), and are not simply due to an affinity change that affects all signaling pathways equally. In other words, the level of TrkA phosphorylation with 7-84-103 is more efficiently transferred to MAPK and Akt activation for survival than it is for differentiation.

The discrimination ratio, or ratio of relative (to wtNGF) EC50 values, was 30-fold based on the relative EC50 values of 100 and 3.3 for differentiation and survival, respectively (Mahapatra et al., 2009). A 30-fold difference in effective EC50 values, in the pathophysiological context of an early cognitively diseased brain, might be sufficient to greatly reduce unwanted neuritic response while still maintaining neuronal viability. Whether the design of these two signal-selective muteins is optimal at this stage, or whether further improvement in discrimination between survival and differentiation pathways is possible, needs to be examined.

5.3 How can a transmembrane receptor be stimulated from the outside of a cell and initiate different kinds of intracellular signals?

The intricacies of intracellular signaling from tyrosine kinase ICDs are just now being elucidated and are more complicated than might be expected from the simple requirement of a receptor dimer to transautophosphorylate tyrosine residues on its ICD domain. Activation subsequent to ligand binding to the ECD typically requires phosphorylation of a tyrosine in a loop in the active site in order to auto-activate the ICD kinase by moving the loop out of its inhibitory position in the active site (Bae & Schlessinger, 2010; Lemmon & Schlessinger, 2010). Then the kinase continues to phosphorylate tyrosine residues in the C-terminal tail of the adjacent ICD of the receptor tyrosine kinase that provide a docking site for SH2 domain adaptor proteins or enzymes (Bae & Schlessinger, 2010; Jura et al., 2011; Lemmon & Schlessinger, 2010). Three distinct molecular mechanisms have been detected: (i) The activation loop interacts directly with the active site of the kinase and blocks access to substrates. (ii) The juxtamembrane region interacts with elements within the active site of the kinase to stabilize an inactive conformation. (iii) The C-terminal tail interacts with the active site of the tyrosine kinase domain to stabilize an inactive conformation. In each case, phosphorylation of the appropriate tyrosine relieves the kinase of its inactivation.

Evidence from crystallographic studies of the EGF receptor ICD has suggested an allosteric mechanism of initiating the signaling cascade (X. Zhang et al., 2006). Two distinct EGFR ICD interactions were described: one being a symmetric interaction and the other an asymmetric interaction that is capable of explaining how the EGF signal is transduced across the cell membrane (X. Zhang et al., 2006). Direct contacts occur between the C-lobe of one ICD, acting as an activator, and the N-lobe of another ICD, acting as a receiver. The activator kinase ICD destabilizes autoinhibitory interactions that involve the activation loop of the receiver ICD. Interactions between the docking proteins, Gab1 and Shc, and the EGFR-ICD generate kinetic discrimination between the unliganded and EGF-liganded states (Fan et al., 2004). The formation of the signal transduction 'signalosome' could well depend upon the intricate relationship of the ICDs with docking proteins and, thus, be susceptible to the manner in which the ligand (neurotrophin mutein or peptidomimetic) brought together two Trk ECDs and their connected ICDs with docking partners. In such a scenario, a larger protein ligand, such as EGF or NGF, would seem to be more capable of having multiple ways to force intracellular interactions in the signalosome than a much smaller peptidomimetic with limited 'hot spots' for interaction.

Thus, to explain the NGF mutein data discussed in Section 5.2 (Mahapatra et al., 2009), the wild-type NGF might orient the two ICDs in a signalosome that generates a "normal" ratio of MAPK to Akt activation. In the survival-selective muteins, 7-84-103 and KKE/7-84-103, the orientation of the ICDs or juxtamembrane regions would have been altered such that the output ratio has been shifted in favor of Akt over MAPK signaling and, hence, survival over neuritogenesis.

6. Neurotrophin peptidomimetics and cell signaling

The use of small molecules is often preferable over the use large proteins as pharmacological agents due to their stability, lower manufacturing costs, ability to pass tissue barriers and good pharmacokinetic profiles. The small molecules can be rationally designed to mimic a region of the ligand that is involved in binding to the receptor or involved in activation of the receptor, thus the term 'peptidomimetics'. Binding of a peptidomimetic to the target receptor may not necessarily result in activation and thus these mimetics may act as antagonists or agonists, depending on their ability to induce a functional response. An inability to induce a functional response would mean that a small molecule with good affinity would be a good inhibitor/antagonist. Two terms that are useful in the design of mimetics are pharmacophore and 'hot spots'. The term 'pharmacophore' relates to the steric and electronic interactions of the mimetic that are necessary to bind to the target receptor, either as an agonist or as an antagonist. The term 'hot spot' refers to the regions on the target protein that specifically interact with a ligand to induce a biological response. Hence, the rational design of mimetics utilizes the information from both the pharmacophore and the hot spots to create libraries of compounds that have subtle structural differences, but significant functional differences (Peleshok & Saragovi, 2006).

6.1 Early neurotrophomimetics

Early studies with cyclized monomeric peptides representing the four loop regions (see Fig. 1B) of NGF (LeSauteur et al., 1995) produced antagonists that competed with NGF for binding and inhibited its activity. The most potent antagonist was derived using amino acids from loop 4 (amino acids 92-97); the peptides designed around loop 2 (amino acids 43-48) or loop 1 (amino acids 30-35) were less effective. As expected, potency was also effected by length and amino acid substitution, with linear peptides showing no activity. Formation of the β-turn is not simply defined by the amino acid sequence and the activity requires mimicking of the 3-dimensional conformation (LeSauteur et al., 1995). Interestingly, in cells expressing both TrkA and p75, the addition of an anti-p75 monoclonal antibody (MC192) that synergizes with NGF caused the antagonistic loop 4 mimetics to behave as agonists with phosphorylation of TrkA and induction of neurites (Maliartchouk et al., 2000). Peptides that formed type I or type γL-αR turns showed greater activity in presence of MC192, suggesting that binding between TrkA and the loop 4 region may require an 'induced fit' mechanism (Beglova et al., 2000).

6.2 Small molecule Trk agonists and antagonists

Other studies, however, reported that cyclized monomeric loop 4 peptide mimetics had to be presented as dimers of cyclized peptides to show agonistic activity (Xie et al., 2000). Their dimeric cyclized peptide, involving amino acids 92-96, showed NGF like activity and induced neurite outgrowth and Akt activation in a TrkA- and ERK- dependent manner. Thus, the dimeric peptide was able to induce an NGF-like signal, by binding to and activating TrkA. Modifications in the peptide sequence abolished the agonistic activity, suggesting specificity conferred by the amino acid sequence (Xie et al., 2000). On the other hand, dimerization of a peptidomimetic does not always behave as expected. Conversion of a monovalent peptidomimetic into a divalent mimetic by chemical coupling resulted, surprisingly, in an antagonist (Brahimi et al., 2010).

Loop 1 peptidomimetics show very unique activity. The loop 1 region (amino acids 30-35) has not only been implicated in activation of TrkA, but amino acids K32, K34 and E35 are extremely important for p75 binding (Ibanez et al., 1992; Ibanez et al., 1993) (see Section 5.1). Therefore, this region influences both TrkA and p75 binding. Cyclized monomeric peptidomimetics designed using the β-turn of NT-3 are good TrkC agonists, however some of the peptides showed partial agonistic response towards TrkA. Interestingly, some of the mimetics were able to induce a neurite outgrowth response through TrkA or TrkC, but failed to induce a survival response on TrkA-only expressing cells (Zaccaro et al., 2005). Neurite outgrowth studies were done using PC12 cells which express both TrkA and p75, whereas survival studies were done using TrkA-only expressing 3T3 cells. The authors, therefore, argued that this peptidomimetic binds to a special 'hot spot' on TrkA that is accessible only when p75 is co-expressed. The co-expression of p75 with TrkA could result in formation of the TrkA-p75 heteroreceptor complex and binding of p75 to TrkA, perhaps, results in conformational changes in the receptor, making the 'hot spot' accessible (Zaccaro et al., 2005). The D3 mimetic in this series was also tested in cognitively impaired aged rats and showed rescue of the cholinergic phenotype in the cortex and nucleus basilis (Bruno, et al., 2004) and to improve learning and reduce β–amyloid in APP mice (Aboulkassim, et al., 2011).

6.3 Small molecule p75 agonists and antagonists

In contrast, Longo's group made loop 1 mimetics (LM11A-24 and LM11A-31) that targeted p75 and were able to induce a survival response through p75 in hippocampal neurons (Massa et al., 2006). Hippocampal neurons express TrkB and p75, but not TrkA; therefore, this survival induced by loop 1 mimetics was suggested to result via p75. They further showed that the survival response was lost in hippocampal neurons from p75-/- mice and that these peptides showed competitive binding to p75 but not TrkA, supporting the interpretation that the activity was through p75. The survival response observed was mediated by NF-κB and the PI3K-Akt pathway (Massa et al., 2006). They further demonstrated that the mimetics were able to rescue the neurons from proNGF-induced (Massa et al., 2006) or Aβ-induced (Yang et al., 2008) cell death, which have implications for Alzheimer's pathogenesis. NGF, even though it can bind p75, was not able to prevent the Aβ-induced neuritic dystrophy. Differences between the signaling by the mimetics vs NGF via p75 were also observed. Both NGF and the mimetics were able to inhibit the ability of Aβ to down regulate Akt signaling; in contrast, the peptidomimetics demonstrated p75-dependent inhibition of Aβ-induced GSK3b and Aβ-induced JNK activation, whereas NGF could not affect these latter two activities. Thus, these loop 1 peptidomimetics induced additional survival promoting cell signaling via p75 in presence of Aβ, not observed with NGF via p75 (Yang et al., 2008). Hence, the selectivity progressed from receptor to signaling pathway. From another laboratory, a different loop1-loop4 mimetic was shown to have some ability to reduce neuropathic pain in a rat model (Colangelo, et al., 2008).

6.4 The prognosis for signal selective mimetics

These studies with NGF peptidomimetics illustrate the advances that have been made as well as outlining the complexities involved. Whether a monovalent or a divalent (dimeric) NGF peptidomimetic is functional and most appropriate for clinical use is, as yet, unresolved. Good NGF mimetics at this stage appear to be D3 or its derivatives and LM11A-24 or LM11A-31, although each may potentially be useful for a distinct purpose. Also being developed are TrkB (O'Leary & Hughes, 2003; Fletcher, et al., 2008; Fletcher & Hughes, 2009) and TrkC (Brahimi, et al., 2009; Chen, et al., 2009; Liu, et al., 2010) antagonists/agonists. BDNF mimetics have made progress toward a useful therapeutic reagent with efficacy studies in rodents (Massa et al., 2010). Some of these neurotrophin reagents show receptor selectivity, as well as selective cellular response, i.e. survival vs differentiation (Saragovi et al., 2009). Whether a small peptidomimetic or a modified, full-length NGF protein will ultimately prove to be the most effective clinical reagent for treatment of AD is an open question at present. The pharmacokinetic advantages of a small molecule mimetic may eventually outweigh the limited information content, relative to the full length protein, provided by such a peptide. In other words, will the chemists be able to design sufficient specificity and selectivity into the peptidomimetics to compete with the potential specificity of a 26 kDa neurotrophin protein with its myriad interaction sites? The answer in some cases for selective signaling appears to be yes (Zaccaro et al., 2005; Longo, et al., 2007; Yang et al., 2008). Conversely, will the means of delivery (intracerebroventricular injection, intranasal inhalation, encapsulation) of a full-length neurotrophin mutein be developed sufficiently to make easy administration to the AD brain competitive with a, perhaps, less effective small molecule that is easily delivered? In either case, exquisite signal selectivity to allow ultra-focus may be most effective and/or desirable.

7. Other growth factors with cellular signaling selectivity

Neurotrophins are not the only ligand-receptor system in which molecular engineering approaches have been employed to improve the therapeutic potential. Mutants of both insulin and tumor necrosis factor (TNFα) have also been developed with enhancement of their therapeutic properties. TNFα was re-designed with the intent of improving its death-inducing targeting toward tumors and reducing its systemic side effects (Wajant, et al., 2005; Gerspach, et al., 2009). This attempt is a true challenge with a multifunctional, pleiotropic cytokine such as TNFα; nevertheless some progress has been made. Similarly, insulin has been engineered to improve its stability as a single chain (Hua, et al., 2008), its stability as a zinc 'stapled' hexamer with even longer lasting attributes (Phillips, et al., 2010), and its selectivity for the insulin receptor over the non-cognate IGF-1 receptor (Zhao, et al., 2009). A reported 3-fold improvement in receptor selectivity has the potential of reducing colorectal cancer risk for diabetic patients using insulin replacement therapy (Zhao, et al., 2009). How well these receptor and/or signal selective mutant cytokines/hormones may work in therapeutic trials is still uncertain.

8. Conclusions and the future

The importance of ligand-receptor interactions in AD and other neurodegenerative conditions is well appreciated. Protein levels and mRNA levels for both TrkA and p75 receptors are reduced in early AD even in the presence of stable NGF expression. A shift from mature NGF to proNGF, which binds p75 and induces apoptosis, has also been observed. Thus, the neurodegeneration in the basal forebrain in AD is aggravated by a reduction in signaling from TrkA receptors coupled with apoptotic signaling by proNGF binding to p75 (see Section 2.2). Animal studies and clinical trials of NGF gene delivery show promise in curtailing neuronal apoptosis in Alzheimer's disease or animal models. However, the CBF in some patients demonstrated a trophic response of immature neuritic processes, i.e. neurite outgrowth where it was not needed or useful. Adult brains with AD possessing an established axonal network may be adversely affected by this type of aberrant neuritogenesis. Survival support for existing neurons is preferable without inducing *de novo* connections that might be dysfunctional. A key goal for future intervention of this type is to promote viability of specific neurons without causing neuritic or axonal overgrowth.

The possibility and potential of designer growth factors has been highlighted in this review. Step-wise mutagenesis of NGF led to the generation of survival-selective muteins that are potentially therapeutic lead candidates for Alzheimer Disease or other neurodegenerative disorders. Two mechanism-selective recombinant NGF muteins show a marked difference in the ratio of survival to neuritogenesis in several assays, including signaling through the Akt survival pathway. Thus, in principle one can separate intracellular signaling pathways for a receptor via modifications to its ligand. Successful parallel studies with molecular engineering of insulin and TNFα support this viewpoint. Structural studies of other receptor systems, e.g., EGF, have provided a logical, molecular basis for understanding how these signals may be separately activated. Progress with small molecule mimetics of NGF that are agonists show some of the same receptor- and signaling- selectivity that receptor- or signal-selective muteins of the parent protein do. The future should provide major advances in this exciting area of improving upon nature and developing novel treatments for AD. Coupling of designer neurotrophins with improved delivery to the brain provides great promise.

9. Acknowledgements

We wish to acknowledge the generous support of the NINDS, NIH, USPHS, USA for nearly 20 years through the grant NS24380. We are grateful to many interesting and challenging discussions with other members of the Neet lab who indirectly contributed to this review. Finally, we would like to acknowledge the collegiality of the investigators in the neurotrophin field and all of their accomplishments that are summarized in this review.

10. Nomenclature

7-84-103, NGF mutein, F7A/H84A/R103A
Aβ, beta amyloid
AD, Alzheimer's disease
APP, amyloid precursor protein
Akt, a ser-thr kinase (also PKB)
BDNF, brain derived neurotrophic factor
BBB, blood brain barrier
CBF, cholinergic basal forebrain
ECD, extracellular domain
EGF, epidermal growth factor
EGFR, EGF receptor
GSK3b, glycogen synthase kinase 3b
ICD, intracellular domain
IGF-1, insulin like growth factor 1
JNK, c-Jun N-terminal kinase
KKE, K32A/K34A/E35A NGF mutein
KKE/7-84-103, hextuple mutein, K32A/K34A/E35A/F7A/H84A/R103A NGF mutein
MAPK, mitogen-activated protein kinase
NF-κB, Nuclear factor kappa-light-chain-enhancer of activated B cells
NGF, nerve growth factor (β-subunit)
NT-3, neurotrophin 3
NT-4, neurotrophin 4
p75, common neurotrophin receptor
PC12, pheochromocytoma 12 cell line
PI3K, phosphoinositide 3-kinase
PLCγ, phospholipase C gamma
proNGF, precursor form of NGF
TNFα, tumor necrosis factor alpha
Trk, tropomyosin related kinase
Δ9/13, NGF mutein with residues 9 through 13 deleted

11. References

Aboulkassim, T., Tong, X.-K., Tse, Y. C., Wong, T.-P., Woo, S. B., Neet, K. E., Brahimi, F., Hamel, E., & Saragovi, H. U. (2011). Ligand-dependent TrkA activity in brain impacts differently on spatial learning and long-term memory. *Molecular Pharmacology*, DOI 10.1124/mol.111.071332 in press.

Alam, M.I., Beg, S., Samad, A., Baboota, S., Kohli, K., Ali, J., Ahuja, A., & Akbar, M. (2010). Strategy for effective brain drug delivery. *European Journal of Pharmaceutical Sciences*, Vol. 40, No. 5, pp. 385-403.

Aloyz, R.S., Bamji, S.X., Pozniak, C.D., Toma, J.G., Atwal, J., Kaplan, D.R., & Miller, F.D. (1998). p53 is essential for developmental neuron death as regulated by the TrkA and p75 neurotrophin receptors. *Journal of Cell Biology*, Vol. 143, No. 6, pp. 1691-1703.

Apfel, S.C. (2002). Nerve growth factor for the treatment of diabetic neuropathy: what went wrong, what went right, and what does the future hold? *International Review of Neurobiology*, Vol. 50, pp. 393-413.

Apfel, S.C., Kessler, J.A., Adornato, B.T., Litchy, W.J., Sanders, C., & Rask, C.A. (1998). Recombinant human nerve growth factor in the treatment of diabetic polyneuropathy. NGF Study Group. *Neurology*, Vol. 51, No. 3, pp. 695-702.

Apfel, S.C., Lipton, R.B., Arezzo, J.C., & Kessler, J.A. (1991). Nerve growth factor prevents toxic neuropathy in mice. *Annals of Neurology*, Vol. 29, No. 1, pp. 87-90.

Bae, J., & Schlessinger, J. (2010). Asymmetric tyrosine kinase arrangements in activation or autophosphorylation of receptor tyrosine kinases. *Molecules and Cells*, Vol. 29, No. 5, pp. 443-448.

Bai, Y., Dergham, P., Nedev, H., Xu, J., Galan, A., Rivera, J. C., ZhiHua, S., Mehta, H. M., Woo, S. B., Sarunic, M. V., Neet, K. E., & Saragovi, H. U. (2010). Chronic and acute models of retinal neurodegeneration of TrkA activity are neuroprotective whereas p75NTR activity is neurotoxic through a paracrine mechanism. *Journal of Biological Chemistry*, Vol. 285, No. 50, pp. 39392-39400.

Bamji, S.X., Majdan, M., Pozniak, C.D., Belliveau, D.J., Aloyz, R., Kohn, J., Causing, C.G., & Miller, F.D. (1998). The p75 neurotrophin receptor mediates neuronal apoptosis and is essential for naturally occurring sympathetic neuron death. *J Cell Biol*, Vol. 140, No. 4, pp. 911-923.

Barrett, G.L., & Bartlett, P.F. (1994). The p75 nerve growth factor receptor mediates survival or death depending on the stage of sensory neuron development. *Proceedings of the National Academy of Sciences, U.S.A.*, Vol. 91, No. 14, pp. 6501-6505.

Bartlett, S.E., Reynolds, A.J., Weible, M., Heydon, K., & Hendry, I.A. (1997). In sympathetic but not sensory neurones, phosphoinositide-3 kinase is important for NGF-dependent survival and the retrograde transport of 125I-betaNGF. *Brain Research*, Vol. 761, No. 2, pp. 257-262.

Beglova, N., Maliartchouk, S., Ekiel, I., Zaccaro, M.C., Saragovi, H.U., & Gehring, K. (2000). Design and Solution Structure of Functional Peptide Mimetics of Nerve Growth Factor. *Journal of Medicinal Chemistry*, Vol. 43, No. 19, pp. 3530-3540.

Benedict, C., Frey, W.H., 2nd, Schioth, H.B., Schultes, B., Born, J., & Hallschmid, M. (2011). Intranasal insulin as a therapeutic option in the treatment of cognitive impairments. *Experimental Gerontology*, Vol. 46, No. 2-3, pp. 112-115.

Bibel, M., & Barde, Y.A. (2000). Neurotrophins: key regulators of cell fate and cell shape in the vertebrate nervous system. *Genes & Development*, Vol. 14, No. 23, pp. 2919-2937.

Bierer, L.M., Haroutunian, V., Gabriel, S., Knott, P.J., Carlin, L.S., Purohit, D.P., Perl, D.P., Schmeidler, J., Kanof, P., & Davis, K.L. (1995). Neurochemical correlates of dementia severity in Alzheimer's disease: relative importance of the cholinergic deficits. *Journal of Neurochemistry*, Vol. 64, No. 2, pp. 749-760.

Bishop, K.M., Hofer, E.K., Mehta, A., Ramirez, A., Sun, L., Tuszynski, M., & Bartus, R.T. (2008). Therapeutic potential of CERE-110 (AAV2-NGF): targeted, stable, and sustained NGF delivery and trophic activity on rodent basal forebrain cholinergic neurons. *Experimental Neurology*, Vol. 211, No. 2, pp. 574-584.

Bottger, D., Ullrich, C., & Humpel, C. (2010). Monocytes deliver bioactive nerve growth factor through a brain capillary endothelial cell-monolayer in vitro and counteract degeneration of cholinergic neurons. *Brain Research*, Vol. 1312, pp. 108-119.

Brahimi, F., Liu, J., Malakhov, A., Chowdhury, S., Purisima, E.O., Ivanisevic, L., Caron, A., Burgess, K., & Saragovi, H.U. (2010). A monovalent agonist of TrkA tyrosine kinase receptors can be converted into a bivalent antagonist. *Biochimica et Biophysica Acta (BBA) - General Subjects*, Vol. 1800, No. 9, pp. 1018-1026.

Brahimi, F., Malakhov, A., Lee, H. B., Pattarawarapan, M., Ivanisevic, L., Burgess, K., & Saragovi, H. U. (2009). A peptidomimetic of NT-3 acts as a TrkC antagonist. *Peptides*, Vol. 30, No. 10, pp. 1833-1839.

Bruno, M. A., Clarke, P. B., Seltzer, A., Quirion, R., Burgess, K., Cuello, A. C., & Saragovi, H. U. (2004). Long-lasting rescue of age-associated deficits in cognition and the CNS cholinergic phenotype by a partial agonist peptidomimetic ligand of TrkA. *Journal of Neuroscience*, Vol. 24, No. 37, pp. 8009-8018.

Calissano, P., Amadoro, G., Matrone, C., Ciafrè, S., Marolda, R., Corsetti, V., Ciotti, M. T., Mercanti, D., Di Luzio, A., Severini, C., Provenzano, C., & Canu, N. (2010a) Does the term trophic actually mean anti-amyloidogenic? The case of NGF. *Cell Death & Differentiation* Vol. 17, No. 7, pp. 1126-33.

Calissano, P., Matrone, C., & Amadoro, G. (2010b). Nerve growth factor as a paradigm of neurotrophins related to Alzheimer's disease. *Developmental Neurobiology*, Vol. 70, No. 5, pp. 372-383.

Canossa, M., Griesbeck, O., Berninger, B., Campana, G., Kolbeck, R., & Thoenen, H. (1997). Neurotrophin release by neurotrophins: implications for activity-dependent neuronal plasticity. *Proceedings of the National Academy of Sciences, U.S.A.*, Vol. 94, No. 24, pp. 13279-13286.

Capsoni, S., Covaceuszach, S., Marinelli, S., Ceci, M., Bernardo, A., Minghetti, L., Ugolini, G., Pavone, F., & Cattaneo, A. (2011). Taking Pain Out of NGF: A "Painless" NGF Mutant, Linked to Hereditary Sensory Autonomic Neuropathy Type V, with Full Neurotrophic Activity. *PLoS ONE*, Vol. 6, No. 2, pp. e17321.

Casaccia-Bonnefil, P., Carter, B.D., Dobrowsky, R.T., & Chao, M.V. (1996). Death of oligodendrocytes mediated by the interaction of nerve growth factor with its receptor p75. *Nature*, Vol. 383, No. 6602, pp. 716-719.

Casademunt, E., Carter, B.D., Benzel, I., Frade, J.M., Dechant, G., & Barde, Y.A. (1999). The zinc finger protein NRIF interacts with the neurotrophin receptor p75(NTR) and participates in programmed cell death. *EMBO Journal*, Vol. 18, No. 21, pp. 6050-6061.

Cattaneo, A., Capsoni, S., & Paoletti, F. (2008). Towards Non Invasive Nerve Growth Factor Therapies for Alzheimer's Disease. *Journal of Alzheimer's Disease*, Vol. 15, No. 2, pp. 255-283.

Chen, D., Brahimi, F., Angell, Y., Li, Y. C., Moscowicz, J., Saragovi, H. U., & Burgess, K. (2009). Bivalent peptidomimetic ligands of TrkC are biased agonists and selectively induce neuritogenesis or potentiate neurotrophin-3 trophic signals. *ACS Chemical Biology*, Vol. 4, No. 9, pp. 769-781.

Chittka, A., & Chao, M.V. (1999). Identification of a zinc finger protein whose subcellular distribution is regulated by serum and nerve growth factor. *Proceedings of the National Academy of Sciences, U.S.A.*, Vol. 96, No. 19, pp. 10705-10710.

Colangelo, A. M., Bianco, M. R., Vitagliano, L., Cavaliere, C., Cirillo, G., De Gioia, L., Diana, D., Colombo, D., Redaelli, C., Zaccaro, L., Morelli, G., Papa, M., Sarmientos, P., Alberghina, L., & Martegani, E. (2008). A new nerve growth factor-mimetic peptide active on neuropathic pain in rats. *Journal of Neuroscience*, Vol. 28, No. 11, pp. 2698-2709.

Cordon-Cardo, C., Tapley, P., Jing, S.Q., Nanduri, V., O'Rourke, E., Lamballe, F., Kovary, K., Klein, R., Jones, K.R., Reichardt, L.F., & Barbacid, M. (1991). The trk tyrosine protein kinase mediates the mitogenic properties of nerve growth factor and neurotrophin-3. *Cell*, Vol. 66, No. 1, pp. 173-183.

Coulson, J., May, L. M., Sykes, A. M., & Hamlin, A. S. (2009). The role of the p75 neurotrophin receptor in cholinergic dysfunction in Alzheimer's disease. *Neuroscientist*, Vol. 15, No. 4, pp. 317-23.

Covaceuszach, S., Capsoni, S., Marinelli, S., Pavone, F., Ceci, M., Ugolini, G., Vignone, D., Amato, G., Paoletti, F., Lamba, D., & Cattaneo, A. (2010). In vitro receptor binding properties of a "painless" NGF mutein, linked to hereditary sensory autonomic neuropathy type V. *Biochemical and Biophysical Research Communications*, Vol. 391, No. 1, pp. 824-829.

Crowder, R.J., & Freeman, R.S. (1998). Phosphatidylinositol 3-kinase and Akt protein kinase are necessary and sufficient for the survival of nerve growth factor-dependent sympathetic neurons. *Journal of Neuroscience*, Vol. 18, No. 8, pp. 2933-2943.

Cuello, A., Bruno, M., Allard, S., Leon, W., & Iulita, M. (2010). Cholinergic Involvement in Alzheimer's Disease. A Link with NGF Maturation and Degradation. *Journal of Molecular Neuroscience*, Vol. 40, No. 1, pp. 230-235.

Cunningham, M.E., & Greene, L.A. (1998). A function-structure model for NGF-activated TRK. *EMBO Journal*, Vol. 17, No. 24, pp. 7282-7293.

Cunningham, M.E., Stephens, R.M., Kaplan, D.R., & Greene, L.A. (1997). Autophosphorylation of activation loop tyrosines regulates signaling by the TRK nerve growth factor receptor. *Journal of Biological Chemistry*, Vol. 272, No. 16, pp. 10957-10967.

Davey, F., & Davies, A.M. (1998). TrkB signalling inhibits p75-mediated apoptosis induced by nerve growth factor in embryonic proprioceptive neurons. *Current Biology*, Vol. 8, No. 16, pp. 915-918.

de Chaves, E.I., Bussiere, M., Vance, D.E., Campenot, R.B., & Vance, J.E. (1997). Elevation of ceramide within distal neurites inhibits neurite growth in cultured rat sympathetic neurons. *Journal of Biological Chemistry*, Vol. 272, No. 5, pp. 3028-3035.

Dechant, G., Barde, Y. A. (2002). The neurotrophin receptor p75(NTR): novel functions and implications for diseases of the nervous system. *Nature Neuroscience*, Vol. 5, No. 11, pp. 1131-1136.

DeKosky, S.T., Ikonomovic, M.D., Styren, S.D., Beckett, L., Wisniewski, S., Bennett, D.A., Cochran, E.J., Kordower, J.H., & Mufson, E.J. (2002). Upregulation of choline acetyltransferase activity in hippocampus and frontal cortex of elderly subjects with mild cognitive impairment. *Annals of Neurology*, Vol. 51, No. 2, pp. 145-155.

Diamond, J., Foerster, A., Holmes, M., & Coughlin, M. (1992). Sensory nerves in adult rats regenerate and restore sensory function to the skin independently of endogenous NGF. *Journal of Neuroscience*, Vol. 12, No. 4, pp. 1467-1476.

Diarra, A., Geetha, T., Potter, P., & Babu, J. R. (2009). Signaling of the neurotrophin receptor p75 in relation to Alzheimer's disease. *Biochemical and Biophysical Research Communications*, Vol. 390, No. 3, pp. 352-356.

Domeniconi, M., Zampieri, N., Spencer, T., Hilaire, M., Mellado, W., Chao, M.V., & Filbin, M.T. (2005). MAG induces regulated intramembrane proteolysis of the p75 neurotrophin receptor to inhibit neurite outgrowth. *Neuron*, Vol. 46, No. 6, pp. 849-855.

Einarsdottir, E., Carlsson, A., Minde, J., Toolanen, G., Svensson, O., Solders, G., Holmgren, G., Holmberg, D., & Holmberg, M. (2004). A mutation in the nerve growth factor beta gene (NGFB) causes loss of pain perception. *Human Molecular Genetics*, Vol. 13, No. 8, pp. 799-805.

Emerich, D.F., Winn, S.R., Harper, J., Hammang, J.P., Baetge, E.E., & Kordower, J.H. (1994). Implants of polymer-encapsulated human NGF-secreting cells in the nonhuman primate: rescue and sprouting of degenerating cholinergic basal forebrain neurons. *Journal of Computational Neurology*, Vol. 349, No. 1, pp. 148-164.

Emilien, G., Maloteaux, J.M., Beyreuther, K., & Masters, C.L. (2000). Alzheimer disease: mouse models pave the way for therapeutic opportunities. *Archives of Neurology*, Vol. 57, No. 2, pp. 176-181.

Eriksdotter Jonhagen, M., Nordberg, A., Amberla, K., Backman, L., Ebendal, T., Meyerson, B., Olson, L., Seiger, Shigeta, M., Theodorsson, E., Viitanen, M., Winblad, B., & Wahlund, L. O. (1998). Intracerebroventricular infusion of nerve growth factor in three patients with Alzheimer's disease. *Dementia and Geriatric Cognitive Disorders*, Vol. 9, No. 5, pp. 246-257.

Fahnestock, M., Michalski, B., Xu, B., & Coughlin, M.D. (2001). The Precursor Pro-Nerve Growth Factor Is the Predominant Form of Nerve Growth Factor in Brain and Is Increased in Alzheimer's Disease. *Molecular and Cellular Neuroscience*, Vol. 18, No. 2, pp. 210-220.

Fan, Y.-X., Wong, L., Deb, T.B., & Johnson, G.R. (2004). Ligand Regulates Epidermal Growth Factor Receptor Kinase Specificity. *Journal of Biological Chemistry*, Vol. 279, No. 37, pp. 38143-38150.

Fjord-Larsen, L., Kusk, P., Tornoe, J., Juliusson, B., Torp, M., Bjarkam, C.R., Nielsen, M.S., Handberg, A., Sorensen, J.C.H., & Wahlberg, L.U. (2010). Long-term Delivery of Nerve Growth Factor by Encapsulated Cell Biodelivery in the Gottingen Minipig Basal Forebrain. *Molecular Therapy*, Vol. 18, No. 12, pp. 2164-2172.

Fletcher, J. M., Morton, C. J., Zwar, R. A., Murray, S. S., O'Leary, P. D., & Hughes, R. A. (2008). Design of a conformationally defined and proteolytically stable circular mimetic of brain-derived neurotrophic factor. *Journal of Biological Chemistry*, Vol. 283, No 48, pp. 33375-33383.

Fletcher, J. M. & Hughes, R. A. (2009). Modified low molecular weight cyclic peptides as mimetics of BDNF with improved potency, proteolytic stability and transmembrane passage in vitro. *Bioorganic Medicinal Chemistry*, Vol. 17, No. 7, pp. 2695-2702.

Friden, P., Walus, L., Watson, P., Doctrow, Kozarich, J., Backman, C., Bergman, H., Hoffer, B., Bloom, F., & Granholm, A. (1993). Blood-brain barrier penetration and in vivo activity of an NGF conjugate. *Science*, Vol. 259, No. 5093, pp. 373-377.

Friedman, W.J., & Greene, L.A. (1999). Neurotrophin signaling via Trks and p75. *Experimental Cell Research*, Vol. 253, No. 1, pp. 131-142.

Funakoshi, H., Risling, M., Carlstedt, T., Lendahl, U., Timmusk, T., Metsis, M., Yamamoto, Y., & Ibanez, C. F. (1998). Targeted expression of a multifunctional chimeric neurotrophin in the lesioned sciatic nerve accelerates regeneration of sensory and motor axons. *Proceedings of the National Academy of Sciences, U.S.A.*, Vol. 95, No. 9, pp. 5269-5274.

Garzon, D.J., & Fahnestock, M. (2007). Oligomeric Amyloid Decreases Basal Levels of Brain-Derived Neurotrophic factor (BDNF) mRNA via Specific Downregulation of BDNF Transcripts IV and V in Differentiated Human Neuroblastoma Cells. *The Journal of Neuroscience*, Vol. 27, No. 10, pp. 2628-2635.

Gerspach, J., Pfizenmaier, K., & Wajant, H. (2009). Improving TNF as a cancer therapeutic: tailor-made TNF fusion proteins with conserved antitumor activity and reduced systemic side effects. *Biofactors*. 35, No. 4, pp. 364-372.

Ginsberg, S.D., Che, S., Wuu, J., Counts, S.E., & Mufson, E.J. (2006). Down regulation of trk but not p75NTR gene expression in single cholinergic basal forebrain neurons mark the progression of Alzheimer's disease. *Journal of Neurochemistry*, Vol. 97, No. 2, pp. 475-487.

Gomez, N., & Cohen, P. (1991). Dissection of the protein kinase cascade by which nerve growth factor activates MAP kinases. *Nature*, Vol. 353, No. 6340, pp. 170-173.

Grewal, S.S., York, R.D., & Stork, P.J. (1999). Extracellular-signal-regulated kinase signalling in neurons. *Current Opinion in Neurobiology*, Vol. 9, No. 5, pp. 544-553.

Grimes, M.L., Beattie, E., & Mobley, W.C. (1997). A signaling organelle containing the nerve growth factor-activated receptor tyrosine kinase, TrkA. *Proceedings of the National Academy of Sciences, U.S.A.*, Vol. 94, No. 18, pp. 9909-9914.

Guo, M., Meyer, S.L., Kaur, H., Gao, J.J., & Neet, K.E. (1996). Mutational studies of conserved residues in the dimer interface of nerve growth factor. *Protein Science*, Vol. 5, No. 3, pp. 447-455.

Hefti, F. (1983). Is Alzheimer disease caused by lack of nerve growth factor? *Annals of Neurology*, Vol. 13, No. 1, pp. 109-110.

Holgado-Madruga, M., Moscatello, D.K., Emlet, D.R., Dieterich, R., & Wong, A.J. (1997). Grb2-associated binder-1 mediates phosphatidylinositol 3-kinase activation and the promotion of cell survival by nerve growth factor. *Proceedings of the National Academy of Sciences, U.S.A.*, Vol. 94, No. 23, pp. 12419-12424.

Hua, Q. X., Nakagawa, S. H., Jia, W., Huang, K., Phillips, N. B., Hu, S. Q., & Weiss, M. A. (2008). Design of an active ultrastable single-chain insulin analog: synthesis, structure, and therapeutic implications. *Journal of Biological Chemistry*, Vol. 283, No. 21, pp. 14703-14716.

Huang, E.J., & Reichardt, L.F. (2003). Trk receptors: roles in neuronal signal transduction. *Annual Review of Biochemistry*, Vol. 72, pp. 609-642.

Hubbard, S.R., Wei, L., Ellis, L., & Hendrickson, W.A. (1994). Crystal structure of the tyrosine kinase domain of the human insulin receptor. *Nature*, Vol. 372, No. 6508, pp. 746-754.

Hughes, A. L., Messineo-Jones, D., Lad, S. P., & Neet, K. E. (2001). Distinction between differentiation, cell cycle, and apoptosis signals in PC12 cells by the nerve growth factor mutant delta9/13, which is selective for the p75 neurotrophin receptor. *Journal of Neuroscience Research*, Vol. 63, No. 1, pp. 10-19.

Hyman, C., Hofer, M., Barde, Y.-A., Juhasz, M., Yancopoulos, G.D., Squinto, S.P., & Lindsay, R.M. (1991). BDNF is a neurotrophic factor for dopaminergic neurons of the substantia nigra. *Nature*, Vol. 350, No. 6315, pp. 230-232.

Ibanez, C.F., Hallbook, F., Ebendal, T., & Persson, H. (1990). Structure-function studies of nerve growth factor: functional importance of highly conserved amino acid residues. *EMBO Journal*, Vol. 9, No. 5, pp. 1477-1483.

Ibanez, C.F., Ebendal, T., & Persson, H. (1991). Chimeric molecules with multiple neurotrophic activities reveal structural elements determining the specificities of NGF and BDNF. *EMBO Journal*, Vol. 10, No. 8, pp. 2105-2110.

Ibanez, C.F., Ebendal, T., Barbany, G., Murray-Rust, J., Blundell, T.L., & Persson, H. (1992). Disruption of the low affinity receptor-binding site in NGF allows neuronal survival and differentiation by binding to the trk gene product. *Cell*, Vol. 69, No. 2, pp. 329-341.

Ibanez, C.F., Ilag, L.L., Murray-Rust, J., & Persson, H. (1993). An extended surface of binding to Trk tyrosine kinase receptors in NGF and BDNF allows the engineering of a multifunctional pan-neurotrophin. *EMBO Journal*, Vol. 12, No. 6, pp. 2281-2293.

Ibanez, C.F. (1994). Structure-function relationships in the neurotrophin family. *Journal of Neurobiolgy*, Vol. 25, No. 11, pp. 1349-1361.

Ilag, L.L., Lonnerberg, P., Persson, H., & Ibanez, C.F. (1994). Role of variable beta-hairpin loop in determining biological specificities in neurotrophin family. *Journal of Biological Chemistry*, Vol. 269, No. 31, pp. 19941-19946.

Ilag, L. L., Curtis, R., Glass, D., Funakoshi, H., Tobkes, N. J., Ryan, T. E., Acheson, A., Lindsay, R. M., Persson, H., Yancopoulos, G. D., DiStefano, P. S. & Ibanez, C. F. (1995). Pan-neurotrophin 1: a genetically engineered neurotrophic factor displaying multiple specificities in peripheral neurons in vitro and in vivo. *Proceedings of the National Academy of Sciences, U.S.A.*, Vol. 92, No. 2, pp. 607-611.

Indo, Y. (2002). Genetics of congenital insensitivity to pain with anhidrosis (CIPA) or hereditary sensory and autonomic neuropathy type IV. Clinical, biological and molecular aspects of mutations in TRKA(NTRK1) gene encoding the receptor tyrosine kinase for nerve growth factor. *Clinical Autonomic Research*, Vol. 12, Suppl 1, pp. I20-32.

Jordão, J.F., Ayala-Grosso, C.A., Markham, K., Huang, Y., Chopra, R., McLaurin, J., Hynynen, K., & Aubert, I. (2010). Antibodies Targeted to the Brain with Image-Guided Focused Ultrasound Reduces Amyloid-β Plaque Load in the TgCRND8 Mouse Model of Alzheimer's Disease. *PLoS ONE*, Vol. 5, No. 5, pp. e10549.

Jura, N., Zhang, X., Endres, Nicholas F., Seeliger, Markus A., Schindler, T., & Kuriyan, J. (2011). Catalytic Control in the EGF Receptor and Its Connection to General Kinase Regulatory Mechanisms. *Molecular Cell*, Vol. 42, No. 1, pp. 9-22.

Kahle, P., Burton, L.E., Schmelzer, C.H., & Hertel, C. (1992). The amino terminus of nerve growth factor is involved in the interaction with the receptor tyrosine kinase p140trkA. *Journal of Biological Chemistry*, Vol. 267, No. 32, pp. 22707-22710.

Kao, S., Jaiswal, R.K., Kolch, W., & Landreth, G.E. (2001). Identification of the mechanisms regulating the differential activation of the mapk cascade by epidermal growth factor and nerve growth factor in PC12 cells. *Journal of Biological Chemistry*, Vol. 276, No. 21, pp. 18169-18177.

Kaplan, D.R., Hempstead, B.L., Martin-Zanca, D., Chao, M.V., & Parada, L.F. (1991). The trk proto-oncogene product: a signal transducing receptor for nerve growth factor. *Science*, Vol. 252, No. 5005, pp. 554-558.

Kaplan, D.R., & Miller, F.D. (2000). Neurotrophin signal transduction in the nervous system. *Current Opinion in Neurobiology*, Vol. 10, No. 3, pp. 381-391.

Katz, D.M., Erb, M., Lillis, R., & Neet, K. (1990). Trophic regulation of nodose ganglion cell development: evidence for an expanded role of nerve growth factor during embryogenesis in the rat. *Experimental Neurology*, Vol. 110, No. 1, pp. 1-10.

Khursigara, G., Orlinick, J.R., & Chao, M.V. (1999). Association of the p75 neurotrophin receptor with TRAF6. *Journal of Biological Chemistry*, Vol. 274, No. 5, pp. 2597-2600.

Korsching, S. (1993). The neurotrophic factor concept: a reexamination. *Journal of Neuroscience*, Vol. 13, No. 7, pp. 2739-2748.

Kullander, K., & Ebendal, T. (1994). Neurotrophin-3 acquires NGF-like activity after exchange to five NGF amino acid residues: molecular analysis of the sites in NGF mediating the specific interaction with the NGF high affinity receptor. *Journal of Neuroscience Research*, Vol. 39, No. 2, pp. 195-210.

Kullander, K., Kaplan, D., & Ebendal, T. (1997). Two restricted sites on the surface of the nerve growth factor molecule independently determine specific TrkA receptor binding and activation. *Journal of Biological Chemistry*, Vol. 272, No. 14, pp. 9300-9307.

Lad, S. P. & Neet, K. E. (2003). Activation of the mitogen-activated protein kinase pathway through p75NTR: a common mechanism for the neurotrophin family. *Journal of Neuroscience Research*, Vol. 73, No. 5, pp. 614-626.

Lad, S.P., Neet, K.E., & Mufson, E.J. (2003a). Nerve growth factor: structure, function and therapeutic implications for Alzheimer's disease. *Current Drug Targets- CNS and Neurological Disorders*, Vol. 2, No. 5, pp. 315-334.

Lad, S.P., Peterson, D.A., Bradshaw, R.A., & Neet, K.E. (2003b). Individual and combined effects of TrkA and p75NTR nerve growth factor receptors. A role for the high affinity receptor site. *Journal of Biological Chemistry*, Vol. 278, No. 27, pp. 24808-24817.

Lane, N.E., Schnitzer, T.J., Birbara, C.A., Mokhtarani, M., Shelton, D.L., Smith, M.D., & Brown, M.T. (2010). Tanezumab for the Treatment of Pain from Osteoarthritis of the Knee. *New England Journal of Medicine*, Vol. 363, No. 16, pp. 1521-1531.

Lemmon, M.A., & Schlessinger, J. (2010). Cell Signaling by Receptor Tyrosine Kinases. *Cell*, Vol. 141, No. 7, pp. 1117-1134.

LeSauteur, L., Wei, L., Gibbs, B.F., & Saragovi, H.U. (1995). Small Peptide Mimics of Nerve Growth Factor Bind TrkA Receptors and Affect Biological Responses. *Journal of Biological Chemistry*, Vol. 270, No. 12, pp. 6564-6569.

Levi-Montalcini, R. (1987). The nerve growth factor 35 years later. *Science*, Vol. 237, No. 4819, pp. 1154-1162.

Liao, G.S., Li, X.B., Zhang, C.Y., Shu, Y.Y., & Tang, S.X. (2001). Pharmacological actions of nerve growth factor-transferrin conjugate on the central nervous system. *Journal of Natural Toxins*, Vol. 10, No. 4, pp. 291-297.

Lindsay, R.M. (1988). Nerve growth factors (NGF, BDNF) enhance axonal regeneration but are not required for survival of adult sensory neurons. *Journal of Neuroscience*, Vol. 8, No. 7, pp. 2394-2405.

Liu, J., Brahimi, F., Saragovi, H. U., & Burgess K. (2010) Bivalent diketopiperazine-based tropomysin receptor kinase C (TrkC) antagonists. *Journal of Medicinal Chemistry*, Vol. 53, No. 13, pp. 5044-5048.

Loeb, D.M., Stephens, R.M., Copeland, T., Kaplan, D.R., & Greene, L.A. (1994). A Trk nerve growth factor (NGF) receptor point mutation affecting interaction with phospholipase C-gamma 1 abolishes NGF-promoted peripherin induction but not neurite outgrowth. *Journal of Biological Chemistry*, Vol. 269, No. 12, pp. 8901-8910.

Longo, F. M., Yang, T., Knowles, J. K., Xie, Y., Moore, L. A., & Massa, S. M. (2007). Small molecule neurotrophin receptor ligands: novel strategies for targeting Alzheimer's disease mechanisms. *Currents in Alzheimer Research*, Vol 4, No. 5, pp. 503-506.

Mahapatra, S. (2008). *Identification of Critical Residues within the Conserved and Specificity Patches of Nerve Growth Factor Leading to Survival or Differentiation*. Ph.D. Thesis, Rosalind Franklin University of Medicine and Science, North Chicago.

Mahapatra, S., Mehta, H., Woo, S.B., & Neet, K.E. (2009). Identification of Critical Residues within the Conserved and Specificity Patches of Nerve Growth Factor Leading to Survival or Differentiation. *Journal of Biological Chemistry*, Vol. 284, No. 48, pp. 33600-33613.

Maliartchouk, S., Debeir, T., Beglova, N., Cuello, A.C., Gehring, K., & Saragovi, H.U. (2000). Genuine Monovalent Ligands of TrkA Nerve Growth Factor Receptors Reveal a Novel Pharmacological Mechanism of Action. *Journal of Biological Chemistry*, Vol. 275, No. 14, pp. 9946-9956.

Massa, S.M., Xie, Y., Yang, T., Harrington, A.W., Kim, M.L., Yoon, S.O., Kraemer, R., Moore, L.A., Hempstead, B.L., & Longo, F.M. (2006). Small, Nonpeptide p75NTR Ligands Induce Survival Signaling and Inhibit proNGF-Induced Death. *The Journal of Neuroscience*, Vol. 26, No. 20, pp. 5288-5300.

Massa, S.M., Yang, T., Xie, Y., Shi, J., Bilgen, M., Joyce, J.N., Nehama, D., Rajadas, J., & Longo, F.M. (2010). Small molecule BDNF mimetics activate TrkB signaling and prevent neuronal degeneration in rodents. *The Journal of Clinical Investigation*, Vol. 120, No. 5, pp. 1774-1785.

McDonald, N.Q., Lapatto, R., Murray-Rust, J., Gunning, J., Wlodawer, A., & Blundell, T.L. (1991). New protein fold revealed by a 2.3-A resolution crystal structure of nerve growth factor. *Nature*, Vol. 354, No. 6352, pp. 411-414.

Mufson, E.J., Conner, J.M., & Kordower, J.H. (1995). Nerve growth factor in Alzheimer's disease: defective retrograde transport to nucleus basalis. *Neuroreport*, Vol. 6, No. 7, pp. 1063-1066.

Mufson, E.J., Counts, S.E., Fahnestock, M., & Ginsberg, S.D. (2007). Cholinotrophic molecular substrates of mild cognitive impairment in the elderly. *Current Alzheimer Research*, Vol. 4, No. 4, pp. 340-350.

Mufson, E.J., Counts, S.E., Perez, S.E., & Ginsberg, S.D. (2008). Cholinergic system during the progression of Alzheimer's disease: therapeutic implications. *Expert Review of Neurotherapeutics*, Vol. 8, No. 11, pp. 1703-1718.

Mufson, E.J., Ma, S.Y., Cochran, E.J., Bennett, D.A., Beckett, L.A., Jaffar, S., Saragovi, H.U., & Kordower, J.H. (2000). Loss of nucleus basalis neurons containing trkA immunoreactivity in individuals with mild cognitive impairment and early Alzheimer's disease. *Journal of Computational Neurology*, Vol. 427, No. 1, pp. 19-30.

Mufson, E.J., Ma, S.Y., Dills, J., Cochran, E.J., Leurgans, S., Wuu, J., Bennett, D.A., Jaffar, S., Gilmor, M.L., Levey, A.I., & Kordower, J.H. (2002). Loss of basal forebrain p75NTR immunoreactivity in subjects with mild cognitive impairment and Alzheimer's disease. *The Journal of Comparative Neurology*, Vol. 443, No. 2, pp. 136-153.

Muller, G., Storz, P., Bourteele, S., Doppler, H., Pfizenmaier, K., Mischak, H., Philipp, A., Kaiser, C., & Kolch, W. (1998). Regulation of Raf-1 kinase by TNF via its second messenger ceramide and cross-talk with mitogenic signalling. *EMBO Journal*, Vol. 17, No. 3, pp. 732-742.

Nagahara, A.H., & Tuszynski, M.H. (2011). Potential therapeutic uses of BDNF in neurological and psychiatric disorders. *Nature Reviews Drug Discovery*, Vol. 10, No. 3, pp. 209-219.

Nicol, G.D., & Vasko, M.R. (2007). Unraveling the Story of NGF-mediated Sensitization of Nociceptive Sensory Neurons: ON or OFF the Trks? *Molecular Interventions*, Vol. 7, No. 1, pp. 26-41.

Nilsson, P., Iwata, N., Muramatsu, S.-i., Tjernberg, L.O., Winblad, B., & Saido, T.C. (2010). Gene therapy in Alzheimer's disease – potential for disease modification. *Journal of Cellular and Molecular Medicine*, Vol. 14, No. 4, pp. 741-757.

Ninkina, N., Grashchuck, M., Buchman, V.L., & Davies, A.M. (1997). TrkB variants with deletions in the leucine-rich motifs of the extracellular domain. *Journal of Biological Chemistry*, Vol. 272, No. 20, pp. 13019-13025.

O'Leary, P. D. & Hughes, R. A. (2003). Design of Potent Peptide Mimetics of Brain-derived Neurotrophic Factor. *Journal of Biological Chemistry*, Vol. 278, No. 28, pp. 25738–25744.

Parain, K., Murer, M.G., Yan, Q., Faucheux, B., Agid, Y., Hirsch, E., & Raisman-Vozari, R. (1999). Reduced expression of brain-derived neurotrophic factor protein in Parkinson's disease substantia nigra. *Neuroreport*, Vol. 10, No. 3, pp. 557-561.

Peleshok, J., & Saragovi, H.U. (2006). Functional mimetics of neurotrophins and their receptors. *Biochemical Society Transactions*, Vol. 34, No. Pt 4, pp. 612-617.

Peng, S., Wuu, J., Mufson, E.J., & Fahnestock, M. (2004). Increased proNGF Levels in Subjects with Mild Cognitive Impairment and Mild Alzheimer Disease. *Journal of Neuropathology & Experimental Neurology*, Vol. 63, No. 6, pp. 641-649.

Peng, S., Wuu, J., Mufson, E.J., & Fahnestock, M. (2005). Precursor form of brain-derived neurotrophic factor and mature brain-derived neurotrophic factor are decreased in the pre-clinical stages of Alzheimer's disease. *Journal of Neurochemistry*, Vol. 93, No. 6, pp. 1412-1421.

Pezet, S., & McMahon, S.B. (2006). Neurotrophins: Mediators and Modulators of Pain. *Annual Review of Neuroscience*, Vol. 29, pp. 507-538.

Phillips, N. B., Wan, Z. L., Whittaker, L., Hu, S. Q., Huang, K., Hua, Q. X , Whittaker, J., Ismail-Beigi, F., & Weiss, M. A. (2010). Supramolecular protein engineering: design of zinc-stapled insulin hexamers as a long acting depot. *Journal of Biological Chemistry*, Vol. 285, No. 16, pp. 11755-11759.

Qian, X., Riccio, A., Zhang, Y., & Ginty, D.D. (1998). Identification and characterization of novel substrates of Trk receptors in developing neurons. *Neuron*, Vol. 21, No. 5, pp. 1017-1029.

Rabizadeh, S., Oh, J., Zhong, L.T., Yang, J., Bitler, C.M., Butcher, L.L., & Bredesen, D.E. (1993). Induction of apoptosis by the low-affinity NGF receptor. *Science*, Vol. 261, No. 5119, pp. 345-348.

Rodriguez-Viciana, P., Warne, P.H., Dhand, R., Vanhaesebroeck, B., Gout, I., Fry, M.J., Waterfield, M.D., & Downward, J. (1994). Phosphatidylinositol-3-OH kinase as a direct target of Ras. *Nature*, Vol. 370, No. 6490, pp. 527-532.

Rydén, M., Hempstead, B., & Ibáñez, C. F. (1997). Differential modulation of neuron survival during development by nerve growth factor binding to the p75 neurotrophin receptor. *Journal of Biological Chemistry*, Vol. 272, No. 26, 16322-16328.

Salehi, A., Ocampo, M., Verhaagen, J., & Swaab, D.F. (2000). P75 neurotrophin receptor in the nucleus basalis of meynert in relation to age, sex, and Alzheimer's disease. *Experimental Neurology*, Vol. 161, No. 1, pp. 245-258.

Salehi, A. H., Xanthoudakis. S., & Barker, P. A. (2002). NRAGE, a p75 neurotrophin receptor-interacting protein, induces caspase activation and cell death through a JNK-dependent mitochondrial pathway. *Journal of Biological Chemistry*, Vol. 277, No. 50, pp. 48043-48050.

Saragovi, H.U., Hamel, E., & Di Polo, A. (2009). A neurotrophic rationale for the therapy of neurodegenerative disorders. *Current Alzheimer Research*, Vol. 6, No. 5, pp. 419-423.

Schecterson, L. C. & Bothwell, M. (2010). Neurotrophin receptors: Old friends with new partners. *Developmental Neurobiology*, Vol. 70, No. 5, pp. 332-338.

Schindowski, K., Belarbi, K., & Buée, L. (2008). Neurotrophic factors in Alzheimer's disease: role of axonal transport. *Genes, Brain and Behavior*, Vol. 7, pp. 43-56.

Schulte-Herbruggen, O., Jockers-Scherubl, M.C., & Hellweg, R. (2008). Neurotrophins: from pathophysiology to treatment in Alzheimer's disease. *Current Alzheimer Research*, Vol. 5, No. 1, pp. 38-44.

Scott, J., Selby, M., Urdea, M., Quiroga, M., Bell, G.I., & Rutter, W.J. (1983). Isolation and nucleotide sequence of a cDNA encoding the precursor of mouse nerve growth factor. *Nature*, Vol. 302, No. 5908, pp. 538-540.

Scott, S.A., Mufson, E.J., Weingartner, J.A., Skau, K.A., & Crutcher, K.A. (1995). Nerve growth factor in Alzheimer's disease: increased levels throughout the brain coupled with declines in nucleus basalis. *Journal of Neuroscience*, Vol. 15, No. 9, pp. 6213-6221.

Segal, R.A. (2003). Selectivity in neurotrophin signaling: theme and variations. *Annual Review of Neuroscience*, Vol. 26, pp. 299-330.

Shih, A., Laramee, G.R., Schmelzer, C.H., Burton, L.E., & Winslow, J.W. (1994). Mutagenesis identifies amino-terminal residues of nerve growth factor necessary for Trk receptor binding and biological activity. *Journal of Biological Chemistry*, Vol. 269, No. 44, pp. 27679-27686.

Simi, A., & Ibanez, C.F. (2010). Assembly and activation of neurotrophic factor receptor complexes. *Developmental Neurobiology*, Vol. 70, No. 5, pp. 323-331.

Soilu-Hanninen, M., Ekert, P., Bucci, T., Syroid, D., Bartlett, P.F., & Kilpatrick, T.J. (1999). Nerve growth factor signaling through p75 induces apoptosis in Schwann cells via a Bcl-2-independent pathway. *Journal of Neuroscience*, Vol. 19, No. 12, pp. 4828-4838.

Soppet, D., Escandon, E., Maragos, J., Middlemas, D.S., Reid, S.W., Blair, J., Burton, L.E., Stanton, B.R., Kaplan, D.R., Hunter, T., Nikolics, K., & Parada L.F. (1991). The neurotrophic factors brain-derived neurotrophic factor and neurotrophin-3 are ligands for the trkB tyrosine kinase receptor. *Cell*, Vol. 65, No. 5, pp. 895-903.

Susen K., Heumann, R., & Blöchl, A. (1999). Nerve growth factor stimulates MAPK via the low affinity receptor p75(LNTR). *FEBS Letters*. Vol. 463, No. 3, pp. 231-234.

Susen, K. & Blöchl, A. (2005). Low concentrations of aggregated beta-amyloid induce neurite formation via the neurotrophin receptor p75. *Journal of Molecular Medicine*, Vol. 83, No. 9, pp. 720-735.

Suter, U., Angst, C., Tien, C., Drinkwater, C., Lindsay, R., & Shooter, E. (1992). NGF/BDNF chimeric proteins: analysis of neurotrophin specificity by homolog-scanning mutagenesis. *The Journal of Neuroscience*, Vol. 12, No. 1, pp. 306-318.

Teng, K. K., Felice, S., Kim, T., & Hempstead, B. L. (2010). Understanding proneurotrophin actions: Recent advances and challenges. *Developmental Neurobiology*, Vol. 70, No. 5, pp. 350-359.

Thoenen, H., & Sendtner, M. (2002). Neurotrophins: from enthusiastic expectations through sobering experiences to rational therapeutic approaches. *Nature Neuroscience*, Vol. 5, No. 11s, pp. 1046-1050.

Tuszynski, M.H., Conner, J., Blesch, A., Smith, D., Merrill, D.A., & Vahlsing, H.L. (2002). New strategies in neural repair. *Progress in Brain Research*, Vol. 138, pp. 401-409.

Tuszynski, M.H., Thal, L., Pay, M., Salmon, D.P., U, H.S., Bakay, R., Patel, P., Blesch, A., Vahlsing, H.L., Ho, G., Tong, G., Potkin, S. G., Fallon, J., Hansen, L., Mufson, E. J., Kordower J. H., Gall, C., & Conner, J. (2005). A phase 1 clinical trial of nerve growth factor gene therapy for Alzheimer disease. *Nature Medicine*, Vol. 11, No. 5, pp. 551-5.

Urfer, R., Tsoulfas, P., O'Connell, L., & Presta, L.G. (1997). Specificity Determinants in Neurotrophin-3 and Design of Nerve Growth Factor-Based trkC Agonists by Changing Central β-Strand Bundle Residues to Their Neurotrophin-3 Analogs. *Biochemistry*, Vol. 36, No. 16, pp. 4775-4781.

Vilar, M., Charalampopoulos, I., Kenchappa, R.S., Reversi, A., Klos-Applequist, J.M., Karaca, E., Simi, A., Spuch, C., Choi, S., Friedman, W.J., Ericson, J., Schiavo, G., Carter, B. D., & Ibáñez, C. F. (2009). Ligand-independent signaling by disulfide-crosslinked dimers of the p75 neurotrophin receptor. *Journal of Cell Science*, Vol. 122, No. 18, pp. 3351-3357.

Wajant, H., Gerspach, J., & Pfizenmaier, K. (2005). Tumor therapeutics by design: targeting and activation of death receptors. *Cytokine Growth Factor Reviews*. Vol. 16, No. 1, pp. 55-76.

Walsh, G.S., Krol, K.M., Crutcher, K.A., & Kawaja, M.D. (1999). Enhanced neurotrophin-induced axon growth in myelinated portions of the CNS in mice lacking the p75 neurotrophin receptor. *Journal of Neuroscience*, Vol. 19, No. 10, pp. 4155-4168.

Wang, J.J., Rabizadeh, S., Tasinato, A., Sperandio, S., Ye, X., Green, M., Assa-Munt, N., Spencer, D., & Bredesen, D.E. (2000). Dimerization-dependent block of the proapoptotic effect of p75(NTR). *Journal of Neuroscience Research*, Vol. 60, No. 5, pp. 587-593.

Wiesmann, C., Ultsch, M.H., Bass, S.H., & de Vos, A.M. (1999). Crystal structure of nerve growth factor in complex with the ligand-binding domain of the TrkA receptor. *Nature*, Vol. 401, No. 6749, pp. 184-188.

Wiesmann, C., & de Vos, A.M. (2001). Nerve growth factor: structure and function. *Cellular and Molecular Life Sciences*, Vol. 58, No. 5-6, pp. 748-759.

Winkler, J., Ramirez, G.A., Kuhn, H.G., Peterson, D.A., Day-Lollini, P.A., Stewart, G.R., Tuszynski, M.H., Gage, F.H., & Thal, L.J. (1997). Reversible Schwann cell hyperplasia and sprouting of sensory and sympathetic neurites after intraventricular administration of nerve growth factor. *Annals of Neurology*, Vol. 41, No. 1, pp. 82-93.

Woo, S.B., Timm, D.E., & Neet, K.E. (1995). Alteration of NH2-terminal residues of nerve growth factor affects activity and Trk binding without affecting stability or conformation. *Journal of Biological Chemistry*, Vol. 270, No. 11, pp. 6278-6285.

Woo, S.B., & Neet, K.E. (1996). Characterization of histidine residues essential for receptor binding and activity of nerve growth factor. *Journal of Biological Chemistry*, Vol. 271, No. 40, pp. 24433-24441.

Wood, J.N. (2010). Nerve Growth Factor and Pain. *New England Journal of Medicine*, Vol. 363, No. 16, pp. 1572-1573.

Xie, Y., Tisi, M.A., Yeo, T.T., & Longo, F.M. (2000). Nerve Growth Factor (NGF) Loop 4 Dimeric Mimetics Activate ERK and AKT and Promote NGF-like Neurotrophic Effects. *Journal of Biological Chemistry*, Vol. 275, No. 38, pp. 29868-29874.

Yang, T., Knowles, J.K., Lu, Q., Zhang, H., Arancio, O., Moore, L.A., Chang, T., Wang, Q., Andreasson, K., Rajadas, J., Fuller, G.G., Xie, Y., Massa, S.M., & Longo, F.M. (2008). Small Molecule, Non-Peptide $p75^{NTR}$ Ligands Inhibit Aβ-Induced Neurodegeneration and Synaptic Impairment. *PLoS ONE*, Vol. 3, No. 11, pp. e3604.

Yeo, T.T., Chua-Couzens, J., Butcher, L.L., Bredesen, D.E., Cooper, J.D., Valletta, J.S., Mobley, W.C., & Longo, F.M. (1997). Absence of p75NTR causes increased basal forebrain cholinergic neuron size, choline acetyltransferase activity, and target innervation. *Journal of Neuroscience*, Vol. 17, No. 20, pp. 7594-7605.

Yoon, S.O., Soltoff, S.P., & Chao, M.V. (1997). A dominant role of the juxtamembrane region of the TrkA nerve growth factor receptor during neuronal cell differentiation. *Journal of Biological Chemistry*, Vol. 272, No. 37, pp. 23231-23238.

Zaccaro, M.C., Lee, H.B., Pattarawarapan, M., Xia, Z., Caron, A., L'Heureux, P.-J., Bengio, Y., Burgess, K., & Saragovi, H.U. (2005). Selective Small Molecule Peptidomimetic Ligands of TrkC and TrkA Receptors Afford Discrete or Complete Neurotrophic Activities. *Chemistry & Biology*, Vol. 12, No. 9, pp. 1015-1028.

Zhang, X., Gureasko, J., Shen, K., Cole, P.A., & Kuriyan, J. (2006). An Allosteric Mechanism for Activation of the Kinase Domain of Epidermal Growth Factor Receptor. *Cell*, Vol. 125, No. 6, pp. 1137-1149.

Zhang, Y., Moheban, D.B., Conway, B.R., Bhattacharyya, A., & Segal, R.A. (2000). Cell surface Trk receptors mediate NGF-induced survival while internalized receptors regulate NGF-induced differentiation. *Journal of Neuroscience*, Vol. 20, No. 15, pp. 5671-5678.

Zhao, M., Wan, Z. L., Whittaker, L., Xu, B., Phillips, N. B., Katsoyannis, P, G., Ismail-Beigi, F., Whittaker, J., & Weiss, M. A. (2009). Design of an insulin analog with enhanced receptor binding selectivity: rationale, structure, and therapeutic implications. *Journal of Biological Chemistry*, Vol. 284, No. 46, pp. 32178-32187.

13

Advances in MicroRNAs and Alzheimer's Disease Research

Francesca Ruberti[1], Silvia Pezzola[2] and Christian Barbato[3]
[1,3]CNR, National Research Council of Italy,
Cell Biology and Neurobiology Institute (IBCN),
IRCCS Fondazione Santa Lucia,
[2,3]EBRI - European Brain Research Institute-
Fondazione EBRI- Rita Levi-Montalcini
Italy

1. Introduction

Molecular and cellular neurobiological studies of the miRNA-mediated gene silencing in Alzheimer's disease represent the exploration of a new frontier of miRNAs biology and the potential development of new diagnostic tests and genetic therapies for this neurodegenerative disease. In few years our understanding of microRNA (miRNA) biogenesis, molecular mechanisms by which miRNAs regulate gene expression, and the functional roles of miRNAs has been expanded. MiRNA are double-stranded RNAs (dsRNAs) ≈22 nucleotides in lenght. These small noncoding RNA molecules operate as guides for RISC (RNA Induced Silencing Complex) to cleave a target mRNA in case of a perfect complementarity (siRNA) or to block the target mRNA translation (miRNA) when there is an imperfect pairing between miRNAs and the targets. In mammalian cells the repression of translation by miRNA is mediated by an imperfect pairing with the 3'UTRs of the mRNA targets. Interestingly, numerous miRNAs are expressed in a spatially and temporally controlled manner in the nervous system, suggesting that mRNA post-transcriptional regulation by microRNAs may be particularly relevant in neural development and function. Individual microRNAs can reduce the production of hundred proteins and miRNAs-mediated post-transcriptional regulation is involved in neuronal differentiation, dendritic spine development and synaptic plasticity. Recently expression profiles of miRNA in Alzheimer's disease brain revealed alterations in many indiviual miRNAs and several in vitro and in vivo studies aimed to the exploration of functional role of miRNA in Alzheimer's disease pathogenesis.

1.1 MicroRNA-mediated gene silencing

MicroRNAs are non-coding single stranded RNA molecules, 18- to 25 nucleotides in lenght, encoded in the genomes of invertebrates, plants and vertebrates. MicroRNA genes represent about 1-2% of the known eukaryotic genomes. The first two miRNAs to be discovered were *lin-4* and *let-7* in *Caenorhabditis elegans,* which regulate expression of *lin-14* and *lin-28* mRNAs, respectively, and are required for larval developmental timing (Lee et al., 1993;

Olsen et al., 1999; Reinhart et al., 2000). Since then, miRNAs have been observed in many contexts and their function involved in numerous regulatory pathways, deserving the attention they are now receiving.

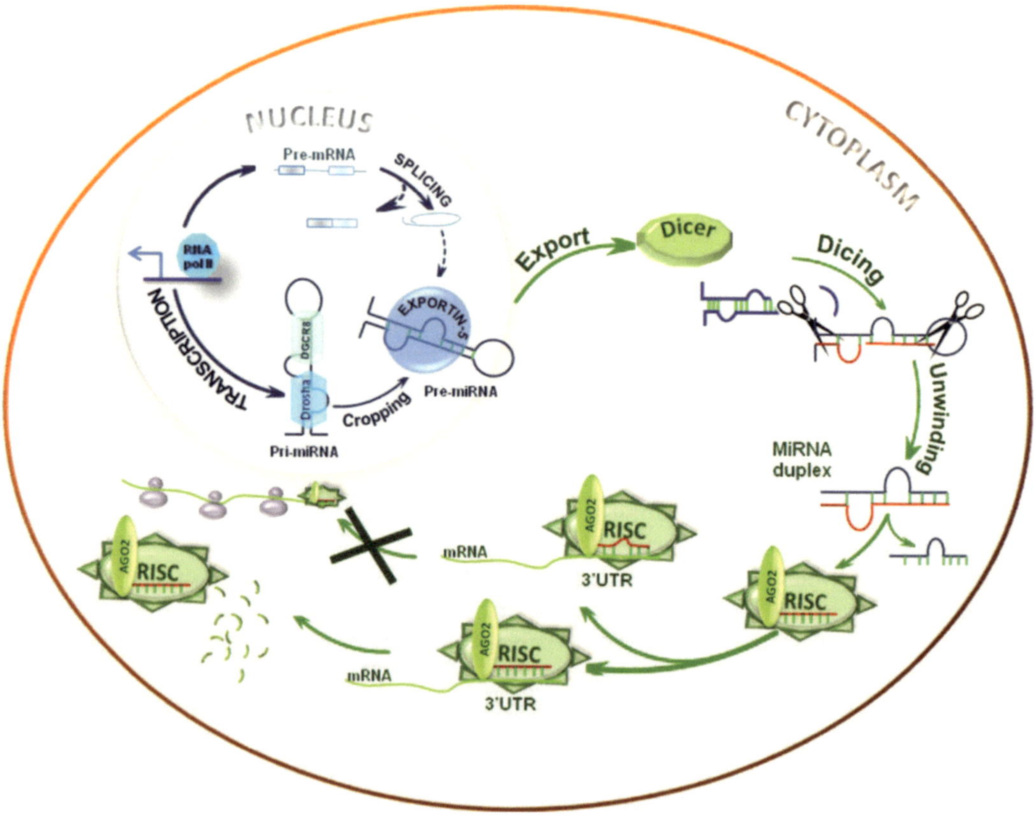

Fig. 1. MicroRNAs biogenesis and activity.

MiRNAs are transcribed by RNA polymerase II (Rodriguez et al., 2004), which mediates the transcription of most miRNA genes to generate an initial transcript, named primary miRNA (pri-miRNA). Pri-miRNAs can be hundreds to thousands nucleotides long, contain several hairpin structures, and undergo capping and polyadenylation (Lee et al., 2003). The first step in miRNA biogenesis occurs in the nucleus and requires the excision of this hairpin structure by a complex containing the RNAse III-endonuclease Drosha enzyme and the RNA binding protein DiGeorge syndrome critical region gene 8 (DGCR8) (Gregory et al., 2004). Apart from canonical intronic miRNAs, a group of intronic miRNAs (named mirtrons), present in the introns of flies and mammals, are derived from small introns that resemble pre-miRNAs and can bypass the Drosha-processing step. The excised hairpin, now called pre-miRNA, is exported to the cytoplasm by a protein heterodimer consisting of the transport factor Exportin-5/RanGTP (Bohnsack et al., 2004), and processed by Dicer, a double-stranded RNA (dsRNA)-specific endonuclease RNaseIII, which removes the loop region of the hairpin, releasing the mature miRNA: miRNA duplex. Dicer interacts with several RNA binding proteins, such as TRBP and PACT, which are not essential for its cleavage activity but are important for miRNA stability and loading of the effector complex RISC (RNA-induced silencing complex) (Chendrimada et al., 2005; Lee et al., 2006). During the assembly of the RISC complex with the miRNA, only one strand of the duplex is loaded, whereas the complementary miRNA* strand is removed and degraded (Kim et al., 2005). The mature miRNA is now ready to direct its activity on a target mRNA, by binding miRNA responsive elements usually located in the 3'UTR of the transcript, which leads to post-transcriptional gene silencing via inhibition of translation initiation or elongation. MicroRNAs associate with Argonaute proteins (Ago1-4, in mammals), which constitute the core of the RISC complex, and mediate post-transcriptional repression of target messenger RNAs. In particular Argonaute proteins are highly basic proteins which contain four domains: the N-terminal, PAZ, Mid and PIWI domains (Hutvagner and Simard, 2008). The PAZ domain binds the single stranded 3'end of miRNAs.

1.2 MicroRNAs in nervous system

The bewildering diversity of neurons, including their distribution in specific functional areas and complex synaptic circuitry, is determined during development and differentiation and is achieved by multiple levels of gene regulation. The transcriptional and post-transcriptional gene regulation mechanisms of development, plasticity and networking might participate in the determination and maintenance of such complexity. Recently, microRNAs are emerging as important players in post-transcriptional regulation in the brain. A major advancement in understanding how miRNAs are involved in this phenomenon comes from studies on miRNAs expression profiles. Several analyses have shown spatially and/or temporally restricted distribution of miRNAs, suggesting that they may control the fine-tuning regulation of neuronal gene expression (Cao et al., 2006; Schratt, 2009).

1.3 MicroRNAs, synaptic plasticity and memory

This section focuses on more relevant works highlighting the relevance of microRNAs post-transcriptional regulation in cellular pathways and functions such as synaptic plasticity and memory. However pathological implications of miRNAs expression associated to cognitive decline in Alzheimer's disease, are still unknown.

1.3.1 MicroRNAs and the dendritic neuronal compartment

Synaptic loss is the major neurobiological substrate of cognitive decline in Alzheimer's disease. The alteration of synaptic integrity occurs very early in AD, and it can be observed in patients with mild cognitive impairment (MCI) (Scheff et al., 2006). Loss of molecular components of presynaptic and postsynaptic membranes, synaptic vescicles, and proteins contributing to the morphological and architectural characteristic of axons and dendrites, is the main feature associated with an impairment of synaptic plasticity in neuronal cells. Neuronal activity is a critical regulator of several nervous system functions, including long-term memory (Malenka and Nicoll, 1999; Sutton and Schuman, 2006). Beyond the reduction of transcripts related to synaptic vesicle trafficking (Coleman and Yao, 2003), it is questionable if there is a post-transcriptional deregulation of mRNAs functionally associated to axonal and dendritic synaptic remodelling in AD. Little is known about the mechanisms that underlie the regulation of protein synthesis in polarized cells like neurons. The synaptic protein synthesis makes necessary the corresponding mRNAs to be transported in the dendritic compartment and to be translated upon site-specific activation. It is generally thought that dendritic mRNAs are transported in a translationally silenced state within ribonucleoprotein complexes (Kiebler and Bassell, 2006). The recent discovery of the existence of a group of molecules regulating gene expression at post-transcriptional levels, named microRNAs, opened a new window on the research of molecular mechanisms of plasticity in the nervous system. Specific sites of protein synthesis are the dendritic spines. In neurons there are thousand of spines throughout multiple arborizations. Spine structures are dinamically regulated (Hotulainen and Hoogenraad, 2010), and functional and structural changes at spines and synapses are proposed as the basis of learning and memory (Kasai et al., 2010). MiRNAs, that are expressed in spatially and temporally controlled manner in the brain, are ideal candidates as modulators of dendritic protein synthesis. MicroRNAs modulate dendritic morphology by regulating expression of proteins involved in the actin cytoskeleton (Vo et al., 2005; Schratt et al., 2006; Siegel et al., 2009; Wayman et al., 2008) mRNA transport (Fiore et al., 2009) and neurotrasmission (Edbauer et al., 2010). The participation of miRNAs in synaptic expression of mRNAs was first observed in *Drosophila melanogaster.* The *Drosophila* ortholog of mammalian fragile X protein, dFmr1 was described to interact with RISC complex, and in particular with the main component Ago2 (Caudy et al., 2002; Ishizuka et al., 2002). Two years later, Warren and collaborators showed that FMRP associates with endogenous miRNAs and Ago1 (Jin et al., 2004). They performed genetic studies in *Drosophila* to find that Ago1 depletion suppresses dFrm1 overexpression phenotype, and that a trans-heterozygote for both AGO1 and dFmrp1 shows an even more pronounced synaptic overgrowth phenotype than the dFmr1 null mutant. This indicates that AGO1 might be a limiting factor in dFmr1 function in synaptogenesis, and suggests that microRNAs might mediate the FMR1 role in silencing of neuronal mRNAs.

1.3.2 RISC, microRNAs and synaptic plasticity

Evidence of miRNAs involvement in synaptic plasticity was first reported by Kunes' laboratory (Ashraf et al., 2006). The regulated disruption of the silencing complex component Armitage, led to the removal of miRNA-mediated repression of CaMKII, an mRNA involved in synaptic plasticity. Putative miRNA binding sites are present within the 3'UTR of CaMKII, as well as within the 3'UTR of the transcripts coding for Staufen and Kinesin-Heavy Chain, two dendritic granule-associated proteins. To test whether these mRNAs are targets of miRNA-silencing activity, their expression levels were assayed in brains from mutants of the RISC pathway. The results indicate that synaptic translation of CaMKII increases in dicer-, armitage-, and aubergine-mutant brains. Indeed, this work suggests an armitage-driven repression of CaMKII expression in drosophila olfactory system. Synaptic activation induces a decrease in the levels of Armitage protein and a correspondent increase in CaMKII abundance. The decrease in Armitage protein is shown to be due to the activity of the proteasome which is known to act at the synaptic level to contribute in modulating synaptic protein content (Bingol and Schuman 2005; 2006). Overall, Ashraf et al. (2006) propose a novel and intriguing regulatory mechanism whereby CaMKII translational repression is driven by miRNAs and in turn is relieved by activity-dependent proteasome-mediated degradation of Armitage (Fig.2)

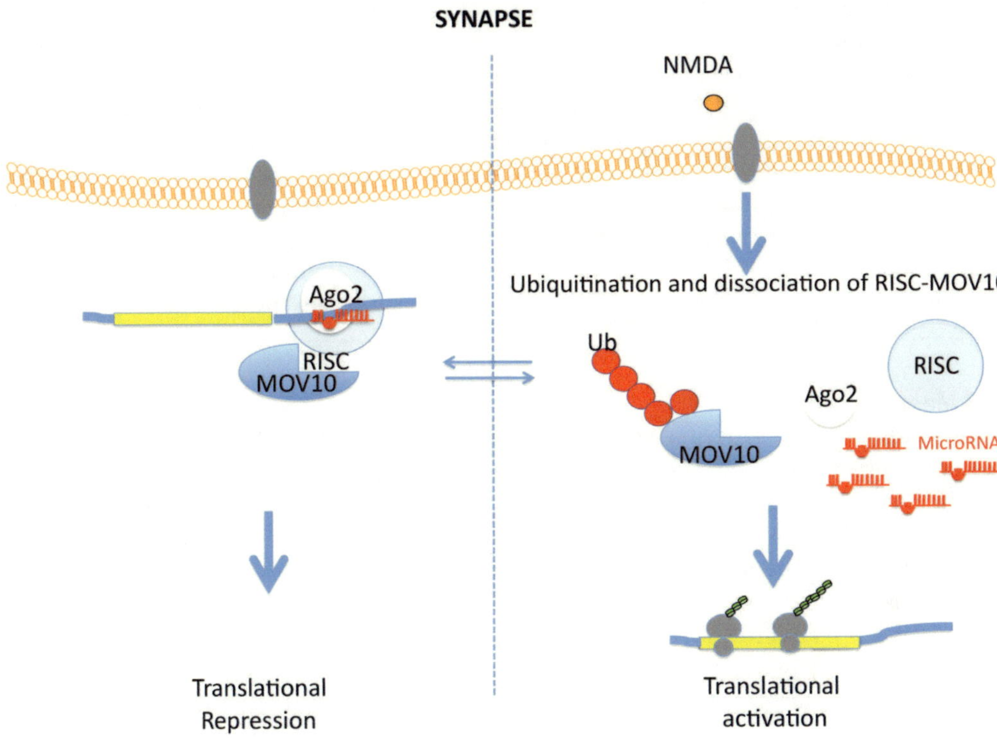

The model depicted here summarizes miRNAs modulation of synaptic protein synthesis and plasticity (Ashraf et al., 2006; Banerjee et al., 2009) MiRNAs are required for the translational silencing of several neuronal mRNAs important for synaptic protein synthesis (see text). Patterns of synaptic activity that induce long-term memory trigger localized proteasome-mediated degradation of MOV10 in mammalian (Armitage in Drosophila RISC) and consequent release of the translational repression guided by miRNAs at synapse.

Fig. 2. RISC regulation in synaptic plasticity.

More recently the silencing of the mammalian ortholog of Armitage, Moloney leukemia virus 10 homolog (MOV10), by RNA interference mediated knockdown, showed the relief of translational repression of miRNA targets. Kosik's group, with the aim to identify dendritic mRNAs under RISC's degradative control, individuated several mRNA localized in the dendrites. They trapped both known RISC-regulated mRNAs, as Limk1 and alfaCaMKII, and novel mRNA Lysophospholipase 1(Lypla1), (also known as acyl protein thioesterase (APT)1), a depalmitoylation enzyme, regulated post-transcriptionally by dendritic miR-138 (Banerjee et al., 2009). Previously Schratt's group showed that in rat hippocampal neurons, miR-138 was enriched at synapses and modulated synaptic development and spine size through the regulation levels of the APT1 (Siegel et al., 2009), followed by depalmitoylation of Ga13, a downstream target of APT1, which is an activator of Rho downstream of G-protein coupled receptor (Kurose et al., 2003). Another finding which associates miRNA function to the synaptic plasticity in mammalian neurons, was made by Schratt and collaborators, with the brain-specific microRNA-134 (Schratt et al., 2006). The overexpression of miR-134 causes a significant reduction in dendritic spine size, whereas its inhibition by 2'-O-methyl antisense oligonucleotides induces a slight increase in spine volume. The mRNA target of miR-134 was identified as Lim-domain containing protein kinase 1 (Limk1). Like to Kunes' laboratory findings (Ashraf et al., 2006), in this case neuronal activation also intervenes to put a brake on miRNA-mediated silencing. MiR-134 repression of Limk1 translation is mitigated upon BDNF stimulation of synaptic activity. In cortical neurons, BDNF induced the translation of the 3'UTR Limk1 mRNA luciferase reporter, but not when neurons were trasfected with a reporter in which miR-134 responsive sequence was mutated. This suggests that the BDNF/miR-134/Limk1 connection plays a role in synaptic plasticity at synaptodendritic compartment of hippocampal neurons (Fig.3). The studies described above, indicate that miRNAs might contribute to fine-tuning regulation of synaptic protein synthesis and plasticity by modulating expression of dendritic mRNAs.

1.3.3 Memory

Dysregulation in the enthorinal cortex and dentate gyrus during the acquisition of memory is one of the hallmarks that occurs early during Alzheimer's neurodegeneration. The loss of coordination between different pathways orchestrating protein expression at synapses, consists in a loss of control of plasticity. The assumption that synaptic plasticity is considered to underlie memory formation (Morris et al., 2003), and the evidence that forms of long-lasting synaptic plasticity depend on protein synthesis (Manahan-Vaughan et al., 2000), suggest that microRNAs may indeed be important for this phenomenon. What are the downstream effectors that mediate such activity? Several observations suggest that the induction of long-term potentiation (LTP) and long-term depression (LTD), two forms of synaptic plasticity, requires microRNAs. Park and Tang (2009) performed the temporal expression profile of sixty hippocampal microRNAs following induction of chemical LTP (C-LTP) and metabotropic glutamate receptor-dependent LTD (mGluR-LTD) in hippocampal slices. They observed that C-LTP or mGluR-LTD evokes changes of the expression levels of most hippocampal miRNAs, suggesting a role for miRNA-mediated translational repression. MiRNAs regulated in both experimental paradigma, displayed distinct temporal expression dynamics. Further, many miRNAs were upregulated at specific time points of C-LTP and mGluR-LTD induction, like to provide an active mechanism to restore the dormant state of mRNA translation after a transient activation (Park and Tang, 2009). Recent studies demonstrated finely regulation of primary and mature miRNA expression by mGluR and NMDAR signaling during LTP induction (Wibrand et al., 2010). Transgenic mouse strain that expresses miR-132 in forebrain neurons, showed an increase in dendritic spine density and a deficits in novel object recognition, suggesting that dysregulation of miR-132 could contribute to an array of cognitive disorders (Hansen et al., 2010). The first evidence that miRNA expression is specifically altered during an in vivo learning paradigm in mammals was carried out by Smalheiser's group, demonstrating that olfactory discrimination training, up-regulates and reorganizes expression of microRNAs in adult mouse hippocampus (Smalheiser et al., 2010). How up-regulation of a subset of miRNAs modulates gene expression pathways during several phases of learning and memory? A new work showing miRNAs as key players in the learning and memory process of mammals, was published by (Konopka et al., 2010). In a mouse model with an inducible disruption of the Dicer1 gene in the adult forebrain, after induction of Dicer1 gene deletion, a progressive loss of a whole set of brain-specific miRNAs was observed. Mice were tested in a battery of both aversively and appetitively motivated cognitive tasks, such as Morris water maze, IntelliCage system, or trace fear conditioning. An enhancement of memory was recorded twelwe weeks after the Dicer1 gene mutation. To date, we can't say a "better memory with less microRNA" or the reverse, but only that microRNAs may modulate memory, that components of long-term potentiation (LTP) require local protein translation, which regulate synaptic plasticity, and that microRNAs have been identified as master regulators of protein synthesis.

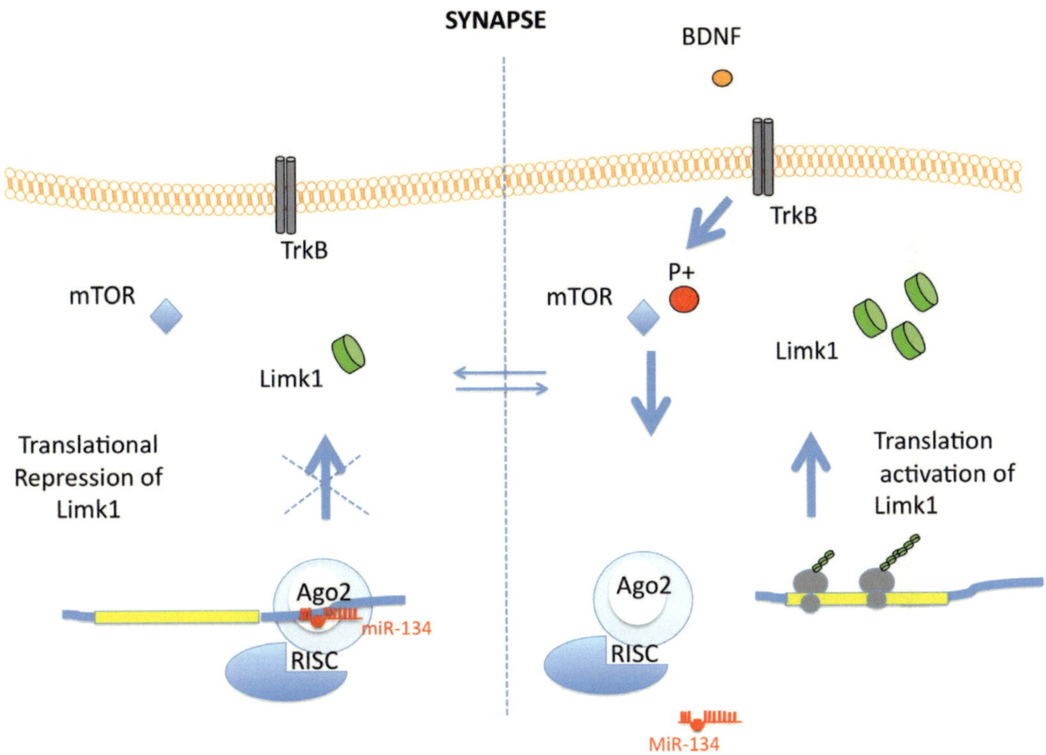

The mechanism unveiled by Schratt et al. (2006) in mammalian neurons is illustrated. Limk1 mRNA is subject to miR-134-mediated repression. Upon synaptic activation, induced by BDNF treatment, the authors observe translational derepression of Limk1 mRNA and an increase in spine size. How synaptic activity might release Limk1 mRNA from miR-134 repression is unclear.

Fig. 3. MicroRNA targets in synaptic plasticity and memory.

2. MicroRNA expression profiles in Alzheimer's disease brain

During the last four years, great strides have been made to profile miRNA expression in several regions of the AD brain. To point out whether miRNA expression may be misregulated in AD, Cogswell and coworkers compared the expression of over 300 miRNAs, isolated from hippocampus, medial frontal gyrus and cerebellum from early and late stage AD, to normal age-matched controls (Cogswell et al., 2008). Tissues were grouped by Braak stage and miRNAs were extracted, quantified and amplified by real-time quantitative PCR assay. Experimental data provide a statistically significant number of under- and over-expressed microRNAs. In particular, hippocampus and medial frontal gyrus, which are the earlier regions affected by AD pathology, were characterized by the major modifications. Expression of twenty-one miRNA (miR-200c, -212, -26a, -27a, -30c, -30e-5p, -34a, 381, -422a, -423, -9, -92, 100, -125b, -132, -145, -146b, -148a, -210, -27b, -425) was altered both in early and in end stages of pathology (Cogswell et al., 2008). The pathological cerebrospinal fluids (CSF) were also analyzed. These samples show a different miRNAs expression between AD and non-affected patients. Both miRNA expression profiles represent the first work aimed to identify specific miRNAs as biomarkers of AD (Cogswell et al., 2008). Several efforts have been made to understand whether miRNAs are also altered in sporadic AD. A microRNA expression profile shows that many miRNAs are potentially involved in the regulation of APP and BACE1 (Hebert et al., 2008). In this study the expression of 328 human miRNAs in the anterior temporal cortex and the cerebellum from five AD patients was monitored and compared with age-matched controls. Among all miRNAs analyzed, 13 were significantly altered and at least 7 were predicted to target the 3′ UTR of BACE1 (miR-15a, 29b-1, -9, and -19b) or APP (let-7, miR101, miR15a, and miR106b) (Hebert et al., 2008). Nunez-Iglesias (2010) used microarrays for the first joint profiling and analysis of miRNAs and mRNAs expression in brain cortex from AD and age-matched control subjects. These data provided the unique opportunity to study the relationship between miRNA and mRNA expression in normal and AD brains. Starting from genome-wide miRNA and mRNA data expression, analysis was carried out to determine the correlation between levels of miRNAs and their target mRNAs (Nunez-Iglesias et al., 2010). The results reveal that most miRNA-mRNA pairs are actually uncorrelated making more difficult to understand the correlation level between miRNAs with their targets. By an elegant analysis performed taking advantage from gene ontology biological processes, RNAs were grouped together. Among the processes most positively correlated with their regulating miRNA, the authors found some specific processes, including metabolism of both carbohydrates and fatty acid, as well as protein refolding which indicate the importance of these processes in the brain. Among the processes most negatively correlated are oxygen transport, cell adhesion, inflammatory response, cytoskeletal organization and dendrite development (Nunez-Iglesias et al., 2010). The method depicted can find active miRNA-mRNA relationships dependent from the tissue context. These authors demonstrate a relationship between the levels of miRNAs and those of their targets in the brain, identyfing a large set of miRNA-mRNA associations that are changed in AD versus control, and AD-specific changes in the miRNA regulatory system. Microarray techniques, based on correlation methods, are proving to be powerful tools for investigation on miRNAs deregulation in AD. The expression of 5-6% of miRNAs was affected by AD at statistical significant level in the studies described above (Hebert et al., 2008; Cogswell et al., 2008; Nunez-Iglesias et al., 2010) suggesting that a substantial number of miRNAs are deregulated in this pathology.

BRAIN AREA	EXPRESSION IN ALZHEIMER'S DISEASE	miRNA	Reference
Gray matter	Upregulated	miR-519e, miR-574-5p, miR-498, miR-518a-5p/miR-527, miR-525-5p, miR-300, miR-576-3p, miR-583, miR-146b-3p, miR-490-3p, miR-549, miR-516a-5p, miR-510, miR-184, miR-516b, miR-298, miR-214, miR-198, miR-451, miR-144, miR-424, let-7e	(Wang et al., 2011)
Gray matter	Downregulated	miR-485-3p, miR-381, miR-124, miR-34a, miR-129-5p, miR-29a, miR-143, miR-36, miR-145, miR-138, miR-129-3p, miR-128, miR-143, miR-136, miR-145, miR-138, miR-129-3p, miR-128, miR-126, miR-411, miR-335, miR-9, miR-378, miR-488, miR-32, miR-127-5p, miR-127-3p, miR-491-5p, miR-376c, miR-377, miR-95, miR-222, miR-29b, miR-329, miR-495, miR-551b, miR-195, miR-125b, miR-30b, miR-221, miR-139-5p, miR-487a, miR-487b, miR-107, miR-146b-5p, miR-29c, miR-30a, miR-582-5p, miR-103, miR-342-3p, miR-331-3p, miR-30c, miR-30d, miR-382, miR-22, miR-125a-5p, miR-425, miR-191, miR-519d, let-7g, miR-98, miR-99a, miR-30e	(Wang et al., 2011)
White matter	Upregulated	miR-509-5p, miR-574-3p, miR-576-5p, miR-302e, miR-220b, miR-208a, miR-215	(Wang et al., 2011)
White matter	Downregulated	miR-491-3p, miR-423-5p, miR-34b, miR-422a, miR-34c-5p, miR-584, miR-219-5p, miR-338-3p, miR-219-2-3p, miR-338-5p, miR-181a, miR-181b, let-7b, miR-151-3p, miR-197, miR-19a, miR-20a, miR-17, miR-106a, miR-32, miR-340, miR-19b, miR-21, miR-151-5p, miR-194, let-7c, miR-330-3p, miR-27b, miR-93, miR-15a, miR-339-5p, miR-193b, miR-106b, miR-16, miR-23b, miR-15b, miR-320d, miR-320b, miR-320c, miR-320a, miR-557, miR-33a, let-7a, miR-374b, miR-140-3p, miR-374a, miR-24, miR-140-5p, miR-26a, miR-513a-5p, miR-212, miR-142-5p, miR-142-3p, miR-26b, miR-520d-5p, miR-193a-3p, miR-92b, miR-330-5p, miR-186, let-7f, miR-223, miR-412, miR-185, miR-148b, miR-101, miR-99b, miR-27a, miR-589, let-7i, miR-361-3p, miR-361-5p, miR-423-3p, miR-190, miR-301a, miR-365, miR-23a, miR-363, miR-326	(Wang et al., 2011)

Hippocampus	Upregulated	miR-26a,miR-27a, miR-30e-5p, miR-34a, miR-92, miR-381, miR-422a, miR-423, miR-27b, miR-125b, miR-145, miR200c	(Cogswell et al., 2008)
		mR-146a	(Cui et al., 2010)
Hippocampus	Downregulated	miR-9,miR-128, miR-125b	(Lukiw, 2007)
		miR-30c, miR-212, miR-132, miR-146b, miR-210, miR-425, miR-9	(Cogswell et al., 2008)
Medial frontal gyrus	Upregulated	miR-27a, miR-30c, miR-30e-5p, miR-34a, miR-92, miR-381, miR-422a, mir-423,miR-27b, miR-100, miR-125b, miR-145, miR-148a, miR-29a, miR-29b, miR-423, miR-145	(Cogswell et al., 2008)
Medial frontal gyrus	Downregulated	miR-26a, miR-200c, miR-212,miR-132, miR-146b, miR-210, miR-425	(Cogswell et al., 2008)

Parietal lobe cortex	Upregulated	miR-30184, miR-617,miR-188,miR-06383, miR-10912,miR-601,miR-23974, miR-10939, miR-19790, miR-35456, miR-134, miR-671, miR-320, miR-575, miR572, miR-45605, miR-765, miR-18895, miR-432, miR-382, miR-185, miR-486, miR-28648	(Nunez-Iglesias et al., 2010)
Parietal lobe cortex	Downregulated	miR-101,miR-20546,miR-29b, miR-181c, miR-08570, miR-42448, miR-44608, miR-02532, miR-12497, miR-582, miR-15a, miR-374, miR-95, miR-05109, miR-30e-5p, miR-148b, miR-130a, miR-598, miR-376a, miR-29c, miR-12504, miR-494, miR-20b, miR-368	(Nunez-Iglesias et al., 2010)
Temporal lobe cortex (Sporadic AD)	Upregulated	miR-197, miR-511, miR-320	(Hebert et al., 2008)
Temporal lobe cortex (Sporadic AD)	Downregulated	miR-210, miR-181c, miR-15a, miR-9, miR-22, miR-101, miR-29b-1, miR-19b, let-7i, miR-106b, miR-26b, miR-363, miR-93	(Hebert et al., 2008)
Temporal lobe cortex	Upregulated	miR-9, miR-125b, miR-146a	(Sethi & Lukiw, 2009)

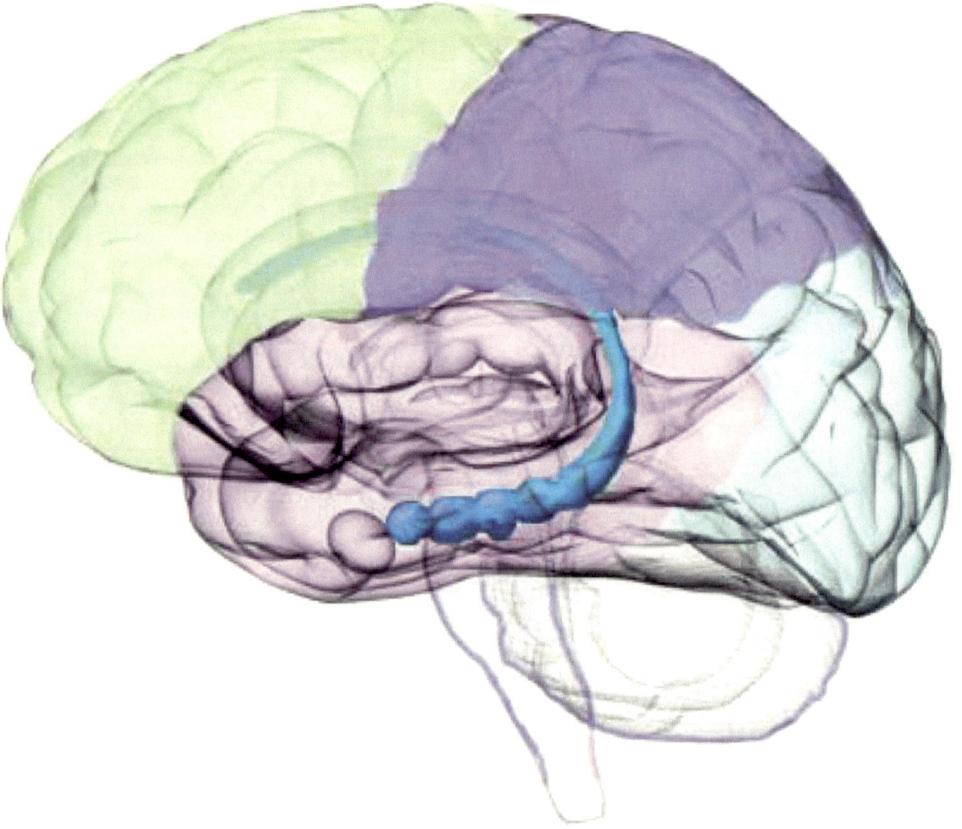

Table 1. Studies reporting changes of miRNAs expression profiles in Alzheimer's disease and in different brain areas.

2.1 Addressing brain tissue complexity

In gene expression studies the heterogeneity of the human cerebral cortex should be considered. For example, former tissue sampling protocols did not segregate white matter from gray matter, increasing variability that reflects differently sample cell population rather than a disease condition (Wang et al., 2011) (Table 1). Nelson's laboratory deals with this question either analyzing different miRNAs expression in human cerebral cortical white matter and gray matter in normal and early AD pathology and using different experimental techniques. MiRNA profiling experiments were performed using a locked nucleic-acid-microarray (LNA-microarray) which highlights a subset of miRNAs that appeared to be strongly expressed and did not appear to be conventional miRNAs (Wang et al., 2011). Using clustering analysis they demonstrated a different miRNA expression pattern between white matter and gray matter and between normal and pathological condition. Further, they found that there was an apparent clustering between samples derived from gray matter relative to those derived from white matter, and also cases with more AD pathology tended to cluster together relative to control cases. Moreover, miRNA expression may be correlated to neuropathological hallmarks in AD: amyloid plaques (with or without degenerating neuritis) and neurofibrillary tangles. Because of the major pathological changes affected gray matter, it is not surprising that a number of miRNAs altered in AD was higher in gray matter than white matter, but a handful of miRNAs was altered specifically in white matter. These data indicate an emerging need: while the expression of individual miRNA may be impactful alone, it is necessary to assess the aggregate impact of multiple miRNAs and the connection between AD pathological features and miRNA alteration (Wang et al., 2011). In fact, miRNA expression profiles highlight almost two altered pathways in AD, which involve inflammatory alteration response and $A\beta_{1\text{-}42}$ production and physiology. However, bioinformatic tools and miRNA expression profile offer a data set that have to be validate in cellular system in order to understand which are the mRNA targets and, eventually the physiopathological implications. Variation in tissue sampling may contribute to heterogeneus results. Banked tissue is essential to the study of neurological diseases but the use of postmortem tissue introduces a number of possible confounds. A variety of antemortem factors may influence the quality of harvested tissue including fever, hypoxia-ischemia and acidosis, while critical postmortem variables include postmortem interval (PMI), brain or cerebrospinal fluid pH, ambient temperature in the postmortem period, harvesting procedures, storage temperature and accidental or systematic thawing and freezing. Interindividual differences in postmortem tissue studies are typically large and often prevent the attainment of statistical significance. Much of interindividual variability may be due to highly variable agonal condition; RNA yield and quality may be affected by the extraction method employed. Many report that global measures of total RNA quality are relatively stable over a wide range of PMIs while some others report a definite loss with increasing time (Birdsill et al., 2010). However, in all extraction techniques employed a negative correlation between PMI and RNA quality-yield is point out. Furthermore, miRNA half-life appears significantly correlated with content of AU and UA dinucleotides in the RNA sequence. MiRNA-9, for example, which has 26.1% of AU in the sequence, has a half-life shorter (c.a 1 h) than miRNA-125b, 9.5% AU rich and 3.5h half-life. These data suggest the importance to compare normal and pathological tissue with similar PMI. In fact, analysis of miRNAs in autopsied brain tissue with post-mortem intervals many-fold greater than the half-lives of miRNAs may lead to inaccurate conclusions concerning their absolute abundance and hence the contribution of miRNAs to gene regulation in the brain during development, aging and in disease processes (Sethi et al., 2009). Studies performed in brain tissues with short PMI indicate that miR-9, miR-146 and miR-125 were significantly upregulated in AD-affected temporal lobe. Importantly comparative expression analysis showed no change of these microRNAs in tissues derived from patients affected with amyotropic lateral sclerosis, Parkinson's disease, schizophrenia. These data suggest that these miRNAs may contribute to the pathogenesis characteristic of AD. Microarray system is suitable to perform miRNA expression profiling but it did not show specific cellular distribution. Instead in situ hybridation (ISH) should be a method to directly understand the specific roles of miRNAs in the human brain at the cellular and sub-cellular levels. ISH is more labor-intensive and "low-throughput" compared to other RNA expression profiling techniques, but allows far greater resolution of given RNA's expression (Nelson et al., 2009). For example, ISH shows important cerebral cortical lamina-specific patterns of miRNA expression that would be lost on most tissue level expression studies, and these lamina-specific patterns may be relevant to human brain disease.

3. Exploring microRNA function in Alzheimer's disease

MiRNA target prediction programs, cell-based functional assays and studies in mouse models have been used to identify some of the molecular and biological functions of microRNAs dysregulated in AD brain tissues.

3.1 miRNAs dysregulated in AD modulate BACE and other targets

The amyloid precursor protein (APP), its proteolytic product amyloid beta (Aβ), generated by beta secretase (BACE) and gamma secretase, are all associated with both familial and sporadic forms of Alzheimer disease (AD) (Fig.4). BACE1 gene was shown post-transcriptionally regulated by miR-107 (Wang et al 2008) and miR-29a/b-1 (Hebert et al 2008). Interstingly miR-107 expression levels decreased during AD pathology progression (Wang et al 2008). On the other hand miR-29 was downregulated in anterior temporal cortex from sporadic AD patients in which BACE 1 protein was abnormally upregulated while BACE 1 mRNA levels were unchanged (Hebert et al 2008). Using BACE1 3'UTR luciferase reporter carrying wild type or mutated miRNA responsive sites BACE1 post-transcriptional regulation by those microRNA was demonstrated. Moreover, upon either overexpression or downregulation of miR-29a/b-1 in human cell culture both BACE1 protein levels and APP cleavage product Aβ were, respectively, reduced and increased (Hebert et al 2008) (Fig.4). Although these studies clearly indicate a relationship of both miR-29 and miR-107 with a gene associated to AD pathology identification of all mRNA targets affected by each microRNA deregulated in AD is the real challenge of future investigations. Indeed other studies indicate that miR-29 may play a more complex role in neurons during AD neurodegeneration. Neuron navigator 3 (NAV3), a regulator of axon guidance, was validated as miR-29 target and by immunohistochemistry NAV3 expression was found enhanced in degenerating pyramidal neurons in the cerebral cortex of AD (Shyoia et al., 2010). Moreover studies in sympathetic neurons have shown that miR-29b function as an inhibitor of neuronal apoptosis (Kole et al., 2011) by inhibition of multiple redundant BH3 only proteins (Bim, Bmf, Hrk, Puma and N-Bak) that are key iniziators of apoptosis. Therefore loss of miR-29 expression may lead to neuron vulnerability and neurodegeneration. Additional roles for miR-107 in AD pathogenesis are demonstrated by studies in a transgenic mouse model of AD which over-expresses human APP carrying familial AD mutations (Yao et al., 2010). In particular reduced levels of miR-103 or miR-107 are associated with elevated cofilin protein levels and formation of rod-like structures in this

AD mouse model. Rod-like structures composed of actin and the actin-binding protein cofilin are also found in Alzheimer's disease (AD) patients (Whiteman et al., 2009).

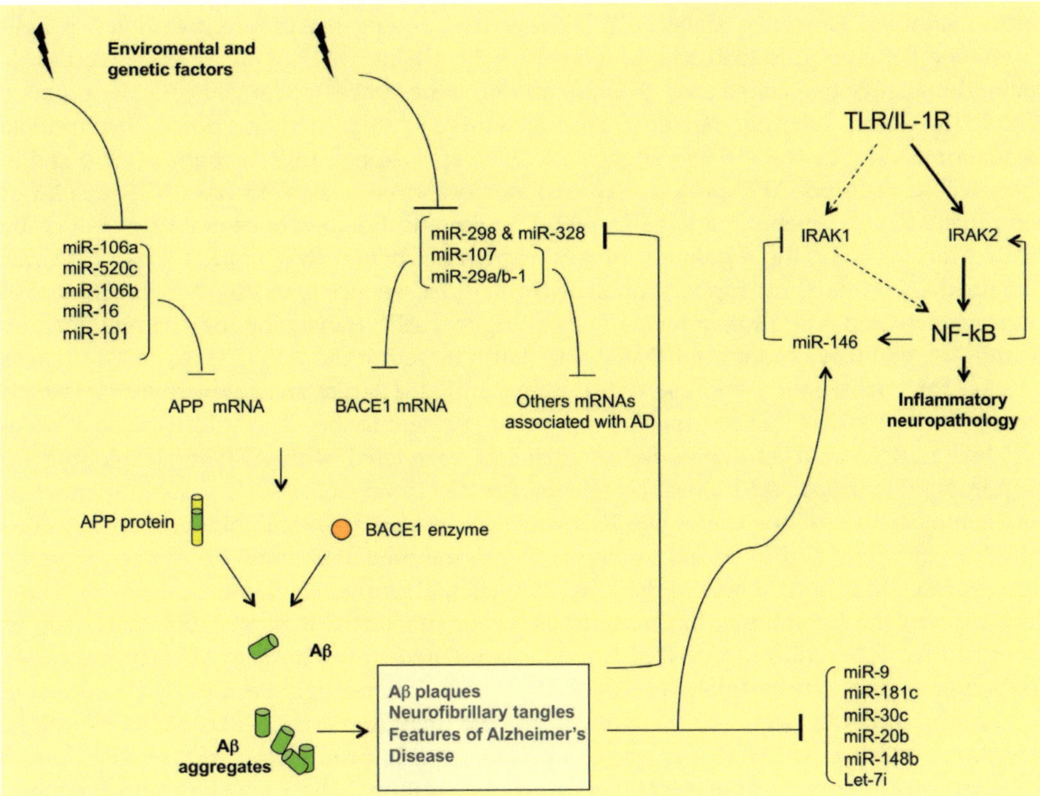

Fig. 4. MiRNAs deregulation in Alzheimer's disease pathology.

3.2 Several miRNAs regulate APP

Among mutations causing familial AD, duplication of the APP gene has also been detected (Rovelet-Lecrux et al., 2006). In addition, individuals with trisomy 21 (the APP gene is located on chromosome 21) are at increased risk of developing AD late in life (Podlisny et al., 1987). Several studies have reported that APP expression is post-transcriptionally regulated by microRNAs. A list of microRNAs: miR-106a and miR-520c, miR-20a family members (including miR-20a, miR-106b and miR-17-5p), miR-16 and miR-101, was demonstrated to downregulate APP expression (Patel et al., 2008; Hebert et al., 2009; Liu et al., 2010; Vilardo et al., 2010). The expression levels of these miRNAs were reduced in AD tissues (Fig. 4). When overexpressed in human cell lines, both miR-106a and miR-520c reduced endogenous APP levels by 50% compared to cells transfected with a non-targeting miRNA (Patel et al., 2008). However, only miR-106a is expressed in neuronal context. Overexpression of miR-20a (and miR-17-5p/106b) post-transcriptionally reduced endogenous APP expression in both non-neuronal and neuronal cells. Moreover, reduction of miR-20a, miR-17-5p and miR-106b levels was correlated with an increase in APP protein levels in developing mouse brain and in primary cultured neurons. Although two putative miR-20 family responsive elements (REs) are predicted within the APP 3'UTR only one RE functionally interacted with miR-20 family miRNAs. When miRNA expression levels in human AD brains were analyzed, miR-106b was significantly reduced with respect to control samples. However, since APP levels varied among the different samples, a tight correlation between miR-106b and APP levels in AD tissues was not obtained (Hebert et al., 2009). In an age-associated AD animal model, senescence-accelerated mouse prone 8 (SAMP8), which has age-related learning and memory deficits post-transcriptional regulation of APP by miR-16 was suggested. Overexpression of miR-16, both in vitro and in vivo, led to reduced APP protein expression. Furthermore, miR-16 and APP displayed complementary expression patterns in SAMP8 mice and BALb/c mice embryos (Liu et al., 2010). More recently, the regulation of APP expression by the RISC/miRNA pathway was examined in primary rat hippocampal neurons. First, silencing of Ago2 in hippocampal neurons increased APP protein levels, suggesting that APP translation may be regulated by an miRNA pathway. Among miRNAs potentially targeting the APP 3'UTR, miR- 101 was selected for further study because two putative miR-101 target sites, which are conserved among the human, rat and murine APP genes, are present in the 3'UTR. MiR-101 is a brain-enriched miRNA and its expression is inversely correlated with APP in developing rat hippocampal neurons and tissues. Using site directed mutagenesis, a functional interaction between miR-101 and one of the two REs was demonstrated. The inhibition of endogenous miR-101 increased APP levels, whereas lentiviral-mediated miR-101 overexpression significantly reduced APP and Aβ load in hippocampal neurons (Vilardo et al., 2010). These data support the hypothesis that miR-101 is a repressor of APP expression. Moreover, as described for other miRNAs, miR-101 is downregulated in the human AD cerebral cortex (Hebert et al 2008; Nunez-Iglesias et al., 2010) (Fig.4). Interestingly besides APP expression regulation, miRNAs were also involved in the regulation of neuronal APP mRNA alternative splicing which also affects β-amyloid peptide production. APP exons 7 and 8 inclusion was observed in postmitotic neurons of conditional Dicer knock-out mice (Hebert et al., 2010), while over-expression of miR-124, an abundant neuronal-specific miRNA, reversed these effects in cultured neurons. Similar results were obtained by depletion of endogenous polypyrimidine tract binding protein 1 (PTBP1) in cells, a recognized miR-124 target gene. Furthermore, PTBP1 levels correlate with the presence of APP exons 7 and 8, while PTBP2 levels correlate with the skipping of these exons during neuronal differentiation. Expression studies in AD brain showed that miR-124 expression was down-regulated (Smith et al., 2011).

3.3 Changes of miRNA in AD are implicated in inflammation, aging and oxidative stress

Inflammatory signaling plays determinant roles in brain homeostasis and neuroprotection however, altered or excessive signaling in these injury defense systems contributes to the irreversible degeneration of brain cells, in neurodegenerative disorders such as Alzheimer disease (AD). The inflammatory processes are involved during progression of AD pathogenesis, and Aβ42 peptides , cytokine IL-1β upregulation and oxidative stress are inflammatory mediators (Lukiw, 2004). A mouse and human brain abundant miRNA-146 was upregulated in AD brain and associated with the down-regulation of complement factor H, an important repressor of inflammatory signaling in the complement cascade, in

AD brain (Lukiw et al 2008). Furthermore in the hippocampus and neocortex of Alzheimer disease (AD) brain as well as in stressed human astroglial (HAG) cells in primary culture, increased expression of an NF-kB-regulated miRNA-146 down-regulates expression of the interleukin-1 receptor-associated kinase-1 (IRAK-1), an essential component of Toll-like/IL-1 receptor signaling (Cui et al 2010). Family of interleukin-1 receptor-associated kinases (IRAKs) in the human genome, including IRAK-1, IRAK-2, IRAK-4, and IRAK-M, are key mediators in the immune pathways utilized by TLR/IL-1R (TIR) signaling. By means of their integral kinase IRAKs initiate diverse downstream signaling processes that can eventually lead to the induction of pro-inflammatory transcription factors such as NF-kB. In control and AD samples a significant up-regulation of miRNA-146a coupled to down-regulation of IRAK-1 and a parallel up-regulation of IRAK-2 was noted. Finally independent regulation of IRAK-1 and IRAK-2 in IL-1β+Aβ42 peptide-stressed HAG cells and inducible, NF-kB-sensitive, miRNA-146a-mediated downregulation of IRAK-1 coupled to an NF-kB-induced up-regulation of IRAK-2 expression was demonstrated (Cui et al., 2010). This regulatory network provides an important basis for a self-perpetuating inflammatory signaling loop (Fig.4). For sporadic Alzheimer's disease, which accounts for the majority of Alzheimer's disease cases, the most important risk factor is aging. Several miRNAs that are modulated in various aging model system, might contribute to AD. It was proposed that an alteration of miRNAs expression control in mid-life may be the putative force inducing molecular frailty in individual cell signaling, and in time leading to tissue-wide dysfunction (Wang, 2007). For example, miR-34a is increased in AD, peripheral blood mononuclear cell, aging mouse liver and *C. elegans* (Cogswell et al., 2008; Schipper et al., 2007; Maes et al., 2008; Ibanez-Ventoso et al., 2006). MiRNA lin-4 has been elegantly shown to influence lifespan and healthspan via its lin-14 mRNA target and the insulin signaling pathway, and several *C. elegans* age-regulated miRNAs have sequence similarity with both fly and human miRNAs (Ibanez-Ventoso & Driscoll, 2009). The question is whether there are evolutionary-conserved homologs of lin-4 and lin-14 that control human longevity and if miRNAs are implicated in many age-associated pathologies. Other miRNAs are upregulated during aging as let-7f, miR-30d, miR -432, miR-517 and downregulated as let-7i and miR-451 (Maes et al., 2009). Are they involved in gene regulation of aging related mechanism in AD? There is a great deal of evidence that suggests that oxidative stress plays a crucial role in the initiation and progression of Alzheimer's disease. In AD peripheral blood mononuclear cells, an impairment in DNA repair and antioxidant gene responses was observed and correlated to the up-regulation of miR-181b, miR-200a, miR-517* and miR-520, that may repress DNA repair and the response to oxidative stress (Shipper et al., 2007).

3.4 Studies in mouse models exploring microRNAs function in Alzheimer's disease

Mouse models have been recently used to investigate microRNA function in AD pathology. Specific deletion of Dicer in the adult forebrain leading to loss of microRNAs, was accompanied by a mixed neurodegenerative phenotype (Hebert et al., 2010). Although neuronal loss was observed in the hippocampus, cellular shrinkage was predominant in the cortex. Interestingly, neuronal degeneration coincides with the hyperphosphorylation of endogenous tau at several epitopes previously associated with neurofibrillary pathology.

Changes of miRNA expression might trigger molecular events inducing AD pathology or generate a feed-forward mechanism during AD progression. Two recent studies performed on mouse models of AD suggest that progression of AD pathology may produce alteration of microRNAs expression (Fig. 4). In APPswe/Psen1 transgenic mice, an AD mouse model which recapitulates some features of the disease, it was observed that BACE1 mRNA decreased and protein levels increased in the hippocampus at 19 months of age (Boissonneault et al., 2009). Two microRNAs, miR-298 and miR- 328, were found to regulate BACE 1 protein expression in mouse cultured neuronal cells. In transgenic mice, the expression of miR- 298 and miR-328 decreased in the granular neurons of the hippocampus during aging. However, while the miR-328 sequence is perfectly conserved between mouse and human, that of miR-298 is only 72% identical. More recently the hypothesis that Aβ itself causes neuronal miRNA deregulation which could contribute to the pathology associated with AD was explored (Schonrock et al 2010). A list of miRNAs, miR-9, miR-181c, miR-30c, miR-20b, miR-148b and Let-7i, was also downregulated in primary hippocampal cell cultures treated with Aβ. The miRNAs changes overlap with those occuring in the hippocampus of APP 23 mice (expressing human APP751 cDNA containing the Swedish double mutation (K651M and N652L) at 7 months of age At this age, mice reach the critical period of Aβ plaque formation where insoluble Aβ42 peptides increase five-fold compared to younger animals and small plaques can be seen in hippocampus and neocortex. In addition, the mice display major cognitive deficits affecting visuo-spatial learning abilities. These deregulated miRNAs overlap also with those found in sporadic human AD brain and potentially affect important biological pathways essential for proper brain function relevant to AD. The overlap between human AD brain and in vitro/in vivo AD models indicates that among the complex AD pathology, downregulation of miR-9, miR-181c, miR-30c, miR-20b, miR-148b and Let-7i could be attributed at least in part to the presence of Aβ (Fig.4).

4. Conclusion

Until now altered expression of miRNAs in Alzheimer's Disease brain tissues was demonstrated, however different studies identified various microRNAs. Increasing the numbers of miRNA expression profiles using large cohort of sporadic AD patients may allow us to better understand whether the variability among different profiles may be due to disease specific interindividual differences. It is difficult to determine if the changes in miRNA expression detected in the brains or CSF of patients are primary or secondary events, or both. Nevertheless early or late in the evolution of the disease, they could contribute to the pathogenesis of the observed lesions and neuronal loss. Unique patterns of miRNA expression profile in the CSF of AD could be useful as molecular biomarkers for disease diagnosis and eventually prediction of therapeutic responses. Target prediction analysis and cell-based assay linked miRNAs dysregulated in AD to APP and BACE1 genes which are associated with the pathology. Now the effort is to identify all targets of individual microRNA and to evaluate the impact that more than one microRNA may play on a specific target. In this regard computational prediction programs may be complemented by experiments in which the changes in transcripts and protein levels due to miRNA induction or knockdown are analysed using microarray platforms and SILAC (stable-isotope labelling with aminoacid in cell culture) and mass spectrometry (Selbach et al 2008). Also the co-immunoprecipitation of mRNA targets with Ago2 combined with microarray analysis of RNA (RIP-Chip assay) represents an alternative approach (Tan et al 2009). As demonstrated for the upregulation of miR-146 by the transcription factor NFkB the charachterization of promoters as well as transcriptional activators and repressors regulating microRNAs expression will be instrumental to delineate the relationship of microRNAs with networks involved in AD pathology. The use of transgenic animal models, manipulated in putative brain-expressed microRNAs associated to high-throughput methodologies, integrating transcriptomic, mirnomic and proteomics, will help to evaluate the potential association between RNA-mediated gene regulation and the pathogenesis of Alzheimer Disease and might indicate unexpected gene networks underlying Alzheimer's Disease.

5. Acknowledgment

This work was supported by Compagnia di San Paolo, Programma Neuroscienze, grant 'MicroRNAs in Neurodegenerative Diseases' (to C.B.), and by CNR grant DG.RSTL.059.012 (to F.R). We thank for graphical assistance -Studio 2CV idee e paesaggi- (www.studio2cv.it).

6. References

Ashraf, SI.; McLoon, AL.; Sclarsic, SM. & Kunes, S. (2006). *Synaptic protein synthesis associated with memory is regulated by the RISC pathway in Drosophila.* Cell 124:191–205

Banerjee, S.; Neveu, P. & Kosik, KS. (2009) *A coordinated local translational control point at the synapse involving relief from silencing and MOV10 degradation.* Neuron. 64(6):871-84

Bingol, B. & Schuman, EM. (2005) *Synaptic protein degradation by the ubiquitin proteasome system.* Curr Opin Neurobiol 15:536– 541

Bingol, B. & Schuman, EM. (2006) *Activity-dependent dynamics and sequestration of proteasomes in dendritic spines.* Nature 441:1144–1148

Birdsill, A.C.; Walker, D. G.; Lue, L.F.; Sue, LI. & Beach, TG. (2010) *Postmortem interval effect on RNA and gene expression in human brain tissue.* Cell Tissue Bank. DOI: 10.1007/s10561-010-9210-8

Bohnsack, M.T; Czaplinski, K. & Gorlich, D. (2004) *Exportin 5 is a RanGTP-dependent dsRNA-binding protein that mediates nuclear export of pre-miRNAs.* RNA 10(2):185–191

Boissonneault, V.; Plante, I.; Rivest, S. & Provost, P. (2009) *MicroRNA-298 and microRNA-328 regulate expression of mouse beta-amyloid precursor protein-converting enzyme 1.* J Biol Chem 284(4):1971-81

Caudy, AA.; Myers, M.; Hannon, GJ. & Hammond, SM. (2002) *Fragile Xrelated protein and VIG associate with the RNA interference machinery.* Genes Dev 16:2491–2496

Cao, X.; Yeo, G.; Muotri, AR., Kuwabara, T. & Gage, FH. (2006) *Noncoding RNAs in the mammalian central nervous system.* Annu Rev Neurosci. 29:77-103.

Chendrimada, TP.; Gregory, RI.; Kumaraswamy, E.; Norman, J. & Cooch, N. et al. (2005) *TRBP recruits the Dicer complex to Ago2 for microRNA processing and gene silencing.* Nature 436(7051): 740–744

Cogswell, J.P.; Ward, J.; Taylor, I.A.; Waters, M.; Shi, Y.; Cannon, B.; Kelnar, K.; Kemppainen, J.; Brown, D.; Chen, C.; Prinjha, C.; Richardson, J.; Saunders, A.M.; Roses, A.D. & Ricards, C.A. (2008). *Identification of miRNA changes in Alzheimerr's Disease brain and CSF yields putative biomarkers insights into disease pathways.* J. Alzheimer's Disease 14: 27-41

Coleman, PD.; & Yao, PJ. (2003) *Synaptic slaughter in Alzheimer's disease.* Neurobiol Aging 24(8):1023-7.

Cui, J.G.; Li, YY., Zhao, Y., Battacharjee, S. & Lukiw, W. (2010). *Differential regulation of interleukin-1 receptor-associated kinase-1 (IRAK-1) and IRAK-2 by microRNA-146a and NF-kB in stressed human astroglial cells and Alzheimer disease.* J. Biol. Chem. 285 (50): 38951-38960

Edbauer, D.; Neilson, JR., Foster, KA., Wang, CF., Seeburg, DP., Batterton, MN., Tada, T., Dolan, BM., Sharp, PA. & Sheng, M. (2010) *Regulation of synaptic structure and function by FMRP-associated microRNAs miR-125b and miR-132.* Neuron 65:373–384

Fiore, R.; Khudayberdiev, S., Christensen, M., Siegel, G., Flavell, SW., Kim, T., Greenberg, ME. & Schratt, G. (2009) *Mef2-mediated transcription of the miR379–410 cluster regulates activity-dependent dendritogenesis by fine-tuning Pumilio2 protein levels.* EMBO J 28:697–710

Gregory, RI.; Yan, KP., Amuthan, G., Chendrimada, TP., Doratotaj, B. et al. (2004) *The microprocessor complex mediates the genesis of microRNAs.* Nature 432(7014):235–240

Hansen, KF; Sakamoto, K., Wayman, GA., Impey, S. & Obrietan, K. (2010) *Transgenic miR132 alters neuronal spine density and impairs novel object recognition memory.* PLoS One. 5(11):e15497.

Hébert, S.; Horré, K., Nicolai, L., Papadopoulou, A., Mandemakers, A. N., Kauppinen, S., Delacourte, A., De Stropper, B. (2008) *Loss of microRNA cluster miR29a/b in sporadic Alzheimer's disease correlates with increased Bace1/β-secretase expression.* PNAS 105(17): 6415-6420

Hébert, S.; Horré, K., Nicolai, L., Bergmans, B., Papadopoulou, A. S., Delacourte, A., De Stropper, B. (2009) *MicroRNA regulation of Alzheimer's amyloid precursor protein expression.* Neurobiol Dis. 33:422-428

Hébert, S.; Papadopoulou, AS., Smith, P., Galas, MC., Planel, E., Silahtaroglu, AN., Sergeant, N., Buée, L. & De Strooper, B. (2010) *Genetic ablation of Dicer in adult forebrain neurons results in abnormal tau hyperphosphorylation and neurodegeneration.* Hum Mol Genet. 19(20):3959-69

Hotulainen, P.; & Hoogenraad, CC. (2010) *Actin in dendritic spines: connecting dynamics to function.* J Cell Biol. 189(4):619-29

Hutvagner, G.; & Simard, MJ. (2008) *Argonaute proteins: key players in RNA silencing.* Nat Rev Mol Cell Biol 9(1):22–32

Ibanez-Ventoso, C.; Yang, M., Guo, S., Robins, H., Padgett, RW. & Driscoll, M. (2006) *Modulated microRNA expression during adult lifespan in Caenorhabditis elegans.* Aging Cell 5:235–246

Ibáñez-Ventoso, C.; & Driscoll, M. (2009) *MicroRNAs in C. elegans Aging: Molecular Insurance for Robustness?* Curr Genomics. 10(3):144-53

Ishizuka, A.; Siomi, MC. & Siomi, H. (2002) *A Drosophila fragile X protein interacts with components of RNAi and ribosomal proteins.* Genes Dev 16:2497–2508

Jin, P.; Zarnescu, DC., Ceman, S., Nakamoto, M., Mowrey, J. et al. (2004) *Biochemical and genetic interaction between the fragile X mental retardation protein and the microRNA pathway.* Nat Neurosci 7:113–117

Kasai, H.; Fukuda M, Watanabe S, Hayashi-Takagi A, Noguchi J. (2010) *Structural dynamics of dendritic spines in memory and cognition.* Trends Neurosci. 33(3):121-9

Kiebler, MA.; & Bassel, GJ. (2006) *Neuronal RNA granules: movers and makers* Neuron. 51(6):685-90

Kim, VN.; (2005) *MicroRNA biogenesis: coordinated cropping and dicing.* Nat Rev Mol Cell Biol 6(5):376–385

Kole, A.; Swhari, V., Hammomnd, S. & Deshmukh, M. (2011) *miR-29b is activated during neuronal maturation and targets BH3-only genes to restrict apoptosis.* Genes Dev 15;25(2):125-30

Konopka, W.; Kiryk, A., Novak, M., Herwerth, M., Parkitna, JR., Wawrzyniak, M., Kowarsch, A. Michaluk, P., Dzwonek, J., Arnsperger, T., Wilczynski, G., Merkenschlager, M., Theis, FJ., Köhr, G., Kaczmarek, L. & Schütz, G. (2010) *MicroRNA loss enhances learning and memory in mice.* J Neurosci. 30(44):14835-42

Kurose, H.; (2003) *Galpha12 and Galpha13 as key regulatory mediator in signal transduction.* Life Sci. 74(2-3):155-61

Lee, RC.; Feinbaum, RL. & Ambros, V. (1993) *The C. elegans heterochronic gene lin-4 encodes small RNAs with antisense complementarity to lin-14.* Cell 75(5):843–854

Lee, Y.; Ahn, C., Han, J., Choi, H., Kim. J et al., (2003) The nuclear Rnase III Drosha initiates microRNA processing. Nature 425(6956): 415–419

Lee, Y.; Hur, I., Park, SY., Kim, YK., Suh, MR. et al. (2006) *The role of PACT in the RNA silencing pathway.* EMBO J 25(3):522–532

Liu, W.; Liu C, Zhu J, Shu P, Yin B, Gong Y, Qiang B, Yuan J, Peng X. (2010) *MicroRNA-16 targets amyloid precursor protein to potentially modulate Alzheimer's-associated pathogenesis in SAMP8 mice.* DOI:10.1016/neurobiolaging.2010.04.034 Neurobiol Aging

Lukiw, WJ.; (2004) *Gene expression profiling in fetal, aged, and Alzheimer hippocampus: a continuum of stress-related signaling.* Neurochem Res 29(6):1287-97

Lukiw, WJ.; (2007) *Micro-RNA speciation in fetal, adult and Alzheimer's disease hippocampus.Neuroreport.* 18(3):297-300

Lukiw, WJ.; Zhao, Y. & Cui, JG. (2008) *An NF-kappaB-sensitive micro RNA-146a-mediated inflammatory circuit in Alzheimer disease and in stressed human brain cells.* J Biol Chem. 283(46):31315-22

Malenka, RC.; & Nicoll, RA. (1999) *Long-term potentiation--a decade of progress?* Science 285(5435):1870-4

Manahan-Vaughan, D.; Kulla, A., & Frey, JU. (2000) *Requirement of translation but not transcription for the maintenance of long-term depression in the CA1 region of freely moving rats.* J Neurosci. 20(22):8572-6

Maes, OC.; An, J., Sarojini, H. & Wang, E. (2008) *Murine microRNAs implicated in liver functions and aging process.* Mech. Ageing Dev 129:534–541

Maes, OC.; Chertkow, HM., Wang, E. & Schipper, HM. (2009) *MicroRNA: Implications for Alzheimer Disease and other Human CNS Disorders.* Curr Genomics. 10(3):154-68

Morris, RG.; (2003) *Long-term potentiation and memory.* Philos Trans R Soc Lond B Biol Sci. 358(1432):643-7

Nelson, PT.; & Wilfred, BN.(2009) *In situ hybridization is a necessary experimental complement to microRNA (miRNA) expression profiling in the human brain.* Neurosci Lett. 4466(2):69-72

Nunez-Iglesias, C.; Lui, C., Morgan, T.E. & Zhou, X.J. (2010) *Joint genome-wide profiling of miRNA and mRNA expression in Alzheimer's disease cortex reveals altered miRNA regulation.* PLoS One 5(2): e8898

Olsen, PH.; & Ambros, V. (1999) *The lin-4 regulatory RNA controls developmental timing in Caenorhabditis elegans by blocking LIN-14 protein synthesis after the initiation of translation.* Dev Biol 216(2):671–680

Park, CS.; & Tang, SJ. (2009) *Regulation of microRNA expression by induction of bidirectional synaptic plasticity.* J Mol Neurosci. 38(1):50-6

Patel, N.; Hoang, D., Miller, N., Ansaloni, S., Huang, Q., Rogers, J. T., Lee, J. C., Saunders, A. J. (2008) *MicroRNA can regulate human APP levels.* Mol Neurodegener 3:10

Podlisny, M.; Lee, G. & Selkoe, DJ. (1987) *Gene dosage of the amyloid beta precursor protein in Alzheimer's disease.* Science 238:669-71.

Reinhart, BJ.; Slack, FJ., Basson, M., Pasquinelli, AE., Bettinger, JC. et al. (2000) *The 21-nucleotide let-7 RNA regulates developmental timing in Caenorhabditis elegans.* Nature 403(6772):901–906

Rodriguez, A.; Griffiths-Jones, S., Ashurst, JL., & Bradley, A. (2004) *Identification of mammalian microRNA host genes and transcription units.* Genome Res 14(10A):1902–1910

Rovelet-Lecrux, A.; Hannequin, D., Raux, G., Le Meur, N., Laquerrie're, A., Vital, A., et al. (2006) *APP locus duplication causes autosomal dominant early-onset Alzheimer disease with cerebral amyloid angiopathy.* Nat Genet 38:24-6

Scheff, S.; & Price, DA.(2006) *Alzheimer's disease-related alterations in synaptic density: neocortex and hippocampus.* J Alzheimers Dis 9(3 Suppl):101-15

Schipper, HM.; Maes, OC., Chertkow, HM. & Wang, E. (2007) *MicroRNA expression in Alzheimer blood mononuclear cells.* Gene Regul. Syst. Bio. 1:263–274

Schonrock, N.; Ke, YD., Humphreys, D., Staufenbiel, M., Ittner, LM., Preiss, T. & Götz, J. (2010) Neuronal microRNA deregulation in response to Alzheimer's disease amyloid-beta. PLoS One. 5(6):e11070

Schratt, GM.; Tuebing, F., Nigh, EA., Kane, CG., Sabatini, ME. et al. (2006) *A brain-specific microRNA regulates dendritic spine development.* Nature 439(7074):283–289

Schratt, G.; (2009) *Fine-tuning neural gene expression with microRNAs.* Curr Opin Neurobiol 19(2):213-9

Selbach, M.; Schwanhäusser, B., Thierfelder, N., Fang, Z., Khanin, R. & Rajewsky, N. (2008) *Widespread changes in protein synthesis induced by microRNAs.* Nature 455(7209):58-63.

Sethi, P.; & Lukiw, WJ. (2009) *Micro-RNA abundance and stability in human brain: specific alterations in Alzheimer's disease temporal lobe neocortex.* Neurosci. Letters 459:100-104.

Shioya, M.; Obayashi, S., Tabunoki, H., Arima, K., Saito, Y., Ishida, T. & Satoh, J. (2010) *Aberrant microRNA expression in the brains of neurodegenerative diseases: miR-29a decreased in Alzheimer disease brains targets neurone navigator 3.* Neuropathology and Applied Neurobiology 36: 320-330

Siegel, G.; Obernosterer, G., Fiore, R., Oehmen, M., Bicker, S., et al.(2009) *A functional screen implicates microRNA-138-dependent regulation of the depalmitoylation enzyme APT1 in dendritic spine morphogenesis.* Nat Cell Biol 11:705–716

Smalheiser, NR.; Lugli, G., Lenon, AL., Davis, JM., Torvik, V. & Larson J. (2010) *Olfactory discrimination training up-regulates and reorganizes expression of microRNAs in adult mouse hippocampus.* ASN Neuro. 2(1):e00028.

Smith, P.; Al Hashimi, A., Girard, J., Delay, C. & Hébert, SS. (2011) *In vivo regulation of amyloid precursor protein neuronal splicing by microRNAs.* 116(2):240-7

Sutton, MA.; & Schuman, EM. (2006) *Dendritic protein synthesis, synaptic plasticity, and memory.* Cell. 2006 Oct 6;127(1):49-58

Tan, LP.; Seinen, E., Duns, G., de Jong, D., Sibon, OC., Poppema, S., Kroesen, BJ., Kok, K., & van den Berg, A. (2009) *A high throughput experimental approach to identify miRNA targets in human cells.*Nucleic Acids Res. 37(20):e137

Vilardo, E.; Barbato, C., Ciotti, MT., Cogoni, C. & Ruberti, F. (2010) *MicroRNA-101 regulates amyloid precursor protein expression in hippocampal neurons.* J Biol Chem 285:18344-51

Vo, N.; Klein, ME., Varlamova, O., Keller, DM., Yamamoto, T. et al. (2005) *A cAMP-response element binding protein-induced microRNA regulates neuronal morphogenesis.* Proc Natl Acad Sci USA 102(45):16426–16431

Wang, E.; (2007) *MicroRNA, the putative molecular control for mid-life decline.* Ageing Res. Rev. 6:1–11

Wang, W.; Rajeev, B., Stromberg, A., Ren, N., Tang., G., Huang, Q., Rigoutsos, I. & Nelson, P.T. (2008). *The Expression of MicroRNA miR-107 Decreases Early in Alzheimer's Disease and may Accelerate Disease Progression through Regulation of β-Site Amyloid Precursor Protein-Cleaving Enzyme 1. J. Neurosci.* 28(5): 1213-1223

Wang, X.; Huang, Q., Hu, Y., Stromberg, A.J. &Nelson, P.T. (2011) *Patterns of microRNA expression in normal and early Alzheimer'disease human temporal cortex: white matter versus gray matter.* Acta Neuropathol 121:193-205

Wayman, GA.; Davare, M., Ando, H., Fortin, D., Varlamova, O., et al. (2008) *An activity-regulated microRNA controls dendritic plasticity by down-regulating p250GAP.* Proc Natl Acad Sci 105:9093–9098

Wibrand, K.; Panja, D., Tiron, A., Ofte, ML., Skaftnesmo, KO., et al. (2010) *Differential regulation of mature and precursor microRNA expression by NMDA and metabotropic glutamate receptor activation during LTP in the adult dentate gyrus in vivo. Eur J Neurosci.* 31(4):636-45

Whiteman, IT.; Gervasio, OL., Cullen, KM., Guillemin, GJ., Jeong, EV., et al. (2009) *Activated actin-depolymerizing factor/cofilin sequesters phosphorylated microtubule- associated protein during the assembly of alzheimer-like neuritic cytoskeletal striations.* J Neurosci 29: 12994–13005

Yao, J.; Hennessey, T., Flynt, A., Lai, E., Beal, MF., et al. (2010) *MicroRNA-related cofilin abnormality in Alzheimer's disease.* PLoS One 5(12):e15546

Part 4

Oxidative Stress, Reactive Oxygen Species, and Heavy Metals

14

Role of Mitochondria in Alzheimer's Disease

Genaro Genaro Gabriel Ortiz[1,2] et al. *
[1]*Lab. Estrés Oxidativo-Mitocondria & Enfermedad. Centro de Investigación Biomédica de Occidente (CIBO). Instituto mexicano del seguro Social (IMSS). Guadalajara, Jalisco,*
[2]*División de Ciencias de la Salud-Escuela de Medicina, Tecnológico de Monterrey, Campus Guadalajara. Zapopan, Jalisco, México*

1. Introduction

Alzheimer's disease is the most common neurodegenerative disorder worldwide characterized by considerable atrophy and an enlargement and coarsening of the sulci, β-amyloid formation in neuritic plaques and brain vessels (amyloid angiopathy), neurofibrillary tangles, and neuronal loss, particularly in the limbic and association cortices. In addition, deficits in cholinergic transmission and associated loss of cholinergic cell bodies, granulovacuolar degeneration and rod-shaped eosinophilic inclusions (Hirano bodies) are common in Alzheimer's disease patients. Clinical symptoms are characterized by progressive worsening of memory, and cognitive impairment accompanied by one of the following symptoms: aphasia, apraxia, agnosia and disorders in the executive function (Selkoe, 2004).

The pathophysiological mechanisms that underlie the neurodegenerative characteristic of Alzheimer's disease are yet to be completely understood, although many factors in disease pathogenesis have been identified, and several theories are emerged. In the last years, mitochondrial dysfunction has been considered as a potential factor implicated at some stage of the pathogenic process (Anandatheerthavarada et al., 2003; Sullivan & Brown, 2005;

---

*Fermín Pacheco-Moisés[3], José de Jesús García-Trejo[4], Roció E. González-Castañeda[5], Miguel A. Macías-Islas[6], José A. Cruz-Ramos[1], Irma E. Velázquez-Brizuela[1], Elva D. Árias Merino[7] and Alfredo Célis de la Rosa[7]

[1]*Lab. Estrés Oxidativo-Mitocondria & Enfermedad. Centro de Investigación Biomédica de Occidente (CIBO). Instituto mexicano del seguro Social (IMSS). Guadalajara, Jalisco, Mexico*

[2]*División de Ciencias de la Salud-Escuela de Medicina, Tecnológico de Monterrey, Campus Guadalajara. Zapopan, Jalisco, México. Mexico*

[3]*Departamento de Química. Centro Universitario de Ciencias Exactas e Ingenierías. Universidad de Guadalajara. Guadalajara, Jalisco, Mexico*

[4]*Departamento de Biología. Facultad de Química. Universidad Nacional Autónoma de México, Mexico*

[5]*Departamento de Neurociencias. Centro Universitario de Ciencias de la Salud. Universidad de Guadalajara. Guadalajara, Jalisco, Mexico*

[6]*Departamento de Neurología. Unidad Médica de Alta Especialidad. Hospital de Especialidades-Centro Médico Nacional de Occidente. IMSS. Guadalajara, Jalisco, Mexico*

[7]*Departamento de Salud Pública. Centro Universitario de Ciencias de la Salud. Universidad de Guadalajara. Guadalajara, Jalisco, Mexico*

Atamna & Frey, 2007: Wang et al., 2008). As essential role players in cellular metabolism, mitochondria are pertinent to cell survival and thus any deviation from their operation is undoubtedly serious. Almost all aspects of mitochondrial function are altered in Alzheimer neurons; particularly it has been reported defects in oxidative phosphorylation (Chandrasekaran et al., 1996; Manczak et al., 2004; Schagger & Ohm, 1995) and both inherited and somatic mitochondrial DNA mutations in certain AD cases (Coskun et al., 2004; Qiu et al., 2001). In addition, changes in the redox status and membrane fluidity have been largely documented in brain and platelets (Mecocci et al., 1996; Zubenko et al., 1999; Mosconi et al., 2008; Ortiz et al., 2008; Su et al., 2008). The extent to which these changes in mitochondrial function represent primary or secondary components of the pathophysiological process are essential in order to understand the basic pathways that lead to the progress of disease. At this regard it has been shown that neurons are particularly vulnerable to any abnormalities of mitochondrial functioning, due to their large energy demand for their survival and specialized function. In this review we will describe the body of evidence supporting the role of mitochondria in the pathogenesis of Alzheimer's disease and discuss mitochondrial alterations in platelets from AD patients, particularly, mitochondrial enzymatic activities and membrane fluidity.

2. Mitochondrial function

2.1 ATP synthesis

Mitochondria are the major site of adenosine triphosphate (ATP) synthesis in most cells by the processes of oxidative phosphorylation. Mitochondria also mediate amino acid biosynthesis, fatty acid oxidation, steroid metabolism, calcium homeostasis, and reactive oxygen species production and detoxification. They synthesize amino acids, pyrimidines, lipids, heme, hormones and other metabolites. Each mitochondrion consists of four main compartments, including the outer membrane, the inner membrane, the inter-membranous space, and the matrix. The outer membrane encloses the entire organelle and is relatively porous, allowing the passage of small molecules. The inner mitochondrial membrane is characterized by a series of complex folds and tubules called cristae, which contain a variety of the enzymes, including those responsible for making ATP, is largely impermeant and forms the major barrier between the cytosol and the mitochondrial matrix. The space between the two membranes is referred to as the intermembrane space. The five complexes of the respiratory chain, complex I (NADH ubiquinone oxidoreductase), complex II (succinate ubiquinone oxidoreductase), complex III (ubiquinone-cytochrome c reductase), complex IV (cytochrome oxidase), and complex V (ATP synthase) are embedded in the inner mitochondrial membrane. The transfer of electrons along the respiratory chain provides the energy to pump protons from the matrix into the intermembrane space, generating the electrochemical gradient required to drive ATP synthesis (Hatefi, 1986).

ATP synthase is an enzyme that works as a rotary motor to carry out ATP synthesis by using Mg^{2+}-ADP complex, inorganic phosphate and a proton electrochemical gradient across energy-transducing membranes. It is composed by two main sectors: F0, a membrane-embedded proton-translocating sector that contains up to 10 different subunits and F1, a soluble catalytic sector comprising five different subunits that is bound through two stalks to F0. The coupling between F1 and F0 is critical for efficient ATP synthesis to occur and a large body of evidence shows that F1 andF0 are structurally and functionally coupled through two stalks. The central stalk forms part of the rotor of the enzyme, and the peripheral stalk is part of the stator that anchors the catalytic sites of F1 to the membrane. The central rotor actually gyrates relative to a stator that holds the catalytic subunits; this rotation induces the alternating binding, catalysis, and product release from three catalytic sites of F1 (Noji & Yoshida, 2001).

Because of thermodynamic and mechanical reversibility, the ATP synthase also hydrolyzes ATP under conditions of partial or total collapse of the proton gradient in all energy-transducing systems. Thus, different subunits and mechanisms have emerged in nature to control the intrinsic rotation of the enzyme to favor the ATP synthase activity over its opposite and commonly wasteful ATPase turnover. A key regulatory subunit of ATP synthase is the mitochondrial inhibitor protein (IF1). Since its first isolation in 1963 (Pullman & Monroy, 1963), this protein was shown to inhibit the hydrolytic activity of the catalytic F1 sector. This protein is therefore crucial to prevent the hydrolysis of newly synthesized ATP in conditions of low membrane potential in mitochondria. Upon membrane energization, IF1 is believed to be relocated from its inhibitory site into an unknown position within (Dreyfus et al., 1981; Sanchez-Bustamante et al., 1982) or outside the F1F0 complex (Schwerzmann & Pedersen 1981; Power et al., 1983), therefore allowing ATP synthesis to occur. In de-energized or uncoupled conditions, IF1 is productively associated with the enzyme, inhibiting the ATPase turnover of the F1I or F1F0I complexes. However, this protein allows the rotational ATP synthesis turnover during energization of mitochondrial membranes. Therefore, IF1 is an important physiological regulator of the functioning of the ATP synthase. Recently, it has been shown that IF1 also contributes to stabilize dimeric and oligomeric forms of the mitochondrial ATP synthase that promote formation of mitochondrial cristae (Minauro-Sanmiguel et al., 2005; García et al., 2006; Campanella et al., 2008), thus adding a further key role of IF1 and dimeric F1F0 in the whole mitochondrial biogenesis (reviewed in García-Trejo & Morales-Ríos, 2008).

2.2 Mitochondrial dynamics

Mitochondrial dynamics implies that mitochondria continuously undergo fission and fusion to generate smaller organelles or elongated, tubular structures, respectively. Thus, mitochondria are not static organelles, but are dynamic bodies that constantly divide and fuse within the cell as the environment demands (Chan, 2006). These processes can facilitate formation of new mitochondria, repair of defective mitochondrial DNA through mixing, and redistribution of mitochondria to sites requiring high-energy production (Frederick & Shaw, 2007; Knott et al., 2008). Both processes effectively lower the percentage of defective mitochondria in the cell and ensure stability in cellular proliferation; indeed, metabolism, energy production, calcium signaling, reactive oxidative species production, apoptosis and senescence all depend on the balance of fission and fusion. Conversely, dynamic distortion (i.e., excessive fragmentation/elongation) results in inefficiencies in cell functioning, if not cell death (Parone et al., 2008; Wang et al., 2009; Chen et al., 2005).

Mitochondrial dynamics is a tightly regulated cellular process, with dedicated molecular machinery involving GTPases. Fission is regulated by at least two proteins: a large GTPase, dynamin-like protein 1, and a small molecule, Fis1, and fusion involves three large mitochondrial transmembrane proteins localized to the outer membrane: mitofusin 1, mitofusin 2, and optic atrophy protein 1 (Chan, 2006; Knott et al., 2008).

Mitochondria structurally abnormal have been reported in Alzheimer´s disease brains, for instance significant alterations in mitochondrial cristae (Hirai et al., 2001), the accumulation of osmiophylic material and significant decreases in mitochondrial size are found predominantly in neurons (Baloyannis, 2006). In addition, mitochondria are redistributed away of axons in the pyramidal (Wang et al., 2009). Electron-microscopic studies have showed an increase in mitochondrial fragmentation in human AD brains (Balayonnis, 2006; Wang et al., 2009). In cell-based experiments, β-amyloidproduction resulted in the appearance of fragmented and abnormally distributed mitochondria (Barsoum et al., 2006; Wang et al., 2008). The dynamic balance of fission and fusion in AD is greatly shifted toward fission, and, as a result, affected neurons contain abnormal mitochondria that are unable to meet the metabolic demands of the cell. Moreover, mitochondrial distribution in AD cells is perinuclear, with few metabolic organelles in the distal processes, where they are normally distributed in healthy cells and are needed for exocytosis, ion channel pumps, synaptic function and other activities.

2.3 Energetic impairment in AD brains

Normal synapse function requires concerted activity of a multitude of metabolic pathways, including the generation of gene products involved in membrane complex formation and maintenance; mitochondrial RNA, protein, and neurotransmitter synthesis and delivery; and most importantly, the maintenance of ion gradients across the plasma membranes, as they are critical for the generation of action potentials. These actions can only be performed efficiently when sufficient energetic substrates are supplied. Glucose metabolism in the brain provides about 95% of the energy required under normal circumstances, with fatty acids only making a minor contribution. This intense demand for energy is continual, even brief periods of oxygen or glucose deprivation result in neuronal death. However, in spite of this high energy requirement, the brain is rather uncompromising in its ability to utilize substrates for energy production (Costantini et al., 2008).
Early evidence for altered glucose metabolism in AD brain comes from *in vivo* fluorodeoxyglucose positron emission tomography measurements of the cerebral metabolic rate for glucose (de Leon et al., 1983). This change in glucose utilization is linked to cognitive performance (Constantini et al., 2008). Reductions up to 45% in cerebral glucose utilization in AD patients have been reported (Ishii K et al., 1997). Other studies have reported low brain's glucose consumption rate in hippocampal and entorhinal cortical regions (Swerdlow, 2007). The posterior cingulate cortex and the neighboring precuneus are metabolically affected in the earliest clinical and preclinical stages of AD and the primary visual cortex is relatively spared (Minoshima et al., 1997; Reiman et al., 1996). That reduction in glucose metabolism is the result of both decreased glucose transport (because of a decrease in the number of synapses) and a decrease in the number of neurons. Therefore, the decreased cerebral metabolism is a true loss of neurons and synapses rather than simply the decreased glucose metabolism expected from a smaller volume of tissue seen in patients with atrophy [Bokde, 2001; Ibanez et al., 1998)]. In addition, in alzheimer´s disease there is a generalized shift from glycolytic energy production toward use of an alternative fuel, ketone bodies. Patients with incipient alzheimer´s disease exhibit a utilization ratio of 2:1 glucose to ketone bodies, whereas comparably aged controls exhibit a ratio of 29:1, whereas young controls exclusively use glucose with a ratio of 100:0 (Hoyer, 1991). On the other hand, *in vitro* analyses of AD autopsy brain show reductions in glycolysis (Swerdlow & Kish, 2002). These findings have been consistently reproduced by a multitude of studies and this pattern of hypometabolism is therefore now widely accepted as a reliable *in vivo* hallmark of Alzheimer's disease, and accurately distinguishes AD from normal aging.

The defects in glucose utilization suggest possible abnormalities in mitochondrial function. In support of this view, a range of reports have shown altered mitochondrial properties in Alzheimer's disease, in particular, the energy extracting mechanisms of the mitochondria. For instance, the temporal and parietal cortical zones consistently exhibits abnormally high oxygen utilization in comparison to the amounts of glucose utilized, and reduced phosphocreatine levels, indicating impairment of the oxidative phosphorylation process in the mitochondria (Benson et al., 1981; Phelps et al., 1982; Friedland et al., 1983 Pettegrew et al, 1994). In addition, AD brain biopsies demonstrated mitochondrial uncoupling, a non-specific abnormality indicative of an impairment in conversion of ADP to ATP (Sims et al., 1987). Interestingly the abnormalities in cerebral metabolism precede the onset of neurological dysfunction as well as gross neuropathology of AD.

In vitro analyses of AD autopsy brain studies have shown that the most consistent defect in mitochondria in AD are the reductions in maximal activities of several key enzymes responsible for oxidative metabolism, including α-ketoglutarate dehydrogenase complex, isocitrate dehydrogenase, and pyruvate dehydrogenase complex, two enzymes involved in the rate-limiting step of tricarboxylic acid cycle (Parker et al., 1994; Gibson et al., 1998; Nagy et al., 1999; Swerdlow & Kish, 2002). In addition, studies have shown reduced cytochrome oxidase activity, the terminal enzyme in the electron transfer chain that is responsible for reducing molecular oxygen (Parker et al., 1994; Gibson et al., 1998; Maurer et al., 2000; Bosetti et al., 2002; Swerdlow & Kish, 2002).

Reductions in maximal activity of cytochrome c oxidase have been reported in several areas of the brain. For instance, it has been found that AD cases had lower cytochrome c oxidase activity than controls in the posterior cingulate cortex. That reduction was significantly greater than that in primary motor cortex (Valla et al., 2001). However, it is unclear to what extent maximal activity reduction reflects reduced COX enzyme expression or a structural change in the enzyme. Numerous studies have linked abnormal mitochondrial protein function to the altered neuronal expression of nuclear and mitochondrial genes encoding subunits of the mitochondrial electron transfer chain. Liang and collaborators (2008) showed that compared to controls, AD cases had the largest proportion (70 percent) of underexpressed genes comprising the nuclear genes encoding for subunits of the mitochondrial electron transfer chain complexes and translocases of the inner and outer mitochondrial membranes in the posterior cingulated cortex, a brain region which positron emission tomography studies found to be metabolically affected in the earliest stages of AD. The visual cortex, on the other hand, a brain region relatively spared in AD, contained significantly less underexpressed genes than the posterior cingulate cortices.

Interestingly, Reddy and Beal (2008) found mitochondrial genes in the NADH ubiquinone oxidoreductase of oxidative phosphorylation system to be downregulated in both early and definite AD brains, whereas complexes ubiquinone-cytochrome c reductase and cytochrome c oxidase showed increased mitochondrial RNA expressions. Several other studies have also reported this phenomenon (Hirai et al., 2001; Strazielle et al., 2003; Manczak et al., 2004; Reddy et al., 2004), which could be interpreted as a compensatory mechanism for the decreased cytochrome c oxidase function and the consequent increase in demand on energy production. As spectral analysis of the enzyme has indicated that cytochrome c oxidase is kinetically altered in AD and lacks one of its two substrate binding sites (Parker & Parks, 1995), altogether the data would imply that cytochrome c oxidase activity is reduced not because the quantity is decreased as a result of down-regulated gene expression, but because in AD, the enzyme is structurally different from that in controls. However, other studies have shown that cytochrome oxidase activity is reduced as a result of decreased mitochondrial RNA expression. Several studies demonstrated decreased mitochondrial RNA expression in NADH ubiquinone oxidoreductase and cytochrome c oxidase (Chandrasekaran et al., 1994, 1996, 1997) and decreased mRNA expression of nuclear-encoded mitochondrial genes in complexes cytochrome c oxidase and ATP synthase in brains of AD patients (Chandrasekaran et al., 1994, 1997; Simonian & Hyman, 1994). Clearly, at this point, it cannot be said whether reduced mitochondrial RNA expression, altered enzyme kinetics or both, contribute to reduced cytochrome c oxidase function in AD. Some studies suggest that mitochondrial DNA and mitochondrial number increase in AD, which would indicate altered cytochrome c oxidase kinetics, while others suggest that mitochondrial DNA and mitochondrial number decline, proposing reduced cytochrome c oxidase expression (De la Monte et al., 2000; Hirai et al., 2001; Baloyannis, 2006). Other studies have reported lowered biosynthesis of beta subunit of the ATP synthase, in the hippocampus and the ubiquinone-cytochrome c reductase core protein 1, respectively (Kim et al., 2000). How these changes in mitochondrial enzymes would translate into loss of specific neuronal populations, including cholinergic neurons in the forebrain, hippocampus, and neocortex is unclear. One possibility is that as yet unknown factors cause an imbalance that favours the generation of reactive oxygen species.

2.4 Mitochondria and oxidative stress

Oxidative stress is a relative increase in the ratio of free radicals to antioxidants. This may originate from an overproduction of reactive oxygen species or from a reduction in antioxidant capacity. Indeed, the activities of the antioxidant enzymes superoxide dismutase and catalase are significantly decreased in the frontal and temporal cortex of AD patients (Marcus et al., 1998). Not only that, antioxidant enzyme activity was shown to be spatially correlated with markers of lipid peroxidation (i.e. oxidative damage) and the brain areas particularly affected by neuronal loss in AD (Takeda et al., 2000). However, increased antioxidant activity in AD brains in response to increased free radical generation has also been reported (Lovell et al., 1995; Lu et al., 2004; Moreira et al., 2009). Thus, one explanation for the studies showing a lack of correlation between impaired mitochondrial function and oxidative stress is that in some AD cases, antioxidant defenses are able to counteract oxidative stress damage, whilst in others they cannot. However, this would automatically mean that in the AD cases with no oxidative stress, other impaired mechanisms must be causing AD.

Some studies show that brain tissue is especially vulnerable to oxidative attack due to its relatively low antioxidant capacity, high consumption of oxygen, high content of polyunsaturated fatty acids, and high content of redox-active transition metals such as iron (Butterfield et al., 2007). Iron can contribute to free radical damage by catalyzing the formation of the hydroxyl radical, inducing secondary initiation of lipid peroxidation and by promoting the oxidation of proteins. The increase in brain iron associated with several neurodegenerative diseases may lead to an increased production of free radicals via the Fenton reaction. Depending on the substrate attacked by the reactive oxygen species, oxidative damage will manifest as protein oxidation, DNA oxidation, or lipid peroxidation products.

Mitochondria are the primary source of cellular oxidants, taking into account that about 2–5% of molecular oxygen is not completely reduced to water at the electron transport chain and, therefore, a prime target of cumulative oxidative damage. Damage to mitochondrial proteins and mitocondrial DNA would be expected to decrease mitochondrial bioenergetics and efficiency (The underlying mechanism of abnormal mitochondrial reactive oxygen species production is the altered redox potential of mitochondrial respiratory chain carriers (due to hyperpolarization of mitochondrial membrane) and an increase in ubisemiquinone anion half-life time, resulting in slower electron transport, producing intermediates that stay reduced longer, thus increasing the chance that the electrons can escape to molecular oxygen, originating the reactive oxygen species (Sullivan & Brown 2005). Ultimately, ATP depletion will lead to necrotic cell death. Other forms of mitochondrial injury may lead to the release of pro-apoptotic factors, particularly of mitochondrial cytochrome c and the initiation of the cascade to apoptotic cell death.

2.5 Studies on platelets

The hypothesis that Alzheimer disease pathology is not brain-limited has led researchers to look for peripheral cells that may harbour changes related to this disease. On one such cell, the platelet, have the following similarities with neurons: 1) contain the amyloid precursor protein and secrete β-amyloid peptide (Di Luca et al., 2000; Sanchez-Gonzalez et al., 2006) 2) express neurotransmitters and some neuron-related proteins, such as NMDA receptors (Dreux & Launay, 1985). Interestingly, several of the enzymatic defects observed in AD brain are also found in noncerebral tissues. In addition, biochemical markers are likely to be important in the study of Alzheimer disease for several reasons. A clinical diagnosis of Alzheimer disease is inaccurate even among experienced investigators in about 10% to 15% of cases, and biomarkers might improve the accuracy of diagnosis. Importantly for the development of putative disease-modifying drugs for Alzheimer disease, biomarkers might also serve as indirect measures of disease severity. Usually biomarkers are assessed in different compartments including cerebrospinal fluid, skin fibroblasts, lymphocytes, blood and urine.

In our group of work we are analyzed platelets from Alzheimer disease patients and healthy subjects. Diagnosis of AD was made by using the: 1) mini mental state evaluation 2) Diagnostic and Statistical Manual of Mental Disorders-IV criteria for dementia and 3) National Institute of Neurological and Communicative Disorders and Stroke and the Alzheimer's Disease and Related Disorders Association criteria for diagnosis of probable dementia of Alzheimer type. Healthy control subjects were free of AD or any other disorder.

2.5.1 ATP synthase and cytochrome c oxidase

To obtain direct evidence that mitochondrial functioning is altered in AD patients; we made measurements of the rate of the hydrolytic activity of ATP synthase and pH gradient driven by ATP hydrolysis, using platelet submitochondrial particles. The hydrolytic activity of ATP synthase in patients with probable AD was 41.7 ± 4.3 nmol min^{-1} (mg protein)$^{-1}$, n =29, whereas in the control subjects was 29.1 ± 1.9 nmol nmol min^{-1} (mg protein)$^{-1}$, n = 29. It is important to note that, in the male population with probable AD, we found that hydrolytic activity of ATP synthase increased as cerebral deterioration progressed. That increase in the hydrolytic activity of ATP synthase was statistically significant. Therefore, we made measurements of the pH gradient driven by ATP hydrolysis determined from the quenching of ACMA fluorescence induced upon 2 mM ATP addition. pH gradient was used as an indication of the enzyme proton channel function and of coupling between transport and catalysis. Data obtained showed a lower pH gradient in the submitochondrial particles of patients with probable AD (0.28 ± 0.08 pH units, n = 25) as compared to the controls (0.5 ± 0.1 pH units, n = 20). This suggests a functional alteration of the ATP synthase. In addition, proton gradient was completely abolished when 1 μM oligomycin was added to the submitochondrial particles. This indicates that the pH gradient was in fact due to the ATP-driven proton translocation through the membrane and that the proton transport activity of the enzyme from AD patients is as sensitive to the inhibitor as the control group (Martínez-Cano et al., 2004).

Functional impairment of mitochondrial ATP synthase can be explained by the following phenomena: If F0 and F1 sectors of the enzyme are separated by physical or kinetic decoupling; for an altered assembly of the regulatory subunits of the enzyme, in particular of the inhibitor protein IF1. Therefore, we made semi quantitative determinations of the inhibitor protein, IF1 in submitochondrial particles of platelets. Densitometric analyses of Western blot experiments indicated a 2-fold decrease of the relative content of the mitochondrial inhibitor protein (IF1) of the ATP synthase in platelets from AD samples compared to control subjects (Figure 1).

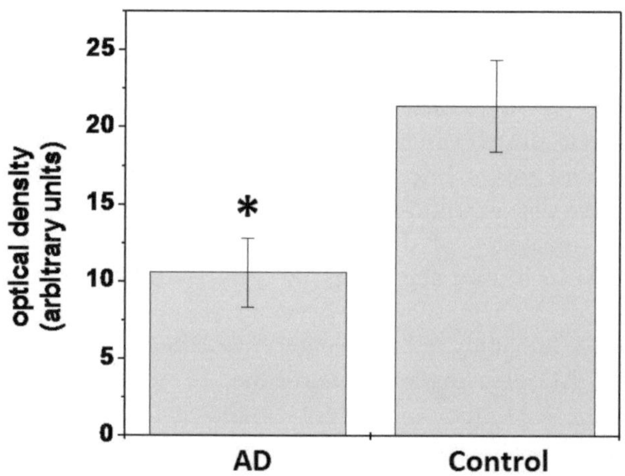

Fig. 1. Densitometric analyses of inhibitor protein IF1 in Alzheimer disease patients and control subjects. Statistical significance was assessed by Dunnett's test. *$P<0.05$ vs control group.

In order to assay the functional association of inhibitor protein IF1 with the ATP synthase in submitochondrial particles from Alzheimer and control group's samples, ATPase activity assays were carried out. Submitochondrial particles were incubated in conditions that induce a progressive release of IF1 to the media, i.e., pH 8.0, KCl 100 mM, and 40 °C. Additional experiments were conducted under conditions that favour the binding of the protein inhibitor of ATP synthase (sucrose medium). Figure 2 shows that the hydrolytic activity of ATP synthase of Alzheimer samples was unaffected by the medium of determination. In contrast, the activity of control samples was increased in a medium with KCl, i.e., in conditions that favours the disotiation of inhibitor protein IF1. Also note that the hydrolytic activity of the ATP synthase of the control samples, in a medium with KCl, did not reach the values of activity of samples from patients with AD, in the same medium. Taken together, these results suggest that that increased hydrolytic activity in patients with AD is partly due to a lower content of the inhibitor protein, IF1.

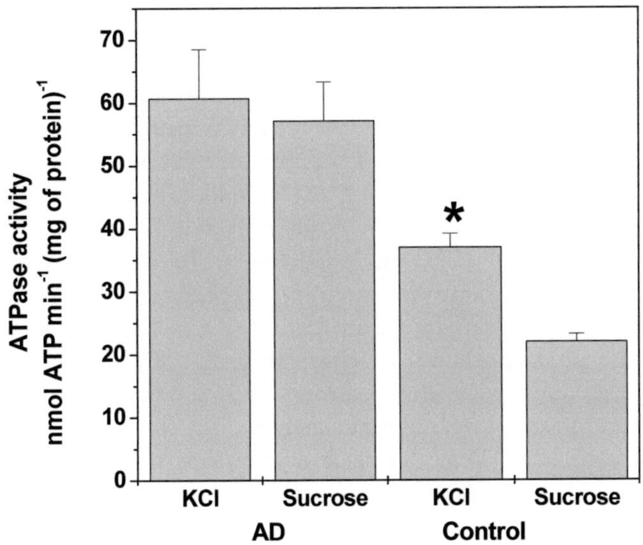

Fig. 2. Hydrolytic activity of ATP synthase in Alzheimer disease and control samples. Enzymatic activity was done at 40 °C, using a potassium chloride or sucrose medium of reaction. Data were subjected to an analysis of variance, and significant differences were assessed by Dunnett's test with $P < 0.05$ for comparison with the sucrose medium.

To our knowledge the hydrolytic activity of ATP synthase in patients with AD has been controversial since it has been reported that ATP hydrolysis activity in platelets was similar in patients with AD and controls (Boseti et al., 2002). Other authors reported a slightly increased in the frontal and occipital brain of AD. These data do not correlate with a 50-60% decrease in the level of mRNA encoding the β subunit of ATP synthase in the temporal cortex of AD patients (Chandrasekaran et al., 1996) or with the reduced amount of ATP synthase in the hippocampus of AD patients (Schagger & Ohm, 1995). Although it is unknown whether the deficiency of mitochondrial enzymes is a cause or an effect of Alzheimer disease, it has been speculated that can be a normal physiological response to a reduction in energy demand in the brains of patients (Jung et al, 2000; Chandrasekaran et al., 1996). So, the functional alterations in key enzymes of mitochondrial metabolism such as ATP synthase, can lead to a decrease in energy generation and can contribute to the neurodegenerative process. Thus, a reduction in cellular ATP concentration can activate specific protein kinases that phosphorylate tau protein, leading to the formation of neurofibrillary tangles (Stanley et al., 1996), and may cause increased susceptibility of neurons to excitatory amino acids, leading to neuronal degeneration by an excitotoxic process (Roder et al., 1993). On the other hand, mitochondrial dysfunction characterized by a combined deficiency of ATP synthase and cytochrome c oxidase can lead to the generation of free radicals that can damage proteins, nucleic acids and membranes and contribute to

aggregation and plaque deposition of β-amyloid and neurofibrillary tangles formation (Beal, 1992; Troncoso et al., 1993).
By restriction analysis we identified the pathogenic mutation of the mitochondrial DNA in the gene encoding the subunit 6 of the ATP synthase. That mutations is T8993G converting the highly conserved leucine to arginine in a transmembrane helix. The mutation causes a severe impairment in the vectorial proton flow through F0 (García et al., 2000) and instability of the monomeric and dimeric forms of the ATP synthase without altering assembly or dimerization of the enzyme (Cortés-Hernández et al., 2007).
On the other hand several mutations in cytochrome c oxidase II gene have been previously described. Sequence chromatogram of mitochondrial cytochrome c oxidase II gene obtained from blood samples of our population revealed that four patients with probable Alzheimer´s disease had a point mutation A8027G (3 of them were identified as early onset, with familial history of the disease). Other four patients with early onset have the following mutations: A8003C, T8082C, C8201T and G7933A, respectively. To our knowledge none of these mutations were found in other neurodegenerative diseases.
It could argue that the mutations found in this work modified the protein conformation, since the different physichochemical characteristics of replaced aminoacids. That conformational change could alter the electrons binding site or the electrons transfer and this contributes to a diminution in enzymatic activity. The diminished cytochrome c activity could cause a decrease in ATP synthesis and diversion of electrons from their normal pathway resulting in increasing in superoxid radical production. Thus, cytochrome oxidase alterations can lead to increased reactive oxygen species generation, oxidative damage to mitochondrial membranes, and increased vulnerability to excitotoxins, and may be important in the pathogenesis of Alzheimer´s disease.

2.5.2 Membrane fluidity

It has been reported that cells of Alzheimer´s disease brains have altered phospholipid metabolism (Blusztajn et al., 1990; Ellison et al., 1987; Klunk et al., 1998; Nitsch et al., 1992) and a diminished unesterified cholesterol:phospholipid mole ratio (Mason et al., 1992), leading to altered membrane fluidity (Mecocci et al., 1996). On the other hand, submitochondrial particles are mainly constituted of inner mitochondrial membrane and are the site of oxidative phosphorylation and other enzymatic systems involved in the transport and utilization of metabolites. Therefore we assessed the membrane fluidity in platelet submitochondrial particles and erythrocyte membranes from Mexican patients with Alzheimer disease. That estimate was achieved from the excimer to monomer fluorescence intensity ratio (Ie/Im) of the fluorescent probe 1,3 dipyrenylpropane incorporated in membranes. That probe at submicromolar concentrations forms intramolecular excimers and its formation in membranes depends mainly of the medium microviscosity and temperature of determination. This method is very simple and does not require higher concentrations of other fluorescent lipophilic probes such as 1,6-diphenyl-1,3,5-hexatriene and its cationic derivative trimethylamino-,6-diphenyl-1,3,5-hexatriene. Thus, the risk of perturbation of the phospholipid phase inherent in the use of all probe molecules is minimized. Intramolecular excimer formation of this probe is related with the membrane fluidity, such the excimer formation depicts mainly the lateral motion of the probe within the membrane (Jurado et al., 1991). The higher the values of the excimer to monomer ratio, the more fluid the membrane, while the lower the ratio, the more rigid the membrane.

Therefore that ratio is directly proportional to membrane fluidity, which is reciprocal to membrane viscosity.

Similarly to the data reported from mitochondria in AD brains fluidity (Mecocci et al., 1996), a reduced fluidity in the platelet inner mitochondrial membrane was found. It can partially be due to increased levels of lipid peroxidation. Reduced membrane fluidity can diminish the activities of the enzymes of oxidative phosphorylation and other transport and receptor proteins, inasmuch as these enzymes are regulated by the physicochemical state of the lipid environment of the membrane. It may diminish significantly the ATP generation from the mitochondria. Interestingly, dysfunctional mitochondria and oxidative damage has been involved in Alzheimer's disease (Bonilla et al., 1999). In agreement with previous reports, membrane fluidity from erythrocyte was not altered in AD (Hajimohammadreza et al., 1990), regardless of increased lipid oxidation in erythrocyte AD patients. This suggests that, in AD, mitochondrial membranes are more sensitive to oxidative stress than erythrocytes.

In contrast to platelet inner mitochondrial membrane, it has been reported an increase in fluidity in whole membranes from platelets of AD patients (Zubenko et al., 1999). This increase results from the elaboration of an internal membrane compartment resembling endoplasmic reticulum that is functionally abnormal (Zubenko et al., 1987). At this regard, it is worth noting that the contribution of mitochondrial membranes to the whole cell membranes in platelets could be minimized since platelets contain few mitochondria (Fukami & Salganicoff, 1973).

On the other hand, Morais Cardoso et al. (2004), using DPH and TMA-DPH as fluorescent probes, found similar fluidity in mitocondrial membranes in platelets from AD patients and controls. That discrepancy with our data may be due to intrinsic differences in the populations tested, the purity of the used mitochondrial fraction and the nature of the probes used. Additionally, it's clear that the lipophilic probes are sensitive to slightly different membrane properties. For instance, DPH and TMA-DPH are rotational probes (Ameloot et al., 1984) and dipyrenylpropane is a lateral diffusion sensitive probe (Zachariasse et al., 1982). In addition, DPH partitions into the interior of the bilayer and its average location has been shown to be about 8 Å from the center of the bilayer. TMA-DPH is oriented in the membrane bilayer with its positive charge localized at the lipid-water interface. Its DPH moiety is localized at about 11 Å from the center of the bilayer and reports the interfacial region of the membrane (Kaiser & London, 1998). Whereas dipyrenylpropane is a highly hydrophobic probe which partitions into the membrane lipid bilayer (Zachariasse et al., 1982). At the moment we do not know whether the diminished membrane fluidity in AD is etiologically significant or a minor result of neurodegeneration

2.5.3 Amyloid precursor protein

Amyloid precursor proteins are transmembrane proteins of about 100 to 130 KDa, located primarily on the cell surface as well as on the endoplasmic reticulum, Golgi apparatus, and endosomes. Amyloid precursor protein may play a role in neuronal trafficking, migration and development (Van Gassen et al., 2000). Although a clear function of amyloid precursor protein has yet to be identified, it is the biochemical pathway leading to *β*-amyloid generation that demonstrates its link to AD pathogenesis. Amyloid precursor protein is subject to cleavage by three proteases, α, β, and γ secretases through two primary pathways. The first pathway involves cleavage of amyloid precursor protein 12 residues N-terminal to the transmembrane sequence by a group of integral membrane enzymes. Termed α-secretase cleavage, this cut creates a large, ectodomain fragment that is released from the cell surface as well asand a smaller C-terminal fragment (83 residues) attached to the membrane. Subsequent cleavage of this membrane-retained fragment by a unique complex of proteins, referred to as γ-secretase, releases a 3-kDa peptide unable to form amyloid fibrils. The second pathway involves an alternative cleavage by β-secretase, located at the N-terminus of the to *β*-amyloid sequence. This releases a unique ectodomain fragment and a C-terminal (C99) membrane-retained fragment. Then, cleavage of C99 by γ-secretase results in formation of to *β*-amyloid. The length of the C-terminal end of to *β*-amyloid varies depending on the specificity of γ-secretase cleavage, resulting in production of Aβ1-40 or a longer, more fibrillogenic *β*-amyloid 1-42/43 (Selkoe, 1998). The longer to *β*-amyloid peptide has a major role in to *β*-amyloid deposition because plaque formation follows a distinct pattern with the 42-43 amino acid peptide detected first followed by the more common to *β*-amyloid 1-40 (Lemere et al., 1996). The balance between α-secretase and β-secretase cleavage of amyloid precursor protein is important for to *β*-amyloid production and AD pathogenesis.

Western blotting experiments of amyloid precursor protein in platelets showed two main bands with molecular weights of 106 to 110 KDa and 130 KDa, respectively. The upper, 130 KDa, band corresponded to the full-length, mature of amyloid precursor protein. The lower, 106–110 KDa, band corresponded to the of amyloid precursor protein immature isoforms. The ratio of amyloid precursor protein isoforms between the 130 Kda amyloid precursor protein and 106–110 KDa amyloid precursor protein and odds ratios were obtained to determine risk factor of this component. Amyloid precursor protein ratio on AD subjects was lower than that of control subjects: 0.36 ± 0.18 vs. 0.67 ± 0.10, respectively. A low amyloid precursor protein ratio (< 0.6) showed an odds ratio of 4.63. When onset of disease was taken into account, an amyloid precursor protein ratio on early onset Alzheimer´s disease subjects of 0.39 ± 0.19 was found vs. 0.34 ± 0.19 on late onset Alzheimer´s disease subjects ($p > 0.05$). This suggests an increased degradation of amyloid precursor protein in AD platelets.

On the other hand we performed *ApoE* genotyping in AD platelets and controls. Data obtained showed that there was no association between amyloid precursor protein ratios and any specific ApoE allele (Sanchez-Gonzalez et al., 2006).

In concordance to previous studies, we observed a significant decreased amyloid precursor protein ratio on AD subjects as compared to that of control subjects (Utermann, 1987; Borroni et al., 2003). This means that an increased degradation of this precursor protein is being performed in peripheral tissues. Whether or not this phenomenon reflects a similar process occurring in the brain of AD subjects is still a matter of controversy. However, the existence of this phenomenon cannot be minimized, for processing and secretion of this precursor protein has been already demonstrated and its importance as a predictor for conversion to dementia of Alzheimer type in subjects with mild cognitive impairment has recently been proved (Borroni et al., 2003).

The precise mechanism of amelioration of amyloid precursor protein concentration is not deciphered yet. Modifications in the splicing mechanism, in the stability of messenger RNA encoding for amyloid precursor protein 751/770 or in the regulation of translation processes are some hypothesis (Di Luca et al., 1996). Our study is consistent with the results of Strittmatter et al., (1993) concerning an increased ApoE ε4 allele frequency in AD patients (Strittmatter & Saunders, 1993). A 4.5-times risk of presenting AD as related to the ApoE ε3/ε4 genotype and a 9.4-times risk related to the ε4 allele was also found. This is in accordance to studies published before showing an increased risk of presenting AD as

related to either ε4 heterozygocity or homozygocity (Amouyel et al., 1993; Anwar et al., 1993; Ben-Shlomo et al., 1993; Czech et al., 1993; Lucotte et al., 1993).
The coexistence of β-amyloid with the ApoE ε4 allele in the pathogenesis of AD has long been thought (Saunders et al., 1993) Increased risk of presenting AD in ApoE ε4 allele porters as well as augmented amyloid precursor protein degradation in platelets led us to consider the probability of relating both factors to determine a combined model for risk factor evaluation. We observed a 5-times risk of presenting the disease when both ε3/ε4 genotype and a low amyloid precursor protein ratio (taken as a ratio below (0.6) were stratified, and a 4-times risk with both the ε4/ε4 genotype and a low amyloid precursor protein ratio. These data confirms the relevance of peripheral amyloid precursor protein altered isoforms as an assessment of risk factor of the disease (Rosenberg et al., 1997). The stratified analysis helped us to exclude the effect of ApoE genotypes on the low amyloid precursor protein ratio. We observed no significant OR amelioration or increase of the low amyloid precursor protein ratio, thus strengthening the importance of a low amyloid precursor protein ratio in peripheral blood as an indicator of the disease.

3. Conclusion

Up to now several hypotheses about the complex etiology of Alzheimer´s disease have been proposed. According to the amyloid hypothesis, abnormal processing, and accelerated deposition of oligomeric forms of beta-amyloid are central mechanisms underlying pathological processes in Alzheimer disease. Although the amyloid hypothesis remains the main pathogenetic model of Alzheimer's disease, its role in the majority of sporadic Alzheimer cases is unclear. Therefore, other innovative proposals have been made in recent years, particularly the association of mitochondrial functional impairment in the development of the Alzheimer's disease. Immunohistochemical, biochemical, neuroimaging, electronic microscopy and molecular studies have demonstrated the existence of signs of mitochondrial impairment in Alzheimer´s disease brain. Interestingly, these changes are evident very early in Alzheimer disease progression. Current evidence shows that oxidative stress, mitochondrial impairment and altered mitochondrial dynamics contribute to the precipitation of Alzheimer´s disease pathology and thus cognitive decline.
On the other hand, using platelets as a model of study we found the following data: 1) an increased degradation of amyloid precursor protein; 2) an increased lipid oxidation products in mitochondria; 3) a dysfunction of mitochondrial ATP syntase; 4) lower levels of inhibitor protein (IF1) of ATP synthase; 5) reduce membrane fluidity in inner mitochondrial membrane; 6) point mutations of the mitochondrially encoded ATP synthase 6 and citochrome oxidase II genes.

4. References

Almeida, L. M.; Vaz, W. L.; Zachariasse, K. A. & Madeira, V. M. (1982). Fluidity of sarcoplasmic reticulum membranes investigated with dipyrenylpropane, an intramolecular excimer probe. *Biochemistry*, Vol. 21, No. 23, (Nov 9 1982), pp. 5972-5977, ISSN 0006-2960

Ameloot, M.; Hendrickx, H.; Herreman, W.; Pottel, H.; Van Cauwelaert, F. & van der Meer, W. (1984). Effect of orientational order on the decay of the fluorescence anisotropy in membrane suspensions. Experimental verification on unilamellar vesicles and lipid/alpha-lactalbumin complexes. *Biophys J*, Vol. 46, No. 4, (Oct 1984), pp. 525-539, ISSN 0006-3495

Amouyel, P.; Brousseau, T.; Fruchart, J. C. & Dallongeville, J. (1993). Apolipoprotein E-epsilon 4 allele and Alzheimer's disease. *Lancet*, Vol. 342, No. 8882, (Nov 20 1993), pp. 1309, ISSN 0140-6736

Anandatheerthavarada, H. K.; Biswas, G.; Robin, M. A. & Avadhani, N. G. (2003). Mitochondrial targeting and a novel transmembrane arrest of Alzheimer's amyloid precursor protein impairs mitochondrial function in neuronal cells. *J Cell Biol*, Vol. 161, No. 1, (Apr 14 2003), pp. 41-54, ISSN 0021-9525

Anantharaman, M.; Tangpong, J.; Keller, J. N.; Murphy, M. P.; Markesbery, W. R.; Kiningham, K. K. & St Clair, D. K. (2006). Beta-amyloid mediated nitration of manganese superoxide dismutase: implication for oxidative stress in a APPNLH/NLH X PS-1P264L/P264L double knock-in mouse model of Alzheimer's disease. *Am J Pathol*, Vol. 168, No. 5, (May 2006), pp. 1608-1618, ISSN 0002-9440

Anwar, N.; Lovestone, S.; Cheetham, M. E.; Levy, R. & Powell, J. F. (1993). Apolipoprotein E-epsilon 4 allele and Alzheimer's disease. *Lancet*, Vol. 342, No. 8882, (Nov 20 1993), pp. 1308-1309, ISSN 0140-6736

Atamna, H. & Frey, W. H., 2nd (2007). Mechanisms of mitochondrial dysfunction and energy deficiency in Alzheimer's disease. *Mitochondrion*, Vol. 7, No. 5, (Sep 2007), pp. 297-310, ISSN 1567-7249

Baloyannis, S. J. (2006). Mitochondrial alterations in Alzheimer's disease. *J Alzheimers Dis*, Vol. 9, No. 2, (Jul 2006), pp. 119-126, ISSN 1387-2877

Barsoum, M.J; Yuan, H.; Gerencser, A. A.; Liot, G.; Kushnareva, Y.; Gräber, S.; Kovacs, I.; Lee, W. D.; Waggoner, J.; Cui, J.; White, A. D.; Bossy, B.; Martinou, J. C.; Youle, R. J.; Lipton, S. A.; Ellisman, M. H.; Perkins, G. A. & Bossy-Wetzel, E. (2006). Nitric oxide induced mitochondrial fission is regulated by dynamin-related GTPases in neurons. *EMBO J*, Vol. 25, No. 16, (Aug 23), pp.3900–3911, ISSN 0261-4189

Beal, M. F. (1992). Does impairment of energy metabolism result in excitotoxic neuronal death in neurodegenerative illnesses? *Ann Neurol*, Vol. 31, No. 2, (Feb 1992), pp. 119-130, ISSN 0364-5134

Benson, D. F.; Kuhl, D. E.; Phelps, M. E.; Cummings, J. L. & Tsai, S. Y. (1981). Positron emission computed tomography in the diagnosis of dementia. *Trans Am Neurol Assoc*, Vol. 106, No. 1981), pp. 68-71, ISSN 0065-9479

Blusztajn, J. K.; Lopez Gonzalez-Coviella, I.; Logue, M.; Growdon, J. H. & Wurtman, R. J. (1990). Levels of phospholipid catabolic intermediates, glycerophosphocholine and glycerophosphoethanolamine, are elevated in brains of Alzheimer's disease but not of Down's syndrome patients. *Brain Res*, Vol. 536, No. 1-2, (Dec 17 1990), pp. 240-244, ISSN 0006-8993

Bokde, A. L.; Pietrini, P.; Ibanez, V.; Furey, M. L.; Alexander, G. E.; Graff-Radford, N. R.; Rapoport, S. I.; Schapiro, M. B. & Horwitz, B. (2001). The effect of brain atrophy on cerebral hypometabolism in the visual variant of Alzheimer disease. *Arch Neurol*, Vol. 58, No. 3, (Mar 2001), pp. 480-486, ISSN 0003-9942

Bonilla, E.; Tanji, K.; Hirano, M.; Vu, T. H.; DiMauro, S. & Schon, E. A. (1999). Mitochondrial involvement in Alzheimer's disease. *Biochim Biophys Acta*, Vol. 1410, No. 2, (Feb 9 1999), pp. 171-182, ISSN 0006-3002

Borroni, B.; Colciaghi, F.; Caltagirone, C.; Rozzini, L.; Broglio, L.; Cattabeni, F.; Di Luca, M. & Padovani, A. (2003). Platelet amyloid precursor protein abnormalities in mild cognitive impairment predict conversion to dementia of Alzheimer type: a 2-year follow-up study. *Arch Neurol*, Vol. 60, No. 12, (Dec 2003), pp. 1740-1744, ISSN 0003-9942

Bosetti, F.; Brizzi, F.; Barogi, S.; Mancuso, M.; Siciliano, G.; Tendi, E. A.; Murri, L.; Rapoport, S. I. & Solaini, G. (2002). Cytochrome c oxidase and mitochondrial F1F0-ATPase (ATP synthase) activities in platelets and brain from patients with Alzheimer's disease. *Neurobiol Aging*, Vol. 23, No. 3, (May-Jun 2002), pp. 371-376, ISSN 0197-4580

Braak, H. & Braak, E. (1991). Neuropathological stageing of Alzheimer-related changes. *Acta Neuropathol*, Vol. 82, No. 4, 1991), pp. 239-259, ISSN 0001-6322

Butterfield, D. A.; Reed, T.; Newman, S. F. & Sultana, R. (2007). Roles of amyloid beta-peptide-associated oxidative stress and brain protein modifications in the pathogenesis of Alzheimer's disease and mild cognitive impairment. *Free Radic Biol Med*, Vol. 43, No. 5, (Sep 1 2007), pp. 658-677, ISSN 0891-5849

Campanella, M.; Casswell, E.; Chong, S.; Farah, Z.; Wieckowski, M. R.; Abramov, A. Y.; Tinker, A.; & Duchen, M. R. (2008). Regulation of mitochondrial structure and function by the F1Fo-ATPase inhibitor protein, IF1. *Cell Metab*, Vol. 8, No. 1 (Jul 2008), pp. 13-25, ISSN 1550-4131

Cardoso, S. M.; Proenca, M. T.; Santos, S.; Santana, I. & Oliveira, C. R. (2004). Cytochrome c oxidase is decreased in Alzheimer's disease platelets. *Neurobiol Aging*, Vol. 25, No. 1, (Jan 2004), pp. 105-110, ISSN 0197-4580

Chan, D. C. (2006). Mitochondria: dynamic organelles in disease, aging, and development. *Cell*, Vol. 125, No. 7, (Jun 30 2006), pp. 1241-1252, ISSN 0092-8674

Chandrasekaran, K.; Giordano, T.; Brady, D. R.; Stoll, J.; Martin, L. J. & Rapoport, S. I. (1994). Impairment in mitochondrial cytochrome oxidase gene expression in Alzheimer disease. *Brain Res Mol Brain Res*, Vol. 24, No. 1-4, (Jul 1994), pp. 336-340, ISSN 0169-328X

Chandrasekaran, K.; Hatanpaa, K.; Brady, D. R. & Rapoport, S. I. (1996). Evidence for physiological down-regulation of brain oxidative phosphorylation in Alzheimer's disease. *Exp Neurol*, Vol. 142, No. 1, (Nov 1996), pp. 80-88, ISSN 0014-4886

Chandrasekaran, K.; Hatanpaa, K.; Rapoport, S. I. & Brady, D. R. (1997). Decreased expression of nuclear and mitochondrial DNA-encoded genes of oxidative phosphorylation in association neocortex in Alzheimer disease. *Brain Res Mol Brain Res*, Vol. 44, No. 1, (Feb 1997), pp. 99-104, ISSN 0169-328X

Chen, H. & Chan, D. C. (2006). Critical dependence of neurons on mitochondrial dynamics. *Curr Opin Cell Biol*, Vol. 18, No. 4, (Aug 2006), pp. 453-459, ISSN 0955-0674

Chen, H.; Chomyn, A. & Chan, D. C. (2005). Disruption of fusion results in mitochondrial heterogeneity and dysfunction. *J Biol Chem*, Vol. 280, No. 28, (Jul 15 2005), pp. 26185-26192, ISSN 0021-9258

Cortés-Hernández, P.; Vázquez-Memije, M.E. & García, J.J. (2007). ATP6 homoplasmic mutations inhibit and destabilize the human F1F0-ATP synthase without preventing enzyme assembly and oligomerization. *J Biol Chem*, Vol. 282, no. 2, (Jan 12), pp. 1051-1058, ISSN 0021-9258

Coskun, P. E.; Beal, M. F. & Wallace, D. C. (2004). Alzheimer's brains harbor somatic mtDNA control-region mutations that suppress mitochondrial transcription and replication. *Proc Natl Acad Sci U S A*, Vol. 101, No. 29, (Jul 20 2004), pp. 10726-10731, ISSN 0027-8424

Costantini, L. C.; Barr, L. J.; Vogel, J. L. & Henderson, S. T. (2008). Hypometabolism as a therapeutic target in Alzheimer's disease. *BMC Neurosci*, Vol. 9 Suppl 2, No. 2008), pp. S16, ISSN 1471-2202

Czech, C.; Monning, V.; Tienari, P. J.; Hartmann, T.; Masters, C.; Beyreuther, K. & Forstl, H. (1993). Apolipoprotein E-epsilon 4 allele and Alzheimer's disease. *Lancet*, Vol. 342, No. 8882, (Nov 20 1993), pp. 1309, ISSN 0140-6736

de la Monte, S. M.; Luong, T.; Neely, T. R.; Robinson, D. & Wands, J. R. (2000). Mitochondrial DNA damage as a mechanism of cell loss in Alzheimer's disease. *Lab Invest*, Vol. 80, No. 8, (Aug 2000), pp. 1323-1335, ISSN 0023-6837

de Leon, M. J.; Ferris, S. H.; George, A. E.; Christman, D. R.; Fowler, J. S.; Gentes, C.; Reisberg, B.; Gee, B.; Emmerich, M.; Yonekura, Y.; Brodie, J.; Kricheff, II & Wolf, A. P. (1983). Positron emission tomographic studies of aging and Alzheimer disease. *AJNR Am J Neuroradiol*, Vol. 4, No. 3, (May-Jun 1983), pp. 568-571, ISSN 0195-6108

Di Luca, M.; Colciaghi, F.; Pastorino, L.; Borroni, B.; Padovani, A. & Cattabeni, F. (2000). Platelets as a peripheral district where to study pathogenetic mechanisms of alzheimer disease: the case of amyloid precursor protein. *Eur J Pharmacol*, Vol. 405, No. 1-3, (Sep 29 2000), pp. 277-283, ISSN 0014-2999

Dreux, C. & Launay, J. M. (1985). [Blood platelets: neuronal model in psychiatric disorders]. *Encephale*, Vol. 11, No. 2, (Mar-Apr 1985), pp. 57-64, ISSN 0013-7006

Dreyfus, G.; Gomez-Puyou, A. & Iuena de Gomez-Puyou, M. (1981). Electrochemical gradient induced displacement of the natural ATPase inhibitor protein from mitochondrial ATPase as directed by antibodies against the inhibitor protein. *Biochem Biophys Res Commun*, Vol. 100, No. 1, (May 15 1981), pp. 400-406, ISSN 0006-291X

Ellison, D. W.; Beal, M. F. & Martin, J. B. (1987). Phosphoethanolamine and ethanolamine are decreased in Alzheimer's disease and Huntington's disease. *Brain Res*, Vol. 417, No. 2, (Aug 11 1987), pp. 389-392, ISSN 0006-8993

Frederick, R. L. & Shaw, J. M. (2007). Moving mitochondria: establishing distribution of an essential organelle. *Traffic*, Vol. 8, No. 12, (Dec 2007), pp. 1668-1675, ISSN 1398-9219

Friedland, R. P.; Budinger, T. F.; Ganz, E.; Yano, Y.; Mathis, C. A.; Koss, B.; Ober, B. A.; Huesman, R. H. & Derenzo, S. E. (1983). Regional cerebral metabolic alterations in dementia of the Alzheimer type: positron emission tomography with [18F]fluorodeoxyglucose. *J Comput Assist Tomogr*, Vol. 7, No. 4, (Aug 1983), pp. 590-598, ISSN 0363-8715

Fukami, M. H. & Salganicoff, L. (1973). Isolation and properties of human platelet mitochondria. *Blood*, Vol. 42, No. 6, (Dec 1973), pp. 913-918, ISSN 0006-4971

García, J.J.; Ogilvie, I.; Robinson, B. & Capaldi, R. A. (2000). Structure, functioning, and assembly of the ATP synthase in cells from patients with the T8993G mitochondrial DNA mutation. Comparison with the enzyme in Rho0 cells completely lacking mtDNA. *J Biol Chem*, Vol. 275, No. 15, (April 14), pp. 11075-11081, ISSN 0021-9258

García, J.J.; Morales-Rios, E.; Cortés-Hernández, P. & Rodríguez-Zavala, J. S. (2006). The inhibitor protein (IF1) promotes dimerization of the mitochondrial F1F0-ATP synthase. *Biochemistry*, Vol. 45, No. 42, (Oct 24), pp. 12695-12703, ISSN 0006-2960

García-Trejo, J. J. & Morales-Ríos, E. (2008). Regulation of the F1F0-ATP synthase rotary nanomotor in its monomeric-bacterial and dimeric-mitochondrial forms. *J Biol Phys*, Vol. 34, No. 1-2, (Apr 2008), pp. 197-212, ISSN: 0092-0606

Hajimohammadreza, I.; Brammer, M. J.; Eagger, S.; Burns, A. & Levy, R. (1990). Platelet and erythrocyte membrane changes in Alzheimer's disease. *Biochim Biophys Acta*, Vol. 1025, No. 2, (Jun 27 1990), pp. 208-214, ISSN 0006-3002

Hatefi, Y. (1985). The mitochondrial electron transport and oxidative phosphorylation system. *Annu Rev Biochem*, Vol. 54, No. 1985), pp. 1015-1069, ISSN 0066-4154

Hirai, K.; Aliev, G.; Nunomura, A.; Fujioka, H.; Russell, R. L.; Atwood, C. S.; Johnson, A. B.; Kress, Y.; Vinters, H. V.; Tabaton, M.; Shimohama, S.; Cash, A. D.; Siedlak, S. L.; Harris, P. L.; Jones, P. K.; Petersen, R. B.; Perry, G. & Smith, M. A. (2001). Mitochondrial abnormalities in Alzheimer's disease. *J Neurosci*, Vol. 21, No. 9, (May 1 2001), pp. 3017-3023, ISSN 0270-6474

Hoyer, S. (1991). Abnormalities of glucose metabolism in Alzheimer's disease. *Ann N Y Acad Sci*, Vol. 640, No. 1991), pp. 53-58, ISSN 0077-8923

Ibanez, V.; Pietrini, P.; Alexander, G. E.; Furey, M. L.; Teichberg, D.; Rajapakse, J. C.; Rapoport, S. I.; Schapiro, M. B. & Horwitz, B. (1998). Regional glucose metabolic abnormalities are not the result of atrophy in Alzheimer's disease. *Neurology*, Vol. 50, No. 6, (Jun 1998), pp. 1585-1593, ISSN 0028-3878

Ishii, K.; Sasaki, M.; Kitagaki, H.; Yamaji, S.; Sakamoto, S.; Matsuda, K. & Mori, E. (1997). Reduction of cerebellar glucose metabolism in advanced Alzheimer's disease. *J Nucl Med*, Vol. 38, No. 6, (Jun 1997), pp. 925-928, ISSN 0161-5505

Jung, C.; Higgins, C. M. & Xu, Z. (2000). Measuring the quantity and activity of mitochondrial electron transport chain complexes in tissues of central nervous system using blue native polyacrylamide gel electrophoresis. *Anal Biochem*, Vol. 286, No. 2, (Nov 15 2000), pp. 214-223, ISSN 0003-2697

Jurado, A. S.; Almeida, L. M. & Madeira, V. M. (1991). Fluidity of bacterial membrane lipids monitored by intramolecular excimerization of 1.3-di(2-pyrenyl)propane. *Biochem Biophys Res Commun*, Vol. 176, No. 1, (Apr 15 1991), pp. 356-363, ISSN 0006-291X

Kaiser, R. D. & London, E. (1998). Location of diphenylhexatriene (DPH) and its derivatives within membranes: comparison of different fluorescence quenching analyses of membrane depth. *Biochemistry*, Vol. 37, No. 22, (Jun 2 1998), pp. 8180-8190, ISSN 0006-2960

Kim, S. H.; Vlkolinsky, R.; Cairns, N. & Lubec, G. (2000). Decreased levels of complex III core protein 1 and complex V beta chain in brains from patients with Alzheimer's disease and Down syndrome. *Cell Mol Life Sci*, Vol. 57, No. 12, (Nov 2000), pp. 1810-1816, ISSN 1420-682X

Klunk, W. E.; Panchalingam, K.; McClure, R. J.; Stanley, J. A. & Pettegrew, J. W. (1998). Metabolic alterations in postmortem Alzheimer's disease brain are exaggerated by Apo-E4. *Neurobiol Aging*, Vol. 19, No. 6, (Nov-Dec 1998), pp. 511-515, ISSN 0197-4580

Knott, A. B.; Perkins, G.; Schwarzenbacher, R. & Bossy-Wetzel, E. (2008). Mitochondrial fragmentation in neurodegeneration. *Nat Rev Neurosci*, Vol. 9, No. 7, (Jul 2008), pp. 505-518, 1471-003X

Lemere, C. A.; Blusztajn, J. K.; Yamaguchi, H.; Wisniewski, T.; Saido, T. C. & Selkoe, D. J. (1996). Sequence of deposition of heterogeneous amyloid beta-peptides and APO E in Down syndrome: implications for initial events in amyloid plaque formation. *Neurobiol Dis*, Vol. 3, No. 1, (Feb 1996), pp. 16-32, ISSN 0969-9961

Liang, W. S.; Reiman, E. M.; Valla, J.; Dunckley, T.; Beach, T. G.; Grover, A.; Niedzielko, T. L.; Schneider, L. E.; Mastroeni, D.; Caselli, R.; Kukull, W.; Morris, J. C.; Hulette, C. M.; Schmechel, D.; Rogers, J. & Stephan, D. A. (2008). Alzheimer's disease is associated with reduced expression of energy metabolism genes in posterior cingulate neurons. *Proc Natl Acad Sci U S A*, Vol. 105, No. 11, (Mar 18 2008), pp. 4441-4446, ISSN 0027-8424

Lovell, M. A.; Ehmann, W. D.; Butler, S. M. & Markesbery, W. R. (1995). Elevated thiobarbituric acid-reactive substances and antioxidant enzyme activity in the brain in Alzheimer's disease. *Neurology*, Vol. 45, No. 8, (Aug 1995), pp. 1594-1601, ISSN 0028-3878

Lu, T.; Pan, Y.; Kao, S. Y.; Li, C.; Kohane, I.; Chan, J. & Yankner, B. A. (2004). Gene regulation and DNA damage in the ageing human brain. *Nature*, Vol. 429, No. 6994, (Jun 24 2004), pp. 883-891, ISSN 0028-0836

Manczak, M.; Park, B. S.; Jung, Y. & Reddy, P. H. (2004). Differential expression of oxidative phosphorylation genes in patients with Alzheimer's disease: implications for early mitochondrial dysfunction and oxidative damage. *Neuromolecular Med*, Vol. 5, No. 2, 2004), pp. 147-162, ISSN 1535-1084

Martinez-Cano, E.; Ortiz-Genaro, G.; Pacheco-Moises, F.; Macias-Islas, M. A.; Sanchez-Nieto, S. & Rosales-Corral, S. A. (2005). [Functional disorders of FOF1-ATPase in submitochondrial particles obtained from platelets of patients with a diagnosis of probable Alzheimer's disease]. *Rev Neurol*, Vol. 40, No. 2, (Jan 16-31 2005), pp. 81-85, ISSN 0210-0010

Mason, R. P.; Shoemaker, W. J.; Shajenko, L.; Chambers, T. E. & Herbette, L. G. (1992). Evidence for changes in the Alzheimer's disease brain cortical membrane structure mediated by cholesterol. *Neurobiol Aging*, Vol. 13, No. 3, (May-Jun 1992), pp. 413-419, ISSN 0197-4580

Maurer, I.; Zierz, S. & Moller, H. J. (2000). A selective defect of cytochrome c oxidase is present in brain of Alzheimer disease patients. *Neurobiol Aging*, Vol. 21, No. 3, (May-Jun 2000), pp. 455-462, ISSN 0197-4580

Mecocci, P.; Cherubini, A.; Beal, M. F.; Cecchetti, R.; Chionne, F.; Polidori, M. C.; Romano, G. & Senin, U. (1996). Altered mitochondrial membrane fluidity in AD brain. *Neurosci Lett*, Vol. 207, No. 2, (Mar 29 1996), pp. 129-132, ISSN 0304-3940

Minauro-Sanmiguel, F.; Wilkens, S. & Garcia, J. J. (2005). Structure of dimeric mitochondrial ATP synthase: novel F0 bridging features and the structural basis of mitochondrial cristae biogenesis *Proc Natl Acad Sci U S A*, Vol. 102, No. 35, (Aug 30 2005), pp. 12356-12358, ISSN 0027-8424

Minoshima, S.; Giordani, B.; Berent, S.; Frey, K. A.; Foster, N. L. & Kuhl, D. E. (1997). Metabolic reduction in the posterior cingulate cortex in very early Alzheimer's disease. *Ann Neurol*, Vol. 42, No. 1, (Jul 1997), pp. 85-94, ISSN 0364-5134

Moreira, P. I.; Duarte, A. I.; Santos, M. S.; Rego, A. C. & Oliveira, C. R. (2009). An integrative view of the role of oxidative stress, mitochondria and insulin in Alzheimer's disease. *J Alzheimers Dis*, Vol. 16, No. 4, 2009), pp. 741-761, ISSN 1387-2877

Mosconi, L.; Brys, M.; Switalski, R.; Mistur, R.; Glodzik, L.; Pirraglia, E.; Tsui, W.; De Santi, S. & de Leon, M. J. (2007). Maternal family history of Alzheimer's disease predisposes to reduced brain glucose metabolism. *Proc Natl Acad Sci U S A*, Vol. 104, No. 48, (Nov 27 2007), pp. 19067-19072, ISSN 0027-8424

Nagy, Z.; Esiri, M. M.; LeGris, M. & Matthews, P. M. (1999). Mitochondrial enzyme expression in the hippocampus in relation to Alzheimer-type pathology. *Acta Neuropathol*, Vol. 97, No. 4, (Apr 1999), pp. 346-354, ISSN 0001-6322

Nitsch, R. M.; Blusztajn, J. K.; Pittas, A. G.; Slack, B. E.; Growdon, J. H. & Wurtman, R. J. (1992). Evidence for a membrane defect in Alzheimer disease brain. *Proc Natl Acad Sci U S A*, Vol. 89, No. 5, (Mar 1 1992), pp. 1671-1675, ISSN 0027-8424

Ortiz, G. G.; Pacheco-Moises, F.; El Hafidi, M.; Jimenez-Delgado, A.; Macias-Islas, M. A.; Rosales Corral, S. A.; de la Rosa, A. C.; Sanchez-Gonzalez, V. J.; Arias-Merino, E. D. & Velazquez-Brizuela, I. E. (2008). Detection of membrane fluidity in submitochondrial particles of platelets and erythrocyte membranes from Mexican patients with Alzheimer disease by intramolecular excimer formation of 1,3 dipyrenylpropane. *Dis Markers*, Vol. 24, No. 3, 2008), pp. 151-156, ISSN 0278-0240

Parker, W. D., Jr.; Parks, J.; Filley, C. M. & Kleinschmidt-DeMasters, B. K. (1994). Electron transport chain defects in Alzheimer's disease brain. *Neurology*, Vol. 44, No. 6, (Jun 1994), pp. 1090-1096, ISSN 0028-3878

Parker, W. D., Jr. & Parks, J. K. (1995). Cytochrome c oxidase in Alzheimer's disease brain: purification and characterization. *Neurology*, Vol. 45, No. 3 Pt 1, (Mar 1995), pp. 482-486, ISSN 0028-3878

Parone, P. A.; Da Cruz, S.; Tondera, D.; Mattenberger, Y.; James, D. I.; Maechler, P.; Barja, F. & Martinou, J. C. (2008). Preventing mitochondrial fission impairs mitochondrial function and leads to loss of mitochondrial DNA. *PLoS One*, Vol. 3, No. 9, 2008), pp. e3257, ISSN 1932-6203

Pettegrew, J. W.; Panchalingam, K.; Klunk, W. E.; McClure, R. J. & Muenz, L. R. (1994). Alterations of cerebral metabolism in probable Alzheimer's disease: a preliminary study. *Neurobiol Aging*, Vol. 15, No. 1, (Jan-Feb 1994), pp. 117-132, ISSN 0197-4580

Phelps, M. E.; Mazziotta, J. C. & Huang, S. C. (1982). Study of cerebral function with positron computed tomography. *J Cereb Blood Flow Metab*, Vol. 2, No. 2, 1982), pp. 113-162, ISSN 0271-678X

Poole, A. C.; Thomas, R. E.; Andrews, L. A.; McBride, H. M.; Whitworth, A. J. & Pallanck, L. J. (2008). The PINK1/Parkin pathway regulates mitochondrial morphology. *Proc Natl Acad Sci U S A*, Vol. 105, No. 5, (Feb 5 2008), pp. 1638-1643, ISSN 0027-8424

Power, J.; Cross, R. L. & Harris, D. A. (1983). Interaction of F1-ATPase, from ox heart mitochondria with its naturally occurring inhibitor protein. Studies using radio-iodinated inhibitor protein. *Biochim Biophys Acta*, Vol. 724, No. 1, (Jul 29 1983), pp. 128-141, ISSN 0006-3002

Pullman, M. E. & Monroy, G. C. (1963). A Naturally Occurring Inhibitor of Mitochondrial Adenosine Triphosphatase. *J Biol Chem*, Vol. 238, No. (Nov 1963), pp. 3762-3769, ISSN 0021-9258

Qiu, X.; Chen, Y. & Zhou, M. (2001). Two point mutations in mitochondrial DNA of cytochrome c oxidase coexist with normal mtDNA in a patient with Alzheimer's disease. *Brain Res*, Vol. 893, No. 1-2, (Mar 2 2001), pp. 261-263, ISSN 0006-8993

Rapoport, S. I.; Hatanpaa, K.; Brady, D. R. & Chandrasekaran, K. (1996). Brain energy metabolism, cognitive function and down-regulated oxidative phosphorylation in Alzheimer disease. *Neurodegeneration*, Vol. 5, No. 4, (Dec 1996), pp. 473-476, ISSN 1055-8330

Reddy, P. H. & Beal, M. F. (2008). Amyloid beta, mitochondrial dysfunction and synaptic damage: implications for cognitive decline in aging and Alzheimer's disease. *Trends Mol Med*, Vol. 14, No. 2, (Feb 2008), pp. 45-53, ISSN 1471-4914

Reddy, P. H.; McWeeney, S.; Park, B. S.; Manczak, M.; Gutala, R. V.; Partovi, D.; Jung, Y.; Yau, V.; Searles, R.; Mori, M. & Quinn, J. (2004). Gene expression profiles of transcripts in amyloid precursor protein transgenic mice: up-regulation of mitochondrial metabolism and apoptotic genes is an early cellular change in Alzheimer's disease. *Hum Mol Genet*, Vol. 13, No. 12, (Jun 15 2004), pp. 1225-1240, ISSN 0964-6906

Reiman, E. M.; Caselli, R. J.; Yun, L. S.; Chen, K.; Bandy, D.; Minoshima, S.; Thibodeau, S. N. & Osborne, D. (1996). Preclinical evidence of Alzheimer's disease in persons homozygous for the epsilon 4 allele for apolipoprotein E. *N Engl J Med*, Vol. 334, No. 12, (Mar 21 1996), pp. 752-758, ISSN 0028-4793

Roder, H. M.; Eden, P. A. & Ingram, V. M. (1993). Brain protein kinase PK40erk converts TAU into a PHF-like form as found in Alzheimer's disease. *Biochem Biophys Res Commun*, Vol. 193, No. 2, (Jun 15 1993), pp. 639-647, ISSN 0006-291X

Roder, H. M. & Ingram, V. M. (1991). Two novel kinases phosphorylate tau and the KSP site of heavy neurofilament subunits in high stoichiometric ratios. *J Neurosci*, Vol. 11, No. 11, (Nov 1991), pp. 3325-3343, ISSN 0270-6474

Rosenberg, R. N.; Baskin, F.; Fosmire, J. A.; Risser, R.; Adams, P.; Svetlik, D.; Honig, L. S.; Cullum, C. M. & Weiner, M. F. (1997). Altered amyloid protein processing in platelets of patients with Alzheimer disease. *Arch Neurol*, Vol. 54, No. 2, (Feb 1997), pp. 139-144, ISSN 0003-9942

Roses, A. D.; Strittmatter, W. J.; Pericak-Vance, M. A.; Corder, E. H.; Saunders, A. M. & Schmechel, D. E. (1994). Clinical application of apolipoprotein E genotyping to Alzheimer's disease. *Lancet*, Vol. 343, No. 8912, (Jun 18 1994), pp. 1564-1565, ISSN 0140-6736

Sanchez-Bustamante, V. J.; Darszon, A. & Gomez-Puyou, A. (1982). On the function of the natural ATPase inhibitor protein in intact mitochondria. *Eur J Biochem*, Vol. 126, No. 3, (Sep 1 1982), pp. 611-616, ISSN 0014-2956

Sanchez-Gonzalez, V. J.; Ortiz, G. G.; Gallegos-Arreola, P.; Macias-Islas, M. A.; Arias-Merino, E. D.; Loera-Castaneda, V.; Martinez-Cano, E.; Velazquez-Brizuela, I. E.; Rosales-Corral, S. A.; Curiel-Ortega, C. R.; Pacheco-Moises, F. & Garcia, J. J. (2006). Altered beta-amyloid precursor protein isoforms in Mexican Alzheimer's Disease patients. *Dis Markers*, Vol. 22, No. 3, 2006), pp. 119-125, ISSN 0278-0240

Saunders, A. M.; Strittmatter, W. J.; Schmechel, D.; George-Hyslop, P. H.; Pericak-Vance, M. A.; Joo, S. H.; Rosi, B. L.; Gusella, J. F.; Crapper-MacLachlan, D. R. & Alberts, M. J. (1993). Association of apolipoprotein E allele epsilon 4 with late-onset familial and sporadic Alzheimer's disease. *Neurology*, Vol. 43, No. 8, (Aug 1993), pp. 1467-1472, ISSN 0028-3878

Schagger, H. & Ohm, T. G. (1995). Human diseases with defects in oxidative phosphorylation. 2. F1F0 ATP-synthase defects in Alzheimer disease revealed by blue native polyacrylamide gel electrophoresis. *Eur J Biochem*, Vol. 227, No. 3, (Feb 1 1995), pp. 916-921, ISSN 0014-2956

Schwerzmann, K. & Pedersen, P. L. (1981). Proton--adenosinetriphosphatase complex of rat liver mitochondria: effect of energy state on its interaction with the adenosinetriphosphatase inhibitory peptide. *Biochemistry*, Vol. 20, No. 22, (Oct 27 1981), pp. 6305-6311, ISSN 0006-2960

Selkoe, D. J. (2004). Cell biology of protein misfolding: the examples of Alzheimer's and Parkinson's diseases. *Nat Cell Biol*, Vol. 6, No. 11, (Nov 2004), pp. 1054-1061, ISSN 1465-7392

Simonian, N. A. & Hyman, B. T. (1994). Functional alterations in Alzheimer's disease: selective loss of mitochondrial-encoded cytochrome oxidase mRNA in the hippocampal formation. *J Neuropathol Exp Neurol*, Vol. 53, No. 5, (Sep 1994), pp. 508-512, ISSN 0022-3069

Sims, N. R.; Finegan, J. M.; Blass, J. P.; Bowen, D. M. & Neary, D. (1987). Mitochondrial function in brain tissue in primary degenerative dementia. *Brain Res*, Vol. 436, No. 1, (Dec 8 1987), pp. 30-38, ISSN 0006-8993

Strittmatter, W. J.; Saunders, A. M.; Schmechel, D.; Pericak-Vance, M.; Enghild, J.; Salvesen, G. S. & Roses, A. D. (1993). Apolipoprotein E: high-avidity binding to beta-amyloid and increased frequency of type 4 allele in late-onset familial Alzheimer disease. *Proc Natl Acad Sci U S A*, Vol. 90, No. 5, (Mar 1 1993), pp. 1977-1981, ISSN 0027-8424

Su, B.; Wang, X.; Nunomura, A.; Moreira, P. I.; Lee, H. G.; Perry, G.; Smith, M. A. & Zhu, X. (2008). Oxidative stress signaling in Alzheimer's disease. *Curr Alzheimer Res*, Vol. 5, No. 6, (Dec 2008), pp. 525-532, ISSN 1567-2050

Sullivan, P. G. & Brown, M. R. (2005). Mitochondrial aging and dysfunction in Alzheimer's disease. *Prog Neuropsychopharmacol Biol Psychiatry*, Vol. 29, No. 3, (Mar 2005), pp. 407-410, ISSN 0278-5846

Swerdlow, R. H. (2007). PET sheds light on Alzheimer's disease genetic risk. *Proc Natl Acad Sci U S A*, Vol. 104, No. 48, (Nov 27 2007), pp. 18881-18882, ISSN 0027-8424

Swerdlow, R. H. & Kish, S. J. (2002). Mitochondria in Alzheimer's disease. *Int Rev Neurobiol*, Vol. 53, No. 2002), pp. 341-385, ISSN 0074-7742

Takeda, A.; Smith, M. A.; Avila, J.; Nunomura, A.; Siedlak, S. L.; Zhu, X.; Perry, G. & Sayre, L. M. (2000). In Alzheimer's disease, heme oxygenase is coincident with Alz50, an epitope of tau induced by 4-hydroxy-2-nonenal modification. *J Neurochem*, Vol. 75, No. 3, (Sep 2000), pp. 1234-1241, ISSN 0022-3042

Troncoso, J. C.; Costello, A.; Watson, A. L., Jr. & Johnson, G. V. (1993). In vitro polymerization of oxidized tau into filaments. *Brain Res*, Vol. 613, No. 2, (Jun 11 1993), pp. 313-316, ISSN 0006-8993

Utermann, G. (1987). Apolipoprotein E polymorphism in health and disease. *Am Heart J*, Vol. 113, No. 2 Pt 2, (Feb 1987), pp. 433-440, ISSN 0002-8703

Valla, J.; Berndt, J. D. & Gonzalez-Lima, F. (2001). Energy hypometabolism in posterior cingulate cortex of Alzheimer's patients: superficial laminar cytochrome oxidase associated with disease duration. *J Neurosci*, Vol. 21, No. 13, (Jul 1 2001), pp. 4923-4930, ISSN 0270-6474

Van Gassen, G.; Annaert, W. & Van Broeckhoven, C. (2000). Binding partners of Alzheimer's disease proteins: are they physiologically relevant? *Neurobiol Dis*, Vol. 7, No. 3, (Jun 2000), pp. 135-151, ISSN 0969-9961

Wang, X.; Su, B.; Lee, H. G.; Li, X.; Perry, G.; Smith, M. A. & Zhu, X. (2009). Impaired balance of mitochondrial fission and fusion in Alzheimer's disease. *J Neurosci*, Vol. 29, No. 28, (Jul 15 2009), pp. 9090-9103, ISSN 0270-6474

Wang, X.; Su, B.; Siedlak, S. L.; Moreira, P. I.; Fujioka, H.; Wang, Y.; Casadesus, G. & Zhu, X. (2008). Amyloid-beta overproduction causes abnormal mitochondrial dynamics via differential modulation of mitochondrial fission/fusion proteins. *Proc Natl Acad Sci U S A*, Vol. 105, No. 49, (Dec 9 2008), pp. 19318-19323, ISSN 0027-8424

Zachariasse, K. A.; Vaz, W. L.; Sotomayor, C. & Kuhnle, W. (1982). Investigation of human erythrocyte ghost membranes with intramolecular excimer probes. *Biochim Biophys Acta*, Vol. 688, No. 2, (Jun 14 1982), pp. 323-332, ISSN 0006-3002

Zubenko, G. S.; Kopp, U.; Seto, T. & Firestone, L. L. (1999). Platelet membrane fluidity individuals at risk for Alzheimer's disease: a comparison of results from fluorescence spectroscopy and electron spin resonance spectroscopy. *Psychopharmacology (Berl)*, Vol. 145, No. 2, (Jul 1999), pp. 175-180, ISSN 0033-3158

Zubenko, G. S.; Malinakova, I. & Chojnacki, B. (1987). Proliferation of internal membranes in platelets from patients with Alzheimer's disease. *J Neuropathol Exp Neurol*, Vol. 46, No. 4, (Jul 1987), pp. 407-418, ISSN 0022-3069

15

Oxidative Stress in Alzheimer's Disease: Pathogenesis, Biomarkers and Therapy

Alejandro Gella and Irene Bolea
Universitat Internacional de Catalunya
Universitat Autònoma de Barcelona
Spain

1. Introduction

Alzheimer's disease (AD) is the most common cause of dementia in the elderly with profound medical and social consequences. The pathogenesis of AD is a complex and heterogeneous process which classical neuropathological hallmarks found in the brain are extracellular deposits of beta-amyloid (Aβ)-containing plaques and intracellular neurofibrillary tangles (NFTs) composed of hyperphosphorylated tau protein. Mutation of *presenilin-1* (PS-1), *presenilin-2* (PS-2), and altered *amyloid precursor protein* (APP) genes has been reported to cause inherited AD. In addition, other genes such as apolipoprotein E-4 (APOE), endothelial nitric oxide synthase-3, and alpha-2-macroglubulin have also been associated with AD. A further number of hypothesis have been proposed for AD mechanism, which include: the amyloid cascade, vascular damage, excitotoxicity, deficiency of neurotrophic factors, mitochondrial dysfunction, trace element neurotoxicity, inflammation and oxidative stress hypothesis.

The oxidative stress (OS) hypothesis of aging postulated by Dr. Denham Harman in 1956 proposed that brain aging is associated to a progressive imbalance between the anti-oxidant defenses and the pro-oxidant species that can occur as a result of either an increase in free radical production or a decrease in antioxidant defence. The fact that age is the main risk factor for AD development provides considerable support to the OS hypothesis since the effects produced by reactive oxygen species (ROS) can accumulate over the years (Nunomura et al., 2001). The link between AD and OS is additionally supported by the finding of decreased levels of antioxidant enzymes, increased protein, lipid and DNA oxidation and advanced glycation end products (AGEs) and ROS formation in neurons of AD patients (Perry et al., 2000; Barnham et al., 2004). It has been reported that the accumulation of the oligomeric form of Aβ, the most toxic form of the peptide, induces OS in neurons (Butterfield, 2002), supporting the hypothesis and suggesting that OS plays a causative role in the development of AD. Then, a large amount of literature has demonstrated that OS is an important feature in AD pathogenesis that deserves to be deeply studied (Perry et al, 2002: Markesbery et al, 1999). In this Chapter, we address the main factors involved in the generation of oxidative stress and provide an overview of the oxidative stress biomarkers status in Alzheimer's disease. The Chapter concludes with a revision of the controversial efficacy of antioxidants as potential treatment in AD therapy as well as an update of the main antioxidant compounds found to have a beneficial effect in AD.

2. Mitochondria as a source of reactive oxygen species

Several years after the postulation of the OS hypothesis, Dr. Harman proposed that life span is determined by the rate of ROS damage to the mitochondria (Harman, 1972) giving for the first time an important role to this organelle in the ageing process and establishing the basis for "mitochondrial theory of ageing". It is important to note that the central nervous system (CNS) is especially vulnerable to oxidative damage as a result of the high oxygen consumption rate (20% of the total oxygen consumption), the abundant content of easily peroxidizable fatty acids, and the relative paucity of antioxidant enzymes compared to other tissues. In aerobic organisms, mitochondria produce semireduced oxygen species during respiration. The initial step of the respiratory chain reaction yields the superoxide radical ($^{\circ}O_2^-$), which produces hydrogen peroxide (H_2O_2) by addition of an electron. The reduction of H_2O_2 through the Fenton reaction produces the highly reactive hydroxyl radical (OH°), which is the chief instigator of oxidative stress damage and reacts indiscriminately with all biomacromolecules (Figure 1). Under normal conditions, damage by ROS is prevented by an efficient antioxidant cascade, including both enzymatic and non-enzymatic entities. The enzymes responsible of the detoxification machinery are the cytosolic copper-zinc superoxide dismutase (CuZnSOD) and the mitochondrial manganese superoxide dismutase (MnSOD), which convert superoxide to O_2 and H_2O_2. Moreover, monoamine oxidases (MAOs) and L-amino acid oxidase can also produce H_2O_2 during its metabolism which is effectively removed by catalase (CAT) and peroxidases (e.g. glutathione peroxidase, GPx). Since CAT is compartmentalized into peroxisomes the detoxification of cytosolic and mitochondrial peroxides depends predominantly on GPx.

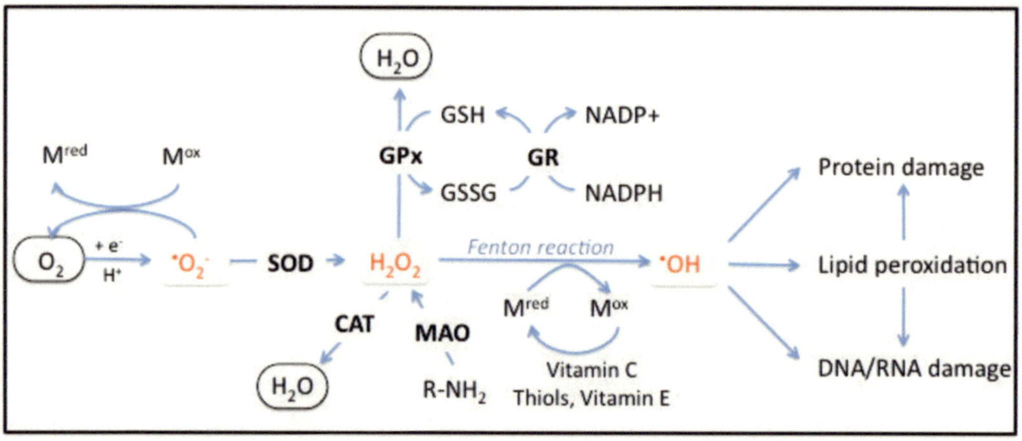

Fig. 1. Schematic illustration of the mechanism involved in reactive oxygen species (ROS) formation and elimination. Glutathione peroxidase (GPx), glutathione reductase (GR), superoxide dismutase (SOD), catalase (CAT), monoamine oxidase (MAO), glutathione (GSH), glutathione disulfide (GSSG).

The non-enzymatic antioxidant defenses include the reduction of the resulting oxidized transition metal ions (usually Fe^{3+} and Cu^{2+}) by cellular reductants such as vitamin C, thiols and perhaps even vitamin E. In this context, SOD can also serve as the reductant of oxidized metal ions for the production of hydroxyl radical from H_2O_2, which coupled with the Fenton reaction, is known as the Haber-Weiss reaction. In AD, this situation is further exacerbated by the fact that redox active transition metals are aberrantly accumulated in cytoplasm of neurons. Moreover, Aβ peptide is considered a strong redox active agent capable of reducing transition metals and allowing for conversion of O_2 to H_2O_2 (Bondy et al, 1998).

3. Biomarkers of oxidative stress in Alzheimer's disease

Biomarkers, as indicators of signalling events in biological systems or samples, can be used as intermediate endpoints or early-outcome predictors of disease development for preventive purposes. Most effort is nowadays focused on the search of reliable and robust biomarkers which would be useful for an earlier AD diagnosis. The emphasis is being placed on the incorporation of oxidative stress biomarkers to study the increased oxidative damage (Lovell & Markesbery, 2007a). It has recently been a significant improvement in assay methods and measurement accuracy for oxidative biomarkers. Nevertheless, it appears imperative that biomarkers of oxidative damage must be validated (Dalle-Donne et al., 2006a) in order to incorporate them into epidemiological studies and provide a better understanding regarding the role of ROS in the pathogenesis and progression of AD, as well as to assess the possible effectiveness of an antioxidant therapy (Griffiths et al., 2002). Strong evidence show that oxidative markers are more prevalent in initial rather than in later stages of the disease, and thus suggesting that targeting the earlier events of the disease may be more successful that targeting the later events (e.g. beta-amyloid (Aβ) plaque deposition and/or intracellular neurofibrillary tangles formation). On the other hand, many studies provided evidence for the deleterious consequences of oxidative stress products on certain cellular targets in AD. Therefore, most highly reactive oxidants react with virtually all biomolecules, including, lipids, DNA/RNA, carbohydrates and proteins. Table 1 summarizes the main OS biomarker candidates for MCI and AD diagnosis.

Biomarker	Specimen	Diagnosis	Reference
Lipid Peroxidation			
4-HNE	Plasma	AD	Mc Grath et al., 2001
	Ventricular fluid	AD	Lovell et al., 1997
F2-Isoprostanes	Urine	AD	Kim et al., 2004
	CSF	AD	Montine et al., 2011
	CSF, plasma and urine	MCI	Pratico et al., 2002
DNA oxidation			
8-OHdG	Peripheral lymphocytes	MCI	Migliore et al., 2005
		AD	Mecocci et al., 2002
AGEs			
CML	CSF	AD	Ahmed et al., 2005
Oxidized Protein			
α-1-antitrypsin	CSF	AD	Puchades et al., 2003
Ig λ light chain	CSF	MCI	Korolainen et al., 2007
α-1-antitrypsin	Plasma	AD	Yu et al., 2003; Choi et al., 2002

Table 1. Potential OS biomarkers under validation for Alzheimer's disease. MCI, mild cognitive impairment; AD, Alzheimer's disease; CSF, cerebrospinal fluid; Ig, immunoglobulin; 4-HNE, 4-hydroxy-2-nonenal; 8-OHdG, 8-oxo-7,8-dihydro-2'-deoxyguanosine; AGEs, Advanced Glycation end products; CML, N-carboxymethyl-lysine.

3.1 Biomarkers of lipid peroxidation

Lipid oxidation (also called lipid peroxidation) has drammatic consequences in ageing and age-related disorders. Phospholipids present in brain membranes are mainly polyunsaturated fatty acids (PUFAs: arachidonic acid, linoleic acid, linolenic acid, docosahexaenoic acid, etc…), which are especially vulnerable to a free radical attack since their double bonds allow an easy removal of hydrogen ions. Oxidation of PUFAs produces a variety of reactive α,β-unsaturated aldehydes such as, acrolein, 4-hydroxy-2-nonenal (4-HNE), 4-oxo-2-nonenal (4-ONE), 4-hydroxy-2-hexanal (4-HHE), 2-hexenal, crotonaldehyde as well as the dialdehydes glyoxal and malondialdehyde (MDA). These species are highly reactive cytotoxic substances than can form stable covalent adducts with free amino groups of proteins (Lys, His and Cys residues) through Michael addition (Calingasan et al., 1999; Carini et al., 2004; Esterbauer et al., 1991; Montine et al., 1997) whick are known as advanced lipoxidation end products (ALEs). 4-HNE is a major and toxic aldehyde generated by free radical attack on PUFAs and is considered a second toxic messenger of oxygen free radicals. Therefore, it has a high biological activity and exhibits numerous cytotoxic, mutagenic, genotoxic, and signalling effects in neurons (Eckl et al., 1993; Williams et al., 2006). In addition, 4-HNE may be an important mediator of OS-induced apoptosis, cellular proliferation and signalling pathways (Uchida, 2003). HNE is permanently formed at basal concentrations under physiologic conditions, but its production is greatly enhanced in the AD brain where increased lipid peroxidation occurs (Butterfield et al., 2010; McGrath et al., 2001). Increased concentrations of 4-HNE, 4-HHE and acrolein have been found in cerebrospinal fluid (CSF) and in multiple brain regions from individuals with mild cognitive impairment and early AD compared with age-matched controls (Bradley et al., 2010a and 2010b; Lovell et al., 1997; Williams et al, 2006). In addition, a positive feedback in the pathogenesis of AD is provoked by HNE that increases Aβ production (Tamagno et al., 2008) which, in turns, induces lipid peroxidation (Butterfield et al., 2002). Furthermore, HNE-adducts have been identified in amyloid plaques and neurofibrillary tangles, the two hallmarks of AD pathogenesis (Sayre et al., 1997; Ando et al., 1998; Wataya et al., 2002).

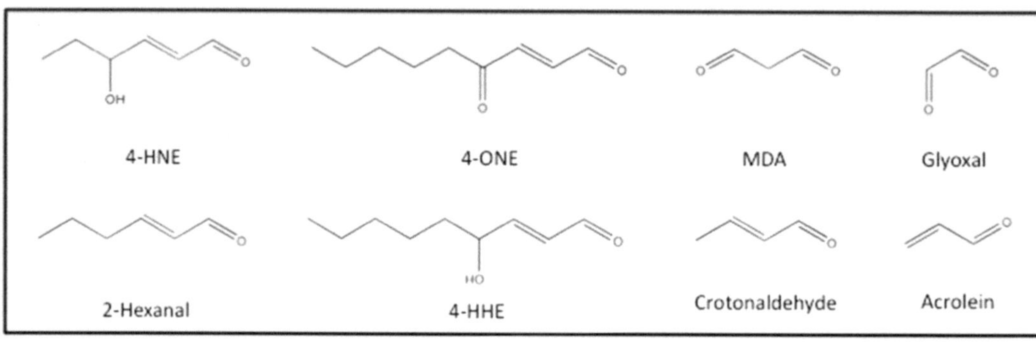

Fig. 2. Lipid peroxidation products. ROS stimulate peroxidation of polyunsaturated fatty acids (PUFA) to generate α-β-unsaturated aldehydes and dialdehydes.

F2-Isoprostanes (F2-IsoPs), which contain an F-type prostane ring, are a group of bioactive prostaglandin-like compounds generated via a non-enzymatic mechanism involving the free radical-initiated peroxidation of esterified arachidonic acid (AA). Then, they are cleaved and released into the circulation by phospholipases before excretion in the urine as free isoprostanes (Basu, 1998). The most studied class of isoprostanes, due to their urine stability, is 8-iso-Prostaglandin F_{2a} (8-iso-PGF$_{2a}$; Figure 3). Urinary F2-IsoPs determination has been proposed as specific, reliable, and non-invasive marker to assess lipid peroxidation in vivo (Cracowski et al., 2002; Montushchi et al., 2004) since an increase in 8-iso-PGF$_{2a}$ levels in CSF and urine have been found in subjects with AD (Montine et al., 1998 and 2011; Kim et al., 2004). On the other hand, oxidation of docosahexanoic acid (DHA) produces F4-neuroprostanes (F4-NeuroPs; Figure 3) (Morrow et al., 1999; Roberts et al., 1998) which levels are elevated in postmortem ventricular CSF of AD patients and are more abundant in the brain that F2-isoprostanes. Nevertheless, plasma F2-IsoPs and F4-NeuroPs do not accurately reflect central nervous system levels and are not reproducibly elevated in body fluids outside of central nervous system in Alzheimer's disease patients (Montine et al., 2002).

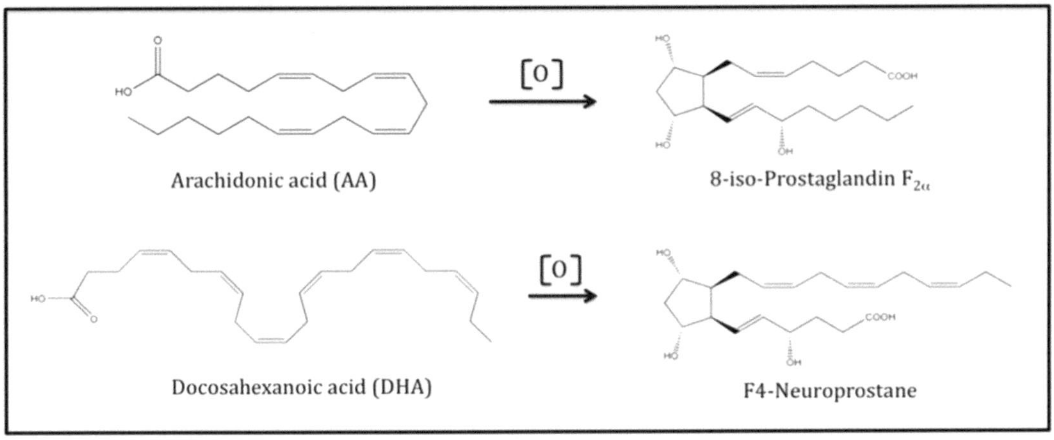

Fig. 3. Chemical structures of F4-neuroprostane and 8-iso-Prostaglandin F_{2a} arising from direct oxidation of docosahexanoic and arachidonic acids, respectively.

3.2 Biomarkers of oxidative DNA damage

Among over 30 nucleobase modifications that have been described, the most extensively studied that reflect oxidative DNA damage is 8-oxo-7,8-dihydro-2′-deoxyguanosine (8-oxodG; also known as 8-OHdG), a product of oxidatively modified DNA base guanine (Figure 4). The detection of this oxidation is important not only due to its abundance but also to its mutagenic potential through GC-to-TA transversion mutations upon replication of DNA (Cheng et al., 1992). Nevertheless, oxidatively damaged DNA can be repaired and released into the bloodstream and consequently appear without further metabolism in the urine (Fraga et al., 1990; Shigenaga et al., 1989). In addition, urinary levels of 8-OHdG have been found to be independent of dietary influence in humans. The modified base 8-oxo-7,8-dihydroguanine (8-oxoGua; Figure 4) and modified nucleoside (8-oxodG; Figure 4), which are found in urine, represent the major repair products of oxidatively damaged DNA in vivo and have been considered to reflect the whole-body oxidative DNA damage (Hamilton et al., 2001; Olinnski et al., 2007). There is considerable evidence supporting that oxidative stress occurs in AD, and increased 8-oxodG levels have been found in DNA isolated from brain tissues, leukocytes and ventricular CSF of AD patients. In contrast, free 8-OHdG was found dramatically decreased in AD samples as compared to the controls (Lovell & Markesbery, 2001; Markesbery & Carney, 1999; Mecocci et al., 2002; Migliore et al., 2005).

Taken together, these data indicate a double insult in AD patients by increasing oxidative damage and decreasing DNA repair mechanisms efficiency. More recent studies showed an elevated 8-OHdG in both nuclear and mitochondrial DNA (mtDNA) isolated from vulnerable brain regions in amnestic mild cognitive impairment (MCI), the earliest clinical manifestation of AD, and thus suggesting that oxidative DNA damage is an early event in AD and is not merely a secondary phenomenon (Lovell & Markesbery, 2007b).
Many methods such as HPLC-ECD, GC-MS, LC-MS, and immunoassay have been established to measure 8-OHdG in biological specimens. In this concern, the European Standards Committee of Urinary (DNA) Lesions Analysis (ESCULA) was formed in 2006 in order to validate the measurement methods of oxidatively damaged DNA and to establish reference urine values (Cooke et al., 2008; Evans et al., 2010). Finally, it is important to mention that DNA can also be modified by products of lipid peroxidation (ALEs). These α-β-unsaturated aldehydes can react with deoxyguanosine through an initial Michael addition of the exocyclic amino group followed by ring closure of N-1 onto the aldehydic group to generate a bulky exocyclic 1-N^2-propanodeoxyguanosine adduct (Liu et al., 2006; Kozekov et al., 2003) and therefore participate in the propagation of the oxidative DNA damage.

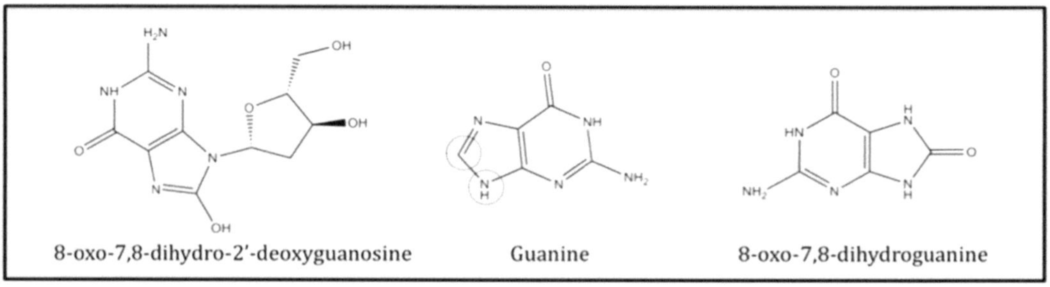

Fig. 4. Chemical structure of 8-oxo-7, 8-dihydro-2'-deoxyguanosine (8-oxodG; 8-OHdG), guanine and 8-oxo-7, 8-dihydroguanine (8-oxoGua).

3.3 Advanced glycation end products

Advanced glycation end products (AGEs), formed by a non-enzymatic reaction of sugars with amino groups in long-lived proteins, lipids, and nucleic acids, are also potent neurotoxins and proinflammatory molecules. Glycation of proteins starts as a non-enzymatic process with the spontaneous condensation of ketone or aldehyde groups of sugars with a free aminoacid group of proteins to form a labile Schiff base, consistent with the classical reaction described by Louis Camille Maillard in 1912 (Figure 5).

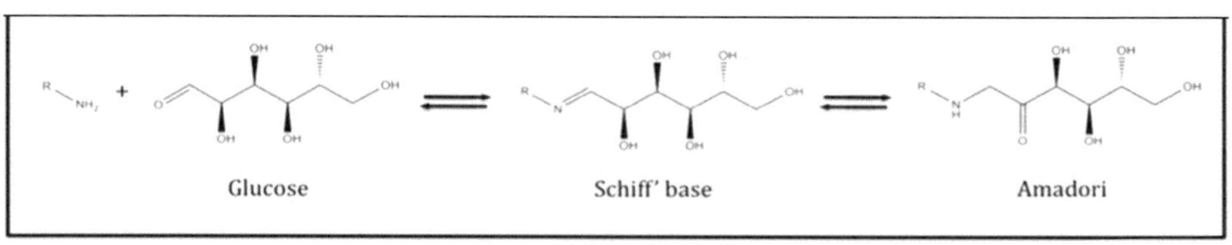

Fig. 5. Non-enzymatic reaction of the carbonyl groups of reducing sugars with primary amino groups produce corresponding Schiff bases, which undergo Amadori rearrangement to give ketoamines.

Glycation is the first step in the cascade of a complex series of very slow reactions in the body known as Amadori reactions, Schiff base reactions and Maillard reactions, all leading to the formation of irreversibly cross-linked heterogeneous aggregates. AGEs are continuously formed in the human body and progressively accumulate with age in plasma and tissues. In diabetes mellitus and AD the rate of AGEs formation is accelerated and consequently, they have been considered potentially useful biomarkers for monitoring the treatment of these disorders. Chemical structures of representative markers of AGEs are summarized in Figure 6. Supporting the argument that AGEs are involved in the pathogenesis of AD, some studies have shown the presence of AGEs in association with two major proteins of AD, Aβ and MAP-tau (Smith et al., 1995; Vitek et al., 1994; Yan et al., 1994). Extracellular AGEs accumulation has been demonstrated in senile plaques in different cortical areas. Intracellular proteins deposits including NFTs, Lewy bodies of patients with Parkinson's disease and Hirano bodies are also crosslinked by AGEs, which may explain their insolubility in detergents and resistance to proteases (Loske et al., 2000). The major component of the NFTs, the microtubuli-associated protein tau (MAP-tau) has been shown to be subject to intracellular AGEs formation. MAP-tau

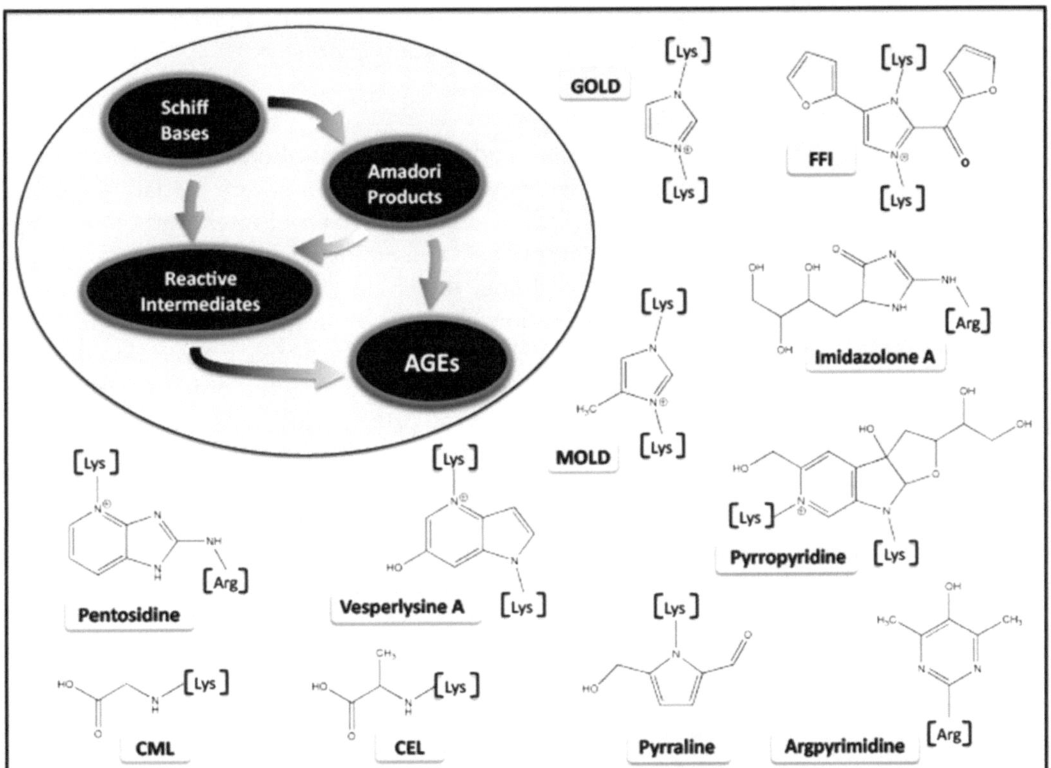

Fig. 6. A variety of highly reactive carbonyl intermediates such as 3-deoxy-glucosone, glyoxal and methyl-glyoxal can be formed by glucose or Schiff's base or Amadori product auto-oxidation which, in turn, can react with free amino groups to form AGE products. N-carboxymethyl-lysine (CML), N- carboxyethyl-lysine (CEL), glyoxal-derived lysine dimer (GOLD), methylglyoxal-derived lysine dimer (MOLD), furoyl-furanyl-imidazole (FFI), Lysine (Lys) and arginine (Arg).

can be glycated in vitro, inhibiting its ability to bind to microtubules. In addition, MAP-tau isolated from brains of AD patients is glycated in the tubulin-binding region, giving rise to the formation of β-sheet fibrils (Ledesma et al., 1998). AGEs accumulate in the human brain during aging (Kimura et al., 1996) and are present in neurofibrillary tangles and senile plaques in patients with AD (Castellani et al., 2001). Furthermore; AGE-modified Aβ peptides accelerate aggregation of soluble nonfibrillar Aβ peptides. In older adults with cerebrovascular disease, elevated N-carboxymethyl-lysine (CML) has been found in cortical neurons and cerebral vessels and has been related to the severity of cognitive impairment (Southern et al., 2007). Brain tissue AGEs can therefore be considered tissue biomarkers for AD, and increased brain AGEs concentrations are reflected in CSF (Ahmed et al., 2005) but no necessarily in plasma (Thome et al., 1996).

A positive feedback loop in the pathogenesis of AD is provoked by AGEs which increase OS and inflammation through binding with AGEs receptor (RAGE). The RAGE signalling pathway, found upregulated in AD brains, can be initiated by a diverse repertoire of pro-inflammatory ligands that include AGEs, S100/calgranulins, amphoterin, and amyloid-β peptide. Ligand binding with RAGE triggers the induction of increased reactive oxygen species, activates NADH oxidase, increases the expression of adhesion molecules, and up-regulates inflammation through NF-kB and other signalling pathways.

3.4 Biomarkers of oxidative protein damage

Carbonylation of proteins is an irreversible oxidative process, often leading to a loss of protein function, which is considered a widespread indicator of severe oxidative damage and disease-derived protein dysfunction (Dalle-Donne et al., 2006). Protein carbonyl groups are introduced to proteins by direct oxidation of several amino acid residues into ketone or aldehyde derivates (particularly lysine, arginine, threonine and proline; Figure 7) or by secondary reaction with the primary oxidation products of sugars (forming AGEs) and lipids (forming ALEs) (Berlett & Stadtman, 1997). Several studies have proved that proteins are major initial cell targets of ROS, leading to earlier formation of the protein carbonyls in biological systems. Detection of increased levels of protein carbonyls in AD has been proposed as a sign of disease-associated dysfunction, suggesting the potentiality as biomarkers for early AD diagnosis.

Recent studies show an increase in protein carbonyls together with NFTs in multiple brain regions of AD subjects (Sultana & Butterfield, 2011). Oxidative modifications of proteins can cause cross-linking of covalent bonds of proteins leading to fibril formation and insolubility. NFTs are characterized by the aggregation and hyperphosphorilation of tau proteins which is linked to oxidation through the microtubule-associated protein kinase pathway and through the activation of the transcription factor NF-kB. A wide number of studies have reported differences in specific carbonated proteins in brain, plasma and CSF of AD patients compared with control group by using 2-dimensional gel electrophoresis in combination with mass spectroscopy techniques (Castegna et al., 2002a, 2002b; Davidsson et al., 2001; Puchades et al., 2003). Some of these studies reveal the presence of specific targets of protein oxidation in AD brain: creatine kinase BB, glutamine synthase, ubiquitin carboxy-terminal hydrolase L-1, dihydropyrimidinase-related protein 2, alpha-enolase and heat shock cognate 71. Glutamine synthase and creatine kinase, both markedly decreased in AD brains, are especially sensitive to oxidative modifications since they may cause alteration of glutamate concentrations (glutamine sinthase), and therefore enhance excitotoxicity, and decrease energy metabolism (creatine kinase). Recently, several oxidized carbonylated proteins have been characterized in frontal cortex (Korolainen et al., 2006), plasma (Yu et al., 2003; Choi et al., 2002) and CSF (Korolainen et al., 2007) of patients suffering from AD by two-dimensional oxyblotting technique.

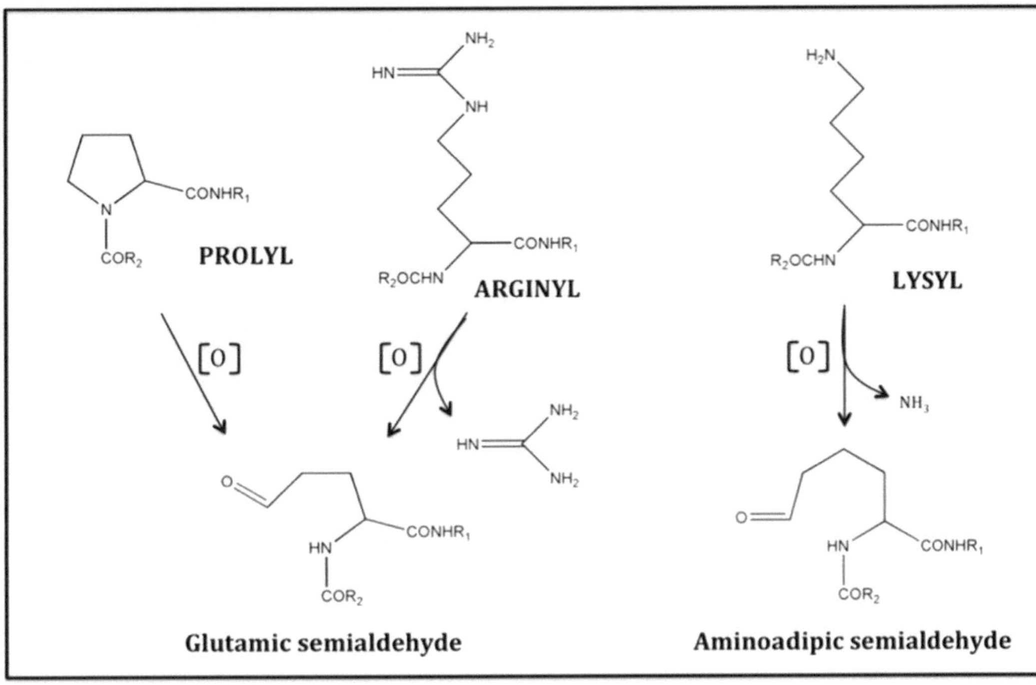

Fig. 7. Chemical structures of protein carbonyls arising from direct oxidation of aminoacid side chains. Glutamic semialdehyde (resulting from direct oxidation of arginyl and prolyl residues) and aminoadipic semialdehyde (resulting from direct oxidation of lysyl residue).

4. Antioxidant therapies in Alzheimer's disease

Currently, the only Food and Drug Administration (FDA) approved treatment for AD is the administration of the cholinesterase inhibitors (AChEI) donepezil, galantamine and rivastigmine and the N-methyl-D-aspartate (NMDA) receptor antagonist, memantine (Birks et al., 2000, 2006; Loy et al., 2004; Areosa et al., 2005). Nevertheless, to date, these drugs have demonstrated to produce only modest symptomatic improvements in some of the patients, but not to cure or stop the disease progression. Moreover, AChEI are expensive and may have side effects resulting from activation of peripheral cholinergic systems (Green et al., 2005). Then, effective treatments are greatly needed. The current therapeutic strategies being investigated for AD include targeting neurotransmission with multifunctional compounds, anti-amyloid and anti-tau therapies, drugs targeting mitochondrial dysfunction, neurotrophins, statins and also other approaches such us PUFAs and antioxidants (for review see Mangialasche et al., 2010). Among them, antioxidant therapies and PUFAs are particularly attractive due to their low toxicity, low cost and their ability to target earlier changes of the disease (e.g oxidative stress) which are linked to cognitive and functional decline. However, there is still much skepticism regarding the likelihood of success with an antioxidant therapy since to date these compounds tested in randomised controlled trials (RCTs) have given controversial results.

4.1 Vitamins

A large amount of literature exists in relation to the potential benefits of vitamins, which act as natural free radical scavengers, in the prevention of AD (Figure 8). Vitamin A has been traditionally considered as antioxidant and it seems essential for learning, memory and cognition. Retinoic acid, a metabolic product of vitamin A, is known to slow cell death and protect from Aβ (Sahin et al., 2005). Thus, since levels of vitamin A decline with age and are found lower in AD individuals (Goodman et al., 2006) vitamin A supplementation might be useful for the treatment of some features in the ageing process. B-vitamins (B_6, B_{12} and folic acid) are lipid soluble antioxidants involved in the methylation of homocysteine (Hcy) which is highly cytotoxic. Cellular catabolism and cellular export mechanisms are the responsible for keeping low intracellular Hcy concentration. AD patients tipically present high levels of Hcy (McIlroy et al., 2002) and low levels of vitamin B_{12} and folate which appear to be associated with an increased rate of cognitive decline (Tucker et al., 2006; Morris et al., 2007). Nevertheless, in a recent study, a combination of vitamins B_{12}, B_6 and folate in mild to moderate AD individuals, although lowering Hcy, did not produce any effect on cognition compared to controls. Vitamin C (ascorbic acid), found in many fruits and vegetables, is the major water-soluble antioxidant and acts as first defence against free radicals in blood and plasma. Bagi et al, 2003, have shown that chronic vitamin C treatment is able to decrease high levels of isoprostanes in animal models. In contrast, other studies have shown that it can also act as pro-oxidant inducing neuronal oxidative stress via its

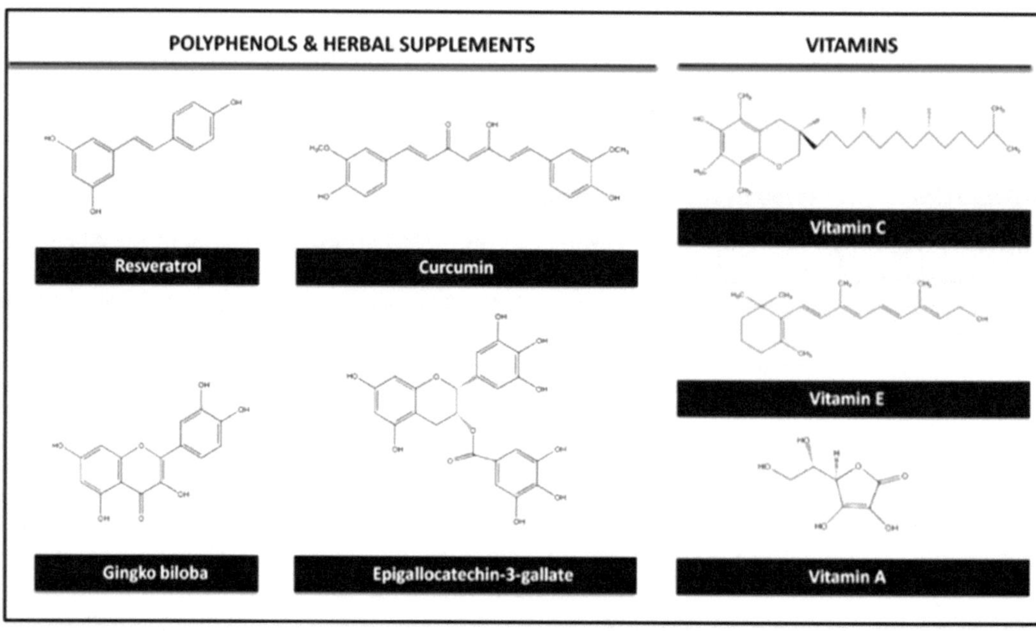

Fig. 8. Chemical structures of the principal polyphenols, herbal suplements and vitamins investigated as promising agents for the treatment of AD.

interaction with metal ions (White et al., 2004). Vitamin E (α-tocopherol), present in whole grains, cereals and vegetable oils, is a lipid-soluble vitamin found in cell membranes and circulating lipoproteins. Its antioxidant capacity acts directly to a variety of ROS. It is found low in AD patients (Jiménez-Jiménez et al., 1997) and although in vitro and animal studies have been encouraging, human trials have produced conflicting results (Berman et al., 2004). A Cochrane study shows that tocopherol is not effective in a prevention trial in mild cognitive impairment (MCI) to reduce progression to AD nor clearly effective in AD patients (Tabet et al., 2000; Luchsinger et al., 2003). Besides, a harmfull effect of tocopherol at high doses has also been suggested (Tucker et al., 2005). However, several studies correlate a reduced risk to AD in elderly persons treated with vitamin E and C alone or in combination (Grundman et al., 2004; Morris et al., 1998; 2002; 2005). On the other hand, brain bioavailability of vitamin E in humans is very low and, as suggested elsewhere may not be enough to quickly inhibit AD neuropathology unless administered as a prophylactic at very early ages. The large amount of contradictory data found in literature about the use of vitamins as antioxidants indicates intricate physiological and pharmacological features of AD and remain questionable its use in human.

4.2 Polyphenols and herbal supplements

Polyphenols are a group of plant-derived chemical substances which protect plants from the stress induced by physical damage, disease, radiation and pests (Figure 8). It has been suggested that curcumin, the yellow pigment extracted from the plant *curcuma longa* (turmeric), may be a promising therapy for AD due to its extended neuroprotective actions (Mishra et al., 2008; Cole et al., 2007), including antioxidant, anti-inflammatory, inhibition of Aβ formation and removal of existing Aβ, as well as cooper and iron chelation. Epigallocathechin-3-gallate (EGCg) is found in green tea and it has been described that prevents Aβ aggregation by directly binding to the unfolded peptide. It also modulates signal transduction pathways, expression of genes regulating cell survival and apoptosis and its actions in mitochondrial function make it a potent antioxidant (Mandel et al., 2008). Resveratrol is present in red wine, peanuts and other plants and it has been found that it reduces OS, inflammation and Aβ deposition, decreases cell death and protects DNA (Mishra et al., 2008; Karuppagounder et al., 2009). A recent study suggests that moderate consumption of red wine reduces the risk of developing AD. Nevertheless, the translation to humans is still somewhat problematic and has some caveats since although polyphenols easily penetrate blood-brain barrier, they show bioavailabity problems such us low absorption, rapid metabolism and quick elimination. Efforts to increase bioavailability have been reviewed (Anand et al., 2007) and the adjuvant use widely extended (Shoba et al., 1998). Indeed, there is currently a clinical trial underway addressing curcumin bioavailability (http://clinicaltrials.gov/NCT01001637). Furthermore, the anti-AD effects of polyphenols may not be mediated solely through their direct antioxidant action but rather indirectly through any other functions. Then, it is still to be clarified whether polyphenols are able to slow the progression of AD. Herbal supplements such us *gingko biloba* have been suggested to possess beneficial properties against AD (Luo et al, 2002). Numerous animal and in vitro studies report that *gingko biloba* extract EGb761 possess neuroprotective benefits (Defeudis et al., 2002) including antioxidant, anti-inflammatory, and regulator of Aβ processing. It has also been described that *gingko* improves cognitive function in mild to moderate AD patients (Oken et al., 1998; Le Bars et al., 2003) and reduces deterioration in subjects with more severe dementia via inhibition of the Aβ induced free radical generation (Napryeyenko et al., 2009; Yao et al., 2001). Nevertheless, a double-blind placebo controlled study found no beneficial effect of *gingko* on dementia in AD patients (Schneider et al, 2005) and DeKosky et al, 2008 showed that gingko was not better than placebo at preventing the onset of dementia. Additionally, there are two more studies finding no correlation between cognitive decline and the use of *gingko biloba* (Snitz et al., 2009; Dodge et al., 2008). Although data is controversial, it then appears that *gingko* may be useful delaying cognition impairment but not preventing the onset of AD. The ongoing clinical trial will help to elucidate this question (http://clinicaltrials.gov/NCT00814346).

4.3 Mitochondrial-related antioxidants

Since mitochondria are the major sources of ROS in the central nervous system, therapeutic strategies have largely focused in targeting mitochondria and mitochondrial-related pathways. There are several compounds showing an in vitro and in vivo antioxidant and neuroprotective action but only a few have been tested in human clinical trials with mixed results.

4.3.1 Quinone family

Ubiquinone (Coenzyme Q, CoQ) and idebenone, a synthetic analog of CoQ, (Figure 9) are the major mitochondrial targets used as therapeutics against ROS-mediated damage. They have demonstrated antioxidant properties in vitro and in animal models (Wadsworth et al., 2008). CoQ has not been yet tested in humans but idebenone has been investigated in clinical trials for its capacity to inhibit lipid peroxidation. Several studies report a significant effect in memory and attention improvements (Gutzmann et al., 2002; Senin et al., 1992; Weyer et al., 1997) but a larger study reported no effect in slowing the disease progression (Thal et al., 2003).

4.3.2 Other mitochondrial antioxidants

Alpha-lipoic acid (LA) is an organosulfur compound derived from octanoic acid and primarily a cofactor in aerobic metabolism for pyruvate dehydrogenase complex. Its reduced bioactive form produced into cells provides its antioxidant properties (Haenen et al., 1991). Acetyl L-carnitine (ALCAR) is formed within mitochondria by carnitine-*O*-acetyltransferase. Both LA and ALCAR (Figure 9) are good candidates for being used therapeutically as mitochondrial antioxidants since it was found that a combination of both decreased mitochondrial dysfunction and its consequent ROS-mediated damage in aged rats, improving cognitive functions (Aliev et al., 2009). Additional neuroprotective functions, including binding to targets involved in Aβ production have been reported (Epis et al., 2008). However, several clinical trials with ALCAR have been conducted with contradictory results: one showed no effectiveness in early onset AD (Thal et al., 2000) whereas another showed a slower deterioration in cognition (Pettergrew et al., 1995). A recent meta-analysis of ALCAR treatment trials showed an improvement in clinical scales in patients with MCI and AD (Montgomery et al., 2003). Dimebon (Figure 9), a non selective antihistamine, possesses several mechanisms of action including the inhibition of Aβ toxicity and the prevention of ROS-mediated damage (Doody et al., 2009; Okun et al., 2010). Several clinical trials have been performed in AD patients with contradictory results: in a phase 2 clinical trial, dimebon improved cognition and behaviour, overall function in MCI and AD (Doody et al., 2008) whereas more recently, a phase 3 CONNECTION trial with AD patients showed no improvement in any parameter (http://clinicaltrials.gov/NCT00675623).

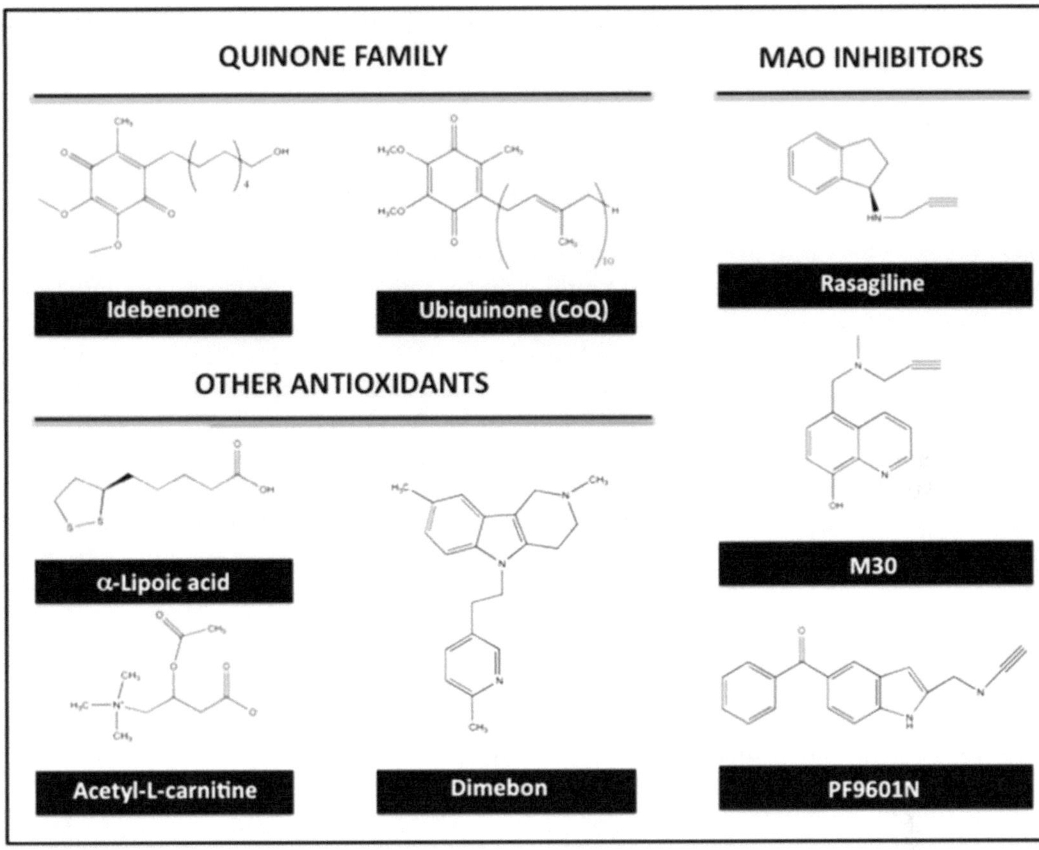

Fig. 9. Chemical structures of mitochondrial-related antioxidants investigated as promising agents for the treatment of AD.

4.3.3 Monoamine oxidase inhibitors

The therapeutic potential of monoamine oxidase inhibitors (MAOIs) for the treatment of AD has been largely reported (Thomas, 2000; Riederer et al., 2004; Youdim et al., 2005) due to their capacity to reduce the formation of toxic metabolites or oxygen radicals by blocking the catalytic activity of monoamine oxidase (MAO), enzyme located in the mitochondrial membrane and responsible of amine metabolism. It has been extensively reported that MAO-B activity besides increasing with age is found in high levels in AD patients. Selegiline, the classic MAO-B inhibitor, and also other propargylamines (Figure 9) possess potent antioxidant properties (Kitani et al., 2000; Sanz et al., 2004). Moreover, it has also been described that propargylamine-derived MAOIs exert neuroprotective effects by acting in very diverse type of targets, including metal chelation (e.g M30), reduction of Aβ aggregation and toxicity (Bar-Am et al., 2009; Youdim et al., 2005) as well as direct actions on diverse mitochondrial-related components. Among this direct functions, propargylamines increase the expression of anti-apoptotic proteins (Akao et al., 2002), prevent citocrom c release and preserve the mitochondrial membrane potential (Mayurama et al., 2000). The great amount of beneficial functions found for MAOIs make them promising molecules for the treatment of AD. Indeed, current pharmacological challenges in AD involve the design and development of multifunctional compounds able to bind to a very diverse type of targets and among them MAO inhibition is strongly recommended.

4.4 PUFAs

The beneficial effects of omega-3 polyunsaturated fatty acids (PUFAs) have been widely reported which make them good candidates for AD therapy (Cole et al., 2005) since they act directly on intracellular pathways and regulate oxidative stress mechanisms. DHA is the major omega-3 fatty acid in the brain. A recent study although showing no effect of DHA on subjects with mild-to-moderate AD it found a slower rate of cognitive decline among those patients without de APO ε4 allele (Quinn et al., 2009). As reviewed by Mangialasche et al, 2010, some studies have reported a beneficial effect of DHA on cognitive function in patients with AD (Yurko-Mauro et al., 2009; Chiu et al., 2008) whereas others did not found a correlation (Quinn et al., 2009). In effect, a recent study showed that treatment of patients with PUFAs did not modify the neuropathology of this disorder in CSF or plasma, nor the biomarkers of inflammation (Freund-Levi et al., 2009) and a randomised control trial in patients with mild to moderate AD did not delay the rate of cognitive decline (Freund-Levi et al., 2006). Some authors suggest that benefits of omega-3 fatty acids are limited to those with very mild cognitive impairment. A phase 2 randomised clinical trial is currently ongoing (http://clinicaltrials.gov/NCT01058941).

4.5 Multiple nutrients

Dietary supplementation with a plethora of nutrients such us apple juice concentrate, red wine, caffeine, fish oil or green tea as well as calorie restriction diets have been conducted. Diverse human studies have shown that multiple formulations improve all measures of cognition, although some authors reported that the increase in memory was not found significant (Chan et al., 2008). A recent study correlates frequent consumption of fruits and vegetables, fish, and omega-3 rich oils with a decreased risk of dementia in AD (Barberger-Gateau et al., 2007). In contrast, interventional trials with antioxidants, B-vitamines and DHA did not give the promising expectations from the epidemiological data. As reported by Von Arnim et al., 2010, although some trials are encouraging, larger randomised clinical trials with combined supplements are needed to draw any conclusion. Supplement composition is still a matter of debate, because high doses of a single antioxidant have been associated with no beneficial effects for AD patients and even with an increase in mortality risk (e.g vitamin E). Many interventional studies are started very late in the disease state, when AD pathology is already at a fulminant level which severely reduces therapeutic effectiveness of tested agents. The multifactorial nature of AD and the necessity to target the earlier production of OS makes important the combination of multiple supplements. Therefore, studies combining nutrients are of particular interest and at present in progress (e.g. T-diet, NKO™, and Memory XL; http://clinicaltrials.gov/NCT01192529, NCT00867828, NCT00903695).

Exposure	Assessment	Design	Case source	Major findings	Reference
EGb 761 (intravenous)	NA	RCT	AD VaD	ADL improvement. Clinical impression of change	Haase et al, 1996
EGb 761 (oral)	NA	RCT	AD VaD	Cognitive improvement	Le Bars et al, 2000
PUFAs	Plasma assay	Cross-sectional	Normal, CI, dementia	Low n-3 and high n-6 associated with CI and AD	Conquer et al, 2000
PUFAs	Plasma assay	Cross-sectional	Normal, CI, dementia	High n-3 associated with CI and AD. Strengthened in ApoEe4 non-carriers	Laurin et al, 2003
PUFAs	Plasma assay	Prospective	Normal	No association between PUFAs and reduced risk of dementia	Kroger et al, 2009
Fish intake	FFQ	Prospective	Normal	Reduced risk of incident dementia	Barberger-Gateau et al, 2002
DHA	Serum assay	Case-control	Normal AD	MMSE and CDR improvement	Tully et al, 2003
Fish oil	FFQ	Prospective	Elderly	Slow rate of decline but not on overall cognitive status	Morris et al, 2005
PUFA	FFQ	Prospective	Elderly	Reduced MMSE decline over 5 years	Van Gelder et al, 2007
β-carotene	NA	Prospective	Elderly	Less cognitive decline only in ApoE4 carriers	Hu et al, 2006
Vitamin E	NA	RCT	MCI	No significant differences compared to placebo or donepezil	Petersen, 2005
α-tocopherol and/or selegiline	NA	RCT	Moderate AD	Longer time to institutionalization in all cases	Sano et al, 1997

Table 2. Studies on antioxidants. EGb 761, Gingko biloba special extract 761; NA, not applicable; VaD, Vascular Disease; ADL, Activities of Daily Living; RCT, Randomised Controlled Trial; ApoE, apolipoprotein E; n-3, omega-3 fatty acids; n-6, omega-6 fatty acids; FFQ, food frequency questionnaire; AD, Alzheimer's Disease; CI, cognitive impairment; MCI, Mild cognitive impairment; DHA, docohexanoic acid; PUFAs, polyunsaturated fatty acids; MMSE, Folstein Mini- Mental State examination; CDR, Clinical Dementia Rating Scale.

5. Conclusions

Oxidative stress increases with ageing and seems to be a consequence of an imbalance between ROS production and antioxidant defences. The accumulation of endogenous oxygen radicals generated in mitochondria and the consequent oxidative modifications of biological molecules have been indicated as responsible for the ageing process. There is therefore an urgent need to identify biomarkers that would help to diagnose and monitor the early AD or "preclinical AD". Indeed, a few CSF proteins (e.g. amyloid-β_{1-42}, total tau and phospho-tau) have already shown promise as diagnostic biomarkers for AD. Nevertheless, these biomarkers are not yet optimal diagnostic tools to identify those MCI patients at higher risk of conversion to AD. Thus, a key objective in the research of OS biomarkers is to identify prodromal stages of the disorder, prior to cognitive decline, for gauging the long-term therapeutic effects of drugs. The contradictory results obtained with diverse antioxidants in clinical trials may be explained by other related differences in health problems as well as due to the fact that most studies are very short and conducted with very few subjects. Methodological problems and poorly matched epidemiological studies have also been pointed as reasons for mixed findings. In fact, very few trials are adequately addressing the effect of antioxidants in AD. Although at this time there is no rationale for recommending antioxidant use for prevention or treatment of AD, the current epidemiologic evidence points toward an important role of nutrition in this pathology. The optimal time for prevention seems to be important and still to be determined. Nevertheless, it seems clear that therapies acting in the beginning of the pathological cascade may be more effective than treatments that act after the fact (e.g., removal of amyloid plaques). Then, therapy should begin as early as possible while reversal of cellular pathologies is still achievable. In conclusion, properly addressed studies with antioxidants are greatly needed to obtain convincing data about its beneficial effects as anti-AD. There is also an urgent need for better formulations with increased bioavailability. Due to the multifactorial nature of AD, it seems imperative that future trials may use drug combinations or even multifunctional molecules, rather than a single compound, able to bind to a very diverse type of target and that an antioxidant capacity may be contemplated.

6. Acknowledgment

The authors gratefully acknowledge Professors Nuria Durany (Universitat Internacional de Catalunya) and Peter Riederer (University of Würzburg).

7. References

Ahmed N, Ahmed U, Thornalley PJ, Hager K, Fleischer G, Münch G. (2005). Protein glycation, oxidation and nitration adduct residues and free adducts of cerebrospinal fluid in Alzheimer's disease and link to cognitive impairment. *J Neurochem,* 92:255-63.

Aliev G, Liu J, Schenk JC et al. (2009). Neuronal mitochondrial amelioration of alpha-lipoic acid and acetyl-L-carnitine. *J Cell Mol Med,* 13:320-333.

Akao I. (2002). Mitochondrial permeability transition mediates apoptosis induced by N-methyl(R)salsolinol, an endogenous neurotoxin, and is inhibited by Bcl-s and rasagiline. *J Neurochem,* 82:913-923.

Anand P, Kunnumakkara AB, Newman RA et al. (2007). Bioavailability of curcumin: problems and promises. *Mol Pharm,* 4:807-818.

Ando Y, Brännström T, Uchida K, Nyhlin N, Näsman B, Suhr O, Yamashita T, Olsson T, El Salhy M, Uchino M, Ando M. (1998). Histochemical detection of 4-hydroxynonenal protein in Alzheimer amyloid. *J Neurol Sci,* Apr 1;156(2):172-6.

Areosa SA, Sheriff F, Mc Shane R. (2005). Memantine for dementia. *Cochrane Database Syst Rev* (2) CD003154 .

Bagi Z, CSeko C, Toth E et al. (2003). Oxidative stress-induced dysregulation of arteriosal wall shear stress and blood pressure in hyperhomocysteinemia is prevented by chronic vitamin C treatment. *Am J Physiol Heart Circ Physiol,* 285:H2277-H2283.

Bar-Am O, Weinreb O, Amit T et al. (2009). The novel cholinesterase-monoamine oxidase inhibitor and antioxidant, ladostigil, confers neuroprotection in neuroblastoma cells and aged rats. *J Mol Neurosci,* 37:135-145.

Barberger-Gateau P, Letenneur L, Deschamps V et al. (2002). Fish, meat, and risk of dementia: cohort study. *BMJ,* 325(7370):932-933.

Barberger-Gateau P, Raffaitin C, Letenneur L et al. (2007). Dietary patterns and risk of dementia : The Three-city chort study. *Neurology,* 69(20):1921-1930.

Barnham KJ, Masters CL, Bush AI. (2004). Neurodegenerative diseases and oxidative stress. *Nat Rev Drug Discov,* Mar;3(3):205-14.

Basu S. Metabolism of 8-iso-prostaglandin F2alpha. (1998). *FEBS Lett.* May 22;428(1-2):32-6.

Berman K & Brodaty H. (2004). Tocopherol (vitamin E) in Alzheimer's disease and other neurodegenerative disorders. *Drugs,* 18:807-825.

Berlett BS, Stadtman ER. (1997). Protein oxidation in aging, disease, and oxidative stress. *J Biol Chem.* Aug 15;272(33):20313-6.

Birks J & Harvey R. (2006). Donepezil for dementia due to Alzheimer's disease. *Cochrane Database Syst Rev* (1) CD001190.

Birks J, Grimley EJ, Iakovidou V et al. (2000). Rivastigmine for Alzheimer's disease. *Cochrane Database Syst Rev* (4) CD001191.

Bondy SC, Guo-Ross SX, Truong AT. (1998). Promotion of transition metal-induced reactive oxygen species formation by beta-amyloid. *Brain Res,* 799:91-96.

Bradley MA, Markesbery WR, Lovell MA. (2010a). Increased levels of 4-hydroxynonenal and acrolein in the brain in preclinical Alzheimer disease. *Free Radic Biol Med,* Jun 15;48(12):1570-6.

Bradley MA, Xiong-Fister S, Markesbery WR, Lovell MA. (2010b). Elevated 4-hydroxyhexenal in Alzheimer's disease (AD) progression. *Neurobiol Aging,* Oct 19.

Butterfield DA, Bader Lange ML, Sultana R. (2010). Involvements of the lipid peroxidation product, HNE, in the pathogenesis and progression of Alzheimer's disease. *Biochim Biophys Acta,* Aug;1801(8):924-9.

Butterfield DA, Castegna A, Lauderback CM, Drake J. (2002). Evidence that amyloid beta-peptide-induced lipid peroxidation and its sequelae in Alzheimer's disease brain contribute to neuronal death. *Neurobiol Aging,* Sep-Oct;23(5):655-64.

Butterfield DA, Griffin S, Munch G, Pasinetti GM. (2002). Amyloid beta-peptide and amyloid pathology are central to the oxidative stress and inflammatory cascades under which Alzheimer's disease brain exists. *J Alzheimers Dis,* Jun;4(3):193-201.

Calingasan NY, Uchida K, Gibson GE. (1999). Protein-bound acrolein: a novel marker of oxidative stress in Alzheimer's disease. *J Neurochem,* Feb;72(2):751-6.

Carini M, Aldini G, Facino RM. (2004). Mass spectrometry for detection of 4-hydroxy-trans-2-nonenal (HNE) adducts with peptides and proteins. *Mass Spectrom Rev*, Jul-Aug;23(4):281-305.

Castegna A, Aksenov M, Aksenova M, Thongboonkerd V, Klein JB, Pierce WM, Booze R, Markesbery WR, Butterfield DA. (2002a). Proteomic identification of oxidatively modified proteins in Alzheimer's disease brain. Part I: creatine kinase BB, glutamine synthase, and ubiquitin carboxy-terminal hydrolase L-1. *Free Radic Biol Med*,. Aug 15;33(4):562-71.

Castegna A, Aksenov M, Thongboonkerd V, Klein JB, Pierce WM, Booze R, Markesbery WR, Butterfield DA. (2002b). Proteomic identification of oxidatively modified proteins in Alzheimer's disease brain. Part II: dihydropyrimidinase-related protein 2, alpha-enolase and heat shock cognate 71. *J Neurochem*, 2002 Sep;82(6):1524-32.

Castellani RJ, Harris PL, Sayre LM, Fujii J, Taniguchi N, Vitek MP, Founds H, Atwood CS, Perry G, Smith MA. (2001). Active glycation in neurofibrillary pathology of Alzheimer disease: N(epsilon)-(carboxymethyl) lysine and hexitol-lysine. Free Radic Biol Med, Jul 15;31(2):175-80.

Chan A, Paskavitz J, Remington R et al. (2008). Efficacy of a vitamin/nutraceutical formulation for early stage Alzheimer's disease: a 1 year, open-label pilot study with a 16-month caregiver extension. *Am J Alzheimer Dis Other Demen*, 23:571-585.

Chen X, Walker DG, Schmidt AM, Arancio O, Lue LF, Yan SD. (2007). RAGE: a potential target for Abeta-mediated cellular perturbation in Alzheimer's disease. Curr Mol Med, Dec;7(8):735-42.

Chiu CC, Su KP, Cheng TC et al. (2008). The effects of omega-3 fatty acids monotherapy in Alzheimer's disease and mild cognitive impairment: a preliminary randomised double-blind placebo controlled study. *Prog Neuropsychopharmacol Biol Psychiatry*, 32:1538-1544.

Cheng KC, Cahill DS, Kasai H, Nishimura S, Loeb LA. (1992). 8-Hydroxyguanine, an abundant form of oxidative DNA damage, causes G----T and A----C substitutions. *J Biol Chem*, Jan 5;267(1):166-72.

Choi J, Malakowsky CA, Talent JM, Conrad CC, Gracy RW. (2002). Identification of oxidized plasma proteins in Alzheimer's disease. *Biochem Biophys Res Commun*, May 24;293(5):1566-70.

Cole GM, Teter B, Frautschy SA. (2007). Neuroprotective effects of curcumin. *Adv Exp Med Biol*, 595:197-212.

Conquer JA, Tierney MC, Zecevic J et al. (2000). Fatty acid analyisis of blood plasma of patients with Alzheimer's disease, other types of dementia, and cognitive impairment. *Lipids*, 35(12):1305-1312.

Cooke MS, Olinski R, Loft S. (2008). European Standards Committee on Urinary (DNA) Lesion Analysis. Measurement and meaning of oxidatively modified DNA lesions in urine. *Cancer Epidemiol Biomarkers Prev*, Jan;17(1):3-14.

Cracowski JL, Durand T, Bessard G. (2002). Isoprostanes as a biomarker of lipid peroxidation in humans: physiology, pharmacology and clinical implications. *Trends Pharmacol Sci*, Aug;23(8):360-6.

CTdotgovdimebon ClinicalTrials.gov study NCT00675623, a safety and efficacy study of oral dimebon in patients with mild-to-moderate Alzheimer's disease (CONNECTION)

Dalle-Donne I, Rossi R, Colombo R, Giustarini D, Milzani A. (2006a). Biomarkers of oxidative damage in human disease. Clin Chem, Apr;52(4):601-23.

Dalle-Donne I, Aldini G, Carini M, Colombo R, Rossi R, Milzani A. (2006b). Protein carbonylation, cellular dysfunction, and disease progression. J Cell Mol Med, Apr-Jun;10(2):389-406.

Davidsson P, Paulson L, Hesse C, Blennow K, Nilsson CL. (2001). Proteome studies of human cerebrospinal fluid and brain tissue using a preparative two-dimensional electrophoresis approach prior to mass spectrometry. *Proteomics*, Mar;1(3):444-52.

Defeudis FV (2002). Bilobalide and neuroprotection. *Pharmacol Res* 46: 565-568.

DeKosky ST, Williamson JD, Fitzpatrick AL et al (2008) Gingko biloba for prevention of dementia: a randomised controlled trial. *JAMA*, 300:2253-2262.

Dodge HH, Zitzelberger T, Oken BS et al. (2008). A randomised placebo-controlled trial of Gingko biloba for the prevention of cognitive decline. *Neurology*, 70:1809-1817.

Doody RS. (2009). Dimebon as a potential therapy for Alzheimer's disease. *CNS Spectrosc*, 14:14-16;discussion 16-18

Doody RS, Gavrilova SI, Sano M et al. (2008). Effect of dimebon on cognition, activities of daily living, behaviour, and global function in patients with mild-to-moderate Alzheimer's disease: a randomised, double-blind, placebo-controlled study. *Lancet* 372:207-215

Epis R, Marcello E, Gardoni F et al. (2008). Modulatory effect of acetyl-L-carnitine on amyloid precursor protein metabolism in hippocampal neurons. *Eur J Pharmacol* 597:51-56

Eckl PM, Ortner A, Esterbauer H. (1993). Genotoxic properties of 4-hydroxyalkenals and analogous aldehydes. *Mutat Res*. Dec;290(2):183-92.

Esterbauer H, Schaur RJ, Zollner H. (1991). Chemistry and biochemistry of 4-hydroxynonenal, malonaldehyde and related aldehydes. *Free Radic Biol M*ed. 11(1):81-128.

Evans MD, Olinski R, Loft S, Cooke MS. (2010). Toward consensus in the analysis of urinary 8-oxo-7,8-dihydro-2'-deoxyguanosine as a noninvasive biomarker of oxidative stress. European Standards Committee on Urinary (DNA) Lesion Analysis, *FASEB J*. Apr;24(4):1249-60.

Freund-Levi Y, Eriksdotter-Jönhagen M, Cederholm T et al. (2006). Omega-3 fatty acids treatment in 174 patients with mild to moderate Alzheimer disease: OmegAD study: a randomised, double-blind trial. *Arch Neurol*, 63(10):1402-1408.

Freund-Levi Y, Hjorth E, Lindberg C et al. (2009). Effects of omega-3 fatty acids on inflammatory markers in cerebrospinal fluid and plasma in Alzheimer's disease: the OmegAD Study. *Dement Geriatr Cogn Disord*, 27:481-490.

Fraga CG, Shigenaga MK, Park JW, Degan P, Ames BN. Oxidative damage to DNA during aging: 8-hydroxy-2'-deoxyguanosine in rat organ DNA and urine. *Proc Natl Acad Sci USA*, 1990 Jun;87(12):4533-7.

Goodman AB. (2006). Retinoid receptors, transporters, and metabolizers as therapeutic targets in late onset Alzheimer disease. *J Cell Physiol*, 209:598-60.

Green C, Picot J, Loveman E et al. (2005). Modelling the cost effectiveness of cholinesterase inhibitors in the management of mild to moderately severe Alzheimer's disease. *Pharmacoeconomics*, 23:1271-1282.

Griffiths HR, Møller L, Bartosz G, Bast A, Bertoni-Freddari C, Collins A, Cooke M, Coolen S, Haenen G, Hoberg AM, Loft S, Lunec J, Olinski R, Parry J, Pompella A, Poulsen H, Verhagen H, Astley SB. (2002). Biomarkers. *Mol Aspects Med*, Feb-Jun;23(1-3):101-208.

Grundman M, Petersen RC, Ferris SH et al. (2004). Mild cognitive impairment can be distinguished from Alzheimer disease and normal aging for clinical trials. *Arch Neurol*, 61:59-66.

Gutzmann H, Khul KP, Hadler D et al. (2002). Safety and efficacy of idebenone versus tacrine in patients with Alzheimer's disease:results of a randomised, double-blind, parallel group multicenter study. *Pharmacopsychiatry*, 35:12-18.

Haase J, Halama P and Horr R. (1996). Effectiveness of brief infusions with Gingko biloba Special Extract EGb 761 in dementia of the vascular and Alzheimer type. *Z Gerontol Geriatr*,29:302-309.

Haenen GR & Bast A. (1991). Scavenging of hypochlorus acid by lipoic acid. *Biochem Pharmacol*, 42:2244-2246.

Hamilton ML, Van Remmen H, Drake JA, Yang H, Guo ZM, Kewitt K, Walter CA, Richardson A. (2001). Does oxidative damage to DNA increase with age? *Proc Natl Acad Sci USA*, Aug 28;98(18):10469-74.

Harman D. (1956). Aging: a theory based on free radical and radiation chemistry. *J Gerontol*, Jul;11(3):298-300.

Harman D. (1972). The biologic clock: the mitochondria?. *J Am Geriatr Soc*, Apr;20(4):145-7.

Hu P, Brestky P, Crimmins EM. (2006). Association between serum beta-carotene levels and decline of cognitive function in high functioning older persons with or without apolipoprotein E 4 alleles: MacArthur studies of successful aging. *J Gerontol A Biol Sci Med Sci*, 61:616-620.

Jiménez-Jiménez FJ, de Bustos F, Molina JA et al. (1997). Cerebrospinal fluid levels of alpha-tocopherol (vitamin E) in Alzheimer's disease. *J Neural Transm*, 104:703-710.

Karuppagounder SS, Pinto JT, Xu H et al. (2009). Dietary supplementation with resveratrol reduces plaque pathology in a transgenic model of Alzheimer's disease. *Neurochem Int*, 54:111-118.

Kim KM, Jung BH, Paeng KJ, Kim I, Chung BC. (2004). Increased urinary F(2)-isoprostanes levels in the patients with Alzheimer's disease. *Brain Res Bull*, Jul 30;64(1):47-51.

Kimura T, Takamatsu J, Ikeda K, Kondo A, Miyakawa T, Horiuchi S. (1996). Accumulation of advanced glycation end products of the Maillard reaction with age in human hippocampal neurons. *Neurosci Lett*, Apr 12;208(1):53-6.

Kitani KA et al. (2000). Common properties for propargylamines of enhancing superoxide dismutase and catalase acivities in the dopaminergic system in the rat: implications for the life prolonging effect of (-)deprenyl. *J Neural Transm*, 60 (Suppl) 139-156.

Korolainen MA, Nyman TA, Nyyssönen P, Hartikainen ES, Pirttilä T. (2007). Multiplexed proteomic analysis of oxidation and concentrations of cerebrospinal fluid proteins in Alzheimer disease. *Clin Chem*, Apr;53(4):657-65.

Korolainen MA, Goldsteins G, Nyman TA, Alafuzoff I, Koistinaho J, Pirttilä T. (2006). Oxidative modification of proteins in the frontal cortex of Alzheimer's disease brain. *Neurobiol Aging*, Jan;27(1):42-53.

Kozekov ID, Nechev LV, Moseley MS, Harris CM, Rizzo CJ, Stone MP, Harris TM. (2003). DNA interchain cross-links formed by acrolein and crotonaldehyde. *J Am Chem Soc*, Jan 8;125(1):50-61.

Kroger E, Verreault R, Carmicael PH et al. (2009). Omega-3 fatty acids and risk of dementia: the Canadian Study of Health and Aging. *Am J Clin Nutr*, 90(1):184-192.

Laurin D, Verreault R, Lindsay J et al. (2003). Omega-3 fatty acids and risk of cognitive impairment and dementia. *J Alzheimers Dis* 5(4):315-322.

Ledesma MD, Pérez M, Colaco C et al (1998) Tau glycation is involved in aggregation of the protein but not in the formation of filaments. *Cell Moll Biol* Nov 44(7):1111-1116.

Liu X, Lovell MA, Lynn BC. (2006). Detection and quantification of endogenous cyclic DNA adducts derived from trans-4-hydroxy-2-nonenal in human brain tissue by isotope dilution capillary liquid chromatography nanoelectrospray tandem mass spectrometry. *Chem Res Toxicol*, May;19(5):710-8.

Le Bars PL, Kieser M and Itil KZ. (2000). A 26-week analysis of a double-blind, placebo-controlled trial of the gingko biloba extract EGb 761 in dementia. *Dement Geriatr Cogn Disord*, 11:230-237.

Le Bars PL. (2003). Response patterns of EGb 761 in Alzhemier's disease: influence of neuropsychological profiles. *Pharmacopsychiatry*, 36 (Suppl 1) S50-S55.

Loske C, Gerdemann A, Schepl W, Wycislo M, Schinzel R, Palm D, Riederer P, Münch G. (2000). Transition metal-mediated glycoxidation accelerates cross-linking of beta-amyloid peptide. Eur J Biochem, Jul;267(13):4171-8.

Lovell MA, Ehmann WD, Mattson MP, Markesbery WR. (1997). Elevated 4-hydroxynonenal in ventricular fluid in Alzheimer's disease. *Neurobiol Aging*, Sep-Oct;18(5):457-61.

Lovell MA, Markesbery WR. (2007a). Oxidative damage in mild cognitive impairment and early Alzheimer's disease. *J Neurosci Res*, Nov 1;85(14):3036-40.

Lovell MA, Markesbery WR. (2007b). Oxidative DNA damage in mild cognitive impairment and late-stage Alzheimer's disease. *Nucleic Acids Res*, 35(22):7497-504.

Lovell MA, Markesbery WR. (2001). Ratio of 8-hydroxyguanine in intact DNA to free 8-hydroxyguanine is increased in Alzheimer disease ventricular cerebrospinal fluid. *Arch Neurol*, Mar;58(3):392-6.

Loy C & Schneider L. (2004). Galantamine for Alzheimer's disease. *Cochrane Database Syst Rev*, (4)CD001747.

Luchsinger JA, Tang MX, Shea S et al. (2003). Antioxidant vitamine intake and risk of Alzheimer disease. *Arch Neurol*, 60:203-208.

Luo Y, Smith JV, Paramasivam V et al. (2002). Inhibition of amyloid beta aggregation and caspase-3 activation by the Gingko biloba extract EGb 761. *Proc Natl Acad Sci USA*, 99-12197-12202.

Mandel SA, Amit T, Kalfon L. (2008). Cell signaling pathways and iron chelation in the neurorestorative activity of green tea polyphenols: special reference to epigallocatechin gallate (EGCG). *J Alzheimer Dis*, 17:681-697.

Mangialasche F, Solomon A, Winblad B et al. (2010). Alzheimer's disease: clinical trials and drug development. *Lancet Neurol* 9:702-716.

Markesbery WR, Lovell MA. (1998). Four-hydroxynonenal, a product of lipid peroxidation, is increased in the brain in Alzheimer's disease. *Neurobiol Aging*, Jan-Feb;19(1):33-6.

Markesbery WR, Carney JM. (1999). Oxidative alterations in Alzheimer's disease. *Brain Pathol*, Jan;9(1):133 46.

Mayurama W, Akao Y, Youdim MB et al. (2000). Transfection-enforced Bcl-2 overexpression and an anti-Parkinson drug, rasagiline, prevent nuclear accumulation of GAPDH induced by an endogenous dopaminergic neurotoxin, N-methyl(R)salsolinol. *J Neurochem*, 78:727-735.

McGrath LT, McGleenon BM, Brennan S, McColl D, McILroy S, Passmore AP. (2001). Increased oxidative stress in Alzheimer's disease as assessed with 4-hydroxynonenal but not malondialdehyde. *QJM*, Sep;94(9):485-90.

McIlroy SP, Dynan KB, Lawson JT et al. (2002). Moderately elevated plasma homocysteine, methylenetetrahydrofolate reductase genotype, and risk for stroke, vascular dementia and Alzheimer disease in Northern Ireland. *Stroke*, 33:2351-2356

Mecocci P, Polidori MC, Cherubini A, Ingegni T, Mattioli P, Catani M, Rinaldi P, Cecchetti R, Stahl W, Senin U, Beal MF. (2002). Lymphocyte oxidative DNA damage and plasma antioxidants in Alzheimer disease. *Arch Neurol*, May;59(5):794-8.

Migliore L, Fontana I, Trippi F, Colognato R, Coppedè F, Tognoni G, Nucciarone B, Siciliano G. (2005). Oxidative DNA damage in peripheral leukocytes of mild cognitive impairment and AD patients. *Neurobiol Aging*, May; 26(5):567-73.

Mishra S & Palanivelu K. (2008). The effect of curcumin (turmeric) on Alzheimer's disease: an overwiew. *Ann Indian Acad Neurol*, 11:13-19.

Montgomery SA, Thal LJ & Amrein R. (2003). Meta-analysis of double-blind randomised controlled clinical trials of acetyl-L-carnitine versus placebo in the treatment of mild conginitive impairment and mild Alzheimer's disease. *Int Clin Psychopharmacol*, 18:61-71.

Montine KS, Kim PJ, Olson SJ, Markesbery WR, Montine TJ. (1997). 4-hydroxy-2-nonenal pyrrole adducts in human neurodegenerative disease. *J Neuropathol Exp Neurol*, 56(8): 866-71.

Montine TJ, Markesbery WR, Morrow JD, Roberts LJ 2nd. (1998). Cerebrospinal fluid F2-isoprostane levels are increased in Alzheimer's disease. *Ann Neurol*, Sep;44(3):410-3.

Montine TJ, Quinn JF, Milatovic D, Silbert LC, Dang T, Sanchez S, Terry E, Roberts LJ 2nd, Kaye JA, Morrow JD. Peripheral F2-isoprostanes and F4-neuroprostanes are not increased in Alzheimer's disease. *Ann Neurol*, 2002 Aug;52(2):175-9.

Montine TJ, Peskind ER, Quinn JF, Wilson AM, Montine KS, Galasko D. Increased Cerebrospinal Fluid F(2)-Isoprostanes are Associated with Aging and Latent Alzheimer's Disease as Identified by Biomarkers. *Neuromolecular Med*, 2011 Mar;13(1):37-43.

Montuschi P, Barnes PJ, Roberts LJ 2nd. Isoprostanes: markers and mediators of oxidative stress. *FASEB J*, 2004 Dec; 18(15):1791-800.

Morris MC, Beckett LA, Scherr PA et al (1998) Vitamin E and vitamin C supplement use and risk of incident Alzheimer disease. *Alzheimer Dis assoc Disord*,12:121-126.

Morris MC, Evans DA, Bienias JL et al (2002) Dietary intake of antioxidant nutrients and the risk of incident Alzheimer disease in a biracial community study. *J Am Med Assoc*, 287:3230-3237.

Morris MC, Evans DA, Bienias JL et al (2003). Consumption of fish and n-3 fatty acids and risk of incident Alzheimer disease. *Arch Neurol*, 60(7):940-946.

Morris MC, Evans DA, Tagney CC (2005) Relation of the tocopherol forms to incident Alzheiemr disese and to cognitive change. *Am J Clin Nutr*, 81:508-514.

Morris MC, Evans DA, Tagney CC et al. (2005). Fish consumption and cognitive decline with age in a large community study. *Arch Neurol*, 62(12):1849-1853.

Morris MS, Jacques PF, Rosenberg IH et al. (2007). Folate and vitamine B12 status in relation to anemia, macrocytosis and cognitive impairment in older Americans in the age of folic acid fortification. *Am J Clin Nutr*, 85:193-200.

Morrow JD, Tapper AR, Zackert WE, Yang J, Sanchez SC, Montine TJ, Roberts LJ. (1999). Formation of novel isoprostane-like compounds from docosahexaenoic acid. *Adv Exp Med Biol*, 469:343-7.

Napryeyenko O, Sonnik G, Tartakovsky I. (2009). Efficacy and tolerability of gingko biloba extract EGb 761 by type of dementia: analyses of a randomised controlled trial. *J Neurol Sci*, 283:224-229.

Nunomura A, Perry G, Aliev G, Hirai K, Takeda A, Balraj EK, Jones PK, Ghanbari H, Wataya T, Shimohama S, Chiba S, Atwood CS, Petersen RB, Smith MA. (2001). Oxidative damage is the earliest event in Alzheimer disease. *J Neuropathol Exp Neurol*, Aug;60(8):759-67.

Oken BS, Storzbach DM, Kaye JA. (1998). The efficacy og Gingko biloba on cognitive function in Alzheimer's disease. *Arch Neurol*, 55:1409-1415.

Okun I, Tkachenko SE, Khvat A et al. (2010). From anti-allergic to anti-Alzheimer's: molecular pharmacology of dimebon. *Curr Alzheimer Res*, 7:97-112.

Olinski R, Siomek A, Rozalski R, Gackowski D, Foksinski M, Guz J, Dziaman T, Szpila A, Tudek B. (2007). Oxidative damage to DNA and antioxidant status in aging and age-related diseases. *Acta Biochim Pol*, 54(1):11-26.

Perry G, Raina AK, Nunomura A, Wataya T, Sayre LM, Smith MA. (2000). How important is oxidative damage? Lessons from Alzheimer's disease. *Free Radic Biol Med*, Mar 1;28(5):831-4.

Perry G, Nunomura A, Cash AD, Taddeo MA, Hirai K, Aliev G, Avila J, Wataya T, Shimohama S, Atwood CS, Smith MA. (2002). *Reactive oxygen: its sources and significance in Alzheimer disease. J Neural Transm Suppl*, (62):69-75.

Petersen RC, Thomas RG, Grudman N et al. (2005). Vitamin E and donepezil for the treatment of mild cognitive impairment. *N Engl J Med* 352:2379-2388,

Pettergrew JW, Klunk WE, Panchalingam K et al, (1995). Clinical and neurochemical effects of acetyl-L-carnitine in Alzheimer's disease. *Neurobiol Aging*, 16:1-4,

Praticò D, Clark CM, Liun F, Rokach J, Lee VY, Troianowski JQ. (2002). Increase of brain oxidative stress in mild cognitive impairment: a possible predictor of Alzheimer disease. *Arch Neurol*, Jun:59(6): 972-6.

Puchades M, Hansson SF, Nilsson CL, Andreasen N, Blennow K, Davidsson P. (2003). Proteomic studies of potential cerebrospinal fluid protein markers for Alzheimer's disease. *Brain Res Mol Brain Res*, Oct 21;118(1-2):140-6.

Quinn JF, Raman R, Thomas RG et al. (2009). A clinical trial of docohexanoic acid (DHA) for the treatment of Alzheimer's disease. *Alzheimers Assoc Int Conf Alzheimer Dis*; July 12.

Riederer P, Danielczyk W, Grünblatt E. (2004). Monoamine oxidase-B inhibition in Alzheimer's disease. *Neurotoxicology*, 25 (1-2):271-277.

Roberts LJ 2nd, Montine TJ, Markesbery WR, Tapper AR, Hardy P, Chemtob S, Dettbarn WD, Morrow JD. (1998). Formation of isoprostane-like compounds (neuroprostanes) in vivo from docosahexaenoic acid. *J Biol Chem*, May 29;273(22):13605-12.

Sahin M, Karauzum SB, Perry G et al. (2005). Retinoic acid isomers protect hippocampal neurons from amyloid-beta induced neurodegeneration. *Neurotox Res*, 7:243-250.

Sano M, Ernesto C, Thomas RG et al. (1997). A controlled trial of selegiline, alpha tocopherol, or both as treatment for Alzheimer's disease. The Alzheimer's disease cooperative study. *N Engl J Med*, 336:1216-1222.

Sanz E, Romera M, Bellik L et al. (2004). Indolalkylamines derivatives as antioxidant and neuroprotective agents in an experimental model of Parkinson's disease. *Med Sci Monit*, 10(12):BR477-484.

Sayre LM, Zelasko DA, Harris PL, Perry G, Salomon RG, Smith MA. (1997). 4-Hydroxynonenal-derived advanced lipid peroxidation end products are increased in Alzheimer's disease. *J Neurochem*, May;68(5):2092-7.

Schneider LS, DeKosky ST, Farlow MR et al. (2005). A randomised, double-bind, placebo controlled trial of two doses of Gongko biloba extract in dementa of the Alzhemier's type. *Curr Alzheimer Res*, 2 541-551.

Senin U, Parnetti L, Barbagallo-Sangiorgi G et al. (1992). Idebenone in senile dementia of Alzheimer type:a multicenter study. *Arch Gerontol Geriatr*, 15:249-260.

Shigenaga MK, Gimeno CJ, Ames BN. (1989). Urinary 8-hydroxy-2'-deoxyguanosine as a biological marker of in vivo oxidative DNA damage. *Proc Natl Acad Sci USA*, Dec;86(24):9697-701.

Shoba G, Joy S, Joseph T et al. (1998). Influence of piperine on the pharmacokinetics of curcumin in animals and human volunteers. *Planta Med*, 64:353-356.

Smith MA, Sayre LM, Monnier VM, Perry G. (1995). Radical AGEing in Alzheimer's disease. Trends Neurosci, Apr;18(4):172-6.

Snitz BE, O'Meara ES, Carlsom MC et al. (2009). Gingko biloba for preventing cognitive decline in older adults: a randomised trial. *JAMA*, 302:2663-2670.

Southern L, Williams J, Esiri MM. (2007). Immunohistochemical study of N-epsilon-carboxymethyl lysine (CML) in human brain: relation to vascular dementia. *BMC Neurol*, Oct 16;7:35.

Sultana R, Butterfield DA. (2011). Identification of the oxidative stress proteome in the brain. *Free Radic Biol Med*, Feb 15;50(4):487-94. Epub 2010 Nov 25.

Tabet N, Birks J, Grimley EF. (2000). Vitamine E for Alhzheimer's disease. *Cochrane database Syst Rev* (4) CD002854.

Tamagno E, Guglielmotto M, Aragno M, Borghi R, Autelli R, Giliberto L, Muraca G, Danni O, Zhu X, Smith MA, Perry G, Jo DG, Mattson MP, Tabaton M. (2008). Oxidative stress activates a positive feedback between the gamma- and beta-secretase cleavages of the beta-amyloid precursor protein. *J Neurochem*, Feb;104(3):683-95.

Thal LJ, Grundman M, Berg J et al. (2003). Idebenone treatment fails to slow cognitive decline in Alzheimer's disease. *Neurology*, 61:1498-1502.

Thal LJ, Calvani M, Amato A et al. (2000). A 1-year controlled trial of acetyl-L-carnitine in early onset AD. *Neurology*, 55:805-810.

Thomas T. (2000). Monoamine oxidase-B inhibitors in the treatment of Alzheimer's disease. *Neurobiol Aging*, 21(2):343-348.

Thome J, Münch G, Muller R, Schinzel R, Kornhuber J, Blum-Degen D et al. (1996). Advanced glycation endproducts-associated parameters in the peripheral blood of patients with Alzheimer's disease. *Neurotox Res*, 4:191-209.

Tucker JM & Townsend DM. (2005). Alpha-tocopherol: roles in prevention and therapy of human disease. *Biomed Pharmacother*, 59 (7):380-387.

Tully AM, Roche HM, Doyle R et al. (2003). Low serum cholesteryl ester-docohexanoic acid levels in Alzheimer's disease: a case-control study. *Br J Nutr*, 89(4):483-489.

Uchida K. (2003). 4-Hydroxy-2-nonenal: a product and mediator of oxidative stress. *Prog Lipid Res*, Jul;42(4):318-43.

Van Gelder BM, Tijhuis M, Kalmijn S et al. (2007). Fish consumption, n-3 fatty acids, and subsequent 5-y cognitive decline in elderly men: the Zutphen Elderly Study. *Am J Clin Nutr*, 85(4):1142-1147.

Vitek MP, Bhattacharya K, Glendening JM, Stopa E, Vlassara H, Bucala R, Manogue K, Cerami A. (1994). Advanced glycation end products contribute to amyloidosis in Alzheimer disease. *Proc Natl Acad Sci USA*, May 24;91(11):4766-70.

Von Arnim CA, Gola U and Biesalski HK. (2010). More than the sumo f its parts? Nutrition in Alzheimer's disease. *Nutrition*, 26(7-8):694-700.

Wadsworth TL, Bishop JA, PAppu AS et al. (2008). Evaluation of Coenzyme Q as an antioxidant strategy for Alzheimer's disease. *J Alzheimer's Dis*, 14:225-234.

Wataya T, Nunomura A, Smith MA, Siedlak SL, Harris PL, Shimohama S, Szweda LI, Kaminski MA, Avila J, Price DL, Cleveland DW, Sayre LM, Perry G. (2002). High molecular weight neurofilament proteins are physiological substrates of adduction by the lipid peroxidation product hydroxynonenal. *J Biol Chem*, Feb 15;277(7):4644-8.

Weyer G, Babej.Dolle RM, Hadler D et al. (1997). A controlled study of 2 doses of idebenone in the treatment of Alzheimer's disease. *Neuropsychobiology*, 36:73-82.

White AR, Barnham KJ, Huang X et al. (2004). Iron inhibits neurotoxicity induced by trace cooper and biological reductants. *J Biol Inorg Chem*, 9:269-280.

Williams TI, Lynn BC, Markesbery WR, Lovell MA. (2006). Increased levels of 4-hydroxynonenal and acrolein, neurotoxic markers of lipid peroxidation, in the brain in Mild Cognitive Impairment and early Alzheimer's disease. *Neurobiol Aging*, Aug;27(8):1094-9.

Yao Z & Drieu V. (2001). Papadopoulos, the Gingko biloba extract Egb 761 rescues the PC12 neuronal cells from beta-amyloid-induced cell death by inhibiting the formation of beta-amyloid-derived diffusible neurotoxic ligands. *Brain Res*, 889:181-190.

Yan SD, Chen X, Schmidt AM, Brett J, Godman G, Zou YS, Scott CW, Caputo C, Frappier T, Smith MA, et al. (1994). Glycated tau protein in Alzheimer disease: a mechanism for induction of oxidant stress. Proc Natl Acad Sci USA, Aug 2;91(16):7787-91.

Youdim BM, Fridkin M and Zheng H. (2005). Bifunctional drug derivates of MAO-B inhibitor rasagiline and iron chelator VK28 as a more effective approach to treatment of brain aging and aging neurodegenerative diseases. *Mech Aging Dev*, 126: 317-326.

Yu HL, Chertkow HM, Bergman H, Schipper HM. (2003). Aberrant profiles of native and oxidized glycoproteins in Alzheimer plasma. *Proteomics*, Nov;3(11):2240-8.

Yurko-Mauro K, McCarthy D, Bailey-Hall E et al. (2009). Results of the MIDAS trial: effects of docohexanoic acid on physiological and safety parameters in age-related cognitive decline. *Alzheimers Assoc Int Conf Alzheimer Dis*; July 12.

16

Impact of Oxidative - Nitrosative Stress on Cholinergic Presynaptic Function

Stefanie A.G. Black and R. Jane Rylett
Molecular Brain Research Group, Robarts Research Institute,
Schulich School of Medicine & Dentistry,
University of Western Ontario, London, ON
Canada

1. Introduction

Cholinergic neurotransmission plays an essential role in a variety of physiological processes in both the central and peripheral nervous systems. Cholinergic neurons use the classical neurotransmitter acetylcholine (ACh) to communicate with their target cells. In the periphery, ACh is the neurotransmitter used at the skeletal neuromuscular junction, at all pre- and postganglionic parasympathetic synapses and at preganglionic sympathetic synapses. In the central nervous system, the actions of ACh are widespread with cholinergic neurotransmission involved in attention, learning and memory, cognition, sleep, wakefulness, and modulation of sensory information (Hasselmo, 2006; Sarter & Parihk, 2005; Woolf & Butcher, 2010). Dysfunction of cholinergic neurotransmission in the central nervous system is apparent in a number of neurological disorders, such as Alzheimer's, Parkinson's, and Huntington's diseases, schizophrenia and amyotrophic lateral sclerosis (Bohnen & Albin, 2010; Mesulam, 2004; Oda, 1999).

Cholinergic neurons innervate almost all areas of the brain, where this can be mediated by either intrinsic interneurons or by extrinsic projection neurons. Cholinergic interneurons localized in the striatum are involved in motor function, cognition, and behavior (Woolf & Butcher, 2010). The basal forebrain, which is comprised of the nucleus basalis of Meynert, medial septum, diagonal band of Broca, the magnocellular preoptic nucleus, and substantia innominata, contains the cell bodies of cholinergic neurons that project to the hippocampus, amygdala, olfactory bulb, and all areas of the cerebral cortex (Woolf & Butcher, 2010). Collectively, basal forebrain cholinergic neuron activity plays a role in attention, learning, memory, perception, and consciousness (Sarter et al., 2003; Woolf, 1998; Woolf & Butcher, 2010). Cholinergic neurons in the mesopontine region (the pedunculopontine and laterodorsal nuclei) project to the thalamus, hypothalamus, basal forebrain, medial frontal cortex, brainstem and spinal cord (Woolf & Butcher, 2010). Descending cholinergic projections from the mesopontine area decrease muscle tone during rapid eye movement sleep while ascending cholinergic projections are involved in cognitive functions and consciousness (Woolf & Butcher, 2010). Cholinergic projections to the interpeduncular nucleus originate from neurons with cell bodies in the medial habenula; these neurons regulate electroencephalogram patterns and rapid eye movement sleep (Woolf & Butcher, 2010).

The cycle of ACh synthesis, storage, release and degradation has been well-characterized at the cellular and molecular levels and is depicted in Figure 1. ACh is synthesized in the cytoplasm of cholinergic neurons from the precursors choline and acetylCoenzyme-A by the enzyme choline acetyltransferase (ChAT), and it is then taken up into synaptic vesicles for storage by the vesicular acetylcholine transporter (VAChT) (Prado et al., 2002). Depolarization of the nerve terminal causes exocytotic fusion of synaptic vesicles with the presynaptic membrane at specialized release sites called active zones (Garner et al., 2000); this is a calcium-dependent process that involves the coordinated actions of many presynaptic proteins such as SNARE and Rab proteins (Sudhof, 2008). When vesicles fuse with the presynaptic membrane, ACh diffuses into the synaptic cleft where it can bind to nicotinic and muscarinic receptors located on both pre- and postsynaptic cells (Gotti et al., 2009; Nathanson, 2008). ACh signalling is terminated by its diffusion away from the synaptic cleft and by its rapid hydrolysis into choline and acetate by acetylcholinesterase (AChE) (Lane et al., 2006). After fusion, synaptic vesicles recycle (S.M. Smith et al., 2008) and are re-filled with neurotransmitter in preparation for another round of depolarization-induced release. The choline derived from ACh hydrolysis is recycled into the presynaptic terminal by the sodium-dependent, high-affinity choline transporter CHT for re-synthesis of ACh (Birks & MacIntosh, 1961; Collier & MacIntosh, 1969; Collier & Katz, 1974; Haga, 1971; Okuda et al., 2000; Yamamura & Snyder, 1972). Mechanistic details of the molecular regulation of these processes in both health and disease are lacking.

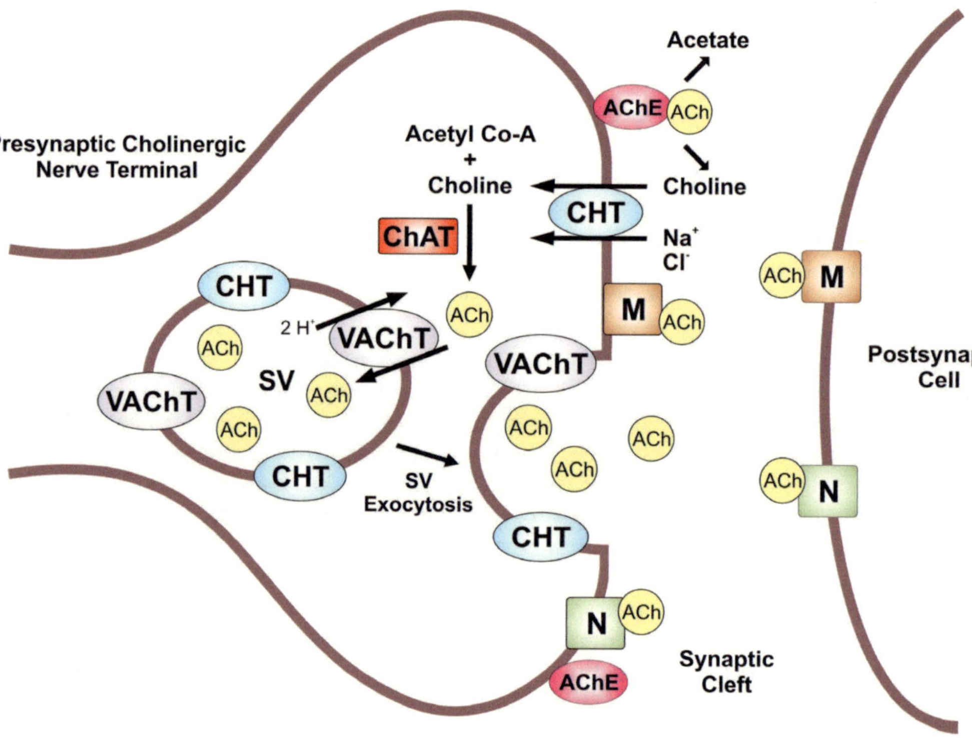

Fig. 1. Mechanisms involved in the synthesis, storage, release and degradation of ACh at the cholinergic synapse. Abbreviations: Acetyl Co-A, acetylCoenzyme-A; ACh, acetylcholine; AChE, acetylcholinesterase; ChAT, choline acetyltransferase; CHT, sodium-dependent, high-affinity choline transporter; M, muscarinic receptor; N, nicotinic receptor; SV, synaptic vesicle; VAChT, vesicular ACh transporter.

Age-related changes in brain that lead to neuronal and vascular pathology frequently compromise synaptic transmission. Many reports associate neurological and cardiovascular diseases with cholinergic neuron dysfunction, and draw parallels between the reduction in cholinergic neurotransmission and cognitive deficits. However, little is known about the actual mechanisms by which these changes impact cholinergic neuron function or the extent to which this can be prevented or reversed. Some of these changes are initiated by oxidative and nitrosative stress which then increases as the pathology progresses. There is also a relationship with altered amyloid precursor protein (APP) metabolism and β-amyloid peptide (Aβ) production that is likely due to changes in the expression or activity of enzymes directing APP into an amyloidogenic pathway. Modified APP/Aβ metabolism is a hallmark of Alzheimer's disease, but is also a result of cardiovascular disease including ischemia (Bennett et al., 2000; Lee et al., 2006; Nihashi et al., 2001; Shi et al., 2000), stroke (Petcu et al., 2008) and hypertension (Gentile et al., 2009; Skoog et al., 1996; Skoog et al., 2006). Age-related increases in soluble oligomeric Aβ acutely modulate synaptic communication at concentrations far below those causing neurodegeneration, and play a central role in Alzheimer's-related synaptic changes (Marcello et al., 2008). The tissue stress response and the generation of reactive oxygen (ROS) and nitrogen species (RNS) in aging brain and early stages of vascular and neuronal disease are attributed partly to increasing Aβ (De Felice et al., 2007). Increased ROS-RNS can initiate changes that result in both reversible and irreversible alterations in protein structure and function. This Chapter focuses on studies of ChAT and CHT structure and function in conditions with altered exposure to ROS-RNS, and the consequences for cholinergic neuron communication related to Alzheimer's disease pathology and potential outcomes related to neuroprotection.

2. Cholinergic neuron function in aging brain

A large literature addresses the role of cholinergic neurons in cognition and attentional processes, and their involvement in Alzheimer's disease (Sarter & Bruno, 1997; Sarter & Bruno, 2004; Schliebs & Arendt, 2006). The current opinion is that while dysfunction of cholinergic neurons is not the cause of this disease, loss of their function is central to changes that occur in brain with normal aging and in a spectrum of disorders that includes mild cognitive impairment (MCI) (Mesulam, 2004). Studies in aging humans and animal models show that some cholinergic pathways have diminished function compared to younger groups. Cognitive decline correlates with elevated oxidative stress in a cohort of normal aging human subjects (Foster, 2006). Also, in aging rats, spatial learning deficits are associated with elevated markers of oxidative stress (Nicolle et al., 2001). However, the small loss of forebrain cholinergic neurons does not relate strongly to cognitive status (McKinney & Jacksonville, 2005) providing compelling evidence that other dynamic cholinergic processes must be affected that are not detected simply by counting the number of neurons.

A comparison of two cholinergic pathways in aged rat brain suggests that neurons in different brain areas can respond differentially to age-related stressors. Basal forebrain cholinergic neurons lose the activity or expression of essential proteins that maintain chemical transmission and their numbers are reduced, whereas brainstem cholinergic neurons in the pontine nuclei are preserved (Baskerville et al., 2006). This is reinforced by the observation that cultured pontine neurons are resistant to ROS-RNS whereas basal forebrain cholinergic neurons are vulnerable (Fass et al., 2000; McKinney et al., 2004). The reasons for this are not known, but age-related oxidative stress in the cortex (Nicolle et al.,

2001) may elevate basal forebrain neuron metabolism. Oxidatively-stressed aged cortex is less responsive to ACh and may compensate for this by requiring enhanced input from basal forebrain neurons thereby causing increased neuron firing rates and/or changes such as increased expression of genes that are involved in energy production (Baskerville et al., 2008; Ongwijitwat et al., 2006; Yang et al., 2006). Alternatively, up-regulation of expression of metabolic genes may be normal and an "adaptive" consequence of aging in basal forebrain neurons that precedes their degeneration (Baskerville et al., 2008). Elevated metabolic activity may also precede increased ROS-RNS levels and, along with pathology such as increased Aβ levels, may mediate their selective vulnerability. It is important to note that basal forebrain cholinergic neurons project to regions with Aβ deposits, whereas pontine cholinergic neurons do not.

A shift in thinking about the timing and nature of changes in cholinergic neuron function in aging and disease came about with reports that ChAT activity is unchanged or even increased in the hippocampus and cortex of subjects with MCI (DeKosky et al., 2002; Ikonomovic et al., 2003; Mufson et al., 2003). This is in sharp contrast to reports of large decreases in cholinergic neuron markers and numbers in Alzheimer's disease (Davies, 1979; Francis et al., 1985; Perry et al., 1977; Rylett et al., 1982; Sims et al., 1983). Mechanisms underlying this apparent increase in cholinergic neuron function are unknown, but it was suggested that basal forebrain cholinergic neurons undergo sprouting in an attempt to maintain neurotransmission or to repair entorhinal cortex damage (Ikonomovic et al., 2003). This has stimulated studies on the functional status of cholinergic neurons in MCI and early Alzheimer's disease; a pivotal study used pharmacological-functional magnetic resonance imaging (fMRI) to document that cholinergic neurotransmission is compromised (Goekoop et al., 2006). It is important to note that most of the studies reported to date have monitored postsynaptic events for insight into the status of cholinergic neurotransmission and to reveal alterations that would result in decreased cholinergic synaptic function and neuron responsiveness in MCI and Alzheimer's disease (Grön et al., 2006). There is a large gap in knowledge about the effects that perturbations such as ROS-RNS, Aβ or altered antioxidant defense mechanisms have on cholinergic presynaptic functions, and the role that this has in compromised neurotransmission. Moreover, most studies have assayed static measures such as neuron numbers or enzyme levels that do not accurately reflect the more dynamic aspects of neurotransmission (Mesulam, 2004), and this may give an incorrect assessment as they do not reveal changes in the capacity for neurotransmitter synthesis and release.

3. Cholinergic neurons have a role in regulation of APP metabolism

A critical link has emerged between cholinergic neurons and APP processing. These neurons are particularly susceptible to the adverse effects of Aβ, and this may partially underlie their vulnerability in amyloidogenic diseases (Auld et al., 1998; Tran el al., 2002). Of note however, cholinergic neurons are also integral in the development of amyloid-based pathology (Auld et al., 1998; Francis et al., 1999; Tran et al., 2002) as they can regulate APP processing and, in turn, Aβ can decrease ACh synthesis and release (Heinitz et al., 2006; Hoshi et al., 1996, 1997; Kar et al., 1996, 1998; Pederson et al., 1996; Pederson & Blusztajn, 1997; Satoh et al., 2001). The stimulation of either nicotinic or muscarinic ACh receptors on cholinoreceptive neurons can promote non-amyloidogenic APP cleavage, thereby potentially decreasing the production of toxic Aβ (Isacson et al., 2002; Seo et al., 2001; Tran et al., 2002; Unger et al., 2005; Verhoeff, 2005). Thus, the activation of either α7- or α4β2-nicotinic receptors (Lahiri et al., 2002; Shimohama & Kihara, 2001; Zamani & Allen, 2001) can decrease Aβ toxicity by protecting neurons through activation of PI3-kinase and increasing levels of Bcl-2 and Bcl-x50. Taken together, the loss of cholinergic neuron innervation may promote Aβ-based pathology, and therapies that would enable cholinergic neurotransmission may indirectly decrease neurodegeneration by reducing Aβ production.

Aβ can assume various physical conformations that may differ in their biological actions. These various Aβ peptides are produced both intracellularly and extracellularly and appear in brain tissue as soluble oligomers and diffusible ligands (Gong et al., 2003; Klein, 2002; Klein et al., 2004) that can aggregate to form insoluble plaques (Kuo et al., 1996; Lue et al., 1999; Walsh et al., 2002a, 2002b; J. Wang et al., 1999). The increased levels of soluble Aβ correlate with synaptic loss and cognitive impairment, and it is now known that synaptic neurotransmission is impacted directly by soluble Aβ with this leading to decreased memory (Klein, 2002). Aβ can bind to a number of different cell surface receptors, modulate synaptic events, lead to generation of ROS-RNS or the release of inflammatory mediators, and disrupt cellular calcium homeostasis (W.W. Smith et al., 2006; Tran et al., 2002). In animal models having chronic delivery of Aβ into rat brain there is increased iNOS expression and disruption of hippocampal cholinergic transmission and memory impairment (Tran et al., 2001).

4. Aβ promotes oxidative stress that can affect neuron function

The inside of cells is normally a reducing environment that maintains proteins in their native reduced states. However, even under these "reducing" conditions some proteins do exist in their *S*-glutathionylated forms (Klatt & Lamas, 2000). Moreover, if ROS-RNS generation exceeds the antioxidant capacity of the cell, then oxidative-nitrosative stress can occur with modification of cellular constituents causing loss of their function. Aβ, particularly the toxic Aβ(1-42), can be involved both directly (Butterfield & Bush, 2004) and indirectly (Lahiri & Greig, 2004) in the generation of ROS-RNS in the brain, thus causing oxidation of lipids and proteins (Qi et al., 2005) and nitration of tyrosine residues in proteins. As it is critical that the oxidative balance inside of the cell is tightly regulated, compensatory mechanisms become upregulated in normal cells that have been exposed to oxidant stress. These adaptive processes are found in the brain, but they can become dysregulated during aging (Mattson & Magnus, 2006) and in pathological states (Mattson, 2004; Zhu et al., 2004). Mitochondria are a source of hydrogen peroxide (H_2O_2), and Aβ in the presence of redox-active ions such as iron and copper can lead to the generation of excess H_2O_2 (Pedersen & Blusztajn, 1997). This ROS may induce cellular damage, particularly by the generation of highly-reactive superoxide radical anion (•$O2^-$) or hydroxyl radical (•OH), the latter being formed in the Fenton reaction in the presence of redox-active iron. However, under some conditions protective mechanisms such as the activation of stress-activated protein kinase (SAPK) pathways are engaged with the induction of downstream antioxidant enzymes (Tamagno et al., 2003). Thus, Aβ alone or in combination with other constituents can lead to the generation of ROS-RNS that can damage macromolecules and result in the modulation of neurotransmission and cause neurotoxicity.

Cholinergic presynaptic function is affected by low levels of Aβ (pM-nM), with the result being decreased pyruvate dehydrogenase activity (Hoshi et al., 1996, 1997), ACh synthesis (Hoshi et al., 1996, 1997; Pederson et al., 1996; Pederson & Blusztajn, 1997) and release (Heinitz et al., 2006; Kar et al., 1996, 1998; Satoh et al., 2001). However, there are conflicting reports on the effects of Aβ on the functions of both ChAT and CHT proteins. Hippocampal ChAT activity is decreased after several days of Aβ administration into rat brain (Nitta et al., 1994, 1997), but this may be due to the loss of neurons rather than to a direct effect on the enzyme. The acute addition of Aβ to neural cells can either reduce ChAT activity (McMillian et al., 1995; Pederson et al., 1996) or have no effect (Hoshi et al., 1996, 1997; Kar et al., 1998); it is difficult to interpret these studies as the Aβ conformation was not determined and it is increasingly clear that the oligomeric, fibrillar or other forms of Aβ have quite different cellular effects. Experiments that involve the use of a variety of model systems indicate that the high-affinity choline uptake activity of CHT can be modulated by Aβ, but the results are also variable. Some reports show that Aβ can actually increase high-affinity choline uptake activity (Bales et al., 2006; Kristofikova et al., 2006), whereas others suggest that Aβ impairs choline uptake (Apelt et al., 2002; Kar et al., 1998; Klingner et al., 2003; Kristofikova et al., 2001, 2008; Opazo et al., 2006; Payette et al., 2007) or that Aβ has no effect on high-affinity uptake of choline (Forgon et al., 1998; Hartmann et al., 2004; Melo et al., 2002). It is known that cholinergic neurochemical function is affected directly by Aβ in a manner that is not related to neuron degeneration, but it is not known to what extent these effects are due to the oxidant stress engaged by increasing Aβ. Unfortunately, for the most part these results are descriptive in nature rather than being mechanistic and do not offer insight into the potential reversibility of the functional changes or information that would be useful for the development of approaches to support cholinergic neuron function.

5. ROS – RNS cause reversible and irreversible modification of proteins

Reactive cysteine (Cys) thiol groups are ionized at physiological pH, and proteins having reactive Cys thiols are found in cells in multiple forms as they are modified by ROS and RNS or form homo- and hetero-protein complexes. Figure 2 shows common modifications that reactive Cys thiols can undergo using ChAT as the model because it is an outstanding example of a protein that has an unusually high number of Cys residues. The modification of reactive Cys thiols during oxidative or nitrosative stress is a key regulator of protein activity (Klatt & Lamas, 2000), and can result in either loss- or gain-of-function (Barrett et al., 1999; Borges et al., 2002; Fukuda et al., 2005; Humphries et al., 2002; Ishii et al., 2005; Jaffrey et al., 2001; Lind et al., 2002; J. Wang et al., 2001). There are cellular mechanisms that protect proteins from irreversible inactivation by oxidation that involve the reversible addition of antioxidant peptides, particularly reduced glutathione (GSH) (Townsend, 2007). The formation of protein-GSH mixed disulphide conjugates can protect vulnerable thiol groups in proteins from further damage during transient oxidative stress (Borges et al., 2002; Jaffreyet al., 2001). A critical point is that protein-GSH mixed disulphide formation is reversible, with the native protein being regenerated as the interior of the cell returns to a more reduced state. However, the more highly oxidized forms of proteins, sulphinic (Pr-SO_2H) and sulphonic (Pr-SO_3H) acids, are not reduced in cells with this leading to irreversible loss-of-function of the target protein. Brain and other tissues can take a double hit during aging by increased ROS–RNS levels and decreased antioxidant mechanisms, with this characterized by a decreased ratio of reduced to oxidized GSH [GSH:GSSG]. This is illustrated in necropsy brain fractions from subjects that were neurologically normal or that had MCI or Alzheimer's disease. The effects of oxidative stress were localized mostly to synaptic regions, with the largest changes seen in presynaptic [synaptosome] fractions as significant decreases in antioxidant levels and increases in markers of oxidative damage (Ansari & Scheff, 2010). These changes occurred early in the disease and the free radical burden increased as an active persistent process in aging and disease (Ansari & Scheff, 2010). Similar findings are seen in aging rodents (Gilmer et al., 2010).

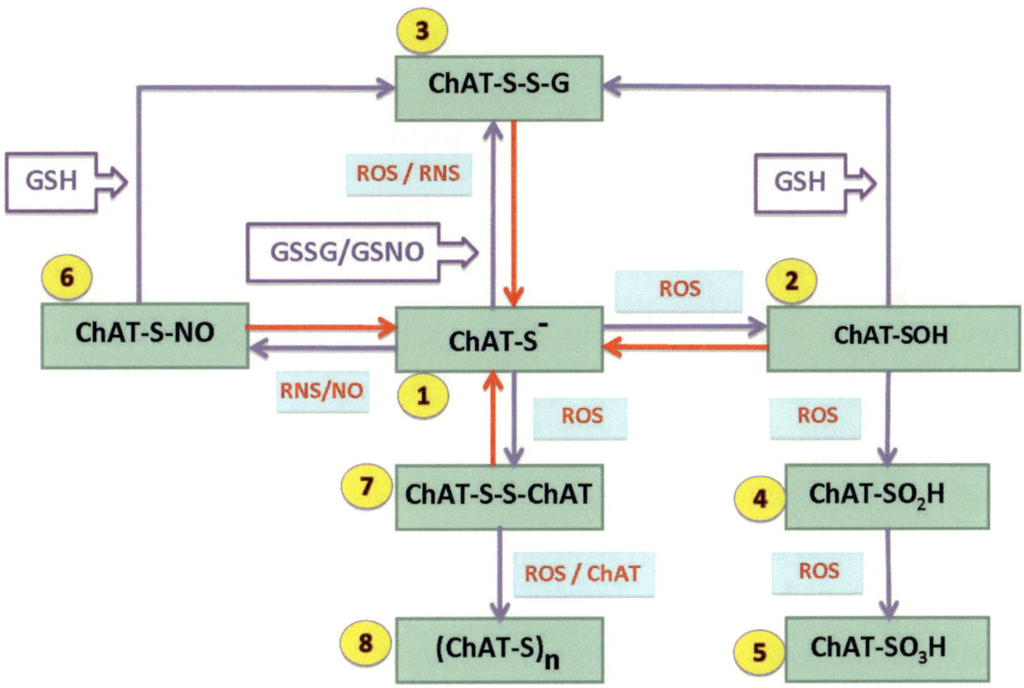

Fig. 2. ROS–RNS can cause reversible and irreversible modification of proteins at reactive cysteine thiol residues. The common modifications that reactive Cys thiols can undergo are shown using ChAT as an example to illustrate that the protein can be found in cells in multiple forms that are modified by ROS and RNS with the potential formation of homo- and hetero-protein complexes. Unmodified ChAT-S$^-$ (1) is oxidized by low levels of H_2O_2 to its sulphenic acid, ChAT-S-OH (2); ChAT-S-OH reacts non-enzymatically with glutathione (GSH) to form ChAT-GSH mixed disulphide, ChAT-S-S-G (3) that protects Cys from further oxidation. ChAT-S-OH (2) is further oxidized by excess ROS to inactive sulphinic ChAT-SO_2H (4) and sulphonic ChAT-SO_3H (5) acids when GSH is depleted. Also, ChAT-S$^-$ (1) can react with NO to form *S*-nitrosylated ChAT, ChAT-S-NO (6) by reaction at reactive Cys thiols. ChAT-S-NO (6) can also react with GSH to give ChAT-S-S-G (3). Alternatively, ChAT-S$^-$ (1) can be converted to ChAT-S-S-G (3) by reaction with *S*-nitrosoglutathione (GSNO). In the absence of GSH, ChAT-S$^-$ (1) can be converted by ROS to intermolecular dimers ChAT-S-S-ChAT (7) or higher-order oligomers (8) that may precipitate from the cytoplasm. [*Adapted from Giustarini et al., 2004*].

6. Effects of oxidative and nitrosative stress alter ChAT activity

It is striking that ChAT contains twenty Cys residues, which is a substantially greater proportion of Cys (3.2%) than is normally found in intracellular proteins (~ 1%). This could make ChAT particularly vulnerable to oxidative-nitrosative stress. Indeed, ChAT activity is decreased by acute exposure of either the purified protein (Guermonprez et al., 2001; Kim et al., 2006; Morris, 1967; Roskoski, 1973) or brain fractions or cells (Liu et al., 1999) to ROS-RNS agents, with some protection being given by the addition of thioreductants (Liu et al., 1999; Morris, 1967). We found that the activity of purified human ChAT is rapidly lost in the absence of reducing agents and that its activity is partially recovered by the addition of fresh reducing agents (Kim et al., 2005). Nitric oxide (NO) donors can also inactivate ChAT with this effect being partially reversed by GSH (Liu et al., 1999). A common site for post-translational modification and redox regulation of proteins is at reactive Cys thiols with this leading to protein *S*-glutathionylation or *S*-nitrosylation. Reactive Cys thiols (Cys-S$^-$) are ionized at physiological pH and are more easily oxidized than are fully-reduced Cys (Cys-SH). ROS-RNS could also cause both reversible and irreversible changes to ChAT resulting in it having altered structure and function. The functional consequences of the oxidation of reactive Cys thiols in ChAT could include regulation or inactivation of catalysis, homo- or hetero-dimerization or oligomerization by disulphide bond formation, altered binding to cellular protein partners, or altered protein stability.

Structural reorganization of a protein can also serve to protect vulnerable reversibly-oxidized Cys residues during acute oxidative stress by the formation of intramolecular disulphide bonds (Cumming & Schubert, 2005). An example of this is seen in protein tyrosine phosphatases where a reactive catalytic Cys residue undergoes reversible oxidation to sulphenic acid, and then participates in the formation of an intramolecular disulphide bond with one of two "backdoor" Cys residues in the catalytic site to protect it from further oxidation to irreversible sulphinic or sulphonic acid species (Chen et al., 2009). The disulphide bond formed is resistant to further oxidation by low levels of ROS and can be re-reduced by GSH. Re-reduction of the catalytic Cys thiolate drives oxidation of the two backdoor Cys causing them to form a disulphide and facilitates regeneration of the active phosphatase. This model is significant with regard to ChAT as there are five Cys residues in its catalytic site, and at least four of these are arranged in a configuration that disulphide bonds may be able to form with only minor changes in side chain torsion angles (Kim et al., 2006).

7. Subcellular trafficking of CHT proteins, an important mode of regulation of high-affinity choline uptake, is altered by nitrosative stress

In many experimental paradigms, high-affinity choline uptake by CHT proteins is the rate-limiting step in the production of ACh, and it is modulated by neuronal activity and dependent upon the sodium electrochemical gradient (Birks & MacIntosh, 1961; Guyenet et al., 1973; Haga, 1971; Simon & Kuhar, 1975; Yamamura & Snyder, 1972). With molecular tools becoming available since the cloning of the CHT gene in the year 2000 (Okuda et al., 2000), the importance of the subcellular trafficking of CHT proteins as a regulatory mechanism for choline uptake, and thus for ACh production, has emerged. CHT proteins are distributed between the plasma membrane and subcellular compartments such as endosomes and synaptic vesicles (Ferguson et al., 2003; Nakata et al., 2004; Ribeiro et al., 2003). It was discovered that CHT proteins are internalized from the plasma membrane to endocytic vesicles via clathrin-mediated endocytosis (Ribeiro et al., 2003), a process that is dependent on a dileucine-like internalization motif located in the cytosolic carboxyl-terminal tail of CHT (Ribeiro et al., 2005); dileucine internalization motifs interact with the adaptor protein 2 complex of the clathrin-mediated endocytosis machinery (Traub, 2009). A subsequent study showed that internalized CHT undergoes constitutive recycling to the plasma membrane; importantly, potassium-mediated depolarization increases the rate of CHT recycling in neural cells, but not in non-neural cells (Ribeiro et al., 2007b). In addition, a recent report indicates that preventing CHT entry into the endosomal compartment using a selective endosomal ablation strategy decreases both CHT levels at the cell surface and choline uptake activity in a time-dependent manner (Ivy et al., 2010).

Since subcellular trafficking of CHT proteins is such a crucial mode of regulation of high-affinity choline uptake, it is important to address the question of how oxidative/nitrosative stress affects the proteins involved in vesicle trafficking. It has been demonstrated by a number of groups that oxidative stress perturbs the dynamic endocytosis of cell surface proteins such as receptors and transporters, with this having key roles in regulating their trafficking and activity. This may involve either the modification of specific amino acids in cargo proteins or be related to changes in the interaction of these receptors or transporters with other cellular proteins involved in their trafficking. For example, the dopamine transporter is inactivated by the RNS peroxynitrite by an action on a Cys residue in its third intracellular loop, with this resulting in toxicity to dopamine neurons (Park et al., 2002). This is prevented, but not reversed, by GSH and some reducing agents. Other studies reveal that the effects of ROS-RNS agents on cell surface proteins can be mediated indirectly by an action on components of the protein trafficking machinery, and this can likely involve changes in both clathrin-mediated and clathrin-independent pathways (Ozawa et al., 2008). Interestingly, this does not always involve inhibition of function of the protein; NO can regulate endocytosis by *S*-nitrosylation of dynamin which then affects endocytic vesicle budding thus facilitating internalization of some membrane proteins (G. Wang et al., 2006). This gain-of-function example illustrates the physiological role for low levels of NO. It has also been demonstrated that peroxynitrite stimulates synaptic vesicle exocytosis and induces the nitration of tyrosine residues in SNARE complex proteins (Di Stasi et al., 2002). However, another recent report showed that the fusion of synaptic vesicles with the presynaptic plasma membrane is impaired by oxidative stress (Arai et al., 2011).

Guermonprez and coworkers (2001) determined that peroxynitrite decreases CHT activity in synaptosomes from *Torpedo marmorata*. We have undertaken studies to identify the mechanisms by which oxidative-nitrosative stress alter choline uptake activity thereby interfering with cholinergic neurotransmission. Thus, we found that peroxynitrite causes a rapid, dose-dependent inhibition of CHT activity that is attenuated specifically by scavengers of peroxynitrite (Pinthong et al., 2008). Other oxidants such as H_2O_2 have no effect on CHT activity (Guermonprez et al., 2001; Pinthong et al., 2008). Importantly, doses of SIN-1, a peroxynitrite-generating molecule, that significantly decrease CHT activity do not compromise membrane integrity or alter cellular membrane potential (Pinthong et al., 2008). The SIN-1-induced decreases in choline uptake activity correlate with decreased CHT cell surface levels that result from accelerated endocytosis of CHT proteins by a clathrin-dependent mechanism (Pinthong et al., 2008).

Based on the important role that neuronal activity has in regulating the levels of CHT that are available at the plasma membrane to take up choline as substrate for ACh synthesis, it is predicted that the reduction in synaptic efficacy that is associated with elevated oligomeric

Aβ levels (Selkoe, 2002) would decrease the movement of CHT to the cell surface as constituents of synaptic vesicles. Thus, under conditions of oxidative-nitrosative stress, this effect of reduced synaptic efficacy associated with increasing oligomeric Aβ could further negatively impact CHT protein levels at the plasma membrane. This in turn would lead to diminished cholinergic signalling, a process found to be crucial in maintaining the cholinergic phenotype and regulating APP metabolism (Isacson et al., 2002; Seo et al., 2001; Tran et al., 2002; Unger et al., 2005; Verhoeff, 2005).

8. ROS-RNS may affect post-translational modifications and protein-protein interactions that regulate CHT and ChAT activities

Post-translational modifications can greatly influence both the function and subcellular localization of proteins. Phosphorylation, the reversible addition of a phosphate group to serine, threonine or tyrosine residues, is an important signalling event that has been shown to regulate both ChAT and CHT proteins. The activities of both ChAT and CHT are altered by treatments that modulate protein kinases or change the levels of protein phosphorylation in the cell (Black et al., 2010; Breer & Knipper, 1990; Cancela et al., 1995; Cooke & Rylett, 1997; Dobransky & Rylett, 2005; Ford et al., 1999; Gates et al., 2004; Guermonprez et al., 2002; Issa et al., 1996; Ivy et al., 2001; Knipper et al., 1992; Vogelsberg et al., 1997). Both ChAT and CHT proteins are phosphorylated in neural cells (Bruce & Hersh 1989; Dobransky et al., 2000; Gates et al., 2004; Habert et al. 1992; Schmidt & Rylett 1993). ChAT is a substrate for protein kinase C (PKC), casein kinase 2 and calcium/calmodulin-dependent kinase II (Dobransky et al., 2000), and CHT activity is modulated by activation of PKC (Black et al., 2010; Gates et al., 2004). Thus, pathological changes in protein kinase levels or functions could affect the functions of ChAT and/or CHT. For example, diminished PKC protein levels and signalling are seen in Alzheimer's disease (Alkon et al., 2007). However, ROS can lead to enhanced PKC activity (Zhao et al., 2011). Since PKC plays an important role in regulation of both ChAT and CHT function, it will be interesting to determine how oxidative stress alters phosphorylation-dependent regulation of ChAT, CHT and ACh synthesis, and the role that this plays in the failure of cholinergic neurotransmission in Alzheimer's disease and related disorders.

Protein-protein interactions are another molecular mode of regulation of protein function and/or subcellular localization, and some protein binding partners for ChAT and CHT have now been identified (Bales et al., 2006; Dobransky et al. 2003; Ribeiro et al., 2007a; B. Wang et al., 2007; Xie & Guo, 2004). In general, the interaction of CHT with other cellular proteins regulates it subcellular distribution. Notably, it has been determined that CHT interacts with the carboxyl-terminus of amyloid precursor protein (APP) family members (B. Wang et al., 2007) and with Aβ peptide (Bales et al., 2006). Mice lacking both APP and APP-like protein 2 have reduced levels of CHT protein at nerve terminals and this is seen as decreased high-affinity choline uptake activity; APP appears to be a modulator of both presynaptic localization and endocytosis of CHT proteins (B. Wang et al., 2007). Recent data indicate that modulation of APP metabolism or processing is an early cellular response to oxidative stress (Recuero et al., 2010). Based on the intimate relationship between oxidative/nitrosative stress and Aβ production, ROS-RNS generation could impact CHT activity by altering the interactions of this transporter with APP or Aβ. However, the mechanisms by which oxidative/nitrosative stress directly affects the interactions of ChAT and CHT with their protein binding partners have not been investigated.

9. Conclusion

The regulation of cellular proteins related to their reactions with ROS and RNS are described by the nitroso- and disulphide proteomes, and this has emerged as a critical modulator of protein function in both physiological and pathological situations (Ghezzi & Benetto, 2003; Lopez-Sanchez et al., 2009; Torta et al., 2008; Yano et al., 2002). A crucial point is that cellular mechanisms of limited capacity are normally in place, such as the formation of protein mixed-disulphides with glutathione (GSH), that transiently protect proteins from detrimental effects of ROS-RNS until redox balance is restored in the cell. *S*-glutathionylation at critical reactive Cys residues may even result in a gain-of-function for some proteins. However, during aging and disease, GSH levels are decreased and this can lead to irreversible oxidation and loss-of-function of vulnerable proteins. Investigations that are combining a range of proteomic, cell biology and *in vivo* experimental approaches have begun to characterize the dynamic responses of cholinergic neurons to the changes in brain that are induced by oxidative-nitrosative stress. A critical outcome of these studies is the identification of conditions that determine if the structural and functional modifications to ChAT and CHT that occur with tissue stress have the potential to be reversible or whether they are persistent. Future studies should focus on defining changes that are consistent with healthy and successful brain aging compared to changes that are associated with the onset of age-related disorders such as Alzheimer's disease. This will give insight into changes that are potentially reversible and that are amenable to intervention, and assist with the identification of therapeutic targets for protection of these proteins in normal aging and in diseases that may involve Aβ-induced / oxidative stress-induced changes.

10. Acknowledgment

Research grants from the Canadian Institutes of Health Research (CIHR) and Alzheimer's Association, USA were awarded to RJR. SAGB is the recipient of a CIHR Doctoral Research Award.

11. References

Alkon, D.L.; Sun, M.K. & Nelson, T.J. (2007). PKC signalling deficits: a mechanistic hypothesis for the origins of Alzheimer's disease. *Trends in Pharmacological Sciences,* Vol. 28, No. 2, (February 2007), pp. 51-60, ISSN 1873-3735

Ansari, M.A. & Scheff, S.W. (2010). Oxidative stress in the progression of Alzheimer disease in the frontal cortex. *Journal of Neuropathology and Experimental Neurology,* Vol. 69, No. 2, (February 2010), pp. 155-167, ISSN 0022-3069

Apelt, J.; Kumar, A. & Schliebs, R. (2002). Impairment of cholinergic neurotransmission in adult and aged transgenic Tg2576 mouse brain expressing the Swedish mutation of human beta-amyloid precursor protein. *Brain Research,* Vol. 953, No. 1-2, (October 2002), pp. 17-30, ISSN 1872-6240

Arai, M.; Saito, M.; Takatsu, H.; Fukui, K. & Urano, S. (2011). Dysfunction of the Fusion of Pre-Synaptic Plasma Membranes and Synaptic Vesicles Caused by Oxidative Stress, and its Prevention by Vitamin E. *Journal of Alzheimer's Disease,* (Feb 2011) [Epub ahead of print], ISSN 1387-2877

Auld, D.S.; Kar, S. & Quirion, R. (1998). Beta-amyloid peptides as direct cholinergic neuromodulators: a missing link? *Trends in Neurosciences,* Vol. 21, No. 1, (January 1998), pp. 43-49, ISSN 1878-108X

Bales, K.R.; Tzavara, E.T.; Wu, S.; Wade, M.R.; Bymaster, F.P.; Paul, S.M. & Nomikos, G.G. (2006). Cholinergic dysfunction in a mouse model of Alzheimer disease is reversed by an anti-A beta antibody. *Journal of Clinical Investigation,* Vol. 116, No. 3, (March 2006), pp. 825-832, ISSN 1558-8238

Barrett, W.C.; DeGnore, J.P.; Konig, S.; Fales, H.M.; Keng, Y.F.; Zhang, Z.Y.; Yim, M.B. & Chock, P.B. (1999). Regulation of PTP1B via glutathionylation of the active site cysteine 215. *Biochemistry,* Vol. 38, No. 20, (May 1999), pp. 6699-6705, ISSN 1520-4995

Baskerville, K.A.; Kent, C.; Nicolle, M.; Gallagher, M. & McKinney, M. (2006). Aging causes partial loss of basal forebrain but no loss of pontine reticular cholinergic neurons. *NeuroReport,* Vol. 17, No. 17, (November 2006), pp. 1819-1823, ISSN 1473-558X

Baskerville, K.A.; Kent, C.; Personett, D.; Lai, W.R.; Park, P.J.; Coleman, P. & McKinney, M. (2008). Aging elevates metabolic gene expression in brain cholinergic neurons. *Neurobiology of Aging,* Vol. 29, No. 12, (December 2008), pp. 1874-1893, ISSN 1558-1497

Bennett, S.A.; Pappas, B.A.; Stevens, W.D.; Davidson, C.M.; Fortin, T. & Chen, J. (2000). Cleavage of amyloid precursor protein elicited by chronic cerebral hypoperfusion. *Neurobiology of Aging,* Vol. 21, No. 2, (March-April 2000), pp 207-214, ISSN 1558-1497

Birks, R. & MacIntosh, F.C. (1961). Acetylcholine metabolism of a sympathetic ganglion. *Canadian Journal of Biochemistry and Physiology,* Vol. 39, pp. 787-827, ISSN 0576-5544

Black, S.A.; Ribeiro, F.M.; Ferguson, S.S. & Rylett, R.J. (2010). Rapid, transient effects of the protein kinase C activator phorbol 12-myristate 13-acetate on activity and trafficking of the rat high-affinity choline transporter. *Neuroscience,* Vol. 167, No. 3, (May 2010), pp. 765-773, ISSN 1873-7544

Bohnen, N.I. & Albin, R.L. (2010). The cholinergic system and Parkinson disease. *Behavioural Brain Research,* (January 2010), doi:10.1016/j.bbr.2009.12.048, ISSN 1872-7549

Borges, C.R.; Geddes, T.; Watson, J.T. & Kuhn, D.M. (2002). Dopamine biosynthesis is regulated by S-glutathionylation. Potential mechanism of tyrosine hydroxylase inhibition during oxidative stress. *Journal of Biological Chemistry,* Vol. 277, No. 50, (December 2002), pp. 48295-48302, ISSN 1083-351X

Breer, H. & Knipper, M. (1990). Regulation of high affinity choline uptake. *Journal of Neurobiology,* Vol. 21, No. 2, (March 1990), pp. 269-275, ISSN 1097-4695

Bruce, G. & Hersh, L.B. (1989). The phosphorylation of choline acetyltransferase. *Neurochemical Research,* Vol. 14, No. 7, (July 1989), pp. 613–620, ISSN 1573-6903

Butterfield, D.A. & Bush, A.I. (2004). Alzheimer's amyloid beta-peptide (1-42): involvement of methionine residue 35 in the oxidative stress and neurotoxicity properties of this peptide. *Neurobiology of Aging,* Vol. 25, No. 5, (May-June 2004), pp. 563-568, ISSN 1558-1497

Cancela, J.M.; Bertrand, N. & Beley, A. (1995). Involvement of cAMP in the regulation of high affinity choline uptake by rat brain synaptosomes. *Biochemical and Biophysical Research Communications,* Vol. 213, No. 3, (August 1995), pp. 944-949, ISSN 1090-2104

Chen, C.Y.; Willard, D. & Rudolph, J. (2009). Redox regulation of SH2-domain-containing protein tyrosine phosphatases by two backdoor cysteines. *Biochemistry,* Vol. 48, No. 6, (February 2009), pp. 1399-1409, ISSN 1520-4995

Collier, B. & MacIntosh, F.C. (1969). The source of choline for acetylcholine synthesis in a sympathetic ganglion. *Canadian Journal of Biochemistry and Physiology,* Vol. 47, pp. 127-135, ISSN 0576-5544

Collier, B. & Katz, H.S. (1974). Acetylcholine synthesis from recaptured choline by a sympathetic ganglion. *Journal of Physiology,* Vol. 238, No. 3, (May 1974), pp. 639-655, ISSN 1469-7793

Cooke, L.J. & Rylett, R.J. (1997). Inhibitors of serine/threonine phosphatases increase membrane-bound choline acetyltransferase activity and enhance acetylcholine synthesis. *Brain Research,* Vol. 751, No. 2, (March 1997), pp. 232-238, ISSN 1872-6240

Cumming, R.C. & Schubert, D. (2005). Amyloid-beta induces disulfide bonding and aggregation of GAPDH in Alzheimer's disease. *FASEB Journal,* Vol. 19, No. 14, (December 2005), pp. 2060-2062, ISSN 1530-6860

Davies, P. (1979). Biochemical changes in Alzheimer's disease-senile dementia: neurotransmitters in senile dementia of the Alzheimer's type. *Research Publications – Association for Research in Nervous and Mental Disease,* Vol. 57, pp. 153-66, ISSN 0091-7443

De Felice, F.G.; Velasco, P.T.; Lambert, M.P.; Viola, K.; Fernandez, S.J.; Ferreira, S.T. & Klein, W.L. (2007). Abeta oligomers induce neuronal oxidative stress through an N-methyl-D-aspartate receptor-dependent mechanism that is blocked by the Alzheimer drug memantine. *Journal of Biological Chemistry,* Vol. 282, No. 15, (April 2007), pp. 11590-11601, ISSN 1083-351X

DeKosky, S.T.; Ikonomovic, M.D.; Styren, S.D.; Beckett, L.; Wisniewski, S.; Bennett, D.A.; Cochran, E.J.; Kordower, J.H. & Mufson, E.J. (2002). Upregulation of choline acetyltransferase activity in hippocampus and frontal cortex of elderly subjects with mild cognitive impairment. *Annals of Neurology,* Vol. 51, No. 2, (February 2002), pp. 145-155, ISSN 1531-8249

Di Stasi, A.M.; Mallozzi, C.; Macchia, G.; Maura, G.; Petrucci, T.C. & Minetti, M. (2002). Peroxynitrite affects exocytosis and SNARE complex formation and induces tyrosine nitration of synaptic proteins. *Journal of Neurochemistry,* Vol. 82, No. 2, (July 2002), pp. 420-429, ISSN 1471-4159

Dobransky, T.; Davis, W.L.; Xiao, G.H. & Rylett, R.J. (2000). Expression, purification and characterization of recombinant human choline acetyltransferase: phosphorylation of the enzyme regulates catalytic activity. *Biochemical Journal,* Vol. 349, No. 1, (July 2000), pp. 141-151, ISSN 1470-8728

Dobransky, T.; Brewer, D.; Lajoie, G. & Rylett, R.J. (2003). Phosphorylation of 69-kDa choline acetyltransferase at threonine 456 in response to amyloid-beta peptide 1–42. *Journal of Biological Chemistry,* Vol. 278, No. 8, (February 2003), pp. 5883–5893, ISSN 1083-351X

Dobransky, T. & Rylett, R.J. (2005). A model for dynamic regulation of choline acetyltransferase by phosphorylation. *Journal of Neurochemistry,* Vol. 95, No. 2, (October 2005), pp. 305-13, ISSN 1471-4159

Fass, U.; Panickar, K.; Personett, D.; Bryan, D.; Williams, K.; Gonzales, J.; Sugaya, K. & McKinney, M. (2000). Differential vulnerability of primary cultured cholinergic neurons to nitric oxide excess. *NeuroReport,* Vol. 11, No. 5, (April 2000), pp. 931-936, ISSN 1473-558X

Ferguson, S.M.; Savchenko, V.; Apparsundaram, S.; Zwick, M.; Wright, J.; Heilman, C.J.; Yi, H.; Levey, A.I. & Blakely, R.D. (2003). Vesicular localization and activity-dependent trafficking of presynaptic choline transporters. *Journal of Neuroscience,* Vol. 23, No. 30, (October 2003), pp. 9697-9709, ISSN 1529-2401

Ford, B.D.; Ivy, M.T.; Mtshali, C.P. & Townsel, J.G. (1999). The involvement of protein kinase C in the regulation of choline cotransport in *Limulus. Comparative Biochemistry and Physiology. Part A, Molecular and Integrative Physiology,* Vol. 123, No. 3, (July 1999), pp. 255-261, ISSN 1095-6433

Forgon, M.; Farkas, Z.; Gulya, K.; Pakaski, M.; Penke, B. & Kasa, P. (1998). Amyloid beta-peptide and its fragments induce acetylcholine release in in vitro basal forebrain tissue slices of rat brain, but do not affect the choline uptake. *Neurobiology (Budapest, Hungary),* Vol. 6, No. 3, pp. 359-361, ISSN 1216-8068

Foster, T.C. (2006). Biological markers of age-related memory deficits: treatment of senescent physiology. *CNS Drugs,* Vol. 20, No. 2, pp. 153-156, ISSN 1172-7047

Francis, P.T.; Palmer, A.M.; Sims, N.R.; Bowen, D.M.; Davison, A.M.; Esiri, M.M.; Neary, D.; Snowden, J.S. & Wilcock, G.K. (1985). Neurochemical studies of early-onset Alzheimer's disease. Possible influence on treatment. *New England Journal of Medicine,* Vol. 313, No. 1, (July 1985), pp. 7-11, ISSN 1533-4406

Francis, P.T.; Palmer, A.M.; Snape, M. & Wilcock, G.K. (1999). The cholinergic hypothesis of Alzheimer's disease: a review of progress. *Journal of Neurology, Neurosurgery, and Psychiatry,* Vol. 66, No. 2, (February 1999), pp. 137-147, ISSN 1468-330X

Fukuda, K.; Davies, S.S.; Nakajima, T.; Ong, B.H.; Kupershmidt, S.; Fessel, J.; Amarnath, V.; Anderson, M.E.; Boyden, P.A.; Viswanathan, P.C.; Roberts, L.J. 2nd & Balser, J.R. (2005). Oxidative mediated lipid peroxidation recapitulates proarrhythmic effects on cardiac sodium channels. *Circulation Research,* Vol. 97, No. 12, (December 2005), pp. 1262-1269, ISSN 0009-7300

Garner, C.C.; Kindler, S. & Gundelfinger, E.D. (2000). Molecular determinants of presynaptic active zones. *Current Opinion in Neurobiology,* Vol. 10, No. 3, (June 2000), pp. 321-327, ISSN 0959-4388

Gates, J. jr.; Ferguson, S.M. & Blakely, R.D. (2004). Regulation of choline transporter surface expression and phosphorylation by protein kinase C and protein phosphatase 1/2. *Journal of Pharmacology and Experimental Therapeutics,* Vol. 310, No. 2, (August 2004), pp. 536-545, ISSN 1521-0103

Gentile, M.T.; Poulet, R.; Di Pardo, A.; Cifelli, G.; Maffei, A.; Vecchione, C.; Passarelli, F.; Landolfi, A.; Carullo, P. & Lembo, G. (2009). Beta-amyloid deposition in brain is enhanced in mouse models of arterial hypertension. *Neurobiology of Aging,* Vol. 30, No. 2, (February 2009), pp. 222-228, ISSN 1558-1497

Ghezzi, P. & Benetto, V. (2003). Redox proteomics: identification of oxidatively modified proteins. *Proteomics,* Vol. 3, No. 7, (July 2003), pp. 1145-1153, ISSN 1615-9861

Gilmer, L.K.; Ansari, M.A.; Roberts, K.N. & Scheff, S.W. (2010). Age-related changes in mitochondrial respiration and oxidative damage in the cerebral cortex of the Fischer 344 rat. *Mechanisms of Ageing and Development,* Vol. 131, No. 2, (February 2010), pp. 133-143, ISSN 0047-6374

Giustarini, D.; Rossi, R.; Milzani, A.; Colombo, R. & Dalle-Donne, I. (2004). S-glutathionylation: from redox regulation of protein functions to human diseases. Journal of Cellular and Molecular Medicine, Vol. 8, No. 2, (April-June 2004), pp. 201-212, ISSN 1582-4934

Goekoop, R.; Scheltens, P.; Barkhof, F. & Rombouts, S.A. (2006). Cholinergic challenge in Alzheimer patients and mild cognitive impairment differentially affects hippocampal activation--a pharmacological fMRI study. *Brain,* Vol. 129, No. 1, (January 2006), pp. 141-157, ISSN 1460-2156

Gong, Y.; Chang, L.; Viola, K.L.; Lacor, P.N.; Lambert, M.P.; Finch, C.E.; Krafft, G.A. & Klein, W.L. (2003). Alzheimer's disease-affected brain: presence of oligomeric A beta ligands (ADDLs) suggests a molecular basis for reversible memory loss. *Proceedings of the National Academy of Sciences of the United States of America,* Vol. 100, No. 18, (September 2003), pp. 10417-10422, ISSN 1091-6490

Gotti, C.; Clementi, F.; Fornari, A.; Gaimarri, A.; Guiducci, S.; Manfredi, I.; Moretti, M.; Pedrazzi, P.; Pucci, L. & Zoli, M. (2009). Structural and functional diversity of native brain neuronal nicotinic receptors. *Biochemical Pharmacology,* Vol. 78, No. 7, (October 2009), pp. 703-711, ISSN 1873-2968

Grön, G.; Brandenburg, I.; Wunderlich, A.P. & Riepe, M.W. (2006). Inhibition of hippocampal function in mild cognitive impairment: targeting the cholinergic hypothesis. *Neurobiology of Aging,* Vol. 27, No. 1, (January 2006), pp. 78-87, ISSN 1558-1497

Guermonprez, L.; Ducrocq, C. & Gaudry-Talarmain, Y.M. (2001). Inhibition of acetylcholine synthesis and tyrosine nitration induced by peroxynitrite are differentially prevented by antioxidants. *Molecular Pharmacology,* Vol. 60, No. 4, (October 2001), pp. 838-846, ISSN 1521-0111

Guermonprez, L.; O'Regan, S.; Meunier, F.M. & Morot-Gaudry-Talarmain, Y. (2002). The neuronal choline transporter CHT1 is regulated by immunosuppressor-sensitive pathways. *Journal of Neurochemistry,* Vol. 82, No. 4, (August 2002), pp. 874-884, ISSN 1471-4159

Guyenet, P.; Lefresne, P.; Rossier, J.; Beaujouan, J.C. & Glowinski, J. (1973). Inhibition by hemicholinium-3 and antiparkinson drugs on (14C)acetylcholine synthesis and (3H)choline uptake in rat striatal synaptosomes. *Brain Research,* Vol. 62, No. 2, (November 1973), pp. 523-529, ISSN 1872-6240

Habert, E.; Birman, S. & Mallet, J. (1992). High-level synthesis and fate of acetylcholine in baculovirus-infected cells: characterization and purification of recombinant rat choline acetyltransferase. *Journal of Neurochemistry,* Vol. 58, No. 4, (April 1992), pp. 1447-1453, ISSN 1471-4159

Haga, T. (1971). Synthesis and release of (14C)acetylcholine in synaptosomes. *Journal of Neurochemistry,* Vol. 18, No. 6, (June 1971), pp. 781-798, ISSN 1471-4159

Hartmann, J.; Erb, C.; Ebert, U.; Baumann, K.H.; Popp, A.; König, G. & Klein, J. (2004). Central cholinergic functions in human amyloid precursor protein knock-in/presenilin-1 transgenic mice. *Neuroscience,* Vol. 125, No. 4, pp. 1009-1017, ISSN 1873-7544

Hasselmo, M.E. (2006). The role of acetylcholine in learning and memory. *Current Opinion in Neurobiology,* Vol. 16, No. 6, (December 2006), pp. 710-715, ISSN 0959-4388

Heinitz, K.; Beck, M.; Schliebs, R. & Perez-Polo, J.R. (2006). Toxicity mediated by soluble oligomers of beta-amyloid(1-42) on cholinergic SN56.B5.G4 cells. *Journal of Neurochemistry,* Vol. 98, No. 6, (September 2006), pp. 1930-1945, ISSN 1471-4159

Hoshi, M.; Takashima, A.; Noguchi, K.; Marayama, M.; Sato, M.; Kondo, S.; Saitoh, Y.; Ishiguro, K.; Hoshino, T. & Imahori, K. (1996). Regulation of mitochondrial pyruvate dehydrogenase activity by tau protein kinase I/glycogen synthase kinase 3beta in brain. *Proceedings of the National Academy of Sciences of the United States of America,* Vol. 93, No. 7, (April 1996), pp. 2719-2723, ISSN 1091-6490

Hoshi, M.; Takashima, A.; Murayama, M.; Yasutake, K.; Yoshida, N.; Ishiguro, K.; Hoshino, T. & Imahori, K. (1997). Nontoxic amyloid beta peptide 1-42 suppresses acetylcholine synthesis. Possible role in cholinergic dysfunction in Alzheimer's disease. *Journal of Biological Chemistry,* Vol. 272, No. 4, (January 1997), pp. 2038-2041, ISSN 1083-351X

Humphries, K.M.; Juliano, C. & Taylor, S.S. (2002). Regulation of cAMP-dependent protein kinase activity by glutathionylation. *Journal of Biological Chemistry,* Vol. 277, No. 45, (November 2002), pp. 43505-43511, ISSN 1083-351X

Ikonomovic, M.D.; Mufson, E.J.; Wuu, J.; Cochran, E.J.; Bennet, D.A. & DeKosky, S.T. (2003). Cholinergic plasticity in hippocampus of individuals with mild cognitive impairment: correlation with Alzheimer's neuropathology. *Journal of Alzheimer's Disease,* Vol. 5, No. 1, (February 2003), pp. 39-48, ISSN 1387-2877

Isacson, O.; Seo, H.; Lin, L.; Albeck, D. & Granholm, A.C. (2002). Alzheimer's disease and Down's syndrome: roles of APP, trophic factors and ACh. *Trends in Neurosciences,* Vol. 25, No. 2, (February 2002), pp. 79-84, ISSN 1878-108X

Ishii, T.; Sakurai, T.; Usami, H. & Uchida, K. (2005). *Biochemistry,* Vol. 44, No. 42, (October 2005), pp. 13893-13901, ISSN 1520-4995

Issa, A.M.; Gauthier, S. & Collier, B. (1996). Effects of the phosphatase inhibitors calyculin A and okadaic acid on acetylcholine synthesis and content of rat hippocampal formation. *Journal of Neurochemistry,* Vol. 66, No. 5, (May 1996), pp. 1924-1932, ISSN 1471-4159

Ivy, M.T.; Newkirk, R.F.; Karim, M.R.; Mtshali, C.M. & Townsel J.G. (2001). Hemicholinium-3 mustard reveals two populations of cycling choline cotransporters in *Limulus. Neuroscience,* Vol. 102, No. 4, pp. 969-978, ISSN 1873-7544

Ivy, M.T.; Newkirk, R.F.; Wang, Y. & Townsel, J.G. (2010). A novel choline cotransporter sequestration compartment in cholinergic neurons revealed by selective endosomal ablation. *Journal of Neurochemistry,* Vol. 112, No. 5, (March 2010), pp. 1295-1304, ISSN 1471-4159

Jaffrey, S.R.; Erdjument-Bromage, H.; Ferris, C.D.; Tempst, P. & Snyder, S.H. (2001). Protein S-nitrosylation: a physiological signal for neuronal nitric oxide. *Nature Cell Biology,* Vol. 3, No. 2, (February 2001), pp. 193-197, ISSN 1476-4679

Kar, S.; Seto, D.; Gaudreau, P. & Quirion, R. (1996). Beta-amyloid-related peptides inhibit potassium-evoked acetylcholine release from rat hippocampal slices. *Journal of Neuroscience,* Vol. 16, No. 3, (February 1996), pp. 1034-1040, ISSN 1529-2401

Kar, S.; Issa, A.M.; Seto, D.; Auld, D.S.; Collier, B. & Quirion, R. (1998). Amyloid beta-peptide inhibits high-affinity choline uptake and acetylcholine release in rat hippocampal slices. *Journal of Neurochemistry,* Vol. 70, No. 5, (May 1998), pp. 2179-2187, ISSN 1471-4159

Kim, A.R.; Doherty-Kirby, A.; Lajoie, G.; Rylett, R.J. & Shilton, B.H. (2005). Two methods for large-scale purification of recombinant human choline acetyltransferase. *Protein Expression and Purification,* Vol. 40, No. 1, (March 2005), pp. 107-117, ISSN 1096-0279

Kim, A.R.; Rylett, R.J. & Shilton, B.H. (2006). Substrate binding and catalytic mechanism of human choline acetyltransferase. *Biochemistry,* Vol. 45, No. 49, (December 2006), pp. 14621-14631, ISSN 1520-4995

Klatt, P. & Lamas, S. (2000). Regulation of protein function by S-glutathiolation in response to oxidative and nitrosative stress. *European Journal of Biochemistry,* Vol. 267, No. 16, (August 2000), pp. 4928-4944, ISSN 1432-1033

Klein, W.L. (2002). Abeta toxicity in Alzheimer's disease: globular oligomers (ADDLs) as new vaccine and drug targets. *Neurochemistry International,* Vol. 41, No. 5, (November 2002), pp. 345-352, ISSN 1872-9754

Klein, W.L.; Stine, W.B. Jr. & Teplow, D.B. (2004). Small assemblies of unmodified amyloid beta-protein are the proximate neurotoxin in Alzheimer's disease. *Neurobiology of Aging,* Vol. 25, No. 5, (May-June 2004), pp. 569-580, ISSN 1558-1497

Klingner, M.; Apelt, J.; Kumar, A.; Sorger, D.; Sabri, O.; Steinbach, J.; Scheunemann, M. & Schliebs, R. (2003). Alterations in cholinergic and non-cholinergic neurotransmitter receptor densities in transgenic Tg2576 mouse brain with beta-amyloid plaque pathology. *International Journal of Developmental Neuroscience,* Vol. 21, No. 7, (November 2003), pp. 357-369, ISSN 1873-474X

Knipper, M.; Kahle, M. & Breer, H. (1992). Regulation of hemicholinium binding sites in isolated nerve terminals. *Journal of Neurobiology,* Vol. 23, No. 2, (March 1992), pp. 163-172, ISSN 1097-4695

Krishnaswamy, A. & Cooper, E. (2009). An activity-dependent retrograde signal induces the expression of the high-affinity choline transporter in cholinergic neurons. *Neuron,* Vol. 61, No. 2, (January 2009), pp. 272-286, ISSN 1097-4199

Kristofiková, Z.; Tejkalová, H. & Klaschka, J. (2001). Amyloid beta peptide 1-40 and the function of rat hippocampal hemicholinium-3 sensitive choline carriers: effects of a proteolytic degradation in vitro. *Neurochemical Research,* Vol. 26, No. 3, (March 2001), pp. 203-212, ISSN 1573-6903

Kristofiková, Z.; Rícný, J.; Kozmiková, I.; Rípová, D.; Zach, P. & Klaschka, J. (2006). Sex-dependent actions of amyloid beta peptides on hippocampal choline carriers of postnatal rats. *Neurochemical Research,* Vol. 31, No. 3, (March 2006), pp. 351-360, ISSN 1573-6903

Kristofiková, Z.; Kopecký, V. Jr.; Hofbauerová, K.; Hovorková, P. & Rípová, D. (2008). Complex of amyloid beta peptides with 24-hydroxycholesterol and its effect on hemicholinium-3 sensitive carriers. *Neurochemical Research,* Vol. 33, No. 3, (March 2008), pp. 412-421, ISSN 1573-6903

Kuo, Y.M.; Emmerling, M.R.; Viog-Pelfrey, C.; Kasunic, T.C.; Kirkpatrick, J.B.; Murdoch, G.H.; Ball, M.J. & Roher, A.E. (1996). Water-soluble Abeta (N-40, N-42) oligomers in normal and Alzheimer disease brains. *Journal of Biological Chemistry,* Vol. 271, No. 8, (February 1996), pp. 4077-4081, ISSN 1083-351X

Lahiri, D.K.; Utsuki, T.; Chen, D.; Farlow, M.R.; Shoaib, M.; Ingram, D.K. & Greig, N.H. (2002). Nicotine reduces the secretion of Alzheimer's beta-amyloid precursor protein containing beta-amyloid peptide in the rat without altering synaptic proteins. *Annals of the New York Academy of Sciences,* Vol. 965, (June 2002), pp. 364-372, ISSN 1749-6632

Lahiri, D.K. & Greig, N.H. (2004). Lethal weapon: amyloid beta-peptide, role in the oxidative stress and neurodegeneration of Alzheimer's disease. *Neurobiology of Aging,* Vol. 25, No. 5, (May-June 2004), pp. 581-587, ISSN 1558-1497

Lane, R.M.; Potkin, S.G. & Enz, A. (2006). Targeting acetylcholinesterase and butyrylcholinesterase in dementia. *International Journal of Neuropsychopharmacology,* Vol. 9, No. 1, (February 2006), pp. 101-124, ISSN 1469-5111

Lee, P.H.; Hwang, E.M.; Hong, H.S.; Boo, J.H.; Mook-Jung, I. & Huh, K. (2006). Effect of ischemic neuronal insults on amyloid precursor protein processing. *Neurochemical Research,* Vol. 31, No. 6, (June 2006), pp. 821-827, ISSN 1573-6903

Lind, C.; Gerdes, R.; Hamnell, Y.; Schuppe-Koistinen, I.; von Lowenhielm, H.B.; Holmgren, A. & Cotgreave, I.A. (2002). Identification of S-glutathionylated cellular proteins during oxidative stress and constitutive metabolism by affinity purification and proteomic analysis. *Archives of Biochemistry and Biophysics,* Vol. 406, No. 2, (October 2002), pp. 229-240, ISSN 1096-0384

Liu, M.; Huang, Y.; Wu, J.; Wang, E. & Wang, Y. (1999). Effect of cysteine residues on the activity of arginyl-tRNA synthetase from *Escherichia coli*. *Biochemistry,* Vol. 38, No. 34, (August 1999), pp. 11006-11011, ISSN 1520-4995

Lopez-Sanchez, L.M.; Muntane, J.; de la Mata, M. & Rodriguez-Ariza, A. (2009). Unraveling the S-nitrosoproteome: tools and strategies. *Proteomics,* Vol. 9, No. 4, (February 2009), pp. 808-818, ISSN 1615-9861

Lue, L.F., Kuo, Y.M.; Roher, A.E.; Brachova, L.; Shen, Y.; Sue, L.; Beach, T.; Kurth, J.H.; Rydel, R.E. & Rogers, J. (1999). Soluble amyloid beta peptide concentration as a predictor of synaptic change in Alzheimer's disease. *American Journal of Pathology,* Vol. 155, No. 3, (September 1999), pp. 853-862, ISSN 1525-2191

Marcello, E.; Epis, R. & Di Luca, M. (2008). Amyloid flirting with synaptic failure: towards a comprehensive view of Alzheimer's disease pathogenesis. *European Journal of Pharmacology,* Vol. 585, No. 1, (May 2008), pp. 109-118, ISSN 1879-0712

Mattson, M.P. (2004). Pathways towards and away from Alzheimer's disease. *Nature,* Vol. 430, No. 7000, (August 2004), pp. 631-639, ISSN 1476-4687

Mattson, M.P. & Magnus, T. (2006). Ageing and neuronal vulnerability. *Nature Reviews. Neuroscience,* Vol. 7, No. 4, (April 2006), pp. 278-294, ISSN 1471-0048

McKinney, M.; Williams, K.; Personett, D.; Kent, C.; Bryan, D.; Gonzalez, J. & Baskerville, K. (2004). Pontine cholinergic neurons depend on three neuroprotection systems to resist nitrosative stress. *Brain Research,* Vol. 1002, No. 1-2, (March 2004), pp. 100-109, ISSN 1872-6240

McKinney, M. & Jacksonville, M.C. (2005). Brain cholinergic vulnerability: relevance to behavior and disease. *Biochemical Pharmacology,* Vol. 70, No. 8, (October 2005), pp. 1115-1124, ISSN 1873-2968

McMillian, M.; Kong, L.Y; Sawin, S.M.; Wilson, B.; Das, K.; Hudson, P.; Hong, J.S. & Bing, G. (1995). Selective killing of cholinergic neurons by microglial activation in basal forebrain mixed neuronal/glial cultures. *Biochemical and Biophysical Research Communications,* Vol. 215, No. 2, (October 1995), pp. 572-577, ISSN 1090-2104

Melo, J.B.; Agostinho, P. & Oliveira, C.R. (2002). Amyloid beta-peptide 25-35 reduces [3H]acetylcholine release in retinal neurons. Involvement of metabolic dysfunction. *Amyloid*, Vol. 9, No. 4, (December 2002), pp. 221-228, ISSN 1744-2818

Mesulam, M. (2004). The cholinergic lesion of Alzheimer's disease: pivotal factor or side show? *Learning and Memory*, Vol. 11, No. 1, (January-February 2004), pp. 43-49, ISSN 1549-5485

Morris, D. (1967). The effect of sulphydryl and other disulphide reducing agents on choline acetyltransferase activity estimated with synthetic acetyl-CoA. *Journal of Neurochemistry*, Vol. 14, No. 1, (January 1967), pp. 19-27, ISSN 1471-4159

Mufson, E.J.; Ginsberg, S.D.; Ikonomovic, M.D. & DeKosky, S.T. (2003). Human cholinergic basal forebrain: chemoanatomy and neurologic dysfunction. *Journal of Chemical Neuroanatomy*, Vol. 26, No. 4, (December 2003), pp. 233-242, ISSN 1873-6300

Nakata, K.; Okuda, T. & Misawa, H. (2004). Ultrastructural localization of high-affinity choline transporter in the rat neuromuscular junction: enrichment on synaptic vesicles. *Synapse*, Vol. 53, No. 1, (July 2004), pp. 53-56, ISSN 1098-2396

Nathanson, N.M. (2008). Synthesis, trafficking, and localization of muscarinic acetylcholine receptors. *Pharmacology and Therapeutics*, Vol. 119, No. 1, (July 2008), pp. 33-43, ISSN 0163-7258

Nicolle, M.M.; Gonzalez, J.; Sugaya, K.; Baskerville, K.A.; Bryan, D.; Lund, K.; Gallagher, M. & McKinney, M. (2001). Signatures of hippocampal oxidative stress in aged spatial learning-impaired rodents. *Neuroscience*, Vol. 107, No. 3, pp. 415-431, ISSN 1873-7544

Nihashi, T.; Inao, S.; Kajita, Y.; Kawai, T.; Sugimoto, T.; Niwa, M.; Kabeya, R.; Hata, N.; Hayashi, S. & Toshida, J. (2001). Expression and distribution of beta amyloid precursor protein and beta amyloid peptide in reactive astrocytes after transient middle cerebral artery occlusion. *Acta Neurochirurgica (Wien)*, Vol. 143, No. 3, pp. 287-295, ISSN 0942-0940

Nitta, A.; Itoh, A.; Hasegawa, T. & Nabeshima, T. (1994). beta-Amyloid protein-induced Alzheimer's disease animal model. *Neuroscience Letters*, Vol. 170, No. 1, (March 1994), pp. 63-66, ISSN 1872-7972

Nitta, A.; Fukuta, T.; Hasegawa, T. & Nabeshima, T. (1997). Continuous infusion of beta-amyloid protein into the rat cerebral ventricle induces learning impairment and neuronal and morphological degeneration. *Japanese Journal of Pharmacology*, Vol. 73, No. 1, (January 1997), pp. 51-57, ISSN 1347-3506

Oda, Y. (1999). Choline acetyltransferase: the structure, distribution and pathologic changes in the central nervous system. *Pathology International*, Vol. 49, No. 11, (November 1999), pp. 921-937, ISSN 1440-1827

Okuda, T.; Haga, T.; Kanai, Y.; Endou, H.; Ishihara, T. & Katsura, I. (2000). Identification and characterization of the high-affinity choline transporter. *Nature Neuroscience*, Vol. 3, No. 2, (February 2000), pp. 120-125, ISSN 1546-1726

Ongwijitwat, S.; Liang, H.L.; Graboyes, E.M. & Wong-Riley, M.T. (2006). Nuclear respiratory factor 2 senses changing cellular energy demands and its silencing down-regulates cytochrome oxidase and other target gene mRNAs. *Gene*, Vol. 374, (June 2006), pp. 39-49, ISSN 1879-0038

Opazo, P.; Saud, K.; de Saint Pierre, M.; Cárdenas, A.M.; Allen, D.D.; Segura-Aguilar, J.; Caviedes, R. & Caviedes, P. (2006). Knockdown of amyloid precursor protein normalizes cholinergic function in a cell line derived from the cerebral cortex of a trisomy 16 mouse: An animal model of down syndrome. *Journal of Neuroscience Research,* Vol. 84, No. 6, (November 2006), pp. 1303-1310, ISSN 1872-8111

Ozawa, K.; Whalen, E.J.; Nelson, C.D.; Mu, Y.; Hess, D.T.; Lefkowitz, R.J. & Stamler, J.S. (2008). S-nitrosylation of beta-arrestin regulates beta-adrenergic receptor trafficking. *Molecular Cell,* Vol. 31, No. 3, (August 2008), pp. 395-405, ISSN 1097-4164

Park, S.U.; Ferrer, J.V.; Javitch, J.A. & Kuhn, D.M. (2002). Peroxynitrite inactivates the human dopamine transporter by modification of cysteine 342: potential mechanism of neurotoxicity in dopamine neurons. *Journal of Neuroscience,* Vol. 22, No. 11, (June 2002), pp. 4399-4405, ISSN 1529-2401

Payette, D.J.; Xie, J. & Guo, Q. (2007). Reduction in CHT1-mediated choline uptake in primary neurons from presenilin-1 M146V mutant knock-in mice. *Brain Research,* Vol. 1135, No. 1, (March 2007), pp. 12-21, ISSN 1872-6240

Pedersen, W.A.; Kloczewiak, M.A. & Blusztajn, J.K. (1996). Amyloid beta-protein reduces acetylcholine synthesis in a cell line derived from cholinergic neurons of the basal forebrain. *Proceedings of the National Academy of Sciences of the United States of America,* Vol. 93, No. 15, (July 1996), pp. 8068-8071, ISSN 1091-6490

Pedersen, W.A. & Blusztajn, J.K. (1997). Characterization of the acetylcholine-reducing effect of the amyloid-beta peptide in mouse SN56 cells. *Neuroscience Letters,* Vol. 239, No. 2-3, (December 1997), pp. 77-80, ISSN 1872-7972

Perry, E.K.; Perry, R.H.; Blessed, G. & Tomlinson, B.E. (1977). Necropsy evidence of central cholinergic deficits in senile dementia. *Lancet,* Vol. 1, No. 8004, (January 1977), p. 189, ISSN 1474-547X

Petcu, E.B.; Sfedel, V.; Platt, D.; Herndon, J.G.; Kessler, C. & Popa-Wagner, A. (2008). Cellular and molecular events underlying the dysregulated response of the aged brain to stroke: a mini-review. *Gerontology,* Vol. 54, No. 1, pp. 6-17, ISSN 1423-0003

Pinthong, M.; Black, S.A.; Ribeiro, F.M.; Pholpramool, C.; Ferguson, S.S. & Rylett, R.J. (2008). Activity and subcellular trafficking of the sodium-coupled choline transporter CHT is regulated acutely by peroxynitrite. *Molecular Pharmacology,* Vol. 73, No. 3, (March 2008), pp. 801-812, ISSN 1521-0111

Prado, M.A.; Reis, R.A.; Prado, V.F.; de Mello, M.C.; Gomez, M.V. & de Mello, F.G. (2002). Regulation of acetylcholine synthesis and storage. *Neurochemistry International,* Vol. 41, No. 5, (November 2002), pp. 291-299, ISSN 1872-9754

Qi, X.L.; Xiu, J.; Shan, K.R.; Xiao, Y.; Gu, R.; Liu, R.Y. & Guan, Z.Z. (2005). Oxidative stress induced by beta-amyloid peptide(1-42) is involved in the altered composition of cellular membrane lipids and the decreased expression of nicotinic receptors in human SH-SY5Y neuroblastoma cells. *Neurochemistry International,* Vol. 46, No. 8, (June 2005), pp. 613-621,ISSN 1872-9754

Ribeiro, F.M.; Alves-Silva, J.; Volknandt, W.; Martins-Silva, C.; Mahmud, H.; Wilhelm, A.; Gomez, M.V.; Rylett, R.J.; Ferguson, S.S.; Prado, V.F. & Prado, M.A. (2003). The hemicholinium-3 sensitive high affinity choline transporter is internalized by clathrin-mediated endocytosis and is present in endosomes and synaptic vesicles. *Journal of Neurochemistry,* Vol. 87, No. 1, (October 2003), pp. 136-146, ISSN 1471-4159

Ribeiro, F.M.; Black, S.A.; Cregan, S.P.; Prado, V.F.; Prado, M.A.; Rylett, R.J. & Ferguson, S.S. (2005). Constitutive high-affinity choline transporter endocytosis is determined by a carboxyl-terminal tail dileucine motif. *Journal of Neurochemistry,* Vol. 94, No. 1, (July 2005), pp. 86-96, ISSN 1471-4159

Ribeiro F.M.; Ferreira, L.T.; Marion, S.; Fontes, S.; Gomez, M.; Ferguson, S.S.; Prado, M.A. & Prado, V.F. (2007a). SEC14-like protein 1 interacts with cholinergic transporters. *Neurochemistry International,* Vol. 50, No. 2, (January 2007), pp. 356-364, ISSN 1872-9754

Ribeiro, F.M.; Pinthong, M.; Black, S.A.; Gordon, A.C.; Prado, V.F.; Prado, M.A.; Rylett, R.J. & Ferguson, S.S. (2007b). Regulated recycling and plasma membrane recruitment of the high-affinity choline transporter. *European Journal of Neuroscience,* Vol. 26, No. 12, (December 2007), pp. 3437-3448, ISSN 1460-9568

Recuero M, Muñoz T, Aldudo J, Subías M, Bullido MJ, Valdivieso F. (2010). A free radical-generating system regulates APP metabolism/processing. *FEBS Letters,* Vol. 584, No. 22, (November 2010), pp. 4611-4618, ISSN 1873-3468

Roskoski, R. (1973). Choline acetyltransferase. Evidence for an acetyl-enzyme reaction intermediate. *Biochemistry,* Vol. 12, No. 19, (September 1973), pp. 3709-3714, ISSN 1520-4995

Ruan, C.J.; Zhang, L.; Chen, D.H.; Li, Z.; Du, G.H. & Sun, L. (2010). Effects of trans-2,4-dimethoxystibene against the neurotoxicity induced by Abeta(25-35) both in vitro and in vivo. *Neuroscience Research,* Vol. 67, No. 3 (July 2010), pp. 209-214, ISSN 1872-8111

Rylett, R.J.; Ball, M.J. & Colhoun, E.H. (1982). Evidence for high affinity choline transport in synaptosomes prepared from hippocampus and neocortex of patients with Alzheimer's disease. *Brain Research,* Vol. 289, No. 1-2, (December 1982), pp. 169-175, ISSN 1872-6240

Sarter, M. & Bruno, J.P. (1997). Cognitive functions of cortical acetylcholine: toward a unifying hypothesis. *Brain Research Reviews,* Vol. 23, No. 1-2, pp. 28-46, ISSN 1872-6321

Sarter, M.; Bruno, J.P. & Givens, B. (2003). Attentional functions of cortical cholinergic inputs: what does it mean for learning and memory? *Neurobiology of Learning and Memory,* Vol. 80, No. 3, (November 2003), pp. 245-56, ISSN 1095-9564

Sarter, M. & Bruno, J.P. (2004). Developmental origins of the age-related decline in cortical cholinergic function and associated cognitive abilities. *Neurobiology of Aging,* Vol. 25, No. 9, (October 2004), pp. 1127-1139, ISSN 1558-1497

Sarter, M. & Parikh, V. (2005). Choline transporters, cholinergic transmission and cognition. *Nature Reviews. Neuroscience,* Vol. 6, No. 1, (January 2005), pp. 48-56, ISSN 1471-0048

Satoh, Y.; Hirakura, Y.; Shibayama, S.; Hirashima, N.; Suzuki, T. & Kirino, Y. (2001). Beta-amyloid peptides inhibit acetylcholine release from cholinergic presynaptic nerve endings isolated from an electric ray. *Neuroscience Letters,* Vol. 302, No. 2-3, (April 2001), pp. 97-100, ISSN 1872-7972

Schliebs, R. & Arendt, T. (2006). The significance of the cholinergic system in the brain during aging and in Alzheimer's disease. *Journal of Neural Transmission,* Vol. 113, No. 11, (November 2006), pp. 1625-1644, ISSN 1435-1463

Schmidt, B.M. & Rylett, R.J. (1993). Phosphorylation of rat brain choline acetyltransferase and its relationship to enzyme activity. *Journal of Neurochemistry,* Vol. 61, No. 5, (November 1993), pp. 1774-1781, ISSN 1471-4159

Selkoe, D.J. (2002). Alzheimer's disease is a synaptic failure. *Science,* Vol. 298, No. 5594, (October 2002), pp. 789-791, ISSN 1095-9203

Seo, J.H.; Kim, S.H.; Kim, H.S.; Park, C.H.; Jeong, A.J.; Lee, J.H.; Choi, K.A.; Rah, J.C.; Koo, J.; Kim, E.M. & Suh, Y.H. (2001). Effects of nicotine on APP secretion and Abeta- or CT(105)-induced toxicity. *Biological Psychiatry,* Vol. 49, No. 3, (February 2001), pp. 240-247, ISSN 1873-2402

Shi, J.; Yang, S.H.; Stubley, L.; Day, A.L. & Simpkins, J.W. (2000). Hypoperfusion induces overexpression of beta-amyloid precursor protein mRNA in a focal ischemic rodent model. *Brain Research,* Vol. 853, No. 1, (January 2000), pp. 1-4, ISSN 1872-6240

Shimohama, S. & Kihara, T. (2001). Nicotinic receptor-mediated protection against beta-amyloid neurotoxicity. *Biological Psychiatry,* Vol. 49, No. 3, (February 2001), pp. 233-239, ISSN 1873-2402

Simon, J.R. & Kuhar, M.G. (1975). Impulse-flow regulation of high affinity choline uptake in brain cholinergic nerve terminals. *Nature,* Vol. 255, No. 5504, (May 1975), pp. 162-163, ISSN 1476-4687

Sims, N.R.; Bowen, D.M.; Allen, S.J.; Smith, C.C.; Neary, D. & Davison, A.N. (1983). Presynaptic cholinergic dysfunction in patients with dementia. *Journal of Neurochemistry,* Vol. 40, No. 2, (February 1983), pp. 503-509, ISSN 1471-4159

Skoog, I.; Lernfelt, B.; Landahl, S.; Palmertz, B.; Andreasson, L.A.; Nilsson, L.; Persson, G.; Odén, A. & Svanborg, A. (1996). 15-year longitudinal study of blood pressure and dementia. *Lancet,* Vol. 347, No. 9009, (April 1996), pp. 1141-1145, ISSN 1474-547X

Skoog, I. & Gustafson, D. (2006). Update on hypertension and Alzheimer's disease. *Neurological Research,* Vol. 28, No. 6, (September 2006), pp. 605-611, ISSN 1743-1328

Smith, S.M.; Renden, R. & von Gersdorff, H. (2008). Synaptic vesicle endocytosis: fast and slow modes of membrane retrieval. *Trends in Neurosciences,* Vol. 31, No. 11, (November 2008), pp. 559-568, ISSN 1878-108X

Smith, W.W.; Gorospe, M. & Kusiak, J.W. (2006). Signaling mechanisms underlying Abeta toxicity: potential therapeutic targets for Alzheimer's disease. *CNS & Neurological Disorders Drug Targets,* Vol. 5, No. 3, (June 2006), pp. 355-361, ISSN 1996-3181

Südhof, T.C. (2008). Neurotransmitter release, In: *Handbook of Experimental Pharmacology,* Vol. 184, T.C. Südhof and K. Starke, (Eds.), pp. 1-21, Springer, ISBN: 978-3-540-74804-5, Berlin, Germany

Tamagno, E.; Parola, M.; Guglielmotto, M.; Santoro, G.; Bardini, P.; Marra, L.; Tabaton, M. & Danni, O. (2003). Multiple signaling events in amyloid beta-induced, oxidative stress-dependent neuronal apoptosis. *Free Radical Biology & Medicine,* Vol. 35, No. 1, (July 2003), pp. 45-58, ISSN 1873-4596

Torta, F.; Usuelli, V.; Malgaroli, A. & Bachi, A. (2008). Proteomic analysis of protein S-nitrosylation. *Proteomics,* Vol. 8, No. 21, (November 2008), pp. 4484-4494, ISSN 1615-9861

Townsend, D.M. (2007). S-glutathionylation: indicator of cell stress and regulator of the unfolded protein response. *Molecular Interventions,* Vol. 7, No. 6, (December 2007), pp. 313-324, ISSN 1543-2548

Tran, M.H.; Yamada, K.; Olariu, A.; Mizuno, M.; Ren, X.H. & Nabeshima, T. (2001). Amyloid beta-peptide induces nitric oxide production in rat hippocampus: association with cholinergic dysfunction and amelioration by inducible nitric oxide synthase inhibitors. *FASEB Journal,* Vol. 15, No. 8, (June 2001), pp. 1407-1409, ISSN 1530-6860

Tran, M.H.; Yamada, K. & Nabashima, T. (2002). Amyloid beta-peptide induces cholinergic dysfunction and cognitive deficits: a minireview. *Peptides*, Vol. 23, No. 7, (July 2002), pp. 1271-1283, ISSN 1873-5169

Traub, L.M. (2009). Tickets to ride: selecting cargo for clathrin-regulated internalization. *Nature Reviews. Molecular Cell Biology*, Vol. 10, No. 9, (September 2009), pp. 583-596, ISSN 1471-0080

Unger, C.; Hedberg, M.M.; Mustafiz, T.; Svedberg, M.M. & Nordberg, A. (2005). Early changes in Abeta levels in the brain of APPswe transgenic mice--implication on synaptic density, alpha7 neuronal nicotinic acetylcholine- and N-methyl-D-aspartate receptor levels. *Molecular and Cellular Neurosciences*, Vol. 30, No. 2, (October 2005), pp. 218-227, ISSN 1095-9327

Verhoeff, N.P. (2005). Acetylcholinergic neurotransmission and the beta-amyloid cascade: implications for Alzheimer's disease. *Expert Review of Neurotherapeutics*, Vol. 5, No. 2, (March 2005), pp. 277-284, ISSN 1744-8360

Vogelsberg, V.; Neff, N.H. & Hadjiconstantinou, M. (1997). Cyclic AMP-mediated enhancement of high-affinity choline transport and acetylcholine synthesis in brain. *Journal of Neurochemistry*, Vol. 68, No. 3, (March 1997), pp. 1062-1070, ISSN 1471-4159

Walsh, D.M.; Klyubin, I.; Fadeeva, J.V.; Cullen, W.K.; Anwyl, R.; Wolfe, M.S.; Rowan, M.J. & Selkoe, D.J. (2002a). Naturally secreted oligomers of amyloid beta protein potently inhibit hippocampal long-term potentiation in vivo. *Nature*, Vol. 416, No. 6880, (April 2002), pp. 535-539, ISSN 1476-4687

Walsh, D.M.; Klyubin, I.; Fadeeva, J.V.; Rowan, M.J. & Selkoe, D.J. (2002b). Amyloid-beta oligomers: their production, toxicity and therapeutic inhibition. *Biochemical Society Transactions*, Vol. 30, No. 4, (August 2002), pp. 552-557, ISSN 1470-8752

Wang, B.; Yang, L.; Wang, Z. & Zheng, H. (2007). Amyloid precursor protein mediates presynaptic localization and activity of the high-affinity choline transporter. *Proceedings of the National Academy of Sciences of the United States of America*, Vol. 104, No. 35, (August 2007), pp. 14140-14145, ISSN 1091-6490

Wang, G.; Moniri, N.H.; Ozawa, K.; Stamler, J.S. & Daaka, Y. (2006). Nitric oxide regulates endocytosis by S-nitrosylation of dynamin. *Proceedings of the National Academy of Sciences of the United States of America*, Vol. 103, No. 5, (January 2006), pp. 1295-1300, ISSN 1091-6490

Wang, J.; Dickson, D.W.; Trojanowski, J.Q. & Lee, V.M. (1999). The levels of soluble versus insoluble brain Abeta distinguish Alzheimer's disease from normal and pathologic aging. *Experimental Neurology*, Vol. 158, No. 2, (August 1999), pp. 328-337, ISSN 1090-2430

Wang, J.; Boja, E.S.; Tan, W.; Tekle, E.; Fales, H.M.; English, S.; Mieyal, J.J. & Chock, P.B. (2001). Reversible glutathionylation regulates actin polymerization in A431 cells. *Journal of Biological Chemistry*, Vol. 276, No. 51, (December 2001), pp. 47763-47766, ISSN 1083-351X

Woolf, N.J. (1998). A structural basis for memory storage in mammals. *Progress in Neurobiology*, Vol. 55, No. 1, (May 1998), pp. 59-77, ISSN 1873-5118

Woolf N.J. & Butcher L.L. (2010). Cholinergic systems mediate action from movement to higher consciousness. *Behavioural Brain Research*, (January 2010), doi:10.1016/j.bbr.2009.12.046, ISSN 1872-7549

Xie, J. & Guo, Q. (2004). Par-4 inhibits choline uptake by interacting with CHT1 and reducing its incorporation on the plasma membrane. *Journal of Biological Chemistry,* Vol. 279, No. 27, (July 2004), pp. 28266-28275, ISSN 1083-351X

Yamamura, H.I. & Snyder, S.H. (1972). Choline: high-affinity uptake by rat brain synaptosomes. *Science,* Vol. 178, No. 61, (November 1972), pp. 626-628, ISSN 1095-9203

Yang, S.J.; Liang, H.L. & Wong-Riley, M.T. (2006). Activity-dependent transcriptional regulation of nuclear respiratory factor-1 in cultured rat visual cortical neurons. *Neuroscience,* Vol. 141, No. 3, (September 2006), pp. 1181-1192, ISSN 1873-7544

Yano, H.; Kuroda, S. & Buchanan, B.B. (2002). Disulfide proteome in the analysis of protein function and structure. *Proteomics,* Vol. 2, No. 9, (September 2002), pp. 1090-1096, ISSN 1615-9861

Zamani, M.R. & Allen, Y.S. (2001). Nicotine and its interaction with beta-amyloid protein: a short review. *Biological Psychiatry,* Vol. 49, No. 3, (February 2001), pp. 221-232, ISSN 1873-2402

Zhao, F.; Ilbert, M.; Varadan, R.; Cremers, C.M.; Hoyos, B.; Acin-Perez, R.; Vinogradov, V.; Cowburn, D.; Jakob, U. & Hammerling, U. (2011). Are zinc-finger domains of protein kinase C dynamic structures that unfold by lipid or redox activation? *Antioxidants and Redox Signaling,* Vol. 14, No. 5, (March 2011), pp. 757-66, ISSN 1557-7716

Zhu, X.; Raina, A.K.; Lee, H.G.; Casadesus, G.; Smith, M.A. & Perry, G. (2004). Oxidative stress signalling in Alzheimer's disease. *Brain Research,* Vol. 1000, No. 1-2, (March 2004), pp. 32-39, ISSN 1872-6240

17

Metals Involvement in Alzheimer's Disease Pathogenesis

Rosanna Squitti[1,2] and Carlo Salustri[3]
[1]*Departement of Neuroscience, AFaR – Fatebenefratelli Hospital, Isola Tiberina, Rome*
[2]*Clinica Neurologica, Università Campus Biomedico, Rome*
[3]*Institute of Cognition Sciences and Technologies (CNR), Fatebenefratelli Hospital, Isola Tiberina, Rome,*
Italy

1. Introduction

When Auguste Deter died in 1906, Alois Alzheimer, who had closely followed her mental degradation over the previous 5 years, obtained her brain and performed a post-mortem study. By using a silver-staining method just developed by Bielschowsky, Alzheimer identified aggregations of fibrils and what he called 'miliary foci'. Alterations of that nature had been already observed by others in post-mortem brains, but Alzheimer was the first to relate them to his patient's dementia. He described the case a year later and Auguste Deter remained in medical history as the first clinical case of what has been ever since referred to as Alzheimer's disease. For an English translation of Alzheimer's 1907 paper, see (Alzheimer et al., 1995).

1.1 General description

Alzheimer's disease (AD) is an irreversible neurodegenerative disorder, characterized by a gradual loss of the cognitive functions inexorably leading to dementia. From an early stage characterized by a mild loss of recent memory, the disease advances to more devastating symptoms such as faulty judgments and even personality changes, to terminate in a complete loss of reasoning ability and self sufficiency. Death normally ensues 8 to 10 years after diagnosis.

AD is often referred to as early- or late-onset depending on whether it appears before or after age 65, and is normally distinguished in familial, i.e., inherited, and sporadic, which is caused by a combination of genetic, lifestyle and environmental factors.

About 75% of AD patients have the sporadic form, which has normally a late-onset. The familial form, which affects the remaining 25%, can have instead either an early-onset (about 5% of all familial cases) or a late-onset.

The early-onset familial AD is attributed to mutations in one of three genes: amyloid precursor protein (APP), Presenilin1 or Presenilin2. The genetic causes of the late-onset familial AD are not fully assessed, although the inheritance of the ε4 allele of the apolipoprotein E (*ApoE4*) has been recognized as a risk factor for both familial and sporadic late-onset AD. Carriers of this allele have a 90% statistical risk of contracting AD if they are heterozygote and a virtual certainty if homozygote (Corder et al., 1993).

All forms share the same alterations that include neuron loss, synapse loss, amyloid plaques, neurofibrillary tangles and microgliosis. However, although it is well established that AD symptoms are due to a compromised neurotransmission originating from these alterations, there is not yet full agreement on what actually initiates the neurodegeneration.

1.2 Diagnosis

Since no single test or biochemical measurement can securely lead to a diagnosis of AD, intellectual deterioration is diagnosed as possible or probable AD on the basis of a careful analysis of the symptoms, the medical history of both patient and his/her relatives, a variety of neuropsychological tests and from the exclusion of alternative conditions, generally attained via neuroimaging. Almost universally physicians today follow the NINCDS-ADRDA Criteria for diagnosis of Alzheimer's disease (McKhann et al., 1984), jointly published in 1984 by the National Institute of Neurological and Communicative Disorders and Stroke and the Alzheimer's Disease and Related Disorders Association, which specify eight cognitive domains that are compromised in AD - memory, language, perceptual skills, attention, constructive abilities, orientation, problem solving and functional abilities - and give guidelines for impairment assessment and diagnosis. NINCDS-ADRDA criteria have proven reliable over the years and have been extensively updated in 2007 to account for recent advances in neuroimaging (Dubois et al., 2007).

1.3 Symptoms

Symptom progression of AD			
Function	**Stage I (mild)**	**Stage II (moderate)**	**Stage III (severe)**
Memory	Mild amnesia (recent memory)	Amnesia (recent and remote)	Not measurable
Language	Quasi-normal, anomia	Sensory aphasia	Severely impaired
Perceptual skills	Mildly impaired	Moderately to severely impaired	Not measurable
Attention	Reduced	Impaired	Not measurable
Constructive abilities	Reduced	Impaired	Not measurable
Orientation	Mildly impaired	Impaired	Not measurable
Problem solving	Mildly impaired	Impaired	Not measurable
Functional abilities	Almost normal, some mistakes	Unreliable	Not measurable
Behavior	Mild changes, signs of withdrawal	Absent	Agitated, delusional
Gait	Normal	Normal	Impaired
Posture	Normal	Normal or flexed	Bedridden
MMSE	25-21	20-11	10-0

Table 1. Symptom progression of AD; MMSE: Mini-mental state examination (Folstein et al., 1975).

1.4 AD pathology

1.4.1 Macroscopic pathology

Atrophy is the major macroscopic characteristic of the AD brain. Ventricles are dilated, gyri appear narrower and sulci wider than in a normal brain. The loss of tissue, which roughly correlates with the degree of cognitive decline, is so severe that an AD brain can weigh less than 1000g. Frontal, parietal and temporal lobes are all involved, the hippocampus in particular being severely affected. The primary sensory-motor cortex appears affected with some delay, whereas the occipital lobe is relatively spared.

1.4.2 Microscopic pathology

The 'miliary foci' and fibril aggregations that Alzheimer observed are today normally referred to as senile plaques (SPs) and neurofibrillary tangles (NTFs), and remain the hallmarks of AD.

SPs are clusters of protein fibrils that form in the extracellular space, made of an amyloidal core, abnormal neurites and glial cells. The amyloidal core is mainly an aggregation of Amyloid-beta (Aβ), a 4 kDa peptide 39 to 43 amino acids long, which is produced by the proteolytic cleavage of the APP, a transmembrane protein present in many cell types and highly concentrated on neuron synapses. Usually, APP is cleaved on the extracellular side of the neuronal membrane by the enzyme α-secretase, but occasionally it can be cleaved by two other enzymes (β- and γ-secretase) at different sites. The result is anyway the production of Aβ segments that are released in the extracellular space and aggregate there in amyloidal plaques. The gene for APP is located on the long arm of chromosome 21.

SPs are roughly spherical with a diameter reaching up to 200 μm, and are normally distinguished in 'diffuse' and 'compact': Diffuse SPs are amorphous deposits of non-fibrillar 'pre-amyloid' Aβ, which produce no alteration of the neuropil. Compact SPs, more often referred to as 'neuritic', show instead an amyloid core surrounded by dystrophic neuritis. The latter appear as clusters of radially oriented neuronal processes.

There are at least 3 subtypes of neuritic SPs: Primitive, which lack the amyloidal core; Classical, in which a dense amyloid core is surrounded by dystrophic neuritis, which in turn appear interconnected by low density amyloidal fibrils; Burned-out, which have only the dense amyloidal core and at most a few neurites. This subdivision mirrors what researches believe is SPs' evolution: after being released, Aβ segments forms diffuse plaques in the extracellular space until elements such as cytokines, ApoE, proteoglycans and others become embedded with the complex causing it to degenerate into neuritic plaques. In other words, SPs start as diffuse and then evolve into neuritic, first primitive, then classical, and finally burned out.

SPs appear to have also an anatomical hierarchy: higher-order association areas have the highest density of SPs, whereas the primary sensory-motor cortex the lowest. Striatum and cerebellum show a rather high density of SPs, but they are all of the diffuse type. The hippocampus appears relatively spared.

Only neuritic SPs are specific to AD, whereas diffuse SPs are found also in the brains of non-demented elderly individuals.

NFTs are aggregates of modified protein tau in the intracellular space. In normal conditions, the protein tau binds to microtubules, contributes to the progress of their formation and is a key element in their stability. In AD, tau undergoes hyper-phosphorylation which causes the protein to aggregate. Moreover, upon hyper-phosphorylation, tau loses its binding capability so that the microtubules disintegrate. Each filament is made of two strands twisted around each other to form a helix, whose period is about 80 nm and diameter either 8 nm or 20 nm.

In AD, the areas most affected by NFTs are hippocampus, sibiculum, amygdala, entorhinal and transentorhinal corteces. In the neocortex, higher-order association areas are more affected than the unimodal association areas, and the primary sensory-motor cortex is relatively spared. NFTs are also numerous in the nucleus basalis, limbic nuclei of the thalamus, locus ceruleus, substantia nigra, and the raphe nuclei of the brainstem.

NFTs' shapes seem to be influenced by the shape of the neuron in which they are. In fact, they look like a flame in pyramidal neurons, as for example in the hippocampus, whereas they appear more globular in rounded neurons, such as those of the nucleus basalis.

NFT develop first into early and then into fully grown tangles. After the death of the neuron some NFTs (often referred to as 'ghost' tangles) are visible also in the extracellular space.

It is important to remember, though, that NFTs are not AD specific and are frequent also in non-demented elderly individuals.

Neuropil threads are another form of neurofibrillary degeneration that in AD is found widely distributed throughout the gray matter, especially in distal dendrites and axons. They owe their name to their appearance which resembles short threads.

As mentioned above, the ultimate result of the presence of plaques and tangles in AD is a severe neuronal loss that can reach 60% in the hippocampus and 80% in the nucleus basalis and in some frontal and temporal areas.

2. Hypotheses on the causes of AD

2.1 Classic hypotheses

There are three major classic hypotheses on the origin of AD. The cholinergic hypothesis (Francis et al., 1999, Rossor 1983), which is the oldest and the one on which the majority of currently available drug therapies are based, proposes that AD is caused by a reduced synthesis of the neurotransmitter acetylcholine. The amyloid hypothesis (Hardy & Allsop, 1991) postulates instead that the fundamental cause of the disease is the deposition of Aβ, which is supported by the evidence that mutations in the gene for APP, which is known to cause Aβ aggregation, are linked to AD. The tau hypothesis, based on a study demonstrating that deposition of Aβ plaques does not correlate well with neuron loss (Schmitz et al., 2004), proposes that abnormalities in the tau protein initiate the disease cascade.

Safety and efficacy of more than 500 pharmaceutical treatments are being investigated in clinical trials worldwide on the basis of these three hypotheses. In 2008, two separate clinical trials showed positive results in modifying the course of the disease in mild to moderate AD: one with the metal complexing agent PBT2 (Lannfelt et al., 2008) and one with methylthioninium chloride (Wischik, 2008), a drug that inhibits tau aggregation, which unfortunately failed to confirm the positive results in its phase III.

2.2 The metal hypothesis

Recently, researchers have uncovered an important role played in AD neurodegeneration by transition metals via their properties to cause oxidative stress. In fact, copper and iron are known to participate in Fenton-type reactions that generate uncontrollable reactive oxygen species (ROS) capable of damaging and destroying molecular and cellular compartments (Atwood et al., 2004).

Authors have widely reported enhanced metal concentrations in specific areas of AD patients' brains, in particular of iron, copper and zinc in cerebrospinal fluid (CSF) (Smith et al., 2010), of iron in the basal ganglia (Bartzokis et al., 2000, Bartzokis & Tishler, 2000), and of both iron and copper within SPs and NFTs (Good et al., 1992, Lovell et al., 1998). It has been also observed that APP possesses selective zinc and copper binding sites which mediate redox activity, causing precipitation of Aβ even at low concentrations (Bush et al., 1994). Also Aβ possesses selective high and low-affinity metal-binding sites. They can bind equimolar amounts of copper and zinc but, in conditions of acidosis, copper completely displaces zinc from Aβ (Atwood et al., 2000). Aβ reduces the metal ions by transferring electrons to O_2 and generating hydrogen peroxide in the process.

If on the one hand Aβ deposition in plaques is an age-dependent phenomenon, on the other hand Aβ production does not appear to increase with age. This seems to indicate that other age-dependent changes, as for example changes in metal homeostasis, may play a key role in Aβ transformation and neurotoxicity. Since copper and zinc are both modulators of the glutamatergic neurotransmission (Bush & Tanzi, 2008), abnormalities in metal homeostasis can have detrimental effects on synaptic processes, such as metal reuptake or storage in the synaptic cleft. All this evidence has eventually led to the proposal of a Metal Hypothesis of AD (Bush & Tanzi, 2008), which is based on the concept that it is the interaction of Aβ with specific metals, especially copper, that drives AD pathogenesis by promoting aggregation and neurotoxicity. By now, this view has become fully accepted and there is general agreement on the existence of a link between AD and oxidative stress phenomena triggered by transition metals. The Metal hypothesis of AD is now supported by the results of numerous clinical studies (Squitti et al., 2006, Squitti et al., 2002a, Squitti et al., 2003, Squitti et al., 2005).

3. Iron

3.1 Iron essentiality

Iron is essential for life. Of the 4-5 grams of iron normally present in a healthy body, about 2.5 g bind to hemoglobin and are used to promote respiration. Normally iron is absorbed from digested food or supplements. Average amounts are 1 mg/day for men, and 1.5-2 mg/day for women (Institute of Medicine Food and Nutrition Board, 2001). The majority is absorbed in the duodenum, where enterocytes of the duodenal lining reduce ferric Fe^{3+} to ferrous Fe^{2+}, which is then transported across the enterocyte's cell membrane into the cell by the divalent metal transporter 1 (DMT1). After completing a number of functions, available Fe^{+2} is transported back out of the cell by ferroportin, which is distributed throughout the duodenum enterocytes. Hephaestin, a ferroxidase found mainly in the small intestine, oxidizes Fe^{2+} back to ferric Fe^{3+}. At this point Fe^{+3} binds transferrin, a protein which takes it into circulation. Our body does not have a way to excrete iron in excess, so that the latter is stored inside another 450 kDa protein, ferritin, which can store up to 4500 atoms of iron per molecule (Fleming & Bacon, 2005).

3.2 Iron toxicity and the role of ceruloplasmin

Transported by transferrin, Fe^{3+} reaches the brain's capillaries and the Blood-Brain-Barrier (BBB), which is made of the brain capillary endothelial cells (BCECs) forming the wall of the

capillaries. The luminal side of the BCECs presents transferrin receptors that pick up the iron-loaded transferrin protein. An endocytosis is initiated and the receptor-transferrin complex is internalized into an endosome. Iron remains inside the endosome while the latter crosses through the BCEC and reaches the abluminal side. Here the endosome fuses with the external membrane, exposing and then releasing Fe^{3+} to the extracellular interstitial space. The apo-transferrin remains attached to the receptor and the two undergo again an endocytosis to travel back to the BCEC luminal side, where apo-transferrin is released into the capillary blood for re-cycling.
In the extracellular space, two Fe^{3+} atoms bind to a passing transferrin molecule, which allows iron to reach the vicinity of a neuron. The neuron membrane displays transferrin receptors, an endocytosis is again initiated and the receptor-transferrin complex is engulfed in an endosome that sinks into the neuron. Differently from the BCECs, though, the neuron possesses DMT1s which allow Fe^{2+} to be released into the neuron's intracellular space, where iron can finally complete its nutritional function.
Unfortunately, a potentially dangerous outcome of this process is the reduction of iron back into Fe^{2+}. Iron is particularly dangerous in this oxidative state since it can easily enter Fenton reactions with H_2O_2:

$$Fe^{2+} + H_2O_2 \rightarrow Fe^{3+} + \bullet OH + OH^- \quad (1)$$

The hydroxyl radical •OH is the most reactive and vicious of all ROS species. Moreover, the above reaction easily proceeds as follows:

$$Fe^{3+} + H_2O_2 \rightarrow Fe^{2+} + \bullet OOH + H^+ \quad (2)$$

Fortunately, the neuron also displays ferroportin molecules on its membrane, which channel Fe^{2+} out into the extracellular space. At this point, a fundamental role in the neuron health is played by ceruloplasmin, a protein present on the astrocytic end-foot. In fact, ceruloplasmin catalyzes the oxidation of $Fe^{2}+$ into $Fe^{3}+$, by way of the following chemical reaction:

$$4\,Fe^{2+} + 4\,H^+ + O_2 \rightarrow 4\,Fe^{3+} + 2\,H_2O \quad (3)$$

Therefore, an unbalance of the ceruloplasmin content or efficiency induces iron-dependent oxidative damage to brain tissues (Patel et al., 2002).
Copper can enter exactly the same reactions, passing through Cu^{2+} to Cu^{1+} oxidative states. This confers to ceruloplasmin a special character as a 'crosstalk' factor linking copper to iron metabolism, which appears disarranged in AD.

4. Copper

4.1 Copper essentiality

Copper is also an essential nutrient for man and is normally ingested via food, although it has been recently proposed that varying degrees of intake originate from drinking water piped through copper plumbing (Brewer, 2010). Copper status in the body is regulated by both duodenal absorption (intestine) and biliary excretion (liver). After crossing the intestinal lumen, copper is transported to the liver via portal circulation. Here, copper is partly stored and partly redistributed to other organs. In the hepatocytes, in particular, copper is incorporated into ceruloplasmin and into low-molecular-weight compounds, and then routed into peripheral circulation or secreted into the bile for excretion. Absorption and excretion interplay in such a way that an occasional over-ingestion in healthy adults normally results in a down-regulation of copper uptake in the duodenum and an up-regulation of biliary excretion.

4.2 Bound and free copper

About 85-95% of copper tightly binds to ceruloplasmin, whereas the remainder loosely binds to and is exchanged among albumin, α2 macroglobulin, amino acids, peptides and several micronutrients. We will refer to the portion that binds to ceruloplasmin as 'bound' copper, and to the portion that binds to the loose compounds as 'free' copper (Linder et al., 1979), following a custom of Wilson's Disease clinical care.

A key difference between bound and free copper lies in the fact that the limited size of the low-molecular-weight compounds and the labile nature of their binding allow free copper to easily cross the BBB (Chutkow, 1978). A recent study (Choi & Zheng, 2009) has in fact shown that the bulk of copper transport into the brain is achieved by free copper ions travelling through the BBB, whereas ceruloplasmin-bound copper represents less than 1% of the brain bound copper. Normal ranges, within which 95% of the normal population falls and which are normally taken as reference values, are 11-22.4 μmol/L for serum copper (corresponding to 70-142.7 μg/dL), 20-60 mg/dL for ceruloplasmin, and 0-1.6 μmol/L for free copper (corresponding to 10 μg/dL) (Jacobs, 2002).

It is generally assumed that normal values are 'healthy', although some authors suggest caution in this regard considering that natural selection works to optimize health and survival only during the reproductive period. Consequently, 'normal' values may not be necessarily optimal after age 50 (Brewer, 2007). In fact, ranges of plasma/serum copper values of healthy elderly individuals reported in the literature are very heterogeneous, adding complexity in the interpretation of their results (Squitti, 2011).

4.3 Copper toxicity

Although copper is an essential nutrient for man, it becomes extremely toxic when its levels loose balance. It is a transition metal and as such takes part in a variety of biological reduction and oxidation (redox) reactions, which make it an important cofactor of many redox enzymes. As mentioned above, copper can easily go into Haber-Weiss and Fenton reactions producing •OH (1), against which the body has no defenses (Gutteridge & Halliwell, 1990). An overload of this metal can easily lead to oxidative reactions resulting in cell damage and death.

Moreover, copper absorption and excretion is regulated by mechanisms controlled by genetic as well as environmental factors. Therefore, a copper toxicosis is generally the result of a failure of one or more of those mechanisms, although sometimes, but infrequently, a copper excess may be due to a clinical disease, such a liver cirrhosis. The genetic origin of copper toxicosis manifests itself most clearly in the failure to express a specific copper transporter, particularly in the liver (see below). Sheep, for example, are easily subject to copper toxicosis since they are not able to increase biliary copper excretion in response to an increased intake. Conversely, pigs are known to tolerate even severe increases of copper intake very well for the opposite reason (Bremner, 1979). However, toxicity per se ultimately stems from copper's ability to catalyze the production of compounds that generate oxidative stress, as expressed in reactions (1), (2), (3) detailed above.

The disruption of the system controlling copper homeostasis has serious consequences for the health and development of the brain. This is well exemplified by two genetic disorders, showing either shortage - Menkes' disease - or excess - Wilson's disease - of systemic copper, but both resulting in neurodegeneration. In these diseases, the genes coding for the two membrane copper transport proteins ATPase7A and ATPase7B are mutated. These two proteins are highly homologous, but with different patterns of tissue expression: ATPase7A (Menkes' protein) is mainly expressed in the intestine and in the BBB, while ATPase7B (Wilson's protein) is primarily found in the liver (Harris, 2000). The mutation impairs the function of the ATPase7A pump and prevents copper absorption at the intestinal level. This causes copper deficiency and reduces the levels of cuproenzymes (Harris, 2000). The location of ATPase7A at the choroid plexes makes this pump crucial for controlling the copper flux into the ventricles of the brain (Qian et al., 1998). Indeed, the copper deficiency in the brain of Menkes' patients is particularly severe because of a decrease in the activity of ATPase7A at the BBB. Defects of ATPase7B in Wilson's disease cause impairment of copper incorporation into ceruloplasmin, with consequent failure of copper release into the bile canalicula for excretion (Iyengar et al., 1988). This produces a copper overload into the hepatocytes, inducing liver cirrhosis as well as slight increased levels of free copper. At the death of the cirrhotic hepatocytes, copper – actually free copper - is released into general circulation in huge amounts and reaches all organs and tissues, including the brain (Choi & Zheng, 2009, Hartter & Barnea, 1988, Iyengar et al., 1988). The holo-active form of ceruloplasmin depends on the ATPase7B activity, which mediates the incorporation of copper atoms into ceruloplasmin during its biosynthesis (Bielli & Calabrese, 2002). ATPase7B absence or impairment prevents copper translocation to the secretory pathway, resulting in 1) secretion of unstable apo-ceruloplasmin which is rapidly degraded in the blood (Bielli & Calabrese, 2002); 2) alteration of copper excretion through the bile via ceruloplasmin (Iyengar et al., 1988); 3) severe hypo-function, which can even cause death, of hepatocytes; 4) release of free copper in general circulation and tissue copper overload or intoxication (Bielli & Calabrese, 2002). During aging, control over copper homeostasis can undergo progressive failure and even "normal" copper values could result in an altered copper burden in the aged brain (Deibel et al., 1996).

4.4 Copper chaperones

Besides the obvious function as means of transportation, chaperones are also the main defense system against copper excess. Copper import into the intestinal epithelial cells is mediated by the membrane protein Copper transporter protein 1 (Ctr1) (Figure 1) (Kim et al., 2008).

Based on its structural and biochemical properties, Ctr1 could be thought of as a Cu^{+1}-specific pore. In hepatocytes, intracellular copper is carried by specific chaperone proteins to Cu-dependent enzymes. So far, researchers have identified three copper chaperones, although new candidates are being investigated: the Human Atox 1 Homologue (HAH1), homologous to the yeast Antioxidant protein 1 (Atox1); the Copper Chaperone for Superoxide Dismutase (CCS); the Cytochrome C Oxidase Assembly Homologue (COX17). HAH1 delivers copper to the two mammalian P-type Cu-transporting ATPases, ATPase7A and ATPase7B. CCS delivers copper to the metal-binding site of Copper-Zinc superoxide dismutase (Cu,Zn SOD). COX17 delivers copper to the mitochondria, where it is ultimately incorporated into the Cytochrome C Oxidase. In a healthy physiological environment, virtually no copper remains unbound (Fig. 1) (Kim, et al., 2008). The chaperone system also includes metallothioneins, a family of proteins, whose expression is regulated by copper and other metals (Palmiter, 1994) and which are active in trapping metals in excess. It has been reported that Metallothionein-3, a member of the family expressed exclusively in the central nervous system and involved in neuronal damage repair through its neuro-inhibitory activity, is significantly down-regulated in AD (Durand et al.,2010 , Meloni et al., 2008, Yu et al., 2001). It was recently proven that this protein protects cultured neurons from toxicity generated by Aβ. A metal swap between Metallothionein-3 and soluble aggregated Aβ 1-40-Cu^{2+} avoids ROS production and consequent cellular toxicity. Finally, Cu,Zn SOD, beside its primary antioxidant function of superoxide dismutation, also plays a role as a buffer of intracellular free copper, since it is stable in its copper-free form (Rossi et al., 1994).

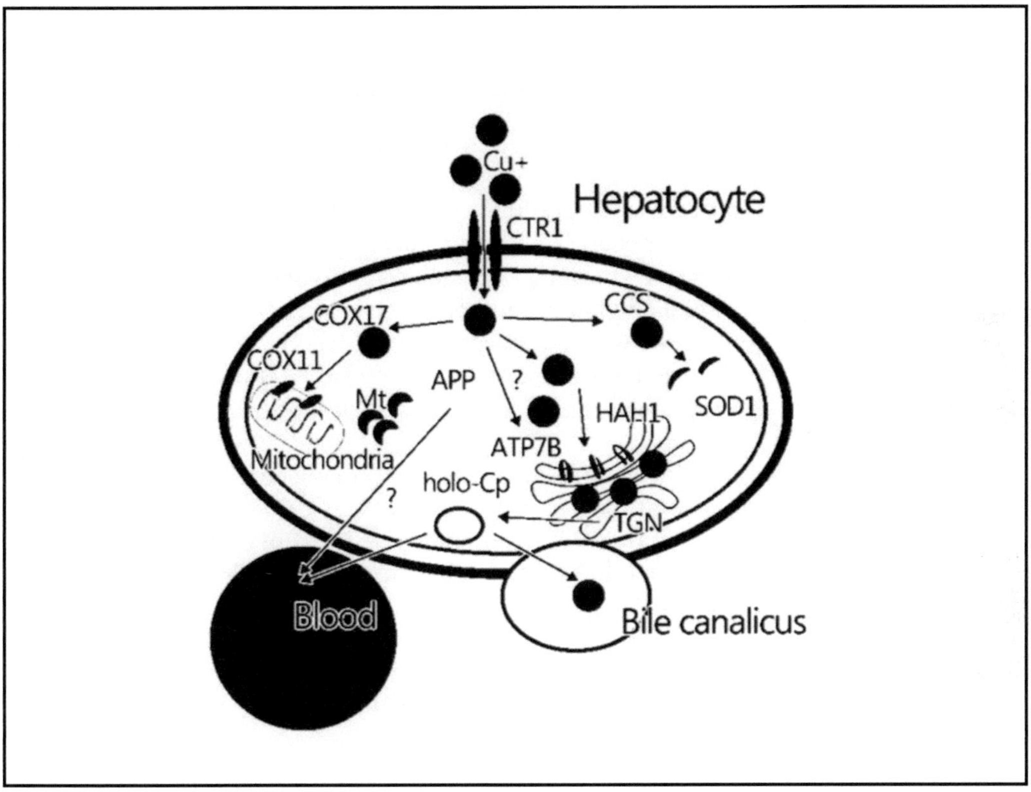

Fig. 1. Copper is metabolically finely regulated by the organism. Once copper crosses the intestinal lumen, it is transported into the liver via portal circulation. In the hepatocytes copper is incorporated into ceruloplasmin, other copper proteins and compounds and then routed into peripheral circulation or secreted into the bile for excretion. Copper in excess from general circulation is excreted through the kidney, in urine. In the hepatocytes, intracellular copper is carried by specific chaperone proteins to Cu-dependent enzymes. Three copper chaperones have been identified to date: the Human Atox 1 Homologue (HAH1), homologous to the yeast Antioxidant protein 1 (Atox1); the Copper Chaperone for Superoxide Dismutase (CCS); the Cytochrome C Oxidase assembly homologue (COX17). The amyloid precursor protein (APP) is deemed to be a new copper chaperone.

4.5 Copper and Aβ

Neurodegenerative metallochemistry has developed on the observation that APP possesses selective zinc and copper binding sequences (Table 1). These sites mediate redox activity and can cause the precipitation of Aβ under mildly acidic conditions, even at very low concentrations (Atwood et al., 1998). Researchers believe that this is what happens in the AD brain (Atwood et al., 1998). Moreover, Aβ reduces the metal ions, producing hydrogen peroxide by transferring electrons to O_2 (Huang et al., 1999a, Huang et al., 1999b). This reduction is the key of Aβ-induced oxidative stress and toxicity, since hydrogen peroxide is a well known pro-oxidant molecule as it triggers Fenton's like reactions (1) (2) that generate hydroxyl radicals (see formulas in iron paragraph).

Milestones	Key Findings
The amyloid precursor protein (APP) is a copper protein	APP has a copper binding domain which reduces Cu(II) to Cu(I) and produces oxidative stress (Barnham et al., 2003b, Multhaup et al., 1996) Depletion of intracellular copper results in a reduction of APP gene expression (Bellingham et al., 2004b)
Zinc and copper interactions with Aβ	Zinc rapidly destabilized human Aβ40 solutions, inducing tinctorial amyloid formation (Bush et al., 1994) Aβ peptide with the sulfur atom of Met-35 oxidized to a sulfoxide is toxic to neuronal cells (Barnham et al., 2003a) Aβ peptide aggregation is induced by copper binding (Atwood et al., 2000) Aβ-Cu interaction generates ROS (Huang et al., 1999b, Multhaup et al., 1996) APP-Cu induced toxicity and oxidative stress in primary neuronal cultures, producing neuronal demise (Huang et al., 1999a, White et al., 1999a)
Solubilization of native Aβ from AD brain, transgenic mice and cell models by metal complexing agents	Solubilization of Aβ from post-mortem brain tissue was significantly increased by the presence of chelators, EGTA, N,N,N*,N*-tetrakis(2-pyridyl-methyl) ethylene diamine, and bathocuproine (Cherny et al., 1999) bis(thiosemicarbazonato) complexes - MII(btsc) examined in chinese hamster ovary cells overexpressing APP increased levels of bioavailable intracellular copper and zinc but also resulted in a dose-dependent reduction of Aβ levels (Donnelly et al., 2008)
Cu-dependent catalytic conversion of dopamine, cholesterol, and biological reducing agents to neurotoxic H_2O_2 *in vitro* and animal models	Aβ binds copper and cholesterol, facilitating copper oxidation of cholesterol to 7-OH cholesterol and to 4-cholestenone, which are extremely toxic to neurons. Cholesterol can catalyse copper-Aβ redox cycling (Opazo et al., 2002, Puglielli et al., 2005) Trace amounts of copper given to cholesterol-fed rabbits induced accumulation of Aβ in senile plaques and impaired the animals' learning capability (Sparks et al., 2006, Sparks & Schreurs, 2003)

Table 2. Milestones of the Evidence of Metal Implication in AD

APP binds copper in two domains, one located in the extracellular N-terminal region and the other in the C-terminal region within the Aβ peptide (review in Squitti & Zito, 2009). It has been proposed that APP reduces Cu^{2+} to Cu^{1+} upon coordination, thus promoting the non-amyloidogenic cleavage pathway (Barnham et al., 2003b). The ablation of APP, which is normally expressed both in the brain and in a limited number of non-neural tissues as platelets, liver, kidney, and heart (Duce et al., 2010, White et al., 1999b) in knockout mice models produces metal dishomeostasis in these organs and tissues. APP-depleted knockout mice have shown a stunning 80% increase of copper concentrations in the liver and a 40% increase in the brain. Recently, Duce et al., (2010) reported that APP ablation causes an iron increase of 26% in the brain, 31% in the liver and 15% in the kidney.
As mentioned above, Aβ is generated from APP cleavage by α-, β- and γ-secretases. β-secretase (BACE1) cleaves at the N terminus, while γ-secretase cleaves at the C terminus of the Aβ sequence. BACE1 is an aspartic protease and may function as a dimer, whereas γ-secretase is a complex of presenilin-1/2, Aph1, Pen2, and Nicastrin (Edbauer et al., 2003). It was reported that BACE1 modulates APP processing and the release of Aβ by interacting with CCS. The concept that copper content can modulate BACE1, i.e. the rate-limiting enzyme in the production of Aβ (Angeletti et al., 2005), is supported by the recent evidence that copper (Cu^{2+}) and manganese (Mn^{2+}) potently increase the expression of both APP and BACE1 in a time- and concentration-dependent manner, whereas zinc (Zn^{2+}), iron (Fe^{2+}) and aluminum (Al^{3+}) do not (Lin et al., 2008). *In vitro* studies have demonstrated that different variants of Aβ (1-40, 1-42) have different affinity for copper, and that higher affinity generates higher toxicity (Crouch et al., 2007). The results of recent *in vitro* studies suggest that Cytochrome C Oxidase, and therefore the energy production of the cell, may be one of the targets of the Cu-Aβ toxic effect (Crouch et al., 2005). Conversely, copper plays a role in the basal regulation of the APP gene. This has been shown in human fibroblasts over-expressing ATPase7A, a condition that causes copper intracellular depletion. Depletion of intracellular copper in these cells results in significant reduction of APP gene expression (Bellingham et al., 2004a, Bellingham et al., 2004b). Moreover, a study of cDNA microarray technology demonstrated an up-regulation of APP and of the normal cellular prion protein (PrPC) in two genetic models of chronic copper overload mutants - fibroblasts from C57BL/6-Atp7aMobr and C57BL/6-Atp7aModap - and in a nutritional model of chronic copper overload (Armendariz et al., 2004).
Overall, this evidence shows that the APP gene harbours a copper response element within its promoter, such that copper depletion leads to a marked decrease in APP expression and supports the evidence that APP is involved in copper homeostasis as a copper detoxification/efflux protein.
Another line of evidence is the effectiveness of copper and iron chelators in hindering redox and toxic activities of Aβ and NTFs, whereas a replacement with those metals fully restores those activities (Sayre et al., 2000).
Regarding genetic risk factors, the *ApoE4*, which is the only well established risk factor for AD, has been demonstrated to interact with copper metabolism at different levels. It has been shown that ApoE protein possesses antioxidant properties which depend on 'bound' copper (Miyata & Smith, 1996, Moir et al., 1999, Sanan et al., 1994). ApoE4 isoform has a lower antioxidant power than ApoE2 or ApoE3, and is therefore the least effective in protecting neurons from the oxidative damage caused by Aβ. In fact, absolute and free copper concentrations are higher in carriers of the *ApoE4* allele than in non-carriers

(Gonzalez et al., 1999, Squitti et al., 2002a, Squitti et al., 2007). In addition, the correlation between typical electroencephalographic (EEG) spectral abnormalities of the AD brain and higher-than-normal serum levels of free copper is stronger in *ApoE4* carriers than in non-carriers (Babiloni et al., 2007b, Zappasodi et al., 2008).
The level of plasma homocysteine is a risk factor for AD (Babiloni et al., 2007a, Gorgone et al., 2009), and it's known that copper mediates Low-Density Lipoprotein (LDL) oxidation by homocysteine (Nakano et al., 2004).
Aβ binds copper and cholesterol, facilitating copper oxidation of cholesterol to 7-0H cholesterol and to 4-cholestenone (Puglielli et al., 2005), which are extremely toxic to neurons (Nelson & Alkon, 2005).
Trace amounts of copper, well below the levels considered safe for humans, given to cholesterol-fed rabbits have induced accumulation of Aβ in senile plaques and impaired the animals' learning capability (Sparks & Schreurs, 2003). Thus, it appears that cholesterol increases Aβ formation and copper promotes Aβ aggregation and toxicity. Furthermore, cholesterol can catalyze copper-Aβ redox cycling (Opazo et al., 2002). The results from the cholesterol-fed rabbit model have been confirmed in transgenic mice (Sparks et al., 2006) and provided the rational for the results of a large community prospective study showing a strong correlation between copper intake from a diet rich in saturated and trans fats and mental decline (Morris et al., 2006). As a result, serious concerns have been raised about a possible relationship between copper overexposure from vitamins or drinking water and cognitive disturbances (Brewer, 2010, Bush et al., 2003). The belief that copper toxicity is involved in the evolution of cognitive disturbances is also supported by recent investigations demonstrating an inverse correlation between cognitive performance and serum copper levels in cohorts of healthy aged individuals (Lam et al., 2008, Salustri et al., 2010a).

5. Metals in AD: A systemic view

The link between metals and AD has been traditionally investigated focusing on local metal accumulations in specific areas of the brain critical for AD. In this frame, authors have reported enhanced iron concentrations in AD brains, both in autopsy brain tissues and in CSF (Smith et al., 2010), in the basal ganglia (Bartzokis et al., 2000, Bartzokis & Tishler, 2000), and around SPs and NFTs (Good et al., 1992, Lovell, et al., 1998). Altered local concentrations of copper (Adlard & Bush, 2006), ceruloplasmin (Castellani et al., 1999, Loeffler et al., 1996), transferrin and ferritin (Connor et al., 1992) have been also reported.
We believe instead that the issue should be approached from the different perspective of systemic, rather than local, alterations. Results of many *in vivo* studies demonstrating correlations between abnormalities in metal homeostasis and specific deficits and markers of AD suggest that local accumulations should be viewed in a wider systemic alteration.

5.1 Iron

Besides of course its own levels in general circulation, typical markers of iron status are the levels of transferrin, ceruloplasmin, ferritin, transferrin saturation, together with the H63D and C282Y mutations of the HFE gene and transferrin's C2 polymorphism (TfC2). Since these gene variants are often associated with a distress of the liver, the classic liver function panel, i.e., albumin, transaminases (aspartate transaminase, AST; alanine transaminase, ALT) and prothrombin time, contribute to the picture.

In a study of 160 AD patients and 79 healthy elderly controls performed by our laboratory (Giambattistelli et al., 2011), we evaluated whether and how all the above listed markers of iron and liver status are interconnected. Our study revealed that AD patients have lower albumin, longer prothrombin time and higher AST/ALT values than controls, indicating a liver distress. Also, transferrin was lower and ferritin higher in AD patients. A multiple logistic regression backward analysis performed to evaluate the effects of these biochemical variables upon the probability to develop AD revealed that a simple one-unit decrease in serum transferrin increases the probability of AD by 80%. A one-unit albumin serum-decrease reduces the AD probability by 20%, while a one-unit increase of AST/ALT ratios generates a fourfold probability increase. The role of genetic mutations is well described by the fact that while healthy controls carriers of the H63D mutation showed a normal iron status, AD patients carriers of the same mutation showed a panel resembling hemochromatosis, i.e., higher levels of iron, lower levels of transferrin and ceruloplasmin. This picture was not found in non-carrier AD patients. These results suggest that carrying the H63D mutation is not itself sufficient to increase the risk of AD. Rather, it is a synergy between iron increase, a condition of liver dysfunction and the genetic mutation that appears to increase the probability of developing AD (Giambattistelli et al., 2011).

In another study, we measured serum levels of iron, ceruloplasmin and transferrin, calculated the transferrin saturation and evaluated the activation of the ceruloplasmin-transferrin (Cp-Tf) system, expressed by the Cp/Tf ratio, in relation to the main cognitive and anatomical deficit of AD, namely MMSE and medial temporal lobe atrophy (Squitti et al., 2010c). Results demonstrated that the values of ceruloplasmin, peroxides and Cp/Tf, besides being elevated, inversely correlated with MMSE scores, while medial temporal lobe atrophy positively correlated with Cp/Tf and negatively with serum iron levels. All these findings demonstrate that the alterations of iron metabolism that accompany the disease are systemic rather than local, and indicate that the role attributed by existing literature to local metal accumulations in brain areas critical for AD should be rather viewed in the frame of a wider systemic alteration, which could be approached taking into account both circulating biochemical markers variations and their genetic makeup. In this line, we recently explored the hypothesis that polymorphisms of ATP7B, the gene encoding the protein that controls the levels of free copper in the body and whose defects cause Wilson's disease, have higher frequencies in AD than in healthy individuals. Two groups of 190 AD patients and 164 controls were studied in order to compare the frequency of alleles for these two polymorphisms using a 'case-control' design. Two polymorphisms previously associated with Wilson's disease - GG genotype in the SNP 2495 A>G (Lys832Arg) (exon 10) and GG in c.1216T>G (Ser406Ala) (exon 2) – showed an association with susceptibility to AD (Bucossi et al., 2010). These polymorphisms also show a link to non-ceruloplasmin copper levels.

5.2 Copper

The existence of systemic copper dysfunctions in AD has been a controversial issue for many years. In fact, many studies have reported an increase of circulating copper in AD patients with respect to healthy controls (Arnal et al., 2010, Bocca et al., 2005, Gonzalez et al., 1999, Smorgon et al., 2004, Squitti et al., 2006, Squitti et al., 2009, Squitti et al., 2002a, Squitti, et al., 2003, Squitti et al., 2007, Zappasodi, et al., 2008), many others no variation (Basun et al., 1991, Baum et al., 2010, Gerhardsson et al., 2008, Jeandel et al., 1989, Kapaki et al., 1989, Molina et al., 1998, Ozcankaya & Delibas, 2002, Snaedal et al., 1998), and two very recent studies even a decrease of copper in plasma (Vural et al., 2010) and serum (Brewer et al., 2010) of AD patients. Moreover, the latter two studies are in line with two older studies showing that low plasma copper concentrations correlate with clinical worsening in AD, one reporting a copper plasma-decrease in more severe vs. less severe patients (Kessler et al., 2006), and the other a direct correlation between low plasma copper concentrations and cognitive decline (Pajonk et al., 2005).

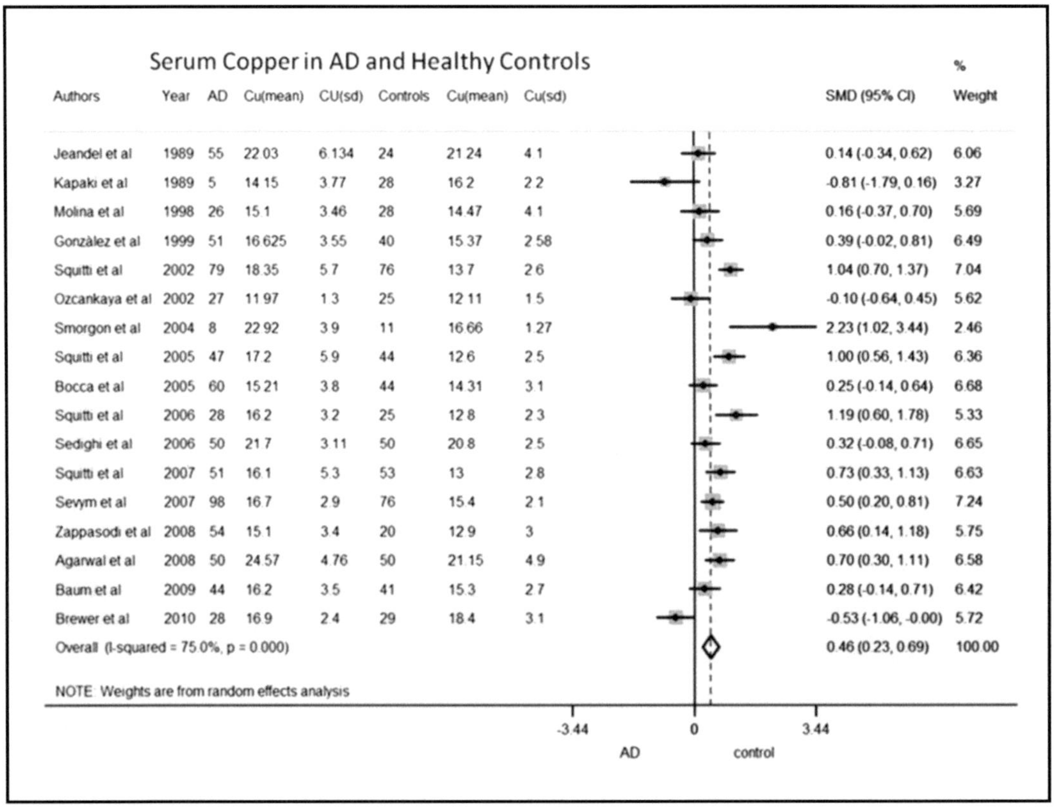

Fig. 2. Standardized mean difference (SMD) in copper serum level. The square represents the SMD between patients and controls. The size of the squares is proportional to the sample size of the study, the whiskers represents the 95% confidence interval. The diamond represents the pooled estimate based one random effects model, with the centre representing the point estimate and the width the associated 95% confidential intervals.

Recently, we have evaluated these heterogeneous results in a meta-analysis, which has analyzed data from all the serum, plasma and CSF studies published since 1983 on AD patients, to gain an objective evaluation of whether systemic copper variation are associated or not with AD. Meta-analysis is a quantitative method that combines the results of independent reports to distinguish between small effects and no effects, random variations, variations in sample used or in different analytical approaches. After an initial selection based on statistical criteria, data from 21 studies on serum copper and 5 studies on plasma copper were merged for a pooled total of 966 AD patients and 831 controls (Bucossi et al., 2010). The analysis concluded that AD patients have actually higher levels of serum copper than healthy controls (Fig. 2). Even though moderate, the assessed copper increase is sufficient to unambiguously distinguish AD patients from healthy controls.

Plasma data did not allow conclusions because of extremely high heterogeneity, but the meta-analysis of the combined serum and plasma studies confirmed higher copper levels in AD. The analysis of CSF data, instead, revealed no difference between AD patients and controls. Previous results from our laboratory are in line with the meta-analysis outcome. When we measured copper, iron, transferrin and copper-enzymes as ceruloplasmin and Cu,Zn SOD, together with total hydro-peroxides and total radical-trapping antioxidant potential (TRAP) levels in the sera of diverse AD patients cohorts (Rossi et al., 2002, Squitti et al., 2006, Squitti et al., 2004, Squitti et al., 2002a, Squitti et al., 2005, Squitti et al., 2007), we found that copper, peroxides and Cu,Zn SOD activity (Rossi et al., 2002) were higher, TRAP was lower and ceruloplasmin and iron did not differ between AD patients and healthy controls. These changes appeared to be specifically referred to the AD patients since they were not present in vascular dementia (VAD) patients, with the exception of TRAP that was lower in VAD patients in comparison to healthy controls (Squitti et al., 2003).

Diverse explanations can be advocated to account for the systemic copper abnormalities in AD. Inflammation can be one reason. In fact, ceruloplasmin, which accounts for 85-95% of circulating copper, is an acute phase reactant, whose levels increase during the inflammatory response. In a previous study (Squitti et al., 2005), our laboratory investigated whether markers of inflammation in general circulation were abnormal in AD, and showed that levels of ceruloplasmin were higher in AD than in healthy controls, though close to the significance threshold. However, it was clear that the level of ceruloplasmin increase could not account for the pronounced rise of serum copper estimated in the patient sample analyzed in that study. In fact, when we performed a deeper analysis by distinguishing between bound and free copper, results revealed that the copper increase in our AD patients was attributable to this latter fraction (Squitti et al., 2006, Squitti et al., 2009, Squitti et al., 2005). It must be remembered, though, that free copper abnormalities should be considered as an additional rather than alternative explanatory variable of copper disturbances in AD (Althaus, 2008, Arnal et al., 2010, Brewer et al., 2010, Hoogenraad, 2007).

5.3 The role of free copper

The considerations above support the notion of a fundamental distinction between the biochemical properties of bound and free copper.

The levels of free copper are higher in AD patients than in healthy individuals. One ultrafiltration study, aimed at finding filterable free copper in AD sera, has also revealed concentrations of free copper 3.7 times higher in AD patients than in controls (Squitti et al., 2006). Free copper levels correlate with AD main cognitive deficits (Squitti et al., 2006, Squitti et al., 2009, Squitti et al., 2004, Squitti et al., 2002a, Squitti et al., 2003, Squitti et al., 2005), with neuro-anatomical (Squitti et al., 2002a) and electrophysiological changes (Babiloni et al., 2007b, Zappasodi et al., 2008), with accepted AD markers (Squitti et al., 2006) and with known genetic risk factors, such as *ApoE4* (Squitti et al., 2002a, Zappasodi et al., 2008). Copper systemic abnormalities in AD resemble those observed in Wilson's disease, where the free fraction transported by micronutrients plays a fundamental role, while ceruloplasmin appears fragmented. Ceruloplasmin fragmentation, revealed by fragments <50 KDa, has been reported in AD patients showing higher-than-normal levels of free copper (Squitti et al., 2008). This suggests impairment in the incorporation of copper into the protein during the biosynthesis (see the "copper chaperones" section). It must be noted, though, that in Wilson's disease the free copper percentage is much higher than the one estimated in AD (Siotto et al., 2010) (Fig. 3).

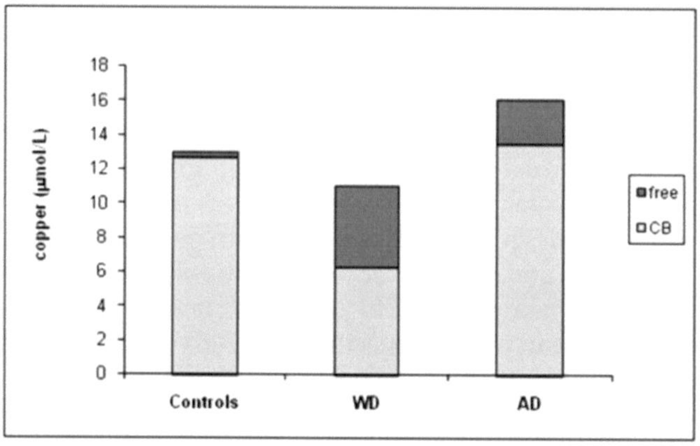

Fig. 3. Free copper in Alzheimer's disease (AD). The figure shows copper distribution its two serum pool - copper bound to ceruloplasmin (CB) and free copper - in healthy controls, Wilson's disease (WD) and AD patients.

Ceruloplasmin fragmentation, together with the free copper rise in AD, is a copper systemic abnormality that could be the cause or the result of a disturbed hepatocyte function, possibly resulting in liver hypo-metabolism. This notion is supported by the results of a clinical study by our laboratory which demonstrated that AD patients with no evidence of additional pathological conditions - including liver diseases - have higher free copper, longer prothrombin time and lower albumin levels than controls matched for age, sex and risk factors for cardiovascular diseases and medication intake (Squitti et al., 2007). Very recently, we reproduced the same evidence in a bigger cohort of AD associated with iron abnormalities (Giambattistelli et al., 2011). The hypothesis that copper, as well as iron (see below) in AD, might be related to liver hypofunction linked to APP metabolism at the hepatocyte level is strongly supported by the evidence that, in the APP knock-out mouse model, the APP ablation causes a massive (80%) copper increase in the liver (White et al., 1999b). More precisely, it could be speculated that, in this mouse model, a perturbation of copper efflux linked to APP at the liver level disrupts normal copper transport, producing a reduction of the liver's efficiency to excrete copper through the bile. This would explain the elevated (40%) copper level found in the brain (White et al., 1999b). A hint towards this interpretation comes from another study of ours, in which we estimated - via a clearance measure - that about 3% of serum free copper is related to CSF copper increase in AD patients, possibly interacting with Aβ (Squitti et al., 2006). This evidence fits very well with previous results in a mouse model of brain uptake of radiocopper [^{67}Cu(II)], as also confirmed by data of a recent study (Choi & Zheng, 2009). In the [^{67}Cu(II)] mouse model, a net brain copper uptake occurs and parallels the free copper increase in the injectate, starting from a concentration of Cu(II) of 3.2 ng/mL, corresponding to 0.05 μmol/L, much lower than the 2.5 μmol/L value that we evaluated in clinical studies on AD patients (Squitti & Salustri, 2009).

The belief that there is a direct interaction between copper and Aβ, based on the strong negative correlation between free copper in serum and Aβ in the CSF (Squitti et al., 2006), is sustained by the negative correlation between copper and Aβ in the CSF found by other authors (Strozyk et al., 2009). This evidence is also supported by the fact that copper detectable in the CSF is not ceruloplasmin-bound, but is bound to a not yet identified ligand (Que et al., 2008).

The occurrence of copper increase or decrease in the brain is a debated issue. Some authors suggested that there is a decrease in bulk tissue levels in AD brains, and particularly in the neocortex (Adlard & Bush, 2006). Loeffer and coworkers (Loeffler et al., 1996) reported instead that ceruloplasmin and copper are actually increased in AD. Deibel and coworkers (Deibel et al., 1996) and Platin and coworkers (Platin et al., 1987) reported lower levels of copper in the amygdala and in the hippocampus of AD brains than controls, however the authors determined nanograms of copper on micrograms of weight tissue, instead of nanograms of copper on micrograms of proteins present in the sample, and it is known that the AD brain tissue has plenty of plaques and not of proteins, so their evaluation at least arises some concerns. Religa's and Squitti's groups (Religa et al. 2006, Squitti et al., 2007) did not find a copper decrease in AD. Also our recent meta-analysis of copper-related literature (Bucossi et al., 2010) revealed no difference in CSF copper between AD patients and healthy controls. So caution is needed when facing this issue. Seminal studies indicate that copper dyshomeostasis in the brain, present in normal aging (Maynard et al., 2002), is substantially more pronounced in the aged AD brain (Lovell et al., 1998). In fact, copper levels in the plaque-free neuropil of an AD brain are approximately 4 times higher than in the neuropil of a healthy brain, and approximately 30% higher in the Aβ plaques than in plaque-free regions.

Our laboratory has started investigating metal involvement in AD as revealed by systemic markers detectable in general circulation, and clinical indices of prognosis or AD conversion. In particular, in order to evaluate whether information on iron or copper abnormalities can help in the AD prognosis, we assessed levels of copper, iron, zinc, transferrin, ceruloplasmin, peroxides, TRAP, free copper and *ApoE4* genotype in 81 mild or moderate AD patients (Squitti et al., 2009). We studied the association of these wide set of parameters with the patients' scores in the MMSE (primary outcome), in the Activities of Daily Living (ADL) and Instrumental of Daily Living (IADL) tests (secondary outcomes), performed at study entry and after 1 year. Our study revealed that free copper can predict the annual change in MMSE, adjusted for the baseline MMSE: it raised the explained variance from 2.4% (with only sex, age and education) to 8.5% ($p = 0.026$). When the annual change in MMSE was divided into <3 or >=3 points, free copper was the only predictor of a more severe decline (predicted probability of MMSE worsening 23%). In other words, this study showed an association between systemic copper deregulation and unfavorable evolution of cognitive function in AD patients, demonstrating that free copper identify those patients at higher risk for a more severe decline (Squitti et al., 2009).

In a very recent study we tested the hypothesis that free copper was increased significantly enough to distinguish also individuals affected by mild cognitive impairment (MCI) from healthy controls (Squitti et al., 2011). To verify this hypothesis a sample of 83 MCI subjects were compared with 100 elderly controls in terms of levels of serum copper, free copper, ceruloplasmin, *ApoE4*, iron, transferrin, and TRAP. The groups were compared also in terms of demographic and cardiovascular risk factors. The comparison with an additional group of 105 mild to moderate AD patients was also evaluated. A multinomial logistic regression analysis demonstrated that *ApoE4* and free copper differentiated MCI from healthy subjects. Chances to acquire MCI increased about 24% for each free copper unit (μmol/L) increment. *ApoE4* and free copper differentiated the MCI group also from the AD group. *ApoE4* and free copper appeared associated to

MMSE worsening, as did age and sex (Squitti et al., 2011). A follow-up study is in progress on MCI subjects, which will test whether free copper can provide information about who, within the MCI subjects, will progress to AD.

In another study we have investigated normal women over age 50 (Salustri et al., 2010a). We studied their free and ceruloplasmin bound copper, and measured MMSE and several other measures of memory and cognition (19 neuropsychological test battery). We found that free (but not ceruloplasmin bound) copper levels correlated inversely with MMSE and certain other measures of memory, that is, the higher the free copper, the poorer the performance on these measures of cognition.

Subsequently, we investigated the relationship between depression, which is advocated as a risk factor of AD, markers of oxidative stress and neurotransmission, as expressed by sensory cortex excitability (Dal Forno et al., 2005, Salustri et al., 2010b). Serum levels of oxidative stress markers and somatosensory magnetic fields, evoked by external galvanic stimulation, were measured in 13 depressed patients and 13 controls. Depressives had higher levels of total and free copper than controls and lower levels of transferrin. They also showed lower sensory cortex excitability, which correlated with copper levels in controls, but not in depressed patients. Transferrin correlated with sensory cortex excitability in both patients and controls, although in opposite ways. Copper level results associated with the patients' clinical status. Pro-oxidant compounds appear to affect neuronal excitability and clinical state of depressed patients, as free copper excess alters their cortical glutamatergic neurotransmission (Salustri et al., 2010a).

6. Treatment of AD with metal complexing agents

Since the '90s, researchers have cultivated the idea that a tuned redistribution of metals (aluminum, iron, selenium, zinc, copper) via metal complexing or ligand agents may positively affect the natural progression of AD. Numerous studies have been published reporting on tests with metal complexing agents as potential therapeutics for AD (Duce & Bush, 2010, Liu et al., 2010, Price et al., 2007), and their pros and cons, as well as the challenges associated with their usage, are under debate (Hegde et al., 2009, Squitti & Salustri, 2009, Squitti & Zito, 2009). The following is a summary of the most promising molecules with metal redistribution properties developed so far, together with a description of their potential or proven applications.

Zinc-induced aggregation of Aβ can be reversed by the divalent metal ion chelator ethilendiamine tetra acetic acid (EDTA)(Huang et al., 1999a). Solubilisation of Aβ derived from AD brains was achieved with N,N,N',N'-tetrakis (2-pyridylmethyl) ethylene diamine (TPEN) and 2,9-dimethyl-4,7-diphenyl-1,10-phenanthroline (bathocuproine) (Cherny et al., 1999). Bathocuproine, bathophenahtroline and diethylenetriamine penta-acetic acid (DTPA) halted Aβ redox activity complexing copper (Atwood et al., 2004).

Another metal ligand molecule [1,2-bis(2-aminophenyloxy)ethane-N,N,N',N'-bis (2-octadecyloxyethyl) ester,N,N'-disodiumsalt] DP-109 (Lee et al., 2004), was found to reduce amyloid plaques and cerebral amyloid angiopathy in Tg2576 mice.

XH1, a lipophilic amyloid-targeting metal chelator designed with amyloid-binding and metal chelating moieties, reduced APP protein expression in human cells and Aβ pathology in APP transgenic mice (Dedeoglu et al., 2004). Similar results were achieved with the lipophilic metal chelator DP-109, which markedly decreased Aβ plaques in APP transgenic mice (Lee et al., 2004).

Ammonium tetrathiomolybdate forms a stable tripartite complex with copper and proteins (Squitti & Salustri, 2009). Given with food, tetrathiomolybdate can complex food copper with food proteins, making all copper, including the endogenously secreted copper in saliva, gastric juice and intestinal secretion completely unabsorbable and thus causing an immediate negative copper unbalance. Given instead separate from food, tetrathiomolybdate is absorbed into the blood, where it forms the tripartite complex, bridging the freely available, and potentially toxic, copper with albumin. This complexed copper cannot be taken up by cells, and is therefore non-toxic, it has no known biological activity, and is largely cleared in the bile (Squitti & Salustri, 2009). A recent study tested the ability of tetrathiomolybdate to reduce Aβ pathology and spatial memory impairment in both a prevention and a treatment paradigm in Tg2576 mice. The study demonstrated that tetrathiomolybdate lowered brain copper concentrations and reduced Aβ levels in the prevention paradigm, but not in the treatment paradigm, suggesting that lowering systemic copper may achieve anti-amyloid effects if initiated early in the disease process (Quinn et al., 2010).

Metal bis(thiosemicarbazonato) complexes - MII(btsc), where M stands for either Copper (II) or Zinc (II) - can affect extracellular levels of Aβ. Treating Chinese hamster ovary cells overexpressing APP with engineered MII(btsc) increased levels of bioavailable intracellular copper and zinc but also resulted in a dose-dependent reduction of Aβ levels (Donnelly et al., 2008).

Iron-regulated APP in Aβ peptide in cell cultures were decreased by (-)-epigallocatechin-3-gallate, the main poliphenol constituent of green tea (Reznichenko et al., 2006). It was demonstrated that this molecule has metal-chelating and radical-scavenging properties that have an effect on iron metabolism in AD.

Nanoparticles conjugated to chelators were shown to easily cross the BBB, chelate metals, and exit through the BBB with their corresponding complexed metal ions (Liu et al., 2010). Early studies from this group (Liu et al., 2005) showed that these nanochelators can effectively remove iron from tissue of AD brain and also from ferritin.

Some studies (Lim et al., 2001, Lin et al., 2008) recently demonstrated the potential application of curcumin, a commonly used spice extracted by turmeric, as an anti-inflammatory and anti-oxidant molecule with neuroprotective properties. Some authors (Cole et al., 2007) demonstrated its metal chelating and neuroprotectant (Jiao et al., 2006) effects. In particular, Lin and coworkers (Lin et al., 2008) demonstrated in PC12 cells that this compound has strong effects on APP and BACE1 transcription up-regulation mediated by copper. The authors suggest that curcumin might have a combined effect on suppressing APP and BACE1 transcriptions, blocking the effect of copper. Due to its multi-functional effect new derivates have been created to improve curcumin brain bioavailability. Clinical studies are currently in progress to verify whether the use of this natural, non-toxic, neuroprotective compound with brain access could offer potential therapeutic benefits against neuronal damage.

Clioquinol (see also below) has been found to reverse the aggregation and redox activity of Aβ (49%) by its low affinity for copper in Tg2576 mice (Cherny et al., 2001).

6.1 Desferrioxamine

Desferrioxamine is a hexadentate chelator that does not cross the BBB. This chelator was tested for AD efficacy in a single-blinded study and it was reported to slow the clinical progression of dementia (Crapper McLachlan et al., 1991). The target metal of the study was aluminum. Iron was administered together with desferrioxamine throughout the whole trial period, with the aim of attenuating the bioavailability of aluminum, but not of iron. A generalized decrease of metal concentration was observed which, together with a decoppering effect, might have been at the basis of the positive clinical outcome.

Rationale	Agent	Type of study	Outcome
Induction of a negative metal balance throughout the whole body, as it happens with D-penicillamine or Zinc compounds in the treatment of Wilson's disease.	Desferrioxamine	One single-blinded study (Crapper McLachlan et al., 1991).	The clinical progression of dementia was reported to slow down.
	D-penicillamine	Prospective, randomized, double blind, parallel, placebo controlled phase II clinical trial (Squitti et al., 2002b).	H_2O_2 levels decreased in a group of AD patients with respect to both their own levels before the treatment and the levels of the AD patients who had taken the placebo
Studies based on the hypothesis that solubilization of Aβ plaques could be achieved by stripping them of their metal content or by facilitating the delivery of metals into the cell	Clioquinol	Prospective, randomized, double blind, parallel, placebo controlled phase II clinical trial (125-375 mg/BID over 36 weeks) (Ritchie et al., 2003).	Slowing of the rate of clinical decline in a subset of AD patients with moderate dementia
	PBT2	Prospective, randomized, double blind, parallel, placebo controlled phase II clinical trial (12-week treatment) (Lannfelt et al., 2008).	Dose-dependent reduction of Aβ concentrations in the CSF and positive impact on two executive functions.
Studies based on the hypothesis that copper supplementation can slow AD progression	Copper	Prospective, randomized, double-blind, placebo-controlled phase II clinical trial. Sixty-eight AD patients were given oral copper supplementation [Cu-(II)-orotate-dihydrate; 8 mg Cu daily, for 12 months (Kessler et al., 2008).	Cu supplementation did not change the rate of clinical decline.
Studies based on the hypothesis that aluminium could cause AD	Zinc aspartate	Preliminary trial with zinc aspartate administrated *per os* and i.v. for three to twelve months to 10 AD patients (Constantinidis, 1992).	Improved memory, understanding and communication in 8 of the 10 patients treated. The 2 patients who did not respond to the treatment had been given zinc aspartate only *per os*.

Table 3. Milestones in the Treatment of AD Patients with Metals or Metal Complexing Agents

The fact that desferrioxamine showed such an effect without crossing the BBB could be explained by the induction of a negative metal balance throughout the whole body, as it happens with D-penicillamine, Zinc compoundsor ammonium tetrathiomolybdate in the treatment of Wilson's disease.

6.2 D-penicillamine

D-penicillamine has been widely used for treatment of Wilson's disease. It functions as a copper chelator, controlling both the reactivity and bioavailability of that metal, ultimately facilitating its disposal through the urine. However, adverse events have been reported which have drastically limited its use.

A study of D-penicillamine tolerability and efficacy in the treatment of AD had to be interrupted before finishing recruitment, due to a number of serious adverse events (Squitti et al., 2002b). Some conclusions were drawn from the patients who had completed the treatment at the moment of interruption (18 patients out of 34). Serum and urine copper were measured together with red blood cells Cu,Zn SOD (Squitti et al., 2002b, Rossi et al., 2002). While serum copper had remained stable, urine copper levels were drastically elevated, indicating that large amounts of copper were indeed being removed from the tissues. Cu,Zn SOD activity was drastically reduced, revealing that this enzyme could be used as an indicator of general depletion of bioavailable copper. A significant reduction was also observed in the hydroperoxide levels.

Despite the positive effect in decreasing the bioavailable copper and the content of hydroperoxides, the clinical relevance of those results could not be fully assessed because of the short duration (24 weeks) of the observation, during which patients in the placebo arm did not worsen, precluding the detection of cognitive differences between the treated and the placebo groups. Crapper McLachlan and colleagues (Crapper McLachlan, et al., 1991) have shown a positive effect of chelation therapy in AD by treating patients for a 24-month period, and Ritchie and coworkers (Ritchie et al., 2003) reported some positive results with clioquinol (see below) after 36 weeks.

6.3 Iodochlorhydroxyquin (clioquinol) drug class

In the early 2000s, clioquinol was tested in man revealing that a treatment of just 21 days resulted in a significant improvement of patients' cognitive performance (Regland et al., 2001). This study was followed by a case report on two AD patients showing that clioquinol could ameliorate focal cerebral glucose metabolism and halt clinical deterioration (Ibach et al., 2005), and by a double-blind placebo-controlled clinical trial, in which 36 patients were treated with 125 mg/day for the first 12 week, then 250 mg/day between week 13 and 24 and finally 375 mg/day in the latest period of weeks 25-36 (Ritchie et al., 2003). The trial revealed that clioquinol slowed the rate of clinical decline in a subset of AD patients having more severe dementia. However, in the subgroup of patients with moderate dementia the difference between clioquinol and placebo did not reach statistical significance. In addition, in this subgroup the drug had no significant effects on the plasma Aβ levels.

As stated by the authors, the results of the clioquinol study supported a proof of concept in humans that a drug targeting Aβ-metal interaction can have a significant effect on slowing the progression of AD.

Clioquinol is capable of crossing the BBB, and it is believed that it solubilizes Aβ plaques by stripping them of their metal content. However, after *in vitro* investigations, it is unclear whether the positive results shown by the clinical trial were related to an attenuated Aβ-metal ion interaction or to some other mechanisms.

In the end, the relevance of the clioquinol conclusions has been severely questioned (Hegde et al., 2009). Arguments against the chelating effectiveness of clioquinol referred mostly to the evidence coming from a study by Treiber and co-workers (Treiber et al., 2004), who, by using a yeast model system, demonstrated that the addition of clioquinol to the culture drastically increased copper concentration within the yeast cells. Thus, they attributed the positive effects of clioquinol on AD patients to an increase of copper uptake into the neural cell, instead of an attenuated Aβ-metal ion interaction outside the cell. However, the authors (Treiber et al., 2004) did not report information about the bioavailability of the intracellular copper-clioquinol complex.

Some information to this regard could be found in a subsequent study demonstrating a decreased intracellular metal bioavailability linked to the accumulation of soluble Aβ outside the cell (White et al., 2006). Clioquinol, by facilitating the delivery of metals (copper and zinc, but not iron) into the cell, seemed to activate the phosphoinositol 3-kinase mediated protein kinase pathways, ultimately leading to an increase in the secretion of matrix metalloproteinases, which can degrade Aβ outside the cell. This is why molecules of the clioquinol drug class have been defined as metal protein attenuating compounds (MPAC), and have been attributed both chelating and ionophoretic properties.

Establishing the exact localization of clioquinol within the cell, or the copper biovailability of the putative clioquinol derivates-copper-complex, could be of help to define the molecular mechanisms either triggered or prevented by this class of molecules. Further clioquinol phase II/III studies were stalled by difficulties in preventing di-iodo 8-hydroxy quinoline contamination upon large-scale chemical synthesis, as well as its citotoxicity profile. In the end, clioquinol was withdrawn from human experimentation.

New compounds were then developed, such as PBT-2, a second-generation compound of the clioquinol drug class, that lacks iodine. PBT-2 has been recently tested on AD patients in a phase II, double-blind, randomized, placebo-controlled 12 week trial. 74 patients completed the trial and well tolerated the 250 mg of PBT-2 daily dosage. This study revealed that PBT2 induced a significant dose-dependent reduction of Aβ concentrations in the CSF, even though no drug effects on either Aβ40 or Aβ42 plasma levels were detected. Moreover, PBT-2 was found to preserve two executive functions, as evaluated via category fluency and trail making tests (Adlard et al., 2008, Lannfelt et al., 2008). This promising MPAC is now been tested in a phase III clinical trial.

6.4 Zinc therapy

Some agents used in anti-copper therapies are specifically aimed at maintaining a state of copper malabsorption (Squitti & Zito, 2009). Zinc acetate and other zinc salts, such as zinc carbonate, zinc sulfate, zinc gluconate, zinc oxide, zinc chloride and zinc stearate, are currently used in the treatment of Wilson's disease (Squitti & Zito, 2009). Zinc antagonizes the absorption of copper in the gut by increasing metallothioneins concentrations in the mucosa up to 25 times. The liver is the main human storage place for copper and metallothioneins are the major copper binding proteins in this organ. Diffusible free copper present in the blood is sequestered in a non-toxic form in the mucosal cells lining the intestine by metallothioneins. In this form copper is then excreted with the stools. The copper body balance becomes negative within 2 weeks when zinc sulphate is administrated in a dose of 600 mg/day. The safety and positive effects shown by zinc compounds, such as zinc sulphate or aspartate, in treating Wilson's disease strongly recommend the testing of these compounds in AD. Encouraging results in this direction were obtained in a preliminary study by Constantinidis (Constantinidis, 1992), who reported improvements in memory, understanding, communication, and social contact in eight out of ten AD patients treated with zinc compounds.

6.5 Side effects of anti-copper complexing agents

The side effects of anti-copper complexing agents and MPAC are primarily limited to anemia and leucopenia, due to bone marrow depletion of copper, and occasionally to liver toxicity. The frequency of occurrence of these effects shows a correlation with dose strength and frequency of drug assumption. For ammonium tetrathiomolybdate, a relatively new copper-lowering agent, these events have been associated with the reduction of serum ceruloplasmin levels, which is assumed to be a marker of copper defective bioavailability. For example, at ceruloplasmin concentrations of 5 mg/dL or less, bone marrow suppression is common; it is somewhat frequent at concentrations between 5 and 10 mg/dL, it is only occasional between 10-18 mg/dL, and very rare above 18.

Clioquinol usage in humans has been halted as it has been related with subacute myelo-optic neuropathy.

Zinc compounds have only minor adverse events, limited to gastrointestinal troubles.

7. Conclusion

The results of the studies described in this chapter should be regarded as single pieces of a complex mosaic of systemic disarrangements which result in severe neurodegeneration via a variety of biochemical phenomena, among which oxidative stress plays a leading role. In this view, systemic metal abnormalities, even if mild but over a long period of time, have disrupting effects on central processes controlling the defenses against metal-induced damage. Glutamatergic synapses definitely represent focal sites where the metal-Aβ toxic action can be promoted resulting in Aβ precipitation (Bush et al., 2003, Bush & Tanzi, 2008). The identification in AD of a free copper serum-level increase, as well as of disturbances of iron homeostasis and the activation of the antioxidant Cp-Tf system, appear coherent with this picture. Not only can free copper cross the BBB and enter reactions promoting Aβ toxicity, but it can systemically activate the Cp-Tf system, promoting iron subtraction from general circulation and its consequent internalization into neural cells. Both pathways converge towards neurodegeneration and neuronal death. In this framework, properly tuning the redistribution of metals via molecules which induce or maintain a state of copper malabsorption, such as zinc compounds or metal complexing agents, may possibly have a positive effect on the natural progression of AD.

8. Acknowledgement

This study was partially supported by the following grants:

Italian Health Department: "Profilo Biologico e Genetico della Disfunzione dei Metalli nella Malattia di Alzheimer e nel 'Mild Cognitive Impairment" [RF 2006 conv.58].

Programma Strategico 2007 conv. PS39; "Ricerca Corrente" grants IRCCS Brescia, Italy.

ERA-Net NEURON (JTC 2008 nEUROsyn), AFaR Foundation - Osp. Fatebenefratelli "AAMS l gioco sicuro".

The author have no conflict of interest.

9. References

Adlard, P.A. & Bush, A.I. (2006). Metals and Alzheimer's disease. *J Alzheimers Dis.* Vol. 10, No. 2-3, pp. 145-63.

Adlard, P.A., Cherny, R.A., Finkelstein, D.I., Gautier, E., Robb, E., Cortes, M., Volitakis, I., Liu, X., Smith, J.P., Perez, K., Laughton, K., Li, Q.X., Charman, S.A., Nicolazzo, J.A., Wilkins, S., Deleva, K., Lynch, T., Kok, G., Ritchie, C.W., Tanzi, R.E., Cappai, R., Masters, C.L., Barnham, K.J. & Bush, A.I. (2008). Rapid restoration of cognition in Alzheimer's transgenic mice with 8-hydroxy quinoline analogs is associated with decreased interstitial Abeta. *Neuron.* Vol. 59, No. 1, pp. 43-55.

Althaus, J., Quinn, J.F. Kaye, J.A., Newsome, D.A., Bisgaier C.L., Kanzer, S.H. (2008). Free copper measured directly in serum using a novel device is elevated in Alzheimer's disease. *Invest Ophthalmol Vis Sci.* Vol. 49(E-abstract), 5218.

Alzheimer, A., Stelzmann, R.A., Schnitzlein, H.N. & Murtagh, F.R. (1995). An English translation of Alzheimer's 1907 paper, "Uber eine eigenartige Erkankung der Hirnrinde". *Clin Anat.* Vol. 8, No. 6, pp. 429-31.

Angeletti, B., Waldron, K.J., Freeman, K.B., Bawagan, H., Hussain, I., Miller, C.C., Lau, K.F., Tennant, M.E., Dennison, C., Robinson, N.J. & Dingwall, C. (2005). BACE1 cytoplasmic domain interacts with the copper chaperone for superoxide dismutase-1 and binds copper. *J Biol Chem.* Vol. 280, No. 18, pp. 17930-7.

Armendariz, A.D., Gonzalez, M., Loguinov, A.V. & Vulpe, C.D. (2004). Gene expression profiling in chronic copper overload reveals upregulation of Prnp and App. *Physiol Genomics.* Vol. 20, No. 1, pp. 45-54.

Arnal, N., Cristalli, D.O., de Alaniz, M.J. & Marra, C.A. (2010). Clinical utility of copper, ceruloplasmin, and metallothionein plasma determinations in human neurodegenerative patients and their first-degree relatives. *Brain Res.* Vol. 1319, No., pp. 118-30.

Atwood, C.S., Moir, R.D., Huang, X., Scarpa, R.C., Bacarra, N.M., Romano, D.M., Hartshorn, M.A., Tanzi, R.E. & Bush, A.I. (1998). Dramatic aggregation of Alzheimer abeta by Cu(II) is induced by conditions representing physiological acidosis. *J Biol Chem.* Vol. 273, No. 21, pp. 12817-26.

Atwood, C.S., Perry, G., Zeng, H., Kato, Y., Jones, W.D., Ling, K.Q., Huang, X., Moir, R.D., Wang, D., Sayre, L.M., Smith, M.A., Chen, S.G. & Bush, A.I. (2004). Copper mediates dityrosine cross-linking of Alzheimer's amyloid-beta. *Biochemistry.* Vol. 43, No. 2, pp. 560-8.

Atwood, C.S., Scarpa, R.C., Huang, X., Moir, R.D., Jones, W.D., Fairlie, D.P., Tanzi, R.E. & Bush, A.I. (2000). Characterization of copper interactions with alzheimer amyloid beta peptides: identification of an attomolar-affinity copper binding site on amyloid beta1-42. *J Neurochem.* Vol. 75, No. 3, pp. 1219-33.

Babiloni, C., Bosco, P., Ghidoni, R., Del Percio, C., Squitti, R., Binetti, G., Benussi, L., Ferri, R., Frisoni, G., Lanuzza, B., Cassetta, E., Anello, G., Gurzi, M., Bartesaghi, S., Lizio, R., Tombini, M. & Rossini, P.M. (2007a). Homocysteine and electroencephalographic rhythms in Alzheimer disease: a multicentric study. *Neuroscience.* Vol. 145, No. 3, pp. 942-54.

Babiloni, C., Squitti, R., Del Percio, C., Cassetta, E., Ventriglia, M.C., Ferreri, F., Tombini, M., Frisoni, G., Binetti, G., Gurzi, M., Salinari, S., Zappasodi, F. & Rossini, P.M. (2007b). Free copper and resting temporal EEG rhythms correlate across healthy, mild cognitive impairment, and Alzheimer's disease subjects. *Clin Neurophysiol*. Vol. 118, No. 6, pp. 1244-60.

Barnham, K.J., Ciccotosto, G.D., Tickler, A.K., Ali, F.E., Smith, D.G., Williamson, N.A., Lam, Y.H., Carrington, D., Tew, D., Kocak, G., Volitakis, I., Separovic, F., Barrow, C.J., Wade, J.D., Masters, C.L., Cherny, R.A., Curtain, C.C., Bush, A.I. & Cappai, R. (2003a). Neurotoxic, redox-competent Alzheimer's beta-amyloid is released from lipid membrane by methionine oxidation. *J Biol Chem*. Vol. 278, No. 44, pp. 42959-65.

Barnham, K.J., McKinstry, W.J., Multhaup, G., Galatis, D., Morton, C.J., Curtain, C.C., Williamson, N.A., White, A.R., Hinds, M.G., Norton, R.S., Beyreuther, K., Masters, C.L., Parker, M.W. & Cappai, R. (2003b). Structure of the Alzheimer's disease amyloid precursor protein copper binding domain. A regulator of neuronal copper homeostasis. *J Biol Chem*. Vol. 278, No. 19, pp. 17401-7.

Bartzokis, G., Sultzer, D., Cummings, J., Holt, L.E., Hance, D.B., Henderson, V.W. & Mintz, J. (2000). In vivo evaluation of brain iron in Alzheimer disease using magnetic resonance imaging. *Arch Gen Psychiatry*. Vol. 57, No. 1, pp. 47-53.

Bartzokis, G. & Tishler, T.A. (2000). MRI evaluation of basal ganglia ferritin iron and neurotoxicity in Alzheimer's and Huntingon's disease. *Cell Mol Biol (Noisy-le-grand)*. Vol. 46, No. 4, pp. 821-33.

Basun, H., Forssell, L.G., Wetterberg, L. & Winblad, B. (1991). Metals and trace elements in plasma and cerebrospinal fluid in normal aging and Alzheimer's disease. *J Neural Transm Park Dis Dement Sect*. Vol. 3, No. 4, pp. 231-58.

Baum, L., Chan, I.H., Cheung, S.K., Goggins, W.B., Mok, V., Lam, L., Leung, V., Hui, E., Ng, C., Woo, J., Chiu, H.F., Zee, B.C., Cheng, W., Chan, M.H., Szeto, S., Lui, V., Tsoh, J., Bush, A.I., Lam, C.W. & Kwok, T. (2010). Serum zinc is decreased in Alzheimer's disease and serum arsenic correlates positively with cognitive ability. *Biometals*. Vol. 23, No. 1, pp. 173-9.

Bellingham, S.A., Ciccotosto, G.D., Needham, B.E., Fodero, L.R., White, A.R., Masters, C.L., Cappai, R. & Camakaris, J. (2004a). Gene knockout of amyloid precursor protein and amyloid precursor-like protein-2 increases cellular copper levels in primary mouse cortical neurons and embryonic fibroblasts. *J Neurochem*. Vol. 91, No. 2, pp. 423-8.

Bellingham, S.A., Lahiri, D.K., Maloney, B., La Fontaine, S., Multhaup, G. & Camakaris, J. (2004b). Copper depletion down-regulates expression of the Alzheimer's disease amyloid-beta precursor protein gene. *J Biol Chem*. Vol. 279, No. 19, pp. 20378-86.

Bielli, P. & Calabrese, L. (2002). Structure to function relationships in ceruloplasmin: a 'moonlighting' protein. *Cell Mol Life Sci*. Vol. 59, No. 9, pp. 1413-27.

Bocca, B., Forte, G., Petrucci, F., Pino, A., Marchione, F., Bomboi, G., Senofonte, O., Giubilei, F. & Alimonti, A. (2005). Monitoring of chemical elements and oxidative damage in patients affected by Alzheimer's disease. *Ann Ist Super Sanita*. Vol. 41, No. 2, pp. 197-203.

Bremner, I., Ed. (1979). Copper toxicity studies using domestic and laboratory animals. In *Copper in the environment*. New York, John Wiley & Sons.

Brewer, G.J. (2007). Iron and copper toxicity in diseases of aging, particularly atherosclerosis and Alzheimer's disease. *Exp Biol Med (Maywood)*. Vol. 232, No. 2, pp. 323-35.

Brewer, G.J. (2010). Toxicity of copper in drinking water. *J Toxicol Environ Health B Crit Rev*. Vol. 13, No. 6, pp. 449-52; author reply 53-9.

Brewer, G.J., Kanzer, S.H., Zimmerman, E.A., Celmins, D.F., Heckman, S.M. & Dick, R. (2010). Copper and ceruloplasmin abnormalities in Alzheimer's disease. *Am J Alzheimers Dis Other Demen*. Vol. 25, No. 6, pp. 490-7.

Bucossi, S., Ventriglia, M., Panetta, V., Salustri, C., Pasqualetti, P., Mariani, S., Siotto, M., Rossini, P.M. & Squitti, R. (2011). Copper in Alzheimer's Disease: A Meta-Analysis of Serum,Plasma, and Cerebrospinal Fluid Studies. *J Alzheimers Dis*. Vol. 24, No, 1, pp. 175-85.

Bush, A.I., Masters, C.L. & Tanzi, R.E. (2003). Copper, beta-amyloid, and Alzheimer's disease: tapping a sensitive connection. *Proc Natl Acad Sci U S A*. Vol. 100, No. 20, pp. 11193-4.

Bush, A.I., Pettingell, W.H., Multhaup, G., d Paradis, M., Vonsattel, J.P., Gusella, J.F., Beyreuther, K., Masters, C.L. & Tanzi, R.E. (1994). Rapid induction of Alzheimer A beta amyloid formation by zinc. *Science*. Vol. 265, No. 5177, pp. 1464-7.

Bush, A.I. & Tanzi, R.E. (2008). Therapeutics for Alzheimer's disease based on the metal hypothesis. *Neurotherapeutics*. Vol. 5, No. 3, pp. 421-32.

Castellani, R.J., Smith, M.A., Nunomura, A., Harris, P.L. & Perry, G. (1999). Is increased redox-active iron in Alzheimer disease a failure of the copper-binding protein ceruloplasmin? *Free Radic Biol Med*. Vol. 26, No. 11-12, pp. 1508-12.

Cherny, R.A., Atwood, C.S., Xilinas, M.E., Gray, D.N., Jones, W.D., McLean, C.A., Barnham, K.J., Volitakis, I., Fraser, F.W., Kim, Y., Huang, X., Goldstein, L.E., Moir, R.D., Lim, J.T., Beyreuther, K., Zheng, H., Tanzi, R.E., Masters, C.L. & Bush, A.I. (2001). Treatment with a copper-zinc chelator markedly and rapidly inhibits beta-amyloid accumulation in Alzheimer's disease transgenic mice. *Neuron*. Vol. 30, No. 3, pp. 665-76.

Cherny, R.A., Legg, J.T., McLean, C.A., Fairlie, D.P., Huang, X., Atwood, C.S., Beyreuther, K., Tanzi, R.E., Masters, C.L. & Bush, A.I. (1999). Aqueous dissolution of Alzheimer's disease Abeta amyloid deposits by biometal depletion. *J Biol Chem*. Vol. 274, No. 33, pp. 23223-8.

Choi, B.S. & Zheng, W. (2009). Copper transport to the brain by the blood-brain barrier and blood-CSF barrier. *Brain Res*. Vol. 1248, No., pp. 14-21.

Chutkow, J.G. (1978). Evidence for uptake of nonceruloplasminic copper in the brain: effect of ionic copper and amino acids. *Proc Soc Exp Biol Med*. Vol. 158, No. 1, pp. 113-6.

Cole, G.M., Teter, B. & Frautschy, S.A. (2007). Neuroprotective effects of curcumin. *Adv Exp Med Biol*. Vol. 595, No., pp. 197-212.

Connor, J.R., Snyder, B.S., Beard, J.L., Fine, R.E. & Mufson, E.J. (1992). Regional distribution of iron and iron-regulatory proteins in the brain in aging and Alzheimer's disease. *J Neurosci Res*. Vol. 31, No. 2, pp. 327-35.

Constantinidis, J. (1992). Treatment of Alzheimer's disease by zinc compounds. *Drug Dev. Res*. Vol. 27, No 1, pp. 1-14.

Corder, E.H., Saunders, A.M., Strittmatter, W.J., Schmechel, D.E., Gaskell, P.C., Small, G.W., Roses, A.D., Haines, J.L. & Pericak-Vance, M.A. (1993). Gene dose of apolipoprotein E type 4 allele and the risk of Alzheimer's disease in late onset families. *Science*. Vol. 261, No. 5123, pp. 921-3.

Crapper McLachlan, D.R., Dalton, A.J., Kruck, T.P., Bell, M.Y., Smith, W.L., Kalow, W. & Andrews, D.F. (1991). Intramuscular desferrioxamine in patients with Alzheimer's disease. *Lancet*. Vol. 337, No. 8753, pp. 1304-8.

Crouch, P.J., Blake, R., Duce, J.A., Ciccotosto, G.D., Li, Q.X., Barnham, K.J., Curtain, C.C., Cherny, R.A., Cappai, R., Dyrks, T., Masters, C.L. & Trounce, I.A. (2005). Copper-

dependent inhibition of human cytochrome c oxidase by a dimeric conformer of amyloid-beta1-42. *J Neurosci*. Vol. 25, No. 3, pp. 672-9.
Crouch, P.J., White, A.R. & Bush, A.I. (2007). The modulation of metal bio-availability as a therapeutic strategy for the treatment of Alzheimer's disease. *Febs J*. Vol. 274, No. 15, pp. 3775-83.
Dal Forno, G., Palermo, M.T., Donohue, J.E., Karagiozis, H., Zonderman, A.B. & Kawas, C.H. (2005). Depressive symptoms, sex, and risk for Alzheimer's disease. *Ann Neurol*. Vol. 57, No. 3, pp. 381-7.
Dedeoglu, A., Cormier, K., Payton, S., Tseitlin, K.A., Kremsky, J.N., Lai, L., Li, X., Moir, R.D., Tanzi, R.E., Bush, A.I., Kowall, N.W., Rogers, J.T. & Huang, X. (2004). Preliminary studies of a novel bifunctional metal chelator targeting Alzheimer's amyloidogenesis. *Exp Gerontol*. Vol. 39, No. 11-12, pp. 1641-9.
Deibel, M.A., Ehmann, W.D. & Markesbery, W.R. (1996). Copper, iron, and zinc imbalances in severely degenerated brain regions in Alzheimer's disease: possible relation to oxidative stress. *J Neurol Sci*. Vol. 143, No. 1-2, pp. 137-42.
Donnelly, P.S., Caragounis, A., Du, T., Laughton, K.M., Volitakis, I., Cherny, R.A., Sharples, R.A., Hill, A.F., Li, Q.X., Masters, C.L., Barnham, K.J. & White, A.R. (2008). Selective intracellular release of copper and zinc ions from bis(thiosemicarbazonato) complexes reduces levels of Alzheimer disease amyloid-beta peptide. *J Biol Chem*. Vol. 283, No. 8, pp. 4568-77.
Dubois, B., Feldman, H.H., Jacova, C., Dekosky, S.T., Barberger-Gateau, P., Cummings, J., Delacourte, A., Galasko, D., Gauthier, S., Jicha, G., Meguro, K., O'Brien, J., Pasquier, F., Robert, P., Rossor, M., Salloway, S., Stern, Y., Visser, P.J. & Scheltens, P. (2007). Research criteria for the diagnosis of Alzheimer's disease: revising the NINCDS-ADRDA criteria. *Lancet Neurol*. Vol. 6, No. 8, pp. 734-46.
Duce, J.A. & Bush, A.I. Biological metals and Alzheimer's disease: implications for therapeutics and diagnostics. *Prog Neurobiol*. Vol. 92, No. 1, pp. 1-18.
Duce, J.A., Tsatsanis, A., Cater, M.A., James, S.A., Robb, E., Wikhe, K., Leong, S.L., Perez, K., Johanssen, T., Greenough, M.A., Cho, H.H., Galatis, D., Moir, R.D., Masters, C.L., McLean, C., Tanzi, R.E., Cappai, R., Barnham, K.J., Ciccotosto, G.D., Rogers, J.T. & Bush, A.I. (2010). Iron-export ferroxidase activity of beta-amyloid precursor protein is inhibited by zinc in Alzheimer's disease. *Cell*. Vol. 142, No. 6, pp. 857-67.
Durand, J., Meloni, G., Talmard, C., Vasak, M. & Faller, P. (2010). Zinc release of Zn-metallothionein-3 induces fibrillar type amyloid-beta aggregates. *Metallomics*. Vol. 2, No. 11, pp. 741-4.
Edbauer, D., Winkler, E., Regula, J.T., Pesold, B., Steiner, H. & Haass, C. (2003). Reconstitution of gamma-secretase activity. *Nat Cell Biol*. Vol. 5, No. 5, pp. 486-8.
Fleming, R.E. & Bacon, B.R. (2005). Orchestration of iron homeostasis. *N Engl J Med*. Vol. 352, No. 17, pp. 1741-4.
Folstein, M.F., Folstein, S.E. & McHugh PR. (1975) "Mini-mental state". A practical method for grading the cognitive state of patients for the clinician. *J Psychiatr Res* Vol. 12, No 3, pp. 189-198.
Francis, P.T., Palmer, A.M., Snape, M. & Wilcock, G.K. (1999). The cholinergic hypothesis of Alzheimer's disease: a review of progress. *J Neurol Neurosurg Psychiatry*. Vol. 66, No. 2, pp. 137-47.
Gerhardsson, L., Lundh, T., Minthon, L. & Londos, E. (2008). Metal concentrations in plasma and cerebrospinal fluid in patients with Alzheimer's disease. *Dement Geriatr Cogn Disord*. Vol. 25, No. 6, pp. 508-15.

Giambattistelli, F., Bucossi, S., Salustri, C., Panetta, V., Mariani, S., Siotto, M., Ventriglia, M., Vernieri, F., Dell'Acqua, M., Cassetta, E., Rossini, P.M. & Squitti, R. (2011). Effects of Hemochromatosis (HFE) and Transferrin gene mutations on iron dyshomeostasis, liver dysfunction and on the risk of Alzheimer's disease. *Neurobiology of Aging, Epub ahead of print.*

Gonzalez, C., Martin, T., Cacho, J., Brenas, M.T., Arroyo, T., Garcia-Berrocal, B., Navajo, J.A. & Gonzalez-Buitrago, J.M. (1999). Serum zinc, copper, insulin and lipids in Alzheimer's disease epsilon 4 apolipoprotein E allele carriers. *Eur J Clin Invest*. Vol. 29, No. 7, pp. 637-42.

Good, P.F., Perl, D.P., Bierer, L.M. & Schmeidler, J. (1992). Selective accumulation of aluminum and iron in the neurofibrillary tangles of Alzheimer's disease: a laser microprobe (LAMMA) study. *Ann Neurol*. Vol. 31, No. 3, pp. 286-92.

Gorgone, G., Ursini F., Altamura C., Bressi F., Tombini M., Curcio G., Chiovenda P., Squitti R., Silvestrini M., Ientile R., Pisani F., Rossini PM. & Vernieri F. (2009). Hyperhomocysteinemia, intima-media thickness and C677T MTHFR gene polymorphism: a correlation study in patients with cognitive impairment. *Atherosclerosis, Vol.* 206, No 1, pp 309-13.

Gutteridge, J.M. & Halliwell, B. (1990). The measurement and mechanism of lipid peroxidation in biological systems. *Trends Biochem Sci*. Vol. 15, No. 4, pp. 129-35.

Hardy, J. & Allsop, D. (1991). Amyloid deposition as the central event in the aetiology of Alzheimer's disease. *Trends Pharmacol Sci*. Vol. 12, No. 10, pp. 383-8.

Harris, E.D. (2000). Cellular copper transport and metabolism. *Annu Rev Nutr*. Vol. 20, No., pp. 291-310.

Hartter, D.E. & Barnea, A. (1988). Evidence for release of copper in the brain: depolarization-induced release of newly taken-up 67copper. *Synapse*. Vol. 2, No. 4, pp. 412-5.

Hegde, M.L., Bharathi, P., Suram, A., Venugopal, C., Jagannathan, R., Poddar, P., Srinivas, P., Sambamurti, K., Rao, K.J., Scancar, J., Messori, L., Zecca, L. & Zatta, P. (2009). Challenges associated with metal chelation therapy in Alzheimer's disease. *J Alzheimers Dis*. Vol. 17, No. 3, pp. 457-68.

Hoogenraad, T. (2007). Measuring hypercupremia in blood of patients with Alzheimer's disease is logical, but the utility of measuring free-copper has to be proven. *Neurologie,* Frijns CJM, Kappelle LJ, Klijn CJM, Wokke JHJ. (Utrechts) Tijdschrift voor, pp. 111-112

Huang, X., Atwood, C.S., Hartshorn, M.A., Multhaup, G., Goldstein, L.E., Scarpa, R.C., Cuajungco, M.P., Gray, D.N., Lim, J., Moir, R.D., Tanzi, R.E. & Bush, A.I. (1999a). The A beta peptide of Alzheimer's disease directly produces hydrogen peroxide through metal ion reduction. *Biochemistry*. Vol. 38, No. 24, pp. 7609-16.

Huang, X., Cuajungco, M.P., Atwood, C.S., Hartshorn, M.A., Tyndall, J.D., Hanson, G.R., Stokes, K.C., Leopold, M., Multhaup, G., Goldstein, L.E., Scarpa, R.C., Saunders, A.J., Lim, J., Moir, R.D., Glabe, C., Bowden, E.F., Masters, C.L., Fairlie, D.P., Tanzi, R.E. & Bush, A.I. (1999b). Cu(II) potentiation of Alzheimer abeta neurotoxicity. Correlation with cell-free hydrogen peroxide production and metal reduction. *J Biol Chem*. Vol. 274, No. 52, pp. 37111-6.

Ibach, B., Haen, E., Marienhagen, J. & Hajak, G. (2005). Clioquinol treatment in familiar early onset of Alzheimer's disease: a case report. *Pharmacopsychiatry*. Vol. 38, No. 4, pp. 178-9.

Institute of Medicine Food and Nutrition Board (2001). *Dietary Reference Intakes for Vitamin A, Vitamin K, Arsenic, Boron, Chromium, Copper, Iodine, Iron, Manganese, Molybdenum, Nickel, Silicon, Vanadium, and Zinc,* National Academy Press, Washington, DC.

Iyengar, V., Brewer, G.J., Dick, R.D. & Chung, O.Y. (1988). Studies of cholecystokinin-stimulated biliary secretions reveal a high molecular weight copper-binding substance in normal subjects that is absent in patients with Wilson's disease. *J Lab Clin Med.* Vol. 111, No. 3, pp. 267-74.

Jacobs, D., Oxley, DK, DeMott, WR (2002). *Laboratory Test Handbook: Concise with Disease Index, 2nd ed.,* Hudson (Cleveland), OH: Lexi-Comp.

Jeandel, C., Nicolas, M.B., Dubois, F., Nabet-Belleville, F., Penin, F. & Cuny, G. (1989). Lipid peroxidation and free radical scavengers in Alzheimer's disease. *Gerontology.* Vol. 35, No. 5-6, pp. 275-82.

Jiao, Y., Wilkinson, J.t., Christine Pietsch, E., Buss, J.L., Wang, W., Planalp, R., Torti, F.M. & Torti, S.V. (2006). Iron chelation in the biological activity of curcumin. *Free Radic Biol Med.* Vol. 40, No. 7, pp. 1152-60.

Kapaki, E., Segditsa, J. & Papageorgiou, C. (1989). Zinc, copper and magnesium concentration in serum and CSF of patients with neurological disorders. *Acta Neurol Scand.* Vol. 79, No. 5, pp. 373-8.

Kessler, H., Pajonk, F.G., Meisser, P., Schneider-Axmann, T., Hoffmann, K.H., Supprian, T., Herrmann, W., Obeid, R., Multhaup, G., Falkai, P. & Bayer, T.A. (2006). Cerebrospinal fluid diagnostic markers correlate with lower plasma copper and ceruloplasmin in patients with Alzheimer's disease. *J Neural Transm.* Vol. 113, No. 11, pp. 1763-9.

Kessler H, Bayer TA, Bach D, Schneider-Axmann T, Supprian T, Herrmann W, Haber M, Multhaup G, Falkai P & Pajonk F.G. (2008). Intake of copper has no effect on cognition in patients with mild Alzheimer's disease: a pilot phase 2 clinical trial. *J Neural Transm.* Vol. 115, No 8, pp. 1181-7.

Kim, B.E., Nevitt, T. & Thiele, D.J. (2008). Mechanisms for copper acquisition, distribution and regulation. *Nat Chem Biol.* Vol. 4, No. 3, pp. 176-85.

Lam, P.K., Kritz-Silverstein, D., Barrett Connor, E., Milne, D., Nielsen, F., Gamst, A., Morton, D. & Wingard, D. (2008). Plasma trace elements and cognitive function in older men and women: the Rancho Bernardo study. *J Nutr Health Aging.* Vol. 12, No. 1, pp. 22-7.

Lannfelt, L., Blennow, K., Zetterberg, H., Batsman, S., Ames, D., Harrison, J., Masters, C.L., Targum, S., Bush, A.I., Murdoch, R., Wilson, J. & Ritchie, C.W. (2008). Safety, efficacy, and biomarker findings of PBT2 in targeting Abeta as a modifying therapy for Alzheimer's disease: a phase IIa, double-blind, randomised, placebo-controlled trial. *Lancet Neurol.* Vol. 7, No. 9, pp. 779-86.

Lee, J.Y., Friedman, J.E., Angel, I., Kozak, A. & Koh, J.Y. (2004). The lipophilic metal chelator DP-109 reduces amyloid pathology in brains of human beta-amyloid precursor protein transgenic mice. *Neurobiol Aging.* Vol. 25, No. 10, pp. 1315-21.

Lim, G.P., Chu, T., Yang, F., Beech, W., Frautschy, S.A. & Cole, G.M. (2001). The curry spice curcumin reduces oxidative damage and amyloid pathology in an Alzheimer transgenic mouse. *J Neurosci.* Vol. 21, No. 21, pp. 8370-7.

Lin, R., Chen, X., Li, W., Han, Y., Liu, P. & Pi, R. (2008). Exposure to metal ions regulates mRNA levels of APP and BACE1 in PC12 cells: blockage by curcumin. *Neurosci Lett.* Vol. 440, No. 3, pp. 344-7.

Linder, M.C., Houle, P.A., Isaacs, E., Moor, J.R. & Scott, L.E. (1979). Copper regulation of ceruloplasmin in copper-deficient rats. *Enzyme*. Vol. 24, No. 1, pp. 23-35.

Liu, G., Garrett, M.R., Men, P., Zhu, X., Perry, G. & Smith, M.A. (2005). Nanoparticle and other metal chelation therapeutics in Alzheimer disease. *Biochim Biophys Acta*. Vol. 1741, No. 3, pp. 246-52.

Liu, G., Men, P., Perry, G. & Smith, M.A. (2010). Nanoparticle and iron chelators as a potential novel Alzheimer therapy. *Methods Mol Biol*. Vol. 610, No., pp. 123-44.

Loeffler, D.A., LeWitt, P.A., Juneau, P.L., Sima, A.A., Nguyen, H.U., DeMaggio, A.J., Brickman, C.M., Brewer, G.J., Dick, R.D., Troyer, M.D. & Kanaley, L. (1996). Increased regional brain concentrations of ceruloplasmin in neurodegenerative disorders. *Brain Res*. Vol. 738, No. 2, pp. 265-74.

Lovell, M.A., Robertson, J.D., Teesdale, W.J., Campbell, J.L. & Markesbery, W.R. (1998). Copper, iron and zinc in Alzheimer's disease senile plaques. *J Neurol Sci*. Vol. 158, No. 1, pp. 47-52.

Maynard, C.J., Cappai, R., Volitakis, I., Cherny, R.A., White, A.R., Beyreuther, K., Masters, C.L., Bush, A.I. & Li, Q.X. (2002). Overexpression of Alzheimer's disease amyloid-beta opposes the age-dependent elevations of brain copper and iron. *J Biol Chem*. Vol. 277, No. 47, pp. 44670-6.

McKhann, G., Drachman, D., Folstein, M., Katzman, R., Price, D. & Stadlan, E.M. (1984). Clinical diagnosis of Alzheimer's disease: report of the NINCDS-ADRDA Work Group under the auspices of Department of Health and Human Services Task Force on Alzheimer's Disease. *Neurology*. Vol. 34, No. 7, pp. 939-44.

Meloni, G., Sonois, V., Delaine, T., Guilloreau, L., Gillet, A., Teissie, J., Faller, P. & Vasak, M. (2008). Metal swap between Zn7-metallothionein-3 and amyloid-beta-Cu protects against amyloid-beta toxicity. *Nat Chem Biol*. Vol. 4, No. 6, pp. 366-72.

Miyata, M. & Smith, J.D. (1996). Apolipoprotein E allele-specific antioxidant activity and effects on cytotoxicity by oxidative insults and beta-amyloid peptides. *Nat Genet*. Vol. 14, No. 1, pp. 55-61.

Moir, R.D., Atwood, C.S., Romano, D.M., Laurans, M.H., Huang, X., Bush, A.I., Smith, J.D. & Tanzi, R.E. (1999). Differential effects of apolipoprotein E isoforms on metal-induced aggregation of A beta using physiological concentrations. *Biochemistry*. Vol. 38, No. 14, pp. 4595-603.

Molina, J.A., Jimenez-Jimenez, F.J., Aguilar, M.V., Meseguer, I., Mateos-Vega, C.J., Gonzalez-Munoz, M.J., de Bustos, F., Porta, J., Orti-Pareja, M., Zurdo, M., Barrios, E. & Martinez-Para, M.C. (1998). Cerebrospinal fluid levels of transition metals in patients with Alzheimer's disease. *J Neural Transm*. Vol. 105, No. 4-5, pp. 479-88.

Morris, M.C., Evans, D.A., Tangney, C.C., Bienias, J.L., Schneider, J.A., Wilson, R.S. & Scherr, P.A. (2006). Dietary copper and high saturated and trans fat intakes associated with cognitive decline. *Arch Neurol*. Vol. 63, No. 8, pp. 1085-8.

Multhaup, G., Schlicksupp, A., Hesse, L., Beher, D., Ruppert, T., Masters, C.L. & Beyreuther, K. (1996). The amyloid precursor protein of Alzheimer's disease in the reduction of copper(II) to copper(I). *Science*. Vol. 271, No. 5254, pp. 1406-9.

Nakano, E., Williamson, M.P., Williams, N.H. & Powers, H.J. (2004). Copper-mediated LDL oxidation by homocysteine and related compounds depends largely on copper ligation. *Biochim Biophys Acta*. Vol. 1688, No. 1, pp. 33-42.

Nelson, T.J. & Alkon, D.L. (2005). Oxidation of cholesterol by amyloid precursor protein and beta-amyloid peptide. *J Biol Chem*. Vol. 280, No. 8, pp. 7377-87.

Opazo, C., Huang, X., Cherny, R.A., Moir, R.D., Roher, A.E., White, A.R., Cappai, R., Masters, C.L., Tanzi, R.E., Inestrosa, N.C. & Bush, A.I. (2002). Metalloenzyme-like activity of Alzheimer's disease beta-amyloid. Cu-dependent catalytic conversion of dopamine, cholesterol, and biological reducing agents to neurotoxic H(2)O(2). *J Biol Chem*. Vol. 277, No. 43, pp. 40302-8.

Ozcankaya, R. & Delibas, N. (2002). Malondialdehyde, superoxide dismutase, melatonin, iron, copper, and zinc blood concentrations in patients with Alzheimer disease: cross-sectional study. *Croat Med J*. Vol. 43, No. 1, pp. 28-32.

Pajonk, F.G., Kessler, H., Supprian, T., Hamzei, P., Bach, D., Schweickhardt, J., Herrmann, W., Obeid, R., Simons, A., Falkai, P., Multhaup, G. & Bayer, T.A. (2005). Cognitive decline correlates with low plasma concentrations of copper in patients with mild to moderate Alzheimer's disease. *J Alzheimers Dis*. Vol. 8, No. 1, pp. 23-7.

Palmiter, R.D. (1994). Regulation of metallothionein genes by heavy metals appears to be mediated by a zinc-sensitive inhibitor that interacts with a constitutively active transcription factor, MTF-1. *Proc Natl Acad Sci U S A*. Vol. 91, No. 4, pp. 1219-23.

Patel, B.N., Dunn, R.J., Jeong, S.Y., Zhu, Q., Julien, J.P. & David, S. (2002). Ceruloplasmin regulates iron levels in the CNS and prevents free radical injury. *J Neurosci*. Vol. 22, No. 15, pp. 6578-86.

Plantin, L.O., Lying-Tunell, U., & Kristensson, K. (1987). Trace elemnts in the human central nervous system studied with neutron activation analysis. *Biochem. Trace Element Research*. Vol 13, pp. 69-75

Price, K.A., Crouch, P.J. & White, A.R. (2007). Therapeutic treatment of Alzheimer's disease using metal complexing agents. *Recent Pat CNS Drug Discov*. Vol. 2, No. 3, pp. 180-7.

Puglielli, L., Friedlich, A.L., Setchell, K.D., Nagano, S., Opazo, C., Cherny, R.A., Barnham, K.J., Wade, J.D., Melov, S., Kovacs, D.M. & Bush, A.I. (2005). Alzheimer disease beta-amyloid activity mimics cholesterol oxidase. *J Clin Invest*. Vol. 115, No. 9, pp. 2556-63.

Qian, Y., Tiffany-Castiglioni, E., Welsh, J. & Harris, E.D. (1998). Copper efflux from murine microvascular cells requires expression of the menkes disease Cu-ATPase. *J Nutr*. Vol. 128, No. 8, pp. 1276-82.

Que, E.L., Domaille, D.W. & Chang, C.J. (2008). Metals in neurobiology: probing their chemistry and biology with molecular imaging. *Chem Rev*. Vol. 108, No. 5, pp. 1517-49.

Quinn, J.F., Harris, C.J., Cobb, K.E., Domes, C., Ralle, M., Brewer, G. & Wadsworth, T.L. A copper-lowering strategy attenuates amyloid pathology in a transgenic mouse model of Alzheimer's disease. *J Alzheimers Dis*. Vol. 21, No. 3, pp. 903-14.

Regland, B., Lehmann, W., Abedini, I., Blennow, K., Jonsson, M., Karlsson, I., Sjogren, M., Wallin, A., Xilinas, M. & Gottfries, C.G. (2001). Treatment of Alzheimer's disease with clioquinol. *Dement Geriatr Cogn Disord*. Vol. 12, No. 6, pp. 408-14.

Religa, D., Strozyk, D., Cherny, R.A., Volitakis, I., Haroutunian, V., Winblad, B., Naslund, J. & Bush, A.I. (2006). Elevated cortical zinc in Alzheimer disease. *Neurology*. Vol. 67, No. 1, pp. 69-75.

Reznichenko, L., Amit, T., Zheng, H., Avramovich-Tirosh, Y., Youdim, M.B., Weinreb, O. & Mandel, S. (2006). Reduction of iron-regulated amyloid precursor protein and beta-amyloid peptide by (-)-epigallocatechin-3-gallate in cell cultures: implications for iron chelation in Alzheimer's disease. *J Neurochem*. Vol. 97, No. 2, pp. 527-36.

Ritchie, C.W., Bush, A.I., Mackinnon, A., Macfarlane, S., Mastwyk, M., MacGregor, L., Kiers, L., Cherny, R., Li, Q.X., Tammer, A., Carrington, D., Mavros, C., Volitakis, I., Xilinas, M., Ames, D., Davis, S., Beyreuther, K., Tanzi, R.E. & Masters, C.L. (2003). Metal-protein attenuation with iodochlorhydroxyquin (clioquinol) targeting Abeta amyloid deposition and toxicity in Alzheimer disease: a pilot phase 2 clinical trial. *Arch Neurol.* Vol. 60, No. 12, pp. 1685-91.

Rossi, L., Ciriolo, M.R., Marchese, E., De Martino, A., Giorgi, M. & Rotilio, G. (1994). Differential decrease of copper content and of copper binding to superoxide dismutase in liver, heart and brain of copper-deficient rats. *Biochem Biophys Res Commun.* Vol. 203, No. 2, pp. 1028-34.

Rossi, L., Squitti, R., Pasqualetti, P., Marchese, E., Cassetta, E., Forastiere, E., Rotilio, G., Rossini, P.M. & Finazzi-Agro, A. (2002). Red blood cell copper, zinc superoxide dismutase activity is higher in Alzheimer's disease and is decreased by D-penicillamine. *Neurosci Lett.* Vol. 329, No. 2, pp. 137-40.

Rossor, M.N. (1983). Focal changes in Alzheimer's disease and cholinergic hypothesis. *Lancet.* Vol. 2, No. 8347, pp. 465.

Salustri, C., Barbati, G., Ghidoni, R., Quintiliani, L., Ciappina, S., Binetti, G. & Squitti, R. (2010a). Is cognitive function linked to serum free copper levels? A cohort study in a normal population. *Clin Neurophysiol.* Vol. 121, No. 4, pp. 502-7.

Salustri, C., Squitti, R., Zappasodi, F., Ventriglia, M., Bevacqua, M.G., Fontana, M. & Tecchio, F. (2010b). Oxidative stress and brain glutamate-mediated excitability in depressed patients. *J Affect Disord.* Vol. 127, No. 1-3, pp. 321-5.

Sanan, D.A., Weisgraber, K.H., Russell, S.J., Mahley, R.W., Huang, D., Saunders, A., Schmechel, D., Wisniewski, T., Frangione, B., Roses, A.D. & et al. (1994). Apolipoprotein E associates with beta amyloid peptide of Alzheimer's disease to form novel monofibrils. Isoform apoE4 associates more efficiently than apoE3. *J Clin Invest.* Vol. 94, No. 2, pp. 860-9.

Sayre, L.M., Perry, G., Harris, P.L., Liu, Y., Schubert, K.A. & Smith, M.A. (2000). In situ oxidative catalysis by neurofibrillary tangles and senile plaques in Alzheimer's disease: a central role for bound transition metals. *J Neurochem.* Vol. 74, No. 1, pp. 270-9.

Schmitz, C., Rutten, B.P., Pielen, A., Schafer, S., Wirths, O., Tremp, G., Czech, C., Blanchard, V., Multhaup, G., Rezaie, P., Korr, H., Steinbusch, H.W., Pradier, L. & Bayer, T.A. (2004). Hippocampal neuron loss exceeds amyloid plaque load in a transgenic mouse model of Alzheimer's disease. *Am J Pathol.* Vol. 164, No. 4, pp. 1495-502.

Siotto, M., Bucossi, S. & Squitti, R. Copper status abnormalities and how to measure them in neurodegenerative disorders. *Recent Pat CNS Drug Discov.* Vol. 5, No. 3, pp. 182-94.

Smith, M.A., Zhu, X., Tabaton, M., Liu, G., McKeel, D.W., Jr., Cohen, M.L., Wang, X., Siedlak, S.L., Dwyer, B.E., Hayashi, T., Nakamura, M., Nunomura, A. & Perry, G. (2010). Increased iron and free radical generation in preclinical Alzheimer disease and mild cognitive impairment. *J Alzheimers Dis.* Vol. 19, No. 1, pp. 363-72.

Smorgon, C., Mari, E., Atti, A.R., Dalla Nora, E., Zamboni, P.F., Calzoni, F., Passaro, A. & Fellin, R. (2004). Trace elements and cognitive impairment: an elderly cohort study. *Arch Gerontol Geriatr Suppl.* Vol., No. 9, pp. 393-402.

Snaedal, J., Kristinsson, J., Gunnarsdottir, S., Olafsdottir, Baldvinsson, M. & Johannesson, T. (1998). Copper, ceruloplasmin and superoxide dismutase in patients with Alzheimer's disease. A case-control study. *Dement Geriatr Cogn Disord.* Vol. 9, No. 5, pp. 239-42.

Sparks, D.L., Friedland, R., Petanceska, S., Schreurs, B.G., Shi, J., Perry, G., Smith, M.A., Sharma, A., Derosa, S., Ziolkowski, C. & Stankovic, G. (2006). Trace copper levels in the drinking water, but not zinc or aluminum influence CNS Alzheimer-like pathology. *J Nutr Health Aging*. Vol. 10, No. 4, pp. 247-54.

Sparks, D.L. & Schreurs, B.G. (2003). Trace amounts of copper in water induce beta-amyloid plaques and learning deficits in a rabbit model of Alzheimer's disease. *Proc Natl Acad Sci U S A*. Vol. 100, No. 19, pp. 11065-9.

Squitti, R. (2011). Metals In Alzheimer's Disease: A Systemic Perspective. *Frontiers in Bioscience, in press.*

Squitti, R., Barbati, G., Rossi, L., Ventriglia, M., Dal Forno, G., Cesaretti, S., Moffa, F., Caridi, I., Cassetta, E., Pasqualetti, P., Calabrese, L., Lupoi, D. & Rossini, P.M. (2006). Excess of nonceruloplasmin serum copper in AD correlates with MMSE, CSF [beta]-amyloid, and h-tau. *Neurology*. Vol. 67, No. 1, pp. 76-82.

Squitti, R., Bressi, F., Pasqualetti, P., Bonomini, C., Ghidoni, R., Binetti, G., Cassetta, E., Moffa, F., Ventriglia, M., Vernieri, F. & Rossini, P.M. (2009). Longitudinal prognostic value of serum "free" copper in patients with Alzheimer disease. *Neurology*. Vol. 72, No. 1, pp. 50-5.

Squitti, R., Cassetta, E., Dal Forno, G., Lupoi, D., Lippolis, G., Pauri, F., Vernieri, F., Cappa, A. & Rossini, P.M. (2004). Copper perturbation in 2 monozygotic twins discordant for degree of cognitive impairment. *Arch Neurol*. Vol. 61, No. 5, pp. 738-43.

Squitti, R., Ghidoni, R., Scrascia, F., Benussi, L., Panetta, V., Pasqualetti, P., Moffa, F., Bernardini, S., Ventriglia, M., Binetti, G. & Rossini, P.M. (2011). Free copper distinguishes mild cognitive impairment subjects from healthy elderly individuals. *J Alzheimers Dis*. Vol. 23, No. 2, pp. 239-48.

Squitti, R., Lupoi, D., Pasqualetti, P., Dal Forno, G., Vernieri, F., Chiovenda, P., Rossi, L., Cortesi, M., Cassetta, E. & Rossini, P.M. (2002a). Elevation of serum copper levels in Alzheimer's disease. *Neurology*. Vol. 59, No. 8, pp. 1153-61.

Squitti, R., Pasqualetti, P., Cassetta, E., Dal Forno, G., Cesaretti, S., Pedace, F., Finazzi-Agro, A. & Rossini, P.M. (2003). Elevation of serum copper levels discriminates Alzheimer's disease from vascular dementia. *Neurology*. Vol. 60, No. 12, pp. 2013-4.

Squitti, R., Pasqualetti, P., Dal Forno, G., Moffa, F., Cassetta, E., Lupoi, D., Vernieri, F., Rossi, L., Baldassini, M. & Rossini, P.M. (2005). Excess of serum copper not related to ceruloplasmin in Alzheimer disease. *Neurology*. Vol. 64, No. 6, pp. 1040-6.

Squitti R, Q.C., Forno GD, Antuono P, Wekstein DR, Capo CR, Salustri C, Rossini PM. (2007). Ceruloplasmin (2-D PAGE) Pattern and Copper Content in Serum and Brain of Alzheimer Disease Patients. *Biomark Insights*. Vol. 7, No. 1, pp. 205-13.

Squitti, R., Quattrocchi, C.C., Salustri, C. & Rossini, P.M. (2008). Ceruloplasmin fragmentation is implicated in 'free' copper deregulation of Alzheimer's disease. *Prion*. Vol. 2, No. 1, pp. 23-7.

Squitti, R., Rossini, P.M., Cassetta, E., Moffa, F., Pasqualetti, P., Cortesi, M., Colloca, A., Rossi, L. & Finazzi-Agro, A. (2002b). d-penicillamine reduces serum oxidative stress in Alzheimer's disease patients. *Eur J Clin Invest*. Vol. 32, No. 1, pp. 51-9.

Squitti, R. & Salustri, C. (2009). Agents complexing copper as a therapeutic strategy for the treatment of Alzheimer's disease. *Curr Alzheimer Res*. Vol. 6, No. 6, pp. 476-87.

Squitti, R., Salustri, C., Siotto, M., Ventriglia, M., Vernieri, F., Lupoi, D., Cassetta, E. & Rossini, P.M. (2010c). Ceruloplasmin/Transferrin ratio changes in Alzheimer's disease. *Int J Alzheimers Dis*. Vol. 2011, No., pp. 231595.

Squitti, R., Ventriglia, M., Barbati, G., Cassetta, E., Ferreri, F., Dal Forno, G., Ramires, S., Zappasodi, F. & Rossini, P.M. (2007). 'Free' copper in serum of Alzheimer's disease patients correlates with markers of liver function. *J Neural Transm*. Vol. 114, No. 12, pp. 1589-94.

Squitti, R. & Zito, G. (2009). Anti-copper therapies in Alzheimer's disease: new concepts. *Recent Pat CNS Drug Discov*. Vol. 4, No. 3, pp. 209-19.

Strozyk, D., Launer, L.J., Adlard, P.A., Cherny, R.A., Tsatsanis, A., Volitakis, I., Blennow, K., Petrovitch, H., White, L.R. & Bush, A.I. (2009). Zinc and copper modulate Alzheimer Abeta levels in human cerebrospinal fluid. *Neurobiol Aging*. Vol. 30, No. 7, pp. 1069-77.

Treiber, C., Simons, A., Strauss, M., Hafner, M., Cappai, R., Bayer, T.A. & Multhaup, G. (2004). Clioquinol mediates copper uptake and counteracts copper efflux activities of the amyloid precursor protein of Alzheimer's disease. *J Biol Chem*. Vol. 279, No. 50, pp. 51958-64.

Vural, H., Demirin, H., Kara, Y., Eren, I. & Delibas, N. (2010). Alterations of plasma magnesium, copper, zinc, iron and selenium concentrations and some related erythrocyte antioxidant enzyme activities in patients with Alzheimer's disease. *J Trace Elem Med Biol*. Vol. 24, No. 3, pp. 169-73.

White, A.R., Du, T., Laughton, K.M., Volitakis, I., Sharples, R.A., Xilinas, M.E., Hoke, D.E., Holsinger, R.M., Evin, G., Cherny, R.A., Hill, A.F., Barnham, K.J., Li, Q.X., Bush, A.I. & Masters, C.L. (2006). Degradation of the Alzheimer disease amyloid beta-peptide by metal-dependent up-regulation of metalloprotease activity. *J Biol Chem*. Vol. 281, No. 26, pp. 17670-80.

White, A.R., Multhaup, G., Maher, F., Bellingham, S., Camakaris, J., Zheng, H., Bush, A.I., Beyreuther, K., Masters, C.L. & Cappai, R. (1999a). The Alzheimer's disease amyloid precursor protein modulates copper-induced toxicity and oxidative stress in primary neuronal cultures. *J Neurosci*. Vol. 19, No. 21, pp. 9170-9.

White, A.R., Reyes, R., Mercer, J.F., Camakaris, J., Zheng, H., Bush, A.I., Multhaup, G., Beyreuther, K., Masters, C.L. & Cappai, R. (1999b). Copper levels are increased in the cerebral cortex and liver of APP and APLP2 knockout mice. *Brain Res*. Vol. 842, No. 2, pp. 439-44.

Wischik, C., Bentham, P, Wischik, DJ, Seng, KM (2008). O3-04-07: Tau aggregation inhibitor (TAI) therapy with rember™ arrests disease progression in mild and moderate Alzheimer's disease over 50 weeks. *Alzheimer's & Dementia*. Vol. 4, No. 4, Supplement, pp. T167.

Yu, W.H., Lukiw, W.J., Bergeron, C., Niznik, H.B. & Fraser, P.E. (2001). Metallothionein III is reduced in Alzheimer's disease. *Brain Res*. Vol. 894, No. 1, pp. 37-45.

Zappasodi, F., Salustri, C., Babiloni, C., Cassetta, E., Del Percio, C., Ercolani, M., Rossini, P.M. & Squitti, R. (2008). An observational study on the influence of the APOE-epsilon4 allele on the correlation between 'free' copper toxicosis and EEG activity in Alzheimer disease. *Brain Res*. Vol. 1215, No., pp. 183-9.

18

Alzheimer's Disease and Metal Contamination: Aspects on Genotoxicity

Lima, P.D.L.[1], Vasconcellos, M.C.[2], Montenegro, R.C.[3] and Burbano, R.R.[3]
[1]*Molecular Biology Laboratory, Center of Biological and Health Sciences, State University of Pará*
[2]*Biological Activities Laboratory, Federal University of Amazonas*
[3]*Human Cytogenetics Laboratory, Institute Biological Institute of Biological Science, Federal University of Pará, Brazil*

1. Introduction

Despite the genetic and environmental factors and the aging process itself, multiple evidence from experimental models and postmortem studies in Alzheimer's disease (AD) brain tissue demonstrate that neurodegeneration is associated with morphological and biochemical features. Considerable evidence suggests a role for oxidative stress/damage (amyloid beta peptide, iron/hydrogen peroxide) or neurotoxic by-products of lipid peroxidation (4-hydroxy-2-nonenal, acrolein) and inflammation, in the pathogenesis of neuron degeneration, which, in turns, are known to cause cell death.

Recently, several reports indicate that, among factors, metal ions (Al, Zn, Cu, Fe, etc) could specifically impair protein aggregation and their oligomeric toxicity. Also, metal-induced (direct) and metal-amyloid-β (indirect) linked neuronal cell death through the formation of reactive oxygen species (ROS) being critical to the understanding of the mechanisms which metal-induced cell death, and thus its role in neurodegenerative disorders.

Some metals are essential for humans and for all forms of life. Even though metals are necessary in biological systems, they are usually required only in trace amounts; in excess, it can be toxic, if not fatal. Environmental metal exposure has been suggested to be a risk factor for AD. High-term exposure to certain metals like manganese (Mn), iron (Fe), aluminum (Al) and many others like copper (Cu), mercury (Hg), zinc (Zn), lead (Pb), arsenic (As), alone or in combination, can increase neurodegenerative process, especially to Alzheimer's disease (AD).

Aluminum is the most widely distributed metal in the environment and is extensively used in daily life that provides easy exposure to human beings. No biological function of the element has been identified, whereas some aspects of its toxicity have been described. It has been suggested that there might be a relationship between high levels of Al and increased risk of a number of pathogenic disorders, such as microcytic anemia, osteomalacia and, possibly, neurodegenerative disorders including dialysis encephalopathy, Parkinson's disease and Alzheimer's disease.

This metal is known to be extremely neurotoxic and in high levels is capable to inhibit the prenatal and post-natal development of the brain. Evidence from clinical and animal studies demonstrated that brain Al content increases with age and that Al generates reactive oxygen species (ROS) that activates signaling pathways which leads to degeneration of neuronal cells. Together with ROS or alone, Al is biochemically attracted to the DNA reveling its genotoxic and mutagenic potential.

Furthermore, high level of Al has been found in brain lesions, such as plaques and tangles, in patients with AD. Several studies demonstrated that among others, Al appears to be the most efficient cation in promoting Aβ aggregation, increasing dramatically cellular neurotoxicity. According to the "amyloid cascade hypothesis", accumulation of Aβ in the brain is the primary event driving AD pathogenesis, increasing the evidences by which Al is involved in AD.

Iron is an essential trace element used by almost all living organisms, being often incorporated into the heme complex, which mediate redox reactions. Disturbances of brain iron homeostasis have been linked to acute neuronal injury. Moreover, iron is toxic to neural tissue, leading to neurodegenerative disorders.

Organic iron (Fe) may increase the genotoxic effects of other compounds when they are combined. Together with aluminum sulfate, at nanomolar concentrations, iron trigger the release of reactive oxygen species (ROS). In high levels, iron can be mutagenic and genotoxic. In AD, iron is an important cause of oxidative stress because of its over-accumulation in the brain and colocalizes with AD lesions, senile plaques and neurofibrillary tangles.

Recent studies also show that homeostasis of essential metals such as copper, iron, selenium and zinc may be altered in the brain of subjects with Alzheimer's disease. It is demonstrated that the plasma concentrations of manganese and total mercury were significantly higher in subjects with AD than in controls, however the concentrations of vanadium, manganese, rubidium, antimony, cesium and lead were significantly lower among subjects with AD cerebrospinal fluid.

The influence of metal ions such as Fe, Cu, and Zn in stimulating Aβ aggregation have been widely studied where they appears to vary depending on tissue pH. It should be noticed that, although there is co-localization of metal ions in the pathological markers of AD, this does not indicate a causative role for these elements in the pathogenesis of the disease. Independently of metals being a primary cause or consequence of the disease mechanism, a change in a single metal ion can cause a significant imbalance on homeostasis in elemental levels in the body (serum, CSF and brain) leading to as a sort of "domino effect". It is clear the need to understand the fundamental biochemical mechanisms linking brain biometal metabolism, environmental metal exposure, genotoxicity and AD pathophysiology. In this review, we discuss the role of metals in Alzheimer disease and its involvement in genotoxicity.

2. Source of metal exposure

Metals have been used throughout human history to make several utensils, machines, jewelry, and so on, where many of then were obtained through mining and smelting, activities that increases their distribution throughout the environment. Furthermore, the use of metals in industry, medicine, agriculture have been increased over the years, which increase the exposure, not only for those workers involved directly in working with metals but also consumers of the products and the general public through environmental contamination (Ferrer, 2003; Ansari *et al.*, 2004).

Metals are among the oldest toxic agents known by humans. Its history starts prior to 2000 BC when it became available as a byproduct of silver smelting. The early Greeks and Romans documented both the toxic as well as the potential healing effects of metals. Theophrastus of Erebus (370-287 BC) and Pliny the Elder (23-79 AD) described the pernicious effects of arsenic and mercury on miners and smelters (Hollenberg, 2010).

In an industrialized world, there are thousands of types of metals in use, and humans are exposed to them at work, or as a result of contamination of food, water and environment. There is abundant evidence indicating an increase of neurodegenerative disorders like AD in industrialized countries (Veldman et al., 1998; Butterworth, 2010). The chronic exposure to metals from several years together with the advance of medical tools may explain why the diagnosis of AD and so its epidemic starts around 1980.

Aluminum is the most widely distributed metal in the environment and is extensively used in a wide variety of products: cans, foils and kitchen utensils, as well as parts of airplanes, rockets and other items that require a strong, light material. It can be deposited on the surface of glass to make mirrors, and also to make synthetic rubies and sapphires for lasers. Al is found in the environment in its natural forms or as a source of human contamination resulting from mining and smelting, activities that increase their distribution throughout the environment. Al occurs naturally only in compounds, never as a pure metal. Because of its strong affinity to oxygen, it is almost never found in the elemental state; instead it is found in oxides or silicates (WHO, 1997; Nayak, 2002).

In nature, this trace element is found in its oxidized state Al^{3+} (soluble toxic form of Al), which binds to others molecules like chloride, forming Aluminum chloride ($AlCl_3$) (Smith, 1996; WHO, 1997). Aluminum chloride ($AlCl_3$) is an important coagulant used in water treatment and purification (WHO, 1997; Zhang e Zhou, 2005) being another source for exposure. Two of the most common compounds are potassium aluminum sulfate ($KAl(SO_4)_2 \cdot 12H_2O$), and aluminum oxide (Al_2O_3).

Although aluminum is a widespread element, almost all metallic aluminium is produced from the ore bauxite ($AlO_x(OH)_{3-2x}$). Bauxite is a complicated mixture of compounds consisting of 55% of aluminum, oxygen, and other elements (WHO, 1997; Nayak, 2002). Large reserves of bauxite are found in Australia, Brazil, Guinea, Jamaica, Russia, and the United States.

No biological function of the element has been identified, whereas some aspects of its toxicity have been described (Berthon, 1996; Corain *et al.*, 1996; Suwalsky *et al.*, 2001). The exposure to this toxic metal occurs through air, food, water and it is also present in medical, cosmetic and environmental products (Berthon, 2002).

Daily consumed of Al by food and beverages is 2.5 to 13 mg, where drinking water can contributes to 0.2 to 0.4 mg of Al daily. Drugs can contribute with increase levels of Al; antiacid drugs (2 tablets) can contribute up to 500 mg of Al (WHO, 1997). As the world becomes more industrialize, the chronic exposure to Al increases, increasing the risk for the development of neurodegenerative disorders like AD and PD.

The period in human history beginning in about 1200 B.C. is called the Iron Age. Iron is a transition metal and normally does not occur as a free element (Meteoric origen) (O´Neil, 1994). The most common ores of iron are hematite, or ferric oxide (Fe_2O_3); limonite, or ferric oxide (Fe_2O_3); magnetite, or iron oxide (Fe_3O_4); and siderite, or iron carbonate ($FeCO_3$). An increasingly important source of iron is taconite. Taconite is a mixture of hematite and silica (sand). The largest iron resources in the world are in China, Russia, Brazil, Canada,

Australia, and Índia. Furthermore, almost all rocks and soils contains at least trace amounts of iron (Sienko, 1977).

Iron is a very reactive metal. Most of then are found as Fe^{2+} which are oxidize to Fe^{3+}. Combines with oxygen in moist air and the product of this reaction is iron oxide (Fe_2O_3) (Cox, 1995). Iron also reacts with very hot water and steam to produce hydrogen gas. It also dissolves in most acids and reacts with many other elements. All of this reaction can be a source for contamination.

Iron is a silvery-white or grayish metal. It is ductile and malleable, very high tensile strength and workable. In general, iron products can be found in automotive, construction, containers, machinery and industrial equipment, railroad tracks, oil and gas industries, electrical tools, appliances and utensils (Ilo, 1997). Furthermore, the fastest growing use of iron compounds is in water treatment systems.

Populations are exposed to iron mainly through foods and beverages. It is available in a number of foods, including meat, milk, eggs, nuts, coffee, tea, fish, grain, soil and raisins. Iron can also be found in fresh water, where recommended levels can not exceed 0.3 mg of iron in 1 liter of water (WHO, 1996). The United State Recommended Daily Allowance (USRDA) for iron is 18 milligrams, being the amount of iron that a person needs to stay healthy. Also, daily recommended doses of Fe varies among age; for children up to 3 months, 1.7 mg/kg/daily are recommended, whereas for adults this is 10 times more (18 mg/kg/daily)(WHO, 1996).

An iron deficiency can cause serious health problems in humans. Also, several alterations have been related to high iron intake where iron is toxic to neural tissue, leading to neurodegenerative disorders like AD (Montgomery, 1995; Campbell & Bondy, 2000; Stankiewicz & Brass, 2009).

Manganese is a transition metal and it took several years to discover the difference between manganese and iron, mainly because it oftens occurs together in the Earth's crust and its similarity properties.

Manganese is a moderately active metal and never occurs as a pure element in nature. It always combines with oxygen in the air to form manganese dioxide (MnO_2) or other elements. It also combines with fluorine and chloride to make manganese difluoride (MnF_2) and manganese dichloride ($MnCl_2$) (WHO, 1999). The most common ores of manganese are pyrolusite (MnO_2), manganite, psilomelane, and rhodochrosite. Manganese is also found mixed with iron ores. The largest producers of manganese ore in the world are China, South Africa, the Ukraine, Brazil, Australia, Gabon, and Kazakstan.

Early artists were familiar with pyrolusite and they used the mineral to give glass a beautiful purple color, and/or to remove color from a glass. By the middle 1700s, chemists proved that pyrolusite contained manganese dioxide. Until now, coloring agents (textiles, paints, inks, glass, and ceramics) still contains manganous chloride.

The most common alloy of manganese is ferromanganese, containing about 48 percent manganese combined with iron and carbon, being the source for making a very large variety steel products, including tools, heavy-duty machinery, railroad tracks, bank vaults, construction components, and automotive parts. Also, manganous chloride ($MnCl_2$), is an additive in animal food for cows, horses, goats, and other domestic animals. In agriculture, manganous chloride are present in fertilizers (Barceloux, 1999).

Manganese is one of the chemical elements that has both positive and negative effects on living organisms because manganese is used by many enzymes in an organism. A very small amount of the element is needed to maintain good health. The absortion of Mn is only

3 to 5%, being food the primary source of this metal. Mn is found in green vegetables, nut, raisins, and also in teas, its main source for human consumption. Low concentrations are found in Milk, meat, fish, eggs and fruits (Barceloux, 1999). Taking all together, soil, fertilizer and food, one can say that humans are exposed to Mn and that excess of manganese can create health problems. Also, a variety of drugs and supplements have Mn in its composition (WHO, 1999).

Human exposure can be also by inhalation. Workers may inhale manganese dust in the air in a factory or mine. Also, human can be exposed by the ingestion of contaminated water with fertilizers and pesticides (WHO, 1999). Exposures to high levels of manganese by ingestion or inhalation can damage the central nervous system. Daily-recommended doses of Mn for children are 0.3 mg/Kg/daily, being 3 times more for adults (10 mg/Kg/daily) (WHO, 1999).

3. Metal neurotoxicity

Abnormal production or clearance of a small peptide, the amyloid β-peptide (Aβ), which is the major constituent of the senile plaques, is a widely accepted causative agent in degenerative disorders like AD (Hardy & Selkoe, 2002; LaFerla et al., 2007; Qiu & Folstein, 2006; Rauk, 2009; Sayre et al., 1997; Selkoe, 2000). Aβ is a 39- to 43-residue peptide cleaved from the C-terminal region of a much larger protein, the amyloid precursor protein (APP), where the most abundant fragments are Aβ (1–40) and Aβ (1–42), being the latter the most neurotoxic (Rauk, 2009).

Several studies have shown that Aβ exerts its toxicity by generating reactive oxidative stress (ROS) molecules, leading to peroxidation of membrane lipids and lipoproteins, induction of H_2O_2 and hydroxynonenal (HNE) in neurons, damages DNA and transport enzymes inactivation (Behl et al., 1994; Kontush et al., 2001; Mark et al., 1997; Mark et al., 1997; Varadarajan et al., 2000; Xu et al., 2001). In addition to a high metabolically levels of ROS, there are other sources that are thought to play an important role in the AD progression. Among them, mitochondrial and metal abnormalities are the major sources of oxidative stress (Su et al., 2008).

Increasing evidences suggest that altered metal homeostasis may contribute to neuronal loss in neurodegenerative diseases (Gerlach et al., 2006; Sayre et al., 2005; Wright, 2008). Given a likely role for metal-associated oxidative stress, herein it is discuss the involvement of metals, such as Al(III), Fe(III) and Mg(II) in neurotoxicity.

3.1 Aluminum and neurotoxicity

Aluminum (Al) is the third most abundant element in the earth's crust and is not an essential trace metal for mammals. However, the concentrations found in the body can be sufficient to modify the activity of several key enzymes and second messenger pathways (Bondy, 2010).

Aluminum is known to be extremely neurotoxic and in high levels is capable to inhibit the prenatal and post-natal development of the brain (Yumoto et al., 2001). Several studies correlated the risk of developing Alzheimer's disease with residing in areas where aluminum concentrations in the drinking water are 100 mg/L or greater (McLachlan et al., 1996; Rondeau et al., 2000).

The hypothesis that there is a link between aluminum and Alzheimer's disease (AD) was first brought out in the 1960s by Terry and Pena (1965) and by Klatzo and colaborators in

1965 (Terry et al., 1969). Early on 1976, high levels of aluminum have been found in brain lesions, such as plaques and tangles, in patients with AD (Crapper et al., 1976), and also in other conditions such as Parkinson's disease (PD), pre-senile dementia, amiotrofic lateral esclerosis, neurofibrilar degeneration, dialysis encephalopathy syndrome and nigroestriatal sindrome (Altschuler, 1999; Gupta et al., 2005; Nayak, 2002; Yasui et al., 1992; Zatta et al., 1991). Elevated aluminum levels have also been reported in other less common neurological disorders such as the Guamanian Parkinsonian-ALS constellation and Hallervorden-Spatz disease (Eidelberg et al., 1987; Garruto et al., 1989).

The most common neurostrutural alterations induced by high levels of aluminum in the brain is: brain ventricle dilatation and thinning of the corpus callosum (Lapresie et al., 1975), reduce neural cell density, degenerative changings like picnosis, vacuolization, chromatin condensation (Varner et al., 1998), increase neural filaments in neuron from the spinal cord and brainstem (Terry et al., 1969), axonal intumescence (Troncoso et al., 1985) and cerebellar disorder with degeneration of the Purkinje cells (Ghetti et al., 1985; Yokel, 1994).

There is some experimental evidence that Al exposure can adversely affect the dopaminergic system. Extended exposure to 100mM Al lactate increased striatal levels of the dopamine metabolite (Li et al., 2008), what, in turns, suggests that exposure to Al may cause increased turnover of dopamine. The development of an encephalopathy, characterized by cognitive deficits, in-coordination, tremor and spinocerebellar degeneration, among workers in the aluminum industry also indicates that exposure to the metal can be profoundly deleterious. Abnormal neurological symptoms have been observed in several patients receiving intramuscular injections of Al-containing vaccines.

There have been many experimental studies on animals and on isolated cells showing that aluminum has toxic effects on the nervous system. In 1991, Guy and colaborators showed that the uptake of aluminum by human neuroblastoma cells display an epitope associated with Alzheimer's diseases. Chronic exposure of animals to aluminum is associated with behavioural, neuropathological and neurochemical changes. Among them, deficits of learning and behavioural functions are most evident (Kummar et al., 2009; Ribes et al., 2010; Sethi et al., 2008). Also, when mice were injected with adjuvants containing aluminum in amounts equivalent to those given to US military service personnel, neuroinflammation and cell loss were found in spinal cord and motor cortex, together with memorial deficits (Petrik et al., 2007).

Several metals interact with β-amyloid (Aβ) in senile plaques. It is interesting to note that, compared to other Aβ-metal complexes (Aβ-Fe, Aβ-Zn, Aβ-Cu), Aβ-Al is unique in promoting a specific form of Aβ oligomerization that has marked neurotoxic effects (Drago et al., 2008).

There are a lot of ways which Al can damage neural cells: (i) interfering with glucose metabolism, leading to low amounts of Acetilcholine (Ach) precursors; (ii) interacting to ATPase Na^+/K^+ and Ca^{2+}/Mg^{2+} -depending, altering excitatory aminoacid release; (iii) inhibition the binding of Ca^{++}; (iv) incresing the production of AMPc; (v) causing changes in the cytoskeleton protein, leading to phosphorilation, proteolysis, transport and synthesis disruption; (vi) interacting directly to genomic structures, and most importantly (vii) inducing oxidative damage by lipid peroxidation (Nayak & Chatterjee, 1999).

Being involved in the production of reactive oxygen species (ROS), aluminum may cause impairments in mitochondrial bioenergetics and may lead to the generation of oxidative stress which may lead to a gradual accumulation of oxidatively modified cellular proteins, lipids and affects endogenous antioxidant enzyme activity, leading to degeneration of neuronal cells (Kummar et al., 2009; Sethi et al., 2008; Wu et al., 2010). In this way, aluminum is a strong candidate for consideration as a subtle promoter of events typically associated with brain aging and neurodegenerative disorders.

3.2 Iron and neurotoxicity

Metal ion homeostasis is maintained through highly regulated mechanisms of uptake, storage, and secretion (Mills et al., 2010). Iron plays a role in oxygen transportation, myelin synthesis, neurotransmitter production, and electron transfers, being a crucial cofactor in normal central nervous (CNS) metabolism. Iron is also abundantly in substantia nigra and globus palladium when compared with other regions and is found to increase with age in humans (Bartzokis et al., 1994; Lee et al., 2010; Zecca et al., 2001). Normally, under healthy conditions, these metal ions are bound to ligands (e.g., transferrin), however when they are found nonbound, iron are potentially harmful mainly due to their redox activities in the synaptic cleft (Salvador et al., 2011).

Free iron catalyzes the conversion of superoxide and hydrogen peroxide into hydroxyl radicals, which promote oxidative stress by the Fenton reaction (Berg et al., 2001). Furthermore, ROS interacts with a variety of molecules, including unsaturated fatty acids, proteins and DNA leading to subsequent cell death/apoptosis, especially on CNS tissue, whereas the antioxidant defenses are rare (Demougeot et al., 2003; Stankiewicz & Brass, 2009; Willmore & Rubin, 1984). Thus, disturbances of brain iron homeostasis have been linked to acute neuronal injury leading to neurodegenerative disorders (Campbell & Bondy, 2000; Montgomery, 1995) such as Alzheimer's (AD), Parkinson's (PD), and Huntington's (HD) diseases as well as amyotrophic lateral sclerosis (ALS) (Connor & Benkovic, 1992; Kell, 2010; Liu et al., 2006; Rouault, 2001; Youdim et al., 2005).

Degradation of the dopaminergic system, where catechols molecules should be produced, may play a role in the extrapyramidal symptoms in PD (Prikhojan et al, 2002; Santiago et al., 2000). *In vitro* studies have shown that iron is accumulated in microglia and astrocytes in the cerebral cortex, cerebellum, substantia nigra, and hippocampus, and it is believed that this metal would be involved in the neuroinflammation observed in AD and PD (Ong & Farooqui, 2005).

Postmortem studies in PD subjects, suggests that accumulation of iron in the substantia nigra stimulates lipid peroxidation, which can lead to cell damage (Nakano, 1993; Riederer et al., 1989). Studies conducted with PD subjects demonstrated that in mild PD, there were no significant differences in the content of total iron between the PD group and control, whereas there was an increase in total iron and iron (III) in substantia nigra of severely affected patients (Riederer et al., 1989). Indeed, lateral substantia nigra pars compacta abnormalities were observed in early PD together with increased iron content.

Within the reduction on glutathione and the change of the iron (II)/iron (III) ratio in favor of iron (III), it is suggest that these changes might contribute to pathophysiological processes underlying PD (Griffiths et al., 1999; Lan & Jiang, 1997; Martin & Wiler, 2008). Interestingly, the increase in iron in the degenerating substantia nigra (SN) occurs only in the advanced stages of the disease, suggesting that these phenomena may be a secondary event, rather than a primary (Double et al., 2000). Patients with diagnosed AD and in normal elderly patients, iron concentrations have been found to be increased in the bilateral hippocampus, parietal cortex, frontal white matter, putamen, caudate nucleus, thalamus, red nucleus, substantia nigra, and dentate nucleus subregions. Particularly in the parietal cortex, at the

early stages of AD, studies have been found to positively correlate with the severity of patients' cognitive impairment (Sullivan et al., 2009; Zhu et al., 2009).
Although extensive evidence links the iron metabolism, aging, and neurodegenerative disorders, relatively little is known about the resulting forms of iron that accumulate in the brain. Numerous techniques have been developed in order to characterize, locate, and quantify iron species and iron- containing compounds in the brain, however, more studies are needed to understand the role of this transition metal in the onset and progression of neurodegenerative diseases and neurological age-related disorders.

3.3 Manganese and neurotoxicity

Manganese is an essential element for many living organisms, especially humans, where some enzymes require (e.g., manganese superoxide dismutase), and some are activated, by manganese (Hurley & Keen, 1987). Excess accumulation of these metal by ingestion or inhalation (mostly in working place) (Agency for Toxic Substances and Disease Registry [ATSDR], 2000) can damage the central nervous system (Winder et al., 2010) most likely due to impaired transport or failure of hepatic detoxification mechanisms, what have deleterious effects on cell function and integrity (Butterworth, 2010).
It is known that astrocytes have a much higher affinity and capacity for manganese uptake compared to neurons and that exposure to manganese results primarily in alterations of astrocyte morphology and function (Aschner et al., 1992). Excessive exposure to Mn can also lead to neural lesion, primarily on the dopaminergic pathway (globus pallidus and substantia nigra pars reticulata), inhibiting dopamine metabolism (Vidal et al., 2005).
Short-term repeated pulmonary exposure to manual metal arc-hard surfacing or gas metal arc-mild steel fumes resulted in selective deposition of Mn in the brain, particularly in dopaminergic brain areas. It is interesting to note that, other constituents of the fumes like Fe, Cr, Ni or Cu did not appear to translocate to the brain despite their large accumulation in the lungs and its associated lymph nodes. Molecular markers of dopaminergic neurotoxicity and injury response can be found in the brain of welding fumes, extended beyond the globus pallidus, considered the primary site of damage in manganism, to broader dopaminergic areas (Sriram et al., 2010).
Neurotoxic effect of Mn can be due to its interaction with detoxification enzymes that protects the cells, and/or its interaction with the redox system. In this way, Mn^{2+} (necessary in the brain) can be oxidize to Mn^{3+}, a toxic compound that enhances the oxidation of dopamine leading to a lots of neurotoxic products (Donaldson et al., 1982). Recent studies reveal that repeated exposure to Mn or Mn-containing welding fumes can cause mitochondrial dysfunction and alterations in the expression of proteins in dopaminergic brain areas, also, events that contribute to dopaminergic neurotoxicity (Sriram et al., 2010). Some evidences indicate that the neurological abnormalities can be found on the striatum and on subthalamic nucleus in the CNS of the monkey receiving $MnCl_2$ by inhalation (Newland et al., 1999). Also, undesirable neurological effects were observed in children who were exposed to excess manganese (Zheng et al., 1998), what can explain the enhanced incidence of neurological symptoms in isolated populations (Florence & Stauber, 1989; Iwami et al., 1994).
Adverse health effects can be caused by inadequate intake or overexposure to manganese. Chronic exposure to high levels of Mn induces a syndrome known as "manganism", characterized by extrapyramidal dysfunction (bradykinesia, rigidity and dystonia) and

neuropsychiatric symptoms that resemble idiopathic Parkinson's disease (Santamaria & Sulsky, 2010).
Although is not completely clear the relationship between Mn and PD patogenesis, or neurodegenerative disorders, it is suggest that this metal accelerates neuronal death and increase the risk of its development (Zheng et al., 1998).

4. Metal contamination and AD developing

Metal are essential for humans and for all forms of life. Even though metals are necessary in biological systems, they are usually required only in trace amounts. As regard to the brain, metals are essential for neuronal activities. However, if not correctly regulated, redox-active can react with molecular oxygen to generate ROS thus causing brain lipid peroxidation and protein oxidation (Salvador et al., 2011; Sayre et al., 1997; Smith et al., 1996; Smith et al., 1997). Also, metal imbalance can lead to aberrant interactions between metals and AD-related proteins, being a potential source of oxidative stress, which is evolved into the "metal hypothesis" of AD (Iqbal et al., 2005).
Protein misfolding associated with Aβ aggregation, is significantly affected by various biological, biophysical and chemical factors including metal ions such as Al, Cu, Zn, and Fe, which have been found in high concentration in the AD brain (Beauchemin et al., 1998; Dong et al., 2003; Lovell et al., 1993; 1998; Miu et al., 2006; Suh et al., 2000;). Also, some metals are able to accelerate the dynamic of Aβ aggregation, thus increasing the neurotoxic effects on neuronal cells (Bush, 2003; House et al., 2004; Maynard et al., 2005; Miu et al., 2006; Morgan et al., 2002; Ricchelli et al., 2005). Kawahara et al. (2001) showed that aluminum induces neuronal apoptosis in vivo as well as in vitro and causes the accumulation of hyperphosphorylated tau protein and Aβ protein in in vivo model.
Several studies have focused on the role of metal ions including Al on the Aβ aggregation properties (House et al., 2004; Kawahara et al., 1994; Pratico et al., 2002; Ricchelli et al., 2005), suggesting that, among various metal ions assessed, Al seems to be the most efficient in promoting Aβ aggregation in vitro, increasing cellular neurotoxicity (Kawahara et al., 2001; Kawahara, 2005; Ricchelli et al., 2005). Also, Al induces the spontaneous increase of Aβ1-42 surface hydrophobicity compared to Aβ alone, which in turns, the complex Aβ1-42-Al reduced the capillary sequestration increasing its permeability through the blood brain barrier resulting intracerebral accumulation as demonstrated by Banks et al. (2006).
Environmental metal exposure has been suggested to be a risk factor for AD. High-term exposure to certain metals like manganese (Mn), iron (Fe), aluminum (Al) and many others, alone or in combination, can increase neurodegenerative process, especially to Alzheimer's disease (AD).
Aluminum (Al) is the most abundant neurotoxic metal on earth, widely bioavailable to humans and repeatedly shown to accumulate in AD-susceptible neuronal foci. Furthermore, several groups reported an increased amounts of Al in neurofibrillary tangles (NFT)-bearing neurons of AD brains, suggesting the association of Al with NFTs (Good et al., 1992; Lovell et al., 1993). Evidence from clinical and animal model studies demonstrated that brain Al content increases with age, suggesting an increased exposure or a decreased ability to remove Al from brain with age (Savory et al., 1999). Furthermore, high levels of Al has been found in brain lesions, such as plaques and tangles, in patients with AD and could be involved in the aggregation of Aβ peptides to form toxic fibrils (Sakae et al., 2009).

Iron is an essential trace element used by almost all living organisms. However, disturbances of brain iron homeostasis have been linked to acute neuronal injury. Increased iron levels were found both in the cortex and cerebellum from the preclinical AD cases (Sullivan et al., 2009; Zhu et al., 2009). Cellular studies have shown that iron is particular accumulated in microglia and astrocytes in the cerebral cortex, cerebellum, substantia nigra, and hippocampus, and it is believed that this metal would be involved in the neuroinflammation found in AD and PD (Ong & Farooqui, 2005; Sullivan et al., 2009; Zhu et al., 2009). It is important to note that these brain iron concentrations, especially in the parietal cortex at the early stages of AD, have been found to positively correlate with the severity of patients' cognitive impairment (Zhu et al., 2009). Interestingly, Aβ insoluble aggregates have been demonstrated to be dissolved by metal chelators (Cherny et al., 1999). Iron itself has been related neurotoxicity, and its accumulation, has been observed to before AD lesions are measurable. In AD, iron is an important cause of oxidative stress because of its over-accumulation in the brain and colocalizes with AD lesions, senile plaques and neurofibrillary tangles. Interestingly, iron has been involved in lipid and protein oxidation and also in DNA damage. Iron is able to oxidize DNA bases, and it has been suggested that the accumulation of this transition metal in some neurodegenerative disorders could act by both increasing oxidative genome damage and also preventing its repair (Hegde et al., 2010).

Manganese (Mn) is an essential element for humans, animals, and plants and is required for growth, development, and maintenance of health, although it has been recognized as a neurotoxic metal for over 150 years (Weiss, 2010). Unbalance of Mn homeostasis has show cognitive deficiencies features that include diminished attention, reduced scores on tests of working memory, lower scores on intelligence tests, impaired learning, and slowed response speed. Also, Weiss (2010) reports that signs of Mn poisoning are impaired coordination, abnormal gait, abnormal laughter, expressionless face, weakness, bradykinesia, somnolence, dysarthria, difficulty walking, clumsiness, lack of balance, muscle pains, and diminished leg power. Furthermore, exposure to high levels of inhaled manganese, as in miners working leads to motor symptoms.

Nonhuman primates can be the most appropriate animal models for studies of manganese neurotoxicity because of their similarities to humans in brain anatomy and neurobehavioral function (Schneider et al., 2009). A recent study by Schneider et al. (2009) demonstrated that trained Cynomologous monkeys for memory test followed by a regimen of intravenous manganese sulfate injections over a period of about 230 days, displayed mild deficits in spatial memory, greater deficits in nonspatial memory, and no deficits in reference memory on animals treated. By analyzing Mn concentrations, the study showed a significant inverse relationship between working memory task performance and Mn levels.

The relationship by Mn exposure and Alzheimer's disease has also been investigated by gene array analysis of frontal cortex from Cynomologous monkeys after Schneider et al. (2009) studies (Guilarte et al., 2010). Amyloid-β Precursor-like Protein 1 (APLP1), a member of the Amyloid Precursor Protein (APP) family was the most expressed out of the 61 upregulated genes. Along with this finding, immunochemistry revealed the presence of Amyloid-β plaques in the brain of subjects with only 6–8 years of age. Thus, these findings links the Mn-induced β-amyloid deposits to impaired memory function what may be extrapolated to human brain and so the features of AD pathogenesis.

5. Metal genotoxicity

Cellular stresses, including DNA damage, have been linked to cell cycle deregulation in neurons (Park et al., 1998; Kruman et al., 2004). Studies on the biological causes of neuronal death in AD have been guided by observations of cell cycle reentry in cellular populations that degenerate in human disease (Busser et al., 1998; Yang et al., 2003). In addition to ectopic cell cycling, AD is also linked to DNA damage; accumulation of DNA damage in neurons is associated with aging (Lu et al., 2004) and is exacerbated in neurodegenerative disorders including AD (Rass et al., 2007). The occurrance of DNA damage was related in astrocytes of AD hippocampus (Myung et al., 2008) and in neurons within the cerebellar dentate nucleus that show the robust DNA damage response (Chen et al., 2010).

The appearance of DNA damage during the course of lateonset neurodegenerative disease has been attributed in part to the fact that neurons exhibit high mitochondrial respiration, which is known to lead to the production of reactive oxygen-species. Over time this oxidative stress results in the accumulated damage of mitochondrial and nuclear DNA (Rass et al., 2007). These findings emphasize the value of using direct markers of neuronal distress, like DNA damage, as neuropathological markers in AD. They augment the classical histopathological picture achieved by staining for amyloid plaques and tau inclusions by providing an early neuronal vulnerability marker (Chen et al., 2010).

As a consequence of industrial production, a large quantity of toxic material is released in the ambient. Due to the elevated concentrations of metals present in different environments, metals are ubiquitous contaminants of ecosystems; therefore, they are among the most intensely studied contaminants. They do not only deteriorate the physicochemical equilibrium of the ecosystems, but they also disrupt the food web and bring about morphological, physiological and cytogenetic changes in the inhabitants (Boge & Roche, 1996). Genotoxic studies have shown that exposure to some metals causes adverse effects to different organisms, especially to humans, and these DNA damages may be implicated in the pathogenesis of some types of cancer and neurodegenerative diseases.

5.1 Genotoxicity of aluminum

Metal-induced genotoxicity is an important pathogenic mechanism whereby toxic metals that riches the nucleus affect the normal structure and function of the genome (Alexandrov et al., 2005; Lukiw, 2001; Sarkander et al., 1983).

There are only few studies in the literature about the genotoxic activities of Al, both in vitro and in vivo. Aluminum is biochemically attracted to interact to the phosphates that form an active part of the DNA. Its mutagenic potential has been studied by micronucleus assay, sister chromatid exchange, Ames and chromosomal aberration analysis, showing a significant genotoxicity in vitro (Banasik et al., 2005; Lankoff et al., 2006). Also, in vivo studies revealed that aluminum could induce in a dose-dependent manner an increase chromosomal aberrations (Roy et al., 1991).

In vitro chromosomal aberrations induction, mostly numeric (anaphasic), was shown first by Moreno et al., (1997), in the Balb c 3T3 cell line exposed to atmospheric dust (20–80 mg/mL), a mixture of particles of potassium aluminum silicates (98%) and sodium dioxide (2%), from Mexicali, Mexico. Other studies (Dovgaliuk et al., 2001a, 2001b) also demonstrated the cytogenetic effects of toxic metal salts including aluminum (Al[NO3]3) in meristematic cells from Allium cepa and the clastogenic and aneugenic effects (disturbances in mitosis and cytokinesis) in these cells.

More recently, the genotoxic potencial of AlCl3 on Vicia faba was investigated using cytogenetic tests, demonstrating that aluminum causes significant increase in the frequencies of micronuclei and anaphase chromosome aberrations in the root cells of Vicia faba (Yi et al., 2009).

Iron and aluminum-sulfate together, at nanomolar concentrations, trigger the release of reactive oxygen species (ROS) in cultures of human brain cells, up-regulating pro-inflammatory and pro-apoptotic genes that redirect cellular fate toward cytoplasmic dysfunction, nuclear DNA fragmentation and cell death (Alexandrov et al., 2005; Lukiw, 2001; Sarkander et al., 1983).

On neural cells from Parkinson´s disease patients, Al treatment did not increase the micronucleus frequency, indicating that Al had no amplified mutagenic effect on these patients (Trippi et al., 2001). Also, chromosome breaks were observed in V79-4 Chinese hamster cells irradiated with low-energy aluminum ions (Botchway et al., 1997). Furthermore, no teratogenic effects on the mouse fetus or genotoxic effects as detected by the Ames assay was observed for aluminum-containing cosmetic formulations (Elmore, 2003).

Lukim & Pogue (2007) first described the neurotoxic effects of aluminum-sulfate and aluminum- plus iron-sulfate on miRNA expression patterns in untransformed human brain cells in primary co-cultures of neurons and glia. Low doses of aluminum have been found to disturb RNA Pol II-directed gene transcription in isolated human brain cell nuclei (Alexandrov et al., 2005; Lukiw, 2001) suggesting an involvement of soluble aluminum- and iron-sulfate in several different aspects of human brain gene expression, specially associated with transcriptional and post-transcriptional control. Synapsin mRNA has been found to be down-regulated in both AD brain and in iron- plus aluminum-sulfate treated primary cell culture (Alexandrov et al., 2005; Lukiw, 2007; Yumei et al., 1998).

On the other hand, studies have demonstrated the mutagenic potential of Al in human cells. For example, genotoxicity of the dust derived from an electrolytic Al plant was evaluated using the Ames assay, unscheduled DNA synthesis test, sister chromatid exchange and micronuclei frequencies in human lymphocytes. The results of these four experiments indicated a high genotoxicity potential of the dust organic extract (Varella et al., 2007). The mutagenic activity of waste material originating from an Al products factory was determined by the Salmonella/microsome assay, where all extracts from the factory had mutagenic activity, especially in the YG1024 yeast strain, suggesting the presence of aromatic amines (WHO, 1997).

Scalon et al (2011) assessed the genotoxic effects in fish exposed to samples from the Sinos River (Rio Grande do Sul - Brazil), and evaluated DNA damage from aluminum, lead, chromium, copper, nickel, iron and zinc contamination. They collected samples of different sites and on differente seasons in the Sinos River, and chemical analysis of the water showed presence of Al and Fe, exceeding the accepted limits in most of the water samples. The index of DNA damage assessed by the comet assay in the peripheral blood of a native fish species demonstrated no significant differences in different seasons or at the different sampling sites. Only the frequency of cells with higher level of DNA damage showed significant difference in comparison to the sampling period. However, the increase in that parameter of genotoxicity does not seem to be related to differences between sampling periods regarding the presence or concentration of the heavy metals analysed.

Garcia-Medina et al (2011) evaluated de genotoxic and cytotoxic effects of Aluminum sulphate on common carp (Cyprinus carpio). They exposed the fishes to 0.05, 120, and 239 mg/L $Al_2 (SO_4)_3 \cdot 7H_2O$ and analysed the cells with the comet assay, flow cytometry, and the TUNEL method. The analyzed cells showed significant increase in the amount of DNA, damage, DNA content increase and ploidy modifications, as well as apoptosis and disturbances of the cell cycle progression and an increase in the amount of apoptotic cells. These results suggests, in a contrary way to the study of Scalon et al (2011), that Al caused deleterious DNA and cellular effects in aquatic organisms.
Recently our research group published a study on the genotoxic, clastogenic and cytotoxic effects of AlCl3 in different phases of the cell cycle using in vitro temporary cultures of human lymphocytes (Lima et al., 2007). Moreover, the mitotic index (MI), chromosomal aberrations (CAs) and DNA damage index were analyzed by the comet assay. The study indicated that AlCl3 induces DNA damage and is cytotoxic during all phases of the cell cycle. Also, the treatment of the cells at G1 phase resulted in polyploidy and endoreduplication, consistent with AlCl3 interacting with the mitotic spindle apparatus (Lima et al., 2007). These data, along with the results of other studies reported in the literature, indicates that AlCl3 is genotoxic and should be used with caution.
More research is needed on this topic, since the use of aluminum cookware, aluminum-containing deodorants and other products are increasing in general population. Moreover, environmental metal contamination contributes with the increase levels of metal exposure (Ansari et al., 2004).

5.2 Genotoxicity of iron

Several studies have been conducted to demonstrate the potential induction of DNA aberrations by iron (Fe) and also by drugs and compounds containing this metal. However, the results are inconclusive, and its toxicity and mutagenic effect is still incompletely understood.
Organic Fe may increase the genotoxic effects of other compounds when they are combined (WHO, 1998). For example, the mutagenic activity by doxorubicin is significantly increased within this metal, as evaluated by the Ames test (Kostoryz & Yourtee, 2001). Furthermore, Jurkat cells simultaneously treated with hydrogen peroxide and desferrioxamine (Fe chelator) significantly inhibit DNA damage, indicating that intracellular Fe, which is a redoxactive metal, plays a role in the induction of DNA strand breaks induced by hydrogen peroxide (Barbouti et al., 2001).
High levels of chromosome and chromatid aberrations were found in human lymphocytes and TK6 lymphoblast cells exposed to high-energy iron ions (56Fe) (Durante et al., 2002; Evans et al., 2001, 2003). Significant DNA damage was detected, by microgel electrophoresis, in differentiated human colon tumor cells (HT29 clone 19A) treated with ferric-nitrilotriacetate (Fe-NTA) (Glei et al., 2002). Mutagenic activity was also found in elemental and salt forms of Fe, evaluated by mutagenicity tests in Salmonella typhimurium and L5178Y mouse lymphoma cells (Dunkel et al., 1999).
Iron compounds have also been reported to be mutagenic in mammalian cells, as detected by the Syrian hamster embryo cell transformation/viral enhancement assay (Heidelberger et al., 1983), sister chromatid exchange (SCE) in hamster cells (Tucker et al., 1993) and base tautomerization in rat hepatocyte cultures (Abalea et al., 1999).
Few or no DNA damage (detected by the comet assay) occurred after treatment of human lymphocytes with ferric chloride (FeCl3) and ferrous chloride (FeCl2), all of them known to

be iron compounds (Anderson et al., 2000a, 2000b). Also, low concentrations of either Fe2+ or Fe3+ were not mutagenic in Chinese hamster ovary cells (CHO-9) treated in vitro, and the mitotic index was also unaffected when compared to negative control. In the other hand, high concentrations of ferrous sulfate, induces significant DNA damage, probably as a consequence of chemical contamination of the metal salt (Antunes et al., 2005).

Mutagenic potential of metallic agents used in dietary supplementation, including iron sulfate, was also investigated by means of the comet assay. The authors reported a genotoxic effect of this metal in mouse blood cells after 24 h of treatment, at all tested concentrations (Franke et al., 2006). Genotoxic effects of Fe were also reported by Garry et al. (2003) in rats treated with iron oxide (Fe_2O_5) for 24 h. They observed that this metal only showed mutagenic potential when the animals were simultaneously treated with benzopyrene.

Furthermore, Hasan et al. (2005) reported that ferritin, an ubiquitously distributed iron storage protein, interacts with microtubules in vitro. In a study conducted by Maenosono et al. (2007) the bacterial reverse mutation assay using S. typhimurium was weakly positive for water-soluble FePt nanoparticles capped with tetramethylammonium hydroxide. Mice subchronically exposed to 33.2 mg/Kg Fe displayed genotoxic effects in whole blood in the alkaline version of the comet assay, with a significant increase in the hepatic level of Fe (Prá et al., 2008).

High-energy iron ions (LET=151 keV/microM) could induce chromosomal aberrations (measured using the fluorescence whole-chromosome painting technique) in normal and repair-deficient human fibroblasts cell lines (George et al., 2009).

Park & Park (2011) screened the potential toxicity of various iron-overloads on human leukocytes using comet assay. Ferric-nitrilotriacetate (Fe-NTA), FeSO(4), hemoglobin and myoglobin were not cytotoxic in the range of 10-1000 microM by trypan blue exclusion assay. The exposure of leukocytes to Fe-NTA (500 and 1000 microM), $FeSO_4$ (250-1000 microM), hemoglobin (10 microM) and myoglobin (250 microM) for 30 min induced significant DNA damage. Iron-overloads generated DNA strand break were rejoined from the first 1h, but no genotoxic effect was observed at 24h.

Recently, our research group conducted an in vitro study aiming to investigate the genotoxic, clastogenic and cytotoxic effects of FeSO4 in different phases of the cell cycle, using short-term cultures of human lymphocytes. The bioactivity parameters tested were the mitotic index, chromosomal aberrations and DNA damage index as detected by the comet assay. Our results showed that Fe induces alterations and inhibition of DNA synthesis, which together explains the concomitant occurrence of mutagenicity and cytotoxicity (Lima et al., 2008).

5.3 Genotoxicity of manganese

Manganese displays an interestingly behavior with regard to its toxicity, since it is relatively non-toxic to the adult organism with an exception to the brain. Even at moderate amounts in a long period of time, when inhaleted can causes Parkinson-like symptoms. Those findings were also observed in animal studies which repeated intravenous Mn administration to monkeys (Olanow et al., 1996) produced a Parkinson-like syndrome characterized by bradykinesia, rigidity, and facial grimacing.

The association of Mn with the risk of developing neurodegenerative processes can be related to DNA damage. Relatively high doses of Mn can disrupt DNA integrity and DNA replication (Beckman et al., 1985; De Meo et al., 1991; Van de Sande et al., 1982) and causes mutations in microorganism (Orgel & Orgel 1965; Rossman et al., 1984; Rossman & Molina, 1986) and mammalian cells although the Ames test does not appear to be particularly responsive to manganese or no suitable to detect toxicity of metal salts (Léonard, 1988).

There are few studies in the literature on the genotoxic action of Mn. Its toxic potential has been studied by in vitro tests in bacteria and by in vivo/in vitro tests in insect and mammalian cells, showing that some chemical forms of this metal have mutagenic potential. Gerber et al. (2002) demonstrated that high doses (0.05 M) of various Mn compounds could affect DNA replication and repair in bacteria. As for mammalian cells, high doses of Mn (compared to the Mn doses recommended for daily consumption) can affect fertilization and are toxic to the embryo and fetus, demonstrating the teratogenic potential of this metal.

Dutta et al. (2006) suggests the manganese dioxide as an established genotoxicant and clastogenic metal that can induce DNA strand breaks, chromosomal aberration and micronucleus in human peripheral lymphocytes. Manganese chloride ($MnCl_2$) was also subjected to the wing spot test of Drosophila melanogaster and was shown to be clearly effective in inducing spots with one or two mutant hairs (small spots) at concentrations over 12 μM (Ogawa et al., 1994).

Concentrations of manganese in the general environment and manufacture products vary widely. Brega et al. (1998) demonstrated that farm workers exposed to pesticides containing Mn, even at a low levels, revealed an increased in the mutagenic potential of those pesticides, as evidenced by an increased number of CAs. It is possible that, at low doses, Mn has genotoxic effects only with long-term exposure, and this may be the reason why Timchenko et al. (1991) did not find CAs in the nasal mucosa of mammals exposed to Mn dioxide aerosol (40–12,000 Hz, 80–100 dB). Furthermore, it is possible that chronic exposure to low doses of Mn can induces CAs over the years.

Studies on eukaryotic cell, revealed that manganese sulfate ($MnSO_4$) did not display mutagenic potential in different strains of Salmonella typhimurium, while, manganese chloride, showed mutagenicity in the TA1537 strain of S. typhimurium as well as in the T7 strain of Saccharomyces cerevisiae (doses over 0.5 mM) (WHO, 1999). In vivo studies have demonstrated that oral doses of manganese sulfate or potassium permanganate (KMnO4) induce CAs in the bone marrow of animals, whereas no CAs have been seemed after oral doses of manganese chloride, even at concentrations over 12 μM (WHO, 1999). These results show that the mutagenic potential of compounds of Mn may be different in permanganate salts and in manganese salts, depending on its chemical formulation, and thus being able to altering their biological availability, activity, and consequently, their toxicity.

De Meo et al. (1991) evaluated the genotoxicity of potassium permanganate ($KMnO_4$), manganese sulfate and manganese chloride using the Ames test within TA97, TA98, TA100 and TA102 strains, with and without metabolic activation. The presence of direct-acting mutagens was detected in all Mn samples in TA102 strain without metabolic activation. Only manganese chloride induced DNA damage in human lymphocytes with a dose-dependent response, as determined by the comet assay.

Animal studies, demonstrated that acute lethality of manganese appears to vary depending on the chemical species. The central nervous system is the chief target of manganese toxicity. Oral doses produced a number of neurological effects in rats and mice, mainly involving alterations in neurotransmitter and enzyme levels in the brain (ATSDR, 2000; Deskin et al., 1980), which can be accompanied to changes in activity level (ATSDR, 2000). Chronic ingestion of manganese (1–2 mg/kg/day) changes appetite and reduces haemoglobin synthesis in different animals (Hurley & Keen, 1987).

Long-term exposure to manganese can cause transient effects on biogenic amine levels and activities of dopamine β-hydroxylase and monoamine oxidase in rat brain (Eriksson et al., 1987; Lai et al., 1984; Nachtman et al., 1986; Subhash & Padmashree, 1990). Also, high doses (1800–2250 mg/kg/day as manganese (II) sulfate) in mice induce hyperplasia, erosion and inflammation in the stomach. Also, number of chromosomal aberrations and micronuclei were observed in rat bone marrow (ATSRD, 2000).

According to WHO (1999) data, other chemical forms of Mn have mutagenic potential, both in vitro and in vivo. Thus, more studies are necessary in order to elucidate the probable mutagenicity of Mn and its chemical forms and their effects on human health.

Erbe et al. (2011) evaluated damage to the genetic material of fish (Astyanax sp. B) exposed to samples of water from a river and a lake located near a hospital waste landfill. Among other parameters, aluminum and manganese were above acceptable levels that have been established in environmental legislation. The comet assay detected significant damage to genetic material in fish that were acutely exposed in the laboratory to these water samples.

Bomhorst et al (2010) evaluated the cytotoxicity and genotoxicity potencial of $MnCl_2$, as well as its impact on the DNA damage response in human cells (HeLa S3) in culture. Whereas up to 10 μM $MnCl_2$ showed no induction of DNA strand breaks after 24 h incubation, manganese strongly inhibited H_2O_2-stimulated poly(ADP-ribosyl)ation at low, completely non-cytotoxic, for certain human exposure, relevant concentrations starting at 1 μM. These results indicate that manganese, under conditions of either overload due to high exposure or disturbed homeostasis can disturb the cellular response to DNA strand breaks, which has been shown before to result in neurological diseases.

Our research group also conducted an in vitro study on the genotoxic, clastogenic and cytotoxic potential of $MnCl_2$-$4H_2O$ (one of the most common forms of Mn) in different phases of the cell cycle, using short-term cultures of human lymphocytes. These effects were determined by the mitotic index (MI), chromosomal aberrations (CAs) and DNA damage index as detected by the comet assay. $MnCl_2$-$4H_2O$ displayed a strong cytotoxicity in all phases of the cell cycle. Genotoxicity was observed at G2 phase of the cell cycle and also in the comet assay, what may be related to the lack of time for the cellular repair system to act. The absence of CAs in the other phases of the cell cycle suggests that Mn-mediated damage may be repaired in vitro (Lima et al., 2008).

6. Conclusion

Metal are essential for humans and for all forms of life. Even though metals are necessary in biological systems, they are usually required only in trace amounts. As regard to the brain, metals are essential for neuronal activities. However, if not correctly regulated, redox-active can react with molecular oxygen to generate ROS thus causing brain tissue damage.

In this chapter, the authors compile several studies that allow to propose that environmental metal exposure are a risk factor for neurodegenerative process. A large quantity of toxic material is released in the ambient as a consequence of industrial production. High-term exposure to certain metals like manganese (Mn), iron (Fe), aluminum (Al) and many others, alone or in combination, can lead to neuronal losts and increase Alzheimer's disease (AD).

In the cellular neurotoxicity, the Al seems to be the most efficient in promoting Aβ aggregation leading to a specific form of Aβ oligomerization that has marked neurotoxic effects. Iron has been found to be accumulated in the substantia nigra and is more related with neurodegenerative disorders, such as Alzheimer's (AD) and Huntington's (HD) diseases and its severity on cognitive impairment aspect (parietal cortex). As for Mn its toxicity has been associated with dopamine metabolism leading to neuropsychiatric symptoms that resemble idiopathic Parkinson's disease.

Our research group published studies on the genotoxic, clastogenic and cytotoxic effects of Al, MN and Fe in different phases of the cell cycle using in vitro temporary cultures of human lymphocytes. The study indicated that these metals induce DNA damage and is cytotoxic during all phases of the cell cycle. Genotoxic studies have shown that exposure to some metals cause adverse effects to humans and may be implicated in the pathogenesis of some types of neurodegenerative diseases as the AD.

Although is not completely clear the relationship between some metals and neurodegenerative disorders, this chapter suggest that Al, Mn and Fe metals can accelerates neuronal death and increase the risk of its development.

7. References

Abalea, V., Cillard, J., Dubos, M.P., Sergent, O., Cillard, P. & Morel, I. (1999). Repair of iron-induced DNA oxidation by the flavonoid myricetin in primary rat hepatocyte cultures. *Free Radical Biology & Medicine*, Vol. 26, No. 11-12, (Jun. 1999), pp. 1457–1466, ISSN 0891-5849.

Aschner, M., Gannon, M., Kimelberg, H.K. (1992). Manganese uptake and efflux in cultured rat astrocytes. *Journal of Neurochemistry*, Vol. 58, No. 2, (Feb. 1992), pp. 730-735, ISSN 0022-3042.

Alexandrov, P.N., Zhao, Y., Pogue, A.I., Tarr, M.A., Kruck, T.P.A., Percy, M.E., Cui, J.G. & Lukiw, W.J. (2005). Synergistic effects of iron and aluminum on stress-related gene expression in primary neural cells. *Journal of Alzheimer's Disease*, Vol. 8, No. 2, (Nov. 2005), pp. 117–127, ISSN 1387-2877.

Altschuler, E. (1999). Aluminum-containing antacids as a cause of idiopathic Parkinson´s disease. *Medical Hypotheses*, 53, 22-23. Vol. 53, No.1 , (Jul. 1999), pp. 22-23, ISSN 0306-9877.

Anderson, D., Yardley-Jones, A., Hambly, R.J., Vives-Bauza, C., Smykatz-Kloss, V., Chua-Anusorn, W. & Webb, J. (2000). Effects of iron salts and haemosiderin from a thalassaemia patient on oxygen radical damage as measured in the comet assay. *Teratogenesis, Carcinogenesis and Mutagenesis*, Vol. 20, No. 1, (Sep. 2000), pp. 11–26, ISSN 0270-3211.

Anderson, D., Yardley-Jones, A., Vives-Bauza, C., Chua-Anusorn, W., Cole, C. & Webb, J. (2000). Effect of iron salts, haemosiderins, and chelating agents on the lymphocytes of a thalassaemia patient without chelation therapy as measured in the comet assay. *Teratogenesis, Carcinogenesis and Mutagenesis*, Vol. 20, No. 5, (May 2000), pp. 251–264, ISSN 0270-3211.

Ansari, T.M., Marr, I.L. & Tariq, N. (2004). Heavy metals in marine pollution perspective - a mini review. *Journal of Applied Sciences*, Vol. 4, No. 1, (Jan. 2004), pp. 1-20, ISSN 1812-5662.

Antunes, L.M.G., Araújo, M.C.P., Dias, F.L. & Takahashi, C.S. (2005). Effects of H_2O_2, Fe^{2+}, and Fe^{3+} on curcumin-induced chromosoma aberrations in CHO cells. *Genetics and Molecular Biology*, Vol. 28, No. 1, (Jan.-Mar. 2005), pp. 161-164, ISSN 1415-4757.

ATSDR. Toxicological profile for manganese. 2000. Atlanta, GA, US Department of Health and Human Services, Public Health Service, Agency for Toxic Substances and Disease Registry.

Banasik, A., Lankoff, A., Piskulak, A., Adamowska, K., Lisowska, H. & Wojcik, A. (2005). Aluminium-induced micronuclei and apoptosis in human peripheral blood lymphocytes treated during different phases of the cell cycle. *Environmental Toxicology* , Vol. 20, No. 4, (Aug. 2005), pp. 402–406, ISSN 1520-4081.

Banks, W.A., Niehoff, M.L., Drago, D. & Zatta, P. (2006). Aluminum complexing enhances amyloid beta protein penetration of blood–brain barrier. *Brain Research,* Vol. 1116, No.1 , (Oct. 2006), pp. 215-221, ISSN 0006-8993.

Barbouti, A., Doulias, P.T., Zhu, B.Z., Frei, B. & Galaris, D. (2001). Intracellular iron, but not copper, plays a critical role in hydrogen peroxide-induced DNA damage. *Free Radical Biology & Medicine,* Vol., 31, No. 4, (Aug. 2001), pp. 490–498, ISSN 0891-5849.

Barceloux, D.G., (1999). Manganese. *Journal of toxicology. Clinical toxicology,* Vol. 37, No, 2, (1999), pp. 293-307, ISSN 0731-3810.

Bartzokis, G., Mintz, J., Sultzer, D., Marx, P., Herzberg, J.S., Phelan, C.K. & Marder, S.R. (1994). In vivo MR evaluation of age-related increases in brain iron. *American Journal of Neuroradiology,* 15, 1129–1138; Vol. 15, No. 6, (Jun. 1994), pp. 1129-1138, ISSN 0306-9877.

Beauchemin, D., Kisilevsky, R. (1998). A method based on ICP-MS for the analysis of Alzheimer's amyloid plaques. *Analytical Chemistry,* Vol. 70, No.5, (Mar. 1998), pp. 026-1029, ISSN 0003-2700.

Beckman, R.A., Mildvan, A.S. & Loeb, L.A. (1985). On the fidelity of DNA replication: manganese mutagenesis in vitro. *Biochemistry,* Vol. 24, No. 21, (Oct. 1985), pp. 5810–17, ISSN 0006-2960.

Behl, C., Davis, J.B., Lesley, R., Schubert, D. (1994). Hydrogen peroxide mediates amyloid beta protein toxicity. *Cell,* Vol. 17, No. 6, (Jun 1994), pp. 817-827, ISSN 0092-8674.

Berg, D., Gerlach, M., Youdim, M.B., Double, K.L., Zecca, L., Riederer, P. & Becker, G. (2001). Brain iron pathways and their relevance to Parkinson's disease. *Journal of Neurochemistry,* Vol.79 , No. 2, (Oct. 2001), pp. 225-236, ISSN 0022-3042.

Berthon G (1996) Chemical speciation studies in relation to aluminium metabolism and toxicity. *Coordination Chemistry Reviews,* Vol. 149, (1996), pp. 241-280, ISSN 0010-8545.

Berthon, G., (2002). Aluminium speciation in relation to aluminium bioavailability, metabolism and toxicity. *Coordination Chemistry Reviews,* Vol. 228, No. 2, (Jun. 2002), pp. 319-341, ISSN 0010-8545.

Bogé, G. & Roche, H. (1996). Cytotoxicity of phenolic compounds on Dicentrarchus labrax erythrocytes. *Bull Environ Contam Toxicol.,* Vol. 57, No. 2, (Mar. 1996), pp. 171-178, ISSN 0007-4861

Bondy, S. C. (2010). The neurotoxicity of environmental aluminum is still an issue. *NeuroToxicology,* Vol.31, No.5, (Sep. 2010), pp. 575-581, ISSN 0161-813X.

Bornhorst, J., Ebert, F., Hartwig, A., Michalke, B. & Schwerdtle T. Manganese inhibits poly(ADP-ribosyl)ation in human cells: a possible mechanism behind manganese-induced toxicity? *J. Environ. Monit.,* Vol. 12, No. 11, (Nov. 2010), pp. 2062-9, ISSN 1464-0325.

Botchway, S.W., Stevens, D.L., Hill, M.A., Jenner, T.J. & O'Neill, P. (1997). Induction and rejoining of DNA double-strand breaks in Chinese hamster V79-4 cells irradiated with characteristic aluminum K and copper L ultrasoft X rays. *Radiation Research,* Vol. 148, No. 4, (Oct. 1997), pp. 317–324, ISSN 0033-7587.

Brega, S.M., Vassilieff, I., Almeida, A., Mercadante, A., Bissacot, D., Cury, P.R. & Freire-Maia, D.V. (1998). Clinical, cytogenetic and toxicological studies in rural workers exposed to pesticides in Botucatu, São Paulo, Brazil. *Reports in Public Health,* Vol. 14, Suppl. 3, (1998), pp. 109–115, ISSN 0102-311X.

Busser, J., Geldmacher, D.S., Herrup, K. (1998). Ectopic cell cycle proteins predict the sites of neuronal cell death in Alzheimer's disease brain. *The Journal of neuroscience : the official journal of the Society for Neuroscience,* Vol. 18, No 8, (Apr. 1998), pp. 2801-2807, ISSN 0270-6474.

Bush, A.I. (2003). The metallobiology of Alzheimer's disease. *Trends Neuroscience,* Vol. 26, No. 4, (Apr. 2003), pp. 207-214, ISSN 0166-2236.

Butterworth, R. F. (2010). Metal Toxicity, Liver Disease and Neurodegeneration. *Neurotoxicity Research,* Vol. 18 , No. 1, (Apr. 2010), pp. 100-105, ISSN 1029-8428.

Campbell, A., Bondy, S.C. (2000). Aluminum induced oxidative events and its relation to inflammation: a role for the metal in Alzheimer's disease. *Cellular and Molecular Biology,* Vol. 46, No. 4, (Jun. 2000), pp. 721-730, ISSN 1098-5549.

Chen, J., Cohen, M.L., Lerner, A.J., Yang, Y. & Herrup, K. (2010). DNA damage and cell cycle events implicate cerebellar dentate nucleus neurons as targets of Alzheimer's disease. *Molecular Neurodegeneration,* Vol. 5, No. 60, (Dec. 2010), pp.1-11, ISSN 1750-1326.

Cherny, R. A., Legg, J. T., McLean, C. A., Farlie, D.P., Huang, X., Atwood, C.S., Beyreuther, K., Tanzi, R.E., Masters, C.L. & Bush, A.L. (1999). Aqueous dissolution of Alzheimer's disease Aβ amyloid deposits by biometal depletion. *Journal of Biological Chemistry,* Vol. 274 , No. 33 , (Aug. 1999), pp. 23223-23228, ISSN 1083-351X.

Connor, J. R., Benkovic, S. A. (1992). Iron regulation in the brain: histochemical, biochemical, and molecular consider- ations. *Annals of Neurology,* Vol. 32 , No. Suppl (1992), pp. S51-S61, ISSN 0364-5134.

Corain, B., Bombi, G.G., Tapparo, A., Perazzolo, M., Zatta, P. (1996). Aluminium toxicity and metal speciation: established data and open questions. *Coordination Chemistry Reviews,* Vol. 149, (May 1996), pp.11-22, ISSN 0010-8545.

Cox, P.A., (1995). *The elements on earth: inorganic chemistry in the environment.* Oxford University Press, ISBN 0198562411, Oxford, New York.

Crapper, D.R., Krishnan, S.S., Quittkat, S. (1976). Aluminium, neurofibrillary degeneration and Alzheimer's disease. *Brain: a Journal of Neurology,* Vol. 99, No.1, (Mar. 1976), pp. 67-80, ISSN 0006-8950.

De Meo, M., Laget, M., Castegnaro, M. & Dumenil, G. (1991). Genotoxic activity of potassium permanganate in acidic solutions. *Mutation Research,* Vol. 260, No. 3, (Jul. 1991), pp. 295–306, ISSN 0027-5107.

Demougeot, C., Methy, D., Prigent-Tessier, A., Garnier, P., Bertrand, N., Guilland, J.C., Beley, A. & Marie C. (2003). Effects of a direct injection of liposoluble iron into rat striatum. Importance of the rate of iron delivery to cells. *Free Radical Research,* Vol. 37, No.1, (Jan. 2003), pp. 59-67, ISSN 1071-5762.

Dennis, J., Selkoe, M.D. (2000). The Origins of Alzheimer Disease. *Journal of American Medical Association*. Vol. 283, No.12 (2000), pp.1615–1617, ISSN 1538-3598.

Deskin R., Bursian S.J. & Edens F.W. (1980). Neurochemical alterations induced by manganese chloride in neonatal rats. *Neurotoxicology*, Vol. 2, No. 1, (Jan. 1980), pp. 65–73, ISSN 0161-813X.

Donaldson, J., McGregor, D., LaBella, F. (1982). Manganese neurotoxicity: A model of free radical mediated neurodegeneration? *Canadian Journal of Physiology and Pharmacology*, Vol. 60, No. 11, (1982), pp. 1398-1405, ISSN 0008-4212.

Dong, J., Atwood, C.S., Anderson, V.E., Siedlak, S.L., Smith, M.A., Perry, G. & Carrey, P.R. (2003). Metal binding and oxidation of amyloid-beta within isolated senile plaque cores: Raman microscopic evidence. *Biochemistry*, Vol. 42, No. 10, (Mar 2003), pp. 2768-2773, ISSN 0264-6021.

Double K.L., Gerlach M., Youdim M.B., Riederer P. (2000). Impaired iron homeostasis in Parkinson's disease. *Journal of Neural Transmission Supplementum*, 60, 37-58. Vol. 60, No.1, (2000), pp. 37-58, ISSN 0303-6995.

Dovgaliuk, A.I., Kaliniak, T.B. & Blium, I.B. (2001b). Cytogenetic effects of toxic metal salts on apical meristem cells of Allium cepa L. seed roots. *TSitologiia i Genetika*, Vol. 35, No. 2, (Mar./Apr. 2001), pp. 3–10, ISSN 0564-3783.

Dovgaliuk, A.I., Kaliniak, T.B., Blium, I.B. (2001a). Assessment of phytoand cytotoxic effects of heavy metals and aluminum compounds using onion apical root meristem. *TSitologiia i Genetika*, Vol. 35, No. 1, (Jan./Feb. 2001), pp. 3–9, ISSN 0564-3783.

Drago, D., Bettella, M., Bolognin, S., Cendron, L., Scancar, J., Milacic, R., Richelli, R., Casini, A., Messori, L., Tagnon, G. & Zatta, P. (2008). Potential pathogenic role of beta-amyloid(1-42)-aluminum complex in Alzheimer's disease. The International Journal of Biochemistry & Cell Biology, Vol. 40, No. 4, (Oct. 2008), pp. 731-746, ISSN 1357-2725.

Dunkel, V.C., San, R.H., Seifried, H.E. & Whittaker, P. (1999). Genotoxicity of iron compounds in Salmonella typhimurium and L5178Y mouse lymphoma cells. *Environmental and Molecular Mutagenesis*, Vol. 33, No. 1 (Feb. 1999), pp. 28-41, ISSN 0893-6692.

Durante, M., Gialanella, G., Grossi, G., Pugliese, M., Scampoli, P.,Kawata, T., Yasuda, N. & Furusawa, Y. (2002). Influence of the shielding on the induction of chromosomal aberrations in human lymphocytes exposed to high-energy iron ions. *Radiation Research*, Vol. 43, Suppl. S, (Dec. 2002), pp. 107–111, ISSN 0449-3060.

Dutta, D., Devi, S.S., Krishnamurthi, K. & Chakrabarti, T. (2006). Anticlastogenic effect of redistilled cow's urine distillate in human peripheral lymphocytes challenged with manganese dioxide and hexavalent chromium. *Biomedical and Environmental Sciences*, Vol. 19, No. 6, (Dec. 2006), pp. 487-494, ISSN 0895-3988.

Eidelberg, D., Sotrel, A., Joachim, C., Selkoe, D., Forman, A., Pendlebury, W.W. & Perl, D.P. (1987). Adult onset Hallervorden-Spatz disease with neurofibrillary pathology. *Brain*, Vol. 110, No. 4, (Aug. 1987), pp. 993-1013, ISSN 1460-2156.

Elmore, A.R. (2003). Final report on the safety assessment of aluminum silicate, calcium silicate, magnesium aluminum silicate, magnesium silicate, magnesium trisilicate, sodium magnesium silicate, zirconium silicate, attapulgite, bentonite, Fuller's earth, hectorite, kaolin, lithium magnesium silicate, lithium magnesium sodium silicate, montmorillonite, pyrophyllite and zeolite. *International Journal of Toxicology*, Vol. 22, Suppl. 1, (2003), pp. 37–102, ISSN 1091-5818.

Erbe, M.C., Ramsdorf, W.A., Vicari, T. & Cestari, M.M. (2011). Toxicity evaluation of water samples collected near a hospital waste landfill through bioassays of genotoxicity piscine micronucleus test and comet assay in fish Astyanax and ecotoxicity Vibrio fischeri and Daphnia magna. *Ecotoxicology*, Vol. 20, No. 2, (Mar. 2011), pp. 320-328, ISSN 0963-9292.

Eriksson, H., Lenngren, S. & Heilbronn, E. (1987). Effect of long-term administration of manganese on biogenic amine levels in discrete striatal regions of rat brain. *Archives of Toxicology*, Vol. 59, No. 6, (Apr. 1987), pp. 426–431, ISSN 0340-5761.

Evans, H.H., Horng, M.F., Ricanati, M., Diaz-Insua, M., Jordan, R. & Schwartz, J.L. (2001). Diverse delayed effects in human lymphoblastoid cells surviving exposure to high-LET (56)Fe particles or low-LET (137)Cs gamma radiation. *Radiation Research*, Vol. 156, No. 3, (Sep. 2001), pp. 259–271, ISSN 0449-3060.

Evans, H.H., Horng, M.F., Ricanati, M., Diaz-Insua, M., Jordan, R. & Schwartz, J.L. (2003). Induction of genomic instability in TK6 human lymphoblasts exposed to 137Cs gamma radiation: comparison to the induction by exposure to accelerated 56Fe particles. *Radiation Research*, Vol. 159, No. 6, (Jun. 2003), pp. 737–747, ISSN 0449-3060.

Ferrer, A. (2003). Metal poisoning. *Anales del Sistema Sanitario de Navarra*, Vol. 26, pp. 141–153., ISSN 1137-6627.

Florence, T.M., Stauber, J.L. (1989). Manganese catalysis of dopamine oxidation. *The Science of the Total Environment*, Vol. 78, No. 1, (Jan. 1989), pp. 233-240, ISSN 0048-9697.

Franke, S.I.R., Prá, D., Giulian, R., Dias, J.F., Yoneama, M.L., Silva, J., Erdtmann, B. & Henriques, J.A.P. (2006). Influence of orange juice in the levels and in the genotoxicity of iron and copper. *Food and Chemical Toxicology* , Vol. 44, No. 3, (Mar. 2006), pp. 425–435, ISSN 0278-6915.

García-Medina, S., Razo-Estrada, C., Galar-Martinez, M., Cortéz-Barberena, E., Gómez-Oliván, L.M., Alvarez-González, I. & Madrigal-Bujaidar, E. (2011). Genotoxic and cytotoxic effects induced by aluminum in the lymphocytes of the common carp (Cyprinus carpio). *Comp. Biochem. Physiol. C. Toxicol. Pharmacol.* Vol. 153, No. 1, (Jan 2011), pp. 113-118, ISSN 1532-0456.

Garruto, R.M., Shankar, S.K., Yanagihara, R., Salazar, A.M., Amyx, H.L., Gajdusek, D.C. (1989). Low- calcium, high-aluminum diet-induced motor neuron pathology in cynomolgus monkeys. *Acta Neuropathologica (Berl)*, Vol. 78, No. 2, (1989), pp. 210-219, ISSN: 0001-6322.

Garry, S., Nesslany, F., Aliouat, E., Haguenoer, J.M. & Marzin, D. (2003). Hematite (Fe(2)O(3)) enhances benzo[a]pyrene genotoxicity in endo-tracheally treated rat, as determined by Comet Assay. *Mutation Research*, Vol. 538, No. 1-2, (Jul. 2003), pp.19–29, ISSN 13835742.

George, K.A., Hada, M., Jackson, L.J., Elliott, T., Kawata, T., Pluth, J.M. & Cucinotta, F.A. (2009). Dose response of gamma rays and iron nuclei for induction of chromosomal aberrations in normal and repair-deficient cell lines. *Radiation Research*, Vol. 171, No. 6, (Jun. 2009), pp. 752-63, ISSN 0033-7587.

Gerber, G.B., Leonard, A. & Hantson, P. (2002). Carcinogenicity, mutagenicity and teratogenicity of manganese compounds. *Critical Reviews in Oncology/Hematology*, Vol. 42, No. 1, (Apr. 2002), pp. 25–34 ISSN 1040-8428.

Gerlach, M., Double, K.L., Youdim, M.B., Riederer, P. (2006). Potential sources of increased iron in the substantia nigra of parkinsonian patients. *The Journal of* Neural Transmission Supplementa, Vol. 70, No. 1, (2006), pp. 133-142, ISSN: 0303-6995.

Ghetti, B., Musicco, M., Morton, J., Bugiani, O. (1985). Nerve cell loss in the progressive encephalopathy induced by aluminum powder: A morphologic and semiquantitative study of the Purkinje cells. *Neuropathology and Applied Neurobiology,* Vol. 11, No. 1, (Jan. - Feb. 1985), pp. 31-53, ISSN: 0305-1846.

Glei, M., Latunde-Dada, G.O., Klinder, A., Becker, T.W., Hermann, U., Voigt, K. & Pool-Zobel, B.l. (2002). Iron-overload induces oxidative DNA damage in the human colon carcinoma cell line HT29 clone 19A. *Mutation Research,* Vol. 519, No. 1-2, (Aug. 2002), pp. 151–161, ISSN 0027-5107.

Good, P.F., Olanow, C.W., Perl, D.P. (1992). Neuromelanin- containing neurons of the substantia nigra accumulate iron and aluminum in Parkinson's disease: a LAMMA study. *Brain Research,* Vol. 593, No. 2, (Oct. 1992), pp. 343-346, ISSN 0006-8993.

Griffiths, P.D., Dobson, B.R., Jones, G.R. & Clarke, D.T. (1999). Iron in the basal ganglia in Parkinson's disease. An in vitro study using extended X-ray absorption fine structure and cryo-electron microscopy. *Brain,* Vol. 122, No. 4, (Nov. 1999), pp. 667-673, ISSN 1460-2156.

Guilarte T. R. (2010.) "APLP1, Alzheimer's-like pathology and neu- rodegeneration in the frontal cortex of manganese-exposed non-human primates". *NeuroToxicology,* Vol.31, No.5, (Sep. 2010), pp. 572-574, ISSN:0161-813X.

Gupta, V.B., Anitha, S., Hegde, M.L., Zecca, L., Garruto, R.M., Ravid, R., Shankar, S.K., Stein, R., Shanmugavelu, P., Jagannatha Rao, K.S. (2005). Aluminium in Alzheimer's disease: are we still at a crossroad? *Cellular and Molecular Life Sciences,* Vol. 62, No.2, (Jan. 2005), pp. 143-158, ISSN 1420-682X.

Guy, S.P., Jones, D., Mann, D.A.M, Itzhaki, R.F. (1991). Human neuroblastoma cells treated with aluminium express an epitope associated with Alzheimer's disease neurofibrillary tangles. *Neuroscience Letters,* Vol. 121, No. 1-2, (Jan. 1991), pp. 166-168, ISSN 0304-3940.

Hardy, J., Selkoe., D.J. (2002). The amyloid hypothesis of Alzheimer's disease: Progress and problems on the road to therapeutics. Science, Vol. 297 , No. 5580 (Jul. 2002), pp. 353-356, ISSN: 1095-9203.

Hasan, M.R., Morishima, D., Tomita, K., Katsuki, M. & Kotani, S. (2005). Identification of a 250 kDa putative microtubule-associated protein as bovine ferritin. Evidence for a ferritin–microtubule interaction. *The FEBS Journal,* Vol. 272, No. 3, (Dec. 2005), pp. 822–831, ISSN 0014-2956.

Hegde, M. L., Hegde, P. M., Holthauzen, L.M.F., Hazra, T. K., Rao, K. S.J., Mitra, S. (2010). Specific inhibition of NEIL-initiated repair of oxidized base damage in human genome by copper and iron: potential etiological linkage to neurodegenerative diseases. *The Journal of Biological Chemistry,* Vol. 285, No. 37, (Jul. 2010), pp. 28812-28825, ISSN 0021–9258.

Heidelberger, C., Freeman, A.E., Pienta, R.J., Sivak, A., Bertram, J.S., Casto, B.C., Dunkel, V.C., Francis, M.W., Kakunaga, T., Little, J.B. & Schechtman, L.M. (1983). Cell transformation by chemical agents - a review and analysis of the literature. A report of the US Environmental Protection Agency Gene-Tox Program. *Mutation Research*, Vol. 114, No. 3, (Apr. 1983), pp. 283–385, ISSN 0027-5107.

Hollenberg P.F. (2010). Introduction: Mechanisms of Metal Toxicity. *Chemical Research in Toxicology*, Vol. 23, No. 15, pp. 292–293, ISSN 0893-228X.

House, E., Collingwod, J., Khan, A., Korchazkina, O., Berthon, G., Exley, C. (2004). Aluminium, iron, zinc and copper influence the *in vitro* formation of amyloid fibrils of Abeta42 in a manner which may have consequences for metal chelation therapy in Alzheimer's disease. *Journal Alzheimer's Disease*, 6: 291-301 Vol. 6, No. 3, (Jun. 2004), pp. 291-301, ISSN 1387-2877.

Hurley, L.S., Keen, C.L. (1987). Manganese. In: *Trace elements in human and animal nutrition*, W. Mertz, (Ed.), Vol. 1. pp. 185–223, Academic Press, New York, NY.

International Labour Organization (ILO), (1997). Encyclopaedia of occupational health and safety. Metals: chemical properties and toxicity. 4th ed. Geneve, 6368 pp, ISBN 978-92-2-109816-4.

Iwami, O., Watanabe, T., Moon, C.S., Nakatsuka, H. & Ikeda, M. (1994). Motor neuron disease on the Kii Peninsula of Japan: excess manganese intake from food coupled with low magnesium in drinking water as a risk factor. *The Science of the Total Environment*, 149(1-2), 121-35. Vol.149, No.1-2, (Jun. 1994), pp. 121-135, ISSN 0048-9697.

Kawahara, M., Muramoto, K., Kobayashi, K., Mori, H. & Kuroda Y., (1994). Aluminum promotes the aggregation of Alzheimer's amyloid beta- protein *in vitro. Biochemical and Biophysical Research* Communication, Vol. 198, No. 2, (Jan. 1994), pp. 531-535, ISSN 0006-291X.

Kawahara, M., Kato, M., Kuroda, Y. (2001). Effects of aluminium on the neurotoxicity of primary cultured neurons and on the aggregation of beta-amyloid protein. *Brain Research Bulletin*, Vol. 55, No. 2, (May 2001), pp. 211-217, ISSN 0361-9230.

Kell, D. B., Towards a unifying, systems biology understand- ing of large-scale cellular death and destruction caused by poorly liganded iron: Parkinson's, Huntington's, Alzheimer's, prions, bactericides, chemical toxicology and others as examples. *Archives of Toxicology*, Vol. 84, No. 11, (Nov. 2010), pp. 825-889, ISSN 1432-0738.

Kontush, A., Berndt, C., Weber, W., Akopyan, V., Arlt, S., Schippling, S. & Beisiegel, U. (2001). Amyloid-beta is an antioxidant for lipoproteins in cerebrospi- nal fluid and plasma. *Free Radical Biology & Medicine*, Vol. 30, No.1, (Dec. 2001), pp. 119-128, ISSN 0891-5849.

Kostoryz, E.L. & Yourtee, D.M. (2001). Oxidative mutagenesis of doxorubicin–Fe(III) complex. *Mutation Research*, Vol. 490, No. 2, (Feb. 2001), pp. 131–139, ISSN 0027-5107.

Kruman, I.I., Wersto, R.P., Cardozo-Pelaez, F., Smilenov, L., Chan, S.L., Chrest, F.J., Emokpae, R., Gorospe, M., Mattson, M.P. (2004). Cell cycle activation linked to neuronal cell death initiated by DNA damage. *Neuron*, Vol. 41, No 4, (Feb. 2004), pp. 549-561, ISSN 1097-4199.

Kumar, V., Gill, K.D. (2009). Aluminium neurotoxicity: neurobehavioural and oxidative aspects. *Archives of Toxicology*, Vol. 83, No. 11, (Nov. 2009), pp. 730-735. ISSN 0340-5761.

LaFerla, F. M., Green, K. N. Oddo, S. (2007). Intracellular amyloid-β in Alzheimer's Disease. *Nature Reviews Neuroscience*, Vol. 7 No. 8 (Jul. 2007), pp. 499– 509, ISSN 1471-003X.

Lai, J.C., Leung T.K. & Lim L. (1984). Differences in the neurotoxic effects of manganese during development and aging: Some observations on brain regional neurotransmitter and non- neurotransmitter metabolism in a developmental rat model of chronic manganese encephalopathy. *NeuroToxicology,* Vol. 5, No. 1, (spring 1984), pp. 37–47, ISSN 0161-813X.

Lan, J., Jiang, D.H. (1997). Excessive iron accumulation in the brain: a possible potential risk of neurodegeneration in Parkinson´s disease. *Journal of Neural Transmission,* Vol. 104, No. 6-7, (1997), pp. 649-660, ISSN 0300-9564.

Lankoff, A., Banasik, A., Duma, A., Ochniak, E., Lisowska, H., Kuszewski, T., Góźdz, S. & Wojcik A. (2006). A comet assay study reveals that aluminium induces DNA damage and inhibits the repair of radiation-induced lesions in human peripheral blood lymphocytes. *Toxicology Letters*, Vol. 161, No. 1, (Feb. 2006), pp. 27–36, ISSN 0378-4274.

Lapresle, J., Duckett, S., Galle, P., Cartier, L. (1975). Clinical, anatomical and biophysical data on a case of encephalopathy with aluminum deposition. *Comptes rendus des séances de la Société de biologie et de ses filiales,* Vol. 169, No. 2, (1975), pp. 282-285, ISSN 0037-9026.

Lee, D.W. Andersen, J.K. (2010). Iron elevations in the aging Parkinsonian brain: a consequence of impared iron homeostasis? *Journal of Neurochemistry*, Vol. 112, No. 2, (Jan. 2010), pp. 332-339. ISSN 0022-3042.

Léonard A. (1988). Mechanisms in metal genotoxicity: the significance of in vitro approaches. *Mutation Research,* Vol. 198, No. 2, (Apr. 1988), pp. 321–6, ISSN 1383-5742.

Li, H., Campbell, A., Ali, S.F., Cong, P., Bondy, S.C. (2008). Chronic exposure to low levels of aluminum alters cerebral cell signaling in response to acute MPTP treatment. Toxicology and Industrial Health, Vol. 23, No. 2, (Jan. 2008), pp. 515-524, ISSN 0748-2377.

Liu G., Huang W., Moir R. D., Vanderburg, C.R,, Lai, B., Peng, Z., Tanzi, R.E., Rogers, J.T. & Huang, X. (2006). Metal exposure and Alzheimer's pathogenesis. *Journal of Structura Biology*, Vol. 155, No. 1, (Jul. 2006), pp. 45-51, ISSN 1047-8477.

Lima, P.D., Leite, D.S., Vasconcellos, M.C., Cavalcanti, B.C., Santos, R.A., Costa-Lotufo, L.V., Pessoa, C., Moraes, M.O. & Burbano, R.R. (2007). Genotoxic effects of aluminum chloride in cultured human lymphocytes treated in different phases of cell cycle. *Food and Chemical Toxicology,* Vol. 45, No. 7, (Jul. 2007), pp. 1154–1159, ISSN 0278-6915.

Lima, P.D., Vasconcellos, M.C., Bahia, M.O., Montenegro, R.C., Pessoa, C.O., Costa-Lotufo, L.V., Moraes, M.O. & Burbano, R.R. (2008). Genotoxic and cytotoxic effects of manganese chloride in cultured human lymphocytes treated in different phases of cell cycle. *Toxicology In Vitro,* Vol. 22, No. 4, (Jun. 2008), pp. 1032-1037, ISSN 0887-2333.

Lima, P.D., Vasconcellos, M.C., Montenegro, R.A., Sombra, C.M., Bahia, M.O., Costa-Lotufo, L.V., Pessoa, C.O., Moraes, M.O. & Burbano, R.R. (2008). Genotoxic and cytotoxic effects of iron sulfate in cultured human lymphocytes treated in different phases of cell cycle. *Toxicology In Vitro*, Vol. 22, No. 3, (Apr. 2008) pp. 723-729, ISSN 0887-2333.

Lovell, M.A., Ehmann, W.D., Markesbery, W.R. (1993). Laser mi- croprobe analysis of brain aluminum in Alzheimer's disease. *Annals of Neurology*, Vol. 33, No. 1, (Jan. 1993), pp. 36-42, ISSN 0364-5134.

Lovell, M.A., Robertson, J.D., Teesdale, W.J., Campbell, J.L. & Markesbery, W.R. (1998). Copper, iron and zinc in Alzheimer's disease senile plaques. *Journal of the Neurological Science*, Vol. 158, No. 1, (Jun. 1998), pp. 47-52, ISSN 0022-510X.

Lu, T., Pan, Y., Kao, S.Y., Li, C., Kohane, I., Chan, J., Yankner, B.A. (2004) Gene regulation and DNA damage in the ageing human brain. *Nature*, Vol. 429, No. 6994, (Jun. 2004), pp. 883-891, ISSN 0028-0836.

Lukiw W.J. & Pogue A.I. (2007). Induction of specific micro RNA (miRNA) species by ROS-generating metal sulfates in primary human brain cells. Journal of Inorganic *Biochemistry*, Vol. 101, No. 9, (Sep. 2007), pp. 1265-1269, ISSN 0162-0134.

Lukiw W.J. (2007). Micro-RNA speciation in fetal, adult and Alzheimer'sdisease hippocampus. *Neuroreport*. Vol. 18, No. 3, (Feb. 2007), pp. 297-300, ISSN 0959-4965.

Lukiw W.J. In: Aluminum and Alzheimer's Disease, the Science that Describes the Link. Exley C, (Ed.), pp. 147–168, Elsevier Publishers, London.

Lukiw, W.J. (2001). Aluminum and Gene Transcription in the Mammalian Central Nervous System—Implications for Alzheimer's Disease, In: *Aluminum and Alzheimer's Disease: the Science that Describes the Link*, Exley, C., pp. 147–68, Elsevier Publishers, ISBN, 978-0-444-50811-9, London.

Maynard, C.J., Bush, A.I., Masters, C.L., Cappai, R. & Li, Q.X. (2005). Metals and amyloid beta in Alzheimer's disease. International Journal of Experimental Pathology, Vol. 86, No. 3, (Jun. 2005), pp. 147-159, ISSN 1365- 2613.

Maenosono, S., Suzuki, T. & Saita, S. (2007). Mutagenicity of water-soluble FePt nanoparticles in Ames test. *The Journal of Toxicological Sciences*, Vol. 32, No. 5, (Dec. 2007), pp. 575-579, ISSN 0388-1350.

Mark, R.J., Lovell, M.A., Markesbery, W.R. Uchida, K., Mattson, M.P. (1997). A role for 4-hydroxynonenal, an aldehydic product of lipid peroxidation, in disruption of ion homeostasis and neuronal death induced by amyloid beta-peptide. *Journal of Neurochemistry*, Vol. 66, No. 1, (Jan. 1997), pp. 255-264. ISSN 0022-3042.

Mark, R.J., Pang, Z., Geddes, J.W., Uchida, K. & Mattson, M.P. (1997). Amyloid beta-peptide impairs glucose transport in hippocampal and cortical neurons: involvement of membrane lipid peroxidation. *The Journal of Neuroscience*, Vol. 17, No. 3, (Feb. 1997), pp. 1046-1054, ISSN 0270-6474.

Martin, W.R.W., Wiler, M. (2008). Midbrain iron content in early Parkinson disease. A potential biomarker of disease status. *Neurology*, Vol. 70, No. 16 pt 2, (Apr. 2008), pp. 1411-1417, ISSN 1473-6551.

McLachlan, D.R.C., Bergeron, C., Smith, J.E., Boomer, D. & Rifat, S.L. (1996). Risk for neuropathologically confirmed Alzheimer's disease and residual aluminum in municipal drinking water employing weighted residential histories. *Neurology*, Vol. 46, No. 2, (Apr. 1996), pp. 401-405, ISSN 1473-6551.

Mills, E., Dong, X. P., Wang, F., Xu, H. (2010). Mechanisms of brain iron transport: insight into neurodegeneration and CNS disorders. *Future Medicinal Chemistry*, Vol. 2, No. 1, (2010), pp. 51-64, ISSN 1756-8919.

Miu, A.C., Benga, O. (2006). Aluminum and Alzheimer's disease: a new look. Journal of Alzheimer's disease, Vol. 10, No. 2-3, (Nov. 2006), pp. 179-201, ISSN 1387-2877.

Montgomery, E.B.J. (1995). Heavy metals and the etiology of Parkinson's disease and other movement disorders. *Toxicology,* Vol. 97, No. 1-3, (Mar. 1995), pp. 3-9, ISSN 0300-483X.

Moreno, E.A., Rojas, G.F., Frenk, F.H., De La Huerta, A.O., Belmares, R.Q. & Vargas, A.R.O. (1997). In vitro induction of abnormal anaphases by contaminating atmospheric dust from the City of Mexicali, Baja California, Mexico. *Archives of Medical Research,* Vol. 28, No. 4, (Dec. 1997), pp. 549–53, ISSN 0188-4409.

Morgan, D.M., Dong, J., Jacob, J., Lu, K., Apkarian, R.P., Thiyagarajan, P. & Lynn, D.G. (2002). Metal switch for amyloid formation: insight into the structure of the nucleus. Journal of the American Chemical Society, Vol. 124, No. 43, (Oct. 2002), pp. 12644-12645, ISSN 0002-7863.

Myung, N.H., Zhu, X., Castellani, R.J., Petersen, R.B., Siedlak, S.L., Perry, G., Smith, M.A., Lee, H.G. (2008). Evidence of DNA damage in Alzheimer disease: phosphorylation of histone H2AX in astrocytes. *Age (Dordrecht, Netherlands),* Vol. 30, No 4, (Apr. 2008), pp. 209-215, ISSN 1574-4647.

Nachtman, J.P., Tubben R.E. & Commissaris, R.L. (1986). Behavioral effects of chronic manganese administration in rats: Locomotor activity studies. *Neurobehavioral Toxicology and Teratology,* Vol. 8, No. 6, (Nov. - Dec. 1986), pp. 711–715, ISSN 0275-1380.

Nakano, M. (1993). A possible mechanism of iron neurotoxicity. *European Neurology,* Vol. 33, No. 1, (1993), pp. 44-51, ISSN 0014- 3022.

Nayak, P. (2002). Aluminum: Impacts and Disease. Environmental Research, Vol. 89, No. 2, (Jun. 2002), pp. 101-115. ISSN 0013-9351.

Nayak, P., Chatterjee, A.K. (1999). Biochemical view of aluminum-induced neurohazards. *Journal of environmental biology,* Vol. 20, No. (1999), pp. 77-84, ISSN 0254-8704.

Newland, M.C., Ceckler, T.L., Kordower, J.H., Weiss, B. (1989). Visualizing manganese in the primate basal ganglia with magnetic resonance imaging. *Expiremental Neurology,* Vol. 106, No. 3, (Dec. 1989), pp. 251-258. ISSN 0014-4886.

Ogawa, H.I., Shibahara, T., Iwata, H., Okada, T., Tsuruta, S., Kakimoto, K., Sakata, K., Kato, Y., Ryo, H. & Itoh, T. (1994). Genotoxic activities in vivo of cobaltous chloride and other metal chlorides as assayed in the Drosophila wing spot test. *Mutation Research,* Vol. 320, No. 1-2, (Jan. 1994), pp. 133–140, ISSN 0027-5107.

Olanow, C.W., Good, P.F., Shinotoh, H., Hewitt, K.A., Vingerhoets, F., Snow, B.J., Beal, M.F., Calne, D.B. & Perl, D.P. (1996). Manganese intoxication in the rhesus monkey: a clinical, imaging, pathologic, and biochemical study. *Neurology,* Vol. 46, No. 2, (Feb. 1996), pp. 492–8 ISSN 0028-3878.

O´Neil, P., (1994). Major elements in the earth´s crust - Iron. In: *Environmental chemistry 2nd ed.,* Chapman and Hall (Eds.), pp. 151-168, ISBN 0045510865, New York,

Ong, W. Y., Farooqui, A. A. (2005). Iron, neuroinflammation, and Alzheimer's disease. *Journal of Alzheimer's Disease,* Vol. 8, No. 2, (Nov. 2005), pp. 183-200, ISSN 1387-2877.

Orgel A. & Orgel L.E. (1965). Induction of mutations in bacteriophage T4 with divalent manganese. *Journal of Molecular Biology,* Vol. 14, No. 2, (Dec. 1965), pp. 453–457, ISSN 0022-2836.

Park, J.H. & Park, E. (2011). Influence of iron-overload on DNA damage and its repair in human leukocytes in vitro. *Mutat. Res.*, Vol. 718, No. 1-2, (Jan. 2011), pp. 56-61, ISSN 1383-5742.

Park, D.S., Morris, E.J., Padmanabhan, J., Shelanski, M.L., Geller, H.M., Greene, L.A. (1998). Cyclin-dependent kinases participate in death of neurons evoked by DNA-damaging agents. *The Journal of cell biology,* Vol. 143, No. 2, (1998), pp. 457-467, ISSN 540-8140.

Petrik, M.S., Wong, M.C., Tabata, R.C., Garry, R.F., Shaw, C.A. (2007). Aluminum adjuvant linked to Gulf War illness induces motor neuron death in mice. *NeuroMolecular Medicine,* Vol. 9, No. 1, (2007), pp. 89-100, ISSN 1559-1174.

Prá, D., Franke, S.I., Giulian, R., Yoneama, M.L., Dias, J.F., Erdtmann, B. & Henriques, J.A. (2008). Genotoxicity and mutagenicity of iron and copper in mice. *Biometals,* Vol. 21, No. 3, (Jun. 2008), pp. 289-297, ISSN 0966-0844.

Pratico, D., Uryu, K., Sung, S., Tang, S., Trojanowski, J.Q., Lee, V.M. (2002). Aluminum modulates brain amyloidosis through oxidative stress in APP transgenic mice. *The FASEB Journal,* Vol. 16, No. 9, (Jul. 2002), pp. 1138-1140, ISSN 0892-6638.

Prikhojan, A., Brannan, T., Yahr, M.D. (2002). Intrastriatal iron perfusion releases dopamine: an in-vivo microdialysis study. *Journal of Neural Transmission,* Vol. 109, No. 5-6, (May 2002), pp. 645-649, ISSN 1435-1463.

Qiu, W.O., Folstein. M. (2006). Insulin, insulin-degrading enzyme and amyloid-β peptide in Alzheimer's disease: review and hypothesis. *Neurobiology of Aging,* Vol. 27 No. 2 (Feb. 2006), pp. 190–198, ISSN 0197-4580.

Rass, U., Ahel, I., West, S.C. (2007). Defective DNA repair and neurodegenerative disease. *Cell,* Vol. 130, No 6, (Sep. 2007), pp. 130:991-1004, ISSN 0092-8674.

Rauk A. (2009). The chemistry of Alzheimer's disease (AD). Chemical Society Reviews, Vol. 38, No. 9, (Aug. 2008), pp. 2698-2715, ISSN 0306-0012.

Ribes, D., Colomina, M.T., Vicens, P., Domingo, J.L. (2010). Impaired spatial learning and unaltered neurogenesis in a transgenic model of Alzheimer's disease after oral aluminum exposure. *Current Alzheimer Research* , Vol. 7, No. 5, (Aug. 2010), pp. 401-408, ISSN 1567-2050.

Ricchelli F, Drago D, Filippi B, Tognon G, Zatta P. (2005). Aluminum- triggered structural modifications and aggregation of beta- amyloids. Cellular and Molecular Life Sciences, Vol. 62, No. 15, (Aug. 2005), pp. 1724-1733, ISSN 1420-9071.

Riederer, P., Sofic, E., Raush, W.D. (1989). Transition metals, ferritin, glutathione, and ascorbic acid in parkinsonian brain. *Journal of Neurochemistry,* 52, 515-520. Vol. 52, No. 2, (Feb. 1989), pp. 515-520. ISSN 0022-3042.

Rondeau, V., Commenges, D., Jacqmin-Gadda, H., Dartigues, J.F. (2001). Relation between aluminum concentrations in drinking water and Alzheimer's disease: an 8-year follow- up study. *American Journal of Epidemiology,* Vol. 154, No. 3, (Aug. 2001), pp. 159- 166, ISSN 1476-6256.

Rossman T.G. & Molina M., 1986. The genetic toxicology of metal compounds: II. Enhancement of ultraviolet light-induced mutagenesis in Escherichia coli WP2. *Environmental Mutagenesis,* Vol. 8, No. 2, (1986), pp. 263–71, ISSN 0192-2521.

Rossman T.G. & Molina M., Meyer L.W. (1984). The genetic toxicology of metal compounds: I. Induction of lambda prophage in E coli WP2s(lambda). *Environmental Mutagenesis,* Vol. 6, No. 1, (1984), pp. 59–69, ISSN 0192-2521.

Rouault, T. A. (2001). Systemic iron metabolism: a review and implications for brain iron metabolism. *Pediatric Neurology, Journal of Neurochemistry,* Vol. 25, No. 2, (Aug. 2001), pp. 130-137, ISSN 1304-2580.

Roy, A.K., Sharma A. & Talukder, G. (1991). Effects of aluminium salts on bone marrow chromosomes in rats in vivo. *Cytobios,* Vol. 66, No. 265 (1991), pp. 105–11, ISSN 0011-4529.

Santiago, M., Matarredona, E.R., Granero, L., Cano, J., Machado, A. (2000). Neurotoxic relationship between dopamine and iron in the striatal dopaminergic nerve terminals. *Brain Research,* Vol. 858, No. 1, (Mar. 2000), pp. 26-32, ISSN 0006-8993.

Sakae, Y., Shigeo, K., Akihiro, O., Akira, I. (2009). Demonstration of aluminum in amyloid fibers in the cores of senile plaques in the brains of patients with Alzheimer's disease. *Journal of Inorganic Biochemistry,* Vol. 103, No. 11, (Nov. 2009), pp. 1579-1584 ISSN 0162-0134.

Salvador, G.A., Uranga, R.M., Giusto, N.M. (2010). Iron and Mechanisms of Neurotoxicity. *International Journal of Alzheimer's Disease,* Vol. 2011, No. 1, (Dec. 2010), pp. 1-9, ISSN 2090-0252.

Santamaria, A.B., Sulsky, S.I. (2010). Risk assessment of an essential element: manganese. *Journal of Toxicology and Environmental Healt A,* Vol. 73, No. 2, (2010), pp. 128-155, ISSN 1087-2620.

Savory, J., Jagannatha Rao K.S., Huang, Y., Letada, P.R. & Herman, M.M. (1999). Age-related hippocampal changes in Bcl-2:Bax ratio, oxidative stress, redox-active iron and apoptosis associated with aluminium- induced neurodegeneration: increased susceptibility with aging. *NeuroToxicology,* Vol. 20, No. 5, (Oct. 2008), pp. 805-818, ISSN 0161-813X.

Sarkander H.I., Balb, G., Schlosser, H., Stoltenburg, G. & Lux, R.M. (1983). In: *Brain Aging: Neuropathology and Neuropharmacology,* Cervos-Navarro, J. & Sarkander, H.I., pp. 259–274, Raven Press, New York

Sayre, L. M., Zagorski, M. G., Surewicz, W. K., Krafft, G. A. & Perry, G. (1997). Mechanism of neurotoxicity associated with amyloid β deposition and the role of free radicals in the pathogenesis of Alzheimer's disease: a critical appraisal. *Chemical Research in Toxicology,* Vol. 10, No. 5 (May 1997), pp.518–526, ISSN 0893-228X.

Sayre, L. M., Zelasko, D.A., Harris, P.L.R., Perry, G., Salomon, R.G. & Smith, M.A. (1997). 4-Hydroxynonenal-derived advanced lipid peroxidation end products are increased in Alzheimer's disease. *Journal of Neurochemistry,* Vol. 68, No. 5, (May 1997), pp. 730-735. ISSN 0022-3042.

Sayre, L.M., Moreira, P.I., Smith, M.A., Perry, G. (2005). Metal ions and oxida- tive protein modification in neurological disease. Annali dell'Istituto Superiore di Sanità, Vol. 41, No. 2, (2005), pp. 143-164, ISSN 0021-2571.

Scalon, M.C., Rechenmacher, C., Siebel, A.M., Kayser, M.L., Rodrigues, M.T., Maluf, S.W., Rodrigues, M.A. & Silva, L.B. (2010). Evaluation of Sinos River water genotoxicity using the comet assay in fish. *Braz. J. Biol.,* Vol. 70, No. 4 (Suppl), (2010), pp. 1217-22, ISSN 1519-6984.

Schneider, J. S., Decamp, E., Clark, K., Bouquio, C., Syversen, T. & Guilarte, T. R. (2009). Effects of chronic manganese exposure on working memory in non-human primates. *Brain Research,* Vol. 1258, No. 3, (Dec. 2009), pp. 86-95, ISSN 0006-8993.

Sethi, P., Jyoti, A., Singh, R., Hussain, E., Sharma, D. (2008). Aluminium-induced electrophysiological, biochemical and cognitive modifications in the hippocampus of aging rats. *NeuroToxicology*, Vol. 29, No.2, (Nov. 2008), pp. 1069-1079, ISSN 0161-813X.

Sienko, M.J., Plane, R.A., (1977). Elementos de transição II. In: *Química 5 ed*, Sienko, M.J., Plane, R.A. (Eds.), pp. 436-454. São Paulo.

Smith, M. A., Tabaton, M., Perry, G. (1996). Early contribution of oxidative glycation in Alzheimer disease. *Neuroscience Letters*, Vol. 217, No. 2-3, (Oct. 1996), pp. 210-211, ISSN 0304-3940.

Smith, M. A., Harris, P. L. R., Sayre, L. M., Perry, G. (1997) Iron accumulation in Alzheimer disease is a source of redox- generated free radicals. *Proceedings of the National Academy of Sciences of the United States of America*, Vol. 94, No. 18, (Sep. 1997), pp. 9866-9868, ISSN 0027-8424.

Sriram, K., Lin G.X., Jefferson, A.M., Roberts, J.R., Chapman, R.S., Chen, B.T., Soukup, J.M., Ghio, A.J. & Antonini, J.M. (2010). Dopaminergic neurotoxicity following pulmonary exposure to manganese-containing welding fumes. *Archives of Toxicology*, Vol. 84, No. 7, (Jul. 2010), pp. 521-540, ISSN 0340-5761.

Stankiewicz, J.M., Brass, S.D. (2009). Role of iron in neurotoxicity: a cause for concern in the elderly? *Current Opinion in Clinical Nutrition and Metabolic Care*, Vol. 12, No. 1, (Jan. 2009), pp. 22-29, ISSN 1363-1950.

Su, B., Wang, X., Nunomura, A., Moreira, P.I., Lee, H.-gon, Perry, G., Smith, M.A. & Zhu., X. (2008). Oxidative Stress Signaling in Alzheimer's Disease. *Current Alzheimer Research*, Vol. 5, No. 6, (Dec. 2008), pp.525-532, ISSN 1567-2050.

Subhash, M.N. & Padmashree, T.S. (1990). Regional distribution of dopamine β-hydroxylase and monoamine oxidase in the brains of rats exposed to manganese. *Food Chemistry and Toxicology*, Vol. 28, No. 8, (Aug. 1990), pp. 567–570, ISSN 0278-6915.

Suh, S.W., Jensen, K.B., Jensen, M.S., Silva, D.S., Kesslak, P.J., Danscher, G. & Frederickson, C.J. (2000). Histochemically-reactive zinc in amyloid plaques, an- giopathy,and degenerating neurons of Alzheimer's diseased brains. *Brain Research*, Vol. 852, No. 2, (Jan. 2000), pp. 274-278, ISSN 0006-8993.

Sullivan, E. V., Adalsteinsson, E., Rohlfing, T., Pfeffer-baum A. (2009). Relevance of iron deposition in deep gray matter brain structures to cognitive and motor on performance in healthy elderly men and women: exploratory findings. *Brain Imaging and Behavior, Journal of Neurochemistry*, Vol. 3, No. 2, (Jun. 2009), pp. 167-175, ISSN 1931-7565.

Suwalsky, M., Ungerer, B., Villena, F., Norris, B., Cardenas, H., Zatta, P., (2001). Effects of AlCl3 on toad skin, human erythrocytes, and model cell membranes. *Brain research bulletin*, Vol. 55, No 2, (May 2001), pp. 205-210, ISSN . 0361-9230.

Terry, R.D., Pena, C. (1965). Experimental production of neurofibrillary degeneration (2) Electron microscopic, phosphatase histochemistry and electron probe analysis. *Journal of Neuropathology and Experimental Neurology*, Vol. 24, No.1, (Apr. 1965), pp. 200-210, ISSN 0022-3069.

Timchenko, O.I., Paran´Ko, N.M., Shantyr, E.E. & Kuz´Menko, S.D. (1991). The cytogenetic effects of separate and combined exposures to a manganese dioxide aerosol and wide-band noise. *Gigiena i Sanitariia*, No. 11, (Nov. 1991), pp. 70–72 , ISSN 0016-9900.

Trippi, F., Botto, N., Scarpato, R., Petrozzi, L., Bonuccelli, U., Latorraca, S., Sorbi, S. & Migliore, L. (2001). Spontaneous and induced chromosome damage in somatic cells of sporadic and familial Alzheimer's disease patients. *Mutagenesis*, Vol. 16, No. 4, (Jul. 2001), pp. 323–327, ISSN 0267-8357.

Troncoso, J.C., Price, D.L., Griffin, J.W. & Perhad, I.M. (1982). Neurofibrillary axonal pathology in aluminum intoxication. *Annals of Neurology*, Vol. 12, No. 3, (Sep. 1982), pp. 278-283, ISSN 0364-5134.

Tucker, J.D., Auletta, A., Cimino, M.C., Dearfield, K.L., Jacobson-Kram, D., Tice, R.R. & Carrano, A.V. (1993). Sister-chromatid exchange: second report of the Gene-Tox Program. *Mutation Research*, Vol. 297, No. 2, (Sep. 1993), pp. 101–180, ISSN 0027-5107.

Van de Sande, J.H., McIntosh, I.P. & Jovin, T.N. (1982). Mn^{2+} and other transition metals at low concentrations at low concentration induce the right-to-left helical transformation of poly d(G–C). *The EMBO Journal*, Vol. 1, No. 7, (1982), pp. 777–782, ISSN 0261-4189.

Varadarajan. S., Yatin, S., Aksenova, M. Butterfield, D.A. (2000). Review: Alzheimer's amyloid beta-peptide-associated free radical oxidative stress and neurotoxicity. *Journal of Structural Biology*, Vol. 130, No. 2-3, (Jun. 2000), pp. 184-208, ISSN 1095-8657.

Varner, J.A., Jensen, K.F., Hovarth, W., Issacson, R.L., (1998). Chronic administration of aluminium fluoride or sodium fluoride to rats in drinking water: Alterations in neuronal and cerebrovascular integrity. *Brain Research*, Vol. 784, No. 16, (Feb. 1998), pp. 284-298, ISSN 0006-8993.

Varella, S.D., Pozetti, G.L., Vilegas, W. & Varanda, E.A. (2004). Mutagenic activity in waste from an aluminum products factory in Salmonella/microsome assay. *Toxicology In Vitro*, Vol. 18, No. 8, (Dec. 2004), pp. 895–900, ISSN 0887-2333.

Veldman, B.A., Widn, A.M., Knoers, N., Pramstra, P., Horstink, M.W., (1998). Genetic and environmental risk factors in Parkinson's disease. *Clinical neurology and neurosurgery*, Vol. 100, No. 1, (Mar. 1998), pp. 295-301, ISSN 0303-8467.

Vidal, L., Alfonso, M., Campos, F., Faro, L.R., Cervantes, R.C. & Duran, R. (2005). Effects of manganese on extracellular levels of dopamine in rat striatum: an analysis in vivo by brain microdialysis. *Neurochemical Research*, Vol. 30, No. 9, (Sep. 2005), pp. 147-1154, ISSN 1573-6903.

Weiss, B. (2010). Lead, Manganese, and Methylmercury as risk factors for neurobehavioral impairment in advanced age. *International Journal of Alzheimer's Disease*, Vol. 2011, No. 27, (Dec. 2010), pp. 1-11 ,ISSN 2090-0252.

Wen-zhen, Z., Wei-de, Z., Wei, W., Chuan-jia, Z., Cheng-yuan, W., Jian-pin, Q., Jian-zhi, W. & Ting, L. (2009). Quantitative MR phase-corrected imaging to investigate increased brain iron deposition of patients with Alzheimer disease. *Radiology*, Vol. 253, No. 2, (Nov. 2009), pp. 497-504, ISSN 1527- 1315.

Willmore, L.J., Rubin, J.J. (1984). The effect of tocopherol and dimethyl sulfoxide on focal edema and lipid peroxidation induced by isocortical injection of ferrous chloride. *Brain Research*, Vol. 296, No. 2, (Apr. 1984), pp. 389-392, ISSN 0006-8993.

Winder, B.S., Salmon, A.G., Marty, M.A. (2010). Inhalation of an essential metal: development of reference exposure levels for manganese. *Regulatory Toxicology and Pharmacology*, Vol. 57, No. 2-3, (Jul. - Aug. 2010), pp. 195-199, ISSN 0273-2300.

Wright, J.A., Brown, D.R. (2008). Alpha-synuclein and its role in metal binding: relevance to Parkinson's disease. *The Journal of Neuroscience Research,* Vol. 86, No. 3, (Feb. 2008), pp. 496-503, ISSN 0360-4012.

World Health Organization (WHO), (1996). Guidelines for drinking - water quality recommendations. 2nd ed. Geneva.

World Health Organization (WHO). (1997). Aluminium. Environmental Health Criteria, N° 194, Geneva.

World Health Organization (WHO). (1998). Trace elements in human nutrition and health.

World Health Organization (WHO), (1999). Manganese and its compounds. Concise International Chemical Assessment Document 12. WHO, Geneva.

Wu, Z., Du, Y., Xue, H., Wu, Y. & Zhou, B. (2010). Aluminum induces neurodegeneration and its toxicity arises from increased iron accumulation and reactive oxygen species (ROS) production. *Neurobiol of Aging.* Jul 29. [Epub ahead of print], ISSN 0197-4580.

Xu J, Chen S, Ahmed SH, Chen H, Ku G, Goldberg MP, Hsu, C.Y. (2001). Amyloid-beta peptides are cytotoxic to oligodendrocytes. *The Journal of Neuroscience,* Vol. 21, No. 1, (Jan. 2001), pp. 1-6, ISSN 0270-6474.

Yang, Y., Mufson, E.J., Herrup, K. (2003). Neuronal cell death is preceded by cell cycle events at all stages of Alzheimer's disease. *The Journal of neuroscience : the official journal of the Society for Neuroscience,* Vol. 23, No. 7, (Apr. 2003), pp. 2557-2563, ISSN 0270-6474.

Yasui, M., Kihira, T., Ota, K. (1992). Calcium, magnesium and aluminum concentrations in Parkinson´s disease. *NeuroToxicology,* Vol. 13, No. 3, (1992), pp. 593-600, ISSN 0161-813X.

Yi, M., Yi, H., Li, H. & Wu, L. (2010). Aluminum induces chromosome aberrations, micronuclei, and cell cycle dysfunction in root cells of Vicia faba. *Environmental Toxicology,* Vol. 25, No. 2, (Apr. 2010), pp. 124-9, ISSN 1520-4081.

Yumei, W., Jinfeng, J., Xiaohong, Z. & Baoshan, Y. (1998). Genotoxicity of the dust organic extract and its fractions derived from an aluminium electrolytic plant. *Toxicology Letters,* Vol. 98, No. 3, (Sep. 1998), pp. 147–153, ISSN 0378-4274.

Yokel, R.A. (1994). Aluminum exposure produces learning and memory deficits, a model of Alzheimer's disease. In: *Toxin-Induced Models of Neurological Disorders,* Woodruff, M.L. and Nonneman, A.J., pp. 301-318, Plenum, ISBN 03064-46146, New York.

Youdim, M. B. H., Fridkin, M., Zheng, H. (2005). Bifunctional drug derivatives of MAO-B inhibitor rasagiline and iron chelator VK-28 as a more effective approach to treatment of brain ageing and ageing neurodegenerative. diseases.*Mechanisms of Ageing and Development,* Vol. 126, No. 2, (Feb. 2005), pp. 317-326, ISSN 0047-6374.

Yumoto, S., Nagai, H., Matsuzaki, H., Matsumura, H., Tada, W., Nagatsma, E., Kobayashi, K. (2001). Aluminium incorporation into the brain of rat fetuses and sucklings. *Brain Research Bulletin,* Vol.55, No. 2, (May 2001), pp. 229-234, ISSN 0361-9230.

Zatta, P.F., Nicolini, M., Corain B. (1991). Aluminum (III) toxicity and blood-brain barrier permeability. In: *Aluminum in Chemistry, Biology and Medicine,* Nicolini, M., Zatta, P.F., Corain, B., pp. 97-12, Cortina International, ISBN 3642105580, Verona.

Zecca, L., Gallorini, M., Schunemann, V., Trautwein, A. X., Gerlach, M., Riederer, P., Vezzoni, P., Tampellini, D. (2001). Iron, neuro- melanin and ferritin content in the substantia nigra of normal subjects at different ages: consequences for iron storage and neurodegenerative processes. *Journal of Neurochemistry*, Vol. 76, No. 6, (Mar. 2001), pp. 1766-1773, ISSN 0022-3042.

Zheng, W., Ren, S., Graziano, J.H., (1998). Manganese inhibits mitochondrial aconitase: a mechanism of manganese neurotoxicity. *Brain Research*, Vol. 799, No. 2, (Jul. 1998), pp. 334-342, ISSN 0006-8993.

Part 5

Metabolic Derangements: Glucose, Insulin, and Diabetes

19

Glucose Metabolism and Insulin Action in Alzheimer's Disease Pathogenesis

Domenico Bosco[1], Massimiliano Plastino[1],
Antonio Spanò[1], Caterina Ermio[2] and Antonietta Fava[3]
[1]Department of Neuroscience, "S. Giovanni di Dio" Hospital, Crotone
[2]Department of Neuroscience, "S. Giovanni Paolo II" Hospital, Lamezia Terme
[3]Clinical Nutrition Unit, Medical School, University of Catanzaro
Italy

1. Introduction

Alzheimer's disease (AD) is a neurological disorder characterized by profound memory loss and progressive dementia. The pathological and histological hallmarks of AD include amyloid plaques, neurofibrillary tangles and amyloidal angiopathy, accompanied by diffuse loss of neurons and synapses [1]. Environmental and genetic factors interact in the development of disease. Type 2 diabetes mellitus (DM) appears to be a significant risk factor for vascular dementia and AD in several epidemiological studies [2, 3]. Recent longitudinal studies have shown that AD and disorder of glucose metabolism are related [4, 5]. One explanation could be that vascular complications of diabetes result in neurodegenerative disease [6]. On the other hand, in addition to its peripheral metabolic effects, insulin also appears have important outcome on brain functions. A recent commentary offers two models of the link between type-2 DM and AD, 1. "central insulin resistance" and 2. inflammation. Both mechanisms influence insulin sensitivity in the brain, finally leading to β-amyloid accumulation and, consequently, to AD [7]. Complex molecular mechanisms, referring to insulin and/or insulin like growth factor-1 (IGF-1) signaling could link DM and AD [8]. In fact, there is evidence that altered insulin and/or IGF-1 signaling to brain cells is probably responsible of amyloid accumulation in AD [9] and several independent effects of insulin on brain functions and cognitive performance have been described [10]. Insulin resistance with associated hyperinsulinemia are the mechanisms suggested to explain the increased AD risk in diabetes [11]. Subsequent investigations demonstrated reduced blood glucose levels and increased insulin levels in patients with late onset AD compared to aged controls or patients with vascular dementia. Although the authors concluded that these findings did not support an association between diabetes and AD [12], the same data were reinterpreted as an increased prevalence of insulin resistance in AD. The latter conclusion contradicts the finding that glucose administration could both increase plasma insulin levels and improve cognition in AD. Working under the assumption that increased insulin rather than glucose was responsible for the improvement in memory, further studies were used to demonstrate that the administration of insulin significantly improved memory performance in AD [8, 13]. Hyperinsulinemic euglycemic clamp studies in humans showed improvement of attention in AD patients and neuroelectric changes in evoked potential induced by insulin [14]. In contrast, increases in plasma glucose that were not accompanied by increases in insulin levels did not influence cognitive performances [15]. The Rotterdam Study was one of the first epidemiology surveys to provide convincing evidence on a relationship between DM and dementia based on a significantly higher prevalence of dementia in patients with insulin-dependent (Type 1) DM compared to non diabetic aged controls [3]. In addition, the possible association between DM-insulin resistance and degree of hippocampal and amygdala atrophy was investigated in vivo by magnetic resonance imaging [16]. The study showed that: 1. Individuals with DM had greater degree of hippocampal and amygdala atrophy compared with subjects who did not have DM; 2. Severity of insulin resistance associated with degree of amygdala atrophy. The inability to convincingly demonstrate a correlation between DM and AD, or find evidence that DM causes neuropathology, led to the alternative hypothesis that diabetes may serve as a co-factor in the pathogenesis of dementia and possibly AD. In this regard, epidemiological studies showed that hyperinsulinemia in patients with APO E_4-negative genotype was correlated with AD-type dementia, whereas in the absence of diabetes, APO E_4+ genotype was also correlated with AD [17], suggesting that APO E_4 genotype and DM contribute independently to the pathogenesis of AD. Correspondingly, post-mortem studies have shown that individuals with DM and APO E_4 genotype had significantly more abundant Aβ deposits and neurofibrillary tangles compared with diabetics who did not have an APO E_4 allele [18]. In this review, we will summarize current evidences supporting the association between insulin action, insulin receptors, IGF-1 and AD, and we will describe the underlying mechanisms.

2. Insulin, IGF-1: Secretion, transport and distribution in human brain

Insulin is almost exclusively synthesized and secreted into the plasma by pancreatic β-cells and has important role in metabolic homeostasis. Although accumulated evidence indicate that insulin is derived from peripheral insulin and transferred by a transporter regulated way through the blood-brain-barrier (BBB), [19, 20] there is also evidence consistent with local synthesis of insulin in the brain. In fact, Schechter et al. demonstrated that insulin can be produced locally in rabbit neuronal cells from culture [21]. besides, Devaskar et al. revealed localization of insulin expressing neurons involved in associative areas of limbic system and areas regulating olfaction [22]. On the other hand, it is now generally thought that insulin synthesis in the brain is restricted is not synthesized to any significant amount in adult developed brain [20]. Over the past few years, it has become clear that insulin and IGF-1 also have intense effects in the central nervous system (CNS), regulating key processes such as energy homeostasis, neuronal survival, longevity, as well as learning and memory. Insulin and IGF-1 bind to tyrosine kinase receptors, the insulin receptor (IR) and IGF-1 receptor (IGF-1R), which share a high degree of identity in their structure and function. Insulin and IR are abundant but selectively distributed in the brain. Rodent studies have shown that insulin binding is highest in the olfactory bulb, cerebral cortex, hippocampus, hypothalamus, amygdala and septum [23, 24]. In the adult mammalian brain, two types of IR were found: a peripheral type and a neuron-specific type [25]. Insulin signaling within the cell is mediated, in general, by two functional cascades, one acting through the phosphatidylinositol-3 (PI3) kinase pathway, and other acting through the mitogen-activated protein kinase pathway [26]. Binding of insulin or IGF-1 induces a conformational change of the receptor and activates tyrosine-kinase which leads to auto-phosphorylation of the intracellular β-subunit [27]. Tyrosine-phosphorylate IR and IGF-1R β-subunits recruit and subsequently phosphorylate tyrosine residues of the intracellular insulin receptor substrates (IRS). The IRS protein family has at least four members, IRS-1 to -4 [28]. IRS proteins are homologue in structure and function but show distinct tissue distribution: IRS-1 and IRS-2 are widely distributed throughout different tissues and the brain, whereas IRS-3 is only expressed in rodent adipose tissue, and IRS-4 is predominantly localized in hypothalamus, thymus, skeletal muscle, heart, kidney, and liver [29]. IR and IGF-1R are also expressed on brain capillaries and mediate the high efficiency translocation of insulin and IGF-1 into the brain across the BBB [30, 31]. Several studies have shown the highest IR density in olfactory bulb, hippocampal formation, hypothalamus, and cerebral cortex [32, 33]. In fact, in postmortem studies in adult humans, Adem et al. showed the highest IGF-1R density in hippocampus, amygdala and parahippocampal gyrus [33]. Whereas the density of brain IR decreases during age, IGF-1R increases, suggesting that specific insulin mediated signals are involved in aging and possibly cause age associated cognitive decline [34, 35]. Insulin has been shown to cross the BBB by different mechanisms: extracellular pathways, non-saturable transmembrane diffusion or saturable active transport [36]. Currently, the majority of studies suggests that the largest proportion of insulin crosses the BBB by receptor-mediated transport [37]. In contrast, insulin IGF-1 is formed within the CNS during the development and, to a lesser extent, in the mature brain [38]. However, Rotwein suggests that IGF-1 might cross the BBB via an analogous mechanism like insulin [39].

3. Insulin and IGF-1 signaling in Alzheimer's disease

In normal physiology, insulin facilitates memory as demonstrated when administration at optimal doses and in contrast of sufficient glucose availability [15]. Type-2-diabetic patients are insulin resistant and have chronic hyperinsulinemia. The peripheral utilization of insulin reduces insulin transport into the brain, ultimately producing brain insulin deficiency [40], and abrogating the beneficial influences of insulin on the brain functions [15]. Different insulin levels have been observed in different brain regions [30, 41], probably linked to multiple insulin actions in CNS. Studies on type-2-DM animal models have shown a reduced uptake of insulin into the brain. It was observed that obese diabetic Zucker rats have a decreased insulin transport into the brain, reduced brain levels of insulin and peripheral hyperglycemia [30, 36, 41]. Recent studies linked diabetes with AD [8, 9, 18] and suggested that the brain may be influenced by changes in insulin levels and sensitivity. The observations that insulin, insulin receptors and C-peptide levels in cerebrospinal fluid (CSF) appears to be reduced in aging [42], along with the finding that AD patients have lower levels of insulin in the CSF, suggest impaired transport of insulin into the brain [43]. However the salutary effect of insulin on brain functions are reserved under conditions that impair its functioning, such as insulin resistance [44]. Frolich et al. found that neuronal tyrosine-kinase activity is decreased in AD patients compared to age-matched controls [35]. The overall expression of IGF-1R is reduced in AD brains dependent on the severity of the disease. Brain IGF-1 mRNA levels diminish in severe AD, whereas IGF-1 serum levels are increased in early stages of the disease, suggesting that IGF-1 resistance plays a role in the pathogenesis of AD [35]. IRS-1/2 protein expression is reduced in AD brains, and inactivating Serine-phosphorylation of IRS-^{312} and Ser^{616} is improved, leading to impaired insulin resistance and IGF-1R signaling [45]. Given that IRS are widely expressed in the hippocampus, the most studied brain region for learning and memory, it seems to be plausible that decline of insulin resistance signaling leads to cognitive impairment [46]. Experiments with adult mice lacking liver IGF-1 production with an up of 85% reduction in circulating IGF-1 showed impaired spatial memory in the Morris water maze task compared to wild type litter mates [46]. These findings might explain the reduction of cognitive functions during aging, since IGF-1 serum levels diminish under physiological conditions [47]. Unpredictably, studies in neuronal-IR-knockout mice (NIRKO) did not provide evidence for impairment in learning and memory, proposing that insulin resistance alone is not a key feature in dementia and neurodegeneration [17].

3.1 Glucose metabolism and Alzheimer's disease

Some of the earliest work on senile dementia, which probably corresponded to AD, vascular dementia, or a combination of both, documented the development of altered brain metabolism soon after the onset of clinical symptoms [48, 49]. The metabolic abnormalities consisted of impaired glucose utilization and energy metabolism, with features that resemble type-2 DM [48]. In addition, several studies confirmed that cerebral metabolism declined prior to the deterioration of cognitive functions, suggesting that energy failure is one of the earliest reversible hallmarks of AD. These observations led to the hypothesis that AD-associated abnormalities in energy metabolism are caused by IR action in the brain, i.e. brain diabetes [49].

3.2 Insulin therapy and Alzheimer's disease

There are conflicting findings regarding the effects of antidiabetic therapy on clinical and neuropathology of AD. The Honolulu-Asia Aging Study demonstrated improvement of cognitive function and memory following induced hyperinsulinemia in patients with AD [2]. Conversely, the Rotterdam Study [3] observed increased risk of dementia in subjects with diabetes treated with insulin. In fact, in this prospective study, DM almost doubled the risk of dementia [Relative Risk (RR) 1.9] and patients treated with insulin were at higher risk of dementia [RR 4.3]. In opposition, recent studies suggest that the combination of insulinic therapy with other diabetes medications is associated to a lower neuritic plaques [50] and to slower cognitive decline in patients with AD [13]. Besides, studies in animals have revealed the beneficial effects of peripheral and cerebroventricular injections of insulin on memory and learning [51]. Several studies have recognized that increasing plasma glucose levels improves memory in patients with AD [14, 15, 30]. Increasing plasma glucose levels also increases endogenous insulin levels, raising the query whether memory improvement is due to changes in insulin, independently of hyperglycemia [14], although the exact mechanism remains unclear. Dense IR distributions have been documented in the dentate gyros, CA1, and CA3 fields of the hippocampus [52]. These regions are known to play a role in declarative memory and they are affected earlier and most severely by the neuropathologic changes of AD [53]. Increased plasma insulin levels result in amplified insulin binding in hippocampus. In turn, increased brain insulin levels results in enlarged glucose utilization in the entorhinal cortex [54]. In contrast to the traditional notion that the brain is not an insulin-sensitive organ, insulin-promoted glucose utilization also results in glycolytic production of acetyl-CoA and subsequent increase in acetylcholine [55], a neurotransmitter closely linked to memory function and severely reduced in AD. Craft et al. confirm that elevated insulin without hyperglycaemia enhances memory in adults with AD, when endogenous insulin was suppressed by concomitant infusion of somatostatin analogues [14]. Moreover, the beneficial effect of insulin appears to be reduced when insulin resistance is present [17]. Craft et al. showed acute effect of hyperinsulinemia in older adults and in patients with AD using a hyperinsulinemic-euglycemic clamps [15]. Low doses of insulin improve memory in normal subjects; AD patients with insulin resistance required higher insulin doses to obtain memory improvement. To date, no genetic risk factors have been identified for these patients, raising the possibility that factors relating to insulin resistance may be important for AD pathogenesis [15].

3.3 Insulin and oxidative stress mechanisms in Alzheimer's disease

Insulin promotes cell membrane expression of N-methyl-D-aspartate (NMDA) receptors, with increased neuronal Ca^{2+} influx [56]. Ca^{2+} influx presumably activates Ca^{2+}dependent enzymes, including α-dependent enzymes and strengthens neuronal synaptic association [10]. A recent study identified a molecular mechanism that protects CNS neurons against β-amyloid-derived-diffusible ligands (ADDL), responsible for synaptic deterioration underlying AD memory failure. The authors found ADDL binding to particular synaptic sites, and the resulting oxidative stress on synapses loss are markedly decreased by the presence of insulin. The protection mechanism does not involve simple competition between ADDLs and insulin, but rather is signaling-dependent down regulation of ADDL binding sites [57]. Another metabolic disturbance of emerging importance in AD involves insulin signaling in the brain. Levels of insulin receptors, glucose-transport proteins, and other insulin pathway components are reduced in some studies of AD brain (central resistance) [30]. Han et al. proposed a central insulin resistance together with decreased brain insulin levels might lead to accumulation of β-amyloid and consequently AD [7]. Insulin and brain derived IGF-1 instigate signals in the brain by activating the phosphatidylinositol-3-kinase-Akt pathway and the mitogen-activated protein kinase-extracellular signal-regulated kinase pathway [58], but it is unclear whether signaling is up-regulated (compensatory) or down-regulated (pathologic) in AD. Aging and life span are also influenced by insulin. Both in AD and in normal aging process mtDNA sustains high levels of oxidative damage **(Figure 1)** [59]. In fact, it was observed the accumulation of Aβ within structural damaged mitochondria isolated from the brains of AD patients [59, 60] and transgenic brains [61], which impair critical mitochondrial enzymes. Dysfunctional mitochondria release oxidizing free radicals, with peroxidation of membrane lipids and output of toxic aldehydes that cause considerable oxidative stress in AD and in normal aging brains [62]. Other essential proteins resulted oxidized, yielding carbonyl and nitrated derivatives, in neuronal cytoplasm in cerebral regions of neurodegeneration, in human brain affected by AD [63]. Subsequently, increased membrane permeability to calcium, and impaired glucose transport aggravate the energy imbalance [64]. Experimental model show that markers of oxidative damage precede pathological changes [65]. Destruction of mitochondria by the oxidation of a dynamic like transporter protein may cause synapse loss in AD [66]. The "receptor for advanced glycation end products" (RAGE) mediates Aβ's pro-oxidant effects on neural, microglial, and cerebrovascular cells [67]. The RAGE receptor is a multi-ligand receptor, and one of its ligands is Aβ [67]. RAGE regulates several intracellular pathways [68], such stimulates expression of b-site Amyloid Precursor Protein (APP)-cleaving enzyme 1 (BACE1) [69], an enzyme that is necessary for Aβ production. Moreover RAGE seems to negatively affect the long term potentiation (LTP) synaptic process of learning and memory [70]. RAGE also exists in a soluble form, structured by alternative splicing [71] or proteolytic cleavage by the metalloprotease 10 (ADAM 10) [72]. Soluble

RAGE (sRAGE) contains the ligand-binding site, but does not have the signaling properties of full-length RAGE (flRAGE). It was observed that flRAGE is engaged in positive feedback mechanisms, enhancing its own production, and limiting sRAGE proposed protective actions. This notion is supported by the finding that flRAGE expression is increased in AD brains [73]. Indeed, studies have shown that sRAGE can inhibit the accumulation and aggregation of Aβ in mice brains [74]. In addition, it has been shown that sRAGE is present at lower levels in the blood and brain of AD patients [75]. Abnormal expression of RAGE in AD brain suggests that it is relevant to the pathogenesis of neuronal dysfunction and death.

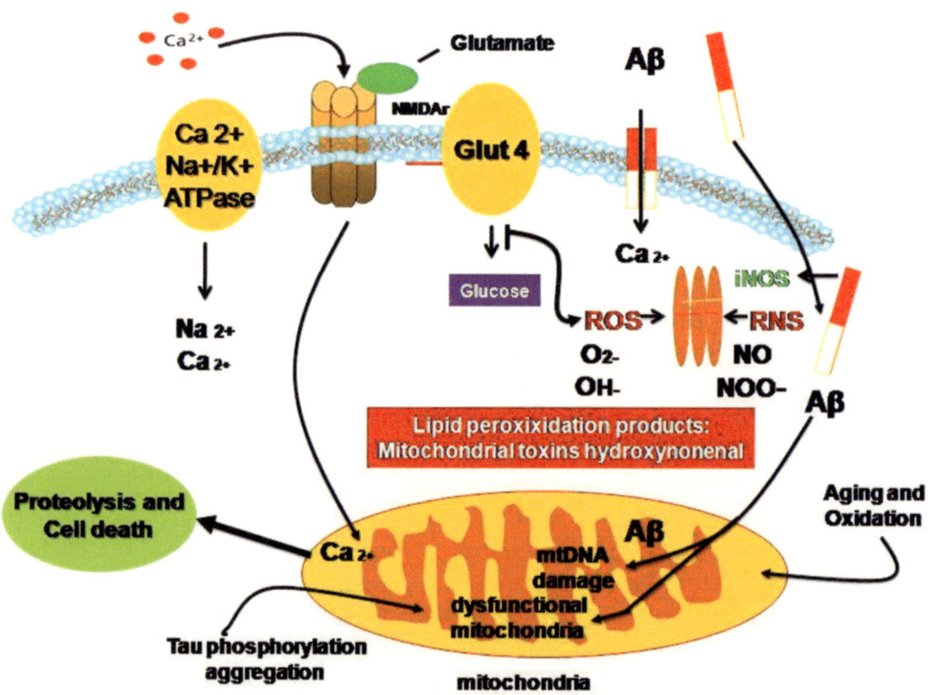

Fig. 1. Oxidative distress

Dysfunctional mitochondria release oxidizing free radicals, and in Alzheimer's disease (AD), they cause significant oxidative stress. Oxidative damage precede pathological changes. Aβ, a strong generator of reactive oxygen species (ROS) and reactive nitrogen species (RNS), is a prime author of this damage. The receptor for advanced glycation end products (RAGE) mediates Aβ's pro-oxidant effects on neural, microglial and cerebrovascular cells. Mitochondrial hydrogen peroxide readily diffuses into the cytosol to contribute in metal-ion-catalyzed hydroxyl radical development. Moved microglia are a major source of the highly diffusible nitric oxide radical. These reactive oxygen species and reactive nitrogen species damage several molecular targets. Peroxidation of membrane lipids yields toxic aldehydes, which impair critical mitochondrial enzymes. Other essential proteins are directly oxidized, yielding carbonyl and nitrated derivates. Consequently, increases in membrane permeability to calcium, other ionic imbalances, and impaired glucose transportation worsen the energy imbalance.

4. The insulin and IGF-1R signaling and Tau phosphorylation

Soluble tau proteins assemble with tubulin to constitute cross bridge between adjacent microtubule and promote stability of microtubules and vesicle transport [76]. Hyperphosphorylation of tau induces abnormal insoluble tau protein [77]. Neurofibrillary tangles are hyperphosphorilated, intracellular polymers of tau proteins. Neurofibrillary tangles are intracellular polymers of tau proteins, observed in cytoplasm of neurons [76] in AD and in other neurodegenerative disorders, such as frontotemporal dementia, Pick's disease, corticobasal degeneration, supranuclear palsy. Several studies [78, 79] supposed that the interaction between Aβ and tau proteins is necessary to cause neuronal loss. When hyperphosphorylated, tau aggregates and interferes with intraneuronal metabolism and transport, leading to neurodegeneration. IR/IGF1 R mediated might be involved in regulation of tau phosphorilation, amyloid precursor protein cleavage, β amyloid transport and degradation, in memory and aging [8]. The phosphorilation of tau is mainly promoted by glycogen syntase kinase (GSK)3β and cyclin dependent kinase(Cdk5).GSK3β is a serine-treonine kinase,regulated by insulin/IGF-1 signaling pathway. GSK-3β is functionally main for regulating glycogen metabolism, proliferation survival, and cell migration [77]. When the IR/IGF-1cascade is activated, GSKβ is phoshorilated by protein kinase AKT at serin leading to its inactivation [80-82] **(Figure 2).** PP2A dephosphorylates tau maintaining an equilibrium of phosphorylation and dephosphorilation of tau [82, 83]. Protein phosphatases 2A (PP2A) is the major phosphatases with 70% activity in human brains [84]. This implies a protective role of PP2A in neurodegeneration which is consistent with the finding that PP2A activity is reduced in AD brains [85]. In vitro studies it was found that insulin influences a regulatory interaction between PP2A and GSK 3β, inducing in activity of both enzymes change in the same direction. This balanced response seemed to preserve equilibrated tau phosphorilation [86, 87]. Several studies on different animal models of insulin resistance showed that impaired IR /IGF-1 signaling and hyperinsulinemia increased tau phosphorylation.[88-89]. In streptozotocina treated mice, model of type 1 diabetes, hyperphosphorilation of tau has be shown, which was reversible after peripheral insulin treatment [90]. Another important physiological role of insulin and IGF-1 in the brain is the regulation of gene transcription by MAP kinase cascade. This pathway leads to activation of extracellular signal-regulated kinase (ERK)-1/-2, involved in long lasting neuronal plasticity, memory consolidation and apoptotic neuronal death [91-93]. Thus, altered IR/IGF-1 signaling as well as lack of insulin might lead to hyperphosphorylation of tau protein and an increased formation of neurofibrillary tangles. These findings suggest that hyperphosphorylation of tau follows an imbalance of insulin regulated tau kinases and phosphatases [94].

Protein phosporylation/dephosphorylation imbalance is generate, at least in part, by a decrease in the activities of tau phosphatases (PP2A), and increase the activities of tau kinase (i.e. cdk5, GSK-3, etc.) affected by insulin. Impaired insulin signaling stimulates GSK-3β activity that increases oxidative stress and tau hyper-phosphorylation, by Cdk-5. Severe or sustained oxidative injury leads to mithocondrial DNA damage, mithocondrial dysfunction, apoptosis and the attendant cell loss and impaired neuronal function lead to dementia. Age reduces membrane fluidity inducing mutations in transmembrane proteins, (i.e. PS1, PS2,..), and vulnerability of the cell membrane to variation in pathological signal transduction.

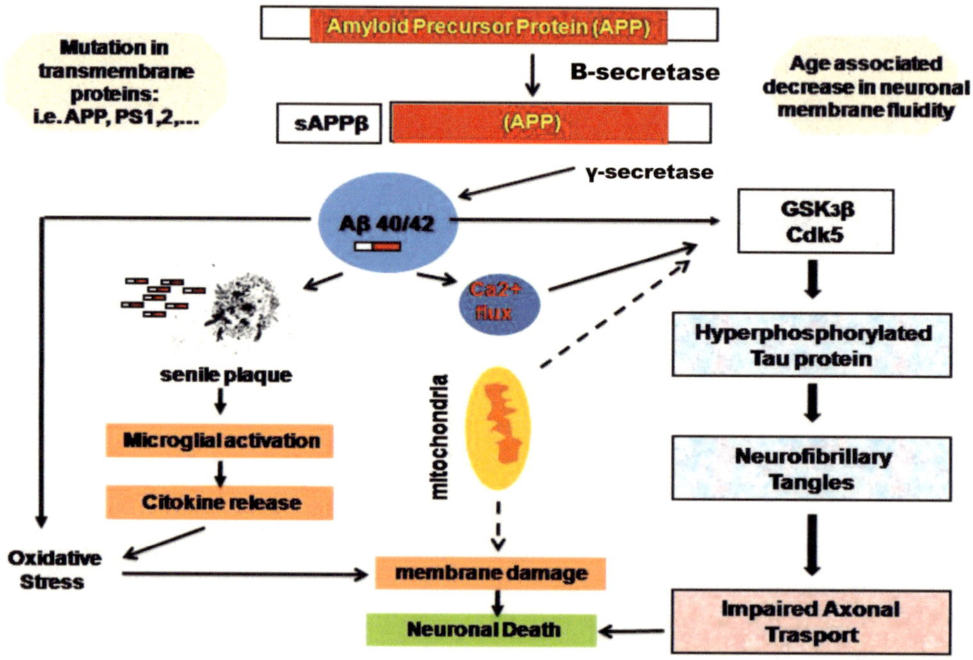

Fig. 2. Dementia and anomalous hyperphosphorylation of tau

4.1 Protein phosphatases A (PPA) processing in Alzheimer's disease

The amyloid plaques is formed by amyloid β (Aβ) peptides organized in fibrils intermixed with non fibrillar forms of this peptide and are surrounded by dystrophic dendrites, axons, reactive astrocytes and activated microglia. Aβ consists of small hydrophobic peptides with N- and C-terminal heterogeneity, i.e. $A\beta_{1-40}$ and $A\beta_{1-42}$ which are proteolytically released from a large type 1 integral membrane glycoprotein, the APP, via sequential cleavage by two aspartyl proteases, the β- and γ-secretases [enzymatic complex, containing nicastrina, presenilina, preselin enhancer-2 (PEN-2), CD_{147}] [95]. Initial β-secretase cleavage generates a soluble fragment from the NH_2-terminus of APP, while the c-terminal fragment (β-CTF) stays membrane bound. Full-length APP can undergo alternative processing by α-secretase, generating a soluble APPsα ectodomain and a membrane-bound carboxy-terminal fragment, APP-CTFα. Processing of APP by α-secretase is postulated to be protective in the context of AD, because the enzyme cleaves within the Aβ-sequence, thereby preventing the production of Aβ. APP, αCTF and βCTF are further cleaved by γ-secretase to generate p83 fragment and Aβ respectively [96]. Multiple lines of biochemical evidence have shown γ-secretases activity to reside in a high molecular weight complex, consisting of at least four components: presenilin (PS, PS1, PS2), nicastrin, anterior pharynx-defective (APH-1) and PEN-2 [97]. The p83 fragment is rapidly degraded and widely believed to possess no important function, if any. γ-secretase-mediated cleavage is unique in that the cleavage takes place within the membrane domain, though the exact site can vary. γ-cleavage can yield both $A\beta_{1-40}$ and to a lesser extent $A\beta_{1-42}$ [96]. Aβ are toxic, and their accumulation is currently seen as a key step in the pathogenesis of AD **(Figure 3).** Closer examination of the amyloidogenic β- and γ-secretates discovered the membrane-anchored aspartyl protease β-site BACE-1, which acts as β-secretase and presenelin 1-2, transmembrane proteins involved in formation of the γ-secretase complex, as the responsible cleavage enzymes. Thus, alteration of their activity might be a possible target for AD treatment [98]. It has been shown that BACE-1 levels are increased in post-mortem brain sections from AD patients [99]. During aging changes in the cerebral expression levels of the neurotrophin receptors, TrkA (tyrosine kinase receptor A) and $p75^{NTR}$ (p75 neurotrophin receptor) have been described. In the human neuroblastoma cell line SHSY5Y as well as primary cultured neurons, chronic treatment with IGF-1 leads to a switch from TrkA to $p75^{NTR}$ expression as seen in aging brains [100]. This switch causes increased β-secretase activity indirectly by activation of neuronal sphingomyelinase which is responsible for hydrolysis of sphingomyelin and active liberation of the second messenger ceramide [101]. Ceramide is responsible for the molecular stabilization of BACE-1, the β-secretase which is rate-limiting for generation of Aβ [102]. This process leads to accumulation of Aβ, connecting IGF-1R signaling to neurotrophin action. These data might provide a molecular link between aging, pathogenesis of AD and neuronal insulin-IGF-1 signaling. Lots of research has been done on the formation and accumulation of Aβ, however, in the last years the mechanisms of amyloid clearance came into focus.

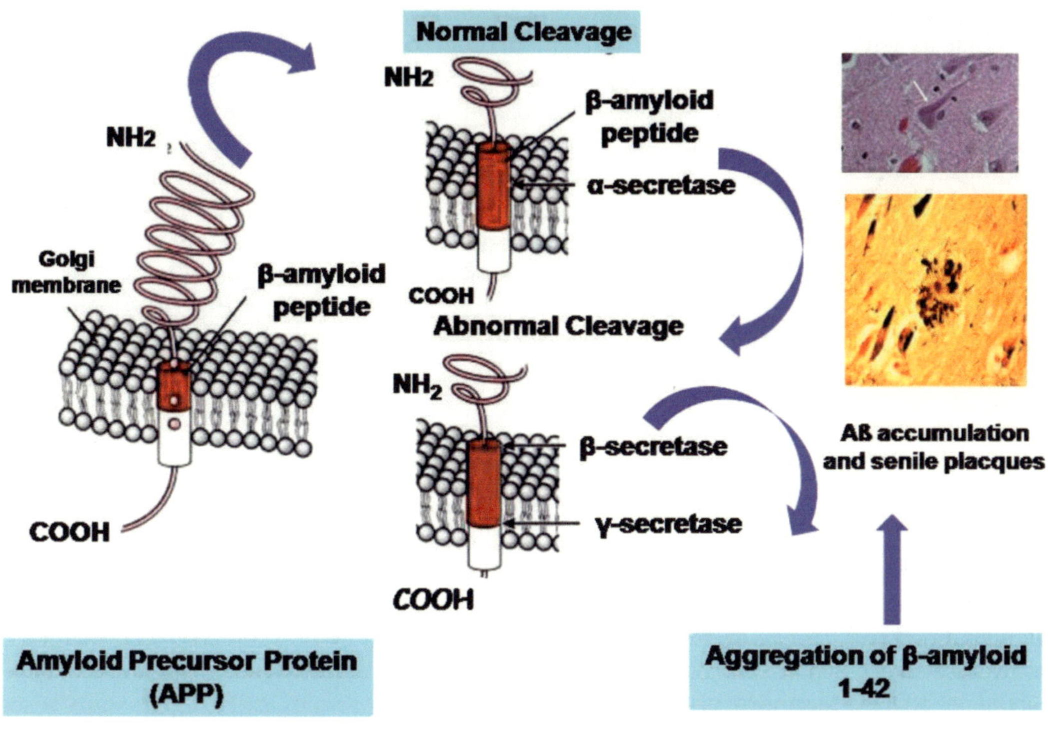

Fig. 3. Amyloid placque formation.

The histological and pathological features of AD are amyloid plaques, neurofibrillary tangles and amyloid angiopathy. The dominant component of the placque core is the the amyloid beta-peptide (Aβ) organized in fibrils of approximately 7-10 nm intermidex with non fibrillar forms of this peptide. Aβ is a a 39-43 aminoacid peptide proteolytically released from a much larger precursor, tha amyloid precursor protein (APP). The generation of Aβ from APP requires the sequential recruitment of two enzymatic activities: β-secretase, also called BACE1 (for beta side APP cleaving enzyme), and γ-secretase , a multicentric protein complex containing presenelin, nicastrina,..Aβ spontaneously self-aggregates into multiple coexisting physical forms, such as oligomers (2 to 6 peptides), transitional assemblies, fibrils that coalesce into β pleated sheets to form insoluble fibers and amyloid plaques. While monomeric Aβ is not neurotoxic, the Aβ oligomers exhibits a marked toxicity (Adapte from Martin JB; 1999).

4.2 Insulin, IGF-1 signaling and β-amyloid in Alzheimer's disease

β-amyloid spontaneously self-aggregates into multiple coexisting physical forms, such as oligomers (2 to 6 peptides), intermediate assemblies, fibrils that coalesce into β pleated sheets to form insoluble fibers and amyloid plaques [103]. While monomeric Aβ is not neurotoxic, the Aβ oligomers exhibits a marked toxicity [104]. Neuronal activation rapidly increase Aβ secretion at the synapse, during the process of neurotransmitters release. Normal levels of Aβ at this site may modulate neuronal transmission and prevent hyperactivity [105]. It was assumed that imbalance between production, aggregation and clearance of peptides, is considered initiating factor in AD [106]. For Aβ clearance several mechanisms have been described: 1. enzymatic degradation by activated microglia or by insulin degrading enzyme (IDE), neprilysin, endothelin converting enzyme (ECE), and angiotensin converting enzyme (ACE); 2. receptor-mediated transport across the BBB by binding to the low-density lipoprotein receptor-related protein (LRP), either directly or after binding to APO E and/or α2-macroglobulin (α2M), to be delivered to peripheral sites of degradation, e.g., liver and kidney [41]. Concerning insulin resistance it has been shown that IDE expression is stimulated by the insulin resistance-IGF-1R cascade [107]. It has been recently reported that membrane associated G protein-coupled receptor kinase-5 (GRK5) deficiency occurs during early AD [108]. In deficient GRK5 mice (tg2576-APPsw) Aß accumulation resulted significantly increased [108]. IGF-1 administration resulted in reduction of cerebral Aβ load in these mice, whereas Aβ was elevated in CSF suggesting an increased Aβ elimination across the BBB or the choroid plexus [109]. Furthermore, it has been shown that the blockade of the IGF-1R in the choroid plexus triggers AD-like pathology. Furthermore, tau phosphorylation did not change significantly following chronic IGF-1 treatment in Tg2576 mice [109]. A possible explanation could be that the chronic increase of IGF-1 by peripheral treatment might down regulate IGF-1R signaling. This hypothesis is supported by the finding that in a cohort of individuals with exceptional longevity serum IGF-1 levels were high but IGF-1R activity was low leading to reduced IGF-1R signaling [110]. However, induction of insulin resistance by high fat diet [111] or intake of sucrose-sweetened water [112] leads to an aggravation of amyloid pathology in mouse models of AD. Furthermore, peripheral injection of supra physiologically high insulin doses but not of physiological doses leads to transient cerebral tau phosphorylation [113], leading to the proposal that there is a dose dependent effect of insulin resistance-IGF-1R signaling in the pathogenesis of AD.

5. Insulin, inflammation and Alzheimer's disease

In recent years inflammatory pathway have been linked to type 2 diabetes mellitus, metabolic syndrome (MS) and neurodegenerative diseases, including AD. Inflammation as able to accelerates the development type2 DM, through its influence on peripheral insulin sensitivity and pancreatic islet function; on the other hand, in addition to impaired insulin signaling, diabetes accelerated the appearance of cerebrovascular inflammation and Aβ deposition, as evidenced by increased levels of proinflammatory cytokines IL6 and TNFα, as well as dense amyloid deposits in blood vessels. [7, 114]. Cerebrovascular and central inflammation, along with increased accumulation of β amyloid, disrupts normal synaptic function, a starting point of AD progression. It was hypothesized the mutual interaction between AD and DM. Takaeda observed increased severity of diabetic phenotype in AD animal models. The reciprocal actions between AD and type-2 DM thus form a vicious cycle, further illustrating the possibility that AD and type-2 DM may share common cellular and molecular mechanisms [114] **(Figure 4).** Peripheral and central inflammation might affect pathogenesis of DM and AD. Elevated concentrations of interleukin (IL) 6 E_2–isoprostane have been observed in CFS of patients with AD [115]. Furthermore, in vitro and animal studies suggest that inflammation interacts with processing and deposit of Aβ [116]. Insulin exerts multiple effects involved in inflammation. In peripheral tissues insulin modulates many aspects of inflammatory network. Low doses of insulin exert anti-inflammatory effects [117]; however, during chronic hyperinsulinemia, insulin may exacerbate inflammatory responses and increase markers of oxidative stress [118]. In human, co-administration of insulin and lipopolysaccharide produces a synergist increase in plasma concentrations of C-reactive protein and proinflammatory cytokines IL-1β, IL-6, TNFα [119]. TNFα has both neurotoxic and neuroprotective effects mediated respectively by two receptor subtypes, TNF-R1 and TNF-R2. TNF-R1 contains a death receptor domain, and has been implicated in pro-apoptotic events, whereas TNF-R2 promotes cell survival. Increased levels of TNF-R1 and decreased levels of TNF-R2 have been observed in AD brain [120]. Abnormal levels of soluble TNF-R1 and R2 have been documented in adults with diabetes and impaired glucose tolerance [121], which reportedly normalize after a 3-weeks low calorie diet [122]. Insulin may also modulate levels of eicosanoids such as F2-isoprostane via regulation of prostaglandin production in adypocites [123]. For example, elevated eicosanoid concentrations have been observed in hyperisulinemic Zucker rats [41]. Furthermore, excessive or chronic hyperinsulinemia inhibits degradation of protein damaged by oxidation and leads to formation of superoxide anions [124]. Insulin may also contribute to inflammation in the CNS, partially through effects on Aβ. In fact, $A\beta_{42}$ interacts with inflammatory agents in a cyclically reinforcing manner, such that Aβ elevations increase pro-inflammatory cytokines [125]. In vitro, soluble Aβ oligomers rapidly increase IL-1β and TNFα levels [126]. Conversely, IL-6 and IL-1β can regulate processing of the APP from which Aβ is derived and increase production of $A\beta_{42}$ [127]. The mutually reinforcing effects of Aβ, TNFα, IL-1β and IL-6 may thus create a "cytokine cycle" [125]. In the periphery, insulin reduces hepatic production of Apo E and regulates its uptake by low-density lipoprotein receptor-related protein [128]. Fishel et al. showed that insulin reduced plasma Apo E levels, an effect that increased with age. In contrast, insulin increased CSF Apo E concentrations for older subjects [129]. Increased brain APO E levels have been reported in AD in association with polymorphisms in the promoter region of the APO E gene that influence protein expression [130]. Recent studies showed that insulin-induced elevations of CSF APO E levels were associated with attenuated increase IL6 and TNFα levels and with higher anti-inflammatory cytokine, IL-1α concentration. This pattern suggests multiple insulin effects that modulate the role of APO E in response to inflammation in CNS [129] .Insulin can regulate CNS norepinephrine [131], an endogenous anti-inflammatory neuromodulator that blocks IL-1β expression [132]. Increased Aβ plaque load in AD has been linked to neuronal loss in the locus coeruleus, the primary source of brain norepinephrine [133]. In human, raising plasma insulin levels while maintain euglycemia increases CSF norepinephine levels [134].Thus, these findings support the notion that insulin action is involved in neutrasmitter modulation and insulin abnormalities might contribute to CNS inflammation.

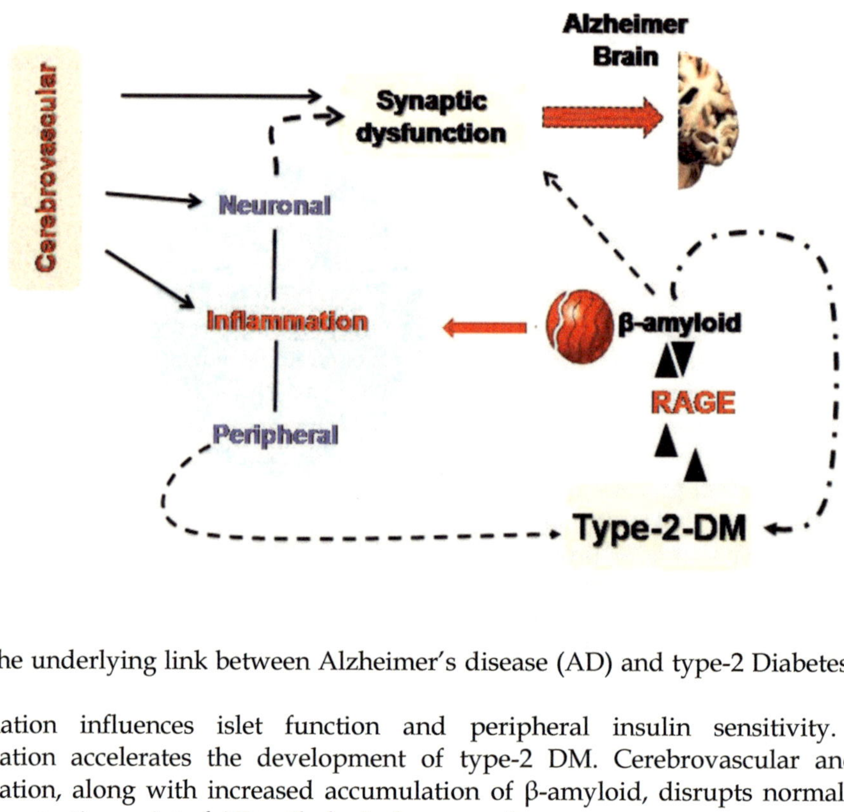

Fig. 4. The underlying link between Alzheimer's disease (AD) and type-2 Diabetes Mellitus (DM).
Inflammation influences islet function and peripheral insulin sensitivity. Besides, inflammation accelerates the development of type-2 DM. Cerebrovascular and central inflammation, along with increased accumulation of β-amyloid, disrupts normal synaptic function, a starting point of AD pathological progression.

6. Conclusion

Mild to moderate impairments of cognitive functioning has been reported both in patients with DM-type1 and in patients with DM-type2. The potential impact of DM on cognitive functions in the elderly is further emphasized by several large epidemiological surveys that report an increased incidence of dementia among DM patients. Several mechanisms may be involved in accelerated cognitive decline in patients with DM. Insulin may affect the metabolism of Aβ and tau, two proteins that represent the building blocks of amyloid plaques and neurofibrillary tangles, the neuropathological hallmarks of AD. Moreover, insulin and its receptor are widely distributed throughout the brain, with particular abundance in defined areas, such as the hypothalamus and the hippocampus. In addition, insulin appears to act as "neuromodulator", that influences the release and reuptake of neurotransmitters, and improves learning and memory. These findings could provide insights to develop a strategy for prevention and treatment of AD. Insulin therapy plays an important role in cognitive processes and could slow dementia in patients with AD and DM. This could be explained by: 1.*molecular mechanisms,* insulin promotes cell membrane expression of NMDA receptors, which increases neuronal Ca2+ influx [56], that activates Ca^{2+}-dependent enzymes, including α-dependent enzymes and strengthens neuronal synaptic association [10]; 2. *glucose metabolism,* low concentrations of exogenous insulin may increase cerebral glucose metabolism and then modulate brain functions such as memory [135]. In fact, insulin has shown a significant effect on global brain glucose metabolism and this effect is mainly expressed in the cerebral cortex; 3. *neurotransmitter modulation,* low doses of insulin can reverse the amnestic effects of cholinergic blockade [136]. Although the concepts of "Cerebral Insulin Resistance" and "insulin-induced amyloid pathology" are an attractive explanation for some of the effects of DM2 on the brain, there are still many loose ends. It is important to point out that definitive conclusions about the value of insulinic treatment in course of AD cannot be established at this time.

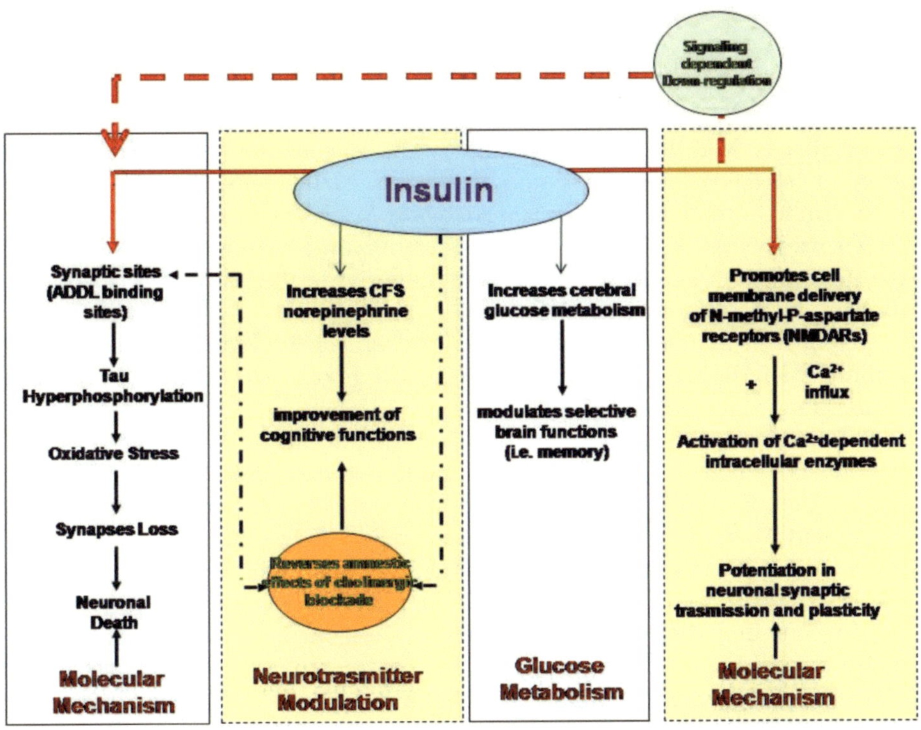

Fig. 5. Schematic representation of molecular mechanism, glucose metabolism and neurotransmitter modulation

Insulin promotes cell membrane expression of NMDA receptors, which increases neuronal Ca^{2-} influx, that activates Ca^{2-} dependent enzymes and strengthens neuronal synaptic association. Besides, diffusible ligands (ADDL) binding to particular synaptic sites and the resulting oxidative stress and synapse loss are markedly decreased by the presence of insulin. This mechanism is associated with a signal dependent down regulation of ADDL binding sites. Low peripheric insulin level may increase cerebral glucose and modulate cognitive functions. Besides, low levels of insulin contributes reverse the anamnestic effects of cholinergic blockade.

7. References

Citron, M. (2002). Alzheimer's disease: treatment in discovery and development. *Nat Neurosci.* 5:1055-7.

Peila, R.; Rodriguez, BL. & Lauren, LJ. (2002). Type-2 diabetes, diabetes, Apo E gene and the risk for dementia and related pathogenesis: the Honolulu-Asia Aging Study. *Diabetes.* 51:1256-62.

Ott, A.; Stolk, RP.; Hofman, A.; Van Harskamp, F.; Pols, HA. & Breteler MM. (1996). Diabetes mellitus and risk of dementia: the Rotterdarm Study. *Neurology* 53(9);1907-9.

Luchsinger, JA.; Tang, MX.; Shea, S. & Mayeux, R. (2004). Hyperinsulinemia and risk of Alzheimer's disease. *Neurology* 63:1187-92.

Janson, J.; Laedtke, T.; Parisi, JE.; O Brien, P.; Petersen, RC. & Butler, PC. (2004). Increased risk of type 2 diabetes in Alzheimer disease. *Diabetes* 53:474-81.

Whitmer, RA.; Sidney, S.; Selby, J.; Johnston, SC. & Yaffe, K. (2005) Midlife cardiovascular risk factors and risk of dementia in late life. *Neurology* 64:277-81

Han, W. & Li, C. (2010) Linking type 2 diabetes and Alzheimer's disease. *Proc Natl Acad Sci USA.* 107:6557-8.

Freude, S.; Schilbach, K & Schubert, M. (2009). The role of IGF-1 receptor and insulin receptor signaling for the pathogenesis of Alzheimer's disease: from model organism to human disease. *Current Alzheimer Research* 6:213-23.

Carro, E. & Torres-Aleman, I. (2004). The role of insulin and insulin-like growth factor I in the molecular and cellular mechanisms underlying the pathology of Alzheimer's disease. *Eur J of Pharmacology* 490:127-33.

Byme, JH. (2003). Learning and memory: basic mechanism. In: Squire LR, Bloom FE, Mc Connel SK, Roberts JL, Spitzer NC, Zigmond MJ, editors. Fundamental neuroscience. *San Diego (CA): Academic Press* 1276–98.

Qiu, WQ. & Folstein, MF. (2006). Insulin, insulin-degrading enzyme and amyloid-beta peptide in Alzheimer's disease: review and hypothesis. *Neurobiol Aging* 27:190-8.

Fisman, M.; Gordon, B.; Feleki, V.; Helmes, T.; Mac Donald & J, Dupre. (1988). Metabolic changes in Alzheimer's disease. *J. Am. Geriatr Soc.* 36:298-300.

Plastino, M.; Fava, A.; Pirritano, D.; Cotronei, P.; Sacco, N.; Sperlì, T.; Spanò, A.; Gallo, D.; Mungari, P.; Consoli, D &, Bosco, D. (2010). Effects of insulinic therapy on cognitive impairment in patients with Alzheimer disease and diabetes mellitus type-2. *J Neurol Sci* 288:112-6.

Craft, S.; Asthana, S.; Newcomer, JW.; Wilkinson, CW.; Matos, IT.; Baker, LD.; Cherrier, K.; Purganan, K.; Wait, C.; Petrova, A.; Plymate, S.; Raskind, M.; Grimwood, K & Veith, RC. (1999). Enhancement of Alzheimer disease with insulin and somatostatin, but not glucose. Arch Gen Psychiatry 56:1135-40.

Craft, S.; Asthana, S.; Cook, DG.; Baker, LD.; Cherrier, K.; Purgan, K.; Wait, C.; Petrova, A.; Latendresse, S.; Watson, GS.; Newcomer, JW.; Schelleenberg, GD & Kreohn, AJ. (2003). Insulin dose-response effects on memory and plasma amyloid precursor protein in Alzheimer's disease: interaction's with Apolipoprotein E genotype. *Psychoneuroendocrinology* 28:809-22.

Den Heijer, T.; Vermeer, SE.; Van Dijk, EJ.; Prins, ND.; Koudstaal, PJ.; Hofman, A & Breteler, MM. (2003). Type 2 diabetes and atrophy of medial temporal lobe structures on brain MRI, *Diabetologia* 46:1604-10.

Craft, S.; Ashana, G.; Schellenberg, G.; Baker, L.; Cherrier, M.; Boyt, AA.; Martins, RN.; Rakind, M.; Peskind, E. & Plymate, S. (2000). Insulin effects on glucose metabolism, memory and plasma amyloid precursor protein in Alzheimer's disease differ according to apolipoprotein-E-genotype. *Ann NY Acad Sci* 903:222-8.

Messier, C. (2003). Diabetes, Alzheimer's disease and apolipoprotein genotype. *Exp Gerontol.* 38:941-6.

Woods, SC.; Seeley, RJ.; Baskin, DG. & Schwartz, MW. (2003). Insulin and the blood brain barrier. *Curr Pharm Des.* 9:795-800.

Banks, WA. (2004). The source of cerebral insulin. *Eur J Pharmacol.* 490:5-12.

Schechter, R.; Whitmire, J.; Wheet, GS.; Beju, D.; Jackson, KW.; Harlow, R. & Gavin, JR. (1994). Immunohistochemical and in situ hybridization study of an insulin-like substance in fetal neuron cell cultures. Brain Res. 636:9-27.

Devaskar, SU.; Giddings, SJ.; Rajakumar, PA.; Carnaghi, LR.; Menon, RK. & Zahm, DS. (1994). Insulin gene expression and insulin synthesis in mammalian neuronal cells. *J Biol Chem.* 269:8445-54.

Havrankova, J.; Schmechel, D.; Roth, J. & Brownstein, M. (1978). Identification of insulin in rat brain. *Proc Natl Acad Sci USA.* 75:5737-41.

Unger, JW.; Livingston, JN. & Moss, AM. (1991). Insulin receptors in the central nervous system: localization, signaling mechanisms and functional aspects. *Prog Neurobiol.* 36:343-62.

Baskin, DG.; Porte, DJ.; Guest, K. & Dorsa, DM. (1983). Regional concentrations of insulin in the rat brain. *Endocrinology.* 112:898-903.

Johnston, AM.; Pirola, L. & Van Obberghen, E. (2003). Molecular mechanisms of insulin receptor substrate protein-mediated modulation of insulin signaling. *FEBS Lett.* 546:32-6.

Kahn, CR.; Bird, KI.; Jarrett, DB. & Flier, JS. (1978). Direct demonstration that receptor cross-linking or aggregation is important in insulin action. *Proc Natl Acad Sci USA.* 75:4209-13.

Sun, XJ.; Rothenberg, P.; Kahn, CR.; Backer, JM.; Araki, E.; Wilden, PA.; Cahill, DA. Goldstein, BJ & White, MF. (1978). Structure of insulin receptor substrate IRS-1 defines a unique signal transduction protein. *Nature* 352:73-7.

Giovannone, B.; Scaldaferri, ML.; Federici, M.; Porzio, O.; Lauro, D.; Fusco, A.; Sbraccia, P.; Borboni, P.; Lauro, R. & Sesti, G. (2000). Insulin receptor substrate (IRS) transduction system: distinct and overlapping signaling potential. *Diabetes Metab Res Rev* 16:434-41

Messier, C. & Teutenberg, K. (2005). The role of insulin, insulin growth factor, and insulin-degrading enzyme in brain aging and Alzheimer's disease. *Neural Plast.* 12:311-28.

Banks, WA.; Jaspan, JB.; Huang, W. & Kastin, AJ. (1997). Transport of insulin across the blood-brain barrier to insulin: saturability at euglycemic doses of insulin. *Peptides.* 1997; 18: 1423-9.

Tchilian, EZ.; Zhelezarov, IE.; Patkov, VV. & Hadjiivanova, CI. (1990). 125I-insulin binding is decreased in olfactory bulbs of aged rats. *Neuropeptides.* 17:193-6.

Adem, A.; Jossan, SS.; D'Argy, R.; Gillberg, PG.; Nordberg, A.; Winblan, B. & Sara, V. (1989). Insulin-like growth factor 1 IGF-1 receptors in the human brain: quantitative autoradiographic localization. *Brain Res.* 503:299-303.

Chung, YH.; Shin, GM.; Joo, KM & Cha, CI. (2002). Region specific alterations in insulin-like growth factor receptor type I in the cerebral cortex and hippocampus of aged rats. *Brain Res* 946:307-13.

Frolic, L.; Blum-Degen, D.; Berstein, HG.; Engelsberger, S.; Humrich, J.; Laufer, S.; Muschner, D.; Thalheimer, A.; Türk, A.; Hoyer, S.; Zöchling, R.; Boissl, KW.; Jellinger, K & Riederer, P. (1998). Brain insulin and insulin receptors in aging and sporadic Alzheimer s disease. *J Neural Transm* 105:423-38.

Banks, WA. & Kastin, AJ. (1985). Peptides and the blood-brain barrier: lipophilicity as a predictor of permeability. *Brain Res Bull.* 15:287-92.

King, GL. & Johnson, SM. (1987). Receptor-mediated transport of insulin across endothelial cells. *Science.* 227:1583-6.

Jialal, I.; King, GL.; Buchwald.; S, Kahn, CR. & Crettaz, M. (1984). Processing of insulin by bovine endothelial cells in culture. Internalization without degradation. *Diabetes.* 33:794-800.

Rotwein, P.; Burgess, SK.; Milbrandt, JD. & Krause, JE. (1988). Differential expression of insulin-like growth factor geneses in rat central nervous system. *Proc Natl Acad Sci USA.* 85:265-9.

Zhao, M.; Cribbs, DH.; Anderson, AJ.; Cummings, BJ.; Su, JH.; Wasserman, AT. & Cotman, CW. (2003). The induction of the TNF alpha death domain signaling pathway in Alzheimer's disease brain. *Neurochem Res* 28:307-18.

Baskin, DG.; Stein, LJ.; Iked, H.; Woods, SC.; Porte, DJ & Dorsa, DM. (2005). Genetically obese Zucker rats have abnormality low brain insulin content. *Life Sci* 36:627-33

Moloney, AM.; Griffin, RJ.; Timmons, S.; O'Connor, R.; Ravid, R. & O'Neill, C. (2010). Defects in IGF-1 receptor, insulin receptor and IRS-1/2 in Alzheimer's disease indicate possible resistance to IGF-1 and insulin signaling. *Neurobiol Aging* 31(2):224-43.

Messier, C & White, NM. (1987). Memory improvement by glucose, fruttose, and two glucose analogs: a possible effect peripheral glucose transport. *Behav Neural Biol* 48:104-27.

Craft, S. (2007). Insulin resistance and Alzheimer's disease. Pathogenesis: potential mechanisms and implications for treatment. *Curr Alzheimer Res.* 4(2):147-52.

Squire, LR. (1986). Mechanisms of memory. *Science.* 232:1612-9.

Svensson, J.; Diez, M.; Engel, J.; Wass, C.; Tivesten, A.; Jansson, JO.; Isaksson, O.; Archer, T.; Hökfelt, T & Ohlsson, C. (2006). Endocrine, liver-derived IGF-1 is of importance for spatial learning and memory in old mice. *J. Endocrinol* 189:617-27.

Dik, MG.; Pluijm, SM.; Jonker, C.; Deeg, DJ.; Lomrcky, MZ & Lips, P. (2003). Insulin-like growth factor-1 (IGF-1) and cognitive decline in older persons. *Neurobiol Aging* 24:573-81.

Hoyer, S. (2000). Brain glucose and energy metabolism abnormalities in sporadic Alzheimer's disease. Causes and consequences: an update. *Exp Gerontol.* 35:1363-72.

Blass, JP.; Gibson, GF. & Hoyer, S. (2002). The role of the metabolic lesion in Alzheimer's disease. *J Alzheimer Dis.* 4:225-32. .

Beeri, MS.; Schmeidler, J.; Silverman, JM.; Gandy, S.; Wysocki, M.; Hannigan, CM.; Purohit, DP.; Lesser, G.; Grossman, HT & Haroutunian, V. (2008). Insulin in combination with other diabetes medication is associated with less Alzheimer neuropathology. *Neurology* 71:750-7.

Craft, S.; Peskind, E.; Schellenberg, G.; Cherrier, M.; Baker, LD.; Newcomer, J.; Plymate, S.; Latendresse, S.; Petrova, A.; Raskind, M.; Peskind, E.; Lofgreen, C. & Grimwood, K. (1999). Cerebrospinal fluid and plasma insulin levels in Alzheimer's disease differs according to apolipoprotein E genotype and gender. *Neuroendocrinology.* 70:146-52.

Adamo, M.; Raizada, MK. & LeRoith, D. (1989). Insulin and insulin growth factors receptors in the nervous system. *Mol Neurobiol.* 3:71-100.

Squire, LR. (1992). Memory and the hippocampus: a synthesis of findings with rats, monkeys, and humans. *Psychol Rev.* 99:195-231.

Hoyer, S.; Henneberg, N.; Knapp, S.; Lannert, H. & Martin, E. (1996). Brain glucose metabolism is controlled by amplification and desensitization of the neuronal insulin receptor. *Ann NY Acad Sci.* 777:374-9.

Messier, C. & Destrade, C. (1994). Insulin attenuates scopolamine-induced memory deficits. *Psychobiology.* 22:16-21.

Skeberdis, VA.; Lan, J.; Zheng, X.; Zukin, RS. & Bennett, MV (2001). Insulin promotes rapid delivery of N-methyl-D-aspartate receptors to the cell surface by exocytosis. *Proc Natl Acad Sci USA.* 98:3561–6.

De Felice, FG.; Vieira, MN.; Bomfirm, TR.; Decker, H.; Velasco, PT.; Lambert, MP.; Viola, KL.; Zhao, WQ.; Ferreira, ST. & Klein WL. (2009). Protection of synapses against Alzheimer's linked toxins: insulin signaling prevents the pathogenic binding of A-beta oligomers. *Proc Natl Acad Sci.* USA 106:1971-6.

De la Monte, SM.; Tong, M.; Lester-Coll, N.; Plater M, Jr.; & Wands, JR. (2006). Therapeutic rescue of neurodegeneration experimental type-3 diabetes: relevance to Alzheimer's disease. *J Alzheimers Dis.* 10:89-109.

Hirai, K.; Aliev, G.; Nunomura, A.; Fujioka, H.; Russell, RL.; Atwood, CS.; Johnson, AB.; Kress, Y.; Vinters, HV.; Tabaton, M.; Shimohama, S.; Cash, AD.; Siedlak, SL.; Harris, PL.; Jones, PK.; Petersen, RB.; Perry, G & Smith, MA. (2001). Mitochondrial abnormalities in Alzheimer's disease. *J Neurosci* 21:3017-23.

Gouras, GK.; Almeida, CG. & Takahashi, RH. (2005). Intraneuronal Abeta accumulation and origin of plaques in Alzheimer's disease. *Neurobiol Aging.* 26:1235-44.

Caspersen, C.; Wang, N.; Yao, J.; Sosunov, A.; Chen, X.; Lustbader, JW.; Xu, HW.; Stern, D.; McKhann, G & Yan, SD. (2005). Mitochondrial Abeta: a potential focal point for neuronal metabolic dysfunction in Alzheimer's disease. *FASEB J.* 19:2040-1.

Smith, MA.; Perry, G.; Richey, PL.; Sayre, LM.; Anderson, VE.; Beal, MF. & Kowall, N. (1996). Oxidative damage in Alzheimer's disease. *Nature* 382: 120-1.

Smith, MA.; Richey Harris, PL.; Sayre, LM.; Beckman, JS. & Perry, G. (1997). Widespread peroxynitrite-mediated damage Alzheimer's disease. *J Neurosci.* 17:2653-7.

Mark, RJ.; Pang, Z.; Geddes, JW.; Uchida, K. & Mattson, MP. (1997). Amyloid-beta peptide impairs glucose transport in hippocampal and cortical neurons: involvement lipid peroxidation. *J Neurosci* 17:1046-54.

Nunomura, A., Perry, G.; Aliev, G.; Hirai, K.; Takeda, A.; Balraj, EK.; Jones, PK.; Ghanbari, H.; Wataya, T.; Shimohama.; S.; Chiba, S.; Atwood, CS.; Petersen, RB. & Smith, MA. (2001). Oxidative damage is the earliest event in Alzheimer's disease. *J Neuropahol Exp Neurol* 60:759-67.

Cho, DH.; Nakamura, T.; Fang, J.; Cieplak, P.; Godzik, A.; Gu, Z. & Lipton, SA. (2009). S-nitrosylation of Drp 1 mediates beta-amyloid-related mithocondrial fissation and neuronal injury. *Science.* 324:102-5.

Yan, SD.; Chen, M.; Zhu, H.; Roher, A.; Slattery, T.; Zhao, L.; Nagashima, M.; Morser, J.; Migheli, A. Nawroth P, Stern, D. & Schmidt, AM. (1996). RAGE and amyloid-beta peptide neurotoxicity in Alzheimer's disease. *Nature* 382:685-91.

Lue, LF.; Walker, DG.; Jacobson, S. & Sabbagh, M. (2009). Receptor for advanced glycation end products: its role in Alzheimer's disease and other neurological diseases. *Future Neurol.* 4:167–77.

Cho, HJ.; Son, SM.; Jin, SM.; Hong, HS.; Shin, DH.; Kim, SJ.; Huh, K. & Mook-Jung, I. (2009). RAGE regulates BACE1 and A-beta generation via NFAT1 activation in Alzheimer's disease animal model. *FASEB J* 23:2639–49.

Martin, SJ.; Grimwood, PD. & Morris, RG. (2000). Synaptic plasticity and memory: an evaluation of the hypothesis. *Annu Rev Neurosci.* 23:649-711.

Ding, Q. & Keller, JN. (2005). Splice variants of the receptor for advanced glycosylation end products (RAGE) in human brain. *Neurosci Lett.* 373:67–72.

Raucci, A.; Cugusi, S.; Antonelli, A.; Barabino, SM.; Monti, L.; Bierhaus, A.; Reiss, K.; Saftig, P. & Bianchi, ME. (2008). A soluble form of the receptor for advanced glycation endproducts (RAGE) is produced by proteolytic cleavage of the membrane-bound form by the sheddase a disintegrin and metalloprotease 10 (ADAM10). *FASEB J.* 22:3716–27.

Lue, LF.; Walker, DG.; Brachova, L.; , Beach, TG.; Rogers, J.; Schmidt, AM.; Stern, DM. & Yan, SD. (2001). Involvement of microglial receptor for advanced glycation endproducts (RAGE) in Alzheimer's disease: identification of a cellular activation mechanism. *Exp Neurol.* 171:29–45.

Deane, R.; Du Yan, S.; Submamaryan, RK.; LaRue, B.; Jovanovic, S.; Hogg, E.; Welch, D.; Manness, L.; Lin, C.; Yu, J.; Zhu, H.; Ghiso, J.; Frangione, B.; Stern, A.; Schmidt, AM.; Armstrong, DL.; Arnold, B.; Liliensiek, B.; Nawroth, P.; Hofman, F.; Kindy, M.; Stern, D. & Zlokovic, B..(2003). RAGE mediates amyloid-beta peptide transport across the blood–brain barrier and accumulation in brain. *Nat Med.* 9:907–13.

Emanuele, E.; D'angelo, A.; Tomaino, C.; Binetti, G.; Ghidoni, R.; Politi, P.; Bernardi, L.; Maletta, R.; Bruni, AC. & Geroldi, D. (2005). Circulating levels of soluble receptor for advanced glycation end products in Alzheimer disease and vascular dementia. *Arch Neurol.* 62: 1734–6.

Lee, VM.; Goedert, M. & Trojanowski, JQ. (2001). Neurodegenerative tauopathies. *Ann Rev Neurosci.* 24:1121-59.

Iqbal, K.; Alonso Adel, C.; Chen, S.; Chohan, MO.; El-Akkad, E.; Gong, CX.; Khatoon, S.; Li, B.; Liu, F.; Rahman, A.; Tanimukai, H. & Grundke-Iqbal, I. (2005).Tau pathology in Alzheimer's disease and other tauopathies. *Biochim Biophys Acta* 1793:198-210.

Delacourte, A.; Sergeant, N.; Champain, D.; Wattez, A.; Maurage, CA.; Lebert, F.; Pasquier, F. & David, JP. (2002). Nonoverlapping but synergetic tau and APP pathologies in sporadic Alzheimer's disease. *Neurology* 59:398-407.

Glenner, GG. & Wong, CW. (1984). Alzheimer disease: initial report of the purification and characterization of a novel cerebrovascular amyloid protein. *Biochem Biophys Res Commun* 120:885-90.

Flaherty, DB.; Soria, JP.; Tomasiewicz, HZ. & Wood, JG. (2000). Phosphorylation of human tau protein by microtubule associated kinases: GSK3β and cdk5 are key partecipants. *J Neurosci Res* 62:463-72.

Stoothoff, WH. & Johnson, GV. (2005). Tau phosphorylation: physiological and pathological consequences. *Biochim Biophys Acta* 1739:280-97.

Millward, TA.; Zolnierowicz, S. & Hemmings, BA. (1999). Regulation of protein kinase cascades by protein phosphatase 2A. *Trends Biochem Sci.* 24:186-91.

Doble, BW. & Woodgett, JR. (2003). GSK-3β: tricks of the trade for a multi-tasking kinase. *J Cell Sci* 116:1175-86.

Avila J. (2008). Tau kinases, phosphatases. *J Cell Mol Med.* 12:258-9.

Liu, R.; Zhou, XW.; Tanila, H.; Bjorkdahl, C., Wang, JZ.; Guan, ZZ.; Cao, Y.; Gustafsson, JA.; Winblad, B. & Pei, JJ. (2008). Phosphorylated PP2A (tyrosine 307) is associated with Alzheimer neurofibrillary pathology. *J Cell Mol Med* 12:241-57.

Hong, M. & Leev, VM. (1997). Insulin and insulin-like growth factor-1 regulate tau phosphorylation in cultured human neurons. *J. Biol. Chem* 272:19547-53.

Meske, V.; Albert, F. & Ohm, TG. (2008). Coupling of mammalian target of rapamyein with phosphoinositide 3-kinase signaling pathway regulates protein phospatase 2A and glycogen synthase kinase-3-dependent phosphorylation of tau. *J. Biol Chem* 283:100-9.

Cheng, CM.; Tseng, V.; Wang, J.; Wang, D.; Matyakhina, L. & Bondy, CA. (2005). Tau is hyperphosporylated in the insulin-like growth factor-I null brain. *Endocrinology* 146:5086-91.

Schubert, M.; Brazil, DP.; Burks, DJ.; Kushner, JA.; Ye, J.; Flint, CL.; Farhang-Fallah, J.; Dikkes, P.; Warot, XM.; Rio, C.; Corfas, G. & White, MF. (2003). Insulin receptor substrate-2 deficiency impairs brain growth and promotes tau phosporylation. *J Neurosc.* 23:7084-92.

Planel, E.; Tatebayashi, Y.; Miyasaka, T.; Liu, L.; Wang, L.; Herman, M.; Yu, WH.; Luchsinger, JA.; Wadzinski, B.; Duff, KE. & Takashima, A. (1997).Insulin dysfunction induces in vivo tau after hyperphosphorylation through distinct mechanisms. *J Neurosci* 27:13635-48.

Kolch, W. (2000). Meaningful relationships: the regulation of the RAS/RAF/MEK/ERK pathway by protein interactions. *Biochem J* 351: 289-305.

Sweatt, JD. (2001). The neuronal MAP kinase cascade: a biochemical signal integration system subserving synaptic plasticity and memory. *J Neurochem* 76:1-10

Zhuang, S. & Schnellmann, RG. (2006). A death-promoting role for extracellular signal-regulated kinase. *J Pharmacol Exp Ther* 319:991-7.

Lesort, M & Johnson, GV. (2000). Insulin-like growth factor-1 and insulin mediate transient site-selective increases in tau phosphorylation in primary cortical neurons. *Neuroscience.* 99:305–16.

Kang, J.; Lemaire, HG.; Unterbeck, A.; Salbaum, JM.; Masters, CL.; Grzeschik, KH.; Multhaup, G.; Beyreuther, K. & Müller-Hill, B. (1987). The precursor of Alzheimer-s disease amyloid A_4 protein resembles a cell-surface receptor. *Nature* 325:733-6.

Zhang, Y.; Thompson, R.; Zhang, H. & Xu, U. (2011). APP processing in Alzheimer's disease. *Mol Brain.* 4: 3.

Kimberly, WT.; LaVoie, MJ.; Ostaszewski, BL; Ye, W.; Wolfe, MS. & Selkoe DJ. (2003). Gamma-secretase is a membrane protein complex comprised of presenilin, nicastrin, Aph-1 and Pen-2. *Proc Natl Acad Sci* USA. 100: 6382-7.

Vassar, R.; Bennett, BD.; Babu-Kahn, S.; Kahn, S.; Mendiaz, EA.; Denis, P.; Teplow, DB.; Ross, S.; Amarante, P.; Loeloff, R.; Luo, Y.; Fisher, S.; Fuller, J.; Edenson, S.; Lile, J.; Jarosinski, MA.; Biere, AL.; Curran, E.; Burgess, T.; Louis, JC.; Collins, F.; Treanor, J.; Rogers, G. & Citron, M. (1999). Beta-secretase cleavage of Alzheimer's amyloid precursor protein by the transmembrane aspartic protease BACE. *Science.* 286:735-41.

Holsinger, RM.; McLean, CA.; Beyreuther, K.; Masters, CL, & Evin, G (2002). Increased expression of the amyloid precursor beta-secretase in Alzheimer's disease. *Ann Neurol.* 51:783-6.

Costantini, C.; Scrable, H. & Puglielli, L. (2006). An aging pathway controls the TrkA to p75NTR receptor switch and amyloid beta-peptide generation. *EMBO J* 25:1997-2006.

Puglielli, L. (2008). Aging of the brain, neurotrophic signaling, and Alzheimer's disease: is IGF-1R the common culprit? *Neurobiol Aging.* 29:795-811.

Puglielli, L.; Ellis, BC.; Saunders, AJ. & Kovacs, DM. (2003). Ceramide stabilizes beta-size amyloid precursor protein-cleaving enzyme I and promotes amyloid beta-peptide biogenesic. *J Biol Chem.* 278:19777-83.

Kayed, RH.; Thompson. JL.; MC Intire, TM.; Milton, SC.; Cotman, CW. & Glabe, CG. (2003). Common structure of soluble amyloid oligomers implies common mechanism of pathogenesis. *Science* 300:486-9.

Hass, C. & Sedkoe, DJ. (2007). Soluble protein oligomers in neuro-degeneration: lessons from the Alzheimer's amyloid beta-peptide. *Nat Rev Mol Cell Bio.* 8:101-2.

Kamenetz, F.; Tomita, T.; Hsieh, H.; Seabrook, G.; Borchelt, D.; Iwatsubo, T.; Sisodia, S. & Malinow, R. (2003). APP Processing and synaptic function. *Neuron.* 37:925-37.

Tanzi, RE.; Moir, RD. & Wagner, SL. (2005). Twenty years of the Alzheimer disease amyloid hypothesis: a genetic perspective. *Cell.* 120:545-55.

Selkoe, DJ. (1999). Translating cell biology in to therapeutic advances in Alzheimer's disease. *Nature.* 399:23-31.

Cheng, S.; Li, L.; He, S.; Liu, J.; Sun, Y.; He, M.; Grasing, K.; Premont, RT. & Suo, WZ. (2010). GRK5 deficiency accelerates ß-amyloid accumulation in Tg2576 mice via impaired cholinergic activity. J Biol Chem. 285:41541-8.

Carro, E.; Trejo, JL.; Spuch, C.; Heard, JM. & Torres-Aleman, I. (2006). Blockade of the insulin-like growth factor I receptor in the choroid plexus originates Alzheimer's like neuropathology in rodents; new cues into the human disease? *Neurobiol Aging* 27:1618-31.

Suh, Y.; Atzomon, G.; Cho, Mo.; Hwang, D.; Liu, B.; Leahy, DJ.; Barzilai, N. & Cohen, P. (2008). Functionally significant insulin-like growth factor I receptor mutations in centenarians. Proc Natl Acad Sci USA. 105:3438-42.

Ho, L.; Qin, W.; Pompl, PN.; Xiang, Z; Wang, J.; Zhao, Z.; Peng, Y.; Cambareri, G.; Rocher, A.; Mobbs, CV.; Hof, PR. & Pasinetti, GM. (2004). Diet-induced insulin resistance promotes amyloidosis in a transgenic mouse model of Alzheimer's disease. *FASEB J* 18:902-4.

Cao, D.; Lu, H.; Lewis, TI. & Li, L. (2007). Intake of sucrose-sweetened water induced insulin resistance and exacerbates memory deficits and amyloidosis in a transgenic mouse model of Alzheimer disease. J Biol Chem. 282:36275-82.

Freude, S.; Plum, L.; Schnitker, J.; Leeser, U.; Udelhoven, M.; Krone, W.; Bruning, JC. & Schubert, M. (2005). Peripheral hyperinsulinemia promotes tau phosphorylation in vivo. *Diabetes* 54:3343-8.

Takeda, S.; Sato, N.; Uchio-Yamada, K.; Sawada, K.; Kunieda, T.; Takeuchi, D.; Kurinami, H.; Shinohara, M.; Rakugi, H. & Morishita, R. (2010). Diabetes accelerated memory dysfunction via cerebrovascular inflammation Aβ deposition in Alzheimer mouse model with diabetes. Proc Natl Acad Sci USA 107:7036-41

Montine, TJ.; Kaye, JA.; Montine, KS.; McFarland, L.; Morrow, JD. & Quinn, JF. (2001). Cerebrospinal fluid abeta-42, tau, and f2-isoprostane concentrations in patients with Alzheimer disease, other dementias, and age-matched controls. *Arch Pathol Lab Med* 125:510-2.

Sheng, JG.; Bora, SH.; Xu, G.; Borchelt, DR.; Price, DL. & Koliatsos, VE. (2003). Lipopolysaccharide-induced-neuroinflammation increase intracellular accumulation of amyloid precursor protein and amyloid beta peptide in APPswe transgenic mice. *Neurobiol Dis* 14:133-45.

Dandona, P. (2002). Endothelium, inflammation and diabetes *Curr Diab Rep.* 2:311-5.

Krogh-Madsen, R.; Plomgaard, P.; Keller, P.; Keller, C. & Pedersen BK. (2004). Insulin stimulates interlukin-6 and tumor necrosis factor-alpha gene expression in human subcutaneous adipose tissue. *Am J Physiol Endocrinol Metab* 286:234-8.

Soop, M.; Duxubury, H.; Agwunobi, AO.; Gibson, JM.; Hopkins, SJ.; Childs, C.; Cooper, RG.; Maycock, P.; Little, RA. & Carlson, GL. (2002). Euglycemic hyperinsulinemia augments the cytokine and endocrine responses in endotoxin in humans. *Am J Physiol Endocrinol Metab* 282:1276-85.

Zhao, M.; Cribbs, DH.; Anderson, AJ.; Cummings, BJ.; Su, JH.; Wasserman, AT. & Cotman, CW. (2003). The induction of the TNF alpha death domain signaling pathway in Alzheimer's disease brain. *Neurochem Res* 28:307-18.

Dzienis-Straczkowski, M.; Szelachowska, M.; Stepien, A.; Kowalska, I. & Kinalska, I. (2003). Soluble tumor necrosis factor-alpha receptors in young obese subjects with normal and impaired glucose tolerance. *Diabetes Care* 26:875-80.

Bastard, JP.; Jardel, C.; Bruckert, E.; Vidal, H. & Hainque, B. (2000). Variations in plasma soluble tumor necrosis factor receptors after diet-induced weight loss in obesity. *Diabetes Obes Metab* 2:323-5.

Axelrod, L. (1991). Insulin, prostaglandins, and the pathogenesis of hypertension. *Diabetes.* 40:1223-7.

Facchini, FS.; Hua, NW.; Reaven, GM. & Stoohs, RA. (2000). Hyperinsulinemia: the missing link among oxidative stress and age-related disease? *Free Radic Biol Med* 29:1302-6.

Mrak, RE. & Griffin, WS. (2001). Interleukin-1, neuroinflammation, and Alzheimer's disease. *Neurobiol Aging.* 22:903-8.

White, JA.; Manelli, AM.; Holmberg, KH.; Van Eldik, LJ. & Ladu, MJ. (2005). Differential effects of oligomeric and fibrillar amyloid-beta 1-42 on astrocyte mediated inflammation. *Neurobiol Dis* 18:459-65.

Papassotiropoulos, A.; Hock, C. & Nitsch, RM. (2001). Genetics of interleukin 6: implications for Alzheimer's disease. *Neurobiol Aging.* 22:863-71.

Descamps, O.; Bilheimer, D. & Herz, J. (1993). Insulin stimulates receptor-mediated uptake of Apo E-enriched lipoproteins and activated alpha 2-macroglobulin in adypocytes. *J Biol Chem.* 268:974-81.

Fishel, MA,.; Watson, GS.; Montine, TJ.; Wang, Q.; Green, PS. & Kulstad, JJ. (2005). Hyperinsulinemia provokes synchronous increases in central inflammation and beta-amyloid in normal adults. *Arch Neurol* 62:1539-44.

Yamada, T.; Kondo, A.; Takamatsu, J.; Tateishi, J. & Goto I (1995). Apolipoprotein E mRNA in the brains of patients with Alzheimer's disease. *J Neurol Sci.* 129:56-61.

Figlewicz, DP.; Bentson, K. & Octrant I. (1993). The effect of insulin on norepinephrine uptake by PC12 cells. *Brain Res* 602:161-4.

Heneka, MT.; Galea, E.; Gavriluyk, V.; Dumitrescu-Ozimek, L.; Daeschner, J.; O'Banion, MK.; Weinberg, G.; Klockgether, T. & Feinstein, DL. (2002). Noradrenergic depletion potentiates beta-amyloid-induced cortical inflammation: implications for Alzheimer's disease. *J Neurosci* 22:2434-42.

Bondareff, W.; Mountjoy, CQ.; Roth, M.; Rossor, MN.; Iversen, LL.; Reynolds, GP. & Hauser, DL. Neuronal degeneration in locus ceruleus and cortical correlates of Alzheimer disease. *Alzheimer Dia Assoc Disord* 1987; 1:256-62.

Watson, GS.; Bernhardt, T.; Reger, MA.; Cholerton, BA.; Baker, LD. & Peskind, ER. (2006). Insulin effects on CSF norepinephrine and cognition in Alzheimer's disease. *Neurobiol Aging* 27:38-41.

Bingham, EM.; Hopkins, D.; Smith, D.; Pernet, A.; Hallett, W. & Reed, L. (2002). The role of insulin in human brain glucose metabolism: an 18fluoro-deoxyglucose positron emission tomography study. *Diabetes* 51:3384–90.

Blanchard, JG. & Duncan, PM. (1997). Effect in combinations of insulin, glucose and scopolamine on radial arm maze performance. *Pharmacol Biochem Behav* 58:209–14.

20

Insulin Resistance, Cognitive Impairment and Neurodegeneration: Roles of Nitrosamine Exposure, Diet and Lifestyles

Suzanne de la Monte, Ming Tong and Jack R. Wands
Rhode Island Hospital and the Warren Alpert Medical School of Brown University
USA

1. Introduction

In Western societies, Alzheimer's disease (AD) is epidemic (de la Monte, Neusner et al. 2009). For decades, the prevailing theories about AD pathogenesis focused on the roles of hyper-phosphorylated and ubiquitinated cytoskeletal proteins in neuronal perikarya and dystrophic fibers, and increased expression and abnormal processing of amyloid-beta precursor protein (AβPP), leading to AβPP-Aβ peptide deposition in neurons, plaques, and vessels, as mediators of neuronal loss, neuritic pathology, synaptic disconnection, and loss of plasticity. Apart from aging, which is the most dominant risk factor, it has not been possible to define convincing roles for AβPP-Aβ or phospho-tau accumulations as principal driving forces of neurodegeneration that could account for all of the protean manifestations of AD, including neuro-inflammation, mitochondrial dysfunction, white matter fiber loss, and neurotransmitter deficiencies. This point is particularly relevant with respect to sporadic AD, which accounts for the vast majority of cases. However, it is entirely possible that the focal points of 30+ years of intense research on the accumulation, abnormal processing, and misfolding of essentially two proteins are somewhat misplaced since these process could be the end-result rather than the cause of the pathophysiological processes that trigger and propagate the neurodegeneration cascade.

Growing evidence supports the concept that AD is actually a metabolic disease in which, neurodegeneration is mediated by impairments in brain glucose utilization and energy production that begin early in the course of disease, and worsen with its progression (Frolich, Blum-Degen et al. 1998; Hoyer 2002; Hoyer 2004; Rivera, Goldin et al. 2005; Steen, Terry et al. 2005). AD-associated reductions in glucose utilization and energy metabolism are accompanied by increased oxidative stress and neuro-inflammation, which appear to be driven by insulin and insulin-like growth factor (IGF) resistance in the brain. AD can be regarded as a brain-specific form of diabetes mellitus, i.e. Type 3 diabetes. This chapter reviews the data showing that sporadic AD in humans is associated with progressive impairments in brain insulin and IGF signaling, and contrasts the roles of peripheral insulin resistance disease states versus primary brain insulin/IGF resistance using data from both human and experimental animal studies. Epidemiological and experimental evidence supporting exposures, particularly to environmental toxins such as nitrosamines, rather than only genetic factors as causal in the pathogenesis of AD are discussed. Dietary and lifestyle changes that could reduce risk for developing insulin resistance diseases, including diabetes mellitus, obesity, non-alcoholic steatohepatitis and neurodegeneration, are discussed as public health strategies that must be considered in earnest.

2. Alzheimer's disease and brain glucose metabolism

Metabolic abnormalities in AD have been linked to deficits in brain insulin and insulin-like growth factor (IGF) signaling through pathways that are critical for maintaining neuronal survival, energy production, gene expression, and plasticity (Frolich, Blum-Degen et al. 1998). Thorough consideration of the pleitropic actions of insulin and IGFs helps to clarify how impairments in these signal transduction networks could account for many, if not all of the critical features of AD-type neurodegeneration, including increased: 1) activity of kinases that aberrantly phosphorylate tau; 2) expression of AβPP and accumulation of AβPP-Aβ; 3) oxidative and endoplasmic reticulum (ER) stress; 4) the generation of reactive oxygen and reactive nitrogen species that damage proteins, RNA, DNA, and lipids; 5) mitochondrial dysfunction; and 6) activation of pro-inflammatory and pro-death cascades. Moreover, impairment or inhibition of insulin/IGF signaling disrupts cholinergic homeostasis, thereby compromising one of the most important neurotransmitter systems utilized for neuronal plasticity, memory, and cognition.

3. Brain insulin and insulin-like growth factor problems in AD

The concept that AD could represent a metabolic disease stemmed from the findings that deficits in cerebral glucose utilization are detectable in the early stages of disease (Adolfsson, Bucht et al. 1980; Fujisawa, Sasaki et al. 1991; Caselli, Chen et al. 2008; Mosconi, Pupi et al. 2008; Mosconi, Mistur et al. 2009; Langbaum, Chen et al. 2010), and as AD progresses, so do the metabolic abnormalities (Hoyer and Nitsch 1989; Hoyer, Nitsch et al. 1991). Although several studies provided initial clues that insulin resistance could be an important feature of AD (Frolich, Blum-Degen et al. 1998; Hoyer 2002; Hoyer 2004), the human postmortem brain studies were critical for definitively establishing that both insulin resistance and insulin deficiency in the brain were consistent and fundamental abnormalities in AD (Rivera, Goldin et al. 2005; Steen, Terry et al. 2005). Gene expression and receptor binding studies showed that in AD, brain insulin gene expression, insulin levels, insulin receptor levels, and insulin receptor binding were all impaired. Insulin resistance is manifested by reduced levels of insulin receptor binding and decreased responsiveness to insulin/IGF stimulation, while the trophic factor deficiency is associated with reduced levels of insulin polypeptide and gene expression in brain and cerebrospinal fluid (Blum-Degen, Frolich et al. 1995; Blass, Gibson et al. 2002; Hoyer 2004; Hoyer 2004; Rivera, Goldin et al. 2005; Steen, Terry et al. 2005). To consolidate these concepts, we proposed that AD be referred to as, "Type 3 diabetes" because it represents the conglomerate effects of Type 1 (insulin deficiency) and Type 2 (insulin resistance) diabetes, whereby the consequential metabolic abnormalities are largely restricted to the brain (Rivera, Goldin et al. 2005; Steen, Terry et al. 2005).

It has been well-established that insulin signaling mechanisms parallel, interact, or cross-talk with related insulin-like growth factor (IGF) pathways in various organ-systems, including the brain (de la Monte and Wands 2005). Despite apparent redundancy, insulin, IGF-1 and IGF-2 stimulations have differential effects on various target cells in the brain, and at different stages of development, maturation, and aging (de la Monte and Wands 2005). Ordinarily, insulin and IGF signaling networks overlap and complement one another, enabling deficits in one pathway to be compensated for by increased activation of one or both of the others, and thereby provide a kind of safety net for supporting critical neuronal and glial functions in the brain. Therefore, with regard to neurodegenerative diseases, it was of interest to determine if the impairments in insulin signaling networks in AD were selective, or whether they broadly affected IGF pathways as well.

The human postmortem studies demonstrated that, like insulin, AD is associated with significant impairments in IGF-1 and IGF-2 signaling mechanisms in the brain, and that as dementia progresses, so do the deficits in IGF signaling networks (Rivera, Goldin et al. 2005; Steen, Terry et al. 2005). AD-associated deficits in IGF signaling are marked by reduced expression of IGF trophic factors and receptors, and decreased binding to IGF receptors, reflecting IGF deficiency and resistance. Since the impairments in IGF signaling mechanisms develop and progress simultaneously with declines in insulin signaling, the scaffolding needed to support a broad range of functions, including cerebral glucose utilization, neuronal survival, myelin maintenance, metabolism, neurotransmitter function, and plasticity gets destroyed, practically en masse. Consequences include reductions in the expression of choline acetyltransferase, tau, and glyceraldehyde-3-phosphate dehydrogenase (GAPDH) genes, which mediate cholinergic/cognitive, neuronal cytoskeletal, and metabolic functions (Rivera, Goldin et al. 2005). Insulin/IGF resistance-mediated impairments in energy metabolism promote oxidative stress, accumulation of reactive oxygen species (ROS), DNA damage, and mitochondrial dysfunction, all of which drive pro-apoptosis, pro-inflammatory, and pro-AβPP-Aβ cascades.

4. Impaired insulin/IGF signaling and tau pathology in AD

Neuronal cytoskeletal lesions that correlate with severity of dementia in AD include, neurofibrillary tangles, dystrophic neurites, and neuropil threads, which contain aggregated and ubiquitinated insoluble fibrillar tau (Duyckaerts, Delatour et al. 2009; Takashima 2009). In AD, hyperphosphorylation of tau, a microtubule-associated protein, is mediated by inappropriate activation of kinases, such as glycogen synthase kinase 3β (GSK-3β). Hyper-phosphorylated tau is rendered highly susceptible to misfolding and self-aggregating into insoluble fibrils, generating dementia-associated cytoskeletal lesions (Iqbal, Liu et al. 2009). These degenerative processes lead to disruption of the neuronal cytoskeletal network and synaptic disconnection (Iqbal, Liu et al. 2009). In addition, pre-fibrillar tau aggregates to form soluble oligomers that are neurotoxic and can cause synaptic disconnection and neuronal death (Takashima 2010). Ubiquitination of hyper-phosphorylated tau (Arnaud, Robakis et al. 2006), along with dysfunction of the ubiquitin-proteasome system (Oddo 2008), result in further accumulation of insoluble fibrillar tau, oxidative stress, ROS generation, and cell loss in AD (Mandelkow, Stamer et al. 2003).

Brain insulin/IGF resistances contribute to the development and accumulation of dementia-associated neuronal cytoskeletal lesions (de la Monte, Ganju et al. 2000; de la Monte, Neely et al. 2001; de la Monte and Wands 2002; Xu, Eun Yeon et al. 2003) because tau gene expression and phosphorylation are regulated by insulin and IGF (Schubert, Brazil et al. 2003; Schubert, Gautam et al. 2004), and brain insulin and IGF resistances decrease signaling through phosphoinositol-3-kinase (PI3K), Akt (Schubert, Brazil et al. 2003; Schubert, Gautam et al. 2004), and Wnt/β-catenin (Doble and Woodgett 2003), which result in increased activation of GSK-3β (Nishimura, Yu et al. 1999; De Ferrari and Inestrosa 2000; Fraser, Yu et al. 2001; Mudher, Chapman et al. 2001; Grilli, Ferrari Toninelli et al. 2003). In addition, tau hyper-phosphorylation in AD is mediated by inhibition of protein phosphatases 1 and 2A (Hanger, Seereeram et al. 2009; Iqbal, Liu et al. 2009; Morales, Farias et al. 2010), which are regulated by insulin/IGF. Besides hyper-phosphorylation, tau pathology in AD is mediated by impaired tau gene expression due to reduced insulin and IGF signaling (de la Monte, Chen et al. 2003). Consequences include failure to generate sufficient amounts of normal soluble tau protein, vis-a-vis accumulation of hyper-phosphorylated insoluble fibillar tau, and attendant exacerbation of cytoskeletal collapse, neurite retraction, and synaptic disconnection.

5. Insulin/IGF resistance and amyloid-beta (Aβ) accumulation and neurodegeneration

Dysregulated expression and processing of amyloid precursor protein (AβPP) results in accumulation of neurotoxic AβPP-Aβ (Aβ) oligomeric fibrils and insoluble aggregated fibrils (plaques) in the brain. These lesions arise secondary to increased AβPP gene expression and abnormal AβPP proteolysis, leading to the generation of 40 or 42 amino acid length Aβ peptides that can aggregate. In sporadic AD, which accounts for 90% or more of the cases, the causes of Aβ accumulation and toxicity are not known, but over the past few years, the role of impaired insulin/IGF signaling has come into consideration. One argument is that Aβ toxicity causes insulin resistance. The opposing argument is that brain insulin resistance with attendant oxidative stress and neuro-inflammation, promotes Aβ accumulation and toxicity. The findings that insulin stimulation promotes trafficking of Aβ from the trans-Golgi network to the plasma membrane, stimulates Aβ secretion (Watson, Peskind et al. 2003), and inhibits Aβ intracellular accumulation (Gasparini, Gouras et al. 2001; Gasparini, Netzer et al. 2002) support the latter position. Moreover, experimental data indicate that impaired insulin signaling disrupts the processing of AβPP and clearance of Aβ (Messier and Teutenberg 2005), which again supports a causal role for brain insulin resistance. On the other hand, it is important to recognize that AD, and all other neurodegenerative diseases represent the effects of cascades that cause diseases to progress over time. Therefore, it is essential that we understand both initiating and propagating factors in disease because treatments can be preventive or interventional. The findings that: 1) Aβ disrupts insulin signaling by competing with insulin, or reducing the affinity of insulin binding to its own receptor (Ling, Martins et al. 2002; Xie, Helmerhorst et al. 2002); 2) AβPP oligomers inhibit neuronal transmission of insulin-stimulated signals by desensitizing insulin receptors; and 3) intracellular AβPP-Aβ interferes with PI3 kinase activation of Akt-mediated survival signaling and increases GSK-3β activation (promoting tau hyper-phosphorylation), suggest that dysregulation of AβPP expression and processing can exacerbate insulin resistance.

6. Insulin/IGF resistance, oxidative stress, and metabolic dysfunction in AD

Deficits in cerebral glucose utilization and energy metabolism occur very early in the course of AD (Iwangoff, Armbruster et al. 1980; Sims, Bowen et al. 1980; Hoyer 2004). Glucose uptake and utilization in brain are dependent upon glucose transport by glucose transporter 4 (GLUT4), which is stimulated by insulin. Therefore, impairments in brain insulin responsiveness could account for the deficits in brain glucose utilization and energy metabolism in AD. Deficiencies in energy metabolism correlate with the increased levels of oxidative stress, mitochondrial dysfunction, and pro-inflammatory cytokine activation in AD brains (Hoyer and Lannert 1999; Hoyer, Lee et al. 2000; de la Monte and Wands 2002). Oxidative stress leads to increased generation and accumulation of reactive oxygen (ROS) and reactive nitrogen species (RNS) that attack subcellular organelles, yielding DNA, RNA, lipid, and protein adducts that further compromise the structural and functional integrity of neurons. Consequences include disruption of the neuronal cytoskeleton, synaptic disconnection, neurotransmitter deficits, impaired neuronal plasticity, and reduced neuronal survival.

Mitochondrial dysfunction reduces ATP production, increases ROS, and triggers neuro-inflammatory responses through the activation of microglia and astrocytes. This cascade is propagated by neuro-inflammation inhibiting insulin/IGF signaling, and increasing stress, organelle dysfunction, pro-apoptosis signaling, AβPP expression, and aberrant AβPP cleavage with AβPP-Aβ deposition and toxic fibril formation (Lorenzo and Yankner 1996; Niikura, Hashimoto et al. 2002; Chen, Xu et al. 2003; Tsukamoto, Hashimoto et al. 2003; Blasko, Stampfer-Kountchev et al. 2004; Eikelenboom and van Gool 2004; Tuppo and Arias 2005). Persistence of oxidative stress leads to constitutive activation of kinases e.g. GSK-3β, that promote hyper-phosphorylation of tau. Therefore, oxidative stress and energy imbalances stemming from brain insulin/IGF resistance contribute to the cascade of neuronal loss, AβPP toxicity, tau cytoskeletal pathology, and neuro-inflammation (de la Monte and Wands 2005; Rivera, Goldin et al. 2005; de la Monte, Tong et al. 2006).

7. Peripheral versus central mediators of brain insulin/IGF deficiency and resistance

The molecular and biochemical abnormalities in AD brains closely mimic those present in diabetes mellitus; however, until recently, the vast majority of sporadic AD cases had no association with diabetes. In fact, prior to 1980, the epidemiological trends for AD (increasing prevalence) were opposite those of diabetes mellitus (declining as a cause of death) (de la Monte, Neusner et al. 2009). Even today, most cases of AD arise in the absence of type 2 diabetes, obesity, or metabolic syndrome, indicating that insulin/IGF resistance and deficiency can selectively involve the brain. Similarly, brain-only insulin and/or IGF resistance with cognitive impairment and AD-type neurodegeneration can be produced by intracerebroventricular (ICV) administration of small interfering (si)-RNA duplexes targeting the insulin or IGF receptors (see below), genetic depletion of insulin/IGF receptors, or ICV treatment with streptozotocin (STZ), which destroys insulin and IGF receptor bearing cells (Biju and Paulose 1998; Lannert and Hoyer 1998; Hoyer, Lannert et al. 1999; Hoyer, Lee et al. 2000; Nitta, Murai et al. 2002; Weinstock and Shoham 2004; Lester-Coll, Rivera et al. 2006; Grunblatt, Salkovic-Petrisic et al. 2007; Labak, Foniok et al. 2010; de la Monte, Tong et al. 2011). These studies support a primary role for brain insulin/IGF resistance and deficiency as the cause of AD-type neurodegeneration.

Within the past 2-3 decades, morbidity and mortality rates have trended upward for diabetes and other insulin resistance diseases, including metabolic syndrome (dyslipidemic states), non-alcoholic steatohepatitis (NASH), and obesity, despite improvements in medical treatment (de la Monte, Neusner et al. 2009). At the same time, the increasing overlap between cognitive impairment or AD and peripheral insulin resistance diseases has raised concerns about the potential contributions or even causal roles of obesity and diabetes mellitus in neurodegeneration and dementia (Qiu, De Ronchi et al. 2007; de la Monte, Neusner et al. 2009). Correspondingly, a number of human and experimental animal studies have demonstrated significant associations between peripheral insulin resistance states, obesity, or diabetes mellitus and brain insulin/IGF resistance, mild cognitive impairment (MCI), dementia, or AD (Craft 2005; Rivera, Goldin et al. 2005; Steen, Terry et al. 2005; Craft 2006; de la Monte, Tong et al. 2006; Lester-Coll, Rivera et al. 2006; Craft 2007). The debate over whether AD and cognitive impairment are caused by peripheral, brain, or both forms of insulin/IGF resistance is on-going, and essentially focused on three main questions: 1) Do T2DM and other peripheral insulin resistance states cause neurodegeneration, including AD? 2) How do T2DM and other peripheral insulin resistance disease states serve as co-factors in cognitive impairment and neurodegeneration? and 3) Is AD fundamentally a brain-specific form of diabetes mellitus? These questions are addressed below.

7.1 Potential roles of obesity and T2DM in cognitive impairment and neurodegeneration

Epidemiologic studies have shown that individuals with glucose intolerance, deficits in insulin secretion, or T2DM have a significantly increased risk for developing mild cognitive impairment (MCI) or AD-type dementia. Longitudinal studies also support roles for T2DM (Pasquier, Boulogne et al. 2006; Verdelho, Madureira et al. 2007) and obesity/dyslipidemic disorders (Martins, Hone et al. 2006) in the development of MCI, dementia, or AD (Haan and Wallace 2004; Luchsinger and Mayeux 2004; Ristow 2004; Launer 2005; Pasquier, Boulogne et al. 2006; Luchsinger, Reitz et al. 2007; Whitmer 2007). Despite these provocative observations, and an independent study demonstrating higher frequencies of peripheral insulin resistance in AD than in normal aging (Janson, Laedtke et al. 2004), postmortem human brain studies detected similar rates of AD among diabetics and controls (Nelson, Smith et al. 2008). Moreover, although experimental chronic high fat diet (HFD) feeding and diet induced obesity (DIO) with T2DM cause cognitive impairment with deficits in spatial learning and memory (Winocur and Greenwood 2005; Winocur, Greenwood et al. 2005), the resulting brain atrophy with brain insulin resistance, neuro-inflammation, oxidative stress, and deficits in cholinergic function are relatively mild and lack most of the important structural lesions that characterize AD pathology (Moroz, Tong et al. 2008; Lyn-Cook, Lawton et al. 2009). Therefore, observations in both humans and experimental models suggest that while obesity or T2DM can be associated with cognitive impairment, brain atrophy, and some aspects of AD-type neurodegeneration, these peripheral insulin resistance disease states are not sufficient to cause AD. Instead, the findings suggest that T2DM, obesity, and probably other peripheral/systemic insulin resistance states serve as co-factors that contribute to the pathogenesis or progression of neurodegeneration. The significance of this conclusion is that therapeutic strategies designed to treat T2DM, obesity, and systemic insulin resistance could help slow the progress or reduce the severity of AD, but will not likely prevent it altogether. Correspondingly, studies have already shown that treatment with hypoglycemic or insulin sensitizer agents can be protective for reducing the incidence and severity of AD (Luchsinger 2010).

7.2 Factors mediating cognitive impairment and neurodegeneration with systemic insulin resistance syndromes

Since it is clear that peripheral insulin resistance disease states can significantly and adversely alter cognitive function and contribute to the progression of AD-type neurodegeneration, efforts should be made to understand which aspects of peripheral insulin/IGF resistance are responsible for these effects. The rationale is that preventive measures could include treatments that ameliorate specific consequences of peripheral insulin resistance diseases, and the use of biomarkers that identify individuals who are at increased risk for developing MCI or AD. Moreover, treatments that restore peripheral insulin responsiveness could be used as neuroprotective agents as well. The ensuing discussion focuses on the roles of cerebral vascular disease and neurotoxic lipids.

7.2.1 Cerebral microvascular disease

How T2DM, obesity, and peripheral insulin resistance contribute to MCI, dementia, and neurodegeneration is not well understood. Factors under investigation include, chronic hyperglycemia, peripheral insulin resistance, oxidative stress, accumulation of advanced glycation end-products, increased expression and activation of insulin degrading enzyme, increased production of pro-inflammatory cytokines, and cerebral microvascular disease (Whitmer 2007). The potential contributions of cerebral microvascular disease require particular attention because chronic ischemic injury is an established mechanism of neurodegeneration, and diabetes mellitus causes significant microvascular disease. Chronic ischemic encephalopathy in AD ranges from multifocal ischemic lesions, to infarcts strategically localized in structures that are typically targeted for AD neurodegeneration, to leukoaraiosis with attrition of white matter fibers (Etiene, Kraft et al. 1998). Magnetic resonance imaging (MRI) studies have shown that lacunes and ischemic atrophy of medial temporal lobe structures (AD targets) increase with duration and progression of T2DM (Korf, White et al. 2006). Hyper-insulinemia and inheritance of the ApoE-ε4 allele also contribute to cerebrovascular disease and increase risk of AD progression. Insulin resistance and hyperinsulinemia can injure blood vessels and cause intimal thickening, scarring, and leakiness (Huang, Zou et al. ; Haudenschild, Van Sickle et al. 1981; Hotta, Taguma et al. 1996; Kubota, Kubota et al. 2003; Kincaid-Smith 2004; Matsumoto, Nakao et al. 2005). A recent study demonstrated that chronic ischemic leukoencephalopathy and leukoaraiosis in cerebral autosomal dominant arteriopathy with subacute infarcts and leukoencephalopathy (CADASIL) is associated with white matter microvascular insulin and IGF resistance (Brennan-Krohn, Salloway et al. 2010). White matter atrophy and fiber degeneration in CADASIL are associated with marked narrowing of vessel lumens, fibrotic destruction of vessel walls, and perivascular tissue attrition. In effect, the loss of vascular elasticity/compliance combined with compromised flow over time lead to chronic ischemic leukoencephalopathy. It is noteworthy that one of the earliest gross abnormalities in AD is white matter atrophy and fiber loss (de la Monte 1989). These findings suggest that, in addition to peripheral insulin resistance, systemic diseases that promote end-arterial resistance, e.g. hypertension could contribute to neurodegeneration by promoting cerebral microvascular disease. In fact, these mechanisms probably underlie the pathophysiology of vascular dementia. Future studies are needed to determine the degree to which reduced cerebral microvascular expression of insulin and IGF receptors correlates with cognitive impairment and neurodegeneration in AD and T2DM.

7.2.2 Neurotoxic lipids and neurodegeneration

Several studies have shown that cognitive impairment and neuropsychiatric dysfunction occur with liver disease caused by various agents, including alcohol abuse, obesity, chronic Hepatitis C virus infection, Reyes syndrome, or nitrosamine exposure (Schmidt, Gallo et al.

2005; Elwing, Lustman et al. 2006; Weiss and Gorman 2006; Karaivazoglou, Assimakopoulos et al. 2007; Loftis, Huckans et al. 2008; Perry, Hilsabeck et al. 2008; Kopelman, Thomson et al. 2009). These disease states are linked by the presence of hepatic steatosis or steatohepatitis with hepatic insulin resistance, endoplasmic reticulum (ER) stress, and increased generation of cytotoxic sphingolipids, including ceramides (de la Monte, Tong et al. 2006; Lester-Coll, Rivera et al. 2006; Moroz, Tong et al. 2008; Lyn-Cook, Lawton et al. 2009; Tong, Neusner et al. 2009; Tong, Longato et al. 2010). Mechanistically, inflammation, superimposed on disease states that promote lipid storage in hepatocytes, results in progressive ER stress, oxidative damage, mitochondrial dysfunction, and lipid peroxidation, which together promote hepatic insulin resistance (Capeau 2008; Kraegen and Cooney 2008). Hepatic insulin resistance stimulates lipolysis (Kao, Youson et al. 1999), and lipolysis leads to increased generation of toxic lipids e.g. ceramides, which further impair insulin signaling, mitochondrial function, and cell viability (Holland and Summers 2008; Kraegen and Cooney 2008; Langeveld and Aerts 2009).

Ceramides are lipid signaling molecules (Summers 2006) that cause insulin resistance (Liu, Obeid et al. 1997; Chalfant, Kishikawa et al. 1999; Arboleda, Huang et al. 2007) by activating pro-inflammatory cytokines (Summers 2006; Van Brocklyn 2007; Bryan, Kordula et al. 2008) and inhibiting signaling through PI3 kinase-Akt (Hajduch, Balendran et al. 2001; Bourbon, Sandirasegarane et al. 2002; Powell, Hajduch et al. 2003; Nogueira, Anhe et al. 2008). With steatohepatitis, hepatic and peripheral insulin resistance are accompanied by local and peripheral increases in ceramide levels (de la Monte, Tong et al. 2006; Lester-Coll, Rivera et al. 2006; Moroz, Tong et al. 2008; Tong, Neusner et al. 2009; Tong, Longato et al. 2010). Further studies showed that in vitro treatments with toxic ceramides cause brain insulin resistance, oxidative stress, and metabolic dysfunction (Tong and de la Monte 2009), and that in vivo administration (i.p.) of toxic ceramides causes cognitive-motor deficits, brain insulin resistance, oxidative stress, and neurodegeneration, similar to the findings in AD-type neurodegeneration. These findings led to the hypothesis that, in the settings of obesity, T2DM, and various peripheral insulin resistance states, cognitive impairment can be mediated via a liver-brain axis of neurodegeneration (de la Monte, Longato et al. 2009; de la Monte, Longato et al. 2009; de la Monte, Tong et al. 2010). We propose that livers with steatohepatitis, insulin resistance, and ER stress produce toxic lipids, in particular ceramides, that traffic through the circulation, and due to their lipid-soluble nature, cross the blood-brain barrier and exert neurotoxic and neurodegenerative effects by impairing brain and cerebral microvascular insulin signaling. This mechanism could account for the parallel and overlapping epidemics of peripheral systemic (T2DM, obesity, non-alcoholic steatohepatitis, metabolic syndrome) and brain (AD) insulin resistance diseases (de la Monte, Neusner et al. 2009).

7.3 Primary brain insulin/IGF resistance as the key pathogenic factor in AD-type neurodegeneration

The above discussion provides ample evidence that peripheral insulin resistance diseases can significantly contribute to the pathogenesis of neurodegeneration mediated through cerebral micro-vascular disease and/or liptoxicity effectuated via a liver-brain axis. However, on the whole, the neuro-behavioral, structural, biochemical, and molecular abnormalities produced by peripheral insulin resistance disease states are relatively modest compared with AD, reinforcing the concept that additional factors are needed to cause the full-blown disease. To better understand the underlying problems associated with AD and why peripheral insulin resistance diseases are themselves not sufficient to cause AD per se, the salient abnormalities in human AD brains requires scrutiny. Moreover, studies designed to produce states of brain but not peripheral insulin resistance must be examined and compared to both AD and the secondary effects of diabetes mellitus and other peripheral insulin resistance diseases.

7.3.1 Alzheimer's is a brain diabetes mellitus (type 3 diabetes)

A convincing argument could be made that AD, in its pure configuration, represents a brain form of diabetes mellitus (Rivera, Goldin et al. 2005; Steen, Terry et al. 2005) given that it is associated with progressive brain insulin/IGF resistance in the absence of T2DM, obesity, or peripheral insulin resistance (Rivera, Goldin et al. 2005; Steen, Terry et al. 2005; Craft 2006; Craft 2007). Moreover, postmortem studies demonstrated that the molecular, biochemical, and signal transduction abnormalities in AD are nearly identical to those that occur in both T1DM and T2DM (Nicolls 2004; Rivera, Goldin et al. 2005; Steen, Terry et al. 2005; Pasquier, Boulogne et al. 2006; Marchesini and Marzocchi 2007; Papandreou, Rousso et al. 2007; Pessayre 2007; Yeh and Brunt 2007). This led us to suggest the term, 'Type 3 diabetes' to better characterize the nature and pathophysiology of AD (Rivera, Goldin et al. 2005; Steen, Terry et al. 2005). These studies beg the question as to whether inhibition of brain insulin/IGF signaling is sufficient to cause neurodegeneration, particularly of the AD type? Alternatively, are factors other than brain insulin/IGF resistance required to mediate neurodegeneration? In this regard, one point that seems to get lost from the discussion is that IGF resistance and deficiency are part of the whole story, as was well documented in the human brain studies. With this in mind, data generated by siRNA inhibition of insulin, IGF-1, or IGF-2 receptor genes are presented to demonstrate the degree to which their adverse effects mimic AD. In addition, results of brain diabetes models produced by administration of streptozotocin are discussed in relation to human sporadic AD.

7.3.2 Experimental targeting of neuronal insulin/IGF receptors — in vitro model of neuronal insulin/IGF resistance

7.3.2.1 Methods

In vitro model. Primary cerebellar granule neuron cultures were generated from postnatal day 6 (P6) Long Evans rats (de la Monte and Tong 2009). Cerebellar granule neurons are a suitable model because the cells are non-transformed, they can be efficiently transfected with non-viral vectors, and they are highly dependent upon insulin and IGF signaling for function. In addition, the cerebellar cortex is a target of neurodegeneration in various diseases including, AD (Cole, Neal et al. 1993; Ishii, Sasaki et al. 1997; Larner 1997; Wegiel, Wisniewski et al. 1999). Freshly isolated cerebellar granule cells were transfected with commercially prepared small interfering RNA duplexes (si-RNA) targeting insulin receptor (siInR) [INSR NM_017071], IGF-1 receptor (siIGF-1R) [IGF1R NM_052807], IGF-2R (siIGF-IIR) [IGF2R NM_012756], or no specific gene sequences (Scrambled; si-Scr) [NM D-001210-01-20] using the Amaxa "v" nucleofector cell line reagents and the Amaxa nucleofector apparatus (Amaxa, Inc. Gaithersburg, MD). With this approach, we achieved 75-90% transfection efficiencies as determined by fluorescence microscopic imaging of cells co-transfected with recombinant plasmid expressing green fluorescent protein (GFP). Cells were seeded into 96-well plates to measure viability, mitochondrial function, and immunoreactivity, or 6-well plates to measure gene expression after 24 or 48 hours in culture. Cell density was determined by labeling the cultures with 10 µg/ml Hoechst H33342 in Tris-buffered saline (TBS), and measuring fluorescence (Ex360 nm/Em460 nm) in a Spectramax M5 microplate reader (Molecular Dynamics, Inc., Sunnyvale, CA). Mitochondrial function was measured using the 3-[4,5-dimethylthiazol-2-yl]-2,5-diphenyltetrazolium bromide (MTT) assay as previously described (de la Monte, Neely et al. 2001). Absorbances were measured at 540 nm in Spectramax M5 microplate reader. Gene expression and immunoreactivity were measured by quantitative reverse transcriptase polymerase chain reaction (qRT-PCR) amplification and cellular enzyme-linked immunosorbant assays.

Gene expression. Gene expression was measured by quantitative reverse transcriptase polymerase chain reaction (qRT-PCR) analysis, as described (Cantarini, de la Monte et al. 2006; Gundogan, Elwood et al. 2008). In brief, cells were lysed in Qiazol reagent and total RNA was isolated using the EZ1 RNA universal tissue kit and the BIO Robot EZ1 (Qiagen, Inc., Valencia, CA). RNA was reverse transcribed using random oligodeoxynucleotide primers and the AMV First Strand cDNA synthesis kit. The cDNA templates were used in qPCR amplifications with gene specific primer pairs published elsewhere (Gundogan, Elwood et al. 2008). Primers were designed using MacVector 10 software (MacVector, Inc., Cary, NC) and their target specificity was verified using NCBI-BLAST (Basic Local Alignment Search Tool). Amplified signals from triplicate reactions were detected and analyzed using the Mastercycler ep realplex instrument and software (Eppendorf AG, Hamburg, Germany). Relative mRNA abundance was calculated from the ng ratios of specific mRNA to 18S rRNA measured in the same samples. Inter-group statistical comparisons were made using calculated mRNA/18S rRNA ratios.

Immunoreactivity. Cellular enzyme-linked immunosorbant assays (ELISAs) were used to measure immunoreactivity directly in fixed cultured cells (96-well plates) (de la Monte, Ganju et al. 1999). The main modification of the original protocol was that immunoreactivity was detected with Amplex Red fluorophor (Ex 579/Em 595) instead of a colorimetric reagent. Cell density was assessed by staining the cells with Hoechst H33342 and measuring fluorescence (Ex360 nm/Em460 nm) in a Spectramax M5 microplate reader. The calculated ratios of fluorescence immunoreactivity (fluorescence light units; FLU) to H33342 were used for inter-group comparisons. Eight replicate cultures were analyzed in each experiment.

Statistics. Inter-group (N=8-12/group) comparisons were made using one-way analysis of variance (ANOVA) with the Tukey post-hoc test. Statistical analyses were performed using the GraphPad Prism 5 software (San Diego, CA) and significant P-values (<0.05) are indicated over the graphs.

Reagents. Rabbit, mouse, or goat generated monoclonal or polyclonal antibodies to tau, phospho-tau (AT8-S199, S202, T205), glial fibrillary acidic protein (GFAP), choline acetyltransferase (ChAT), Amyloid-β precursor protein (AβPP), AβPP-amyloid-β peptide (AβPP-Aβ), acetylcholinesterase (AChE), and Hu (neuronal marker) were purchased from Chemicon (Tecumsula, CA), CalBiochem (Carlsbad, CA), Molecular Probes (Eugene, OR), Invitrogen (Carlsbad, CA), or Abcam (Cambridge, MA). All other immunodetection reagents were purchased from Vector Laboratories (Burlingame, CA) or Molecular Probes (Eugene, OR). Histochoice fixative was purchased from Amresco, Inc (Solon, OH). QIAzol Lysis Reagent for RNA extraction and QuantiTect SYBR Green PCR Mix were obtained from Qiagen, Inc (Valencia, CA). The AMV 1st Strand cDNA Synthesis kit was purchased from Roche Applied Science (Indianapolis, IN). Synthetic oligonucleotides used in quantitative polymerase chain reaction (qPCR) assays were purchased from Sigma-Aldrich Co (St. Louis, MO). Fine chemicals were purchased from CalBiochem (Carlsbad, CA) or Sigma-Aldrich (St. Louis, MO).

7.3.2.2 Results

si-RNA targeting of insulin/IGF receptors broadly inhibited expression of insulin and IGF polypeptide and receptor genes. The qRT-PCR analyses demonstrated that cells transfected with si-InR, si-IGF-1R, or si-IGF-2R had significantly reduced expression of the insulin and insulin receptor mRNA transcripts relative to si-Scr transfected control cells (Figures 1A, 1B). In contrast, cells transfected with si-InR had significantly increased expression of IGF-1 and IGF-1R relative to si-Scr transfected cells (Figures 1C, 1D). si-InR transfected cells also had significantly higher levels of IGF-1R relative to both si-IGF-1R and si-IGF-2R transfected cells (Figure 1C).

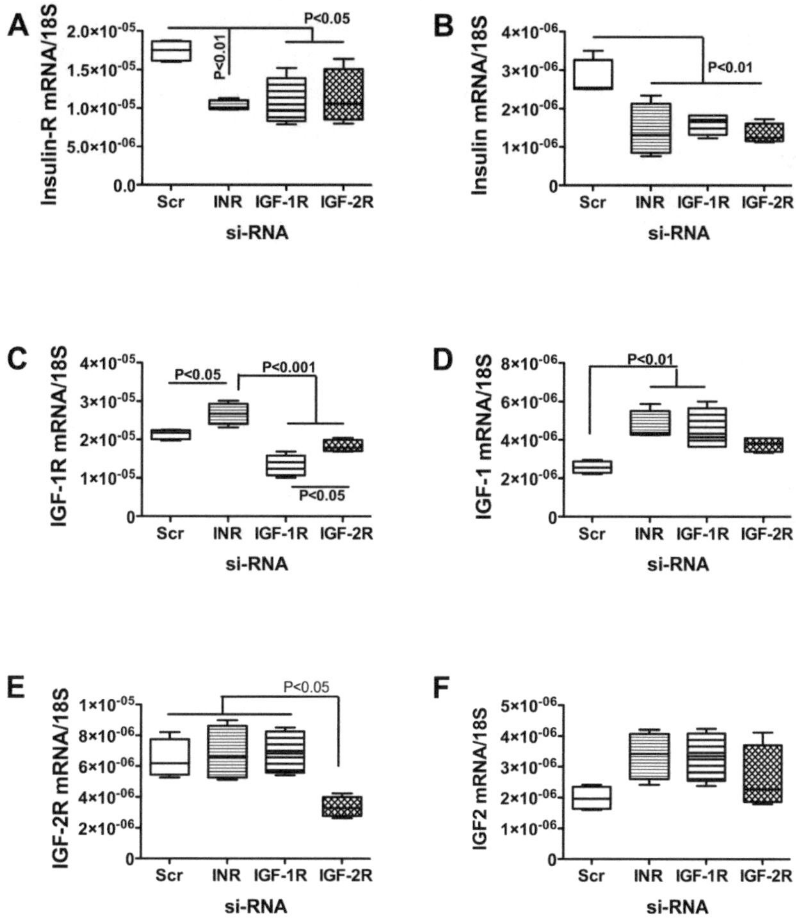

Fig. 1. Effects of si-RNA treatments on expression of insulin receptor, IGF-1, and IGF-2 receptors and polypeptide genes. mRNA levels of (A) InR, (B) insulin, (C) IGF-1R, (D) IGF-1, (E) IGF-2R, or (F) IGF-2 were measured by qRT-PCR with data normalized to 18S rRNA (N=8 per group). Inter-group comparisons were made by ANOVA and the Tukey post hoc test. P values are shown.

Cells transfected with si-IGF-1R had significantly reduced levels of IGF-1R relative to all other groups (Figure 1C) and higher levels of IGF-1 relative to si-Scr controls (Figure 1D). Cells transfected with si-IGF-2R had significantly lower mean levels of IGF-2R compared with the other groups (Figure 1E). IGF-1 (Figure 1D) and IGF-2 (Figure 1F) polypeptide expressions were generally higher in the experimental si-RNA groups relative to control, but the differences were only statistically significant with respect to IGF-1 mRNA levels in si-InR and si-IGF-1R transfected cells. Therefore, InR and insulin gene expression were inhibited in CNS neurons that were transfected with si-RNA targeting insulin, IGF-1, or IGF-2 receptors, while IGF-1R expression was selectively suppressed by transfection with si-IGF-1R, and IGF-2R expression was selectively inhibited in cells transfected with si-IGF-2R. With regard to the polypeptide genes, as noted, insulin gene expression was suppressed by si-InR, si-IGF-1R, or si-IGF-2R, whereas IGF-1 and IGF-2 mRNAs were generally increased relative to control. The latter could reflect a compensatory response to down regulation of the receptors. The aggregate results suggest that in cerebellar granule neurons, InR expression overlaps with IGF-1R and IGF-2R, and that some sub-populations express of IGF-1R and IGF-2R, while others may only express IGF-2R. Moreover, the findings suggest that the insulin polypeptide gene is expressed in insulin receptor bearing cells, whereas IGF-1 and IGF-2 are probably expressed in several different neuronal populations.

si-RNA targeting InR or IGF-2R impairs cell survival and mitochondrial function in neuronal cultures. Mitochondrial function was measured with the MTT assay, and cell density was measured by Hoechst H33342 fluorescence. MTT activity, corrected for cell density, was significantly lower in si-InR and si-IGF-2R relative to si-Scr transfected cultures (Figure 2A). In addition, the mean cell densities in cultures transfected with si-InR or si-IGF-2R were reduced relative to si-Scr transfected control cells (Figure 2B). Therefore, inhibition of signaling through the insulin or IGF-2 receptors impairs CNS neuronal viability and mitochondrial function.

Effects of si-RNA transfection on neuronal and astrocytic biomarkers. We used qRT-PCR analysis to measure gene expression corresponding to Hu and glial fibrillary acidic protein (GFAP), reflecting neuronal and astrocyte cell populations. The higher levels of Hu relative to GFAP reflect the predominantly neuronal nature of the cells isolated from cerebella (Figures 3A and 3B). Hu expression in si-InR, si-IGF-1R, and si-IGF-2R transfected cultures was similar to that measured in si-Scr control cells (Figure 3A). In contrast, GFAP expression was significantly reduced in si-InR transfected relative to all other groups, and in si-IGF-2R relative to si-IGF-1R transfected cells (Figure 3B). GFAP expression in cells transfected with si-IGF-1R was similar to control.

Inhibition of insulin and IGF receptor gene expression mediate neurodegeneration. We investigated the extent to which neuronal transfection with si-RNA targeting insulin, IGF-1 or IGF-2 receptor altered Tau, ChAT, AβPP, or AChE gene expression, as occur in AD. Tau gene expression was significantly reduced in cells transfected with si-IGF-2R relative to control (Figure 3C), corresponding with the somewhat reduced expression of Hu in the same cells (Figure 3A). In addition, AβPP mRNA was increased in si-InR transfected cells, and reduced in si-IGF-1R and si-IGF-2R transfected relative to si-Scr and si-InR transfected cells (Figure 3D). ChAT and AChE mRNA levels were significantly reduced in si-InR, si-IGF-1R, and si-IGF-2R transfected relative to si-Scr controls (Figure 3E and 3F).

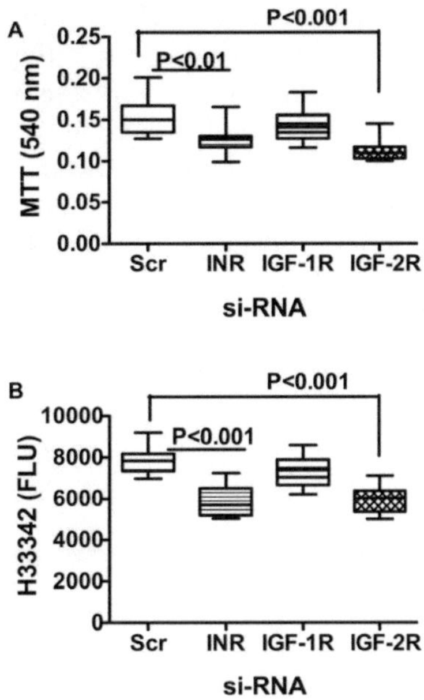

Fig. 2. Effects of siRNA treatments on mitochondrial function (MTT assay) and cell survival (H33342 fluorescence). N=8 cultures/group. Data were analyzed by ANOVA.

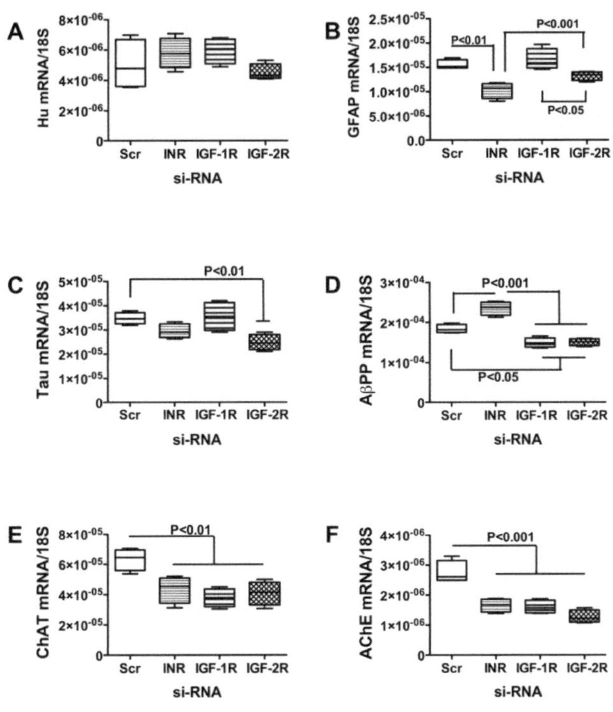

Fig. 3. Effects of siRNA treatments on expression of neuronal and glial genes shown by qRT-PCR. N=8 group. Data were analyzed by ANOVA.

Cellular ELISAs demonstrated similar mean levels of Tau and pTau among all groups, except in the si-InR relative to siScr transfected controls (Figures 4A and 4B). In addition, AβPP was significantly higher in cells transfected with si-IGF-1R or si-IGF-2R relative to si-Scr controls (Figure 4C), and AβPP-Aβ immunoreactivity was significantly increased in si-IGF-1R and si-IGF-2R relative to si-Scr and si-InR transfected cells (Figure 4D). Finally, corresponding with the qRT-PCR results, ChAT immunoreactivity was significantly lower in si-InR, si-IGF-1R, and si-IGF-2R transfected relative to controls (Figure 4E). AChE immunoreactivity was also significantly reduced in si-InR and si-IGF-1R transfected relative to control (Figure 4F).

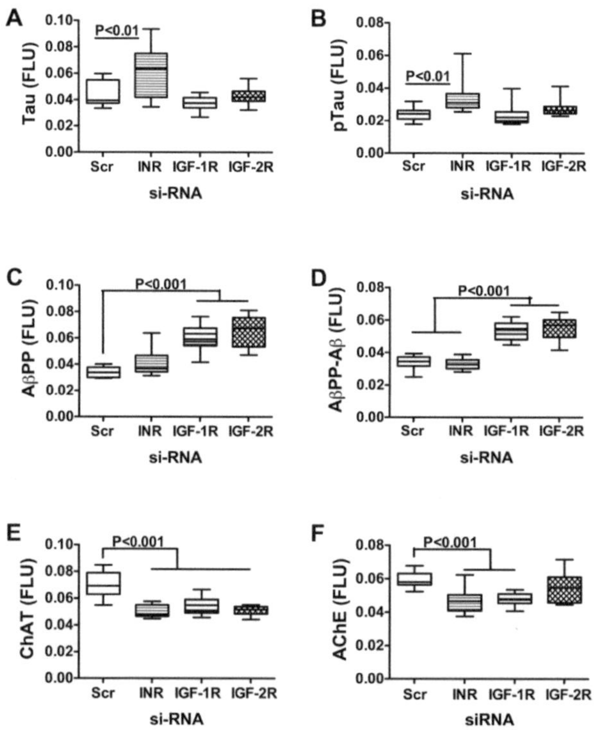

Fig. 4. Effects of siRNA treatments on expression of neuronal proteins pertinent to neurodegeneration shown by cellular ELISA. N=8 group. Data were analyzed by ANOVA.

7.3.2.3 Discussion

These studies demonstrate that transfection of CNS neurons with si-RNA targeting InR, IGF-1R, or IGF-2R leads to impaired neuronal survival, reduced mitochondrial function, and several abnormalities in gene or protein expression that occur in AD. Cells transfected with si-InR or si-IGF-2R were more adversely affected than those transfected with si-IGF-1R. The finding of increased pTau in si-InR transfected cells supports the concept that brain insulin resistance promotes Tau hyper-phosphorylation. The higher levels of AβPP and AβPP-Aβ in si-IGF-1R or si-IGF-2R transfected cells suggests that IGF resistance is an important mediator of AβPP-Aβ deposition and accumulation in brain. Cells transfected with si-InR, si-IGF-1R, or si-IGF-2R had reduced expression of AChE and/or ChAT. Altogether, these findings provide new evidence that molecular inhibition of insulin or IGF signaling in CNS neurons causes cellular, molecular, and biochemical abnormalities similar to those present in AD brains. Moreover, the findings suggest that signaling through the insulin and IGF receptors has distinct but overlapping effects; therefore, differential impairment of their functions produces different pathological and neurodegenerative effects, e.g. pTau levels increase with brain insulin resistance, AβPP expression increases and its protein is aberrantly processed with IGF-1 or IGF-2 resistance, and ChAT inhibition occurs with brain insulin and/or IGF resistance.

The overlapping inhibitory effects of the si-RNA transfections suggest that insulin and IGF-2 receptors are co-expressed in many of the same cells, and that IGF-1 and IGF-2 receptors are co-expressed in cells that have relatively low levels of insulin receptor. In addition, the reductions in insulin gene expression observed in cells that were transfected with si-InR, si-IGF-1R, or si-IGF-2R suggest that insulin polypeptide gene is expressed in insulin receptor bearing cells in the brain, and that endogenous insulin stimulation may be effectuated via autocrine or paracrine loops. Reduced cell density and mitochondrial function produced by si-InR or si-IGF-2R transfection suggest that signaling through the insulin and IGF-2 receptors is critical for CNS neuronal viability and metabolism. Moreover, the reduced Hu expression in si-InR- and si-IGF-2R- but not si-IGF-1R- transfected cells suggests that insulin and IGF-2 receptors are abundantly expressed in CNS neurons, as previously suggested (Xu, Eun Yeon et al. 2003; Soscia, Tong et al. 2006), and that signaling through either or both receptors supports neuronal survival and function. Sharply reduced levels of GFAP were detected in cells transfected with si-InR or si-IGF-2R. Since GFAP is expressed by astrocytes, the findings suggest that signaling through InR- or IGF-2R-regulated pathways is critical to glial cell survival and function. Therefore, inhibition of insulin or IGF-2 receptor signaling impairs neuronal and astrocyte survival and function, whereas inhibition of the IGF-1 receptor alone is not detrimental to CNS cell survival or energy metabolism.

We investigated the degree to which molecular abnormalities characteristically associated with AD are produced by inhibiting insulin, IGF-1, or IGF-2 receptor expression in CNS neurons. Cells transfected with si-InR, si-IGF-1R, or si-IGF-2R each had reduced levels of ChAT, corresponding with an earlier finding that ChAT is regulated by insulin and IGF (Soscia, Tong et al. 2006). ChAT generates acetylcholine, which has an important role in cognitive and motor functions (Dineley-Miller and Patrick 1992; Deutsch, Urbano et al. 2010; Peeyush, Savitha et al. 2010; Pepeu and Giovannini 2010). Since inhibition of neuronal insulin, IGF-1, or IGF-2 receptors leads to deficits in ChAT expression, impairments in cognition can be attributed to CNS insulin/IGF resistance (Rivera, Goldin et al. 2005; Lester-Coll, Rivera et al. 2006; Soscia, Tong et al. 2006; de la Monte and Wands 2008; de la Monte 2009; de la Monte, Longato et al. 2009; Lyn-Cook, Lawton et al. 2009; Tong, Longato et al. 2010). AChE expression was suppressed by the same si-RNA treatments. Although the down--regulation of AChE could represent a compensatory neuroprotective response (Noh, Koh et al. 2009) to decreased ChAT, instead it could represent a damaging effect leading to increased apoptosis (Greenberg, Toiber et al. 2010).

Transfection of CNS neurons with si-InR or si-IGF-2R inhibited Tau gene expression, while si-InR increased pTau immunoreactivity. These results corroborate previous reports that tau expression is stimulated by insulin and IGFs, while increased tau phosphorylation is mediated by impaired signaling through the insulin receptor and activation of kinases such as GSK-3β (Hong and Lee 1997). The increased levels of AβPP and AβPP-Aβ immunoreactivity in cultures transfected with si-IGF-1R and si-IGF-2R suggest that intact signaling through the IGF-1 and IGF-2 receptors may be important for regulating metabolism of AβPP and clearance of AβPP-Aβ. Since si-IGF-2R reduced expression of GFAP, astrocytes may play important roles in AβPP and AβPP-Aβ processing and clearance in the brain. On the other hand, cultures transfected with si-InR had increased AβPP gene expression, similar to the findings in AD (Rivera, Goldin et al. 2005; Steen, Terry et al. 2005). This effect could be mediated by increased oxidative stress caused by reduced energy metabolism and increased phospho-tau. Previous studies showed that oxidative stress was sufficient to increase CNS neuronal phospho-Tau and AβPP-Aβ (Chen, Xu et al. 2003). Together, the findings herein suggest that inhibition of insulin, IGF-1, and IGF-2 receptor expression and function have complimentary but overlapping roles in mediating the molecular pathogenesis of neurodegeneration, including AD. In addition, the results suggest that therapeutic measures should target all 3 receptors, since impairments of their signaling pathways would likely mediate distinct but overlapping components of the neurodegeneration cascade.

7.3.3 Experimental targeting of neuronal insulin/IGF receptors — in vivo model of brain insulin/IGF resistance

7.3.3.1 Methods

In vivo siRNA delivery. To evaluate the roles of insulin and IGF receptor resistance in relation to neurodegeneration in vivo, we generated a model in which P2 Long Evans rats were given a single intracerebroventricular (ICV) injection of si-InR [INSR NM_017071], si-IGF-1R [IGF1R NM_052807], si-IGF-2R [IGF2R NM_012756], or si-Scr (negative control) [NM D-001210-01-20]. For each rat, 0.4 nmol si-RNA plus 100 ng recombinant green fluorescent protein (GFP) expressing plasmid were combined with 10 μl of Dharmafect reagent, and injected into the right frontal region over the lateral ventricle using a Hamilton syringe with a 26-gauge needle as previously described (de la Monte, Jhaveri et al. 2007). GFP expression, which was under the control of a CMV promoter, was used to monitor success of the transfections. All rats survived the procedure, and none of them exhibited aberrant behaviors or adverse effects such as failure to thrive, poor grooming, reduced physical activity, or weight loss.

To monitor effectiveness of the transfections, rats (N=4 per group) were sacrificed at regular intervals after ICV gene delivery, and GFP expression was measured in whole brain by qRT-PCR analysis. Those studies demonstrated peak levels of GFP expression 2-3 days after ICV gene delivery, followed by a gradual decline in GFP mRNA levels. However, GFP expression persisted over the time course of the experiment as previously reported (de la Monte, Jhaveri et al. 2007). Gene expression and histological studies were performed with temporal lobe tissue. Upon sacrifice, temporal lobes were either immersion fixed in Histofix, embedded in paraffin, and used to make hematoxylin and eosin (H&E) stained histological sections (5 μm-thick), or they were snap-frozen in a dry ice/methanol bath and stored at -80°C for mRNA and protein studies. Our protocol was approved by the Institutional Animal Care and Use Committee at Lifespan-Rhode Island Hospital, and it conforms to guidelines set by the National Institutes of Health.

Morris water maze testing. We used Morris water maze tests to assess long-term effects of ICV si-InR, si-IGF-1R and si-IGF-2R on spatial learning and memory, corresponding to hippocampal function (Hamm, Dixon et al. 1992; McLay, Freeman et al. 1999; Gomez-Pinilla, So et al. 2001). Beginning on P24, rats were subjected to 3 daily trials in which latency (seconds) required to locate and land on the platform was recorded. On Day 1, the platform was visible, but on Days 2-4, the platform was submerged. On Days 3 and 4, the water entry quadrants were randomized for each trial. The data were analyzed using area-under-the-curve (AUC) calculations corresponding to performance over the 3 trials each day (de la Monte, Tong et al. 2006; Lester-Coll, Rivera et al. 2006).

Gene and protein expression. Gene and protein expression were measured by qRT-PCR analysis (see above) and direct binding ELISA. For ELISAs, temporal lobe homogenates were prepared in radioimmunoprecipitation assay (RIPA) buffer containing protease and phosphatase inhibitors (Lester-Coll, Rivera et al. 2006). Protein concentrations were determined using the BCA assay. 50 ng protein samples in Tris buffered saline, pH 7.4 (TBS) were adsorbed to flat-bottom surfaces of 96-well polystyrene plates, overnight at 4°C. Non-specific binding sites were masked by a 3-hour room temperature incubation with 300 µl/well of TBS + 0.05% Tween 20 + 3% BSA. Samples were then incubated with 0.1-0.5 µg/ml primary antibody for 1 h at 37°C. Immunoreactivity was detected with horseradish peroxidase (HRP)-conjugated secondary antibody and Amplex Red soluble fluorophore (de la Monte and Tong 2009). Fluorescence was measured (Ex 530/Em 590) in a SpectraMax M5 microplate reader. Parallel negative control assays had primary, secondary, or both antibodies omitted. Between steps, reactions were rinsed 3 times with TBS + 0.05% Tween 20 using a Nunc ELISA plate washer. Levels of immunoreactivity were normalized to protein content in the wells, which was measured using NanoOrange reagent.

Statistical analysis. Inter-group comparisons were made using repeated measures one-way ANOVA and the Dunnett post-hoc significance test for comparisons with the si-Scr control group. Statistical analyses were performed using the GraphPad Prism 5 software (San Diego, CA) and P<0.05 was considered significant.

7.3.3.2 Results

ICV si-RNA targeting the insulin or IGF receptors impaired spatial learning and memory. On Day 1 of testing, the mean latencies were longer for all experimental groups relative to control. However, the differences were significant only for si-InR- and si-IGF-1R-treated rats (Fig 5A). On Day 2, when the platform was submerged but entry was from a fixed position, the 95% confidence limits were broad for the 3 experimental groups, and inter-group differences were statistically significant only for the si-InR and si-IGF-1R-treated relative to controls (Figure 5B). On Day 3, the first day of randomized entry into the maze, the si-InR treated rats had significantly longer mean latencies for locating the hidden platform relative to control, whereas mean performance among si-IGF-1R and si-IGF-2R treated rats did not significantly differ from control (Figure 5C). However, performance among the si-IGF-1R treated rats was highly variable, as evidenced by the broad overlap with the si-InR and si-Scr treated groups. On Day 4, mean performances among the 4 groups were similar (Figure 5D). Therefore, the si-InR and si-IGF-1R treatments mainly impaired performance on spatial learning and memory tasks during the acquisition phases.

ICV treatment with si-InR, si-IGF-1R, or si-IGF-2R caused hippocampal hyopotrophy. Histological sections of temporal lobe, including the hippocampus, revealed normal architecture in siScr-treated controls, and pronounced hypotrophy of both the hippocampal formation and temporal cortex in rats treated with si-InR, si-IGF-1R or si-IGF-2R (Figure 6). The most striking abnormalities occurred in si-IGF-2R, followed by si-InR-treated rats, in which there were marked reductions in overall size of the temporal lobes, accompanied by conspicuously decreased neuropil volume rather than cell density (Figure 6). Since neuropil contains mainly interconnecting cell processes, the major adverse effects ICV si-InR, si-IGF-1R, and si-IGF-2R were to impair neuritic growth and synapse formation.

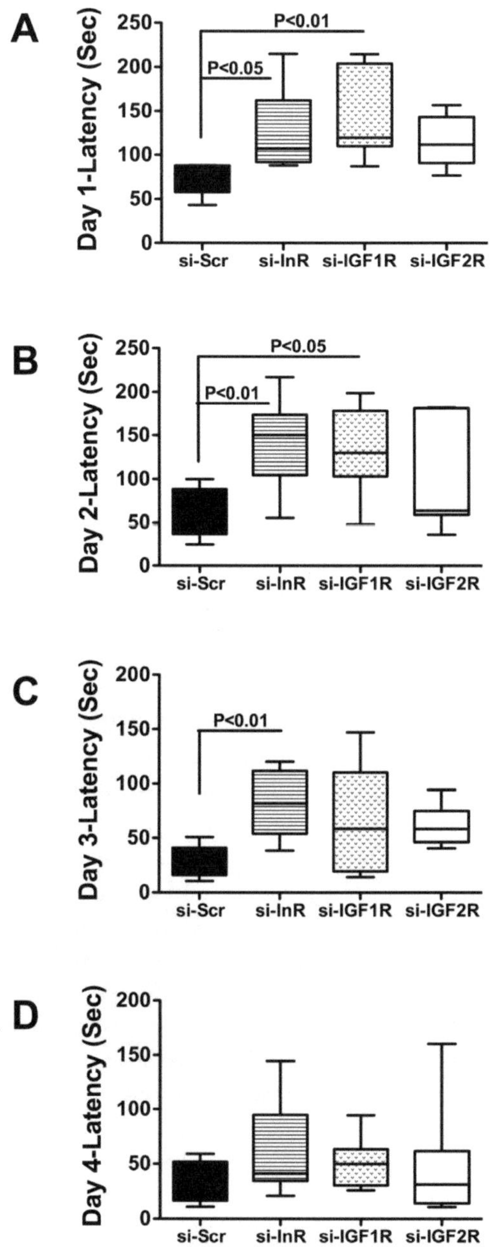

Fig. 5. Effects of ICV si-InR, si-IGF-1R, and si-IGF-2R on spatial learning and memory. P2 Long Evans rats were given ICV si-RNA targeting InR, IGF-1R, IGF-2R, or no specific gene (si-Scr). Morris Water Maze tests were performed on 4 consecutive days, beginning on P24. Data from the 3 trials/day were used to calculate area under the curve for latency. Comparisons were made by ANOVA and the Dunnett post-hoc test. Significant P values are indicated.

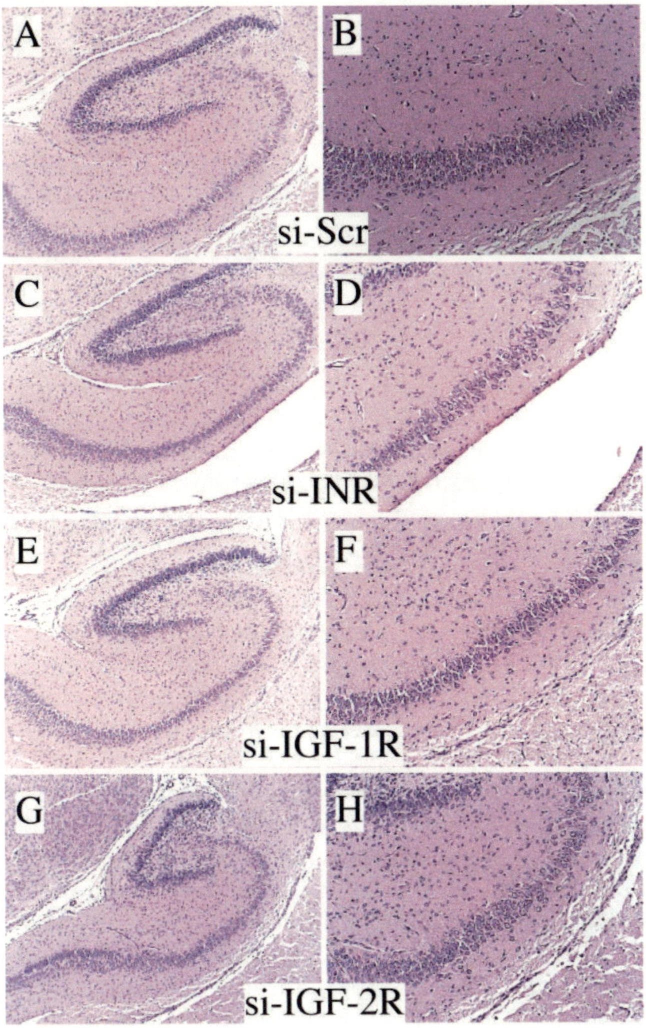

Fig. 6. ICV si-InR, si-IGF-1R, or si-IGF-2R causes hippocampal hypotrophy. Brains were harvested on P30, immersion fixed, and embedded in paraffin. Histological sections of temporal lobe, including the hippocampi, were stained with H&E. Panels A,C,E, G depict 40x original magnification images of temporal lobe and hippocampus, and Panels B,D,F,H show 100x original magnification images of the hippocampus from (A,B) si-Scr, (C,D) si-InR, (E,F) si-IGF-1R, or (G,H) si-IGF-2R transfected brains. Note extreme hypotrophy of the temporal lobe and hippocampus in si-IGF-2R and si-INR treated relative si-Scr treated controls.

Short-term effects of ICV si-InR, si-IGF-1R, and si-IGF-2R on insulin, IGF, and neurotrophin signaling (Table 1). Gene expression analysis performed on P9, i.e. 7 days after the ICV treatments, demonstrated significantly reduced temporal lobe levels of InR in the si-InR, si-IGF-1R, and si-IGF-2R treated groups (P=0.003). In addition, IGF-1R and IGF-2R expression were reduced in brains transfected with si-InR, si-IGF-1R or si-IGF-2R, although the inter-group differences were only significant for IGF-1R (P=0.008).

mRNA	si-Scr	si-InR	si-IGF-1R	si-IGF-2R	P-Value
Insulin R	15.3 ± 1.8	10.4 ± 0.6*	9.4 ± 0.8**	9.9 ± 1.1**	0.003
IGF-1R	8.3 ± 0.6	7.5 ± 0.8	7.0 ± 0.5	5.4 ± 0.4**	0.008
IGF-2R	7.9 ± 0.7	6.9 ± 0.5	6.5 ± 0.6	5.8 ± 0.6	
Insulin	0.19 ± 0.03	0.17 ± 0.04*	0.15 ± 0.02	0.16 ± 0.02	
IGF-1	2.4 ± 0.09	3.1 ± 0.17	2.6 ± 0.13	3.0 ± .29	0.008
IGF-2	49.5 ± 7.5	59.9 ± 9.4	49.1 ± 7.0	65.5 ± 5.0	
BDNF	1.6 ± 0.2	2.1 ± 0.3	1.3 ± 0.1	2.2 ± 0.3	
NGF	0.04 ± 0.004	0.06 ± 0.005	0.06 ± 0.009	0.08 ± 0.02*	0.0003
P75	14.5 ± 1.1	7.5 ± 0.8	8.2 ± 1.4	12.5 ± 2.5	0.008
NRTK	0.17 ± 0.06	0.24 ± 0.06	0.11 ± 0.04	0.16 ± 0.03	0.043
18S	2.9 ± 0.2	2.4 ± 0.7	2.8 ± 0.1	3.0 ± 0.2	

Gene expression was measured by qRT-PCR analysis. mRNA levels correspond to the mean ratio relative to 18S rRNA x10^{-6} ± S.E.M. Inter-group comparisons were made using repeated measures one-way ANOVA and the Dunnett post-hoc test for comparison with control (si-Scr). *P<0.05; **P<0.01

Table 1. Effects of siRNA targeting insulin and IGF receptors on receptor and trophic factor gene expression- P9 temporal lobe

Although insulin polypeptide gene expression was reduced in all experimental groups relative to control, the differences were not statistically significant due to the large variances and very low levels of insulin gene expression in the brain. In contrast, IGF-1 polypeptide gene expression was higher in the experimental groups relative to control (P=0.008). There were no significant inter-group differences in the mean levels of IGF-2 expression in the brain.

Neurotrophins and their receptors mediate structural and functional aspects of neuronal plasticity in the brain, their genes are regulated in part by insulin/IGF stimulation expression. Therefore, it was of interest to characterize the effects of ICV si-InR, si-IGF-1R and si-IGF-2R treatment on the expression of brain derived neurotrophic factor (BDNF), nerve growth factor (NGF), P75, and neuronal receptor tyrosine kinase (nRTK) by qRT-PCR. On P9, the mean levels of BDNF were similar among the groups, whereas for NGF (P=0.0003), P75 (P=0.008), and nRTK (P=0.043), the inter-group differences were statistically significant (Table 1). The mean levels of NGF mRNA were higher in all experimental groups relative to control, and the post hoc Dunnett test demonstrated significantly higher NGF expression in si-IGF-2R relative to si-Scr transfected brains (P<0.05). In contrast, the mean levels of P75 were lower in all experimental groups relative to control, and the post hoc Dunnett test showed that the differences were significant for the ICV si-InR and si-IGF-1R treated rats (both P<0.05). For nRTK, the mean mRNA levels were somewhat higher in the si-InR, and lower in the si-IGF-1R group relative to control, but the post hoc tests did not reach statistical significance (Table 1).

Sustained effects of ICV treatments on insulin, IGF, and neurotrophin signaling molecules in brain (Table 2). In P30 rats, 4 weeks after the ICV treatments, the mean levels of InR, IGF-1R, and IGF-2R expression were either similar, or somewhat elevated relative to si-Scr controls, but none of the inter-group differences were statistically significant. In contrast, insulin polypeptide gene expression was reduced (P=0.027), while IGF-1 expression was increased (P=0.011) in the 3 experimental groups. The mean levels of IGF-2 mRNA were also higher in experimental relative to control brains, but the differences did not reach statistical significance.

mRNA	si-Scr	si-InR	si-IGF-1R	si-IGF-2R	P-Value
Insulin R	9.9 ± 0.8	12.8 ± 1.3	11.5 ± 1.3	10.5 ± 1.1	
IGF-1R	7.1 ± 0.6	8.2 ± 0.9	8.4 ± 0.8	6.9 ± 0.7	
IGF-2R	7.0 ± 0.5	8.1 ± 0.9	7.5 ± 0.8	7.0 ± 0.7	
Insulin	0.23 ± 0.02	0.13 ± 0.02**	0.17 ± 0.03	0.16 ± 0.02	0.027
IGF-1	2.4 ± 0.09	3.4 ± 0.3**	2.8 ± 0.15	3.1 ± 0.28	0.011
IGF-2	49.5 ± 7.5	67.7 ± 12.5	52.8 ± 7.2	66.9 ± 5.0	
BDNF	1.6 ± 0.2	2.6 ± 0.3**	1.4 ± 0.14	2.5 ± 0.26*	0.0003
NGF	0.04 ± 0.003	0.07 ± 0.004	0.07 ± 0.01**	0.08 ± 0.01	<0.0001
P75	11.9 ± 1.8	9.1 ± 1.3	12.9 ± 3.5	15.5 ± 4.7	
NRTK	0.06 ± 0.01	0.28 ± 0.07**	0.12 ± 0.04	0.19 ± 0.02	0.0032

Gene expression was measured by qRT-PCR analysis. mRNA levels correspond to the mean ratio relative to 18S rRNA x10^{-6} ± S.E.M. Inter-group comparisons were made using repeated measures one-way ANOVA and the Dunnett post-hoc test for comparison with control (si-Scr). *P<0.05; **P<0.01

Table 2. Effects of siRNA targeting insulin and IGF receptors on receptor and trophic factor gene expression- P30 temporal lobe

Significant inter-group differences were observed with respect to BDNF (P=0.0003), NGF (P<0.0001), and nRTK (P=0.0032), but not P75 (Table 2). BDNF expression was significantly elevated in the si-InR (P<0.01) and si-IGF-2R (P<0.05) treated relative to control brains. The mean NGF mRNA levels were higher in all 3 experimental groups relative to control, and the post hoc Dunnett test demonstrated the differences to be significant for si-IGF-2R relative to si-Scr controls (P<0.01). Similarly, nRTK expression was higher in all three experimental groups relative to control, and the Dunnett post hoc test demonstrated the difference from control to be significant for the si-InR-treated group (P<0.01).
Sustained effects of ICV delivery of si-InR, si-IGF-1R, and si-IGF-1R on neuronal, cytoskeletal, cholinergic, and neurotrophin protein expression (Table 3): In P30 rats, Tau immunoreactivity was higher in brains transfected with si-InR or si-IGF-1R relative to control (P=0.0077).

mRNA	si-Scr	si-InR	si-IGF-1R	si-IGF-2R	P-Value
Tau	19195 ± 2951	26872 ± 1200*	23532 ± 2328	16110 ± 1946	0.008
pTau	3297 ± 467	2814 ± 164	2857 ± 128	2525 ± 119	
Actin	56026 ± 3356	63245 ± 1033*	63514 ± 997*	59794 ± 1373	0.0003
GAPDH	5244 ± 228	4856 ± 164	5214 ± 451	5172 ± 319	
ChAT	20244 ± 1863	15514 ± 606*	16660 ± 658	17375 ± 847	0.033
AChE	29347 ± 982	32767 ± 297*	34190 ±590***	31688 ± 1095	0.0013
BDNF	15932 ± 650	15563 ± 607	15353 ± 390	15936 ± 793	
NGF	38604 ± 3334	49538±1521***	45705 ± 816*	43071 ± 936	<0.0001
NT3	16714 ± 1178	11879±290***	13468 ± 499*	15528 ± 959	0.0004
NT4	7378 ± 378	9074 ± 1189	8197 ± 440	8357 ± 904	

Immunoreactivity was measured by ELISA and results were normalized to protein content in the wells. Inter-group comparisons were made by repeated measures one-way ANOVA and the Dunnett post-hoc test for comparison with control (si-Scr). *P<0.05; **P<0.01; ***P<0.001.

Table 3. Effects of siRNA targeting insulin and IGF receptors on neuronal structural and neurotrophin protein expression- P30 temporal lobe.

β-actin expression was higher in si-InR and si-IGF-1R relative to si-Scr transfected brains (P=0.0003). ICV delivery of si-InR, si-IGF-1R, or si-IGF-2R reduced temporal lobe levels of ChAT (P=0.036). In contrast, AChE immunoreactivity was elevated in si-InR, si-IGF-1R, and si-IGF-2R transfected brains (P=0.0013).
Corresponding with the qRT-PCR analyses, NGF expression was increased in the si-InR, si-IGF-1R, and si-IGF-2R treated relative to control brains (P<0.0001). The mean levels of NT3 immunoreactivity were lower in the 3 experimental groups relative to control (P=0.0004). There were no significant inter-group differences in the mean levels of pTau, GAPDH, BDNF, or NT4 in P30 rat brains.

7.3.3.3 Discussion

We used ICV injections to transfect brains with si-RNA duplex molecules targeting InR, IGF-1R, IGF-2R, or no specific genes (si-Scr). Previously, we used the same approach to generate a model of neurodegeneration, and demonstrated sustained transgene expression throughout the brain and in all cell types (de la Monte, Jhaveri et al. 2007).
Morris water maze tests demonstrated significant impairments in spatial learning in the si-InR, si-IGF-1R, and si-IGF-2R treated rats. Histopathological studies showed that the deficits in spatial learning were associated with reduced sizes of the hippocampi and temporal lobes, and hypotrophy of the neuropil, which contains interconnecting cell processes and synapses. Major abnormalities in AD include dendritic spine atrophy and synapse disruption. Since insulin and IGFs modulate neuronal plasticity and neurite outgrowth (de la Monte 2009), these findings suggest that AD-associated impairments in spatial learning and memory could be mediated by brain insulin and IGF resistance.
Gene expression studies showed that, in addition to reducing expression of the target genes, ICV si-InR, si-IGF-1R and si-IGF-2R each inhibited expression of the other two non-targeted receptors. The most likely explanation for this phenomenon is that cells in the temporal lobe express all 3 receptors at once. The inhibitory effects of the si-RNA treatments were most pronounced for si-InR. This finding, together with fact that all 3 experimental treatments resulted in hypotrophy of the temporal lobe and hippocampus, suggest that the adverse effects of the si-RNA treatments were mainly due to inhibition of insulin signaling.
Although GFP expression persisted in the brains due to continued presence of the plasmid, it is unlikely that the si-RNA molecules remained intact 1 or 2 days after transfection. The absence of any significant reduction in InR, IGF-1R, or IGF-2R expression at P30 indicates that the effects of the si-RNA treatments were transient with respect to gene expression. Therefore, the sustained effects of the si-RNA treatments on temporal lobe structure and function were mediated by short-term inhibition of gene expression during the critical postnatal period of synaptic plasticity and development. The relatively modest inhibitory effects on insulin and IGF polypeptides indicate that the structural and functional impairments caused by ICV si-InR, si-IGF-1R, or si-IGF-2R were mediated by insulin/IGF resistance rather than withdrawal of endogenously produced trophic factors.
We investigated the effects of the si-RNA treatments on neurotrophin and neurotrophin receptor expression because these molecules mediate neurite outgrowth, plasticity, neuronal survival, and other function, and insulin/IGF modulate expression and function of neurotrophins in brain (Maisonpierre, Belluscio et al. 1990; Cowansage, LeDoux et al. 2010). The studies demonstrated that the main adverse effect of the si-RNA treatments was to reduce expression of p75 neurotrophin receptor on P9. Otherwise, BDNF, NGF, p75 neurotrophin receptor, and nRTK were either increased or similarly expressed compared

with si-Scr controls. ELISA studies demonstrated similar or increased expression of BDNF, NGF, and neurotrophin 4 (NT4) in P30 temporal lobes of experimental si-RNA treated rats, but significantly reduced expression of NT3 in both si-InR and si-IGF-1R treated rats. Since all neurotrophins, including NGF, BDNF, NT3 and NT4/5 function by binding to the p75 neurotrophin receptor (Frebel and Wiese 2006), early inhibition of p75 expression would have impaired neurotrophin signaling and could account for both the spatial learning deficits and hypotrophy of the temporal lobe/hippocampus in the si-RNA treated rats. NT3 regulates neuronal survival, synaptic plasticity, and neurotransmission, particularly in the hippocampus (Pae, Marks et al. 2008). Therefore, persistent reductions in NT3 expression represent local trophic factor withdrawal, which could have contributed to the cognitive impairment detected by Morris water maze testing. Although insulin/IGF regulation of neurotrophin and neurotrophin expression has not yet been characterized, the findings herein suggest that neurotrophin expression and function may be downstream of insulin/IGF signaling pathways in the brain.

In previous studies, inhibition of brain insulin and IGF signaling reduced expression of tau, ChAT, and GAPDH, increased pTau, and had variable effects on AChE expression (Soscia, Tong et al. 2006; de la Monte and Wands 2008; Tong, Longato et al. 2010). Corresponding with the normalized levels of InR and IGF-1R expression at P30, tau and GAPDH were not reduced, and pTau was not increased, but the impairments in cholinergic homeostasis were sustained in temporal lobes of si-InR and/or si-IGF-1R treated rats. ChAT is a major neurotransmitter that mediates cognitive function and plasticity throughout life (Perry, Piggott et al. 1993), and evidence suggests that besides insulin/IGF stimulation (Shi, Rabin et al. 1998), cholinergic function can be regulated by neurotrophins, including NT3 (Robertson, Baratta et al. 2006). It is noteworthy that in both si-InR and si-IGF-1R, ChAT and NT3 expression were reduced to greater extents than in si-IGF-2R treated brains.

These in vivo experiments demonstrate that sustained structural and functional developmental abnormalities can be produced by transient ICV transfection with siRNA molecules targeting insulin, IGF-1, or IGF-2 receptors. The long-term effects include deficits in spatial learning and memory, striking abnormalities in temporal lobe structure, and inhibition of mechanisms needed for cholinergic homeostasis. While these results are exciting and very much validate a role for primary brain insulin and IGF resistance as mediators of neurodegeneration and dementia, the structural changes in neurons and disorganization of the cortical laminar architecture that characterize AD-type neurodegeneration were not detected. This suggests that additional factors such as ongoing oxidative injury, are likely required to propagate the neurodegeneration cascade.

8. Experimental type 3 diabetes

The human studies provide convincing evidence that AD is associated with progressive insulin and IGF resistance and deficiency, accompanied by oxidative stress, deficits in energy metabolism, cholinergic function, neuronal survival, and synaptic plasticity in the brain. Given the fact that most cases of sporadic AD are not associated with obesity or diabetes mellitus, the said abnormalities must originate primarily in the brain. The siRNA experiments targeting the insulin or IGF receptors showed that inhibition of signaling through these receptors is sufficient to cause neurodegeneration and significantly impair a range of functions as observed in AD. On the other hand, the deficits, although sustained, were relatively static rather than progressive, suggesting that another "hit" was needed to propagate the cascade of neurodegeneration.

8.1 Toxin-induced brain diabetes mimics sporadic Alzheimer's disease

Analysis of postmortem human brains demonstrated progressive insulin and IGF resistance and deficiency with increasing severity of AD and dementia, which correlated with increased indices of oxidative stress and DNA damage, and reduced cholinergic homeostasis. Neuroinflammation and AβPP gene expression were increased early in the course of AD, but they either stabilized or declined as disease progressed. None of the subjects in those studies had diabetes mellitus, non-alcoholic steatohepatitis, or obesity. Perhaps the best model of sporadic AD is the one generated by ICV streptozotocin (STZ) treatment. STZ is a pro-diabetes drug that when injected systemically causes Type 1 diabetes mellitus (insulin deficiency) with higher doses, and Type 2 diabetes (insulin resistance) at lower doses. The i.p. or i.v. administration of STZ also causes mild hepatic steatosis and neurodegeneration (Biju and Paulose 1998; Szkudelski 2001; Bolzan and Bianchi 2002; Koulmanda, Qipo et al. 2003), but low dose ICV STZ treatment causes cognitive impairment with brain insulin resistance, brain insulin deficiency, and AD-type neurodegeneration, and not diabetes mellitus or hepatic steatosis (Biju and Paulose 1998; Hoyer, Lannert et al. 1999; Nitta, Murai et al. 2002; Weinstock and Shoham 2004; Lester-Coll, Rivera et al. 2006). STZ-induced neurodegeneration is characterized by impairments in brain insulin and IGF signaling, brain atrophy, impaired energy metabolism, mitochondrial dysfunction, oxidative stress, DNA damage, and increased AβPP, expression, AβPP-Aβ accumulation, neuroinflammation, and tau phosphorylation. Therefore, limited exposure to a single pro-diabetes drug causes neurodegeneration with all of the characteristic features of AD. Moreover, depending upon dose and route of administration, STZ treatment produces insulin resistance diseases that target the CNS, liver, pancreas, or skeletal muscle with variable degrees of overlap, or else the brain could represent the primary focus of disease.

8.2 Environmental/dietary causes of insulin/IGF resistance syndromes: Nitrosamine exposures mediate Alzheimer's, diabetes mellitus, and hepatic steatosis

Sporadic AD or Type 3 diabetes is overwhelmingly a brain-specific disease that leads to total body wasting and eventual arrival at a vegetative state. The closest experimental model of sporadic AD is that produced by ICV STZ, which does not cause systemic diabetes mellitus, i.e. Type 1 or Type 2. This very point begs the question of, what relevance could STZ possibly have in relation to the pathogenesis AD, diabetes, or hepatic steatosis in humans? After all, human are not generally exposed to STZ. The probable answer was uncovered by the realization that STZ is a nitrosamine-related compound, and that over the past several decades, Western societies have been assaulted by continuous and growing exposures to environmental and food-related nitrosamines. The epidemiological trends for AD, diabetes mellitus, obesity, and non-alcoholic steatohepatitis all show substantial increases in incidence, prevalence, morbidity, and mortality rates that correspond more with exposures than genetics as underlying causes (de la Monte, Neusner et al. 2009). For unclear reasons, although the connection between nitrosamine exposure and diabetes was entertained years ago (Berne, Gunnarsson et al. 1974; Portha, Giroix et al. 1980; Helgason, Ewen et al. 1984; Boucher, Ewen et al. 1994; Dahlquist 1994; Essien and Akpan 2006), that concept seems to have been missed, and therefore has not yet been incorporated into the conceptualization about the origins of our insulin resistance diseases epidemic.

We conducted experiments to determine if low, sub-mutagenic doses of nitrosamines that are found in processed foods, e.g. N-nitrosodiethylamine (NDEA), could cause insulin resistance diseases. The results were alarming because low-dose and very limited exposures to NDEA cause T2DM, non-alcoholic steatohepatitis, visceral obesity, cognitive impairment, and AD-type neurodegeneration with peripheral, hepatic, and brain insulin resistance (Tong, Neusner et al. 2009; Tong, Longato et al. 2010), similar to the effects of STZ. Therefore, depending on the structure of the compound, dose, and route of administration, exposures to nitrosamine-related chemicals can cause insulin resistance diseases in multiple different target organs, including brain. In addition to providing evidence that the relatively recent epidemics of sporadic AD, T2DM, and non-alcoholic steatohepatitis/metabolic syndrome could be mediated by environmental or dietary exposures (de la Monte, Neusner et al. 2009), these studies demonstrate that insulin resistance diseases with essentially the same underlying cellular abnormalities, can develop in various organs and tissues. This phenomenon could account for the overlapping increases in prevalence rates of various insulin resistance diseases within the past several decades, as well as the very frequent but incomplete overlap between AD and obesity, T2DM, and NASH (Janson, Laedtke et al. 2004), which did not exist prior to 1980, and is not accounted for by aging of the population (de la Monte, Neusner et al. 2009).

8.3 The liver-brain-axis of neurodegeneration hypothesis

Experiments with STZ and NDEA provided clear evidence that low dose exposures to nitrosamines can reproduce the molecular, biochemical, neuropathological, and neurobehavioral abnormalities observed in human sporadic cases of AD, and also cause a broad spectrum of peripheral insulin resistance diseases, including visceral obesity, diabetes, and non-alcoholic steatohepatitis (de la Monte, Tong et al. 2006; Lester-Coll, Rivera et al. 2006; de la Monte and Tong 2009; Tong, Neusner et al. 2009). Subsequent studies showed that, the adverse effects of NDEA were exacerbated by chronic high fat diet feeding (de la Monte, Tong et al. 2009; Tong, Longato et al. 2010), and that i.p. treatment with NDEA was more effective in causing neurodegeneration than ICV NDEA. Further consideration of the data revealed that the degrees of steatohepatitis, and the levels of toxic lipids, i.e. ceramides produced in liver following NDEA ± high fat diet exposures were critical variables in the equation. These findings led us to the liver-brain- axis of neurodegeneration hypothesis (de la Monte, Longato et al. 2009; de la Monte, Longato et al. 2009), which states that, chronic injury to the liver that results in steatohepatitis, hepatic insulin resistance, and ER stress, leads to dysregulated lipid metabolism and attendant elaboration of toxic lipids, including ceramides and other sphingolipids. The toxic lipids get released into the circulation due to impaired membrane integrity or cell death. Their lipid-soluble nature enables the toxic lipids to cross the blood brain barrier and exert their adverse effects on brain insulin signaling pathways that mediate neuronal and glial survival, energy metabolism, neurotransmitter function, and synaptic plasticity. This hypothesis is supported by preliminary data showing that the same profiles of sphingolipids in steatotic livers are represented in peripheral blood, and that lipids isolated from peripheral blood in insulin-resistance disease states, when applied to brain slice cultures, cause neurodegeneration with insulin resistance. Experimental in vitro and in vivo exposures to chemically defined toxic ceramides also cause neurodegeneration with brain insulin resistance (Tong and de la Monte 2009; de la Monte, Tong et al. 2010). In addition to providing a mechanism whereby environmental toxins in processed and preserved foods, and agricultural products grown with heavy doses of nitrate-containing fertilizers may be responsible for our current and growing insulin resistance diseases epidemic that is becoming pandemic with exportation of our diets and lifestyles, the liver-brain-axis hypothesis suggests how the lipotoxicity associated with visceral obesity, type 2 diabetes, and NASH could serve as co-factors in the pathogenesis of AD-type neurodegeneration.

9. Western diet and insulin/IGF resistance mediated neurodegeneration

Since aging is essential and unequivocally the most dominant risk factor for AD, critical changes associated with the loss of youthful compensatory and protective mechanisms must be responsible for the acquired permissiveness to neurodegeneration. Mechanisms of aging are still under investigation. However, strong data from organisms that span the phylogenetic tree, indicate a role for caloric restriction as preventive, and excess caloric intake as a promoter of aging. One image I find impossible to dismiss, is the one displaying two primates of approximately the same age, side by side: one monkey was chronically fed with a low calorie diet, and the other was maintained on a high calorie diet. The differences in appearance and behavior were striking. The lean monkey appeared youthful and spunky, whereas the obese monkey looked aged and sluggish (Colman, Anderson et al. 2009). In addition to obesity, high caloric intake increased the rates of diabetes, cardiovascular disease, cancer, and brain atrophy in the colony (Colman, Anderson et al. 2009; Cruzen and Colman 2009). Moreover, diets high in trans fatty acids, which are abundantly present in processed foods, caused abdominal obesity and insulin resistance (Kavanagh, Jones et al. 2007). Similar effects of nutrient poor, calorically dense diets have been demonstrated in humans (Hodge, Dowse et al. 1995; Tran, Komatsu et al. 2001; Hursting, Lavigne et al. 2003; Newby, Muller et al. 2003). In humans, caloric restriction also retards aging and reduces rates of chronic disease; therefore, this simple measure may also help to reduce risk for neurodegeneration (Qin, Chachich et al. 2006; Kim, Nguyen et al. 2007; Wang, Fivecoat et al. 2010).

Beyond avoidance of excessive caloric intake, growing evidence suggests that the source of calories is also of concern. A number of reports suggest that aging and pathophysiological states that contribute to chronic diseases are promoted by diets low in nutrient value, and high in simple sugars (fructose), starches, and trans fatty acids. Added to this is the problem associated with consumption of heavily processed foods and exposure to nitrosamines. Unfortunately, the vast majority of foods consumed in the USA are processed and contain preservatives, and over time, our exposures to nitrosamines through food processing and preservation and the heavy use of fertilizers in agriculture have increased sharply and in parallel with the insulin resistance disease epidemics (de la Monte, Neusner et al. 2009). The implications with regard to strategies for disease prevention are obvious. The implementation of measures to protect citizens of this country while not destroying lifestyle conveniences brought by modernization of culture is possible for those who are informed and proactive, but will be challenging for individuals who are unwilling to make proper choices. The larger concern is the rapid rate in which our insulin resistance disease epidemic is becoming pandemic secondary to the exportation of inexpensive Western convenience foods.

10. Sedentary lifestyles contribute to brain insulin/IGF resistance

Attempts to curb the obesity epidemic and associated health risks have focused on implementing lifestyle changes that promote healthful eating and regular exercise. Cross-cultural studies have shown that adoption of Western, go-easy lifestyles with reduced physical activity results in higher rates of obesity (Hodge, Dowse et al. 1995), and increased obesity correlates with progressive hyperlipidemia (Berns, de Vries et al. 1989). In addition, sedentary lifestyles among children lead to increased energy intake in the forms of fat, sweets, salty snacks, and carbonated beverages, and reduced intake of fruits and vegetables (Coon and Tucker 2002). In contrast, increased physical activity in the form or aerobic exercise prevents the long-term weight gain that is associated with aging (Littman, Kristal et al. 2005), and reduces risk for both cardiovascular events and cognitive impairment (Nash and Fillit 2006). More recently, clinical research demonstrated that regular physical exercise can reduce the risks for cognitive impairment and neurodegeneration (Radak, Hart et al.), or help maintain (Plassman, Williams et al. ; Deslandes, Moraes et al. 2009) or improve (Rolland, Abellan van Kan et al. ; Weih, Abu-Omar et al. 2009; Baker, Frank et al. 2010) cognitive function in the elderly. Experimentally, physical exercise was demonstrated to reduce the AβPP-Aβ burden in transgenic mouse brains (Adlard, Perreau et al. 2005), although other studies suggest that improved cognitive performance and neurotrophin function were mediated by physical activity with environmental enrichment (Wolf, Kronenberg et al. 2006). These results provide convincing evidence that regular aerobic physical exercise can help prevent neurodegeneration and preserve cognitive function. The therapeutic effects of aerobic physical exercise are likely mediated by weight loss with reduced peripheral insulin resistance, increased cerebrovascular insulin/IGF responsiveness with attendant improvements in blood flow, nutrient delivery, and metabolism, and decreased production of toxic lipids that promote neurodegeneration and brain insulin resistance.

11. Conclusions

After 30+ years of intense research, new data have emerged supporting the concept that AD is heterogeneous in nature, and mediated by brain insulin and IGF resistance with reductions in glucose utilization and energy metabolism, increased oxidative stress, and neuro-inflammation. Impairments in brain insulin and IGF signaling contribute to neuronal loss, synaptic disconnection, tau hyperphosphorylation, AβPP-Aβ accumulation, and metabolic disturbances. Peripheral insulin resistance disease states, including diabetes mellitus, obesity, and non-alcoholic steatohepatitis, contribute to brain insulin/IGF resistance and neurodegeneration, but alone, they are not sufficient to cause AD. This conclusion is supported by experiments in which brain insulin or IGF resistance were produced by ICV delivery of siRNA duplexes targeting the insulin or IGF receptors. AD fundamentally represents a brain-specific form of diabetes i.e. Type 3 diabetes that can, and often does overlap with peripheral insulin resistance diseases. Analysis of experimental streptozotocin (STZ) treatment models showed that insulin resistance and insulin deficiency states could be produced in peripheral organs, including liver, and/or the brain. The realization that STZ is a nitrosamine, led to further studies revealing that NDEA, which is one of the nitrosamines present in processed and preserved foods, or can be produced in our bodies by exposure to nitrites, also causes the full spectrum of insulin resistance diseases that are epidemic in the USA. Moreover, experimental results showed that when combined with chronic high fat dietary intake, the severity and extent of insulin resistance diseases are worsened substantially. Due to the common link of steatohepatitis with increased dysregulation of lipid metabolism and generation of toxic lipids, we proposed that AD-type neurodegeneration in the context of peripheral insulin resistance diseases is mediated via a liver-brain axis. In essence, toxic lipids generated in liver, enter the circulation, cross the blood-brain barrier, and cause brain insulin resistance by inhibiting signal transduction through the insulin receptor. This concept provides a mechanism whereby peripheral insulin resistance diseases could serve as co-factors in the pathogenesis of AD and cognitive impairment. Dietary and lifestyle measures to prevent insulin resistance diseases, including sporadic AD, were discussed, with particular emphasis on avoiding processed and preserved foods that permeate Western diets.

12. Acknowledgements

The work in our laboratory is been generously supported by grants AA-11431, AA-12908, and AA-16260 from the National Institutes of Health. The author has no competing financial interests.

13. References

Adlard, P. A., V. M. Perreau, et al. (2005). "Voluntary exercise decreases amyloid load in a transgenic model of Alzheimer's disease." J Neurosci 25(17): 4217-4221.

Adolfsson, R., G. Bucht, et al. (1980). "Hypoglycemia in Alzheimer's disease." Acta Med Scand 208(5): 387-388.

Arboleda, G., T. J. Huang, et al. (2007). "Insulin-like growth factor-1-dependent maintenance of neuronal metabolism through the phosphatidylinositol 3-kinase-Akt pathway is inhibited by C2-ceramide in CAD cells." Eur J Neurosci 25(10): 3030-3038.

Arnaud, L., N. K. Robakis, et al. (2006). "It may take inflammation, phosphorylation and ubiquitination to 'tangle' in Alzheimer's disease." Neurodegener Dis 3(6): 313-319.

Baker, L. D., L. L. Frank, et al. (2010). "Effects of aerobic exercise on mild cognitive impairment: a controlled trial." Arch Neurol 67(1): 71-79.

Berne, C., R. Gunnarsson, et al. (1974). "Letter: Diabetogenic nitrosamines?" Lancet 1(7849): 173-174.

Berns, M. A., J. H. de Vries, et al. (1989). "Increase in body fatness as a major determinant of changes in serum total cholesterol and high density lipoprotein cholesterol in young men over a 10-year period." American journal of epidemiology 130(6): 1109-1122.

Biju, M. P. and C. S. Paulose (1998). "Brain glutamate dehydrogenase changes in streptozotocin diabetic rats as a function of age." Biochem Mol Biol Int 44(1): 1-7.

Blasko, I., M. Stampfer-Kountchev, et al. (2004). "How chronic inflammation can affect the brain and support the development of Alzheimer's disease in old age: the role of microglia and astrocytes." Aging Cell 3(4): 169-176.

Blass, J. P., G. E. Gibson, et al. (2002). "The role of the metabolic lesion in Alzheimer's disease." J Alzheimers Dis 4(3): 225-232.

Blum-Degen, D., L. Frolich, et al. (1995). "Altered regulation of brain glucose metabolism as a cause of neurodegenerative disorders?" J Neural Transm Suppl 46: 139-147.

Bolzan, A. D. and M. S. Bianchi (2002). "Genotoxicity of streptozotocin." Mutat Res 512(2-3): 121-134.

Boucher, B. J., S. W. Ewen, et al. (1994). "Betel nut (Areca catechu) consumption and the induction of glucose intolerance in adult CD1 mice and in their F1 and F2 offspring." Diabetologia 37(1): 49-55.

Bourbon, N. A., L. Sandirasegarane, et al. (2002). "Ceramide-induced inhibition of Akt is mediated through protein kinase Czeta: implications for growth arrest." J Biol Chem 277(5): 3286-3292.

Brennan-Krohn, T., S. Salloway, et al. (2010). "Glial Vascular Degeneration in CADASIL." Journal of Alzheimer's disease : JAD.

Bryan, L., T. Kordula, et al. (2008). "Regulation and functions of sphingosine kinases in the brain." Biochim Biophys Acta 1781(9): 459-466.

Cantarini, M. C., S. M. de la Monte, et al. (2006). "Aspartyl-asparagyl beta hydroxylase over-expression in human hepatoma is linked to activation of insulin-like growth factor and notch signaling mechanisms." Hepatology 44(2): 446-457.

Capeau, J. (2008). "Insulin resistance and steatosis in humans." Diabetes Metab 34(6 Pt 2): 649-657.

Caselli, R. J., K. Chen, et al. (2008). "Correlating cerebral hypometabolism with future memory decline in subsequent converters to amnestic pre-mild cognitive impairment." Arch Neurol 65(9): 1231-1236.

Chalfant, C. E., K. Kishikawa, et al. (1999). "Long chain ceramides activate protein phosphatase-1 and protein phosphatase-2A. Activation is stereospecific and regulated by phosphatidic acid." J Biol Chem 274(29): 20313-20317.

Chen, G. J., J. Xu, et al. (2003). "Transient hypoxia causes Alzheimer-type molecular and biochemical abnormalities in cortical neurons: potential strategies for neuroprotection." J Alzheimers Dis 5(3): 209-228.

Cole, G., J. W. Neal, et al. (1993). "The distribution of amyloid plaques in the cerebellum and brain stem in Down's syndrome and Alzheimer's disease: a light microscopical analysis." Acta Neuropathol 85(5): 542-552.

Colman, R. J., R. M. Anderson, et al. (2009). "Caloric restriction delays disease onset and mortality in rhesus monkeys." Science 325(5937): 201-204.

Coon, K. A. and K. L. Tucker (2002). "Television and children's consumption patterns. A review of the literature." Minerva pediatrica 54(5): 423-436.

Cowansage, K. K., J. E. LeDoux, et al. (2010). "Brain-derived neurotrophic factor: a dynamic gatekeeper of neural plasticity." Curr Mol Pharmacol 3(1): 12-29.

Craft, S. (2005). "Insulin resistance and cognitive impairment: a view through the prism of epidemiology." Arch Neurol 62(7): 1043-1044.

Craft, S. (2006). "Insulin resistance syndrome and Alzheimer disease: pathophysiologic mechanisms and therapeutic implications." Alzheimer Dis Assoc Disord 20(4): 298-301.

Craft, S. (2007). "Insulin resistance and Alzheimer's disease pathogenesis: potential mechanisms and implications for treatment." Curr Alzheimer Res 4(2): 147-152.

Cruzen, C. and R. J. Colman (2009). "Effects of caloric restriction on cardiovascular aging in non-human primates and humans." Clinics in geriatric medicine 25(4): 733-743, ix-x.

Dahlquist, G. (1994). "Non-genetic risk determinants of type 1 diabetes." Diabete & metabolisme 20(3): 251-257.

De Ferrari, G. V. and N. C. Inestrosa (2000). "Wnt signaling function in Alzheimer's disease." Brain Res Brain Res Rev 33(1): 1-12.

de la Monte, S. M. (1989). "Quantitation of cerebral atrophy in preclinical and end-stage Alzheimer's disease." Ann Neurol 25(5): 450-459.

de la Monte, S. M. (2009). "Insulin resistance and Alzheimer's disease." BMB Rep 42(8): 475-481.

de la Monte, S. M., G. J. Chen, et al. (2003). "Neuronal thread protein regulation and interaction with microtubule-associated proteins in SH-Sy5y neuronal cells." Cell Mol Life Sci 60(12): 2679-2691.

de la Monte, S. M., N. Ganju, et al. (2000). "Partial rescue of ethanol-induced neuronal apoptosis by growth factor activation of phosphoinositol-3-kinase." Alcohol Clin Exp Res 24(5): 716-726.

de la Monte, S. M., N. Ganju, et al. (1999). "Microtiter Immunocytochemical ELISA Assay: A Novel and Highly Sensitive Method of Quantifying Immunoreactivity." Biotecniques 26(6): 1073-1076.

de la Monte, S. M., A. Jhaveri, et al. (2007). "Nitric oxide synthase 3-mediated neurodegeneration after intracerebral gene delivery." J Neuropathol Exp Neurol 66(4): 272-283.

de la Monte, S. M., L. Longato, et al. (2009). "The liver-brain axis of alcohol-mediated neurodegeneration: role of toxic lipids." Int J Environ Res Public Health 6(7): 2055-2075.

de la Monte, S. M., L. Longato, et al. (2009). "Insulin resistance and neurodegeneration: roles of obesity, type 2 diabetes mellitus and non-alcoholic steatohepatitis." Curr Opin Investig Drugs 10(10): 1049-1060.

de la Monte, S. M., T. R. Neely, et al. (2001). "Ethanol impairs insulin-stimulated mitochondrial function in cerebellar granule neurons." Cell Mol Life Sci 58(12-13): 1950-1960.

de la Monte, S. M., A. Neusner, et al. (2009). "Epidemilogical Trends Strongly Suggest Exposures as Etiologic Agents in the Pathogenesis of Sporadic Alzheimer's Disease, Diabetes Mellitus, and Non-Alcoholic Steatohepatitis." J Alzheimers Dis.

de la Monte, S. M. and M. Tong (2009). "Mechanisms of Nitrosamine-Mediated Neurodegeneration: Potential Relevance to Sporadic Alzheimer's Disease." J Alzheimers Dis.

de la Monte, S. M., M. Tong, et al. (2011). "si-RNA inhibition of brain insulin or insulin-like growth factor receptors causes developmental cerebellar abnormalities: relevance to fetal alcohol spectrum disorder." Molec Brain: (In Press).

de la Monte, S. M., M. Tong, et al. (2009). "Nitrosamine exposure exacerbates high fat diet-mediated type 2 diabetes mellitus, non-alcoholic steatohepatitis, and neurodegeneration with cognitive impairment." Mol Neurodegener 4: 54.

de la Monte, S. M., M. Tong, et al. (2006). "Therapeutic rescue of neurodegeneration in experimental type 3 diabetes: relevance to Alzheimer's disease." J Alzheimers Dis 10(1): 89-109.

de la Monte, S. M., M. Tong, et al. (2010). "Ceramide-mediated insulin resistance and impairment of cognitive-motor functions." J Alzheimers Dis 21(3): 967-984.

de la Monte, S. M. and J. R. Wands (2002). "Chronic gestational exposure to ethanol impairs insulin-stimulated survival and mitochondrial function in cerebellar neurons." CMLS, Cell Mol Life Sci 59: 882-893.

de la Monte, S. M. and J. R. Wands (2005). "Review of insulin and insulin-like growth factor expression, signaling, and malfunction in the central nervous system: relevance to Alzheimer's disease." J Alzheimers Dis 7(1): 45-61.

de la Monte, S. M. and J. R. Wands (2008). "Alzheimer's disease is type 3 diabetes-evidence reviewed." J Diabetes Sci Technol 2(6): 1101-1113.

Deslandes, A., H. Moraes, et al. (2009). "Exercise and mental health: many reasons to move." Neuropsychobiology 59(4): 191-198.

Deutsch, S. I., M. R. Urbano, et al. (2010). "Cholinergic abnormalities in autism: is there a rationale for selective nicotinic agonist interventions?" Clin Neuropharmacol 33(3): 114-120.

Dineley-Miller, K. and J. Patrick (1992). "Gene transcripts for the nicotinic acetylcholine receptor subunit, beta4, are distributed in multiple areas of the rat central nervous system." Brain Res Mol Brain Res 16(3-4): 339-344.

Doble, B. W. and J. R. Woodgett (2003). "GSK-3: tricks of the trade for a multi-tasking kinase." J Cell Sci 116(Pt 7): 1175-1186.

Duyckaerts, C., B. Delatour, et al. (2009). "Classification and basic pathology of Alzheimer disease." Acta Neuropathol 118(1): 5-36.

Eikelenboom, P. and W. A. van Gool (2004). "Neuroinflammatory perspectives on the two faces of Alzheimer's disease." J Neural Transm 111(3): 281-294.

Elwing, J. E., P. J. Lustman, et al. (2006). "Depression, anxiety, and nonalcoholic steatohepatitis." Psychosom Med 68(4): 563-569.

Essien, A. D. and J. O. Akpan (2006). "Diabetogenic property of charred meat on litters of pregnant albino rats." Nigerian journal of physiological sciences : official publication of the Physiological Society of Nigeria 21(1-2): 37-41.

Etiene, D., J. Kraft, et al. (1998). "Cerebrovascular Pathology Contributes to the Heterogeneity of Alzheimer's Disease." J Alzheimers Dis 1(2): 119-134.

Fraser, P. E., G. Yu, et al. (2001). "Presenilin function: connections to Alzheimer's disease and signal transduction." Biochem Soc Symp(67): 89-100.

Frebel, K. and S. Wiese (2006). "Signalling molecules essential for neuronal survival and differentiation." Biochem Soc Trans 34(Pt 6): 1287-1290.

Frolich, L., D. Blum-Degen, et al. (1998). "Brain insulin and insulin receptors in aging and sporadic Alzheimer's disease." J Neural Transm 105(4-5): 423-438.

Fujisawa, Y., K. Sasaki, et al. (1991). "Increased insulin levels after OGTT load in peripheral blood and cerebrospinal fluid of patients with dementia of Alzheimer type." Biol Psychiatry 30(12): 1219-1228.

Gasparini, L., G. K. Gouras, et al. (2001). "Stimulation of beta-amyloid precursor protein trafficking by insulin reduces intraneuronal beta-amyloid and requires mitogen-activated protein kinase signaling." J Neurosci 21(8): 2561-2570.

Gasparini, L., W. J. Netzer, et al. (2002). "Does insulin dysfunction play a role in Alzheimer's disease?" Trends Pharmacol Sci 23(6): 288-293.

Gomez-Pinilla, F., V. So, et al. (2001). "Spatial learning induces neurotrophin receptor and synapsin I in the hippocampus." Brain Res 904(1): 13-19.

Greenberg, D. S., D. Toiber, et al. (2010). "Acetylcholinesterase variants in Alzheimer's disease: from neuroprotection to programmed cell death." Neuro-degenerative diseases 7(1-3): 60-63.

Grilli, M., G. Ferrari Toninelli, et al. (2003). "Alzheimer's disease linking neurodegeneration with neurodevelopment." Funct Neurol 18(3): 145-148.

Grunblatt, E., M. Salkovic-Petrisic, et al. (2007). "Brain insulin system dysfunction in streptozotocin intracerebroventricularly treated rats generates hyperphosphorylated tau protein." J Neurochem 101(3): 757-770.

Gundogan, F., G. Elwood, et al. (2008). "Impaired placentation in fetal alcohol syndrome." Placenta 29(2): 148-157.

Haan, M. N. and R. Wallace (2004). "Can dementia be prevented? Brain aging in a population-based context." Annu Rev Public Health 25: 1-24.

Hajduch, E., A. Balendran, et al. (2001). "Ceramide impairs the insulin-dependent membrane recruitment of protein kinase B leading to a loss in downstream signalling in L6 skeletal muscle cells." Diabetologia 44(2): 173-183.

Hamm, R. J., C. E. Dixon, et al. (1992). "Cognitive deficits following traumatic brain injury produced by controlled cortical impact." J Neurotrauma 9(1): 11-20.

Hanger, D. P., A. Seereeram, et al. (2009). "Mediators of tau phosphorylation in the pathogenesis of Alzheimer's disease." Expert Rev Neurother 9(11): 1647-1666.

Haudenschild, C. C., W. Van Sickle, et al. (1981). "Response of the aorta of the obese Zucker rat to injury." Arteriosclerosis 1(3): 186-191.

Helgason, T., S. W. Ewen, et al. (1984). "N-nitrosamines in smoked meats and their relation to diabetes." IARC scientific publications(57): 911-920.

Hodge, A. M., G. K. Dowse, et al. (1995). "Modernity and obesity in coastal and Highland Papua New Guinea." International journal of obesity and related metabolic disorders : journal of the International Association for the Study of Obesity 19(3): 154-161.

Holland, W. L. and S. A. Summers (2008). "Sphingolipids, insulin resistance, and metabolic disease: new insights from in vivo manipulation of sphingolipid metabolism." Endocr Rev 29(4): 381-402.

Hong, M. and V. M. Lee (1997). "Insulin and insulin-like growth factor-1 regulate tau phosphorylation in cultured human neurons." J Biol Chem 272(31): 19547-19553.

Hotta, O., Y. Taguma, et al. (1996). "Possible relationship between hyperinsulinemia and glomerular hypertrophy in nephrosclerosis." Ren Fail 18(2): 271-278.

Hoyer, S. (2002). "The brain insulin signal transduction system and sporadic (type II) Alzheimer disease: an update." J Neural Transm 109(3): 341-360.

Hoyer, S. (2004). "Causes and consequences of disturbances of cerebral glucose metabolism in sporadic Alzheimer disease: therapeutic implications." Adv Exp Med Biol 541: 135-152.

Hoyer, S. (2004). "Glucose metabolism and insulin receptor signal transduction in Alzheimer disease." Eur J Pharmacol 490(1-3): 115-125.

Hoyer, S. and H. Lannert (1999). "Inhibition of the neuronal insulin receptor causes Alzheimer-like disturbances in oxidative/energy brain metabolism and in behavior in adult rats." Ann N Y Acad Sci 893: 301-303.

Hoyer, S., H. Lannert, et al. (1999). "Damaged neuronal energy metabolism and behavior are improved by Ginkgo biloba extract (EGb 761)." J Neural Transm 106(11-12): 1171-1188.

Hoyer, S., S. K. Lee, et al. (2000). "Inhibition of the neuronal insulin receptor. An in vivo model for sporadic Alzheimer disease?" Ann N Y Acad Sci 920: 256-258.

Hoyer, S. and R. Nitsch (1989). "Cerebral excess release of neurotransmitter amino acids subsequent to reduced cerebral glucose metabolism in early-onset dementia of Alzheimer type." J Neural Transm 75(3): 227-232.

Hoyer, S., R. Nitsch, et al. (1991). "Predominant abnormality in cerebral glucose utilization in late-onset dementia of the Alzheimer type: a cross-sectional comparison against advanced late-onset and incipient early-onset cases." J Neural Transm Park Dis Dement Sect 3(1): 1-14.

Huang, K., C. C. Zou, et al. "Carotid intima-media thickness and serum endothelial marker levels in obese children with metabolic syndrome." Arch Pediatr Adolesc Med 164(9): 846-851.

Hursting, S. D., J. A. Lavigne, et al. (2003). "Calorie restriction, aging, and cancer prevention: mechanisms of action and applicability to humans." Annual review of medicine 54: 131-152.

Iqbal, K., F. Liu, et al. (2009). "Mechanisms of tau-induced neurodegeneration." Acta Neuropathol 118(1): 53-69.

Ishii, K., M. Sasaki, et al. (1997). "Reduction of cerebellar glucose metabolism in advanced Alzheimer's disease." J Nucl Med 38(6): 925-928.

Iwangoff, P., R. Armbruster, et al. (1980). "Glycolytic enzymes from human autoptic brain cortex: normal aged and demented cases." Mech Ageing Dev 14(1-2): 203-209.

Janson, J., T. Laedtke, et al. (2004). "Increased risk of type 2 diabetes in Alzheimer disease." Diabetes 53(2): 474-481.

Kao, Y., J. H. Youson, et al. (1999). "Effects of insulin on lipid metabolism of larvae and metamorphosing landlocked sea lamprey, Petromyzon marinus." Gen Comp Endocrinol 114(3): 405-414.

Karaivazoglou, K., K. Assimakopoulos, et al. (2007). "Neuropsychological function in Greek patients with chronic hepatitis C." Liver Int 27(6): 798-805.

Kavanagh, K., K. L. Jones, et al. (2007). "Trans fat diet induces abdominal obesity and changes in insulin sensitivity in monkeys." Obesity 15(7): 1675-1684.

Kim, D., M. D. Nguyen, et al. (2007). "SIRT1 deacetylase protects against neurodegeneration in models for Alzheimer's disease and amyotrophic lateral sclerosis." EMBO J 26(13): 3169-3179.

Kincaid-Smith, P. (2004). "Hypothesis: obesity and the insulin resistance syndrome play a major role in end-stage renal failure attributed to hypertension and labelled 'hypertensive nephrosclerosis'." J Hypertens 22(6): 1051-1055.

Kopelman, M. D., A. D. Thomson, et al. (2009). "The Korsakoff syndrome: clinical aspects, psychology and treatment." Alcohol Alcohol 44(2): 148-154.

Korf, E. S., L. R. White, et al. (2006). "Brain aging in very old men with type 2 diabetes: the Honolulu-Asia Aging Study." Diabetes Care 29(10): 2268-2274.

Koulmanda, M., A. Qipo, et al. (2003). "The effect of low versus high dose of streptozotocin in cynomolgus monkeys (Macaca fascilularis)." Am J Transplant 3(3): 267-272.

Kraegen, E. W. and G. J. Cooney (2008). "Free fatty acids and skeletal muscle insulin resistance." Curr Opin Lipidol 19(3): 235-241.

Kubota, T., N. Kubota, et al. (2003). "Lack of insulin receptor substrate-2 causes progressive neointima formation in response to vessel injury." Circulation 107(24): 3073-3080.

Labak, M., T. Foniok, et al. (2010). "Metabolic changes in rat brain following intracerebroventricular injections of streptozotocin: a model of sporadic Alzheimer's disease." Acta Neurochir Suppl 106: 177-181.

Langbaum, J. B., K. Chen, et al. (2010). "Hypometabolism in Alzheimer-affected brain regions in cognitively healthy Latino individuals carrying the apolipoprotein E epsilon4 allele." Arch Neurol 67(4): 462-468.

Langeveld, M. and J. M. Aerts (2009). "Glycosphingolipids and insulin resistance." Prog Lipid Res.

Lannert, H. and S. Hoyer (1998). "Intracerebroventricular administration of streptozotocin causes long-term diminutions in learning and memory abilities and in cerebral energy metabolism in adult rats." Behav Neurosci 112(5): 1199-1208.

Larner, A. J. (1997). "The cerebellum in Alzheimer's disease." Dement Geriatr Cogn Disord 8(4): 203-209.

Launer, L. J. (2005). "Diabetes and brain aging: epidemiologic evidence." Curr Diab Rep 5(1): 59-63.

Lester-Coll, N., E. J. Rivera, et al. (2006). "Intracerebral streptozotocin model of type 3 diabetes: relevance to sporadic Alzheimer's disease." J Alzheimers Dis 9(1): 13-33.

Ling, X., R. N. Martins, et al. (2002). "Amyloid beta antagonizes insulin promoted secretion of the amyloid beta protein precursor." J Alzheimers Dis 4(5): 369-374.

Littman, A. J., A. R. Kristal, et al. (2005). "Effects of physical activity intensity, frequency, and activity type on 10-y weight change in middle-aged men and women." International journal of obesity 29(5): 524-533.

Liu, B., L. M. Obeid, et al. (1997). "Sphingomyelinases in cell regulation." Semin Cell Dev Biol 8(3): 311-322.

Loftis, J. M., M. Huckans, et al. (2008). "Depressive symptoms in patients with chronic hepatitis C are correlated with elevated plasma levels of interleukin-1beta and tumor necrosis factor-alpha." Neurosci Lett 430(3): 264-268.

Lorenzo, A. and B. A. Yankner (1996). "Amyloid fibril toxicity in Alzheimer's disease and diabetes." Ann N Y Acad Sci 777: 89-95.

Luchsinger, J. A. (2010). "Type 2 diabetes, related conditions, in relation and dementia: an opportunity for prevention?" J Alzheimers Dis 20(3): 723-736.

Luchsinger, J. A. and R. Mayeux (2004). "Cardiovascular risk factors and Alzheimer's disease." Curr Atheroscler Rep 6(4): 261-266.

Luchsinger, J. A., C. Reitz, et al. (2007). "Relation of diabetes to mild cognitive impairment." Arch Neurol 64(4): 570-575.

Lyn-Cook, L. E., Jr., M. Lawton, et al. (2009). "Hepatic ceramide may mediate brain insulin resistance and neurodegeneration in type 2 diabetes and non-alcoholic steatohepatitis." J Alzheimers Dis 16(4): 715-729.

Maisonpierre, P. C., L. Belluscio, et al. (1990). "NT-3, BDNF, and NGF in the developing rat nervous system: parallel as well as reciprocal patterns of expression." Neuron 5(4): 501-509.

Mandelkow, E. M., K. Stamer, et al. (2003). "Clogging of axons by tau, inhibition of axonal traffic and starvation of synapses." Neurobiol Aging 24(8): 1079-1085.

Marchesini, G. and R. Marzocchi (2007). "Metabolic syndrome and NASH." Clin Liver Dis 11(1): 105-117, ix.

Martins, I. J., E. Hone, et al. (2006). "Apolipoprotein E, cholesterol metabolism, diabetes, and the convergence of risk factors for Alzheimer's disease and cardiovascular disease." Mol Psychiatry 11(8): 721-736.

Matsumoto, H., T. Nakao, et al. (2005). "Insulin resistance contributes to obesity-related proteinuria." Intern Med 44(6): 548-553.

McLay, R. N., S. M. Freeman, et al. (1999). "Tests used to assess the cognitive abilities of aged rats: their relation to each other and to hippocampal morphology and neurotrophin expression." Gerontology 45(3): 143-155.

Messier, C. and K. Teutenberg (2005). "The role of insulin, insulin growth factor, and insulin-degrading enzyme in brain aging and Alzheimer's disease." Neural Plast 12(4): 311-328.

Morales, I., G. Farias, et al. (2010). "Neuroimmunomodulation in the pathogenesis of Alzheimer's disease." Neuroimmunomodulation 17(3): 202-204.

Moroz, N., M. Tong, et al. (2008). "Limited Alzheimer-type neurodegeneration in experimental obesity and Type 2 diabetes mellitus." J Alzheimers Dis 15(1): 29-44.

Mosconi, L., R. Mistur, et al. (2009). "FDG-PET changes in brain glucose metabolism from normal cognition to pathologically verified Alzheimer's disease." Eur J Nucl Med Mol Imaging 36(5): 811-822.

Mosconi, L., A. Pupi, et al. (2008). "Brain glucose hypometabolism and oxidative stress in preclinical Alzheimer's disease." Ann N Y Acad Sci 1147: 180-195.

Mudher, A., S. Chapman, et al. (2001). "Dishevelled regulates the metabolism of amyloid precursor protein via protein kinase C/mitogen-activated protein kinase and c-Jun terminal kinase." J Neurosci 21(14): 4987-4995.

Nash, D. T. and H. Fillit (2006). "Cardiovascular disease risk factors and cognitive impairment." Am J Cardiol 97(8): 1262-1265.

Nelson, P. T., C. D. Smith, et al. (2008). "Human cerebral neuropathology of Type 2 diabetes mellitus." Biochim Biophys Acta.

Newby, P. K., D. Muller, et al. (2003). "Dietary patterns and changes in body mass index and waist circumference in adults." The American journal of clinical nutrition 77(6): 1417-1425.

Nicolls, M. R. (2004). "The clinical and biological relationship between Type II diabetes mellitus and Alzheimer's disease." Curr Alzheimer Res 1(1): 47-54.

Niikura, T., Y. Hashimoto, et al. (2002). "Death and survival of neuronal cells exposed to Alzheimer's insults." J Neurosci Res 70(3): 380-391.

Nishimura, M., G. Yu, et al. (1999). "Presenilin mutations associated with Alzheimer disease cause defective intracellular trafficking of beta-catenin, a component of the presenilin protein complex." Nat Med 5(2): 164-169.

Nitta, A., R. Murai, et al. (2002). "Diabetic neuropathies in brain are induced by deficiency of BDNF." Neurotoxicol Teratol 24(5): 695-701.

Nogueira, T. C., G. F. Anhe, et al. (2008). "Involvement of phosphatidylinositol-3 kinase/AKT/PKCzeta/lambda pathway in the effect of palmitate on glucose-induced insulin secretion." Pancreas 37(3): 309-315.

Noh, M. Y., S. H. Koh, et al. (2009). "Neuroprotective effects of donepezil through inhibition of GSK-3 activity in amyloid-beta-induced neuronal cell death." Journal of neurochemistry 108(5): 1116-1125.

Oddo, S. (2008). "The ubiquitin-proteasome system in Alzheimer's disease." J Cell Mol Med 12(2): 363-373.

Pae, C. U., D. M. Marks, et al. (2008). "Does neurotropin-3 have a therapeutic implication in major depression?" Int J Neurosci 118(11): 1515-1522.

Papandreou, D., I. Rousso, et al. (2007). "Update on non-alcoholic fatty liver disease in children." Clin Nutr 26(4): 409-415.

Pasquier, F., A. Boulogne, et al. (2006). "Diabetes mellitus and dementia." Diabetes Metab 32(5 Pt 1): 403-414.

Peeyush, K. T., B. Savitha, et al. (2010). "Cholinergic, dopaminergic and insulin receptors gene expression in the cerebellum of streptozotocin-induced diabetic rats: functional regulation with Vitamin D3 supplementation." Pharmacol Biochem Behav 95(2): 216-222.

Pepeu, G. and M. G. Giovannini (2010). "Cholinesterase inhibitors and memory." Chem Biol Interact 187(1-3): 403-408.

Perry, E. K., M. A. Piggott, et al. (1993). "Transmitters in the developing and senescent human brain." Ann N Y Acad Sci 695: 69-72.

Perry, W., R. C. Hilsabeck, et al. (2008). "Cognitive dysfunction in chronic hepatitis C: a review." Dig Dis Sci 53(2): 307-321.

Pessayre, D. (2007). "Role of mitochondria in non-alcoholic fatty liver disease." J Gastroenterol Hepatol 22 Suppl 1: S20-27.

Plassman, B. L., J. W. Williams, Jr., et al. "Systematic review: factors associated with risk for and possible prevention of cognitive decline in later life." Ann Intern Med 153(3): 182-193.

Portha, B., M. H. Giroix, et al. (1980). "Diabetogenic effect of N-nitrosomethylurea and N-nitrosomethylurethane in the adult rat." Annales de la nutrition et de l'alimentation 34(5-6): 1143-1151.

Powell, D. J., E. Hajduch, et al. (2003). "Ceramide disables 3-phosphoinositide binding to the pleckstrin homology domain of protein kinase B (PKB)/Akt by a PKCzeta-dependent mechanism." Mol Cell Biol 23(21): 7794-7808.

Qin, W., M. Chachich, et al. (2006). "Calorie restriction attenuates Alzheimer's disease type brain amyloidosis in Squirrel monkeys (Saimiri sciureus)." J Alzheimers Dis 10(4): 417-422.

Qiu, C., D. De Ronchi, et al. (2007). "The epidemiology of the dementias: an update." Curr Opin Psychiatry 20(4): 380-385.

Radak, Z., N. Hart, et al. "Exercise plays a preventive role against Alzheimer's disease." J Alzheimers Dis 20(3): 777-783.

Ristow, M. (2004). "Neurodegenerative disorders associated with diabetes mellitus." J Mol Med 82(8): 510-529.

Rivera, E. J., A. Goldin, et al. (2005). "Insulin and insulin-like growth factor expression and function deteriorate with progression of Alzheimer's disease: link to brain reductions in acetylcholine." J Alzheimers Dis 8(3): 247-268.

Robertson, R. T., J. Baratta, et al. (2006). "A role for neurotrophin-3 in targeting developing cholinergic axon projections to cerebral cortex." Neuroscience 143(2): 523-539.

Rolland, Y., G. Abellan van Kan, et al. "Healthy brain aging: role of exercise and physical activity." Clin Geriatr Med 26(1): 75-87.

Schmidt, K. S., J. L. Gallo, et al. (2005). "The neuropsychological profile of alcohol-related dementia suggests cortical and subcortical pathology." Dement Geriatr Cogn Disord 20(5): 286-291.

Schubert, M., D. P. Brazil, et al. (2003). "Insulin receptor substrate-2 deficiency impairs brain growth and promotes tau phosphorylation." J Neurosci 23(18): 7084-7092.

Schubert, M., D. Gautam, et al. (2004). "Role for neuronal insulin resistance in neurodegenerative diseases." Proc Natl Acad Sci U S A 101(9): 3100-3105.

Shi, B., S. J. Rabin, et al. (1998). "Dexamethasone induces hypertrophy of developing medial septum cholinergic neurons: potential role of nerve growth factor." J Neurosci 18(22): 9326-9334.

Sims, N. R., D. M. Bowen, et al. (1980). "Glucose metabolism and acetylcholine synthesis in relation to neuronal activity in Alzheimer's disease." Lancet 1(8164): 333-336.

Soscia, S. J., M. Tong, et al. (2006). "Chronic gestational exposure to ethanol causes insulin and IGF resistance and impairs acetylcholine homeostasis in the brain." Cell Mol Life Sci 63(17): 2039-2056.

Steen, E., B. M. Terry, et al. (2005). "Impaired insulin and insulin-like growth factor expression and signaling mechanisms in Alzheimer's disease--is this type 3 diabetes?" J Alzheimers Dis 7(1): 63-80.

Summers, S. A. (2006). "Ceramides in insulin resistance and lipotoxicity." Prog Lipid Res 45(1): 42-72.

Szkudelski, T. (2001). "The mechanism of alloxan and streptozotocin action in B cells of the rat pancreas." Physiol Res 50(6): 537-546.

Takashima, A. (2009). "Amyloid-beta, tau, and dementia." J Alzheimers Dis 17(4): 729-736.

Takashima, A. (2010). "[Drug development for tauopathy and Alzheimer's disease]." Nihon Shinkei Seishin Yakurigaku Zasshi 30(4): 177-180.

Tong, M. and S. M. de la Monte (2009). "Mechanisms of ceramide-mediated neurodegeneration." J Alzheimers Dis 16(4): 705-714.

Tong, M., L. Longato, et al. (2010). "Early limited nitrosamine exposures exacerbate high fat diet-mediated type2 diabetes and neurodegeneration." BMC Endocr Disord 10(1): 4.

Tong, M., A. Neusner, et al. (2009). "Nitrosamine Exposure Causes Insulin Resistance Diseases: Relevance to Type 2 Diabetes Mellitus, Non-Alcoholic Steatohepatitis, and Alzheimer's Disease." J Alzheimers Dis.

Tran, T. M., T. Komatsu, et al. (2001). "Blood pressure, serum cholesterol concentration and their related factors in urban and rural elderly of Ho Chi Minh City." Journal of nutritional science and vitaminology 47(2): 147-155.

Tsukamoto, E., Y. Hashimoto, et al. (2003). "Characterization of the toxic mechanism triggered by Alzheimer's amyloid-beta peptides via p75 neurotrophin receptor in neuronal hybrid cells." J Neurosci Res 73(5): 627-636.

Tuppo, E. E. and H. R. Arias (2005). "The role of inflammation in Alzheimer's disease." Int J Biochem Cell Biol 37(2): 289-305.

Van Brocklyn, J. R. (2007). "Sphingolipid signaling pathways as potential therapeutic targets in gliomas." Mini Rev Med Chem 7(10): 984-990.

Verdelho, A., S. Madureira, et al. (2007). "Differential impact of cerebral white matter changes, diabetes, hypertension and stroke on cognitive performance among non-disabled elderly. The LADIS study." J Neurol Neurosurg Psychiatry 78(12): 1325-1330.

Wang, J., H. Fivecoat, et al. (2010). "The role of Sirt1: at the crossroad between promotion of longevity and protection against Alzheimer's disease neuropathology." Biochim Biophys Acta 1804(8): 1690-1694.

Watson, G. S., E. R. Peskind, et al. (2003). "Insulin increases CSF Abeta42 levels in normal older adults." Neurology 60(12): 1899-1903.

Wegiel, J., H. M. Wisniewski, et al. (1999). "Cerebellar atrophy in Alzheimer's disease-clinicopathological correlations." Brain Res 818(1): 41-50.

Weih, M., K. Abu-Omar, et al. (2009). "[Physical activity and prevention of Alzheimer's dementia: current evidence and feasibility of an interventional trial]." Fortschr Neurol Psychiatr 77(3): 146-151.

Weinstock, M. and S. Shoham (2004). "Rat models of dementia based on reductions in regional glucose metabolism, cerebral blood flow and cytochrome oxidase activity." J Neural Transm 111(3): 347-366.

Weiss, J. J. and J. M. Gorman (2006). "Psychiatric behavioral aspects of comanagement of hepatitis C virus and HIV." Curr HIV/AIDS Rep 3(4): 176-181.

Whitmer, R. A. (2007). "Type 2 diabetes and risk of cognitive impairment and dementia." Curr Neurol Neurosci Rep 7(5): 373-380.

Winocur, G. and C. E. Greenwood (2005). "Studies of the effects of high fat diets on cognitive function in a rat model." Neurobiol Aging 26 Suppl 1: 46-49.

Winocur, G., C. E. Greenwood, et al. (2005). "Memory impairment in obese Zucker rats: an investigation of cognitive function in an animal model of insulin resistance and obesity." Behav Neurosci 119(5): 1389-1395.

Wolf, S. A., G. Kronenberg, et al. (2006). "Cognitive and physical activity differently modulate disease progression in the amyloid precursor protein (APP)-23 model of Alzheimer's disease." Biol Psychiatry 60(12): 1314-1323.

Xie, L., E. Helmerhorst, et al. (2002). "Alzheimer's beta-amyloid peptides compete for insulin binding to the insulin receptor." J Neurosci 22(10): RC221.

Xu, J., J. Eun Yeon, et al. (2003). "Ethanol impairs insulin-stimulated neuronal survival in the developing brain: Role of PTEN phosphatase." J Biol Chem 278(29): 26929-26937.

Yeh, M. M. and E. M. Brunt (2007). "Pathology of nonalcoholic fatty liver disease." Am J Clin Pathol 128(5): 837-847.

21

The Relations Between the Vitamins and Alzheimer Dementia

Emel Koseoglu
Erciyes University, Medicine Faculty, Neurology Department, Kayseri Turkey

1. Introduction

The number of people suffering from dementia might triple over the next 50 years, measures for treatment and prevention of dementia are crucial. As vitamins are involved in many biochemical processes, they are essential for good health. They can possibly take role more probably in the prevention and treatment of dementia. For this reason, the relations between the vitamins and dementia, especially Alzheimer Dementia (AD) have been studied for many years.

Until the 1900s, vitamins were obtained solely through food intake, and changes in diet can alter the types and amounts of vitamins ingested. Vitamins have been produced as commodity chemicals and made widely available as inexpensive pills for several decades, allowing supplementation of dietary intake.

There are many observational studies indicating associations of vitamin deficiencies with cognitive dysfunction. Most of the studies in the subject are cross sectional studies. Nevertheless, these type of studies can not prove whether a nutritional deficit is the cause or the result of an impaired cognitive status. Longitudinal prospective observational studies and interventional studies are more suitable to releave causal relationships. Interventional studies with long follow up periods are preferred, since short follow up time can not be enough to evaluate the effects. There are some individual studies reporting promising, positive results about vitamin supplementation in prevention and treatment of dementia.

Vitamin A, C and E have antioxidant activity, which have been investigated for its prevention from neuronal death and improving neuronal function through maintaining mitochondrial homeostasis. Vitamin E may modulate signal transduction pathways and participate in the synthesis pathways of neurotransmitters. Several epidemiological studies have indicated a relationship between blood concentrations of antioxidant micronutrients and cognitive impairment. Though not sufficient, there are some prospective longitudinal and interventional studies indicating the useful effects of antioxidant vitamins in prevention and treatment of dementia.

Deficiencies of several B vitamins, including thiamine (B1), riboflavin (B2), niacin (B3), pyridoxine (B6), folate (B9) and cobalamin (B12) have been reported to be associated with cognitive dysfunction in many studies. In some studies, pathophysiological models have been formulated, including the association of B vitamin deficiencies with metabolic disturbances in the structural constituents of cerebral tissue, such as phospholipids and myelin, as well as in signaling molecules, such as neurotransmitters. More recently, the association between the deficiency of B vitamins, particularly folate and cobalamin, and cognitive impairment has been investigated in relation to hyperhomocysteinemia. It was shown that plasma homocysteine is a better correlate of cognitive function than the serum folate or cobalamin concentrations themselves. Homocysteine is a well established risk factor for vascular disease, but some epidemiological and cross sectional studies have also suggested that it may play a role in cognitive performance and pathophysiology of dementia in older people, possibly as the metabolic link between micro-vascular disease and Alzheimer dementia. Some prospective longitudinal and interventional studies have reported the useful effects of some B vitamins, though there existed contradictory results also. Furthermore, there was a large heterogenity among present vitamin B interventional studies with cognitive assessments in terms of dosage, routes of intervention (for vitamin B12), age and cognitive function assessments. It seems that it will be worthwhile to perform new larger studies, especially considering the results of the studies reporting recovering effect of folate supplementation on cognition.

The most recent reported vitamins related to cognitive functioning are vitamin D and vitamin K. Vitamin D has been reported to be critical to healthy brain development and function. Vitamin D in sufficient amounts seemed to protect brain cells and reduce inflammation according to some biological evidence. Some epidemiological and cross-sectional studies showed the association of vitamin D deficiency with Alzheimer disease and dementia. To disclose if there is a causal relationship between them, prospective longitudinal studies are needed in the subject. Vitamin K is also required for normal brain development and function. Some authors proposed a possible role of vitamin K deficiency in the pathogenesis of Alzheimer disease. It is obviously useful to do experimental animal and case controlled human studies in the first step to clarify the role of vitamin K in the pathogenesis of dementia.

In this section, we will try to discuss the relations of AD with the antioxidant vitamins, B vitamins and lastly vitamin D and K with the help of cross-sectional or longitudinal prospective observational studies, and interventional studies. Nevertheless, the subject has many aspects. As vitamin deficiencies can cause cognitive impairment, cognitive impairment can also determine changes in dietary habits and consequently cause vitamin deficiencies. Vitamin intake through food or supplementation forms can have different effects. There is also a possibility that vitamins have useful effects in different subgroups of people, based on age, nutritional status or vitamin level. Multivitamin supplementation may be more useful. Detailed investigations about these aspects will be informative.

2. Antioxidant vitamins

2.1 Pathophysiological mechanisms

Brain tissue is particularly vulnerable to free-radical damage because of its low level of endogenous antioxidants (Reiter, 1995). Neuropathological studies documented typical lesions from exposure to free radicals in the brains of patients with AD (Behl, 1997; Christen, 2000; Pratico & Delanty, 2000; Varadarajan et al., 2000). Lipid peroxidation seems to be especially susceptible to oxidative stress (Knopman, 1998; Pitchumoni et al., 1998; Sinclair et al., 1998). Increasing evidence also implicates neuronal membrane associated oxidative stress (for example, consequent to deposition of amyloid β-peptide (Aβ)) and alteration of membrane lipid metabolism (and consequent accumulation of ceramides and cholesterol) as pathogenetic factors of synaptic dysfunction and neuronal degeneration (Cutler et al., 2004; Hyun et al., 2010; L.J. Miller & Chacko, 2004). Antioxidant treatment improved neuronal function through maintaining mitochondrial homeostasis. In a canine model of human aging, it was shown that aged canine mitochondria showed significant increases in reactive oxygen species production and a reduction in NADH-linked respiration. Mitochondrial function was improved selectively in aged dogs treated with antioxidant diet (Head et al., 2009).

Vitamin A levels in brain decline with age and lower still in individuals with AD (Goodman, 2006).A metabolic product of vitamin A, retinoic acid, is known to slow cell death and offer protection from Aβ (Sahin et al., 2005). In addition to its antioxidant activity, vitamin E may modulate signal transduction pathways and participate in the synthesis pathways of neurotransmitters (Azzi et al., 1992; Martin et al., 1997; Meydani et al., 1997). Plasma vitamin C level was decreased in AD in addition to vitamin A and E (Foy et al., 1999). Vitamin C enhances the effect of medications used to treat dementia allowing the drugs to pass more easily into the brain and therefore to cause a greater effect. As a conflicting result, in the analysis of the association between the level of serum antioxidants and memory performance in an elderly, multiethnic sample of 4809 subjects; Perkins et al (Perkins et al., 1999) found a decreased serum level of vitamin E consistently associated with memory deficit after adjustment for age, education, income and vascular risk factors. Serum levels of other antioxidants (vitamins A and C, β-carotene and selenium) did not correlate with memory performance.

2.2 Studies

SENECA study reported a positive, although weak, correlation between plasma concentrations of lycopene, α- carotene, β-carotene, total carotenes, β-cryptoxanthin, α-tocopherol and Mini Mental State Examination (MMSE) scores (Haller et al., 1996). In the elderly population studied by Ortega et al., dietary intake of vitamin C, β-carotene and vitamin E were associated with a better cognitive function (Ortega et al., 2002). Perrig et al. (Perrig et al., 1997) showed that higher plasma ascorbic acid and β-carotene concentrations were associated with better memory performance in older people, both cross-sectionally and longitudinally over a 22 year period. In another cohort study performed on 455 elderly people with a duration of 7 year, high β-carotene levels were associated with less cognitive decline in APOE4 carriers but not in APOE4 negatives (Hu et al., 2006). Rats given dietary supplements of fruit and vegetable extracts for 8 months, beginning at 6 months of age, slowed age-related declines in neuronal and cognitive functions (Joseph et al., 1998). More importantly, these rats were able to reverse age-related deficits in several neuronal and behavioral parameters when administration was started at 19 months of age (Joseph et al., 1999). In another study investigating the effects of acute, short and long term pre-training administration of ascorbic acid on passive avoidance learning and memory in rats, it was concluded that short- and long-term supplementation with ascorbic acid (vitamin C) had facilitatory effects on acquisition and retrieval processes of passive avoidance learning and memory in rats (Shadidi et al., 2008).

Vitamin C supplements were shown to protect against cognitive decline in a 4 year follow up study (Paleologos et al., 1998). In Rotterdam Study (Engelhart et al., 2002), the cohort study of dietary antioxidants with a duration of 6 years, high intakes of vitamin C and E were found to be associated with lower risk of AD. In a recent study on 5395 participants older than 54 years of age and free of dementia with a mean follow up period of 9.6 years, it was shown that participants in the highest tertile of vitamin E intake were 25% less likely to develop dementia compared with those in the lowest tertile of the intake. Dietary intake levels of vitamin C, beta carotene, and flavonoids were not related with dementia risk after multivariate adjustments. Results were similar when risk for AD was specifically assessed (Devore et al., 2010). In CHAP cohort study, on 815 elderly residents free of AD at baseline with a follow up period of 3.9 years, it was found that dietary vitamin E was associated with decreased risk for AD, while intakes of vitamin C, β-carotene and vitamin E from supplements were not associated at all (M.C. Morris et al., 2002). In another study investigating the effects of high dietary intake of vitamin E on prevention from AD, it was found that α-tocopherol alone may not be as protective as the combined tocopherols (M.C. Morris et al., 2005a). In addition, the risk of AD was inversely related to the intake of α, γ and δ but not β tocopherol. It was found that higher levels of dietary vitamin E lowered the risk of AD and slowed cognitive decline over the six-year course of the investigation.

In Cache County study, performed on 3227 subjects older than 64 years of age with a follow-up period of 3 years, vitamin E and C supplements in combination were associated with reduction in AD incidence, but not in users of those supplements alone (Zandii et al., 2004). Likewise, in another cohort study with a 5 year follow-up period, conducted on 894 elderly subjects, combined use of vitamins E and C supplements were associated with less cognitive decline (Maxwell et al., 2005); while in another study performed on 2969 elderly participants without cognitive impairment at baseline, the use of supplemental vitamin E and C, alone or in combination, did not reduce risk of AD or overall dementia over 5.5 years of follow-up period (Gray et al., 2008). In spite of the successful results of dietary intake of vitamin E on the prevention, supplemental use of it alone (2000 IU/day) was not shown to have an effect on progression of minimal cognitive impairment to AD and on mean cognitive change in randomised controlled studies respectively (Kang et al., 2006; Petersen et al., 2005). In a randomised controlled study performed on 341 patients with moderate AD, the patients treated with selegiline, α-tocopherol supplement or combination of them had longer time to institutionalization (Sano et al., 1997). However, no significant benefit was shown in cognitive tests.

About the role of vitamin E in treatment, there is a safety problem other than analying its effectiveness. Recent meta-analyses of randomized trials involving vitamin E in cardiac patients and other patient groups suggest a slightly higher mortality risk associated with vitamin E treatment (Bjelokovic et al., 2007; E.R. Miller et al., 2005; Vivekananthan et al., 2003). One meta -analysis (E.R. Miller, 2005) concluded that the mortality rate associated with vitamin E treatment increased in a nonlinear dose-dependent manner, with the relative risk beginning to rise above 1 at doses ≥ 400 IU/day. In a study about this subject performed on 847 probable or mixed AD patients with a follow up period up to 15 years, there was no evidence that treatment with high doses of vitamin E (2000 IU/day)had an adverse effect on survival. In fact, patients whose regimens included vitamin E tended to survive longer than those taking no drug or a choline esterase inhibitor alone. It is noteworthy that the survival benefit to those taking vitamin E did not become apparent until after 4 or more years of follow up. In light of the potential for beneficial effects on vitamin E and mixed clinical trial evidence, these results emphasize the need for additional research on vitamin E supplementation in AD using a dose range that extends above 400 IU per day.

2.3 Comments

In conclusion, there are positive results about the use of antioxidant vitamins on mostly prevention of AD and mostly through diet. There is not sufficient evidence about their use in the treatment. In recent years, it seems that the researches on vitamin E and C have dominated. This can be due to the relation of these vitamins to the structure and physiology of brain and, more consistent finding of association between serum levels of vitamin E and memory performance in the studies. However, vitamin A is also a good candidate for more future studies.

The intake of vitamins through diet or supplementation forms and the number or quantity of different vitamins and presence of other ingredients in the supplementation forms can change the effect. For example, in the manufactured capsules of vitamin E, only α-tocopherol is present. But at real, vitamin E is composed of 4 different tocopherol forms and 4 corresponding tocotrienols. This may cause ineffectiveness of vitamin E supplementation found in some studies. Also, the interaction of antioxidant vitamins with other antioxidants like flavonoids and other chemicals present in fruits and vegetables can provide benefit in the dietary intake of vitamins.

3. B vitamins

3.1 Pathophysiological mechanisms

Deficiencies of several B vitamins, including thiamine (B1), riboflavin (B2), niasin (B3), pyridoxine (B6), folate (B9) and cobalamin (B12), have been related with cognitive dysfunction in many observational study (Riedel et al., 1998). In some studies, pathophysiological models have been formulated, including the association of B vitamin deficiencies with metabolic disturbances in the structural constituents of cerebral tissue, such as phospholipids and myelin, as well as in signaling molecules, such as neurotransmitters (Rampersaud et al., 2003). In particular, thiamine deficiency has been associated with lactic acid accumulation, reduction in oxygen uptake, decrease in transketolase activity, and an impairment in cholinergic activity, leading to the loss of memory and other cognitive functions (Micheau et al., 1985). Cobalamin is essential for neuronal generation and its deficiency can cause degeneration of the nervous system (Herrmann & Obeid, 2007). Various cobalamines were shown to have intracellular antioxidant activity in vitro. The compounds inhibited intracellular peroxide production, maintained intracellular glutathione levels, and prevented apoptotic and necrotic cell death (Birch et al., 2009). Folic acid plays an important role in neuroplasticity and in the maintenance of neuronal integrity (Kronenberg et al., 2009). It enhances the plasma concentrations of docosahexaenoic acid (DHA) and eicosapentaenoic acid (EPA). EPA, DHA, and arachidonic acid are of benefit in dementia by up-regulating gene expression concerned with neurogenesis, neurotransmission and connectivity, improving endothelial nitric oxide (eNO) generation, enhancing brain acetylcholine levels, suppressing the production of proinflammatory cytokines and precursing to anti-inflammatory compounds that protect neurons from cytotoxic action of various noxious stimuli, oxidative stress and neuronal apoptosis (Das, 2008).

Recently, the association between the deficiency of B vitamins, particularly folate and cobalamin, and cognitive impairment has been investigated in relation to hyperhomocysteinemia (hHcy). Several epidemiological studies have also suggested that hHcy may play a role in the cognitive performance (Prins ND, 2002) and pathophysiology of dementia in older people (Bell et al, 1992; Nilsson et al., 1996; Wahlin et al., 1996), possibly as the metabolic link between micro-vascular disease and old-age dementia (M.S. Morris et al., 2001; Parnetti et al., 1997). Feeding mice with a B-vitamin deficient diet for 10 weeks induced hHcy, significantly impaired learning and memory, and caused a significant rarefaction of hippocampal microvasculature unrelated to gliosis and neurodegeneration (Troen et al., 2008).

Homocystein (Hcy) is an aminoacid entirely derived from the body's intermediary metabolism (Fekkes et al., 1998; Pietrzik & Bronstrup, 1997), which can be converted to either methionine or cysteine. Both folate and cobalamin participate in the methylation of Hcy to methionine and in the remethylation and synthesis of S-adenosylmethionine (Bottiglieri, 1996; Parnetti et al., 1997). The other metabolic pathway, which converts Hcy to cysteine requires the active form of vitamin B6 (pyridoxal phosphate) (Pietrzik & Bronstrup, 1997). The most common cause of hHcy is accepted to be a deficiency of folate or cobalamin (Selhub, 2000). Almost two-thirds of the prevalance of hHcy is attributable to low vitamin B status or intake (Selhub J, 2008). Although the catabolic rate of Hcy results from the interaction between genetic make-up and B vitamin status, it is generally accepted that elevated plasma Hcy concentrations are a sensitive marker for folate and cobalamin tissue deficiency (Bottiglieri, 1996; Joosten et al., 1993; Lokk, 2003; McCaddon et al., 1998; Nilsson et al., 1996; Nilsson et al., 1999; Parnetti et al., 1997).

Folate and vitamin B12 are essential cofactors for the methionine/Hcy cycle in the brain. These vitamins mediate the remethylation of Hcy, which affects the production of the universal methyl donor, S-adenosylmethionine, in the brain among other organs. Hypomethylation, caused by low B-vitamin and hHcy, is linked to key pathomechanisms of dementia (Obeid et al., 2007). Also, Hcy is recognised to be proatherogenic and protrombotic (Hassan et al., 2004) and accepted to be an independent risk for developing occlusive arterial diseases (Refsum et al., 1998; Ueland & Refsum, 1989). hHcy exerts an inhibitory effect on adult mouse brain neurogenesis (Rabaneda et al., 2008). Low folate status and elevated Hcy increase the generation of reactive oxygen species and contribute to excitotoxicity and mitochondrial dysfunction which may lead to apoptosis (Kronenberg et al., 2009). hHcy is also proposed to be one of the effects of the oxidation of vitamin B12, as a result of oxidative stress (McCaddon et al., 2002). Furthermore, experimental studies in cell cultures have shown that Hcy is neurotoxic, possibly by activating N-methyl-D-aspartate receptors (Lipton et al., 1997) or DNA damage and consequent apoptosis (Kruman et al., 2000). In a population based study on 1779 subjects, hHcy has been reported to be an independent risk factor for dementia and cognitive impairment without dementia (Haan et al., 2007).

Depending on the used marker, 3-60 % of the elderly are classified as vitamin B12 deficient and about 29 % as folate deficient. Predominantly, the high prevalance of poor cobalamin status is caused by the increasing prevalance of atrophic gastritis type B, which occurs with a frequency of approximately 20-50% in elderly subjects (Wolters et al., 2004). Another cause of atropfic gastritis is long term treatment with proton pump inhibitors (Kuipers et al., 1995,1996; Lundell et al., 2006). Atrophic gastritis results in declining gastric acid and pepsinogen secretion, and hence decreasing intestinal digestion and absorption of both B vitamins. Such patients with atrophic gastritis require parenteral supplements. Folic acid intake among elderly subjects is generally well below the recommended dietary reference values (Wolters et al., 2004). So, folic acid deficiency is primarily caused by dietary deficiency. Meanwhile, vitamin B12 deficiency is due to two main causes, food cobalamin malabsorption and pernicious anemia (Andres et al., 2004).

3.2 Studies

Many epidemiological, cross-sectional and case control studies reported the association of dementia with low blood levels of vitamin B12 and folate or hHcy. Hovewer, these studies are unable to exclude the possibility that such associations of hHcy or vitamin B deficiencies are rather a result than a cause of the disease.

Kivipelto M et al (Kivipelto et al., 2009), in their prospective study found that persons with high Hcy had more than twice as high a risk of developing AD than persons with low Hcy, even after adjusting for confounding or mediating factors, suggesting that Hcy is involved in the development of dementia and AD. Vitamin B12 itself seemed not to be directly involved, because holo-transcobalamin showed no association with dementia. In some cohort studies, hHcy was found to be correlated with decline in constructional praxis and recall memory (Tucker et al., 2005) and increased risk for dementia (Dufoil et al., 2003; Haan et al., 2007; Ravaglia et al., 2005; Seshadri et al., 2002; McCaddon et al., 2001), while in some others it was not correlated with cognitive decline (Clarke et al., 2007; Kalmijn et al., 1999; Luchsinger et al., 2004; Mooijaart et al., 2005; Teunissen et al., 2003). In the cohort studies, low plasma level of folate was found to be associated with decline in constructional praxis and lower cognitive function regardless of Hcy respectively (de Lau et al., 2007; Tucker et al., 2005). In another cohort study performed on 370 non demented persons older than 74 years of age, persons with low serum level of vitamin B12 or folate had the risk of developing AD (Wang et al., 2001). In addition to low folate and high Hcy plasma levels, low plasma concentration of vitamin B12 was also associated with decline of constructional praxis in a 3 year cohort study (Tucker et al., 2005).

Cohort studies of dietary intake of B vitamins in healthy elderly persons revealed conflicting results. In one of them, dietary intake was found to be not related with the risk of developing AD (MC Morris, 2006a). In another, the highest quartile of total folate intake was related to lower risk of AD (Luchsinger et al., 2007), while the other reported that rate of cognitive decline among persons in the top folate intake was more than twice that of those in the lowest fifth of intake (MC Morris et al., 2005b).

Despite potential benefits of vitamin B supplementation for lowering Hcy, the positive contribution of this supplementation to cognitive function among demented and non-demented persons remains debatable. There was a large heterogeneity among present vitamin B interventional studies with cognitive assessments in terms of dosage, routes of intervention (for vitamin B12), age and cognitive function assessments.

It has been proven that folate supplementation reduces plasma Hcy levels. This was observed by Jacques et al. in the Framingham Offspring Study cohort, after the folate fortification of grain in the Unites States started in January 1998 (Jacques et al., 1999). Nevertheless, the relationship between dietary folic acid intakes and plasma Hcy concentrations seems to be characterized by a threshold effect (Selhub, 1993): above a certain dosage of folate supplementation, there is no additional effect on lowering circulating Hcy. It is not clear where this threshold stands: a metanalysis of 12 randomized controlled trials assessed that the minimum dosage of folate capable of determining a maximum reduction (about %25) of circulating Hcy was 0.5 mg/day. More recent randomized trials determined this threshold at 0.8 mg/day (Wald et al., 2001) or 0.4 mg/day (van Oort et al., 2003). The differences are possibly explained by population selection biases (van Oort et al., 2003).

Some randomised controlled trials, including persons with normal cognitive function, cognitive impairment and dementia, evaluated the effect of folate supplementation on cognitive function. Among cognitively impaired subjects (n=30) with low folate serum levels, Fioravanti et al (Fioravanti et al., 1998) observed a significant improvement of some scores of the Randt Memory Test in the folate treated group compared with the placebo group after 60 days of treatment. In another trial using a mixed factorial design in normal subjects (n=211), the authors observed that folate-treated older women's cognitive test scores (Rey Auditory-Verbal Learning Test) improved (Bryan et al., 2002). Controversially, in another small study including 7 subjects with dementia reported no statistically significant differences between the supplemented group and the control group, and noted a negative trend in specific test scores of the supplemented group (Sommer et al., 2003). Because of the small number of subjects, study results need to be interpreted cautiously. Finally, the 3-year randomised controlled FACIT trial included 818 older subjects (older than 60 years) with augmented plasma total Hcy and normal serum vitamin B12 levels. The effect of folic acid supplementation on cognition was the secondary end point. The 3-year change in memory, information processing speed and sensorimotor speed were significantly improved in the folic acid group in comparison to the placebo group (Durga et al., 2007). Folic acid potentiated the effect of memantine on spatial learning and neuronal protection in an AD transgenic model (Chen et al., 2010).

Some other randomised controlled studies assessed the effect of vitamin B12 intervention on cognitive functions in humans. There is a large heterogeneity among trials regarding the cognitive status of participants, the doses and administration routes of vitamin B12, the duration of supplementation and the applied cognitive function assessment instruments. Sample sizes ranged from 18 to 78 subjects receiving vitamin B12, and the duration of supplementation ranged from 4 weeks to 6 months. For most cognitive tests, there was no significant improvement in vitamin B12 supplemented patients as compared with the placebo group (Eussen et al., 2006; Hvas et al., 2004; Stoot et al., 2008). However, Bryan J et al found that healthy younger, middle-aged and older women (n=211) who took vitamin B12 (or either of folate and vitamin B6) for 35 days showed better performance on some measures of memory performance compared to placebo (Bryan et al., 2002). Interestingly, a statistically significant worsening of cognitive tests was reported in two studies. In 195 vitamin B12 deficient subjects of normal and impaired cognition, Eussen et al (Eussen et al., 2006) observed that improvement of the cognitive test score in the placebo group was significantly more marked than that of the vitamin B12 group. Similarly, another study reported a significant worsening of the '12 words learning test' score in a vitamin B12 treated population of 140 old patients with cognitive impairment and methylmalonic acidemia, in comparison to the placebo group (Hvas et al., 2004). For reasons of heterogeneity of these controlled trials, no reasonable conclusion can be drawn regarding the effects of vitamin B12 on cognition. In addition, several uncontrolled cohort studies assessed the effects of vitamin B12 intervention on cognitive function in humans with conflicting results.

A few studies (Lewerin et al., 2005; McMahon et al., 2006; Stott et al., 2005; van Uffelen et al., 2007) reported data of combined B vitamin intervention on cognition, in subjects with normal cognition, dementia or vascular disease (17-409 participants). Trial durations ranged from 12 weeks to 2 years. One study found a significant improvement in one of eight cognitive tests (Reitan trail-making test, part B) (McMahon et al., 2006). In a recent randomized, double-blind controlled study in 271 individuals over 70 years old with mild cognitive deficit, high dose B vitamins lowering Hcy level slowed the rate of accelerated brain atrophy, which was found to be major determinant of cognitive decline in this population (Smith et al., 2010). It was reported that trials were needed to see if the same treatment will delay the development of AD (Smith et al., 2010).

3.3 Comments

Most studies reporting associations between cognitive function and Hcy or B vitamins have used a cross-sectional or case-control design and have been unable to exclude the possibility that such associations are a result of the disease rather than being causal. The prospective study indicating that persons with high Hcy have more than twice as high as developing AD than persons with low Hcy, even after adjusting for confounding or mediating factors, is an important one. The Hcy hypothesis of dementia has attracted considerable interest, as Hcy can be easily lowered by folic acid and vitamin B12, raising the prospect that B-vitamin supplementation could lower the risk of dementia (Clarke et al., 2008). While some trials assessing effects on cognitive function have used folic acid alone, vitamin B12 alone or a combination, few trials have included a sufficient number of participants to provide reliable evidence. Among these studies, FACIT Trial (Durga et al., 2007) is an outstanding one. This large, randomised and controlled trial on elderly participants with high plasma Hcy and normal vitamin B12 serum level have showed that folic acid supplementation improved several cognitive domains that tend to decline with advancing age. Therefore, folate supplementation may be an interesting approach to prevent cognitive decline in elderly people. New trials with larger number of participants are needed to test the importance of vitamin B intake through diet or supplementation forms in the prevention and treatment of AD.

4. Vitamin D

Vitamin D exhibits functional attributes that may prove neuroprotective through antioxidative mechanisms, neuronal calcium regulation, immunomodulation, enhanced nerve conduction and detoxification mechanisms. Compelling evidence supports a beneficial role for the active form of vitamin D in developing brain as well as in adult brain function. The vitamin D receptor and, biosynthetic and degredative pathways for the hydroxylation of vitamin D have been found in the rodent brain; more recently these findings have been confirmed in humans. The vitamin D receptor and catalytic enzymes are colocalized in the areas of the brain involved in complex planning, processing, and the formation of new memories. These findings potentially implicate vitamin D in neurocognitive function (Buell & Dawson-Hughes, 2008).

Treatment with 1,25 $(OH)_2D_3$ attenuated hippocampal atrophy and protected neuron density (a marker for neuronal death) in aging rats (Landfield & Cadwalleder-Neal, 1998). Data in human subjects with AD revealed a reduction in VDR mRNA in specific regions of the hippocampus (CA1 and CA2) compared to controls (Sutherland et al., 1992) and a higher frequency of VDR polymorphisms were found in Alzheimer's brains than age-matched controls (Gezen-Ak et al., 2007).

Low serum levels of 25(OH)D have been associated with increased risk for cardiovascular diseases, diabetes mellitus, depression, dental caries, osteoporosis, and periodontal disease, all of which are either considered risk factors for dementia or have preceded incidence of dementia. There is a higher prevalence of falls and fractures in patients with AD (Buchner & Larson, 1987) and community studies have shown that residents with AD and dementia had lower serum concentrations of 25(OH)D (Kipen et al., 1995). While the temporal associations of these findings remains unclear, in a study in patients with AD, 25(OH)D concentrations were significantly elevated after year-round sun exposure. Additionally, the sun- exposed cohort had a reduced risk of falls and fractures compared to the unexposed (Sato et al., 2005).

Data from the Nutrition and Memory in Elderly study (NAME) (Scott et al., 2004) supported these findings. In subjects (n=318) who completed a full neurological and psychiatric examination, in addition to magnetic resonance imaging, it was observed that vitamin D concentrations were lower in patients with dementia than those without. Additionally, vitamin D concentrations lesser than 50 nmol/L were associated with a higher prevalence of a diagnosis of possible or probable AD. In a recent cross-sectional investigation of vitamin D, dementia and MRI measures of cerebrovascular disease among 318 participants, mean vitamin D concentrations were lower in subjects with dementia. There was a higher prevalence of dementia, large vessel infarcts and increased white matter hyperintensity volume among participants with vitamin D insufficiency. After adjustment for age, race, sex, bodymass index, and education, vitamin D insufficiency was associated with more than twice the odds of all cause dementia, AD and stroke (Buell et al., 2010). Based on increasing number of studies linking the risk factors of AD with vitamin D deficiency, Grant WB (Grant, 2009) states that there are established criteria for causality in a biological system. The important criteria include strength of association, consistency of findings, determination of the dose-response relation, an understanding of the mechanisms, and experimental verification. Grant WB (Grant, 2009) suggests that further investigation of possible direct or indirect linkages between vitamin D and dementia is needed. Studies of incidence of dementia with respect to prediagnostic serum 25(OH)D or of vitamin D supplementation are warranted. In addition, since the elderly are generally vitamin D deficient and since vitamin D has so many health benefits, those over the age of 60 years should consider having their serum 25(OH)D tested, looking for a level of at least 30 ng/ml but preferably over 40 ng/ml, and supplementing with 1000-2000 IU/day of vitamin D3 or increased time in the sun spring, summer, and fall if below those values (Grant, 2009).

5. Vitamin K

Vitamin K is necessary for the liver functioning. Vitamin K dependent γ-carboxylation of glutamate takes part in formation of the coagulation factors 2, 7, 9 and 10. More recently, it has been established that vitamin K dependent γ-carboxylation of glutamate occurs also in extrahepatic sites and modifies proteins with other functions. One of these sites is brain. Allison AC (Allison, 2001) proposed a possible role of vitamin K deficiency in the pathogenesis of AD and in augmenting brain damage associated with cerebrovascular disease, based on the potential actions of vitamin K in the brain and through a link to the apolipoprotein E genotype. The apolipoprotein E4 allele, an established risk factor for AD (Mattson, 2004), strongly influences plasma vitamin K levels (Kohlmeier M, 1996; Saupe J, 1993). Thus, carriers of apolipoprotein E4 allele could also those with the lowest vitamin K concentrations, an association that has not yet been investigated. Vitamin K is required for normal brain development and function. The maternal exposure to coumarin derivatives is associated with abnormalities of the central nervous system (Pauli & Haun, 1979). Vitamin K deficiency is associated with decrased sulfation in the brain. Keratan sulfate is dramatically decreased in cerebral cortex of AD patients (Lindahl, 1996). Considering keratan sulfate proteoglycan being the major protein of synaptic vesicles (Scranton et al., 1993), one manifestation of decreased sulfation can be abnormal structure and function of the major protein of synaptic vesicles (Allison, 2001). Likewise, addition of vitamin K to the chick embriyo increases tyrosine phosphorylation in the brain adhesion and cytoskletal proteins (Saxena et al., 1997), suggesting that vitamin K plays an role in the development of the

central nervous system. Another vitamin K dependent protein in the brain is Gas 6, a product of growth arrest specific gene 6. Both Gas 6 and its tyrosine kinase receptor are widely distributed throughout the central nervous system (Prieto et al., 1999). Interaction of these plays an important role in preventing neurons from apoptosis (Allen et al., 1999). Cell culture studies have shown that Gas 6 can rescue cortical neurons from Aβ induced apoptosis (Yagami et al., 2002) and provided evidence that vitamin K can have a protective role against oxidative injury in developing oligodendrocytes and neurons (Denisova & Booth, 2005).
Considering that a relative deficiency of vitamin K, affecting the extrahepatic functions of the vitamin, is common in aging men and women; Allison AC (Allison, 2001) suggests that it is obviously useful to do experimental animal and case controlled human studies in the first step to clarify the role of vitamin K in the pathogenesis of dementia. In a likely study, low vitamin K intakes in 31 community-dwelling elders at an early stage of AD was detected in comparison to 31 age and sex matched cognitively intact control subjects (Presse et al., 2008).

6. Multi-intervention

Due to the fact that the interventional trials with antioxidants and B-vitamins did not hold the expectations, studies combining micronutriens are of particular interest. To date, a few prospective studies estimating the effect of nutrition and vitamin supplementation exist. One of these studies (Wolters et al., 2005) was performed on 220 healthy, free living women older than 60 years of age. After taking multivitamins (containing 8 vitamins and 4 minerals) for 6 months daily, no change on cognitive performance was observed as compared to placebo. The intervention period of only 6 months may be too short for improving cognitive performance in well-educated elderly women without dementia. Another study (McNeill et al., 2007) was performed on 910 healthy men and women aged 65 years and over. Four hundred and fifty six of them were on active daily treatment with 11 vitamins and 5 minerals for 12 months, while the remaining ones took placebo. Benefit was detected only on verbal fluency tests in the subgroups of participants aged over 74 years or those with increased risk of micronutrient deficiency. In a 12 month, open label trial with 14 mild AD patients, the efficacy of a multi-component formulation showed promising results regarding neuropsychiatric inventory and activities of daily living (Chan et al., 2008). This was confirmed by placebo-controlled data from 12 institutionalized patients with moderate to severe AD showing improvement in cognition, mood, and daily function (Remington et al., 2009). As a result, to draw any conclusion, larger randomized controlled studies with combined supplements are needed, especially in the context that multi-component dietary approaches such as Mediterranean diet or fruit and vegetable (or juice) consumption have been shown to be successful (Barberger-Gateau et al, 2007; Dai et al., 2006; MC Morris et al., 2006b; Scarmeas et al., 2006, 2009).

7. Conclusion

There is a relationship of levels of antioxidant vitamins and B vitamins to vascular dementia. Nevertheless, if this relationship is based on causality, it is not so clear after performed longitudinal and interventional studies. New trials with larger number of participants will be more clarifying. Recently, vitamin D deficiency has been found to be related with AD. Longitudinal and interventional studies, especially with long follow up period, will be informative about its role. Additionally, vitamin K is thought to have a possible role in the pathogenesis of dementia.

The subject has multiple aspects. As vitamin deficiencies can cause cognitive impairment, cognitive impairment can also determine changes in dietary habits and consequently cause vitamin deficiencies. Vitamin intake through diet or supplementation forms can have different effects. There is also a possibility that vitamins have useful effects in different subgroups of people, based on age, nutritional status or vitamin level. Multivitamin supplementation may be more useful. The roles of vitamins in dementia are not clear yet as those of macronutrients in spite of the reports expressing the benefits of caloric restriction and intake of higher unsaturated fatty acids on cognitive functions. Presence of relationships between macronutrients and vitamins is also possible. Detailed investigations about these aspects will be informative.

8. References

Allen MP, Zeng C, Schneider K, Xiong X, Meintzer MK, Bellosta P, Basilico C, Varnum B, Heidenreich KA & Wierman ME. (1999). Growth arrest-specific gene 6 (gas6)/adhesion related kinase (Ark) signaling promotes gonadotropin-releasing hormone neuronal survival via extracellular signal related kinase (ERK) and Akt. *Mol Endocrinol*, Vol.13, No.2, (February 1999), pp. 191-201, ISSN 0888-8809.

Allison AC. (2001). The possible role of vitamin K deficiency in the pathogenesis of Alzheimer's disease and in augmenting brain damage associated with cardiovascular disease. *Medical Hypothesis*, Vol.57, No.2, (August 2001), pp. 151-5, ISSN 0306-9877.

Andres E, Loukili NH, Noel E, Kaltenbach G, Abdelgheni MB, Perrin AE, Noblet-Dick M, Maloisel F, Schlienger JL & Blickle JF. (2004). Vitamin B12 (cobalamin) deficiency in elderly patients. *CMAJ*, Vol.171, No.3, (August 2004), pp. 251-9, ISSN 0820-3946.

Azzi A, Boscoboinik D & Hensey C. (1992). The protein kinase C family. *Eur J Biochem*, Vol.208, No.3, (September 1992), pp. 547-57, ISSN 0014-2956.

Barberger-Gateau P, Raffaitin C, Letenneur L, Berr C, Tzourio C, Dartigues JF & Alperovitch A. (2007). Dietary patterns and risk of dementia: the three-city cohort study. *Neurology*, Vol.69, No.20, (November 2007), pp. 1921-30, ISSN 0028-3878.

Behl C. (1997). Amyloid beta-protein toxicity and oxidative stres in Alzheimer's disease. *Cell Tissue Res*, Vol.290, No.3, (December 1997), pp. 471-80, ISSN 0302-766X.

Bell IR, Edman JS, Selhub J, Morrow FD, Marby DW, Kayne HL & Cole JO. (1992). Plasma homocysteine in vascular disease and in non-vascular dementia of depressed elderly people. *Acta Psychiatr Scand*, Vol.86, No.5, (November 1992), pp. 386-90, ISSN 0001-690X.

Birch CS, Brach NE, McCaddon A & Williams JH. (2009). A novel role for vitamin B(12): Cobalamins are intracellular antioxidants in vitro. *Free Radic Biol Med*, Vol.47, No.2, (July 2009), pp.184-8, ISSN 0891-5849.

Bjelakovic G, Nikolova D, Gluud LL, Simonetti RG & Gluud C. (2007). Mortality in randomized trials of antioxidant supplements for primary and secondary prevention: systematic review and meta-analysis. *JAMA*, Vol.297, No.8, (February 2007), pp. 842-57, ISSN 0098-7484.

Bottiglieri T. (1996). Folate, vitamin B12, and neuropsychiatric disorders. *Nutr Rev*, Vol.54, No.12, (December 1996), pp. 382-90, ISSN 0029-6643.

Bryan J, Calvaresi E & Hughes D. (2002). Short-term folate, vitamin B-12 or vitamin B-6 supplementation slightly affects memory performance but not mood in women of various ages. *J Nutr*, Vol.132, No.6, (June 2002), pp. 1345-56, ISSN 0022-3166.

Buchner DM & Larson EB. (1987). Falls and fractures in patients with Alzheimer-type dementia. *JAMA*, Vol.257, No.11, (March 1987), pp. 1492-5, ISSN 0098-7484.

Buell JS & Dawson-Hughes B. (2008). Vitamin D and neurocognitive dysfunction: Preventing Decline? *Molecular Aspects of Medicine*, Vol.29, No.6, (December 2008), pp. 415-22, ISSN 0098-2997.

Buell JS, Dawson-Hughes B, ScottTM, Weiner DE, Dallal GE, Qui WQ, Bergethon P, Rosenberg IH, Folstein MF, Patz S, Bhadelia RA & Tucker KL. (2010). 25-Hydroxyvitamin D, dementia, and cerebrovascular pathology in elders receiving home services. *Neurology*, Vol.74, No.1, (January 2010), pp. 18-26, ISSN 0028-3878.

Chen TF, Huang RF, Lin SE, Lu JF, Tang MC & Chiu MJ. (2010). Folic acid potentiates the effect of memantine on spatial learning and neuronal protection in an Alzheimer's disease transgenic model. *J Alzheimers Dis*, Vol.20, No.2, pp.607-15, ISSN 1387-2877.

Christen Y. (2000). Oxidative stress and Alzheimer disease. *Am J Clin Nutr*, Vol.71, No.2, (February 2000), pp.S621-9, ISSN 0002-9165.

Clarke R, Birks J, Nexo E, Ueland PM, Schneede J, Scott J, Molloy A & Evans JG. (2007). Low vitamin B-12 status and risk of cognitive decline in older adults. *Am J Clin Nutr*, Vol.86, No.5, (November 2007),pp. 1384-91, ISSN 0002-9165.

Cutler RG, Kelly J, Storie K, Pedersen WA, Tammara A, Hatanpaa K, Troncoso JC, Mattson MP. (2004). Involvement of oxidative stres-induced abnormalities in ceramide and cholesterol metabolism in brain aging and Alzheimer's disease. *Proc Natl Acad Sci USA*, Vol.101, No.9, (February 2009), pp. 2070-5, ISSN 0027-8424.

Dai Q, Borenstein AR, Wu Y, Jackson JC & Larson EB. (2006). Fruit and vegetable juices and Alzheimer's disease: the Kame Project. *Am J Med*, Vol.119, No.9, (September 2006), pp. 751-9, ISSN 0002-9343.

Das UN. (2008). Folic acid and polyunsaturated fatty acids improve cognitive function and prevent depression, dementia, and Alzheimer's disease-but how and why? *Prostaglandins Leukot Essent Fatty Acids*, Vol.78, No.1, (January 2008), pp. 11-9, ISSN 0952-3278.

de Lau LM, Refsum H, Smith AD, Johnston C & Breteler MM. (2007). Plasma folate concentration and cognitive performance: Rotterdam Scan Study. *Am J Clin Nutr*, Vol.86, No.3, (September 2007), pp. 728-34, ISSN 0002-9165.

Denisova NA, Booth SL. (2005). Vitamin K and sphingolipid metabolism: Evidence to date. *Nutr Rev*, Vol.63, No.4, (July 2010), pp. 111-21, ISSN 0029-6643.

Devore EE, Grodstein F, van Rooij FJA & Hofman A. (2010). Dietary antioxidants and long term risk of dementia. *Arch Neurol*, Vol.67, No.7, (July 2010), pp. 819-25, ISSN 0002-9262.

Dufouil C, Alperovitch A, Ducros V & Tzourio C. (2003). Homocysteine, white matter hyperintensities, and cognition in healthy elderly people. *Ann Neurol*, Vol.53, No.2, (February 2003), pp. 214-21, ISSN 0364-5134.

Durga J, van Boxtel MP, Schouten EG, Kok FJ, Jolles J, Katan MB & Verhoef P. (2007). Effect of 3-year folic acid supplementation on cognitive function in older adults in the FACIT trial: a randomised, double blind, controlled trial. *Lancet*, Vol.369, No.9557, (January 2007), pp. 208-16, ISSN 0140-6736.

Engelhart MJ, Geerlings MI, Ruitenberg A, van Switen JC, Hofman A, Witteman JC & Breteler MM. (2002). Dietary intake of antioxidants and risk of Alzheimer disease. *JAMA*, Vol.287, No.24, (June 2002), pp. 3223-9, ISSN 0098-7484.

Eussen SJ, de Groot LC, Joosted LW, Bloo RJ, Clarke R, Ueland PM, Schneede J, Blom HJ, Hoefnagels WH & van Staveren WA. (2006). Effect of oral vitamin B-12 with or without folic acid on cognitive function in older people with mild vitamin B-12 deficiency: a randomised, placebo controlled trial. *Am J Clin Nutr*, Vol.84, No.2, (August 2006), pp. 361-70, ISSN 0002-9165.

Fekkes D, van der Cammen TJ, Van Loon CP, Verschoor C, van Harskamp F, de KI, Schudel WJ & Pepplinkhuizen L. (1998). Abnormal amino acid metabolism in patients with early stage Alzheimer dementia. *J Neural Transm*, Vol.105, No.2-3, pp. 287-94, ISSN 0300-9564.

Fioravanti M, Ferrario E, Massaia M, Cappa G, Rivolta G, Grossi E & Buckley AE. (1998). Low folate levels in the cognitive decline of elderly patients and the efficacy of folate as a treatment for imprpving memory deficits. *Arch Gerontol Geriatr*, Vol.26, No.1, (January-February 1998), pp. 1-13, ISSN 0167-4943.

Foy CJ, Passmore AP, Vahidassr MD, Young IS & Lawson JT. (1999). Plasma chain-breaking antioxidants in Alzheimer's disease, vascular dementia and Parkinson's disease. *Q J Med*, Vol.92, No.1, (January 1999), pp. 39-45, ISSN 0033-5622.

Gezen-Ak D, Dursun E, Ertan T, Hanagasi H, Gürvit H, Emre M, Eker E, Ozturk M, Engin F & Yilmazer S. (2007). Association between vitamin D receptor gene polymorphism and Alzheimer's disease. *Tohoku J Exp Med*, Vol.212, No.3, (July 2007), pp. 275-82, ISSN 0040-8727.

Goodman AB. (2006). Retinoid receptors, transporters, and metabolizers as therapeutic targets in late onset Alzheimer disease. *J Cell Physiol*, Vol.209, No.3, (December 2006), pp. 598-603, ISSN 0021-9541.

Grant WB. (2009). Does vitamin D reduce the risk of dementia? *J Alzheimers Dis*, Vol.17, No.1, pp. 151-9, ISSN 1387-2877.

Gray SL, Anderson ML, Crane PK, Breitner JC, McCormick W, Bowen JD, Teri L & Larson E. (2008). Antioxidant vitamin supplement use and risk of dementia or Alzheimer's disease in older adults. *J Am Geriatr Soc*, Vol.56, No.2, (February 2008), pp. 291-5, ISSN 0002-8614.

Haan MN, Miller JW, Aiello AE, Whitmer RA, Jagust WJ, Mungas DM, Allen LH & Green R. (2007). Homocysteine, B vitamins, and the incidence of dementia and cognitive impairment: results from the Sacramento Area Latino Study on Aging. *Am J Clin Nutr*, Vol.85, No.2, (February 2007), pp. 511-7, ISSN 0002-9165.

Haller J, Weggemans RM, Lammi-Keefe CJ & Ferry M. (1996). Changes in the vitamin status of elderly Europeans: plasma vitamins A, E, B-6, B-12, folic acid and carotenoids. *Eur J Clin Nutr*, Vol.50, No. Suppl 2, (July 1996), pp. S32-36, ISSN 0954-3007.

Hassan A, Hunt BJ, O'Sullivan M, Bell R, D'Souza R, Jeffery S, Bamford JM, Markus HS. (2004). Homocysteine is a risk factor for cerebral small vessel disease acting via endothelial function. *Brain*, Vol.127, No.1, (January 2004), pp. 212-9, ISSN 0006-8950.

Head E, Nukala VN, Fenoglio KA, Muggenburg BA, Cotman CW & Sullivan PG. (2009). Effects of age, dietary, and behavioral enrichment on brain mitochondria in a canine model of human aging. *Exp Neurol,* Vol.220, No.1, (November 2009), pp. 171-6, ISSN 0014-4886.

Herrmann W, Obeid R. (2007). Biomarkers of folate and vitamin B(12) status in cerebrospinal fluid. *Clin Chem Lab Med,* Vol.45, No.12, pp. 1614-20, ISSN 1434-6621.

Hu P, Bretsky P, Crimmins EM, Guralnik JM, Reuben DM & Seeman TE. (2006). Association between serum beta-carotene levels and decline of cognitive function in high-functioning older persons with or without apolipoprotein E4 alleles: MacArthur studies of successful aging. *J Gerontol A Biol Sci Med Sci,* Vol.61, No.6, (June 2006), pp. 616-20, ISSN 1079-5006.

Hvas AM, Juul S, Lauritzen L, Nexo E & Ellegaard J. (2004). No effect of vitamin B-12 treatment on cognitive function and depression: a randomized placebo controlled study. *J Affect Disord,* Vol.81, No.3, (September 2004), pp. 269-73, ISSN 0165-0327.

Hyun DH, Mughal MR, Yang H, Lee JH, Ko EJ, Hunt ND, de Cabo R, Mattson MP. (2010). The plasma membrane redox system is impaired by amyloid β-peptide in the hippocampus and cerebral cortex of 3xTgAD mice. *Exp Neurol,* Vol.225, No.2, (October 2010), pp. 423-9, ISSN 0014-4886.

Jacques PF, Selhub J, Bostom AG, Wilson PW & Rosenberg IH. (1999). The effect of folic acid fortification on plasma folate and total homocysteine concentrations. *N Eng J Med,* Vol.340, No.19, (May 1999), pp. 1449-54, ISSN 0028-4793.

Joosten E, van den BA, Riezler R, Naurath HJ, Lindenbaum J, Stabler SP & Allen RH. (1993). Metabolic evidence that deficiencies of vitamin B-12 (cobalamin), folate, and vitamin B-& occur commonly in elderly people. *Am J Clin Nutr,* Vol.58, No.4, (October 1993), pp. 468-76, ISSN 0002-9165.

Joseph JA, Shukitt-Hale B, Denisova NA, Prior RL, Cao G, Martin A, Taglialatela G & Bickford PC. (1998). Long- term dietary strawberry, spinach, or vitamin E supplementation retards the onset of age- related neuronal signal transduction and cognitive behavioral deficits. *J Neurosci,* Vol.18, No.19, (October 1998), pp. 8047-55, ISSN 0270-6474.

Joseph JA, Shukitt-Hale B, Denisova NA, Bielinski D, Martin A, McEwen JJ & Bickford PC. (1999). Reversals of age-related declines in neuronal signal transduction, cognitive, and motor behavioral deficits with blueberry, spinach, or strawberry dietary supplementation. *J Neurosci,* Vol.19, No.18, (September 1999), pp. 8114-21, ISSN 0270-6474.

Kalmijn S, Launer LJ, Lindemans J, Bots ML, Hofman A & Breteler MM. (1999). Total homocysteine and cognitive decline in a community-based sample of elderly subjects: the Rotterdam study. *Am J Epidemiol,* Vol.150, No.3, (August 1999), pp. 283-9, ISSN 0002-9262.

Kang JH, Cook N, Manson J, Buring JE & Grodstein F. (2006). A randomized trial of vitamin E supplementation and cognitive function in women. *Arch Intern Med,* Vol.166, No.22, (December 2006), pp. 2462-8, ISSN 0003-9926.

Kipen E, Helme RD, Wark JD & Flicker L. (1995). Bone density, vitamin D nutrition, and parathyroid hormone levels in women with dementia. *J Am Geriatr Soc,* Vol.43, No.10, (October 1995), pp. 1088-91, ISSN 0002-8614.

Kivipelto M, Annerbo S, Hultdin J, Backman L, Viitanen M, Fratiglioni L & Lokk J. (2009). Homocysteine and holo-transcobalamin and the risk of dementia and Alzheimers disease: a prospective study. *Eur J Neurol,* Vol.16, No.7, (July 2009), pp. 808-13, ISSN 1351-5101.

Knopman DS. (1998). Current pharmacotherapies for Alzheimer's disease. *Geriatrics,* Vol.53, No. Suppl.1, (September 1998), pp. S31-4, ISSN 0016-867X.

Kohlmeier M, Solomon A, Saupe J & Shearer MJ. (1996). Transport of vitamin K to bones in humans. *J Nutr,*Vol. 126, No.4 Suppl1, (April 1996), pp. S1192-6, ISSN 0022-3166.

Kronenberg G, Colla M & Endres M. (2009). Folic acid, neurodegenerative and neuropsychiatric disease. *Curr Mol Med,* Vol.9, No.3, (April 2009), pp. 315-23, ISSN 1566-5240.

Kruman II, Culmsee C, Chan SL, Kruman Y, Guo Z, Penix L & Mattson MP. (2000). Homocysteine elicits a DNA damage response in neurons that promotes apoptosis and hypersensitivity to excitotoxicity. *J Neurosci,* Vol.20, No.18, (September 2000), pp. 6920-6, ISSN 0270-6474.

Kuipers EJ, Uyterlinde AM, Pena AS, Hazenberg HJ, Bloemena E, Lindeman J, Klinkenberg-Knol EC & Meuwissen SG. (1995). Increase of Helicobacter pylori-associated corpus gastritis during acid suppressive therapy: implications for long term safety. *Am J Gastroenterol,* Vol.90, No.9, (September 1995), pp. 1401-6, ISSN 0002-9270.

Kuipers EJ, Lundell L, Klinkenberg-Knol EC, Havu N, Festen HP, Liedman B, Lamers CB, Jansen JB, Dalenback J, Snel P, Nelis GF &Meuwissen SG. (1996). Atrophic gastritis and Helicobacter pylori infection in patients with reflux esophagitis treated with omeprazol or fundoplication. *N Engl J Med,* Vol.334, No.16, (April 1996), pp. 1018-22, ISSN 0028-4793.

Landfield PW & Cadwallader-Neal L. (1998). Long term treatment with calcitriol (1,25 (OH)2 vit D3) retardsa biomarker of hippocampal aging in rats. *Neurobiol Aging,* Vol.19, No.5, (September-October 1998), pp. 469-77, ISSN 0197-4580.

Lewerin C, Matousek M, Steen G, Johansson B, Steen B & Nilsson-Ehle H. (2005). Significant correlations of plasma homocysteine and serum methylmalonic acid with movement and cognitive performance in elderly subjects but no improvement from short-term vitamin therapy: a placebo-controlled randomized study. *Am J Clin Nutr,* Vol.81, No.5, (May 2005), pp. 1155-62, ISSN 0002-9165.

Lindahl B, Eriksson L, Spillmann D, Caterson B & Lindahl U. (1996). Selective loss of cerebral keratan sulfate in Azheimer's disease. *J Biol Chem,* Vol.271, No.29, (July 1996), pp. 16991-4, ISSN 0021-9258.

Lokk J. (2003). News and views on folate and elderly persons. *J Gerontol A Biol Sci Med Sci,* Vol.58, No.4, (April 2003), pp. 354-61, ISSN 1079-5006.

Luchsinger JA, Tang MX, Shea S, Miller J, Green R & Mayeux R. (2004). Plasma homocysteine levels and risk of Alzheimer disease. *Neurology,* Vol.62, No.11, (June 2004), pp. 1972-6, ISSN 0028-3878.

Lundell L, Havu N, Miettinen P, Myrvold HE, Wallin L, Julkunen R, Levander K, Hatlebakk JG,

Liedmann B, Lamm M, Malm A & Walan A: Nordic Gerd Study Group. (2006). Changes of gastric mucosal architecture during long-term omeprazole therapy: results of a randomized clinical trial. *Aliment Pharmacol Ther,* Vol.23, No.5, (March 2006), pp. 639-47, ISSN 0269-2813.

Martin A, Foxall T, Blumberg JB & Meydani M. (1997). Vitamin E inhibits low-density lipoprotein-induced adhesion of monocytes to human aortic endothelial cells in vitro. *Arterioscler Thromb Vasc Biol,* Vol.17, No.3, (March 1997), pp. 429-36, ISSN 1079-5642.

Mattson MP. (2004). Pathways towards and away from Alzheimer's disease. *Nature,* Vol.430, No.7000, (August 2004), pp. 631-9, ISSN 0028-0836.

Maxwell CJ, Hicks MS, Hogan DB, Basran J & Ebly EM. (2005). Supplemental use of antioxidant vitamins and subsequent risk of cognitive decline and dementia. *Dement Geriatr Cogn Disord,* Vol.20, No.1, pp. 45-51, ISSN 1420-8008.

McCaddon A, Davies G, Hudson P, Tandy S & Cattell H. (1998). Total serum homocysteine in senile dementia of Alzheimer type. *Int J Geriatr Psychiatry,* Vol.13, No.4, (April 1998), pp. 235-9, ISSN : 0885-6230.

McCaddon A, Hudson P, Davies G, Hughes A, Williams JH & Wilkinson C. (2001). Homocysteine and cognitive decline in healthy elderly. *Dement Geriatr Cogn Disord,* Vol.12, No.5, (September-October 2001), pp. 309-13, ISSN 1420-8008.

McCaddon A, Regland B, Hudson P & Davies G. (2002). Functional vitamin B (12) deficiency and Alzheimer disease. *Neurology,* Vol.58, No.9, (May 2002), pp. 1395-9, ISSN 0028-3878

McMahon JA, Green TJ, Skeaff CM, Knight RG, Mann JI & Williams SM. (2006). A controlled trial of homocysteine lowering and cognitive performance. *N Eng J Med,* Vol.354, No.26, (June 2006), pp. 2764-72, ISSN 0028-4793.

McNeill G, Avenell A, Campbell MK, Cook JA, Hannaford PC, Kilonzo MM, Mile AC, Ramsay CR, Seymour DG, Stephen AI & Vale LD. (2007). Effect of multivitamin and multimineral supplementation on cognitive function in men and women aged 65 years and over: a randomised controlled trial. *Nutr J,* Vol.2, No.1, (May 2007), pp. 6-10, ISSN 1475-2891.

Meydani SN, Meydani M, Blumberg JB, Leka LS, Siber G, Loszewski R, Thompson C, Pedrosa MC, Diamond RD & Stollar BD. (1997). Vitamin E supplementation and in vivo immune response in healthy elderly subjects. A randomised controlled trial. *J Am Med Assoc,* Vol.277, No.17, (May 1997), pp. 1380-6, ISSN 0002-9955.

Micheau J, Durkin TP, Destrade C, Rolland Y & Jaffard R. (1985). Chronic administration of sulbutiamine improves long term memory formation in mice: possible cholinergic mediation. *Pharmacol Biochem Behav,* Vol.23, No.2, (August 1985), pp. 195-8, ISSN 0091-3057.

Miller ER 3rd, Pastor-Barriuso R, Dala D, Riemersma RA, Appel LJ & Guallar E. (2005). Meta-analysis: high- dosage vitamin E supplementation may increase all-cause mortality. *Ann Intern Med,* Vol.142, No.1, (January 2005), pp. 37-46, ISSN 0003-4819.

Miller LJ & Chacko R. (2004). The role of cholesterol and statins in Alzheimer's disease. *Ann Pharmacother,* Vol.38, No.1, (January 2004), pp. 91-8, ISSN 1060-0280.

Mooijaart SP, Gussekloo J, Frölich M, Jolles J, Stott DJ, Westendorp RG & de Craen AJ. (2005). Homocysteine, vitamin B-12, and folic acid and the risk of cognitive decline in old age: the Leiden 85-Plus study. *Am J Clin Nutr,* Vol.82, No.4, (October 2005), pp. 627-35, ISSN 0002-9165.

Morris MS, Jacques PF, Rosenberg IH & Selhub J. (2001). Hyperhomocysteinemia associated with poor recall in the third National Health and Nutrition Examination Survey. *Am J Clin Nutr,* Vol.73, No.5, (May 2001), pp. 927-33, ISSN 0002-9165.

Morris MC, Evans DA, Bienias JL, Tangney CC & Wilson RS. (2002). Vitamin E and cognitive decline in older persons. *Arch Neurol,* Vol.59, No.7, (July 2007), pp. 1125-32, ISSN 0003-9942.

Morris MC, Evans DA, Tangney CC, Bienias JL, Wilson RS, Aggarwal NT & Scherr PA. (2005a). Relation of tocopherol forms to incident Alzheimer disease and to cognitive change. *Am J Clin Nutr,* Vol.81, No.2, (February 2005), pp. 508-14, ISSN 0002-9165.

Morris MC, Evans DA, Bienias JL, Tangney CC, Hebert LE, Scherr PA & Schneider JA. (2005b). Dietary folate and vitamin B12 intake and cognitive decline among community-dwelling older persons. *Arch Neurol,* Vol.62, No.4, (April 2005), pp. 641-5, ISSN 0003-9942.

Morris MC, Evans DA, Schneider JA, Tangney CC, Bienias JL & Aggarwal NT. (2006a). Dietary folate and vitamins B-12 and B-6 not associated with incident Alzheimer's disease. *J Alzheimers Dis,* Vol.9, No.4, (August 2006), pp. 435-43, ISSN 1387-2877.

Morris MC, Evans DA, Tangney CC, Bienias JL & Wilson RS. (2006b). Associations of vegetable and fruit consumption with age-related cognitive change. *Neurology,* Vol.67, No.8, (October 2006), pp. 1370-6, ISSN 0028-3878.

Nilsson K, Gustafson L, Faldt R, Andersson A, Brattstrom L, Lindgren A, Israelson B & Hultberg B. (1996). Hyperhomocysteinaemia- a common finding in psychogeriatric population. *Eur J Clin Invest,* Vol.26, No.10, (October 1996), pp. 8534-9, ISSN 0014-2972.

Nilsson K, Gustafson L & Hultberg B. (1999). Plasma homocysteine is a sensitive marker for tissue deficiency of both cobalamines and folates in a psychogeriatric population. *Dement Geriatr Cogn Disord,* Vol.10, No.6, (November-December 1999), pp. 476-82, ISSN 1420-8008.

Obeid R, McCaddon A & Herrman W. (2007). The role of hyperhomocysteinemia and B-vitamin deficieny in neurological and psychiatric diseases. *Clin Chem Lab Med,* Vol.45, No.12, pp. 1590-606, ISSN 1434-6621.

Ortega RM, Requejo AM, Lopez-Sobaler AM, Andres P, Navia B, Perea JM & Robles F. (2002). Cognitive function in elderly people is influenced by Vitamin E status. *J Nutr,* Vol.132, No.7, (July 2002), pp. 2065-8, ISSN 0022-3166.

Paleologos M, Cumming RG & Lazarus R. (1998). Cohort study of Vitamin C intake and cognitive impairment. *Am J Epidemiol,* Vol.148, No.1, (July 1998), pp. 45-50, ISSN 0002-9262.

Parnetti L, Bottiglieri T & Lowenthal D. (1997). Role of homocysteine in age related vascular and non-vascular disease. *Aging (Milano),* Vol.9, No.4, (August 1997), pp. 241-57, ISSN 0011-3662.

Pauli RM & Haun JM. (1979). Warfarin embryopathy. *Lancet,* Vol.2, No.8134, (July 1999), pp. 144, ISSN 0140-6736.

Perkins AJ, Hendrie HC, Callahan CM, Gao S, Unverzagt FW, Xu Y, Hall KS & Hui SL. (1999). Association of antioxidants with memory in a multiethnic elderly sample using the Third National Health and Nutrition Examination Survey. *Am J Epidemiol,* Vol.150, No.1, (July 1999), pp. 37-44, ISSN 0002-9262.

Perrig WJ, Perrig P & Stahelin HB. (1997). The relation between antioxidants and memory performence in the old and very old. *J Am Geriatr Soc,* Vol.45, No.6, (June 1997), pp. 718-24, ISSN 0002-8614.

Petersen RC, Thomas RG, Grundman M, Bennett D, Doody R, Ferris S, Galasko D, Jin S, Kaye J, Levey A, Pfeiffer E, Sano M, van Dyck CH & Thal LJ. (2005). Vitamin E and donepezil for the treatment of mild cognitive impairment. *N Eng J Med,* Vol.352, No.23, (June 2005), pp. 2379-88, ISSN 0028-4793.

Pietrzik K & Bronstrup A. (1997). Causes and consequences of hyperhomocyst(e)inemia. *Int J Vitam Nutr Res,* Vol.67, No.5, pp. 389-95, ISSN 0300-9831.

Pitchumoni SS & Doraisway PM. (1998). Current status of antioxidant therapy for Alzheimer's Disease. *J Am Geriatr Soc,* Vol.46, No.12, (December 1998), pp. 1566-72, ISSN 0002-8614.

Pratico D & Delanty N. (2000). Oxidative injury in diseases of the central nervous system: focus on Alzheimer's disease. *Am J Med,* Vol.109, No.7, (November 2000), pp. 577-85, ISSN 0002-9343.

Presse N, Shatenstein B, Kergoat MJ & Ferland G. (2008). Low vitamin K intakes in community-dwelling elders at an early stage of Alzheimer's disease. *J Am Diet Assoc,* Vol.108, No.12, (December 2008), pp.2095-9, ISSN 0002-8223.

Prieto AL, Weber JL, Tracy S, Heeb MJ & Lai C. (1999). Gas 6, a ligand for the receptor tyrosine kinase tyro 3, is widely expressed in the central nervous system. *Brain Res,* Vol.816, No.2, (January 1999), pp. 646-61, ISSN 0006-8993.

Prins ND, Den Heijer T, Hofman A, Koudstaal PJ, Jolles J, Clarke R & Breteler MM. (2002). Homocysteine and cognitive function in the elderly: Rotterdam Scan Study. *Neurology,* Vol.59, No.9, (November 2002), pp. 1375-80, ISSN 028-3878.

Rabaneda LG, Carrasco M, Lopez-Toledano MA, Murillo-Carretero M, Ruiz FA, Estrada C & Castro C. (2008). Homocysteine inhibits proliferation of neuronal precursors in the mouse adult brain by impairing the basic fibroblast growth factor signaling cascade and reducing extracellular regulated kinase-dependent cyclin E expression. *FASEB J,* Vol.22, No.11, (November 2008), pp. 3823-35, ISSN 0892-6638.

Rampersaud GC, Kauwell GP & Bailey LB. (2003). Folate: a key to optimizing health and reducing disease risk in the elderly. *J Am Coll Nutr,* Vol.22, No.1, (February 2003), pp. 1-8, ISSN 0731-5724.

Ravaglia G, Forti P, Maioli F, Martelli M, Servadei L, Brunatti N, Porcellini E & Licastro F. (2005). Homocysteine and folate as risk factors for dementia and Alzheimer disease. *Am J Clin Nutr,* Vol.82, No.3, (September 2005), pp. 636-43, ISSN 0002-9165.

Refsum H, Ueland PM, Nygard O & Vollset SE. (1998). Homocysteine and cardiovascular disease. *Annu Rev Med,* Vol.49, No.1, pp. 31-62, ISSN 0066-4219.

Reiter R.J. (1995). Oxidative processes and antioxidative defence mechanisms in the aging brain. *FASEB J,* Vol.9, No.7, (April 1995), pp. 526-33, ISSN 0892-6638.

Remington R, Chan A, Paskavitz J & Shea TB. (2009). Efficacy of a vitamin/nutriceutical formulation for moderate-stage to later stage Alzheimer's disease: a placebo-controlled pilot study. *Am J Alzheimers Dis Other Demen,* Vol.24, No.1, (February-March 2009), pp. 27-33, ISSN 1533-3175.

Riedel WJ, Jorissen B & Nutrients L. (1998). Age and cognitive function. *Curr Opin Clin Nutr Metab Care,* Vol.1, No.6, (November 1998), pp. 579-85, ISSN 163-1950.

Sahin M, Karauzum SB, Perry G, Smith MA & Aliciguzel Y. (2005). Retinoic acid isomers protect hippocampal neurons from amyloid-beta induced neurodegeneration. *Neurotox Res,* Vol.7, No.3, pp. 243-50, ISSN 1029-8428.

Sano M, Ernesto C, Thomas RG, Klauber MR, Schafer K, Grundman M, Woodbury P, Growdon J, Cotman CW, Pfeiffer E, Schneider LS & Thal LJ. (1997). A controlled trial of selegiline, alpha-tocopherol, or both as treatment for Alzheimer's disease. The Alzheimer's Disease Cooperative Study. *N Eng J Med,* Vol.336, No.17, (April 1997), pp. 1216-22, ISSN 0028-4793.

Sato Y, Iwamoto J, Kanoko T & Satoh K. (2005). Amelioration of osteoporosis and hypovitaminosis D by sunlight exposure in hospitalized, elderly women with Alzheimer's disease: a randomized controlled trial. *Journal of Bone&Mineral Research,* Vol.20, No.8, (August 2005), pp. 1327-33, ISSN 0884-0431.

Saupe J, Shearer MJ & Kohlmeier M. (1993). Phylloquinone transport and its influence on y-carboxyglutamate residues of osteocalcin in patients on hemodialysis. *Am J Clin Nutr,* Vol.58, No.2, (August 1993), pp. 204-8, ISSN 0002-9165.

Saxena SP, Fan T, Li M, Israels ED & Israels LG. (1997). A novel role for vitamin K, in a tyrosine phosphorylation cascade during chick embryogenesis. *J Clin Invest,* Vol.99, No.4, (February 1997), pp. 602-7, ISSN 0021-9738.

Scarmeas N, Stern Y, Tang MX, Mayeux R & Luchsinger JA. (2006). Mediterranean diet and risk for Alzheimer's disease. *Ann Neurol,* Vol.59, No.6, (June 2006), pp. 912-21, ISSN 0364-5134.

Scarmeas N, Stern Y, Mayeux R, Manly JJ, Schupf N & Luchsinger JA. (2009). Mediterranean diet and mild cognitive impairment. *Arch Neurol,* Vol.66, No.2, (February 2009), pp. 216-25, ISSN 0003-9942.

Scott TM, Peter I, Tucker KL, Arsenault L, Bergethon P, Bhadelia R, Buell J, Collins L, Dashe JF, Griffith J, Hibberd P, Leins D, Liu T, Ordovas JM, Patz S, Price LL, Qiu WQ, Sarnak M, Selhub J, Smaldone L, Wagner C, Wang L, Weiner D, Yee J, Rosenberg I & Folstein M. (2006). The Nutrition, Aging, and Memory in Elders (NAME) study: design and methods for a study of micronutrients and cognitive function in a homebound elderly population. *Int J Geriatr Psychiatr,* Vol.21, No.6, (June 2006), pp. 519-28, ISSN 0885-6230.

Scranton TW, Iwata M & Carlson SS. (1993). The SV-2 protein of synaptic vesicles is a keratan sulfate proteoglycan. *J Neurochem,* Vol.61, No.1, (July 1993), pp. 29-44, ISSN 0022-3042.

Selhub J, Jacques PF, Wilson PW, Rush D & Rosenberg IH. (1993). Vitamin status and intake as primary determinants of homocysteinemia in an elderly population. *J Am Med Assoc,* Vol.270, No.22, (December 1993), pp. 2693-8, ISSN 0002-9955.

Selhub J, Bagley LC, Miller J & Rosenberg IH. (2000). B vitamins, homocysteine, and neurocognitive function in the elderly. *Am J Clin Nutr,* Vol.71, No.2, (February 2000), S614-20, ISSN 0002-9165.

Selhub J. (2008). Public health significance of elevated homocysteine. *Food Nutr Bull,* Vol.29, No.2 Suppl), pp. S116-25, ISSN 0379-6721.

Seshadri S, Beiser A, Selhub J, Jacques PF, Rosenberg IH, D'Agostino RB, Wilson PW & Wolf PA. (2002). Plasma homocysteine as a risk factor for dementia and Alzheimer's disease. *N Eng J Med,* Vol.346, No.7, (February 2002), pp. 476-83, ISSN 0028-4793.

Shahidi S, Komaki A, Mahmoodi M, Atrvash H & Ghodrati M. (2008). Ascorbic acid supplementation could affect passive avoidance learning and memory in rats. *Brain Res Bull,* Vol.76, No.1-2, (May 2008), pp.109-13, ISSN 0361-9230.

Sinclair AJ, Bayer AJ, Johnston J, Warner C & Maxwell SR. (1998). Altered plasma antioxidant status in subjects with Alzheimer's disease and vascular dementia. *Int J Geriatr Psychiatry,* Vol.13, No.12, (December 1998), pp. 840-5, ISSN 0885-6230.

Smith AD, Stephen MS, de Jager CA, Whitbread P, Johnston C, Agacinski G, Oulhaj A, Bradley KM, Jacoby R & Refsum H. (2010). Homocysteine-lowering by B vitamins slows the rate of accelerated brain atrophy in mild cognitive impairment: a randomized controlled trial. In: *PLoS ONE,* 5(9), 17.05.2011, Available from e12244. doi:10.1371/journal.pone.0012244.

Sommer BR, Hoff AL & Costa M. (2003). Folic acid supplementation in dementia: a preliminary report. *J Geriatr Psychiatry Neurol,* Vol.16, No.3, (September 2003), pp. 156-9, ISSN 0891-9887.

Stott DJ, MacIntosh G, Lowe GD, Rumley A, McMahon AD, Langhorne P, Tait RC, O'Reilly DS, Spilg EG, MacDonald JB, MacFarlane PW, Westendorp RG. (2005). Randomized controlled trial of homocysteine-lowering vitamin treatment in elderly patients with vascular disease. *Am J Clin Nutr,* Vol.82, No.6, (December 2006), pp. 1320-6, ISSN 0002-9165.

Sutherland MK, Somerville MJ, Yoong LK, Bengeron C, Haussler MR & McLachlan DR. (1992). Reduction of vitamin D hormone receptor mRNA levels in Alzheimer as compared to Huntington hippocampus: correlation with calbindin -28k mRNA levels. *Brain Res Mol Brain Res,* Vol.13, No.3, (April 1992), pp. 239-50, ISSN 0169-328X.

Teunissen CE, Blom AH, Van Boxtel MP, Bosma H, de Bruijn C, Jolles J, Wauters BA, Steinbusch HW & de Vente J. (2003). Homocysteine: a marker for cognitive performance? A longitudinal follow-up study. *J Nutr Health Aging,* Vol.7, No.3, pp. 153-9, ISSN 1279-7707.

Troen AM, Shea-Budgell M, Shukitt-Hale B, Smith DE, Selhub J & Rosenberg IH. (2008). B-vitamin deficiency causes hyperhomocysteinemia and vascular cognitive impairment in mice. *Proc Natl Acad Sci USA,* Vol.105, No.34, (August 2008), pp. 12474-9, ISSN 0027-8424.

Tucker KL, Qiao N, Scott T, Rosenberg I & Spiro A 3rd. (2005). High homocysteine and low B vitamins predict cognitive decline in aging men: the Veterans Affairs Normative Aging Study. *Am J Clin Nutr,* Vol.82, No.3, (November 2005), pp. 627-35, ISSN 0002-9165.

Ueland PM & Refsum H. (1989). Plasma homocysteine, a risk factor for vascular disease: plasma levels in health, disease, and drug therapy. *J Lab Clin Med,* Vol.114, No.5, (November 1989), pp. 473-501, ISSN 0022-2143.

van Oort FV, Melse-Boonstra A, Brouwer IA, Clarke R, West CE, Katan MB & Verhoef P. (2003). Folic acid and reduction of plasma homocysteine concentrations in older adults: a dose-response study. *Am J Clin Nutr,* Vol.77, No.5, (May 2003), pp. 1318-23, ISSN 0002-9165.

van Uffelen JG, Chin A, Paw MJ, Hopman-Rock M & van Mechelen W. (2007). The effect of walking and vitamin B supplementation on quality of life in community-dwelling adults with mild cognitive impairment: a randomized, controlled trial. *Qual Life Res,* Vol.16, No.7, (September 2007), pp. 1137-46, ISSN 0962-9343.

Varadarajan S, Yatin S, Aksenova M & Butterfield DA. (2000). Review: Alzheimer's amyloid beta-peptide-associated free radical oxidative stress and neurotoxicity. *J Struct Biol*, Vol.130, No.2-3, (June 2000), pp. 184-208, ISSN 1047-8477.

Vivekananthan DP, Penn MS, Sapp SK, Hsu A & Topol EJ. (2003). Use of antioxidant vitamins for the prevention of cardiovascular disease: meta-analysis of randomised trials. *Lancet*, Vol.361, No.9374), pp. 2017-23, ISSN 0140-6736.

Wahlin A, Hill RD, Winblad B & Backman L. (1996). Effects of serum vitamin B12 and folate status on episodic memory performance in very old age: a population- based study. *Psychol Aging*, Vol.11, No.3, (September 1996), pp. 487-96, ISSN 0882-7974.

Wald DS, Bishop L, Wald NJ, Law M, Hennessy E, Weir D, McPartlin J & Scott J. (2001). Randomized trial of folic acid supplementation and serum homocysteine levels. *Arch Intern Med*, Vol.161, No.5, (March 2001), pp. 695-700, ISSN 0003-9926.

Wang HX, Wahlin A, Basun H, Fastbom J, Winblad B & Fratiglioni L. (2001). Vitamin B(12) and folate in relation to the development of Alzheimer's disease. *Neurology*, Vol.56, No.9, (May 2001), pp. 1188-94, ISSN 0028-3878.

Wolters M, Strohle A & Hahn A. (2004). Age-associated changes in the metabolism of vitamin B (12) and folic acid: prevalance, aetiopathogenesis and pathophysiological consequences. *Z Gerontol Geriatr*, Vol.37, No.2, (April 2004), pp. 109-35, ISSN 0948-6704.

Wolters M, Hickstein M, Flintermann A, Tewes U & Hahn A. (2005). Cognitive performance in relation to vitamin status in healthy elderly German women-the effect of 6-month multivitamin supplementation. *Prev Med*, Vol.41, No.1, (July 2005), pp. 253-9, ISSN 0091-7435.

Yagami T, Ueda K, Asakura K, Sakaeda T, Nakazato H, Huroda T, Hata S, Sakaguchi G, Itoh N, Nakano T, Kambayashi Y & Tsuzuki H. (2002). Gas6 rescues cortical neurons from amyloid β protein-induced apoptosis. *Neuropharmacology*, Vol.43, No.8, (December 2002), pp. 1289-96, ISSN 0028-3908.

Zandi PP, Anthony JC, Khachaturian AS, Stone SV, Gustafson D, Tschanz JT, Norton MC, Weish-Bohmer KA, Breitner JC. (2004). Reduced risk of Alzheimer disease in users of antioxidant vitamin supplements. *Arch Neurol*, Vol.61, No.1, (January 2004), pp. 82-8, ISSN 0003-9942.

Part 6

Additional and Novel Concepts

22

Hypotension in Subcortical Vascular Dementia, a New Risk Factor – Wasn't It Hypertension?

Rita Moretti, Francesca Esposito, Paola Torre,
Rodolfo M. Antonello and Giuseppe Bellini
Medicina Clinica, Ambulatorio Complicanze Internistiche Cerebrali, Dipartimento Universitario Clinico di Scienze Mediche Tecnologiche e Traslazionali, Università degli Studi di Trieste,
Italy

1. Introduction

The identification of additional genetic susceptibility genes in the etiology of AD and the metabolic mechanisms leading to differences in age of onset and disease pathogenesis are active areas of current susceptibility. Although all the contributing factors may never be known, scientists have identified several common threads. They include: age (more than 65 years old), sex (women are more likely than men are to develop the disease, in part because they live longer), toxicity (such as overexposure to certain trace metals, such as aluminum), head injury (serious traumatic injury to the head, for example, a concussion with a prolonged loss of consciousness) may be a risk factor for Alzheimer's), hormone replacement therapy (the exact role hormone replacement therapy may play in the development of dementia isn't yet clear; throughout the 1980s and '90s, evidence seemed to show that estrogen supplements given after menopause could reduce the risk of dementia; results from the large-scale Women's Health Initiative Memory Study indicated an increased risk of dementia for women taking estrogen after age 65: the verdict is not yet in on whether estrogen affects the risk of dementia if given at an earlier age), lifestyle (the same factors that put you at risk of heart disease, such as high blood pressure and high cholesterol, may also increase the likelihood that you'll develop Alzheimer's disease, poorly controlled diabetes is another risk factor). Atrial fibrillation, systolic hypertension, and angina have been associated with more rapid decline in cognition, while history of coronary artery bypass graft surgery, diabetes, and antihypertensive medications were associated with a slower rate of decline, and may represent modifiable risk factors for secondary prevention in Alzheimer disease. There was an age interaction such that systolic hypertension, angina, and myocardial infarction were associated with greater decline with increasing baseline age. The attenuated decline for diabetes and coronary artery bypass graft surgery may be due to selective survival. Some of these effects appear to vary with age (Mielke et al., 2007). There is an overlap of risk factors between VaD and AD, so much so that it raises some serious questions about vascular contributions to AD. Recognition that cerebrovascular disease causing dementia may be modified by treatment of cerebrovascular risk factors serves as an important tool for investigating various treatments aimed at secondary prevention of vascular cognitive impairment (Moretti et al., 2008). Some individuals presenting cerebrovascular pathology probably have some component of Alzheimer's Disease (AD) pathology as part of their dementia; this relationship supports the possible interaction between cerebrovascular disease, aging and the degenerative process (see data and Literature in: Brookmeyer et al., 1998). Various factors may influence the nature and severity of brain degeneration. The degree of cerebral grey matter damage, neuronal death, and survival will be dictated by the multiplicity, size, and laterality of the tissue injury or the extent of vascular disease (Kalaria, 1996; Kalaria, 2010). Anatomical features of the circulation, including the size of vessels and vascular wall cellular elements, e.g., arterioles versus capillaries, are important factors in defining the pathology. The distribution territories of the anterior, posterior, and middle cerebral and the lenticulo-striate arteries affect different structures, including the angular gyrus, the caudate nucleus and medial thalamus in the dominant hemisphere, the amygdala, and the hippocampus, all structures implicated in forms of cognitive impairment (Kalaria, 2010; Ferrer et al, 2008). The origin and degree of vascular occlusion or injury and whether this results in ischemic or hemorrhagic lesions are further factors that define the extent and severity of damage. Alterations in specific genes associated with systemic disease or brain-specific proteins and environmental or lifestyle factors may further modify the course of degeneration. On the other hand, vascular dementia is defined simply as the syndrome of dementia due to brain vascular disease (Hebert et al., 2003). Numerous epidemiological studies show a high prevalence of vascular brain injury amongst the elderly (Wolf et al., 1991; Wu et al., 2002) and recent evidence supports a strong association between vascular risk factors and dementia (Vermeer et al, 2003; Chui, 1989). Overall in the Western world, vascular disease is the second most common cause of dementia (Skoog et al., 1993). However in the very elderly, aged 85 years and older, there is a high risk of both stroke and Alzheimer's disease, and the prevalence of VaD is reported to be slightly higher than that of Alzheimer's disease (46.9% and 43.5%, respectively, with some patients possibly having mixed forms of dementia) (Skoog et al., 1993). Vascular dementia is a heterogeneous syndrome, grouping together a broad category of patients in whom various manifestations of cognitive decline are attributed to cerebral- or cardio-vascular disease. The National Institute of Neurological Disorders and Stroke and the Association Internationale pour la Recherche et l'Enseignement en Neurosciences (NINDS-AIREN) (Roman et al, 1993) elaborated a clinical and diagnostic tool, the so- called NINDS-AIREN criterium. It lists different pathologies, in order to identify patients with different subtypes of VaD: multi-infarct dementia (multiple large and complete infarcts); post-hemorrhage dementia, and subcortical VaD (small-vessel disease). According to NINDS-AIREN, the subcortical VaD (sVaD) is mainly due to lacunar infarct, occurring in distribution of small arteriole, usually in the white matter, basal ganglia, thalamus and pons, or to microinfarct - not seen on macroscopic examination, small area of cystic or non-cystic necrosis surrounded by astrocytes. Incomplete infarct may also be present, due to a selective loss of neurons, myelin, and oligodendrocytes, without cystic necrosis, occurring in the periphery of major artery distribution infarcts (e.g., penumbra) or in deep white matter. Incomplete white matter infarcts are associated with myelin pallor, astrocytosis, and a variable degree of axonal loss. Subcortical VaD now incorporates the old entities 'lacunar state' and 'Binswanger disease' and relates to small vessel disease and hypoperfusion resulting in focal and diffuse ischaemic white matter lesions and incomplete ischaemic injury (Erkinjuntti et al 1997; Pantoni et al., 2000). Assaying cerebrovascular risk factors probably can't be used for diagnosis of microvascular VaD, but the more risk factors there are might have some predictive value. There is an uncanny overlap of risk factors between VaD and AD, so much so that it raises some serious questions about vascular contributions to AD. Hypertension has often been observed to be a risk factor for VaD (Brookmeyer et al., 1998; Hebert et al., 2000) and sometimes for AD (Posner et al., 2002; LAuner et al., 1995; Morris et al. 2001) although not always (van Dijck et al., 2004). Hypertension leads to changes in arterioles and eventually to arteriolar occlusive disease and then on to infarction. Hypertension's effects on the brain in VaD or AD could also be related to changes in blood flow or blood-brain-barrier integrity. In fact, a number of epidemiological studies show strong associations between elevations in middle-life blood pressure and the prevalence of later life cognitive impairment and dementia. Increase in systolic blood pressure levels has been associated with more severe periventricular and subcortical white matter lesions (van Dijck et al., 2004). People with poorly controlled hypertension had a higher risk of severe white matter lesions than those without hypertension. But, it clearly merged that a potential negative effect of decreasing diastolic blood pressure level on the occurrence of severe periventricular white matter lesions should be taken into account. Recent large observational studies have suggested that high blood pressure may also play a role in Alzheimer's disease and in the so-called mixed forms of dementia, also defined as overlapping syndromes (vascular/degenerative dementia). The mechanisms linking hypertension to Alzheimer's disease remain to be elucidated, but white matter lesions seen on cerebral magnetic resonance imaging appear to be a good marker of this association (Brookmeyer et al., 1998; Ferrer et al., 2008; Tzourio, 2007). Hypertension leads to changes in arterioles and eventually to arteriolar occlusive disease and then on to infarction, and consequent brain parenchima degeneration (Skoog et al., 1993; 1Hebert et al., 2000; Posner et al., 2002). A large number of epidemiological studies show strong associations between elevations in middle-life blood pressure and the prevalence of later life cognitive impairment and dementia. Early evidence suggest that treatment hypertension in the elderly may be quite successful in reducing incident dementia. In the Syst-Eur trial (Forette et al., 1998), given the high percentage of elderly suffering with untreated hypertension, are that secondary prevention treatment trials such as Syst-Eur might have a substantial impact on cognitive impairment. Indeed, high blood pressure may accelerate cerebral white matter lesions (Yamamoto et al., 1998; Schmidt et al., 1999), but white matter lesions have been found to be facilitated also by excessive fall in blood pressure, (Kario et al., 1996; Nakamura et al., 1995; Watanabe et al., 1996; Chamorro et al., 1997), including orthostatic dysregulation (Matsubayashi et al., 1997) and postprandial hypotension (Kohara et al., 1999). The traditional general practice teaches that "the lower the blood pressure is, the better is the prognosis"; nevertheless, low blood pressure as a predictor of increased mortality has been described in a 5-year prospective study in Finland (Mattila et al. 1988) as well as paradoxical survival of elderly men with high blood pressure (Brookmeyer et al., 1988; 33Langer et al., 1989). Notwithstanding all of this, interpretations of these so-called J-shaped curves between blood pressure, and mortality have always been viewed with caution and skepticism by epidemiologists and statisticians (Fletcher & Bulpitt, 1992; Glynn et al., 1995). Chronic low blood pressure has been positively associated with a number of clinical symptoms and psychosomatic distress—including unexplained fatigue, depression, and anxiety—and with minor psychiatric morbidity (de Buyzere et al., 1998). A causal relationship between low blood pressure and low mood remains uncertain, but a vicious circle should not be excluded (de Buyzere et al., 1998). Zhu et al. (1998) observed that there was a correlation between systolic pressure reduction and cognitive decline in women, which was not accounted for by other factors. Baseline blood pressure level was not significantly related to cognitive decline in that sample with initial good cognition. The Authors speculated that blood pressure reduction might be an early change of the dementing process (see also literature in Gorelick, 1997), even if no clear statement merges on this point (Ferrer et al., 2008). Ruitenberg et al. (2001) found out that lower systolic and diastolic blood pressures at baseline were associated with a higher risk of dementia at follow-up. This association was observed across all age strata, in men as well in woman and both in Alzheimer's disease and vascular dementia. Subjects with incident dementia also decreased more in blood pressure level than in persons without dementia, even if not significantly (Ruitenberg et al., 2001). This may reflect that low blood pressure causes or contributes to dementia or that incipient dementia leads a drop in blood pressure (Ruitenberg et al., 2001). The authors suggested that for the first part of the proposition, they observed an inverse association between blood pressure and dementia mainly in subjects, who used antihypertensive medication (Ruitenberg et al., 2001). This may indicate that their hypertension was longer lasting, and perhaps that these patients were more susceptible to pressure drops, causing inadequate cerebral blood flow. That would be particularly important in vulnerable areas, such as watershed zones and white matter. A second explanation given by the authors (Ruitenberg et al., 2001) was that low pressure might be a consequence of an incipient dementia. The Authors found that blood pressure was lower in subjects with manifest dementia, and those with dementia, who presented lower pressure, declined more rapidly. The possible explanation given by these Authors (Ruitenberg et al., 2001) is that several areas are involved in pressure regulation; Burke et al. (1994) reported a strong correlation between the decrease of the number of C1 neurones in the medulla oblongata and blood pressure dysregulation in Alzheimer patients. Guo et al. (1999) examined whether initially low blood pressure is related to the incidence of dementia and showed that individuals with baseline systolic pressure of 140 mmHg or less had a significantly higher risk of dementia and Alzheimer's disease. That was the first study that has reported clearly an association between relatively low systolic pressure and increased incidence of dementia with a particular presumable sufferance of brain parenchima, generally hypoperfused in dementia patients (Brown & Frackowiak, 1991), related to an impairment of the cerebral autoregulation, secondary to the degenerative disorder. The direct consequence would be a sequential ulterior reduction of blood pressure, due to dysregulation, which might accelerate the lowering of blood perfusion, altered regulation flow capacity, and therefore the underlying degenerative process (Forette et al., 1998 Bolster et al., 2001; Nilsson et al., 2007). Starting from these studies, we would like to prove if hypotension is a key point in vascular dementia patients, and if this aspect reflects its importance in the daily living assistance.

2. Subjects and methods

2.1 Patients

Study subjects were men and women aged 68–94 years, entering in Cognitive Disorder Unit Evaluation of the University of Trieste, with Mini-Mental State Examination (MMSE) scores of at least 14 (Folstein et al., 1975) and satisfying the fourth edition of the Diagnostic and Statistical Manual of Mental Disorders (APA, 2000) for dementia, recruited from June 1st

2007 to December 31st 2010. We have examined 2657 patients, who have been diagnosed as suffering from Mild Cognitive Impairment, Alzheimer's Disease, Frontal Lobe Dementia, Lewy Body Dementia and Parkinson - dementia complex. 1047 patients suffered from vascular dementia: 183 have been diagnosed as Multi-Infarct Dementia. 864 patients suffered from subcortical vascular dementia: these study subjects satisfied the criteria for probable VaD in accordance with the NINDS-AIREN criteria (Roman et al., 1993). A patient was diagnosed as having subcortical VaD (sVaD) when the CT/MRI scan showed moderate to severe ischemic white matter changes (Erkinjunnti et al., 2000) and at least one lacunar infarct. Brain CT-scans or MRI images were randomized and assessed independently, after the radiologist's opinion, by neurologists (RM, PT). Patients were not included in the study if they showed signs of normal pressure hydrocephalus, previous brain tumors, previous diagnosis of major stroke or brain hemorrhage. We did not include patients with white matter lesions, caused by specific etiologies, such as multiple sclerosis, brain irradiation, collagen vascular disease, and genetic forms of vascular dementia (such as CADASIL or CARASIL). Patients with previous major psychiatric illness (i.e. schizophrenia, bipolar disorders, psychosis, compulsive-obsessive disorders, etc) or central nervous system disorders and alcoholism were excluded too.

2.2 Study design

This was a prospective cohort study, designed to investigate gait (balance and equilibrium) disorders, behavioral alterations, drug intake of a subcortical dementia population. Study subjects were 646 men and women, diagnosed as previously stated as subcortical vascular dementia (sVaD), not bedridden, aged 68-94 years outpatients, recruited from June, 1st 2007 to December, 31st 2010, who underwent a standardized baseline assessment that included a detailed history, a physical examination, laboratory tests and psychiatric evaluations. The physical examination included evaluations of pulse rate and rhythm, blood pressure, heart size and sounds, peripheral pulses, retinal vessel and carotid artery evaluation, electrocardiographic evaluation, and chest X-ray. The physical examination was repeated at every visit; electrocardiographic evaluation and laboratory tests were repeated every 3 months. Caregivers have been instructed to measure blood pressure 3 times/week, baseline and after two minutes in hortostatism and write the evaluation in a diary, which we checked at each visit. Patients in both groups were allowed to continue any previous therapy (e.g. cholinesterase inhibitors, antihypertensive, antidyslipidemic, antidiabetic drugs). (Table 1). Patients were divided in two groups: those with hypertension history and at baseline, who progressively registered low blood pressure (415 patients) and those with hypertension history, who maintained elevated values of systolic/diastolic pressure (398 patients). From this point, the former will be defined as group A, the latter as group B. All patients were followed with periodical neurological and neuropsychological examinations. Visits were scheduled to take place every four months. A complete neuropsychological examination was conducted at baseline, and every 6 months; every 12 months' results were compared. The trial was conducted in accordance with the Declaration of Helsinki and with the Ethics Guidelines of the Institute.

2.3 Outcome measures

Global performance was assessed using the Ten Point Clock test (Manos, 1997) at every visit. Behavioral symptoms were assessed using the Neuropsychiatric Inventory (NPI)

(Cummings et al., 1994) at every visit. In particular, we have examined sub-item "apathy", from the complex of NPI evaluation system. The Complex activities of daily living were evaluated by the Instrumental activity of Daily living (IADL) (Lawton & Brody, 1969). Frontal Battery has been evaluated every three months (Dubois et al., 1997). Mobility problems were assessed by the Tinetti scale for equilibrium/balance and gait (Tinetti, 1986) at every visit. Hachinski Ischemic score (HIS) was done (Hachinski et al., 1973). Patients were registered for their medical intake and for their blood pressure diaries.

2.4 Statistical analyses

Statistical analyses were performed using the Statistical Package for the Social Sciences (SPSS, version 16.0). Within- and between -group changes from baseline to 12, 24 and 36 months were tested using the Wilcoxon Signed Ranks test. This was done for the overall scores for each efficacy variable. Spearman's rank correlation analyses were performed between behavioral outcome measures (NPI), Tinetti scale, Ten Point Clock Test (TPCT), FAB assessment score, Apathy, and BI. Results are presented as mean changes from baseline with standard deviations, and P-values are presented where appropriate.

3. Results

We have examined 2657 patients, who have been diagnosed as suffering from Mild Cognitive Impairment, Alzheimer's Disease, Frontal Lobe Dementia, Lewy Body Dementia and Parkinson - dementia complex. 1047 patients suffered from vascular dementia: 183 have been diagnosed as Multi-Infarct Dementia. 864 patients suffered from subcortical vascular dementia. These patients, 415 men and 449 women, were included in the study (Table 1).

Age in years (mean ± SD)	72.4 ± 5.8
Gender (male/female)	401/412
Education level in years (mean ± SD)	10.4 ± 2.3
Concomitant illnesses (N.+ % patients)	
Essential hypertension	794 (97.6%)
Diabetes mellitus, type 2	236 (29.1%)
Ischaemic cardiopathy/valvular failure/arrythmias	413 (50.8%)
Chronic obstructive bronchopathy	205 (25.2%)
Neoplasia	36 (4.4%)

Table 1. Baseline characteristics of patients.

Their mean age was 72.4 + 5.8 years, and they had a mean education level of 10.4 + 2.3 years. The diagnosis was based on historical information and neuropsychological assessment and supported by findings on structural (CT or magnetic resonance) imaging. Subsequent follow-up of subjects has reinforced the clinical diagnoses in all cases. Brain CT-scans or MRI images were available for all the 864 selected patients; all the patients attended CT scans, 246 patients did, moreover, MRI studies. These 246 patients were requested by us to complete their diagnostic route with MRI sequences, in case of not adequate imaging acquisition, or not convincing data. Thirty one patients died during follow-up; twenty patients did not have a caregiver, who could guarantee adequate compliance, and therefore have been excluded, after the first year from the study. All the other 813 patients (401 men and 412 women) completed the full 36-month study. Patients were allowed to continue any previous therapy (e.g. antihypertensive, antidyslipidemic, antidiabetic drugs) (Table 2).

Drug utilization mg/day	baseline	12 months	24 months	36 months
ACE inhibitor	**412 patients**	**292 patients**	**203 patients**	173 patients
Sartan	**283 patients**	**169 patients**	**179 patients**	143 patients
Calcium antagonists	**345 patients**	**172 patients**	**167 patients**	158 patients
Two or more (Antihypertensive) drugs together	**246 patients**	**0**	**0**	**0**
Antidiabetic medication	**186 patients**	**251 patients**	**198 patients**	105 patients
Antiplatetelet drugs	**321 patients**	**349 patients**	**430 patients**	349 patients
ASA	**247 patients**	**344 patients**	**376 patients**	389 patients
Digoxin	**223 patients**	**215 patients**	**175 patients**	125 patients
Diuretics	**153 patients**	**187 patients**	**178 patients**	196 patients
Thiazide diuretics	**165 patients**	**143 patients**	**189 patients**	110 patients
Lipid lowering drugs	**156 patients**	**189 patients**	**265 patients**	311 patients
Nitroglycerine or analogue	**234 patients**	**254 patients**	**209 patients**	148 patients
Bronchodilators	**121 patients**	**87 patients**	**97 patients**	104 patients
A combination of the above therapies	**512 patients**	**683 patients**	**545 patients**	**631patients**

Table 2. A synopsis of the drugs employed by the two groups of patients at baseline

During the follow-up, the patients were prescribed neuroleptics and/or benzodiazepines (Table 3).

Drug utilization	baseline	12 months	24 months	36 months
Benzodiazepines	**144 patients**	**289 patients**	**276 patients**	314 patients
Typical neurolpetics	**78 patients**	**356 patients**	**498 patients**	577 patients
Atypical neurolpetics	**24 patients**	**115 patients**	**167 patients**	345 patients
Two or more drugs	203 patients	345 patients	406 patients	567 patients

Table 3. A synopsis of the SNC drugs employed by the patients

The patients were homogeneously recruited and no demographical/social/ cultural/clinical difference distinguish from each other. Patients were divided in two groups: those with hypertension history and at baseline, who progressively registered low blood pressure (415 patients), and those with hypertension history, who maintained elevated values of systolic/diastolic pressure (398 patients). From this point, the former will be defined as group A, the latter as group B. Two neurologists of the group revised all the imaging, employing the Blennow et al. (1991) scale for CT scans and the Scheltens et al. (1993) scale for MRI imaging. There was 94.2% inter-rater agreement for the independent assessment of the scans (kappa=0.76). Considering the global health conditions, there was an obvious deterioration in the patients as evidenced by the increase of the daily drug uptake (Table 3). Main scores obtained by the patients, during the follow-up have been reported in table 4 as mean and SD . Particularly, the results obtained in the FAB scale, Tinetti Scale, apathy (as sub-score of NPI) have been reported in table 4a which reports the differences within Group A, in the follow-up; in table b, it has been reported the differences within Group B during follow-up; in table 4c it has been reported the differences between the two groups in the follow-up. According to a Wilcoxon Signed Ranks test, there was a general worsening of the cognitive, behavioral and instrumental capacities of the patients observed in the 36 months of follow-up within the two groups (table 4a and 4b). It has been showed that there was an evident difference between groups, as evidenced in table 4c: no significant difference has been registered between the two groups at baseline, a part from the performance obtained at the FAB test ($p<0.05$). At twelve, twenty four and thirty six months, the differences between the two groups were significant ($p<0.01$) as demonstrated by table 4c.

Tests	Baseline		12 months		24 months		36 months	
	Group A	Group B	Group A	Group B	Group A	Group B	Group A	Group B
TPCT	7.7 ± 0.2	7.4 ± 0.5	6.1 ± 0.1	6.8 ± 0.3	5.4 ± 0.2	6.1 ± 0.5	4.1 ± 0.1	5.9 ± 0.6
NPI	24.5 ± 3.2	23.5 ± 2.4	41.4 ± 2.1	34.5 ± 3.2	66.4 ± 1.1	64.5 ± 2.7	86.3 ± 9.1	74.5 ± 3.2
Apathy (NPI)	6.6± 0.2	6.2 ± 0.4	8.3 ± 0.1	6.8 ± 0.6	9.2 ± 0.5	7.9 ± 0.7	11.1± 0.2	9.6± 0.1
FAB	13.3 ± 1.2	14.1 ± 1.1	10.3 ± 0.5	11.1 ± 1.1	9.3 ± 0.9	10.8 ± 1.3	8.4 ± 0.2	10.1 ± 0.9
Barthel Index	89.1 ± 5.3	87.1 ± 6.2	81.1 ± 1.2	83.1 ± 2.4	76.8 ± 6.1	81.1 ± 4.1	61.1 ± 7.3	69.1 ± 4.3
Tinetti score	21.8 ± 1.8	22.1 ± 1.1	18.3 ± 1.4	21.4 ± 1.4	17.7 ± 1.5	21.1 ± 0.5	15.7 ± 1.6	19.1± 1.1
Hachinski Ischemic Score	7.6 ± 0.1	8.1 ± 0.3	6.4 ± 0.11	7.9 ± 0.1	6.2 ± 0.3	7.3 ± 0.1	6.2 ± 0.1	6.9 ± 0.3

Table 4. Tests results in the patients observed during follow-up

Tests	12 months vs baseline	24 months vs baseline	36 months vs baseline
TPCT	0.9 ± 0.3 p<0.01	5.4 ± 0.1 p<0.01	3.6 ± 0.2 p<0.01
NPI	-16.9 ± 1.3 p<0.01	-41.9 ± 4.3 p<0.01	-61.8 ± 2.1 p<0.01
Apathy (NPI)	-1.7 ± 0.4 p<0.01	-2.6 ± 0.3 p<0.01	-4.5 ± 0.1 p<0.01
FAB	3.2 ± 0.7 p<0.01	4.3 ± 0.3 p<0.01	4.9 ±1.0 p<0.01
Barthel Index	8± 9.3 p<0.01	12.3 ± 5.1 p<0.01	28 ± 4 p<0.01
Tinetti score	3.5 ± 0.4 p<0.01	4.1 ± 1.3 p<0.01	6.1 ± 0.2 p<0.01
Hachinski Ischemic Score	0.8 ± 0.3 p<0.01	1.4 ± 0.2 p<0.01	1.4 ± 0.1 p<0.01

Table 4 a. Tests results in the patients observed during follow-up in Group A

Tests	12 months vs baseline	24 months vs baseline	36 months vs baseline
TPCT	0.6 ± 0.1 p<0.05	1.3 ± 0.1 p<0.05	1.5 ± 0.2 p<0.01
NPI	-11 ± 1.2 p<0.05	-41 ± 0.3 p<0.05	-51 ± 2.1 p<0.01
Apathy (NPI)	-0.6 ± 0.2 p<0.05	-1.3 ± 0.2 p<0.05	-3.4 ± 0.3 p<0.01
FAB	3 ± 0.1 p<0.05	3.3 ± 0.2 p<0.05	4 ±0.2 p<0.01
Barthel Index	4 ± 2.8 p<0.05	6 ± 2.1 p<0.05	26 ± 1.5 p<0.01
Tinetti score	0.7 ± 0.2 p<0.05	1.1 ± 0.6 p<0.05	6.4 ± 1.4 p<0.01
Hachinski Ischemic Score	0.2 ± 0.2 p<0.05	1 ± 0.2 p<0.05	1.2 ± 0.3 p<0.01

Table 4 b. Tests results in the patients observed during follow-up in Group B

Tests	baseline	12 months vs baseline	24 months vs baseline	36 months vs baseline
TPCT	-0.3 ±0.2 ns	-0.8 ±0.2 p<0.05	0.6 ±0.3 p <0.01	1.8 ±0.5 p<0.01
NPI	-1 ±0.8 ns	6.9 ±1.1 p <0.05	1.9 ±1.6 p <0.01	-11.38 ±5.9 p <0.01
Apathy (NPI)	-0.4 ±0.2 ns	1.5 ±0.5 p <0.01	2.7 ±0.2 p <0.01	-1.5 ±0.1 p <0.01
FAB	-0.8 ±0.2 p<0.05	-1.2 ±0.6 p <0.05	-1.5 ±0.4 p <0.01	1.7 ±0.5 p <0.01
Barthel Index	-2 ±1.7 ns	-2.1 ±1.2 p <0.05	-4.3 ± 2 p <0.01	8.0 ±3.0 p <0.01
Tinetti score	-0.3 ±0.7 ns	-3.1 ±0.1 p <0.05	3.4 ± 1 p <0.01	4.6 ±0.5 p <0.01
Hachinski Ischemic Score	-0.5 ±0.2 ns	-1.5 ±0.1 p <0.05	-1.1 ±0.2 p <0.01	0.37 ±0.2 p <0.01

Table 4 c. Tests results in the patients observed during follow-up B vs A

In group A, blood pressure mean values are 130/80 ± 6.5 mm Hg at baseline, and then a decrease of 10.4 ± 7.5 mm Hg at twelve months, 15.6 ± 6.7 mm Hg at twenty four months, and

18.7 ± 5.3 mm Hg at thirty six months. In group B, blood pressure mean values are 150/85 ± 10.2 mm Hg at baseline, and then a decrease of 8.4 ± 3.5 mm Hg at twelve months, 7.6 ± 3.5 mm Hg at twenty four months, and 11. 2 ± 5.3 mm Hg at thirty six months. In group A, there was a dramatic decrease of anti-hypertensive drugs prescriptions. In group B, patients maintained their original prescriptions, though under strict medical follow-up. Spearman's rank correlation analyses indicated that there was a significant correlation between NPI scores and Tinetti score over 24 months (NPI= 56.84 ±12.11, r=0.81, p<0.01), over 36 months (NPI= 66.03 ±8.81, r=0.87, p<0.01), in both group. Though it has been evidenced a significant decrease of Tinetti score in Group A, with low blood pressure than in Group B (see table 4, 4 1, b and c). We have found a correlation between benzodiazepines and neuroleptics intake and Tinetti score at 12, 24 and 36 months (respectively r=0.77, p<0.05; r=0.78, p<0.05; r=0.67, p<0.05 at 12 months; r=0.81, p<0.01; r=0.77, p<0.05; r=0.84, p<0.01 at 24 months; r=0.81, p<0.01; r=0.82, p<0.01; r=0.89, p<0.01 at 36 months) in both Groups. We have observed a positive correlation between apathy and NPI total scores in both the groups over 12, 24 and 36 months (respectively r=0.78, p<0.05; r=0.8, p<0.05 at baseline; r=0.82, p<0.01; r=0.67, p<0.05; at 12 months; r=0.86, p<0.01; r=0.77, p<0.05 at 24 months; r=0.91, p<0.01; r=0.82, p<0.01 at 36 months). Finally, we did observe a positive correlation between apathy scores and FAB scores only in Group A at every session; in Group B at 24 and at 36 months (respectively r=0.78, p<0.05 at baseline; r=0.82, p<0.01 at 12 months, only for Group A; r=0.86, p<0.01; r=0.77, p<0.05 at 24 months; r=0.91, p<0.01; r=0.82, p<0.01 at 36 months, respectively).

4. Discussion

We have studied well selected 864 patients, for three years, suffering from subcortical vascular dementia. Our aim has been to prove if hypotension is a key point in vascular dementia patients, and if this aspect reflects its importance in the daily living assistance. What we have observed are different points. Subcortical vascular dementia is related somehow to hypertension, mainly because) all the patients recruited have been diagnosed hypertension, during their life. Curiously, some of them (n=415; group A), during the follow-up, registered a dramatic decrease of their blood pressure values, constantly during the entire follow-up, even if the anti-hypertensive drugs have been interrupted; some other (n=398; group B), who had a hypertension history, but maintained elevated values of systolic/diastolic pressure during the entire follow-up. These patients have been studied, and what merged is that the two groups did not differ from a neurological, behavioral, and general drug intake at baseline; there was only a significant difference in cognition performance, as far as group A frontal functions (implementation of strategies, executive function, judgment capability, abstract reasoning, go/no go strategies and auto-inhibition) appear significantly worse (p<0.05) than those of Group B. During follow-up, both patients did worse, in their life functions, as far as cognition, behavior, gait, functional independence; but, during the entire follow-up, Group A did worse in all the items when compared to Group B. In particular, these patients were referred as more apathic, abulic, with less frontal performances, with major walking impairment and with lower independence. In other words, it seems that given a selected population, in which hypertension has been correctly established and treated, it might have led to a well-defined white-matter deterioration (the previously called Binswanger' disease); then, when dementia has been diagnosed, the sudden modification of blood pressure regulation, changed in hypotension, led to a poorer life expectance, due to a worse performance in cognition (as above mentioned), behavior (more apathy and abulia), walking strategies. All these aspects reflect a functional sufference of frontal subcortical neural pathways: it is not known the reason, but frontal lobes have a metabolism rate under basal condition that is 20% more than that of the other brain areas (Moretti, 2006). And it is also well known that age cognitive modifications are related to frontal dysfunctions (Levine et al., 1997; Esposito, 1999; Kramer et al., 1999), due to a reduction of brain reserve capacity. This brings an aged individual closer to the level of insufficiency where only minor additional lesions may be required to precipitate dementia. The degenerative aging changes, though milder, repeat much of the pathology of Alzheimer's disease. In vascular dementia, especially in subcortical vascular type, there is an accentuate expression of what is found in old age (Moretti, 2006). The complete and incomplete white matter infarction, frequently coexisting, would, by virtue of their high prevalence, be the underlying substrate in the recognition of white matter disease (Capizzano Aristides et al., 2007), leuko-encephalopathy or leuko-araiosis (Hachinski, 1994). Having this point stated, it should be consider another question: why are these patients so sensitive to hypotension? And another major problem is: why do these patients change their historical profile and suddenly have low blood pressure, having a positive history of hypertension and not clear signs of new concomitant pathologies, which can determine, *per se*, low blood pressure? The hypothesis here are suggestive, but not at all conclusive. The small artery vessels of an hypertensive patient show a degeneration of the smooth muscle layer, which is replaced by collagen in a hyaline fibrosis, leading to a subtotal luminal occlusion. These arterioles share traits with non-hypertensive lipohyalinosis (Zhang et al, 1994), as well as with hypertensive arteriolosclerosis, and may concur with hypertensive changes. Anatomically, the smaller resistance blood vessels undergo degenerative changes consisting of thickening and fibrosis of the media (in muscular arteries) and intima, and patchy degeneration of smooth muscle cells producing luminal narrowing and increased vascular resistance. Although the resting CBF is the same in normotensive and hypertensive individuals, these structural changes limit the capacity of the resistance vessels for maximal vasodilatation and impair tolerance of lower blood pressures, while improving tolerance to hypertension through vasoconstriction of these same vessels. Long-term antihypertensive treatment can reverse these adaptive changes and shift the auto-regulation curve back to its normal range, although only limited reversibility occurs in elderly hypertensive patients (Moretti et al., 2008). Moreover, it has been observed that there is another possible explanation which might be related to the sudden dys-regulation observed in these patients. Relatively low blood pressure seems to be correlated with dementia even in a preclinical stage. Different Authors (Guo et al., 1991) started from the speculation that cerebral blood flow is reduced in dementia patients (Brown & Frackowiak, 1991). That was generally thought to be related with reduced metabolic activity of the brain or with a major vascular lesion. The authors hypothesized that the reduction of cerebral blood flow might be related to the impairment of the cerebral autoregulation, secondary to the degenerative disorder. The direct consequence would be a sequential ulterior reduction of blood pressure, due to dys-regulation, which might accelerate the lowering of blood perfusion and therefore the underlying degenerative process (Yamamoto et al., 1998; Bolster et al., 2001; Nilsson et al., 2007; Mehagnoul-Schipper et al., 2002). Moreover, the authors interpreted these results as a potential expression of the frailty and deteriorated vitality of the oldest old, in keeping constantly the auto-regulation capabilities of the normal brain, and expressed their concern, due to this frailty, on the real impact of lowering pressure in oldest age (Nilsson et al., 2007). An age-related impairment of the vascular auto-regulation due to impaired functioning of the autonomic nervous system can lead to symptoms derived from blood pressure altered dysregulation in the elderly. Additionally, age-related arteriolar changes, including endothelial changes, have been suggested to reduce the baroreflex activity and thereby predispose for deleterious blood pressure falls (Salloway, 2003). The prevalence of orthostatic and non-orthostatic hypotension reached 50% in clinically evaluated VaD cases (Salloway et al., 2003; Mirski, 2005). The possible *liaison* that relates lower blood pressure, dysregulation of cerebral blood flow, vascular dementia, (and eventual AD dementia) might be the pivotal role of acetylcholine (Ach). Ach regulates the cerebral blood flow through the parasympathetic innervation of the circle of Willis and of the pial vessels (Vasquez & Purve, 1979), and it causes significant arterial relaxation by promoting the synthesis of vasodilator agents (Vanhoutte, 1989). Preclinical research using the spontaneously hypertensive stroke-prone rat model of VaD has shown a significant reduction in the levels of acetylcholine (ACh) and choline in the cortex, hippocampus and cerebrospinal fluid compared with normal rats (Kimura et al., 2000). When compared with normal rats, spontaneously hypertensive stroke-prone rats have significantly lower levels of acetylcholine in the cerebrospinal fluid (CSF) (Togashi et al., 1994). In the latter study, the differences in CSF levels between normal rats and stroke prone rats increased with age, suggesting progressive deterioration of central cholinergic function in hypertensive stroke prone rats. The cholinesterase inhibitor epistigmine has been shown to improve blood flow in the Sprague-Dawley rat with tandem occlusion of left middle cerebral and common carotid arteries. Epistigmine also enhanced the ischaemia-induced rostral shift of cerebral blood flow maximum in the contralateral hemisphere and the redistribution of cerebral blood flow, a phenomenon possibly related to recovery of function (Scremin et al., 1997). Very recently, to prove the role of acetylcholine in vessel regulation muscarinic receptors, M5, have been studied. The M5 muscarinic receptor is the most recent member of the muscarinic acetylcholine receptor family (M1-M5) to be cloned. Because M5 receptor mRNA has been detected in several blood vessels, Yamada et al. (2001) investigated whether the lack of M5 receptors led to changes in vascular tone by using several in vivo and in vitro vascular preparations in knockout mice. Strikingly, acetylcholine, a powerful dilator of most vascular beds, virtually lost the ability to dilate cerebral arteries and arterioles in M5R_/_ mice. This effect was specific for cerebral blood vessels, because acetylcholine-mediated dilation of extra-cerebral arteries remained fully intact in M5R_/_ mice. Therefore, as often happens in neurological studies, the more hypotheses, the more questions: why should patients with the same pathology (subcortical vascular dementia) respond so differently to blood pressure regulation? What is the role of blood pressure dysregulation in sVAD patients, without a previous history of hypertension? Should we consider the possibility to treat differently patients with dementia and hypertension? More studies should consider these fundamental points, in order to implement knowledge and eventfully ameliorate treatment options for vascular dementia.

5. Conclusions

In conclusion, we could state:

1. low flow states are critical to the pathogenesis of ischemic leuko-encephalopathy; in particular this is particularly true in subcortical vascular dementia, where the cerebral frontal subcortical regions are particularly sensitive to hypo-perfusion
2. We do not know several points: is hypotension a primary event in vascular dementia or is it secondary to the degeneration of brain structure? What is the role of acetylcholine in blood flow dys-regulation? Why do patients with dementia have such different response to blood pressure control?
3. Taking into considerations all these points, we strictly recommend to the clinicians who face every day these patients that they should check strictly blood pressure, and that they should taper anti-hypertensive medications according to aging-associated declines in BP and tendency toward orthostasis? The neurological concept of "tailored therapy" should begin with the most huge and wide-spread diffused drugs, such as hypertensive drugs
4. In frail patients, such as the old patients with dementia, clinicians should consider the concept of the minimization of ancillary drugs, e.g. anti-diabetes, bronchodilators, diuretics, anty-arythmics, and so on. The entire drug set should be reconsidered at every visit, taking into account the real state of the patients, updated at the moment
5. Benzodiazepines and other meds that could lower BP in the elderly should be prescribed when necessary, without doubts, but the prescriptions should be followed during the time course of the life span of the demented patients.

6. References

American Psychiatric Association. 2000. *Diagnostic and Statistical Manual of Mental Disorders-R*. 4th edition. American Psychiatric Association. ISBN: 0890420246. Washington DC

Blennow K, Wallin A, Uhlemann C, Gottfries CG. 1991. White matter lesions on CT in Alzheimer patients: relation to clinical symptomatologic and vascular factors. *Acta Neurol Scand*. 83, pp 187-193. ISSN 0065-1427

Bolster BD, Serfaty JM, Atalar E. 2001. In vivo measurements of pulse wave in small vessels using intravenous MR. *Magn. Resonance Med.* 45, pp 53-60. ISSN: 1522-2594

Brookmeyer, R., S. Gray, Kawas C. 1998. Projections of Alzheimer's disease in the United States and the public health impact of delaying disease onset. *Am J Public Health*. 88, (9), pp 1337-1342. ISSN: 0090-0036

Brown WD, Frackowiak RSJ. 1991. Cerebral blood flow and metabolism studies in multi-infarct dementia. *Alzh Dis Assoc Dis*. 5,pp 131-143. ISSN:0893-0341

Burke WJ, Coronado PG, Schmitt CA, Gillespie KM, Chung HD. 1994. Blood pressure regulation in Alzheimer's disease. *J. Auton. Nerv. Syst.* 48, pp 65-71. ISSN: 0165-1838

Capizzano Aristides A, Schuff Norbert, Amend Diane L, Tanabe Jody L, Norman David, Maudsley Andrew A, Jagust William, Chui Helena C, Fein George, Segal Mark R, Weiner Michael W. 2007. Subcortical Ischemic Vascular Dementia: Assessment with Quantitative MR Imaging and 1H MR Spectroscopy. *AJNR Am J Neuroradiol.* 16, 21(4), pp 621–630. ISSN: 0195-6108

Chamorro A, Pujol J, Saiz A, Vila N, Vilanova JC, Alday M, Blanc R. 1997. Periventricular white matter lucencies in patients with lacunar stroke: a marker of too high or too low blood pressure? *Arch Neurol.* 54, pp 1284–1288. ISSN: 0003-9942

Chui HC. Dementia. 1989. A review emphasizing clinico-pathologic correlation and brain-behaviour relationships. *Arch. Neurol.* 46, ,7, pp 806-814. ISSN: 0003-9942

Cummings JL, Mega M, Gray K. 1994. The Neuropsychiatric Inventory: comprehensive assessment of psychopathology in dementia. *Neurology* 44, pp 2308–2314. ISSN: 10158618

De Buyzere M, Clement DL, Duprez D. 1998. Chronic Low Blood Pressure: A Review. *Cardiovascular Drugs and Therapy* 12, pp 29–35. ISSN: 1573-7241

Dubois B, Pillon B, Slachevsky A, Litvan I. 1997. *Frontal Assessment Battery (FAB).* Retrieved from: Documents and Settings\UK\Documenti\PSICO\Test-Scales\FAB.doc

Erkinjuntti T, Inzitari D, Pantoni L, Wallin A, Scheltens P, Rockwood K, Desmond DW. 2000. Limitations of clinical criteria for the diagnosis of vascular dementia in clinical trials. Is a focus on subcortical vascular dementia a solution? *Ann NY Acad Sci* 903, pp 262–272. ISSN: 0077-8923

Erkinjuntti T. 1997. Vascular dementia: challenge of clinical diagnosis. *Int Psychogeriatr.* 9, 77–83. ISSN: 1041-6102

Esposito G. 1999. Context-dependent, neural system-specific neuropsychological concomitants of aging: mapping PET correlates during cognitive activation. *Brain,* 122: 963-979. ISSN 0006-8950

Ferrer I, Kaste M, Kalimo H. Vascular diseases.2008. In: *Greenfield's Neuropathology* Love S, Louis D, Ellison D, (eds.). pp 121–240. Oxford University Press. ISBN: 978-0-0340906820 Oxford

Fletcher AE, Bulpitt CJ. 1992. How far should blood pressure be lowered? *N Engl J Med* 326, 251–254. ISSN 0028-4793

Folstein M, Folstein S, McHugh P. 1975. Mini-Mental state. A practical method for grading the cognitive state of patients for the clinician. *J Psychiatr Res.* 12, 189–198. ISSN: 1049-8931

Forette, F., Seux M.L., Staessen J.A., Thijs L., Birkenhager W.H., Babarskiene M.R., et al. 1998. Prevention of dementia in randomised double-blind placebo-controlled Systolic Hypertension in Europe (Syst-Eur) trial. *Lancet* 352, 9137, pp. 1347-1351. ISSN: 0140-6736

Glynn RJ, Field TS, Rosner B, Hebert PR, Taylor JO, Hennekens CH. 1995. Evidence for a positive linear relation between blood pressure and mortality in elderly people. *Lancet* 345, pp. 825–829. ISSN: 0140-6736

Gorelick PB. 1997. Status risk factors for dementia associated with stroke. Stroke. 28, pp 459-463. ISSN: 00392499

Guo Z, Vintanen M, Winblad B, Fratiglioni L.1999. Low blood pressure and incidence of dementia in a very old sample: dependent on initial cognition. *J. Am. Ger. Soc.* 47, pp 723-726. ISSN: 0002-8614

Hachinski V. 1994. Vascular dementia: a radical redefinition. *Dementia* 5, pp. 130-132. ISSN: 1471-3012

Hachinski VC, Iliff LD, Zhilka E. 1975. Cerebral blood flow in dementia. *Arch. Neurol.* 32, pp. 632-637. ISSN 0003-9942

Hebert R, Lindsay J, Verreault R, Rockwood K, Hill G, Dubois MF. 2000. Vascular dementia : incidence and risk factors in the Canadian study of health and aging. *Stroke* 31, pp 1487-1493. ISSN: 00392499

Hebert LE, Scherr PA, Bienias JL, Bennett DA, Evans DA. 2003. Alzheimer disease in the US population: prevalence estimates using the 2000 census. *Arch Neurol* 60, 8, pp. 1119-22. ISSN 0003-9942

Kalaria RN. 2010. Vascular basis for brain degeneration: faltering controls and risk factors for dementia *Nutrition Reviews*. 68 (Suppl. 2), pp S74–S87. ISSN 0029-6643

Kalaria RN. 1996. Cerebral vessels in ageing and Alzheimer's disease. *Pharmacol Ther.* 72, pp 193–214. ISSN: 0163-7258

Kario K, Matsuo T, Kobayashi H, Imiya M, Mastuo M, Shimada K. 1996. Nocturnal fall of blood pressure and silent cerebrovascular damage in elderly hypertensive patients: advanced silent cerebrovascular damage in extreme dippers. *Hypertension.* 27, pp 130–135. ISSN: 1062-4821.

Kimura S, Saito H, Minami M. 2000. Pathogenesis of vascular dementia in stroke-prone spontaneously hypertensive rats. *Toxicology* 153, pp 167–87. ISSN: 0378-4274

Kohara K, Jiang Y, Igase M, Takata Y, Fukuoka T, Okura T, Kitami Y, Hiwada K. 1999. Postprandial hypotension is associated with asymptomatic cerebrovascular damage in essential hypertensive patients. *Hypertension.* 33, pp 565–568. ISSN: 1062-4821.

Kramer AE, Hahn S., Gopher D. 1999. Task coordination and aging: explorations of executive control processes in the task switching paradigm. *Acta Psychol.*, 101, pp 339-378. ISSN: 0439-755X

Langer RD, Ganiato TG, Barrett-Conner E. 1989. Paradoxical survival of elderly men with high blood pressure. *Br Med J* 298, pp 1356–1358. ISSN: 09598138

Launer LJ, Masaki K, Petrovitch H, Foley D, Havlik RJ. 1995. The association between midlife blood pressure levels and late-life cognitive function. The Honolulu-Asia Aging Study. *JAMA* 274, pp 1846-1851. ISSN 0098-7484

Lawton MP, Brody EM. 1969. Assessment of older people: self-maintaining and instrumental activities of daily living. *Gerontologist* 9, pp 179-186. ISSN: 0016-9013

Levine B, Stuss DT, Milberg WP. 1997. Effects of aging on conditional associative learning: process analyses and comparison with focal frontal lesions. *Neuropsychology* 11, pp 367-381. ISSN: 1380-3395

Manos PJ. 1997. The utility of the ten-point clock test as a screen for cognitive impairment in general hospital patients. *Gen Hosp Psych* 8, pp 469–476. ISSN: 0163-8343

Matsubayashi K, Okumiya K, Wada T, Osaki Y, Fujisawa M, Doi Y, Ozawa T.1997. Postural dysregulation in systolic blood pressure is associated with worsened scoring on neurobehavioral function tests and leukoaraiosis in the older elderly living in a community. *Stroke* 28, pp 2169–2173. ISSN: 00392499

Mattila K, Haavisto M, Rajala S, Heikinheimo R. 1988. Blood pressure and five years survival in the very old. *Br Med J* 296:887–889. ISSN: 09598138

Mehagnoul-Schipper DJ, Colier WN, Hoefnagels WH, Verheugt FW, JANser RW. 2002. Effects of furosemide versus captopril on post-prandial and orthostatic blood pressure and on cerebral oxygenation in patients ≥ 70 years old of age with heart failure. *Am. J. Cardiol.* 90, pp 596-600, ISSN 0002-9149

Mielke MM, Rosenberg PB, Tschanz J, Cook L, Corcoran C, Hayden KM, Norton M, Rabins PV, Green RC, Welsh-Bohmer KA, Breitner JC, Munger R, Lyketsos CG. 2007. Vascular factors predict rate of progression in Alzheimer disease. *Neurology* 6, 69, 19, pp 1850-1858. ISSN: 10158618

Mirski MA. 2005. *Pharmacology of blood pressure management during cerebral ischemia.* American Academy of Neurology lecture collections (AAN) on CD-ROM. Miami, 5PC-004, pp. 456-469.

Moretti R. (Ed.) 2006. *Subcortical vascular dementia,* NovaPublisher Editorials. New York. ISBN 1-59454-996-6.

Moretti R, Torre P, Antonello RM. 2008. Alzheimer's Dementia and Vascular Risk Factors. In: *Alzheimer's Disease: New Research.* Visser AM (Ed). Pp. 193-209. NovaPublishers Editorials. ISBN: 978-1-60456-481-5. New York.

Morris MC, Scherr PA, Hebert LE, Glynn RJ, Bennett DA, Evans DA. 2001. Association of incident Alzheimer disease and blood pressure measured from 13 years before to 2 years after diagnosis in a large community study. *Arch Neurol* , 58, pp 1640-1646. ISSN 0003-9942

Nakamura K, Oita J, Yamaguchi T. 1995. Nocturnal blood pressure dip in stroke survivors: a pilot study. *Stroke,* 26, pp 1373–1378. ISSN: 00392499

Nilsson SE, Read S, Berg S, Johansson B, Melander A, Lindblad V. 2007. Low systolic blood pressure is associated with impaired cognitive function in the oldest old: longitudinal observations in a population-based sample 80 years and older. *Aging Clin. Exp. Res.* 19, pp 41-47. ISSN: 1594-0667

Pantoni L, Rossi R, Inzitari D. 2000. Efficacy and safety of nimodipine in subcortical vascular dementia: a subgroup analysis of the Scandinavian Multi-Infarct Dementia Trial. *J Neurol Sci* 175:124–34. ISSN: 0022-510X

Posner HB, Tang MX, Luchsinger J, Lantigua R, Stern Y, Mayeux R. 2002. The relationship of hypertension in the elderly to AD, vascular dementia, and cognitive function. *Neurology* 58, pp 1175-1181. ISSN: 10158618

Roman GC, Tatemichi TK, Erkinjuntti T. 1993. Vascular dementia: diagnostic criteria for research studies. Report of the NINDS-AIREN international work group. *Neurology* 43, pp 250-260. ISSN: 10158618

Ruitenberg A, Skoog I, Ott Am Aevarsson O, Witteman JCM, Lernfelt B, vanHarskamp F, Hofman A, Bretler MMB. 2001. Blood pressure and risk of dementia: results from the Rotterdam Study and the Gothenburg H-70 study. *Dem.Ger. Cog. Dis.* 12, pp 33-39. ISSN: 1420-8008

Salloway S. *Subcortical vascular dementia: Binswanger's and CADASIL.* American Academy of Neurology (AAN) lecture collections on CD-ROM. 2003; Honolulu: 8AC.006-2, pp. 1-29.

Scheltens Ph., Barkhof F, Leys D. 1993. A semiquantitative rating scale for the assessment of signal hyperintensities on magnetic resonance imaging. *J. Neurol. Sci.* 114, pp 7-12. ISSN: 0022-510X

Schmidt R, Fazekas F, Kappeller P, Schmidt H, Hartung HP. 1999. MRI white matter hyperintensities: three-year follow up of the Austrian Stroke Prevention Study. *Neurology* 53, pp 132–139. ISSN: 10158618

Scremin OU, Li MG, Scremin AM, Jenden DJ.1997. Cholinesterase inhibition improves blood flow in the ischemic cerebral cortex. *Brain Res Bull* 42, pp 59–70. ISSN: 0361-9230

Skoog I, Nilsson L, Palmertz B. 1993. A population-based study of dementia in 85-year olds. *NEJM* 328, pp 153–158. ISSN 1533-4406

Tinetti ME.1986. Performance-oriented assessment of mobility problems in elderly patients. *J. Am. Ger. Soc.* 34, pp 119-126. ISSN: 0002-8614.

Togashi H, Matsumoto M, Yoshioka M, Hirokami M, Minami M, Saito H. 1994. Neurochemical profiles in cerebrospinal fluid of stroke-prone spontaneously hypertensive rats. *Neurosci Lett.* 17, 166,1, pp 117-20. ISSN 0304-3940

Tzourio C. 2007. Hypertension, cognitive decline, and dementia: an epidemiological perspective. *Dialog. Clin Neurosci.* 9, 1, pp 61-70. ISSN:1294-8322

van Dijck EJ, Breteler M, Schmidt R, Berger K, Nilsson LG, Oudkerk M, Pajak A, Sans S, de Ridder M. 2004. The association between blood pressure, hypertension, and cerebral white matter lesions. *Hypertension* 44, pp 625- 650, ISSN: 0194911X.

Vanhoutte PM. 1989. Endothelium and control of vascular function. State of the art. *Hypertension* 13, pp 658–667. ISSN: 0194911X.

Vasquez J, Purve MJ. 1979. The cholinergic pathway to cerebral blood vessels. I. Morphological studies. *Pflugers Arch* 379, pp 157–163. ISSN: 1432-2013

Vermeer SE, Prins ND, den Heijer T, Hofman A, Koudstaal PJ, Breteler MM. 2003. Silent brain infarcts and the risk of dementia and cognitive decline. *NEJM*, 348, 13, pp 1215-22. ISSN 1533-4406

Watanabe N, Imai Y, Nagai K, Tsuji I, Satoh H, Sakuma M, Sakuma H, Kato J, Onodera-Kikuchi H, Yamada M, Abe F, Hisamichi S, Abe K.1996. Nocturnal blood pressure and silent cerebrovascular lesions in elderly Japanese. *Stroke* 27, pp 1319–1327. ISSN: 00392499.

Wolf PA, D'Agostino RB, Belanger AJ, Kannel WB. 1991. Probability of stroke: a risk profile from the Framingham Study. Stroke, 1991. 22(3): p. 312-8. ISSN: 00392499

Wu CC, Mungas D, Petkov CI, Eberling JL, Zrelak PA, Buonocore MH, Brunberg JA, Haan MN, Jagust WJ. 2002. Brain structure and cognition in a community sample of elderly Latinos. *Neurology* 59, 3, pp. 383-391. ISSN: 10158618

Yamada M, Lamping KG., Duttaroy A , Zhang W , Cui Y , Bymaster FP. , McKinzie DL., Felder CC, Deng CX, Faraci FM, Wess J. 2001. Cholinergic dilation of cerebral blood vessels is abolished in M5 muscarinic acetylcholine receptor knockout mice. *PNAS*, 98, 24, pp 14096–14101. ISSN: 1091-6490

Yamamoto Y, Akiguchi I, Oiwa K, Hayashi M, Kimura J. 1998. Adverse effect of nighttime blood pressure on the outcome of lacunar infarct patients. *Stroke* 29, pp 570–576 . ISSN: 00392499

Zhang WW, Badonic T, Höög A, Jiang MH, Ma KC, Nie JX, Olsson Y, Sourander P. 1994. Structural and vasoactive factors influencing intracerebral arterioles in cases of vascular dementia and other cerebrovascular disease: a review. *Dementia* 5, pp 153-62. ISSN: 1471-3012

Zhu L, Viitanen M, Guo Z, Winblad B, Fratiglioni L. 1998. Blood pressure reduction, cardiovascular disease, and cognitive decline in the Mini-Mental State Examination in a community population of normal very old people: a three year follow-up. J. Clin Epidem. 51, 5, pp 385-391. ISSN: 0895-4356

23

Autophagy-Derived Alzheimer's Pathogenesis

Daijun Ling and Paul M. Salvaterra
Beckman Research Institute of City of Hope,
USA

1. Introduction

Alzheimer's disease (AD) is an incurable terminal neurodegenerative disorder primarily affecting the elderly. Even after a century of intensive investigation, its pathogenic mechanism still remains enigmatic. Many hypotheses have been advanced to interpret the disease pathogenesis; however none are able to provide an integrated mechanistic view that can unify the numerous superficially disconnected aspects of AD etiology and pathology. Extracellular amyloid plaques and intracellular neurofibrillary tangles are the two prominent hallmarks of AD neuropathology. It remains unclear what pathogenic events link aggregated proteins such as amyloid beta peptides (Aβ) and/or phosphorylated tau to neuronal damage and death. It is also important to know more precisely how advancing age triggers the disease pathogenesis and how other modifiers affect the disease process. The absence of this basic knowledge is a major barrier not only for understanding of the disease but also for development of effective AD therapies.

Autophagy, or specifically macroautophagy, is a subcellular process participating in membrane trafficking and intracellular degradation and functions in the turnover of damaged organelles and unfavorable proteins through the lysosomal machinery. The autophagy-lysosomal system plays an important role in maintaining intracellular homeostasis and also participates in the pathophysiology of many diseases including cancer, infectious and neurodegenerative diseases (Mizushima et al., 2008). Abnormal autophagic structures have been reported to be extensively involved in AD pathology in brains of human patients as well as animal models (Nixon et al., 2005; Shacka et al., 2008). However, it remains unclear how autophagy contributes to the disease.

Numerous review papers are available that summarize the current knowledge regarding the molecular and cellular aspects of autophagy and its extensive involvement in various diseases. In this chapter, we focus on the concept of an "autophagy-lysosomal cascade" as a key mechanistic insight into AD pathogenesis. This disease hypothesis is based on recent work from our laboratory as well as growing evidence from other AD research groups. The autophagy-lysosomal cascade hypothesis has the capability to integrate many seemingly disconnected aspects of AD pathophysiology into a common cellular framework. We believe that further characterization of the details of autophagic participation in AD will be important for development of anti-Alzheimer's therapies.

2. Autophagy-derived Alzheimer's pathogenesis: Signs, lesions and causes

Autophagy-lysosomal involvement in AD and other related animal models has been extensively documented. However, it remains enigmatic if autophagy plays a causative role or is a consequence of the disease process. It is also unclear if autophagy is protective or detrimental with respect to the disease pathogenesis. AD has a multifactorial etiology and also exhibits heterogeneous pathological signs. Correspondingly, numerous disease hypotheses have been proposed primarily based on one or few particular pathological features; currently, no hypothesis can provide a unified mechanistic connection to the hierarchical changes in AD pathogenesis. Practically, an accurate disease mechanism is expected to be attributable to different aspects of the disease etiology and also interpretable to the development of different pathological features of the disease. Here we introduce an autophagy-lysosomal cascade in AD pathogenesis and discuss how this pathogenic cascade is initiated by or contributes to the different aspects of the causes, the signs and the lesions of AD pathophysiology.

2.1 Granulovacuolar degeneration and autophagy-lysosomal neuropathology

Granulovacuolar degeneration (GVD) along with plaques and tangles are the earliest described and also the most prominent histopathologic signs of AD (Anderton, 1997; Ball, 1982; Burger & Vogel, 1973; Funk et al., 2011; Okamoto et al., 1991). Granulovacuolar structures were initially reported for AD in 1911. They are characterized as large translucent vacuoles containing electron-dense granule cores appearing in cytoplasm (Shacka et al., 2008) and are often found in pyramidal neurons of the hippocampus. GVD bodies are double membrane enclosed partially digested cytoplasmic contents (Okamoto et al., 1991), suggesting an autophagic origin for the GVD. This autophagic association is further confirmed by positive immunostaining for LC3 and p62 (autophagic markers), LAMP1 (lysosome-associated membrane protein 1) and CHMP2B (charged multivesicular body protein 2B) to the GVD bodies (Funk et al., 2011; Yamazaki et al., 2010). These studies suggest that the GVD bodies are enlarged vesicles derived from autophagy and endocytosis. GVD may also appear in the normal aging brains where plaques and tangles are sparse (Anderton, 1997).

One of the earliest pathological signs observed in patients with AD is the appearance of numerous enlarged autophagic and endosomal vesicles accumulating in perikarya, neurites and synaptic terminals (Nixon et al., 2005; Nixon et al., 2008; Shacka et al., 2008) due to defective autophagy-lysosomal degradation. The defect was initially thought to result from a putative blockage of vesicle fusion among autophagosomes, endosomes and lysosomes thus leading to the failure for autophagosomes to acquire lysosomal catabolic enzymes necessary for cargo digestion (Boland et al., 2008; Nixon, 2007; Nixon et al., 2005; Yu et al., 2005). This view was primarily based on distinguishing autophagosomes in electron micrographs. The identification of pre- and post-lysosomal autophagic or endosomal vesicles in electron micrographs may be misleading. Distinct types of vesicles can dynamically fuse with each other and thus form diverse highly polymorphic structures. These heterogeneous vesicles are hard to be identified with certainty, especially when compromised as part of the disease process. Failure of lysosomal acidification was also proposed as an alternative mechanism responsible for defective autophagic degradation (Lee et al., 2010). By direct expression of human $A\beta_{1-42}$ in *Drosophila* brains, we found that some dysfunctional autophagic vesicles have clearly fused with lysosomes and are acidified (Ling et al., 2009). Thus the massive accumulation of autophagy-lysosomal vesicles in brains apparently results from the vesicular storage of indigestible cargo including $A\beta_{1-42}$ aggregates and other contents. Lysosomal-derived secondary lesions caused by the vesicular leakage of the autophagy-lysosomal contents into cytosol may further activate autophagy and exacerbate vesicle accumulation as discussed in the next section.

Direct $A\beta_{1-42}$ expression in *Drosophila* brains induces age-dependent neurodegeneration through an autophagy-lysosomal injury (Ling et al., 2009). Many degenerative neurons exhibit typical granulovacuolar features (Fig. 1), reflecting the reliability of the *Drosophila* model as an important tool to dissect AD pathogenic mechanisms. In addition to the prominent GVD, the neuronal autophagy-lysosomal machinery may also contribute to the development of amyloid plaques (our unpublished observation) as well as other disease-associated phenotypes such as tangle formation, neurite atrophy, synapse loss, etc as discussed in the following sections. Taken together, autophagy-lysosomal involvement in AD is an early histopathologic sign that has been well recapitulated in different animal models of AD.

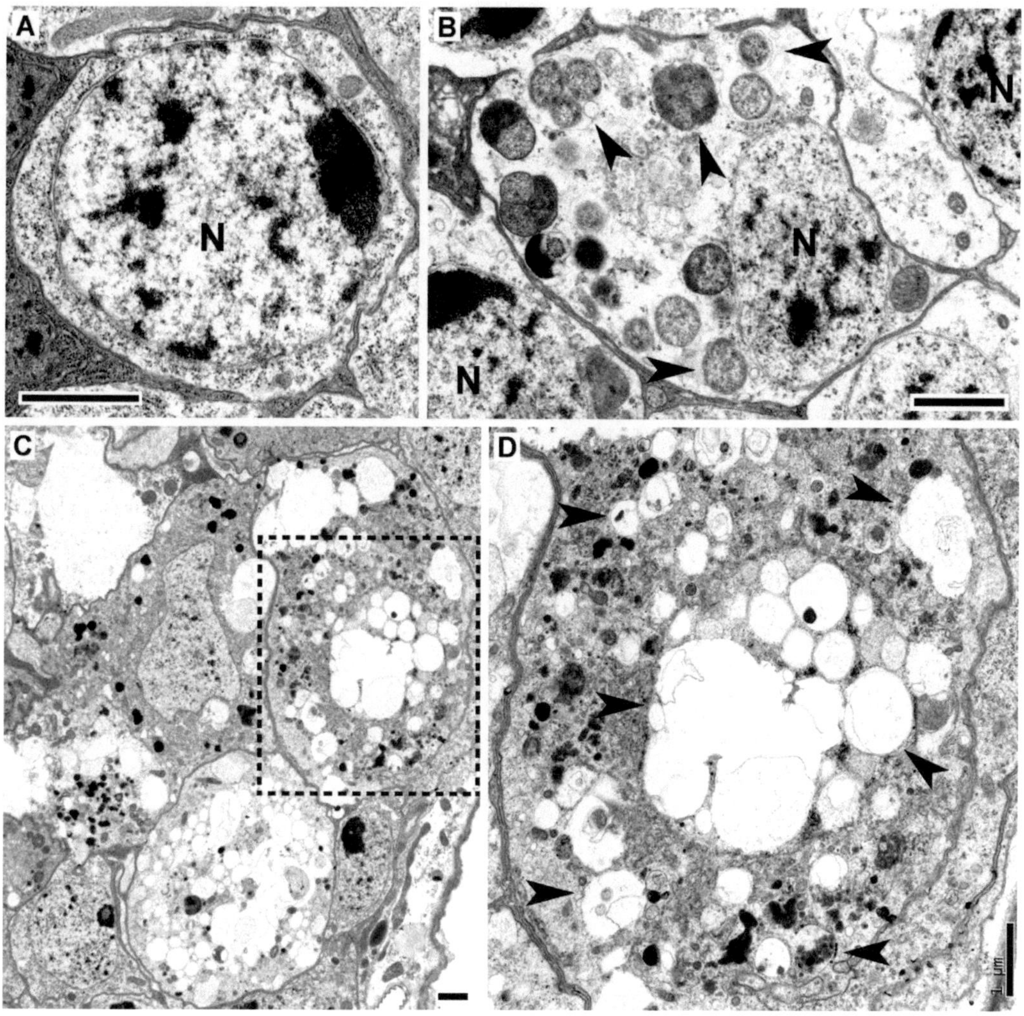

Fig. 1. The GVD morphology recapitulated in a *Drosophila* AD model with neuron-limited expression of human $A\beta_{1-42}$. (A) A normal morphology of neuronal soma. (B) An affected neuron accumulates numerous autophagy-lysosomal vesicles. (C) Extensive neurodegeneration occurs with GVD feature. (D) A higher magnification of view of the neuronal soma in the square area in (C). Arrowheads, autophagy-lysosomal vesicles; N, nuclei. Scale bars = 1μm.

2.2 The pathogenic lesions of AD are a result of the autophagy-lysosomal injury

AD exhibits heterogeneous features in its clinical symptoms, histopathology and neurochemistry. Besides the GVD discussed above, other well-documented neuropathological changes include widespread neuron loss, extracellular plaques, intraneuronal tangles, Hirano bodies, defective mitochondria, neurite atrophy, synapse loss, calcium dyshomeostasis, oxidative stress, neuroinflammation, cerebral amyloid angiopathy, etc. The cause-effect relationships between or among these changes have never been clearly established. To clarify the cause-effect relationships among these changes related to neuronal autophagy, we classify them here as pathological signs or pathogenic lesions. A pathological sign is defined as any detectible pathological event not resulting in additional downstream pathological events; whereas a pathogenic lesion is defined as any detectible pathological event causing other downstream pathological events. Previously we proposed a central role of autophagy-lysosomal system in AD pathogenesis (Ling & Salvaterra, 2009). Here we discuss how a primary autophagy-lysosomal injury in neurons might sit at the top of a pathogenic hierarchy and initiate the secondary and tertiary lesions such as mitochondrial dysfunction, oxidative stress, intracellular Ca^{2+} dyshomeostasis, membrane and organelle damage, all of which eventually develop into the plethora of heterogeneous neuropathologic signs including neurological defects, extracellular diffuse Aβ deposition, amyloid plaques, intracellular tangles, Hirano bodies, neurite and synapse atrophy, extensive neuronal death, etc.

2.2.1 Amyloid deposition and autophagy-lysosomal machinery

A widely held view is that Aβ is produced via APP proteolysis at the surface of neuronal cytoplasmic membranes and released into extracellular spaces. Diffusely distributed extracellular Aβ then assembles into toxic oligomers, aggregates and eventually condenses into senile plaques over a long period of time (Armstrong, 1998; Marchesi, 2005; Torp et al., 2000). However, emerging evidence has demonstrated that a large fraction of Aβ is generated in intracellular compartments rather than at cell surfaces (Gouras et al., 2005; LaFerla et al., 2007). Several subcellular loci have been suggested for intracellular Aβ production including rough endoplasmic reticulum (ER), Golgi apparatus, endosomes, autophagosomes and lysosomes. However, it is unclear how intracellular Aβ is subsequently transported to extracellular spaces and how Aβ deposits into the focal amyloid plaques (Fiala, 2007; Gouras et al., 2005).

The intracellular Aβ may be sequestered by autophagy-lysosomal machinery along with damaged organelles where Aβ is generated. We previously showed that autophagy-sequestered $A\beta_{1-42}$, in turn, decreases the capacity of autophagy-lysosomal degradation (Ling & Salvaterra, 2011a; Ling et al., 2009). $A\beta_{1-42}$-induced dysfunction of lysosomal vesicles may retain indigestible $A\beta_{1-42}$ along with $A\beta_{1-40}$. In support of this possibility, highly concentrated intracellular Aβ has been identified in various autophagic and endosomal vesicles (Petanceska et al., 2000; Takahashi et al., 2002). Autophagy-lysosomal compartments also function in secretion (Gerasimenko et al., 2001; Griffiths, 2002; Luzio et al., 2007; Manjithaya & Subramani, 2011; Pfeffer, 2010). It is plausible therefore that some of lysosomal vesicles may secret their stored monomeric or oligomeric Aβ peptides into extracellular spaces. Consistent with this, some early observations showed that Aβ is secreted by intracellular secretory compartments (Probst et al., 1991; Rajendran et al., 2006). Highly concentrated $A\beta_{1-42}$ aggregates stored in enlarged autophagy-lysosomal vesicles may contribute to the development of amyloid plaques during aging or neurodegeneration (our unpublished observation). Thus the neuronal autophagy-lysosomal pathway appears to play a central role in amyloid deposition associated with either AD or normal brain aging.

2.2.2 Lysosome-derived chemical lesions and subcellular damage

Aβ (especially $A\beta_{1-42}$) is an amphipathic molecule known to disturb biological membranes (Eckert et al., 2010; Gibson Wood et al., 2003). The membranes of lysosome-related vesicles with an acidic microenvironment are especially sensitive to Aβ disturbance (Ditaranto et al., 2001; McLaurin & Chakrabartty, 1996). This membrane disruption is thought to result from the direct interaction between the hydrophobic C-terminus of Aβ peptides and the lipid bilayer of the membrane (Marchesi, 2005). The interaction also appears to be important for membrane-associated Aβ assembly into higher ordered structures (Friedman et al., 2009; Sureshbabu et al., 2010). Compromised membrane integrity greatly increases membrane conductance that has been attributed to a putative ionic channel formed by Aβ peptides (Jang et al., 2010).

$A\beta_{1-42}$ expressed in *Drosophila* brains induces a deterioration and compromise of autophagy-lysosomal vesicles (Ling et al., 2009). The vesicle compromise and subsequent leakage is a primary causative event that results in secondary pathogenic lesions as evident by extensive membrane disruption occurring in cytoplasmic, nuclear and other organelle membranes. In electron micrographs, disrupted membranes are discontinuous with large gaps or exhibit irregularly multilamellar or indistinct cloud-like morphology (Fig. 2), suggesting that membrane disruption results from structural destabilization likely due to an altered intracellular microenvironment rather than direct interaction between $A\beta_{1-42}$ and lipid bilayers. Furthermore, affected neurons are consistently associated with cytoplasmic acidification. Because numerous autophagy-lysosomal vesicles are dramatically enlarged and retained in affected neurons, once their membranes are compromised, a leakage of their contents will significantly alter the chemical microenvironment of the cytosol causing an intraneuronal chemical lesion. Thus the autophagy-lysosomal injury may be the cause of multiple downstream pathogenic events (Ling & Salvaterra, 2009; Reddy & Beal, 2008).

Mitochondrial deficits are a prominent pathogenic lesion in AD (Moreira et al., 2010a; Moreira et al., 2010b; Reddy & Beal, 2008). Lysosomal-derived chemical lesions may be the proximate cause of these deficits. Electron micrographs show a host of morphological changes including decreased size, abnormal cristae and accumulation of osmiophilic materials in brain tissues from AD patients (Baloyannis, 2006). These morphological features are consistent with our observations using the *Drosophila* model of AD (Ling et al., 2009). Mitochondria provide the energy necessary to support various cellular activities many of which are quite demanding in neurons such as active maintenance of ionic gradients. At the same time, mitochondria also produce free radicals and other oxidative molecules that are intimately involved in the aging process (Balaban et al., 2005). Indeed, metabolic defects, energy deficiency and increased oxidative stress are common pathogenic lesions found in AD (Baloyannis, 2006). In addition to being the major source of intracellular reactive oxygen species, mitochondria are also particularly vulnerable to oxidative damage. Oxidative stress may thus result in a self-amplifying pathogenic lesion. Oxidative stress induces additional compromise of autophagy-lysosomal and mitochondrial membranes and the later will produce more free radicals and further exacerbate the pathogenic lesion.

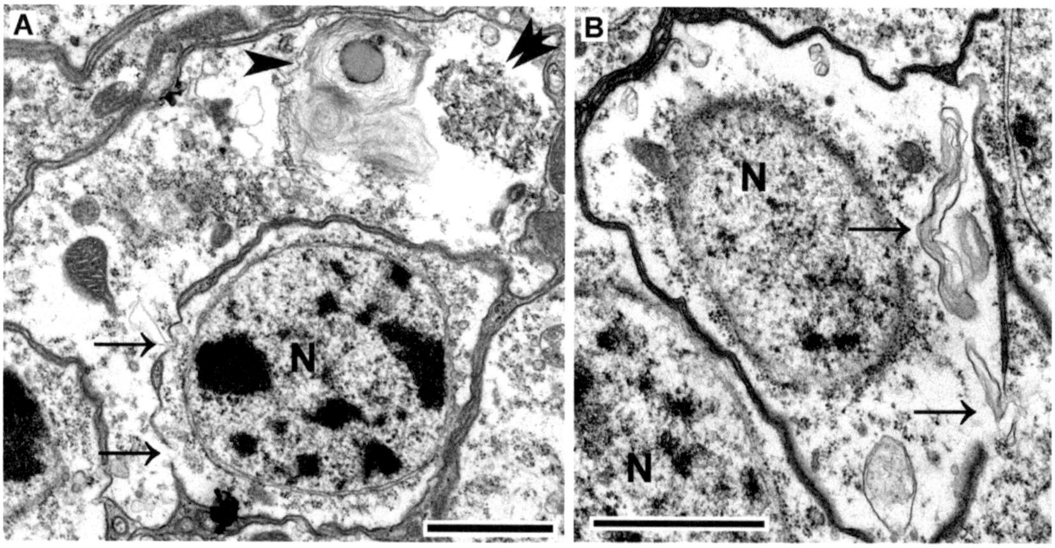

Fig. 2. $A\beta_{1\text{-}42}$ expression causes membrane disruption due to a lysosome-derived chemical lesion. (A) The plasma membranes of an affected and adjacent neuronal somas exhibit discontinuity (arrows). The arrowhead points to a damaged autophagy-lysosomal vesicle; Double arrowheads point to $A\beta_{1\text{-}42}$ aggregate. (B) The plasma and intracellular membranes exhibit multilamellar or cloudy morphology (arrows). N, nuclei. Scale bars = 1µm. The image in (B) was previously published (Ling et al., 2009).

Lysosomal-derived chemical lesions may also destabilize membranes of ER, nuclei and various transport vesicles that will release Ca^{2+} into the cytosol. Neuronal Ca^{2+} is normally stored in membrane compartments such as ER, mitochondria, nuclear envelope and neurotransmitter vesicles (Verkhratsky & Petersen, 1998). Compromise of these membrane-bounded organelles results in a loss of homeostatic intracellular Ca^{2+} control, another prominent chemical lesion in AD pathogenesis (LaFerla, 2002; Supnet & Bezprozvanny, 2010). Cytoplasmic Ca^{2+} is a pivotal neuronal signal regulating multiple intraneuronal activities, neural functions and synaptic plasticity. In vitro application of synthetic Aβ can elevate intracellular Ca^{2+} levels that make cultured neurons more vulnerable to glutamate excitotoxicity (Mattson et al., 1992). Disturbances in neuronal Ca^{2+} may also affect mitochondrial function and vesicular trafficking and, in turn, exacerbate the neurodegenerative cascade.

Lysosomal-derived chemical lesions can destabilize the cytoskeleton, a subcellular component essential for axonal transport, maintenance of normal structure and function of neurites and synapses as well as other cellular activities. Elevated intracellular Ca^{2+} alone was observed to be sufficient to destabilize microtubules and accelerate tau phosphorylation (Mattson et al., 1991), thus linking this chemical lesion with the formation of neurofibrillary tangles. Lysosomal-derived chemical lesions are also associated with the formation of Hirano bodies, rod-shaped and paracrystalline intracellular aggregates composed of actin and cofilin (Maciver & Harrington, 1995). Many neurodegenerative conditions induce the rapid formation of cofilin-actin rod-like inclusions that occur primarily in axons and neurites (Minamide et al., 2000). Cytoskeletal destabilization will disrupt axonal transport of mitochondria and neurotransmitter vesicles as well as many other important subcellular activities in neurons (McMurray, 2000; Stokin et al., 2005). Tau hyperphosphorylation and microtubule destabilization will also accelerate neurite and synapse atrophy due to the crucial role of microtubules in supporting neuronal terminals and maintaining synaptic integrity (Harada et al., 1994). Thus lysosomal-derived chemical lesions may initiate multiple downstream pathogenic lesions via oxidative stress, Ca^{2+} aberration, cytoplasmic acidification, etc leading to a self-exacerbating and vicious cycle.

Membrane integrity is essential for implementation of neuronal function because the conduction of nerve impulses depends on the maintenance of stable ionic gradients. After an electrical signaling event, restoration of active membrane properties requires an intact membrane to restore proper ionic gradients. Normal neuronal function also relies on the integrity of neurites that extend far from cell bodies. Thus the abnormally elevated Ca^{2+} levels, destabilized microtubules and other cytoskeletal elements, defects in axonal transport, degenerating neurites and synapses resulting from lysosome-derived chemical lesions will cause a decline in neuronal functional performance that may contribute to impairment in the encoding or retrieval of new memories, one of the earliest signs of AD (Selkoe, 2002).

2.2.3 Autophagy-lysosomal injury contributes to neurite and synapse atrophy

Alzheimer's dementia is believed to start from synaptic alterations that correlate more robustly with cognitive decline, memory loss and neurodegeneration than the traditional pathological markers such as plaques and tangles (Selkoe, 2002). Synapse loss and neurite atrophy is critically dependent on cortical Aβ levels. Direct expression of Aβ in *Drosophila* neurons is sufficient to induce synaptic neuropathy (Zhao et al., 2010). However it has never been clear how Aβ induces synapse and neurite damage. Recent evidence demonstrates that neurite atrophy is associated with autophagy activation; and autophagy inhibition protects neurites from degeneration (Wang et al., 2006; Yang et al., 2007). Brain traumatic injury elevates neuronal autophagy and also exhibits axonal degeneration (Chu et al., 2009), supporting an association between the two. Degenerating axons have autophagosome accumulation and cytoplasmic vacuolization along with intracellular Ca^{2+} elevation and cytoskeletal alterations (Knoferle et al., 2010), indicating that lysosomal-derived chemical lesions may contribute to neurite and synapse degeneration. Consistent with this, manipulation of autophagy activity or intracellular Ca^{2+} levels affects the severity of axonal degeneration (Knoferle et al., 2010). In addition, implementation of neuronal function intimately relies on endocytic recycling of neurotransmitters and their receptors at synaptic terminals. Thus subtle changes in the autophagy-lysosomal system may affect synapse construction, maintenance and remodeling (Rowland et al., 2006).

2.2.4 Widespread neuronal loss and autophagy-derived necrosis

A major unanswered question in Alzheimer's pathogenesis is to identify the execution pathway responsible for widespread neuronal death. Apoptosis, a well-controlled and self-regulated programmed cell death, has been widely considered to be the relevant cell death mechanism in many neurodegenerative disorders. However, this appealing mechanism is problematic when applied to Alzheimer's pathogenesis (Graeber & Moran, 2002). Apoptosis is characterized by DNA fragmentation, chromatin condensation, caspase activation, cell shrinking and plasma membrane blebbing. DNA fragmentation detected by the TUNEL method is widespread in AD type neuronal death; however apoptotic morphology is rare

(Jellinger & Stadelmann, 2000). DNA fragmentation, phosphatidylserine exposure on the cell surface as well as mitochondrial dysfunction also exist in other non-apoptotic types of cell death, raising the concern that the widely used TUNEL or annexin V staining alone is not sufficient to validate apoptosis as a particular cell death mechanism.

Autophagy, while generally viewed as a cell survival mechanism, is also thought to cause autophagic cell death (Bursch, 2001), another type of programmed cell death characterized by an abundance of autophagic vesicles in dying cells (Chen et al., 2010). Autophagy over-activation in *Drosophila* larval fat body results in a significant cell loss suggesting that this pathway is capable of inducing cell death (Scott et al., 2007). Neuronal death after hypoxic and ischemic brain injury is also associated with a dramatic increase of autophagic vesicles; furthermore, mice with *Atg7* deficiency show nearly complete protection from neuronal death, suggesting that autophagy plays an essential role in executing neuronal death after hypoxic and ischemic injury (Koike et al., 2008). Cellular models for Parkinson's disease using the 1-methyl-4-phenylpyridium (MPP+) neurotoxin show that induced autophagic toxicity leads to neuronal death (Chu et al., 2007). Even with these observations, it is still controversial whether the presence of autophagy morphology is a cause or a result of cell death.

Either brain aging or $A\beta_{1\text{-}42}$ production causes a chronic deterioration of the neuronal autophagy-lysosomal system leading to accumulation of inefficient and enlarged autophagy-lysosomal vesicles in neurons (Ling & Salvaterra, 2011a). Lysosomal compartments are known for membrane permeabilization that release lysosomal cathepsins and other hydrolases into the cytosol; however, the process and the extent of the leakage are usually regulable or may activate a controlled mode of cell death (i.e. apoptosis) (Boya & Kroemer, 2008; Guicciardi et al., 2004). Intriguingly, we found that $A\beta_{1\text{-}42}$-induced lysosomal leakage causes uncontrollable intraneuronal necrotic destruction (Ling et al., 2009). Some dying neurons lose their normal cytosolic structures but maintain a relatively normal shape for the plasma membrane forming balloon cells (Fig. 3). Necrotic cell death usually stimulates a powerful inflammatory response. Indeed, neuroinflammation is a prominent pathological feature of AD (Sastre et al., 2011). These data indicate that autophagy-derived necrosis is likely to be the primary cell death execution pathway responsible for the widespread neuronal loss in AD pathogenesis.

2.3 Causative connections between AD risk factors and autophagy-lysosomal injury

The firmly established risk factors of AD are increasing age, the ε4 allele of the apolipoprotein E (*ApoE*) gene, familial history of AD and Down syndrome. Down syndrome-associated AD neuropathology is thought to be a consequence of the over dosage of the *APP* gene. Familial history as a risk factor is particularly associated with early-onset familial AD and is attributable to various inheritance-acquired mutations predominantly located in three genes: *APP, PSEN1* and *PSEN2* (Bertram & Tanzi, 2008). The *ApoE* ε4 allele is associated with sporadic AD (Bertram & Tanzi, 2008) and may account for 50% of AD cases in United States (Raber et al., 2004). Thus among the 4 firmly-established AD associated genes, *APP, PSEN1* and *PSEN2* are causative genes for familial AD; whereas *ApoE* is a susceptibility gene for sporadic AD. Among various AD risk factors, advancing age is the most prominent as evident by a dramatically increased prevalence of AD as people get older. The incidence of AD in the American population raises from 2% at 65–74 years old to 19% at 75–84 and 42% or more in individuals over 85 years old (see Alzheimer's Disease Facts and Figures 2007, Alzheimer's Association). Besides aging, other less prominent risk factors include traumatic brain injuries, increased cholesterol levels and other lifestyle and pathophysiological conditions such as high blood pressure, heart disease, stroke and diabetes (Flicker, 2010; Lahiri & Maloney, 2010; McDowell, 2001; Martins et al., 2006; Rosendorff et al., 2007). It is currently unknown how those causative and susceptibility genes, aging, various environmental and lifestyle risk factors interact to affect the disease onset. Here we consider how the autophagy-lysosomal injury establishes a pathological connection between the main etiological factors and AD onset. Other risk factors that could also be attributable to AD pathogenesis through direct or indirect connection to the autophagy-lysosomal injury are not discussed here due to space limitations.

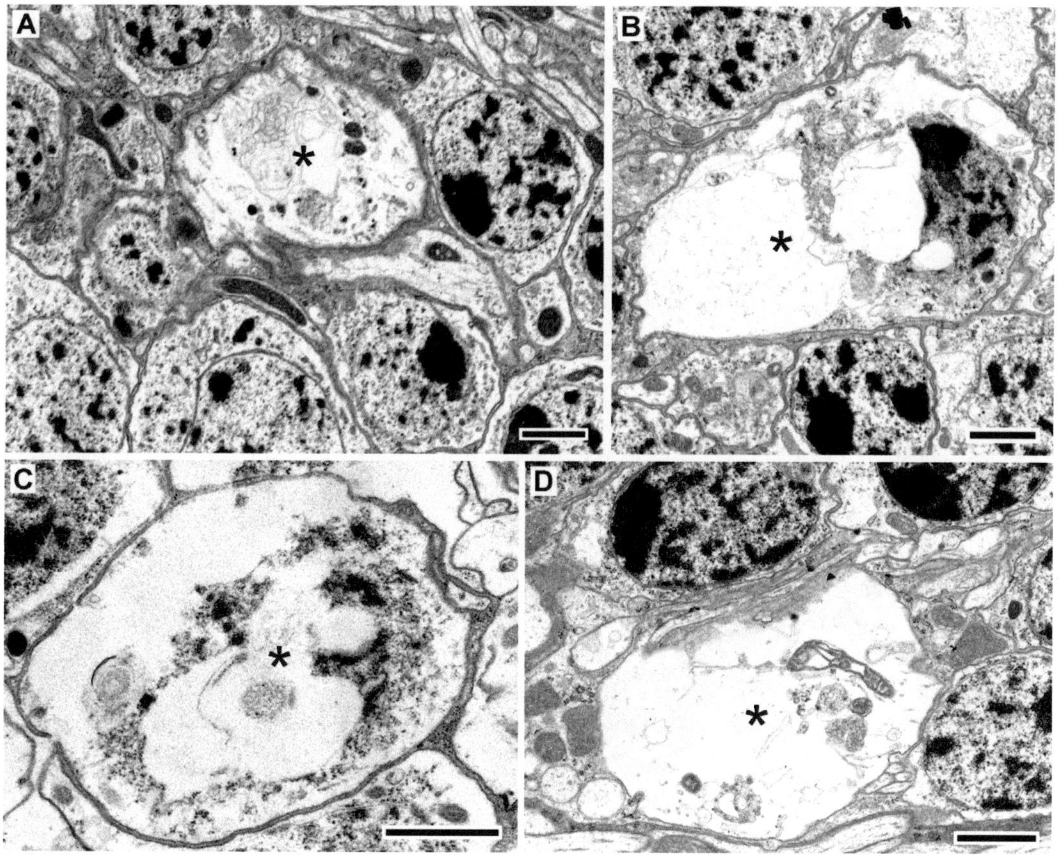

Fig. 3. The morphology of balloon cells results from $A\beta_{1\text{-}42}$-induced neurodegeneration. (A) A balloon cell of degenerated neuronal soma surrounded by relatively normal neuronal somas. (B-C) Necrotic intracellular destruction causes the formation of balloon cells. (D) A balloon cell is electron lucent with partially digested mitochondria and other organelles. Stars (*), balloon cells. Scale bars = 1μm.

2.3.1 Genetic determinants and autophagy-lysosomal Aβ degradation

Amyloid deposition formed by Aβ aggregates is a pathological hallmark of AD. Familial AD-associated mutations on *APP*, *PSEN1* and *PSEN2* genes mostly favor production of hyperaggregatable $A\beta_{1\text{-}42}$ rather than $A\beta_{1\text{-}40}$. More AD susceptibility loci recently identified are also associated with Aβ metabolism (Sleegers et al., 2010). $A\beta_{1\text{-}42}$ in its fibrillary or oligomeric form is believed to be the main causative agent of AD. Aβ overproduction causes a dementia-like phenotype in transgenic animals (McGowan et al., 2006). Direct $A\beta_{1-42}$ expression in *Drosophila* brains induces age-dependent neurodegeneration (Finelli et al., 2004; Iijima et al., 2004; Crowther et al., 2005; Ling et al., 2009), suggesting that overproduction of $A\beta_{1-42}$ alone is sufficient to initiate neurodegenerative cascade. Even though $A\beta_{1-42}$ is the most widely accepted causative agent for AD, brain amyloid load does not correlate strictly with the severity of dementia. In an interrupted clinical trial, anti-Aβ immuno-therapy resulted in decreased brain amyloidosis but exhibited subtle cognitive benefits (Gilman et al., 2005). Furthermore, Aβ is a normal component of serum and cerebrospinal fluid in individuals with no disease symptoms. These observations complicate the cause-effect relationship between Aβ and AD. However, these seemingly paradoxical aspects of Aβ and AD are compatible with the self-exacerbating autophagy-lysosomal cascade that is initiated by but then independent of further $A\beta_{1-42}$ production as discussed in the next section.

$A\beta_{1-42}$-induced neurodegeneration via an autophagy-lysosomal injury does not conflict with the general protective function of the autophagy-lysosomal machinery. The protective or detrimental effect of neuronal autophagy is primarily dependent on the efficiency of lysosomal degradation of disease-associated aggregate-prone proteins and damaged organelles. Not all aggregate-prone proteins are amenable to autophagic degradation (Wong et al., 2008). Human $A\beta_{1-40}$ and $A\beta_{1-42}$ expressed in *Drosophila* brain have differential effects on neuronal autophagy-lysosomal degradation (Ling et al., 2009). $A\beta_{1-42}$ induces an age-dependent functional defect as well as a structural compromise in autophagy-lysosomal vesicles. These deteriorated vesicles massively accumulate in affected neurons and their size is dramatically enlarged. $A\beta_{1-40}$, in contrast, does not produce any detectible changes in either the neuronal autophagy-lysosomal machinery or neurological defects in animals, suggesting that $A\beta_{1-40}$ may be amenable to autophagic removal and thus lack significant neurotoxicity. The differential autophagic responses to $A\beta_{1-40}$ vs. $A\beta_{1-42}$ is consistent with the paradoxical observations that APP proteolysis primarily generates $A\beta_{1-40}$ (Hartmann et al., 1997), while it is $A\beta_{1-42}$ that predominantly accumulates in neurons (Gouras et al., 2005). The early-onset deterioration of neuronal autophagy-lysosomal machinery specific to $A\beta_{1-42}$ but not $A\beta_{1-40}$ is also consistent with the causative role of $A\beta_{1-42}$ in AD pathogenesis.

2.3.2 The risk factors of ApoE and cholesterol

ApoE and cholesterol, known to have a strong impact on development of cardiovascular disease (Purnell et al., 2009), are also important modifiers of AD onset (Lahiri et al., 2004; Sambamurti et al., 2004). The underlying mechanism linking ApoE and cholesterol with AD pathogenesis is still not completely understood. Cholesterol is a normal membrane component that modifies membrane fluidity. Accumulating evidence shows that cholesterol modulates Aβ production and aggregation through its effect on lipid rafts. Membrane-embedded APP undergoes amyloidogenic proteolysis by beta-secretase (BACE1) or non-amyloidogenic proteolysis by alpha-secretase. Lipid rafts, the cholesterol- and sphingolipid-enriched membrane microdomains (Simons & Toomre, 2000), play an essential role in amyloidogenic APP proteolysis, because the lipid raft enhances accessibility of BACE1 to APP (Ehehalt et al., 2003; Rushworth & Hooper, 2010; Vetrivel & Thinakaran, 2010). Lipid rafts may also facilitate Aβ aggregation (Rushworth & Hooper, 2010) and extracellular Aβ internalization (Lai & McLaurin, 2010). Increased cholesterol accelerates APP localization into lipid rafts and enhances Aβ generation (Kosicek et al., 2010; Michikawa, 2003); consistent with observations that elevated dietary cholesterol uptake or hypercholesterolemia is associated with increased formation of amyloid plaques (Kivipelto et al., 2001). In addition, cholesterol depletion inhibits neuronal Aβ generation (Sambamurti et al., 2004); and cholesterol-reducing statin drugs appear to reduce the risk of dementia (Gibson Wood et al., 2003).

ApoE is the major carrier of lipids, including cholesterol, in the brain. Lipidated ApoE has been shown to inhibit Aβ transport across blood-brain-barrier and facilitate its degradation (Fan et al., 2009). The ε4 allele of *ApoE* gene was observed to contribute to Aβ deposition (Jones et al., 2011; Raber et al., 2004), favor cerebral amyloid angiopathy (Kumar-Singh, 2008) and promote earlier AD onset (Roses, 1996). So ApoE and cholesterol may affect the onset of AD likely through modification of Aβ production and aggregation and thus indirectly influence the neuronal autophagy-lysosomal machinery. It is also plausible that there is a direct interaction between ApoE/cholesterol and the efficiency of autophagic-lysosomal turnover as a potential mechanism for the altered risk of AD. ApoE/cholesterol modifies membrane fluidity that could directly affect the trafficking of lysosomal vesicles as well as their degradation. ApoE in neurons is actively recycled by endocytosis (DeKroon & Armati, 2001) but not amenable to intracellular degradation (Rensen et al., 2000). ApoE ε4 also appears to accentuate abnormal changes in early endosomes at preclinical stages of AD (Cataldo et al., 2000), impair endocytosis of extracellular Aβ internalization, prevent lysosomal degradation of Aβ (Yamauchi et al., 2002) and increase intracellular $A\beta_{1\text{-}42}$ accumulation (Yu et al., 2010; Zerbinatti et al., 2006).

2.3.3 Brain aging and autophagy-lysosomal catabolism

AD exhibits multiple neuropathological signs and clinical symptoms that distinguish it from normal brain aging. However, normal aging brains undergo similar histopathologic changes seen in AD including the presence of plaques, tangles, Hirano bodies, GVD, neurite and synapse deficit, shrinkage in overall brain volume, decreased brain weight and enlargement of brain ventricles (Anderton, 1997; Drachman, 2007). The differences in these changes comparing AD with normal aging appear to be quantitative rather than qualitative (Ball, 1982). Even after a century of intensive studies, the pathogenic connection between normal aging and AD remains elusive.

Human $A\beta_{1\text{-}42}$ expression in *Drosophila* brains results in a massive accumulation of enlarged dysfunctional autophagy–lysosomal vesicles that become increasingly compromised with age leading to deterioration of neuronal integrity and necrotic intraneuronal destruction (Ling et al., 2009). Intriguingly, the process of normal aging undergoes similar pathogenic changes in wild-type *Drosophila* brains without expression of any disease-associated proteins (Ling & Salvaterra, 2011a). The only difference between $A\beta_{1\text{-}42}$ expression and normal brain aging is the time scale of the neuropathological progression. $A\beta_{1\text{-}42}$ induces an early-onset autophagy-lysosomal neuropathology which progresses rapidly; whereas normal aging has a late-onset neuropathology which progresses at a slower rate. These data are consistent with observations that low levels of abnormal autophagy-lysosomal vesicles, characterized as typical granulovacuolar degeneration, are also observed in hippocampal neurons from brains of mentally normal patients (Ball & Lo, 1977), suggesting that brains normally undergo deterioration of the autophagy-lysosomal machinery during aging. Thus normal brain aging accompanies neurodegeneration via an autophagy-lysosomal neuropathology that may occur at a slow enough rate or on a small enough scale. Any cognitive decline associated with normal aging-associated neurodegeneration will go unnoticed. Consistent with this possibility, individuals with normally measured cognitive function undergo an age-dependent reduction in overall brain volume and weight as well as an age-dependent enlargement of brain ventricles due to neuron loss (Anderton, 1997).

Autophagy-lysosomal machinery maintains intracellular homeostasis and thus protects neurons from degeneration. Basal levels of neuronal autophagy are believed to decrease with age (Komatsu et al., 2007); however, direct evidence supporting this view is absent. In *Drosophila* brains autophagy activity during normal aging appears to be stable based on observations that no significant changes occurs in expression levels for several autophagy-related genes (Ling & Salvaterra, 2011b). Moreover, induction of neuronal autophagy in a conditional *Drosophila* model is protective in young animals, but likely detrimental in older animals (Ling & Salvaterra, 2011a). Therefore it is reasonable to propose that the autophagy–lysosomal machinery likely shifts from a functional and protective status to a pathological and deleterious status during brain aging. Consistent with this, autophagic function is known to decline with age (Bergamini et al., 2007). Taken together, either brain aging or $A\beta_{1-42}$ proteotoxicity contributes to the chronic deterioration of the neuronal autophagy-lysosomal system. The deterioration of this catabolic machinery appears to be a key pathogenic event that converts normal brain aging into pathological aging leading to Alzheimer's neurodegeneration.

3. Autophagy-lysosomal cascade: A hypothesis for AD pathogenesis

Remarkable progress has been made in studying many aspects of AD. Unfortunately, this has not resulted in the successful development of effective treatments, primarily because of the absence of a definite pathogenic mechanism. Numerous hypotheses have been advanced to address AD pathogenesis including the amyloid cascade, membrane disruption/Aβ ion channel, mitochondrial abnormalities, energy deficits, glutamate excitotoxicity, cerebrovascular dysfunction, neuroinflammation, oxidative stress, Ca^{2+} dyshomeostasis and cytoskeletal aberrations. Each of these ideas were proposed and developed based on one or few particular pathological features of AD. As a consequence most of the currently favored hypotheses provide only a limited view rather than a more global perspective of the pathogenic mechanism. It also remains unclear what initial event(s) trigger the pathogenic cascade and how so many different pathological insults can be attributed to the key pathogenic event.

Extensive autophagy involvement in AD has been well documented (Nixon et al., 2005; Shacka et al., 2008; Suzuki & Terry, 1967). However, it remains unsettled if autophagy plays a causative role, a protective role or is a consequence of the disease process itself (Ling & Salvaterra, 2009). Among the various signs and lesions of AD neuropathology, compromised autophagy-lysosomal vesicles and their resultant injuries appear to play a central role in initiating the pathogenic cascade leading to disease progression. Based on *Drosophila* models of AD and brain aging as well as growing evidence in this field, we have proposed an autophagy-derived neurodegenerative cascade initiated by $A\beta_{1-42}$ and enhanced by aging (Ling & Salvaterra, 2009, 2011a; Ling et al., 2009).

APP proteolysis and Aβ production occurs at membrane surfaces facing the lumen of membrane compartments including ER, Golgi apparatus and endosomal vesicles (Fiala, 2007; Gouras et al., 2005). Aβ is constitutively produced in human brains throughout the normal lifespan. Apparently the levels of newly generated Aβ peptides may not be sufficient to initiate a pathogenic cascade in healthy neurons; however, due to their amphipathic property, they may disturb local membranes and the functional execution of host organelles. These organelles, if damaged, will be sequestered by autophagy. However, Aβ particularly $A\beta_{1-42}$ cannot be efficiently degraded in autophagy-lysosomal vesicles especially under chronic deterioration of this machinery during advancing age (Ling & Salvaterra, 2011a). Other indigestible proteins and lipids (for example lipofuscin) may synergistically contribute to the deterioration of autophagy-lysosomal machinery causing cargo storage in enlarged vesicles. Consistent with this view, intracellular Aβ peptides predominantly accumulate within autophagic and endosomal vesicles (Nixon, 2004; Takahashi et al., 2002; Yu et al., 2005) and AD-like neuropathological phenotypes are also seen in some lysosomal storage diseases (Bahr & Bendiske, 2002; Ohm et al., 2003; Jin et al., 2004; Settembre et al., 2008).

Numerous lysosomal vesicles in cytosol would represent a large source of acidic contents and lysosomal hydrolases. The enlarged size and long-term retention of these vesicles may make them easily compromised especially when $A\beta_{1-42}$ becomes concentrated within them. Compromised vesicles result in leakage of their acidic contents into cytosol. This will destabilize other intracellular structures and organelles including ER and mitochondria leading to oxidative stress and Ca^{2+} dyshomeostasis. The resultant damage from this altered intracellular microenvironment will further activate autophagy causing additional pathogenic stress. Thus a self-exacerbated pathogenic cascade is formed through initiation, dysfunction, compromise of autophagic vesicles and the resultant cytosolic chemical lesions. This neurodegenerative cascade is initiated by $A\beta_{1-42}$ and enhanced by aging and eventually results in necrotic neuronal death. Once initiated, the cascade would likely become independent of continuous Aβ production since cytosolic chemical lesions would drive it as a progressive and irreversible pathogenic pathway. This autophagy-lysosomal-derived neurodegenerative cascade provides a common cellular framework for a detailed mechanistic understanding of the heterogeneous aspects of AD neuropathology as the signs, the lesions and the causes of the disease.

4. Conclusion

Alzheimer's disease is an incurable terminal neurodegenerative disorder with multifactorial etiology and heterogeneous pathology. The clearer we understand the pathogenic mechanism(s) regarding its causes, lesions and signs, the better we should be able to develop effective treatments for mitigating or even preventing this disastrous disorder. The autophagy-lysosomal system, a bulk process for removal of intracellular toxic proteins and damaged organelles, appears to play a central role in the disease pathogenesis. Based on our recent work and a large volume of previous studies from other groups, we propose an autophagy-lysosomal cascade that is attributable to various AD etiologies, and responsible for the hierarchical pathological signs and pathogenic lesions. One of the prominent features of this pathogenic mechanism is its potential for self-exacerbation. Once progressing to an uncontrollable stage, this cascade is likely to be independent of initial contributions from causative factors and will continue to develop progressively and irreversibly. This feature fits well with the onset of pathological and clinical AD. It has never been clear when the disease pathology actually starts; however, once diagnosed, the disease develops progressively and relentlessly. This feature emphasizes the importance of preventative strategies applied to the at-risk individuals prior to the actual occurrence of this disease.

The autophagy-lysosomal cascade for AD pathogenesis appears to provide a unified cellular framework for understanding the disease; however, therapeutic development targeting autophagy-lysosomal pathway is far from maturation. Our knowledge of the autophagy-lysosomal system is fast growing (Klionsky, 2007). Many basic aspects of the pathway are still waiting for detailed characterization. A beneficial outcome from manipulation of autophagy activity under neurodegenerative conditions is still uncertain. Even though basal autophagy is protective and autophagy induction has prosurvival effects observed in some disease models (Rubinsztein et al., 2007), detrimental effects of increased autophagy are also associated with certain pathological conditions (Cherra et al., 2010; White & DiPaola, 2009). Our studies, however, emphasize that enhancing the maintenance of an integrated and efficient autophagy–lysosomal system in brain rather than simply induction of autophagy activity would be a promising therapeutic direction for anti-aging or prevention of AD.

5. Acknowledgements

The work in our laboratory has been generously supported by grants from the American Health Assistant Foundation (AHAF) and the Sidell-Kagan Foundation. DL was partially supported by postdoctoral fellowships from the John Douglas French Alzheimer's Foundation (2005-2007) and the American Federation for Aging Research (2009-2010). The authors thank all other authors making contributions to the studies cited in this manuscript and apologize to those who made similar contributions in work not being cited due to space limitation. The authors have no competing financial interests.

6. References

Anderton, B.H. (1997). Changes in the ageing brain in health and disease. *Philosophical transactions of the Royal Society of London* 352, 1781-1792.

Armstrong, R.A. (1998). Beta-amyloid plaques: stages in life history or independent origin? *Dementia and geriatric cognitive disorders* 9, 227-238.

Bahr, B.A. & Bendiske, J. (2002). The neuropathogenic contributions of lysosomal dysfunction. *Journal of neurochemistry* 83, 481-489.

Balaban, R.S., Nemoto, S. & Finkel, T. (2005). Mitochondria, oxidants, and aging. *Cell* 120, 483-495.

Ball, M.J. (1982). Alzheimer's disease: a challenging enigma. *Archives of pathology & laboratory medicine* 106, 157-162.

Ball, M.J. & Lo, P. (1977). Granulovacuolar degeneration in the ageing brain and in dementia. *Journal of neuropathology and experimental neurology* 36, 474-487.

Baloyannis, S.J. (2006). Mitochondrial alterations in Alzheimer's disease. *Journal of Alzheimer's disease* 9, 119-126.

Bergamini, E., Cavallini, G., Donati, A. & Gori, Z. (2007). The role of autophagy in aging: its essential part in the anti-aging mechanism of caloric restriction. *Annals of the New York Academy of Sciences* 1114, 69-78.

Bertram, L. & Tanzi, R.E. (2008). Thirty years of Alzheimer's disease genetics: the implications of systematic meta-analyses. *Nature Reviews Neuroscience* 9, 768-778.

Boland, B., Kumar, A., Lee, S., Platt, F.M., Wegiel, J., Yu, W.H. & Nixon, R.A. (2008). Autophagy induction and autophagosome clearance in neurons: relationship to autophagic pathology in Alzheimer's disease. *Journal of Neuroscience* 28, 6926-6937.

Boya, P. & Kroemer, G. (2008). Lysosomal membrane permeabilization in cell death. *Oncogene* 27, 6434-6451.

Burger, P.C. & Vogel, F.S. (1973). The development of the pathologic changes of Alzheimer's disease and senile dementia in patients with Down's syndrome. *The American journal of pathology* 73, 457-476.

Bursch, W. (2001). The autophagosomal-lysosomal compartment in programmed cell death. *Cell death and differentiation* 8, 569-581.

Cataldo, A.M., Peterhoff, C.M., Troncoso, J.C., Gomez-Isla, T., Hyman, B.T. & Nixon, R.A. (2000). Endocytic pathway abnormalities precede amyloid beta deposition in sporadic Alzheimer's disease and Down syndrome: differential effects of APOE genotype and presenilin mutations. *The American journal of pathology* 157, 277-286.

Chen, Y., Azad, M.B. & Gibson, S.B. (2010). Methods for detecting autophagy and determining autophagy-induced cell death. *Canadian journal of physiology and pharmacology* 88, 285-295.

Cherra, S.J., 3rd, Dagda, R.K. & Chu, C.T. (2010). Autophagy and neurodegeneration: survival at a cost? *Neuropathology and applied neurobiology* 36, 125-132.

Chu, C.T., Plowey, E.D., Dagda, R.K., Hickey, R.W., Cherra, S.J., 3rd & Clark, R.S. (2009). Autophagy in neurite injury and neurodegeneration: in vitro and in vivo models. *Methods in enzymology* 453, 217-249.

Chu, C.T., Zhu, J. & Dagda, R. (2007). Beclin 1-independent pathway of damage-induced mitophagy and autophagic stress: implications for neurodegeneration and cell death. *Autophagy* 3, 663-666.

Crowther, D.C., Kinghorn, K.J., Miranda, E., Page, R., Curry, J.A., Duthie, F.A., Gubb, D.C. & Lomas, D.A. (2005). Intraneuronal Abeta, non-amyloid aggregates and neurodegeneration in a *Drosophila* model of Alzheimer's disease. *Neuroscience* 132, 123-135.

DeKroon, R.M. & Armati, P.J. (2001). The endosomal trafficking of apolipoprotein E3 and E4 in cultured human brain neurons and astrocytes. *Neurobiology of disease* 8, 78-89.

Ditaranto, K., Tekirian, T.L. & Yang, A.J. (2001). Lysosomal membrane damage in soluble Abeta-mediated cell death in Alzheimer's disease. *Neurobiology of disease* 8, 19-31.

Drachman, D.A. (2007). Rethinking Alzheimer's disease: the role of age-related changes. *Current neurology and neuroscience reports* 7, 265-268.

Eckert, G.P., Wood, W.G. & Muller, W.E. (2010). Lipid membranes and beta-amyloid: a harmful connection. *Current protein & peptide science* 11, 319-325.

Ehehalt, R., Keller, P., Haass, C., Thiele, C. & Simons, K. (2003). Amyloidogenic processing of the Alzheimer beta-amyloid precursor protein depends on lipid rafts. *The Journal of cell biology* 160, 113-123.

Fan, J., Donkin, J. & Wellington, C. (2009). Greasing the wheels of Abeta clearance in Alzheimer's disease: the role of lipids and apolipoprotein E. *BioFactors (Oxford, England)* 35, 239-248.

Fiala, J.C. (2007). Mechanisms of amyloid plaque pathogenesis. *Acta neuropathologica* 114, 551-571.

Finelli, A., Kelkar, A., Song, H.J., Yang, H. and Konsolaki, M. (2004). A model for studying Alzheimer's Abeta42-induced toxicity in Drosophila melanogaster. *Molecular and Cellular Neurosciences* 26: 365–375.

Flicker, L. (2010). Modifiable lifestyle risk factors for Alzheimer's disease. *Journal of Alzheimer's disease* 20, 803-811.

Friedman, R., Pellarin, R. & Caflisch, A. (2009). Amyloid aggregation on lipid bilayers and its impact on membrane permeability. *Journal of molecular biology* 387, 407-415.

Funk, K.E., Mrak, R.E. & Kuret, J. (2011). Granulovacuolar Degeneration Bodies of Alzheimer's Disease Resemble Late-stage Autophagic Organelles. *Neuropathology and applied neurobiology* 37, 295-306.

Gerasimenko, J.V., Gerasimenko, O.V., and Petersen, O.H. (2001). Membrane repair: Ca(2+)-elicited lysosomal exocytosis. *Current Biology* 11, R971-974.

Gibson Wood, W., Eckert, G.P., Igbavboa, U. & Muller, W.E. (2003). Amyloid beta-protein interactions with membranes and cholesterol: causes or casualties of Alzheimer's disease. *Biochimica et biophysica acta* 1610, 281-290.

Gilman, S., Koller, M., Black, R.S., Jenkins, L., Griffith, S.G., Fox, N.C., Eisner, L., Kirby, L., Rovira, M.B., Forette, F., *et al.* (2005). Clinical effects of Abeta immunization (AN1792) in patients with AD in an interrupted trial. *Neurology* 64, 1553-1562.

Gouras, G.K., Almeida, C.G. & Takahashi, R.H. (2005). Intraneuronal Abeta accumulation and origin of plaques in Alzheimer's disease. *Neurobiology of aging* 26, 1235-1244.

Graeber, M.B. & Moran, L.B. (2002). Mechanisms of cell death in neurodegenerative diseases: fashion, fiction, and facts. *Brain pathology (Zurich, Switzerland)* 12, 385-390.

Griffiths, G. (2002). What's special about secretory lysosomes? *Seminars in cell & developmental biology* 13, 279-284.

Guicciardi, M.E., Leist, M. & Gores, G.J. (2004). Lysosomes in cell death. *Oncogene* 23, 2881-2890.

Harada, A., Oguchi, K., Okabe, S., Kuno, J., Terada, S., Ohshima, T., Sato-Yoshitake, R., Takei, Y., Noda, T. & Hirokawa, N. (1994). Altered microtubule organization in small-calibre axons of mice lacking tau protein. *Nature* 369, 488-491.

Hartmann, T., Bieger, S.C., Bruhl, B., Tienari, P.J., Ida, N., Allsop, D., Roberts, G.W., Masters, C.L., Dotti, C.G., Unsicker, K., *et al.* (1997). Distinct sites of intracellular production for Alzheimer's disease A beta40/42 amyloid peptides. *Nature medicine* 3, 1016-1020.

Iijima, K., Liu, H.P., Chiang, A.S., Hearn, S.A., Konsolaki, M., et al. (2004). Dissecting the pathological effects of human Abeta40 and Abeta42 in Drosophila: a potential model for Alzheimer's disease. *Proceedings of the National Academy of Sciences of the United States of America* 101, 6623–6628.

Jang, H., Arce, F.T., Ramachandran, S., Capone, R., Azimova, R., Kagan, B.L., Nussinov, R. & Lal, R. (2010). Truncated beta-amyloid peptide channels provide an alternative mechanism for Alzheimer's Disease and Down syndrome. *Proceedings of the National Academy of Sciences of the United States of America* 107, 6538-6543.

Jellinger, K.A. & Stadelmann, C. (2000). Mechanisms of cell death in neurodegenerative disorders. *Journal of neural transmission* 59, 95-114.

Jin, L.W., Shie, F.S., Maezawa, I., Vincent, I., and Bird, T. (2004). Intracellular accumulation of amyloidogenic fragments of amyloid-beta precursor protein in neurons with

Niemann-Pick type C defects is associated with endosomal abnormalities. *The American journal of pathology* 164, 975-985.

Jones, P.B., Adams, K.W., Rozkalne, A., Spires-Jones, T.L., Hshieh, T.T., Hashimoto, T., von Armin, C.A., Mielke, M., Bacskai, B.J. & Hyman, B.T. (2011). Apolipoprotein E: Isoform Specific Differences in Tertiary Structure and Interaction with Amyloid-beta in Human Alzheimer Brain. *PloS One* 6, e14586.

Kivipelto, M., Helkala, E.L., Laakso, M.P., Hanninen, T., Hallikainen, M., Alhainen, K., Soininen, H., Tuomilehto, J. & Nissinen, A. (2001). Midlife vascular risk factors and Alzheimer's disease in later life: longitudinal, population based study. *British Medical Journal (Clinical research ed.)* 322, 1447-1451.

Klionsky, D.J. (2007). Autophagy: from phenomenology to molecular understanding in less than a decade. *Nature reviews* 8, 931-937.

Knoferle, J., Koch, J.C., Ostendorf, T., Michel, U., Planchamp, V., Vutova, P., Tonges, L., Stadelmann, C., Bruck, W., Bahr, M., *et al.* (2010). Mechanisms of acute axonal degeneration in the optic nerve in vivo. *Proceedings of the National Academy of Sciences of the United States of America* 107, 6064-6069.

Koike, M., Shibata, M., Tadakoshi, M., Gotoh, K., Komatsu, M., Waguri, S., Kawahara, N., Kuida, K., Nagata, S., Kominami, E., *et al.* (2008). Inhibition of autophagy prevents hippocampal pyramidal neuron death after hypoxic-ischemic injury. *The American journal of pathology* 172, 454-469.

Komatsu, M., Ueno, T., Waguri, S., Uchiyama, Y., Kominami, E. & Tanaka, K. (2007). Constitutive autophagy: vital role in clearance of unfavorable proteins in neurons. *Cell death and differentiation* 14, 887-894.

Kosicek, M., Malnar, M., Goate, A. & Hecimovic, S. (2010). Cholesterol accumulation in Niemann Pick type C (NPC) model cells causes a shift in APP localization to lipid rafts. *Biochemical and biophysical research communications* 393, 404-409.

Kumar-Singh, S. (2008). Cerebral amyloid angiopathy: pathogenetic mechanisms and link to dense amyloid plaques. *Genes, brain, and behavior* 7 Suppl 1, 67-82.

LaFerla, F.M. (2002). Calcium dyshomeostasis and intracellular signalling in Alzheimer's disease. *Nature Review Neuroscience* 3, 862-872.

LaFerla, F.M., Green, K.N. & Oddo, S. (2007). Intracellular amyloid-beta in Alzheimer's disease. *Nature Review Neuroscience* 8, 499-509.

Lahiri, D.K. & Maloney, B. (2010). The "LEARn" (Latent Early-life Associated Regulation) model integrates environmental risk factors and the developmental basis of Alzheimer's disease, and proposes remedial steps. *Experimental gerontology* 45, 291-296.

Lahiri, D.K., Sambamurti, K. & Bennett, D.A. (2004). Apolipoprotein gene and its interaction with the environmentally driven risk factors: molecular, genetic and epidemiological studies of Alzheimer's disease. *Neurobiology of aging* 25, 651-660.

Lai, A.Y. & McLaurin, J. (2010). Mechanisms of amyloid-Beta Peptide uptake by neurons: the role of lipid rafts and lipid raft-associated proteins. *International journal of Alzheimer's disease* 2011, 548380.

Lee, J.H., Yu, W.H., Kumar, A., Lee, S., Mohan, P.S., Peterhoff, C.M., Wolfe, D.M., Martinez-Vicente, M., Massey, A.C., Sovak, G., *et al.* (2010). Lysosomal proteolysis and autophagy require presenilin 1 and are disrupted by Alzheimer-related PS1 mutations. *Cell* 141, 1146-1158.

Ling, D. & Salvaterra, P.M. (2009). A central role for autophagy in Alzheimer-type neurodegeneration. *Autophagy* 5, 738-740.

Ling, D. & Salvaterra, P.M. (2011a). Brain aging and Abeta (1-42) neurotoxicity converge via deterioration in autophagy-lysosomal system: a conditional *Drosophila* model linking Alzheimer's neurodegeneration with aging. *Acta neuropathologica* 121, 183-191.

Ling, D. & Salvaterra, P.M. (2011b). Robust RT-qPCR data normalization: validation and selection of internal reference genes during post-experimental data analysis. *PloS One* 6, e17762

Ling, D., Song, H.J., Garza, D., Neufeld, T.P. & Salvaterra, P.M. (2009). Abeta42-induced neurodegeneration via an age-dependent autophagic-lysosomal injury in *Drosophila*. *PloS One* 4, e4201.

Luzio, J.P., Pryor, P.R. & Bright, N.A. (2007). Lysosomes: fusion and function. *Nature reviews* 8, 622-632.

Maciver, S.K. & Harrington, C.R. (1995). Two actin binding proteins, actin depolymerizing factor and cofilin, are associated with Hirano bodies. *Neuroreport* 6, 1985-1988.

Manjithaya, R. & Subramani, S. (2011). Autophagy: a broad role in unconventional protein secretion? *Trends in cell biology* 21, 67-73.

Marchesi, V.T. (2005). An alternative interpretation of the amyloid Abeta hypothesis with regard to the pathogenesis of Alzheimer's disease. *Proceedings of the National Academy of Sciences of the United States of America* 102, 9093-9098.

Martins, I.J., Hone, E., Foster, J.K., Sunram-Lea, S.I., Gnjec, A., Fuller, S.J., Nolan, D., Gandy, S.E., and Martins, R.N. (2006). Apolipoprotein E, cholesterol metabolism, diabetes, and the convergence of risk factors for Alzheimer's disease and cardiovascular disease. *Molecular psychiatry* 11, 721-736.

Mattson, M.P., Cheng, B., Davis, D., Bryant, K., Lieberburg, I. & Rydel, R.E. (1992). Beta-Amyloid peptides destabilize calcium homeostasis and render human cortical neurons vulnerable to excitotoxicity. *Journal of Neuroscience* 12, 376-389.

Mattson, M.P., Engle, M.G. & Rychlik, B. (1991). Effects of elevated intracellular calcium levels on the cytoskeleton and tau in cultured human cortical neurons. *Molecular and chemical neuropathology* 15, 117-142.

McDowell, I. (2001). Alzheimer's disease: insights from epidemiology. *Aging (Milan, Italy)* 13, 143-162.

McGowan, E., Eriksen, J. & Hutton, M. (2006). A decade of modeling Alzheimer's disease in transgenic mice. *Trends in Genetics* 22, 281-289.

McLaurin, J. & Chakrabartty, A. (1996). Membrane disruption by Alzheimer beta-amyloid peptides mediated through specific binding to either phospholipids or gangliosides. Implications for neurotoxicity. *The Journal of biological chemistry* 271, 26482-26489.

McMurray, C.T. (2000). Neurodegeneration: diseases of the cytoskeleton? *Cell death and differentiation* 7, 861-865.

Michikawa, M. (2003). The role of cholesterol in pathogenesis of Alzheimer's disease: dual metabolic interaction between amyloid beta-protein and cholesterol. *Molecular neurobiology* 27, 1-12.

Minamide, L.S., Striegl, A.M., Boyle, J.A., Meberg, P.J. & Bamburg, J.R. (2000). Neurodegenerative stimuli induce persistent ADF/cofilin-actin rods that disrupt distal neurite function. *Nature cell biology* 2, 628-636.

Mizushima, N., Levine, B., Cuervo, A.M. & Klionsky, D.J. (2008). Autophagy fights disease through cellular self-digestion. *Nature* 451, 1069-1075.

Moreira, P.I., Carvalho, C., Zhu, X., Smith, M.A. & Perry, G. (2010a). Mitochondrial dysfunction is a trigger of Alzheimer's disease pathophysiology. *Biochimica et biophysica acta* 1802, 2-10.

Moreira, P.I., Santos, R.X., Zhu, X., Lee, H.G., Smith, M.A., Casadesus, G. & Perry, G. (2010b). Autophagy in Alzheimer's disease. *Expert review of neurotherapeutics* 10, 1209-1218.

Nixon, R.A. (2004). Niemann-Pick Type C disease and Alzheimer's disease: the APP-endosome connection fattens up. *The American journal of pathology* 164, 757-761.

Nixon, R.A. (2007). Autophagy, amyloidogenesis and Alzheimer disease. *Journal of cell science* 120, 4081-4091.

Nixon, R.A., Wegiel, J., Kumar, A., Yu, W.H., Peterhoff, C., Cataldo, A. & Cuervo, A.M. (2005). Extensive involvement of autophagy in Alzheimer disease: an immuno-electron microscopy study. *Journal of neuropathology and experimental neurology* 64, 113-122.

Nixon, R.A., Yang, D.S. & Lee, J.H. (2008). Neurodegenerative lysosomal disorders: a continuum from development to late age. *Autophagy* 4, 590-599.

Ohm, T.G., Treiber-Held, S., Distl, R., Glockner, F., Schonheit, B., Tamanai, M. & Meske, V. (2003). Cholesterol and tau protein--findings in Alzheimer's and Niemann Pick C's disease. *Pharmacopsychiatry* 36 Suppl 2, S120-126.

Okamoto, K., Hirai, S., Iizuka, T., Yanagisawa, T. & Watanabe, M. (1991). Reexamination of granulovacuolar degeneration. *Acta neuropathologica* 82, 340-345.

Petanceska, S.S., Seeger, M., Checler, F. & Gandy, S. (2000). Mutant presenilin 1 increases the levels of Alzheimer amyloid beta-peptide Abeta42 in late compartments of the constitutive secretory pathway. *Journal of neurochemistry* 74, 1878-1884.

Pfeffer, S.R. (2010). Unconventional secretion by autophagosome exocytosis. *The Journal of cell biology* 188, 451-452.

Probst, A., Langui, D., Ipsen, S., Robakis, N. & Ulrich, J. (1991). Deposition of beta/A4 protein along neuronal plasma membranes in diffuse senile plaques. *Acta neuropathologica* 83, 21-29.

Purnell, C., Gao, S., Callahan, C.M. & Hendrie, H.C. (2009). Cardiovascular risk factors and incident Alzheimer disease: a systematic review of the literature. *Alzheimer disease and associated disorders* 23, 1-10.

Raber, J., Huang, Y. & Ashford, J.W. (2004). ApoE genotype accounts for the vast majority of AD risk and AD pathology. *Neurobiology of aging* 25, 641-650.

Rajendran, L., Honsho, M., Zahn, T.R., Keller, P., Geiger, K.D., Verkade, P. & Simons, K. (2006). Alzheimer's disease beta-amyloid peptides are released in association with exosomes. *Proceedings of the National Academy of Sciences of the United States of America* 103, 11172-11177.

Reddy, P.H. & Beal, M.F. (2008). Amyloid beta, mitochondrial dysfunction and synaptic damage: implications for cognitive decline in aging and Alzheimer's disease. *Trends in molecular medicine* 14, 45-53.

Rensen, P.C., Jong, M.C., van Vark, L.C., van der Boom, H., Hendriks, W.L., van Berkel, T.J., Biessen, E.A. & Havekes, L.M. (2000). Apolipoprotein E is resistant to intracellular degradation in vitro and in vivo. Evidence for retroendocytosis. *The Journal of biological chemistry* 275, 8564-8571.

Rosendorff, C., Beeri, M.S. & Silverman, J.M. (2007). Cardiovascular risk factors for Alzheimer's disease. The American journal of geriatric cardiology *16*, 143-149.

Roses, A.D. (1996). Apolipoprotein E alleles as risk factors in Alzheimer's disease. *Annual review of medicine* 47, 387-400.

Rowland, A.M., Richmond, J.E., Olsen, J.G., Hall, D.H. & Bamber, B.A. (2006). Presynaptic terminals independently regulate synaptic clustering and autophagy of GABAA receptors in Caenorhabditis elegans. *Journal of Neuroscience* 26, 1711-1720.

Rubinsztein, D.C., Gestwicki, J.E., Murphy, L.O. & Klionsky, D.J. (2007). Potential therapeutic applications of autophagy. *Nature Reviews Drug Discovery* 6, 304-312.

Rushworth, J.V. & Hooper, N.M. (2010). Lipid Rafts: Linking Alzheimer's Amyloid-beta Production, Aggregation, and Toxicity at Neuronal Membranes. *International journal of Alzheimer's disease 2011*, 603052.

Sambamurti, K., Granholm, A.C., Kindy, M.S., Bhat, N.R., Greig, N.H., Lahiri, D.K. & Mintzer, J.E. (2004). Cholesterol and Alzheimer's disease: clinical and experimental models suggest interactions of different genetic, dietary and environmental risk factors. *Current drug targets* 5, 517-528.

Sastre, M., Richardson, J.C., Gentleman, S.M. & Brooks, D.J. (2011). Inflammatory Risk Factors and Pathologies Associated with Alzheimer's Disease. *Current Alzheimer research* 2011 Feb 23 [Epub ahead of print].

Scott, R.C., Juhasz, G. & Neufeld, T.P. (2007). Direct induction of autophagy by Atg1 inhibits cell growth and induces apoptotic cell death. *Current Biology* 17, 1-11.

Selkoe, D.J. (2002). Alzheimer's disease is a synaptic failure. *Science* 298, 789-791.

Settembre, C., Fraldi, A., Jahreiss, L., Spampanato, C., Venturi, C., Medina, D., de Pablo, R., Tacchetti, C., Rubinsztein, D.C. & Ballabio, A. (2008). A block of autophagy in lysosomal storage disorders. *Human molecular genetics* 17, 119-129.

Shacka, J.J., Roth, K.A. & Zhang, J. (2008). The autophagy-lysosomal degradation pathway: role in neurodegenerative disease and therapy. *Frontiers in bioscience* 13, 718-736.

Simons, K. & Toomre, D. (2000). Lipid rafts and signal transduction. *Nature reviews* 1, 31-39.

Sleegers, K., Lambert, J.C., Bertram, L., Cruts, M., Amouyel, P. & Van Broeckhoven, C. (2010). The pursuit of susceptibility genes for Alzheimer's disease: progress and prospects. *Trends in Genetics* 26, 84-93.

Stokin, G.B., Lillo, C., Falzone, T.L., Brusch, R.G., Rockenstein, E., Mount, S.L., Raman, R., Davies, P., Masliah, E., Williams, D.S., *et al.* (2005). Axonopathy and transport deficits early in the pathogenesis of Alzheimer's disease. *Science* 307, 1282-1288.

Supnet, C. & Bezprozvanny, I. (2010). Neuronal calcium signaling, mitochondrial dysfunction, and Alzheimer's disease. *Journal of Alzheimer's disease* 20 Suppl 2, S487-498.

Sureshbabu, N., Kirubagaran, R., Thangarajah, H., Malar, E.J. & Jayakumar, R. (2010). Lipid-induced conformational transition of amyloid beta peptide fragments. *Journal of Molecular Neuroscience* 41, 368-382.

Suzuki, K. & Terry, R.D. (1967). Fine structural localization of acid phosphatase in senile plaques in Alzheimer's presenile dementia. *Acta neuropathologica* 8, 276-284.

Takahashi, R.H., Milner, T.A., Li, F., Nam, E.E., Edgar, M.A., Yamaguchi, H., Beal, M.F., Xu, H., Greengard, P. & Gouras, G.K. (2002). Intraneuronal Alzheimer abeta42 accumulates in multivesicular bodies and is associated with synaptic pathology. *The American journal of pathology* 161, 1869-1879.

Torp, R., Head, E., Milgram, N.W., Hahn, F., Ottersen, O.P. & Cotman, C.W. (2000). Ultrastructural evidence of fibrillar beta-amyloid associated with neuronal membranes in behaviorally characterized aged dog brains. *Neuroscience* 96, 495-506.

Verkhratsky, A.J. & Petersen, O.H. (1998). Neuronal calcium stores. *Cell calcium* 24, 333-343.

Vetrivel, K.S. & Thinakaran, G. (2010). Membrane rafts in Alzheimer's disease beta-amyloid production. *Biochimica et biophysica acta* 1801, 860-867.

Wang, Q.J., Ding, Y., Kohtz, D.S., Mizushima, N., Cristea, I.M., Rout, M.P., Chait, B.T., Zhong, Y., Heintz, N. & Yue, Z. (2006). Induction of autophagy in axonal dystrophy and degeneration. *Journal of Neuroscience* 26, 8057-8068.

White, E. & DiPaola, R.S. (2009). The double-edged sword of autophagy modulation in cancer. *Clinical Cancer Research* 15, 5308-5316.

Wong, E.S., Tan, J.M., Soong, W.E., Hussein, K., Nukina, N., Dawson, V.L., Dawson, T.M., Cuervo, A.M. & Lim, K.L. (2008). Autophagy-mediated clearance of aggresomes is not a universal phenomenon. *Human molecular genetics* 17, 2570-2582.

Yamauchi, K., Tozuka, M., Hidaka, H., Nakabayashi, T., Sugano, M. & Katsuyama, T. (2002). Isoform-specific effect of apolipoprotein E on endocytosis of beta-amyloid in cultures of neuroblastoma cells. *Annals of clinical and laboratory science* 32, 65-74.

Yamazaki, Y., Takahashi, T., Hiji, M., Kurashige, T., Izumi, Y., Yamawaki, T. & Matsumoto, M. (2010). Immunopositivity for ESCRT-III subunit CHMP2B in granulovacuolar degeneration of neurons in the Alzheimer's disease hippocampus. *Neuroscience letters* 477, 86-90.

Yang, Y., Fukui, K., Koike, T. & Zheng, X. (2007). Induction of autophagy in neurite degeneration of mouse superior cervical ganglion neurons. *The European journal of neuroscience* 26, 2979-2988.

Yu, C., Nwabuisi-Heath, E., Laxton, K. & Ladu, M.J. (2010). Endocytic pathways mediating oligomeric Abeta42 neurotoxicity. *Molecular neurodegeneration* 17, 19.

Yu, W.H., Cuervo, A.M., Kumar, A., Peterhoff, C.M., Schmidt, S.D., Lee, J.H., Mohan, P.S., Mercken, M., Farmery, M.R., Tjernberg, L.O., *et al.* (2005). Macroautophagy--a novel Beta-amyloid peptide-generating pathway activated in Alzheimer's disease. *The Journal of cell biology* 171, 87-98.

Zerbinatti, C.V., Wahrle, S.E., Kim, H., Cam, J.A., Bales, K., Paul, S.M., Holtzman, D.M. & Bu, G. (2006). Apolipoprotein E and low density lipoprotein receptor-related protein facilitate intraneuronal Abeta42 accumulation in amyloid model mice. *The Journal of biological chemistry* 281, 36180-36186.

Zhao, X.L., Wang, W.A., Tan, J.X., Huang, J.K., Zhang, X., Zhang, B.Z., Wang, Y.H., YangCheng, H.Y., Zhu, H.L., Sun, X.J., *et al.* (2010). Expression of beta-amyloid induced age-dependent presynaptic and axonal changes in *Drosophila*. *Journal of Neuroscience* 30, 1512-1522.

Plasmalogen Deficit: A New and Testable Hypothesis for the Etiology of Alzheimer's Disease

Paul L. Wood, M. Amin Khan, Rishikesh Mankidy,
Tara Smith and Dayan B. Goodenowe
Phenomenome Discoveries,
Canada

1. Introduction

Alzheimer's disease (AD) is a complex cognitive disorder for which the single greatest risk factor is age. The pathophysiological basis for AD is still a matter of debate with no current hypothesis explaining all of the complex pathological changes observed. These include neurofibrillary tangles, amyloid plaques, neuroinflammation, hypomyelination, neuronal shrinkage (eg. N- basalis cholinergic neurons, resulting in a dramatic cholinergic deficit), ocular pathology, microvascular pathology and liver peroxisomal dysfunction. The hypothesis that we are presenting, namely peroxisomal dysfunction resulting in decreased supply of critical ethanolamine plasmalogens to the brain, eye and vascular endothelium, is the first hypothesis that can potentially explain all of these complex pathologies in AD. The value of this hypothesis is that it is imminently testable via resupply of critical ether lipid precursors of plasmalogens. PPI-1011 is such a drug candidate and will be presented after a review of the basis of this hypothesis.

2. Plasmalogens in aging and AD

Advancing age remains the largest risk factor for the development of AD. Pathologically, AD is primarily defined by the accumulation of amyloid plaques (AP) and neurofibrillary tangles (NFT), whereas clinically, AD is primarily defined as the progressive deterioration of mental function the earliest symptoms of which are reduced memory functions. Epidemiologically, these three features exhibit essentially superimposable age-severity plots [compare (Braak and Braak 1997) to (Bachman et al., 1992)], yet the mechanism behind this association remains elusive. In this section we attempt to peel back one more layer of the AD onion and put forward the hypothesis that age-related decline in the peripheral synthesis of ethanolamine plasmalogens (PlsEtn), a critical component of both neuronal membranes and myelin sheaths, is responsible for both the pathological and clinical AD cascade. The underlying cause behind peripheral PlsEtn depletion is currently unknown and therefore represents yet another layer to be uncovered in the future.
The time course of the presence and severity of the pathological features of AD was described in detail (Braak and Braak 1997) using a large population of non-selected post-mortem human

brains (ages 26-95, n= 2661). In regards to amyloid deposition, they reported that initial amyloid patches appear in temporal areas such as the perirhinal and/or ectorhinal fields (Stage A) followed by spreading to adjoining neocortical areas and hippocampus (Stage B), and that the primary areas of the neocortex were the last regions to exhibit plaques (Stage C). Of the three stages, only the prevalence of stage C increases with age. This increase begins in the last half of the 6th decade of life. In regards to NFT, six stages are defined. The earliest signs are observed in the transentorhinal region (temporal lobe) (Stage I), then into the entorhinal region (Stage II), then to the hippocampus and temporal proneocortex (Stage III) then the adjoining proneocortex (Stage IV). The lesions then spread superolaterally (Stage V) and finally into the primary regions of the neocortex (Stage VI). In interpreting their data, Braak and Braak commented that the sequence of pathological progression is the inverse of the sequence of cortical myelination and that poorly myelinated areas were the first affected. This observation is of interest in that white matter, but not gray matter appears to exhibit an appreciable age-related degeneration as well (Meier-Ruge et al., 1992; Bartzokis, 2004). These findings have led some researchers to put forward the hypothesis that age-related myelin degeneration is a causative feature in AD (Bartzokis, 2004; Braak and Del Tredici, 2004). PlsEtn but not phosphatidylethanolamines (PtdEtn) exhibit an age-related decline after age 50-69 (Figure 1).

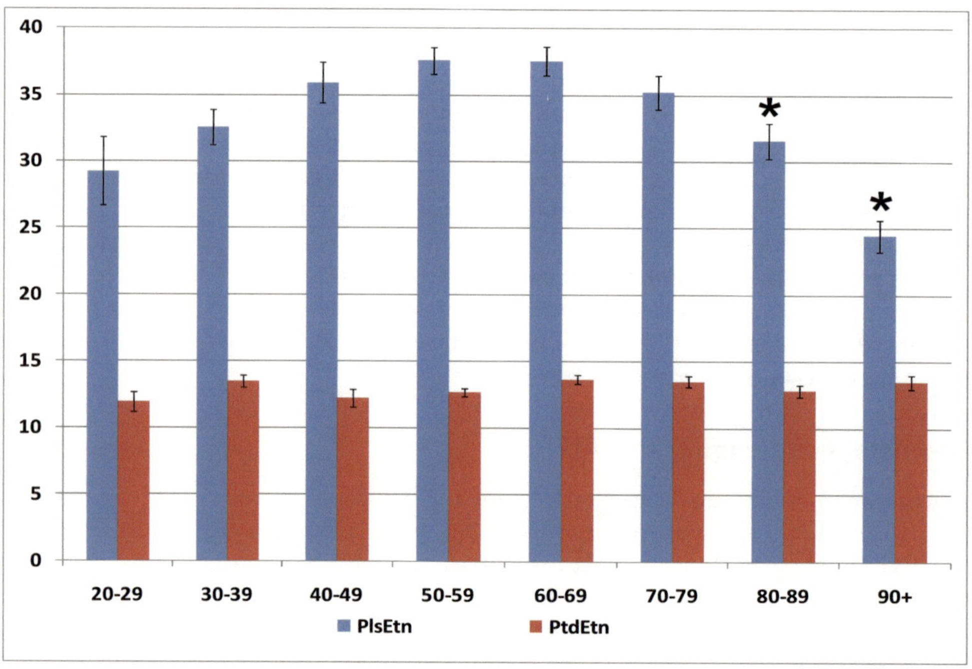

Fig. 1. Effect of age on total serum PlsEtn and PtdEtn. Total PlsEtn and PtdEtn is the sum of 15 sn1/sn2 combinations sn1: 16:0, 18:0, 18:1; sn2: 18:1, 18:2, 18:3, 20:4, 22:6. each normalized to PtdEtn 16:0/18:0. *, $p < 0.05$. Serum samples for the age-association study (Figures 1-2) were provided as anonymized reference samples comprising a random population of 990 control subjects aged 11-99 collected at the provincial clinical testing lab in Regina, Saskatchewan, Canada from the Saskatchewan Disease Control Lab (SDCL) in accordance with SDCL policies and under a protocol approved by the Ethics Department of the University of Saskatchewan. PlsEtn and PlsEtn analyses performed as per Goodenowe et al., 2007.

Interestingly, when the PlsEtn/PtdEtn pairs of the key white matter (18:1) and gray matter (22:6) PlsEtn are compared, the peak age of PlsEtn as a percentage of the ethanolamine phospholipid pool is 50-59. Docosahexaenoic acid (DHA, 22:6) shows the most precipitous decline with age (Figure 2). If PtdEtn and PlsEtn were co-regulated, these ratios should be constant with age. However, this is clearly not the case, indicating that selective plasmalogen decline occurs with age. This age effect is analogous to the above mentioned white matter depletion and AP/NFT accumulation. In addition, DHA-PlsEtn levels decrease in both post-mortem brain and pre-mortem serum samples with increasing Braak scale (Figure 3). These results are consistent with the dementia severity dependent decrease in DHA-PlsEtn in post-mortem brain previously reported (Han et al., 2001). A pharmacologically induced reduction of serum plasmalogens in healthy mice using cuprizone (a molecule that does not cross the blood-brain barrier), preferentially depletes DHA-PlsEtn in the serum and kidney but 18:1-PlsEtn in the CNS, the most abundant PlsEtn of myelin (Figure 4). These data support the hypothesis that a peripheral decline in PlsEtn can cause CNS PlsEtn depletion.

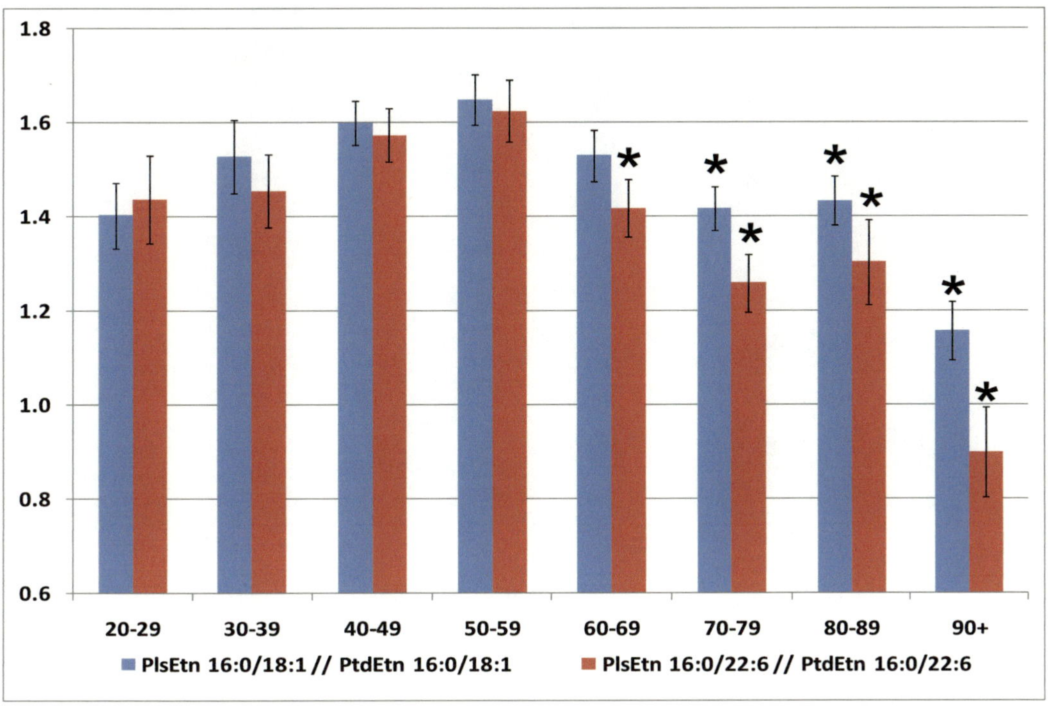

Fig. 2. Effect of age on the relative ratio of specific PlsEtn / PtdEtn species pairs in serum. *, $p < 0.05$.

We have previously reported extensively on the role of plasmalogens in cognition and the association between serum DHA-PlsEtn levels and AD (Goodenowe et al., 2007; Wood et al., 2010). In brief, when compared to cognitively confirmed, age and gender-matched controls (MMSE 29-30, age 77+/-0.8, n=68), subjects with low (ADAS cog 5-19, age 79.3+/-0.8, n=78), moderate (ADAS cog 20-39, age 79.1+/-0.7, n=112), and severe (ADAS cog 40-70, age 82.1+/-1, n=66) dementia had increasingly lower levels of DHA-PlsEtn in their serum (74%, p=3.0e-4; 66%, p=1.3e-7; 53%, p=3.9e-11, respectively). This finding was confirmed in pre-mortem serum samples collected from subjects later confirmed pathologically to have AD and in Japanese subjects with mild AD (Goodenowe et al., 2007). Subsequently, the effect of serum DHA-PlsEtn levels at enrollment on the rate of cognitive decline over 12 months was investigated (Wood et al., 2010). It was observed that only subjects with serum DHA-PlsEtn of 75% or less of normal levels exhibited cognitive decline over a 12 month period. Using samples collected from Rush University's Memory and Aging Program (Bennett et al., 2006) we investigated the predictability of pre-mortem MMSE scores (within 12 months of death) on post-mortem pathology (Figure 5).

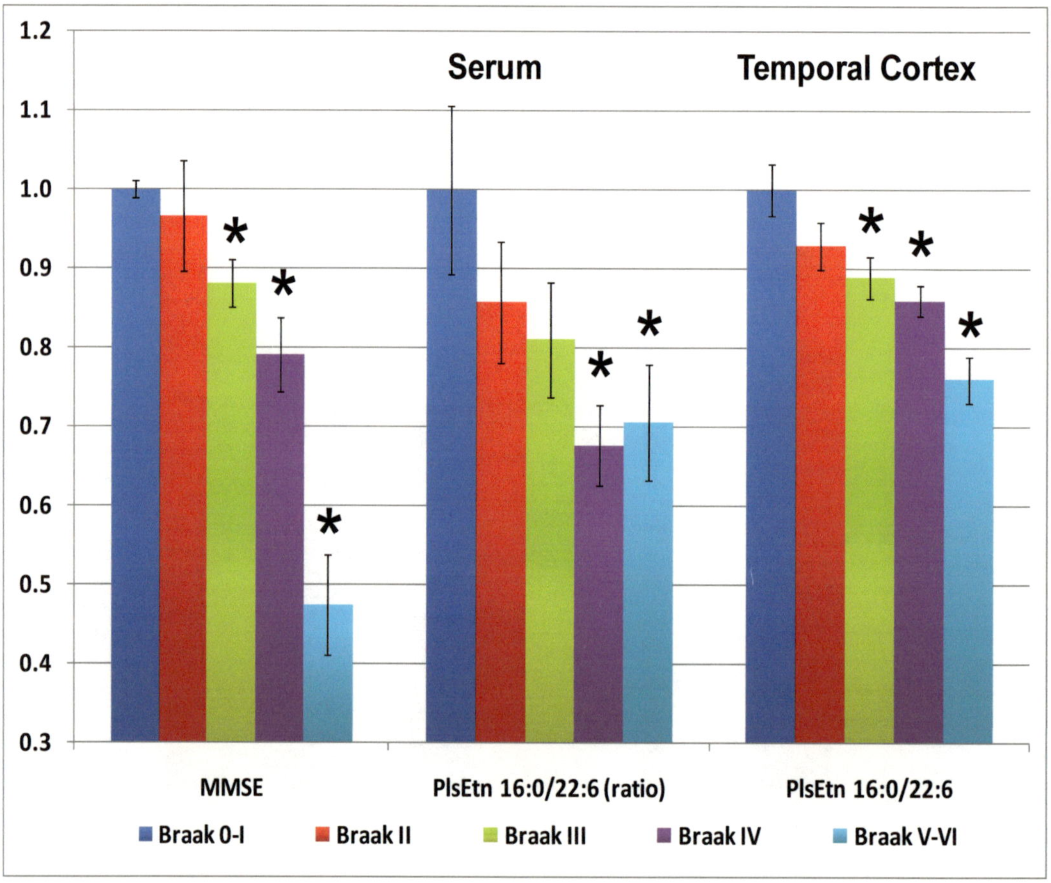

Fig. 3. Effect of Braak Stage on pre-mortem MMSE and Serum DHA-PlsEtn, and post-mortem temporal cortex DHA-PlsEtn levels. Serum levels are normalized to PtdEtn 16:0/18:0, * p<0.05. Braak 0-I (n=11, age 82.9+/-2.6, MMSE=28+/-0.5, 4F); Braak II (n=8, age 86.0+/-1.9, MMSE=25.4+/-3.6, 3F); Braak III (n=23, age 88.2+/-1.0, MMSE 23.9+/-1.2, 14F); Braak IV (n=23, age 91.1+/-0.8, MMSE 22.4+/-1.7, 9F); Braak V-VI (n=21, age 89.1+/-1.0, MMSE 12.5+/-2.1, 14F).

These data indicate that pre-mortem MMSE scores of 25 or less are predictive of increased Braak stage and decreased DHA-PlsEtn levels, whereas MMSE scores of 20 or less are needed to be predictive of increased Aβ-42 (the key protein in amyloid plaques) levels. Further support for the role of DHA-PlsEtn in cognition is the observation that deficient liver biosynthesis of DHA correlates with cognitive impairment in AD (Astarita et al., 2010) and that phospholipid linked DHA (containing significant levels of plasmalogen) has a positive cognition effect whereas triglyceride linked DHA has a minimal effect (Hiratsuka et al., 2009).

The biosynthesis of DHA and plasmalogens occurs exclusively in peroxisomes (Nagan and Zoeller, 2001), however, it does not appear that the brain is a significant producer of these molecules. The key dietary metabolic precursor of DHA (alpha-linolenic acid) is converted to DHA in the liver, not the brain, and then transported to the brain pre-packaged on phospholipids. Peroxisomal function, as a whole, is known to decline with age (Munn et al., 2003; Mandel et al., 1998). Decreased peroxisomal function leads to decreased synthesis of PlsEtn and DHA (Zoeller and Raetz, 1986; Martinez, 1990). DHA synthesis involves chain elongation and desaturation of 18:3 n-3 fatty acids to 24:6 in the ER. The final step of DHA synthesis, β-oxidation to DHA, occurs in the peroxisome (Voss et al., 1991). Both DHAP synthase (Andre et al., 2006) and β-oxidase (Perichon and Bourre, 1995), exhibit decreased function with age and DHA containing PlsEtn are selectively decreased with age (Favreliere et al., 2000) In addition, the activity of catalase, the principal peroxisomal enzyme responsible for detoxifying H_2O_2 also decreases in activity with age (Perichon and Bourre, 1995; Favreliere et al., 2000; Rao et al., 1990), and is believed to be associated with increased lipid peroxidation with age. Accordingly, there is ample evidence of impaired plasmalogen synthesis and/or increased degradation with increasing age, however, the underlying causes and relative contribution of these processes are currently unknown.

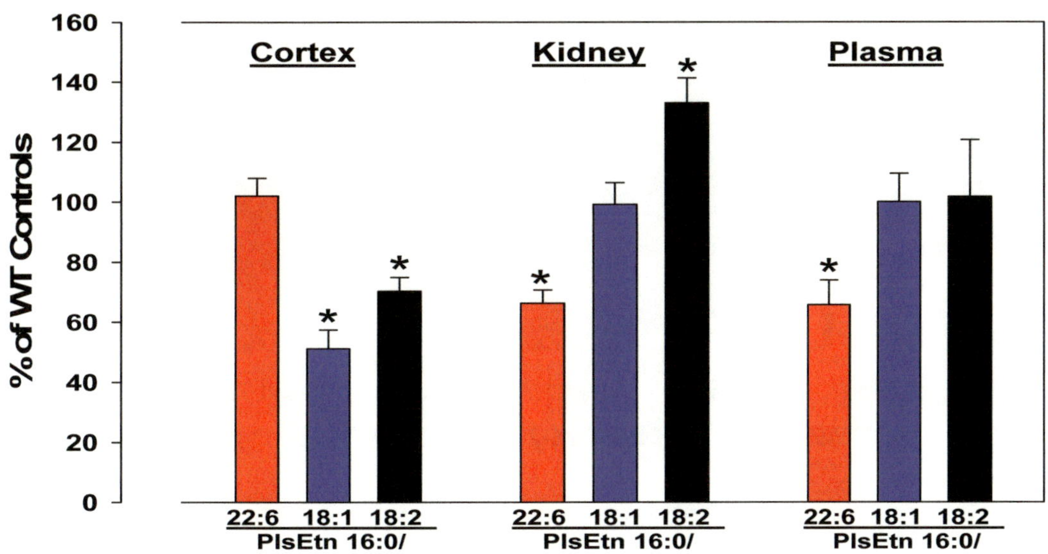

Fig. 4. Effect of cuprizone on plasma, kidney, and cortex 16:0 (sn-1) ethanolamine plasmalogen levels. * $p<0.05$ versus untreated. See PPI-1011 section for methodological description.

3. Plasmalogen biochemistry and its role in AD

The fundamental role of PlsEtn is as a membrane lipid. PlsEtn constitute over 80 mol% of the ethanolamine phospholipid pool in non-neuronal brain membranes and over 60 mol% in neurons and synaptosomes (Han et al., 2001). PlsEtn found in white matter contain predominately 18:1, 20:1 and 22:4 fatty acids at the sn-2 position, whereas in gray matter, 22:6, 20:4, and 22:4 are found in highest concentration (Horrocks and Sharma, 1982). These differences result in dramatically different membrane structures. A high percentage of monounsaturates at *sn*-2 results in very compact and stable membrane conformations (Han and Gross, 1990; 1991) which is consistent with the function of the myelin sheath. A high percentage of polyunsaturates results in more fluid membrane structures that are required for membrane fusion (Lohner et al., 1991; Lohner, 1996; Glaser and Gross, 1994; 1995), which is consistent with the functions performed by neurons. Plasmalogen deficient cells exhibit decreased transmembrane protein function (Perichon et al., 1998) and membrane related intra-cellular (Munn et al., 2003) and extra-cellular (Mandel et al., 1998) cholesterol transport.

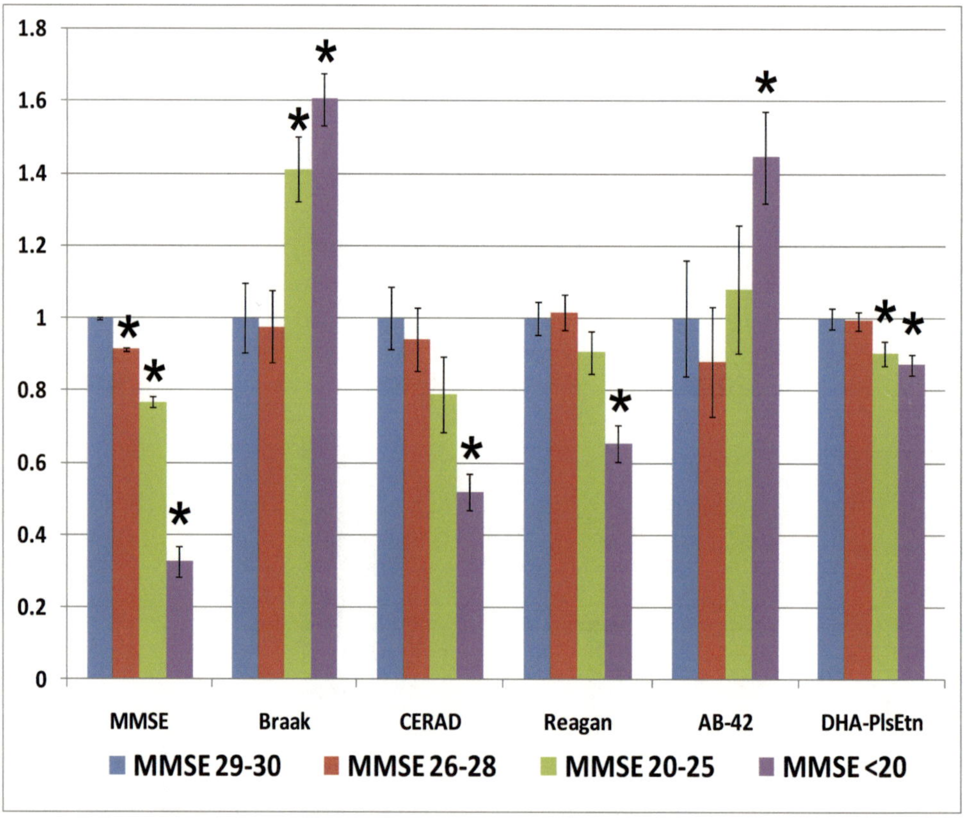

Fig. 5. Effect of pre-mortem MMSE on post-mortem pathology in the temporal cortex. * $p<0.05$. MMSE 29-30 (n=22, age 86.4+/-1.3, 11F); MMSE 26-28 (n=29, age 87.6+/-1.2, 15F); MMSE 20-25 (n=19, age 90.5+/-1.0, 11F); MMSE <20 (n=29, age 89.9 ± 1.0, 14F). MMSE scores obtained <365 days before death. Cognition analysis and pathology analyses as per Bennett et al., 2006. DHA-PlsEtn analyses performed as per Goodenowe et al., 2007; AB-42 by ELISA as per manufacturer (Covance Laboratories, Princeton, NJ)

Abnormal cholesterol regulation has been extensively implicated in AD. One plausible theory that explains the sporadic accumulation of Aβ peptides in AD is a disruption in amyloid precursor protein (APP) processing due to increased membrane cholesterol levels (Puglielli et al., 2003). This theory is supported by evidence that membrane cholesterol increases with age in both rats and humans (Hegner, 1980) and that a high cholesterol diet can increase deposition of Aβ (Refolo et al., 2000) and Aβ accumulation is closely related to the processing of the cholesterol transport protein ApoE (Refolo et al., 2000; Pratico et al., 2001) Furthermore, membrane lipid analyses of post-mortem AD subjects have shown that AD severity is positively correlated with membrane cholesterol (Cutler et al., 2004).

PlsEtn deficient cells have been previously shown to have impaired HDL-mediated cholesterol efflux (Mandel et al., 1998) and impaired intracellular LDL-mediated transport (Munn et al., 2003). In both of these studies, normal functionality was restored by PlsEtn replacement (Munn et al., 2003). Using 1-O-alkyl, 2-acyl glycerols the peroxisomal biosynthesis of plasmalogens can be bypassed and specific classes of plasmalogens selectively enhanced or restored (Figure 6), (Mankidy et al., 2010) and the effect of such manipulations on cholesterol regulation investigated. In brief, we observed that plasmalogen deficient cells (N-Rel) had reduced levels of esterified cholesterol and increased levels of free and total cholesterol in the membrane (Figure 7). We further observed that selective restoration of polyunsaturated rather than saturated PlsEtns was more effective at increasing cholesterol esterification and lowering total and free cholesterol in plasmalogen deficient cells (Table 1, Figure 7).

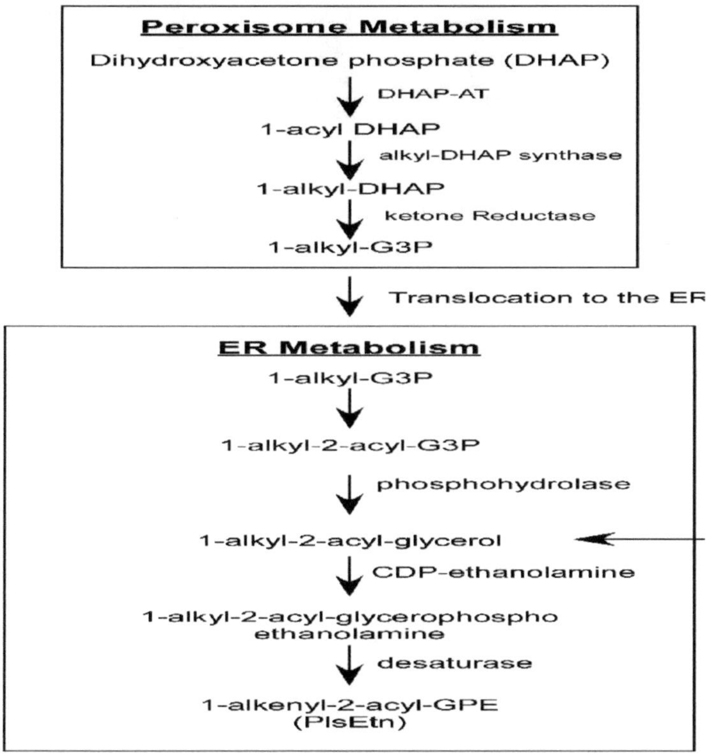

Fig. 6. Plasmalogen biosynthetic pathway. Arrow represents the entry point of sn-2 selective plasmalogen precursors.

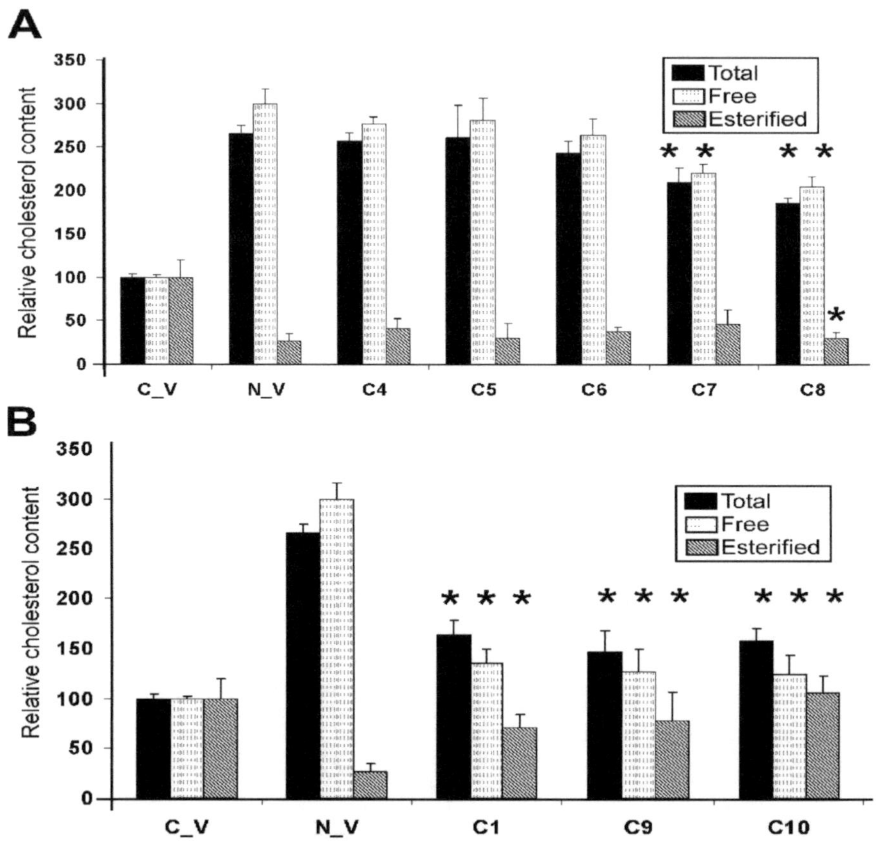

Fig. 7. Effect of plasmalogen deficiency and selective restoration on total, free, and esterified cholesterol levels in N-Rel (N) cells relative to control CHO (C) cells. * $p<0.05$ versus untreated N-Rel cells. Structures of the lipids C1, C9 and C10 are presented in Table 1.

	Compound	sn-1	sn-2	sn-3
1	cis-(±)-2-*O*-docosahexaenoyl-1-*O*-hexadecylglycerol	**16:0 (alkyl)**	**DHA**	**OH**
2	cis-(±)-2-*O*-docosahexaenoyl-1-*O*-octadecylglycerol	**18:0 (alkyl)**	**DHA**	**OH**
3	cis-(±)-2-*O*-docosahexaenoyl-1-*O*-octadec-9-enylglycerol	**18:1 (alkyl)**	**DHA**	**OH**
4	cis-(±)-2-*O*-docosahexaenoyl-1-*O*-palmitoylglycerol	**16:0 (acyl)**	**DHA**	**OH**
5	cis-(±)-2-*O*-docosahexaenoyl-1-*O*-stearoylglycerol	**18:0 (acyl)**	**DHA**	**OH**
6	cis-(±)-2-*O*-stearoyl-1-*O*-hexadecylglycerol	**16:0 (alkyl)**	**18:0**	**OH**
7	cis-(±)-2-*O*-oleoyl-1-*O*-hexadecylglycerol	**16:0 (alkyl)**	**18:1**	**OH**
8	cis-(±)-2-*O*-linoleyl-1-*O*-hexadecylglycerol	**16:0 (alkyl)**	**18:2**	**OH**
9	cis-(±)-2-*O*-α-linolenoyl-1-*O*-hexadecylglycerol	**16:0 (alkyl)**	**18:3**	**OH**
10	cis-(±)-2-*O*-arachidonoyl-1-*O*-hexadecylglycerol	**16:0 (alkyl)**	**20:4**	**OH**

Table 1. Structures of the lipids used in Figures 7-12. See Mankidy et al., 2010 for additional details.

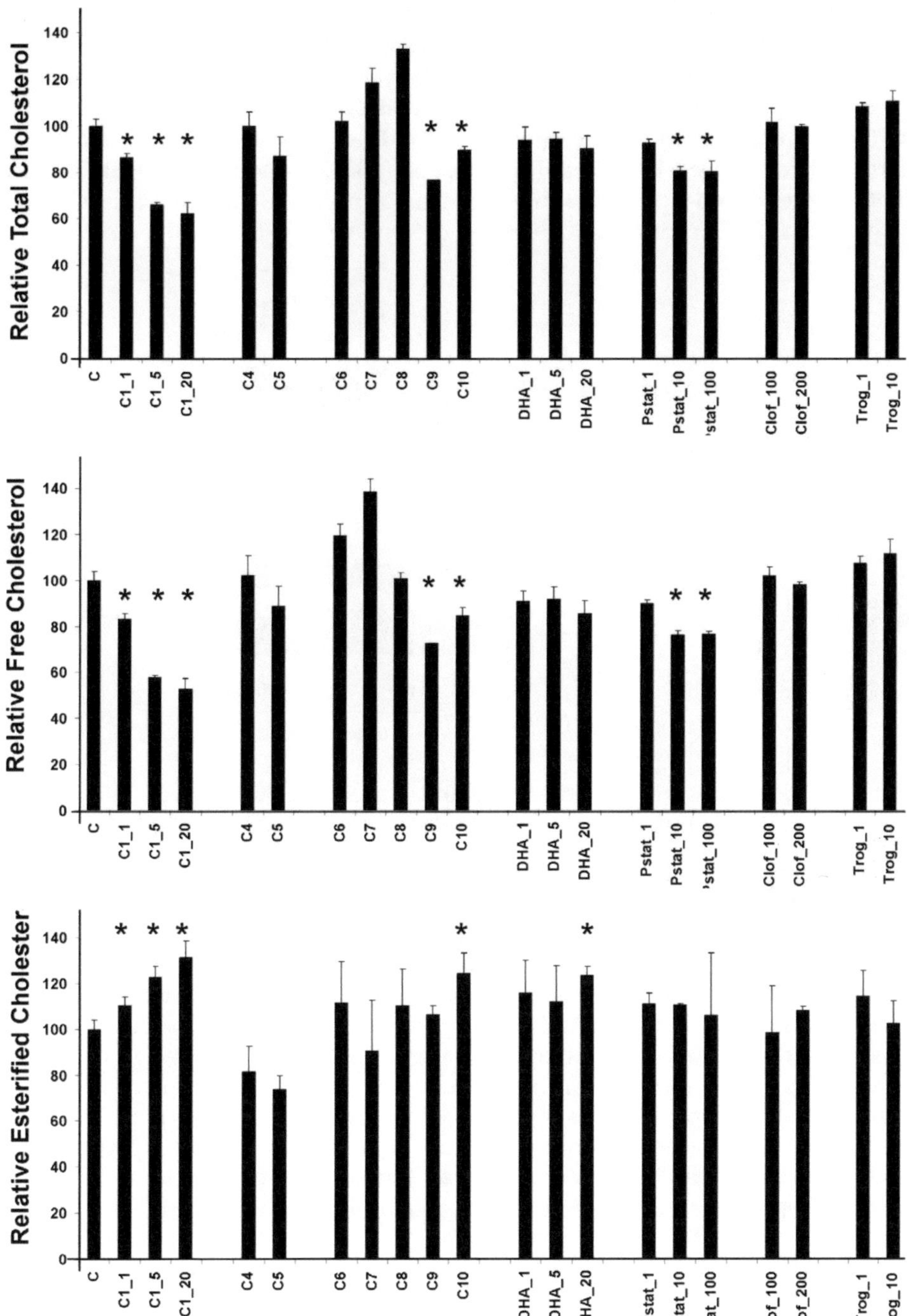

Fig. 8. Effect of plasmalogen precursors on total, free, and esterified cholesterol levels in HEK 293 cells [37]. * $p<0.05$ versus untreated controls. Structures of the lipids C1 to C10, are presented in Table 1. Clof, clofibrate; DHA, docosahexaenoic acid; Pstat, pravastatin; Trog, troglitazone. The numbers for DHA, Clof, Pstat and Trog are μM concentrations.

This effect on cholesterol regulation was also observed in plasmalogen normal, HEK293 cells (Figure 8). The observed increase in cholesterol esterification was further determined to be due to increased levels of sterol-O-acetyltransferase (SOAT) and that this increase was not cholesterol related (no effect of escalating pravastatin dose; Figure 9). These observations explain the increase in esterified cholesterol and an elevated rate of HDL-mediated cholesterol efflux reported by others (Munn et al., 2003; Mandel al., 1998). These effects could not be reproduced by either PPAR agonists or by HMG-CoA reductase antagonists. Clearly membrane PlsEtn composition is a key determiner of cholesterol regulation.

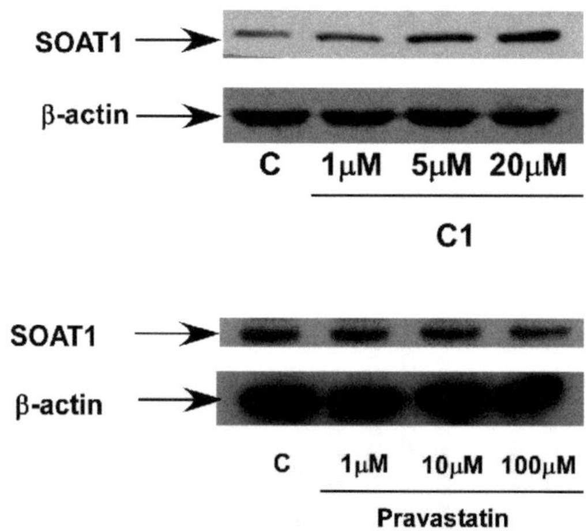

Fig. 9. Effect of the plasmalogen precursor C1 and pravastatin SOAT levels in HEK293 cells (Mankidy et al., 2010). The structures of the lipids C1 is presented in Table 1.

The role of membrane composition on amyloid precursor protein (APP) processing has also been a topic of vigorous experimentation (Puglielli et al., 2003; Chauhan, 2003). The focus of these studies has been on the role of membrane cholesterol. In brief, APP when processed via the β-secretase pathway leads to the pathological accumulation of Aβ peptides. However, under normal conditions, less than 5% of APP is processed via this pathway. The vast majority of APP is processed via the non-pathological α-secretase pathway. Alpha-secretase is located in a phospholipid-rich membrane domain, whereas β-secretase is located in cholesterol-rich lipid rafts. Both of these enzymes are sensitive to changes in membrane cholesterol. When membrane cholesterol is increased, α-secretase activity is decreased (Kojro et al., 2001) and β-secretase activity is increased (Cordy et al., 2003). A similar set of experiments as that described above for cholesterol processing was carried out focusing on APP processing. Consistent with previously published findings, cholesterol loaded HEK293 cells exhibited increased AB42 secretion which was blocked by pravastatin treatment (Figure 10). Interestingly, C1 was observed to dose dependently decrease AB42 secretion. When the proteins involved in APP processing were investigated, it was observed that cholesterol elevated β-secretase levels, but had no effect on α-secretase. C1, on the other hand dose-dependently increased α-secretase levels and decreased β-secretase levels only at the high dose. Levels of sAPPα correlated with α-secretase levels. The effect of C1 versus pravistatin on α-secretase levels was further investigated in HEK293 cells under normal conditions (Figure 11) and it was observed that only C1 was effective at modulating α-secretase levels. Clearly membrane PlsEtn composition is also a key determiner of APP processing.

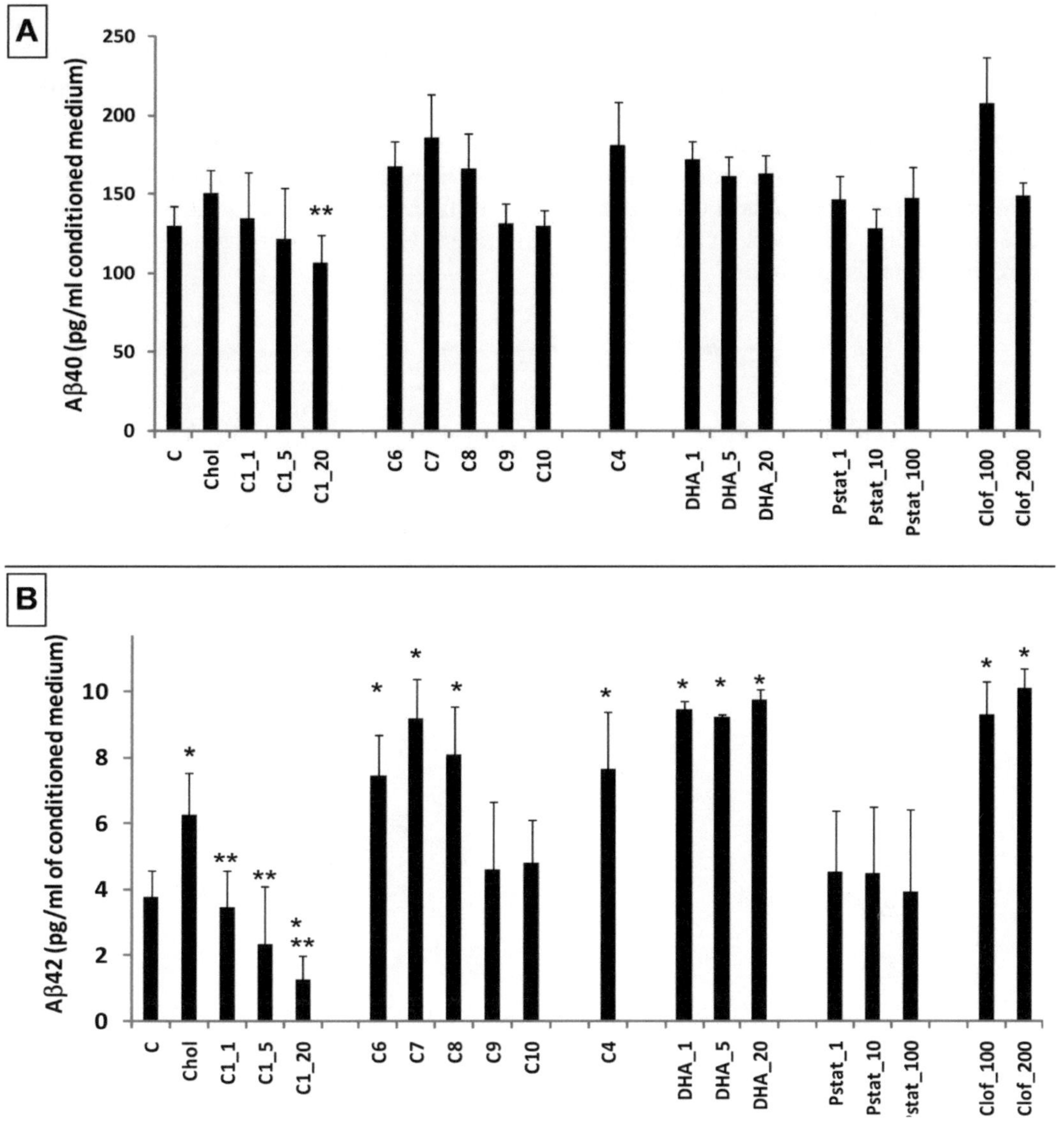

Fig. 10. Effect of various lipid mediators on AB40 and AB42 levels in HEK293 cells. Cell systems prepared as per Mankidy et al., 2010. AB levels determined using ELISA as per manufacturer's instructions (Covance Laboratories, Princeton, NJ). Structures of the lipids C1 to C10, are presented in Table 1. Chol, cholesterol; Clof, clofibrate; DHA, docosahexaenoic acid; Pstat, pravastatin; Trog, troglitazone. The numbers after compound abbreviations are μM concentrations.

In regards to cognition, the most consistent neurochemical observation in AD is decreased choline acetyltransferase (ChAT) activity in the neocortex and hippocampus (Bennett et al., 2006; Perry et al., 1978; Wilcock et al., 1982; DeKosky et al., 1992; Behl et al., 2006). Reductions in cortical ChAT activity, monitored by biopsy or in autopsy samples, correlate with the extent of intellectual impairment in AD patients. In addition, these cortical cholinergic deficits have been found in patients examined within a year of onset of symptoms and cholinesterase inhibitors which potentiate residual cholinergic transmission, slow the decline in executive memory functions in AD patients (Behl et al., 2006). Furthermore, the inhibition of postsynaptic acetyl-choline (ACh) activity can directly induce cognitive dysfunction in healthy humans (Etienne et al., 1986). Studies of ChAT levels in the N. basalis and cortex in the same autopsy samples have shown that in 50% of AD patients there is a marked loss of cortical ChAT with no reduction in N. basalis ChAT suggesting abnormal axonal transport in AD and that the neurodegeneration originated at the axon terminal, not in the cell body.

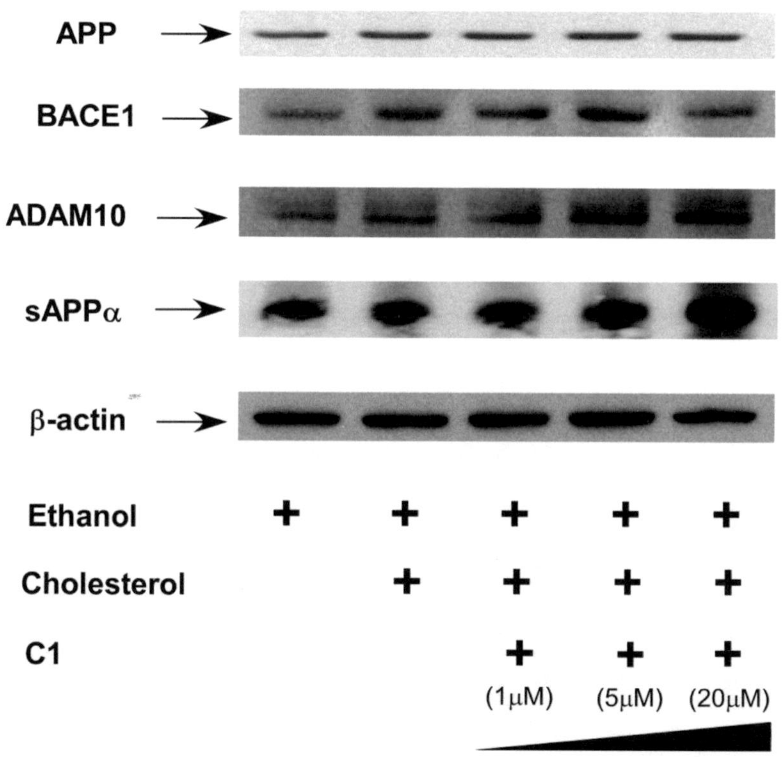

Fig. 11. Effect of escalating dose of C1 on APP, β-secretase (BACE), α-secretase (ADAM10), and sAPPα in cholesterol loaded HEK293 cells. Immunoblotting performed as per Mankidy et al., 2010.

PlsEtn are unique among neuronal lipids in that they have a high propensity to form an inverse hexagonal phase which is the essential transitory phase for successful membrane fusion events (Horrocks and Sharma, 1982). Optimal vesicular fusion is very sensitive to the amount and type of PlsEtn content. Relatively small reductions in either the vinyl ether content and/or the polyunsaturated fatty acid content of vesicles dramatically reduces the number of successful membrane fusion events (Han and Gross, 1991; Lohner et al., 1991). Therefore, this mechanism alone is sufficient to explain the correlation between decreased membrane PlsEtn and the severity of cognitive dysfunction in AD. However, in regards to cholinergic neurons there is yet a second mechanism of importance and that is pre-synaptic ACh synthesis. When a cholinergic nerve terminal releases ACh into the synaptic cleft during a depolarization event, the released ACh is ultimately degraded to choline and acetate by acetylcholineesterase (AChE). This extracellular choline in the synaptic cleft is then rapidly re-absorbed into the presynaptic terminal by the choline high affinity transporter (CHT). The reabsorbed choline is preferentially utilized by ChAT to re-synthesize ACh, which is then transported into vesicles by an ACh transporter protein and stored for future depolarizing events. Brain slice studies have shown that as long as the CHT is functioning normally, the cholinergic terminal can maintain ACh release for extended periods of time by utilizing membrane stores of PtdCho and PtdEtn (Ulus et al., 1989) and by the extraction of choline from surrounding cells (Farber et al., 1996). This occurs even in the absence of exogenous choline. However, in the presence of the CHT inhibitor, HC-3, the ability to sustain release of ACh is dramatically reduced, even in the presence of exogenous supplied choline (Maire and Wurtman, 1985). These data indicate that the proper functioning of the CHT is essential for the sustained release of ACh from cholinergic neurons. Recently, Ferguson *et al.* made a landmark finding where they showed that the CHT is localized on pre-synaptic vesicles, not constituently expressed on the pre-synaptic membrane (Ferguson et al., 2003; 2004). This finding indicates that the dynamic regulation of choline uptake via the CHT occurs by an increased density of CHTs at the synapse following a nerve impulse and subsequent deactivation by vesicular endocytosis. Impaired vesicular fusion as a result of a PlsEtn deficiency would be expected to have a similar effect on choline uptake as the presence of HC-3, albeit via a different mechanism.

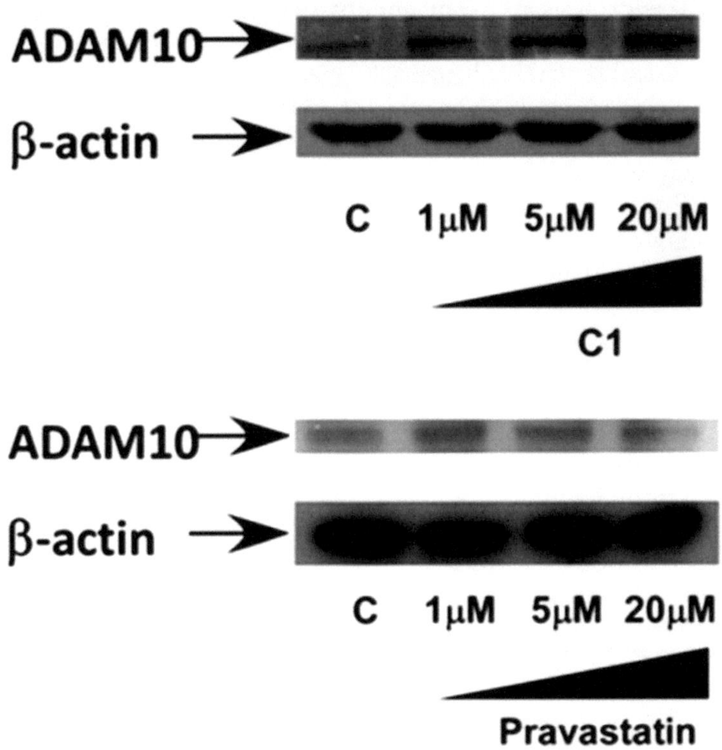

Fig. 12. Effect of escalating dose of C1 (Table 1) and pravastatin on α-secretase (ADAM10) levels in HEK293 cells. Immunoblotting performed as per Mankidy et al., 2010.

In summary, a deficiency in polyunsaturated PlsEtn in the CNS would be expected to reduce non-pathogenic APP processing, impair membrane cholesterol clearance, reduce vesicular release of neurotransmitters, and selectively impair pre-synaptic ACh replenishment following a nerve impulse. Accordingly, a therapeutic strategy aimed at developing an orally bioavailable DHA-PlsEtn precursor warrants clinical investigation in AD.

4. Plasmalogen replacement therapy for Alzheimer's disease

The goal of our research program was to design an orally bioavailable DHA-plasmalogen precursor drug that bypasses age- and disease-sensitive peroxisomal biosynthetic pathways for both plasmalogens and DHA, thereby effectively restoring and/or enhancing DHA-plasmalogen-dependent synaptic and membrane functions that are diminished in AD, and which correlate with both clinical and pathological features of AD.

Since brain plasmalogens are supplied by the liver and intestinal mucosa, we established a research program to design an orally bioavailable ether lipid precursor that would bypass the requirement for peroxisomes to generate the ether lipid linkage at sn-1 of the glycerol backbone. Additionally, the decreased ability of the AD liver to synthesize DHA, along with decreased circulating plasma levels of DHA in AD patients, prompted us to substitute DHA as the fatty acid at sn-2 of the glycerol backbone. A sn-3 substituent was required to stabilize the DHA substitution at sn-2. The requirements for this substitution were: 1) A substituent that did not hinder hydrolysis at sn-3 by gut lipases to provide the alkyl-acyl-glycerol to the gut mucosa for addition of phosphoethanolamine at sn-3; 2) The released sn-3 substituent should be non-toxic and preferably beneficial; 3) Stabilization of the drug product; 4) Ease of synthesis and low cost of goods. A number of candidates were examined and lipoic acid was found to meet all of these criteria, as embodied in the drug development candidate PPI-1011

4.1 PPI-1011: Chemistry

PPI-1011 is an ether lipid plasmalogen precursor possessing palmitic acid at sn-1 of the glycerol backbone; DHA at sn-2 and lipoic acid at sn-3. That lipoic acid at sn-3 was the best moiety for both stabilizing the drug during storage and for synthetic purity.

For the synthesis of PPI-1011, solketal **1** was alkylated using cetyl bromide under phase transfer conditions (TBAB / aq. NaOH) to furnish **2**. Acidic hydrolysis of the ketal in **2** gave 1-cetyl glycerol **3** in good yield. The primary hydroxyl at sn-3 position was selectively protected as a TBS ether to give **4.** DHA was activated as its acid chloride using oxalyl chloride and then treated with **4** under basic conditions to furnish **5.** Desilyation of **5** using equimolar mixture of TBAF / acetic acid proceeded smoothly to give **6** as the major product. Initial efforts to carry out the esterification of **6** with R-lipoic acid *via* the acid chloride route did not proceed well, giving low yields of the required product. Esterification under Yamaguchi conditions involving the mixed anhydride of R-lipoic acid afforded the desired lipoic acid conjugate **PPI-1011** in 54% yield.

The scheme was further modified to decrease the number of steps and increase the overall yield of the product. The primary alcohol in diol **3** was coupled with R-Lipoic under EDC/DMAP conditions to give **6** as the major product. Bis lipoic acid product formed as the minor product was easily separated by column chromatography. Esterification of the sn-2 position in **6** with DHA was also carried out under EDC/DMAP conditions to give **PPI-**

1011. This route is superior to the previous route in the following ways: i) Protection-deprotection steps are avoided ii) Compound **6** can directly be carried forward for Step 2 (purification can be attempted after step 2) iii) This route is economically viable, easily scalable and can serve as a general protocol for the synthesis of analogues.

Molecular Formula: $C_{49}H_{82}O_5S_2$
Molecular Weight: 815.3
Dosage Form: Gelatin capsule
Glycerol sn-1 : Palmitic acid (alkyl linkage)
Glycerol sn-2 : DHA (acyl linkage)
Glycerol sn-3 : Lipoic acid (acyl linkage)

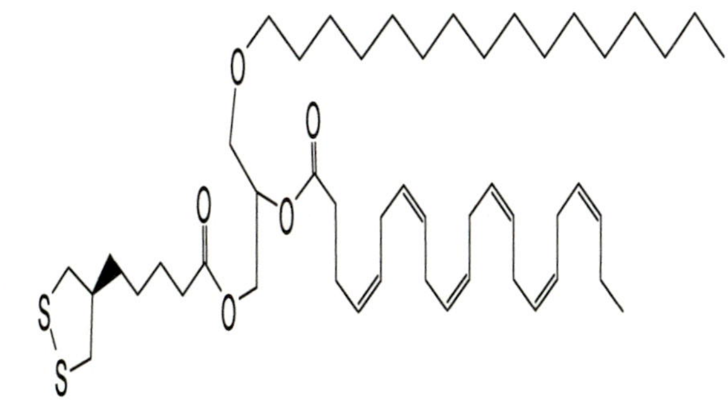

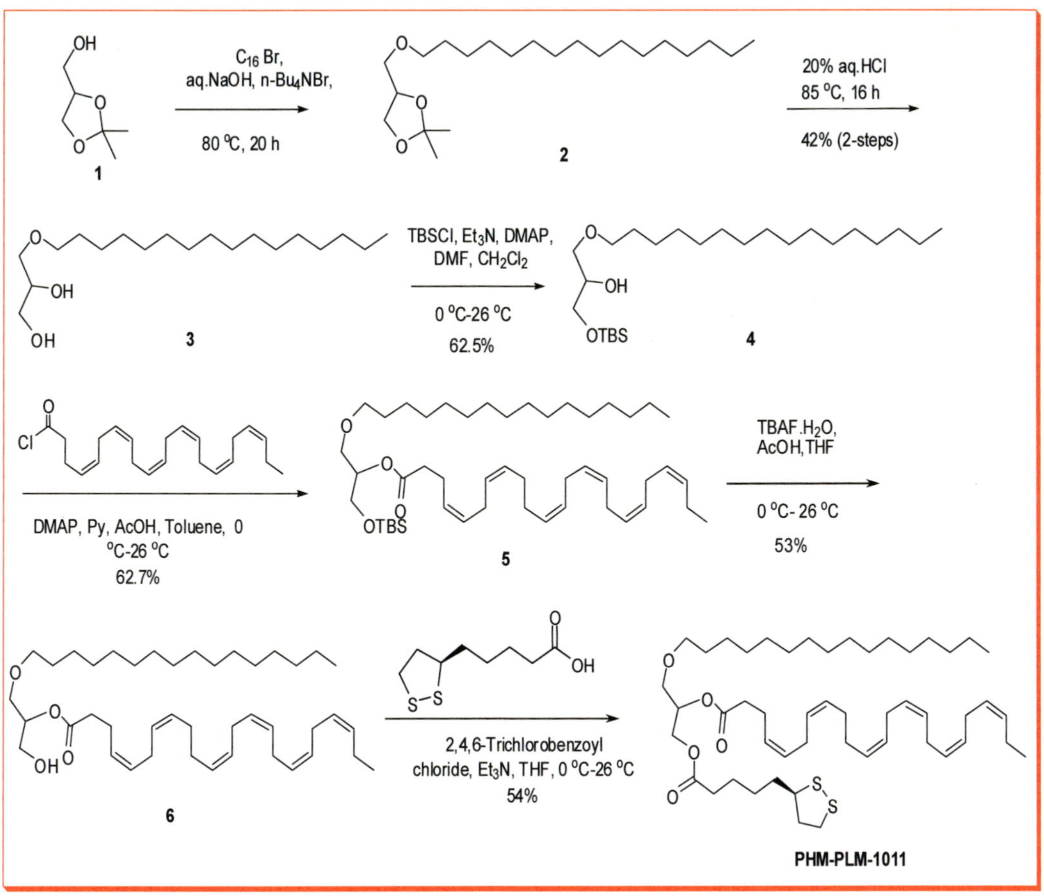

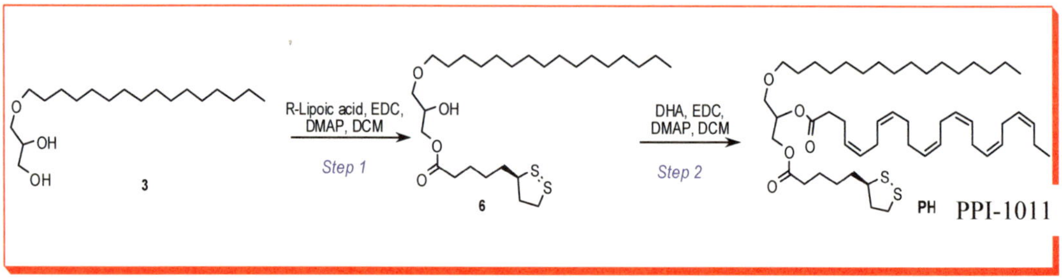

4.2 PPI-1011: In vitro data

In vitro studies with PPI-1011 have demonstrated that PPI-1011 can restore the target PlsEtn 16:0/22:6 in N-Rel cells which lack the peroxisomal enzymes required to generate ether lipids. These mutant Chinese hamster ovary (CHO) cells have plasmalogen levels that are 5 to 10% of control CHO cells, both at the whole cell level and in isolated mitochondria. The target plasmalogen 16:0/22:6 generated by PPI-1011undergoes lipid remodeling with sn-2 deacylation/reacylation thereby restoring other cellular plasmalogens. The released lipoic acid rather than being a prodrug waste product may provide some neuroprotective actions in AD patients (Maczurek et al., 2008).

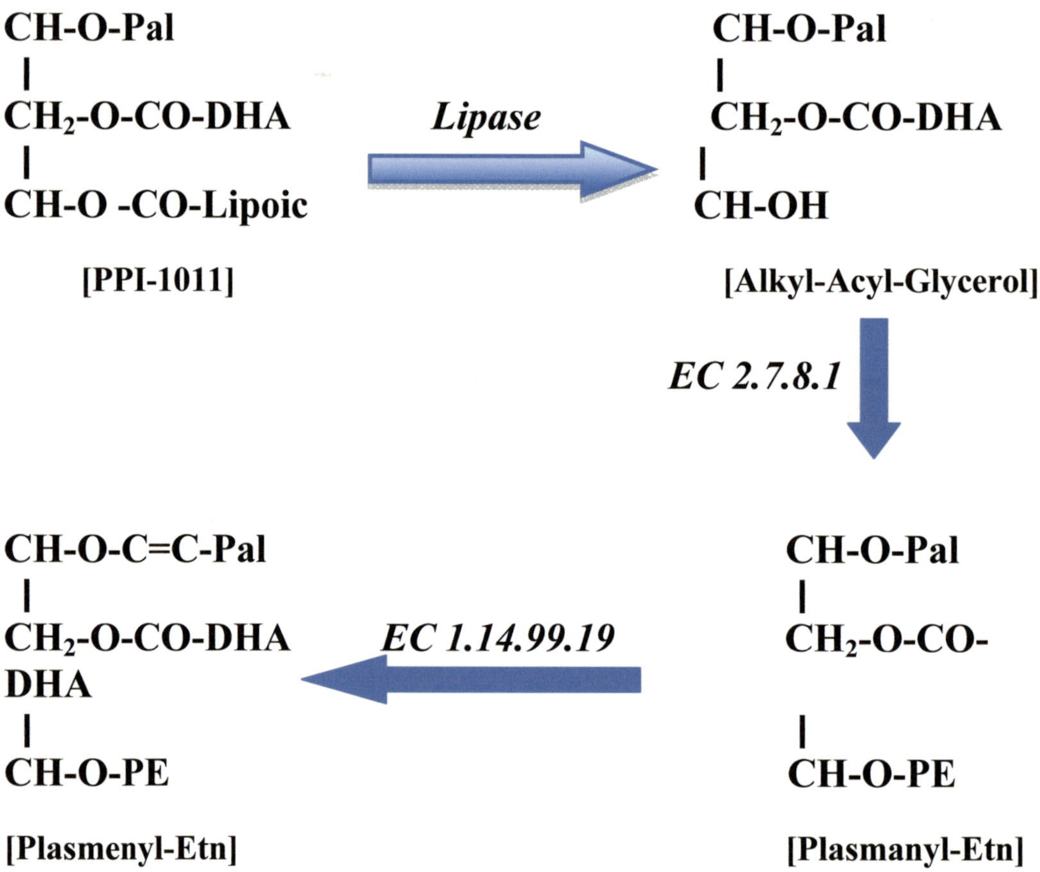

The *in vitro* effects of PPI-1011 on ethanolamine plasmalogen levels were determined using N-Rel cells which possess a deficiency in DHAPT, a peroxisomal membrane protein, which catalyses the first step in plasmalogen biosynthesis (Nagan et al., 1998). The DHAPT deficiency causes a severe decrease in ethanolamine plasmalogens. However, N-Rel cells do continue to have otherwise functional peroxisomes. N-Rel cells were initially created as a mutagenized cell population of CHO cells. Cell experiments were set up with an n=5 for the control, vehicle and treatment groups. Figure 13 demonstrates the ability of PPI-1011 to bypass peroxisomes and generate the target PlsEtn 16:0/22:6 which undergoes lipid remodeling to also resupply PlsEtns 16:0:20:4, 16:0/18:1 and 16:0/18:2.

The deacylation of DHA (22:6) from the *sn*-2 position of PPI-1011 and reacylation at *sn*-2 with oleic acid (18:1), linoleic acid (18:2), or arachidonic acid (20:4) was observed following PPI-1011 cell treatment. Increases in plasmalogens were both concentration and time-dependent with maximal increases by 72 hr at 100 μM. Utlizing the Alamar blue assay, PPI-1011 was not cytotoxic at 100, 300, 600, 900, 1200, 1500 and 2100 μM with 72 hr incubations. Analyzing whole cell plasmalogen levels, PPI-1011 augmented PlsEtn levels while DHA supplementation was ineffective (Figure 14). These data demonstrate that DHA supplementation is critically dependent upon ether lipids supplied by peroxisomes to effectively augment PlsEtns.

Restoring normal plasmalogen levels in plasmalogen-deficient cells with PPI-1011 also has been demonstrated to have the functional benefit of restoring cholesterol efflux and reducing cellular cholesterol levels in N-Rel cells (Nagan and Zoeller, 2001) as previously reported with other ether lipid precursors (Mankidy et al., 2010).

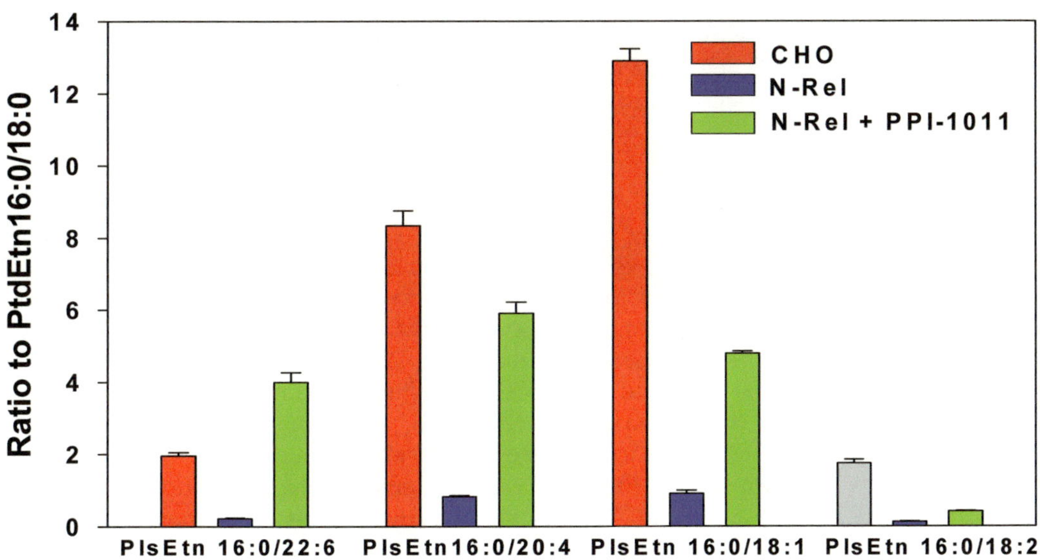

Fig. 13. Augmentation of N-Rel mitochondrial plasmalogens after a 72 hr incubation with 100 μM PPI-1011. Data are expressed as a ratio of the plasmalogen to the housekeeping metabolite phosphatidylethanolamine 16:0/18:0. N= 5; Mean ± SEM. PPI-1011 significantly (p <0.01) restored all 16:0/x plasmalogens.

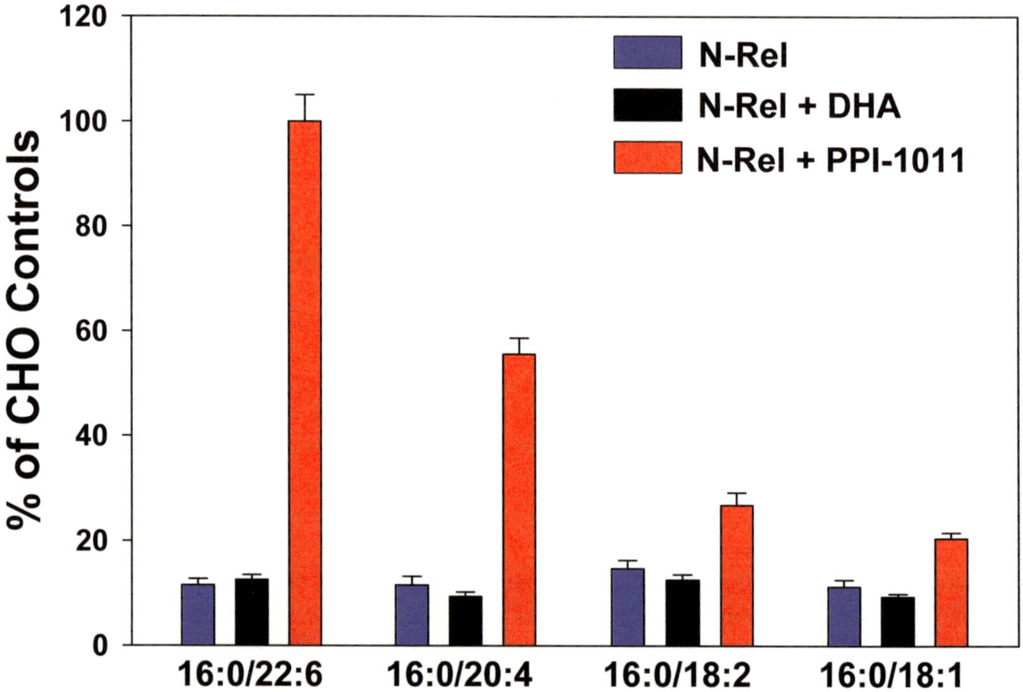

Fig. 14. Augmentation of cellular plasmalogens in N-Rel cells after a 72 hr incubation with PPI-1011 (100 µM) but not with DHA (100 µM; Martek). Data are presented as % of CHO control cells. N= 5; Mean ± SEM. PPI-1011 significantly ($p < 0.01$) restored all 16:0/x plasmalogens. All bars are significantly less than control ($p < 0.01$), except for the 16:0/22:6 in PPI-1011 treated cells.

4.3 PPI-1011: In vivo data

Oral dosing of rabbits (manuscript in preparation) with PPI-1011 in gelatin capsules demonstrated dose (10 to 200 mg/kg)- and time (0 to 48 hr)-dependent augmentation of DHA-containing plasmalogens with further increases in doses (500 and 1000 mg/kg) not further augmenting circulating plasmalogen levels. DHA was also released, via deacylases, with peak plasma DHA levels at 6 hours and maximal plasma levels at a dose of 500 mg/kg rather than 200 mg/kg as observed with plasmalogens. These data support once daily dosing of PPI-1011 and demonstrate that circulating plasmalogens are auto-regulated thereby limiting the potential for toxicity from excess levels.

The critical *in vivo* evaluation of PPI-1011 was to demonstrate restoration of deficient plasmalogens in an animal model. To this end we investigated the murine cuprizone model of extensive cortical demyelination (Skripuletz et al., 2008). C57BL/6J mice were separated into 3 treatment groups: control, cuprizone and cuprizone + PPI-1011 (n=7). Standard rodent chow was ground and 0.3% cuprizone (bis-cyclohexanone oxaldihydrazone) was added to the ground diet of the treated animals. Control or 0.3% cuprizone chow and water were provided to animals *ad libtum*. Diets were fed to the treatment groups for a total of 7 weeks. For the last 2 weeks the cuprizone + PPI-1011 group was given 100 mg/kg/day of PPI-1011 suspended in soybean oil by oral gavage.

Upon completion of the study animals were anesthetized with isoflurane and plasma, kidney and neocortex collected for analyses.

Total RNA was isolated from approximately 2 µg of pulverized cortex tissue using the RNeasy Mini Kit (Qiagen) as per the manufacture's protocol. RNA was quantified by optical density with the NanoVue spectrophotometer (GE Healthcare Life Sciences). Reverse transcription reactions were performed on 800ng RNA using the qScript cDNA SuperMix (Quanta Biosciences). Each cortex samples was analyzed to determine expression of reelin (sense 5′-cccagcccagacagacagtt-3′; antisense 5′-ccaggtgatgccattgttga-3′), as well as the myelin markers myelin basic protein (sense-5' cctcaaagacaggccctcag 3'; antisense-5' cctgtcaccgctaaagaagc 3') and 2',3'-cyclic-nucleotide 3'-phosphodiesterase (EC 3.1.4.37; sense-5' catcctcaggagcaaaggag 3'; antisense-5' tgaatagcgtcttgcactcg 3') and the housekeeping gene β-actin (sense-5' agccatgtacgtagccatcc 3'; antisense-5' ctctcagctgtggtggtgaa 3' (Mack et al., 2007; Heinrich et al., 2006). Specificity of each primer set was determined by analysis of the dissociation curve. Quantitative real-time PCR was carried out in triplicate using the Fast SYBR Green Master Mix (Applied Biosystems) on the StepOne Plus Real-Time PCR System (Applied Biosystems). Thermocycling conditions were: 95°C for 20s followed by 40 cycles of 95°C for 3s and 60°C for 30s. For plasmalogen analyses, 10 mg of tissue powder in 5 mL screw cap tubes were polytroned in 1 mL of PBS + 0.5 mL MeOH. In the case of plasma, 100 µL were vortexed with 1 mL of PBS + 0.5 mL MeOH. Next, 2 mL tert-butylmethylether were added to the plasma samples and tissue homogenates and the samples capped and shaken (1400 rpm) for 15 min at room temperature. The samples were then centrifuged for 8 min in a clinical centrifuge and 1 ml of the upper organic layer isolated for LC-MS/MS analyses of DHA, ethanolamine plasmalogens and phosphatidylethanolamines as reported previously (Wood et al., 2010). For cholesterol and myoinositol analyses, 2 mg of tissue powder in 5 ml screw cap tubes were polytroned in 1.2 ml of acetonitrile:MeOH:formic acid (800:200:2.4) containing [$^2H_7$]cholesterol and [$^2H_6$]myoinositol (Cambridge and CDN Isotopes) as internal standards. The homogenates were transferred to 1.5 ml screw top microtubes and centrifuged at 4°C and 25,000xg for 30 min. Next, 200 µL of the supernatant were dried in a Savant centrifugal evaporator. Trimethylsilylation of the samples was conducted at 80°C for 1 hr with 100 µL acetonitrile and 100 µL of N,O-bis(trimethylsilyl)trifluoro-acetamide and TMCS (10/1). The TMS derivatives were analyzed by GC-MS with the $[M-72]^+$ cations 386.3 and 393.3 monitored under ammonia PCI for cholesterol and [$^2H_7$]cholesterol, respectively and the $[MH]^+$ cations of 613.2 and 619.2 monitored for myoinositol and [$^2H_6$]myoinositol, respectively.

Analysis of plasma phosphatidylethanolamines and ethanolamine plasmalogens revealed selective 20 to 40% decrements in free DHA and DHA containing phospholipids in cuprizone treated mice (Figure 15). Additionally, oral administration of PPI-1011 for 2 weeks fully restored these plasma decrements (Figure 15).

Cuprizone toxicity also resulted in significant decrements in kidney PlsEtns (Figure 16). PPI-1011 treatment restored kidney tissue levels of DHA-containing plasmalogens (PlsEtn 16:0/22:6, 18:0/22:6, 18:1/22:6) and augmented free DHA levels. PlsEtn18:1/18:2 was also restored with PPI-1011 treatment (Figure 16). In the cuprizone model, decrements in circulating and kidney DHA and DHA-containing plasmalogens are most likely the result of cuprizone toxicity in the liver (Heinrich et al., 2006). PPI-1011 clearly demonstrated oral bioavailability in that it was able to fully reverse these effects of cuprizone on circulating and kidney plasmalogens.

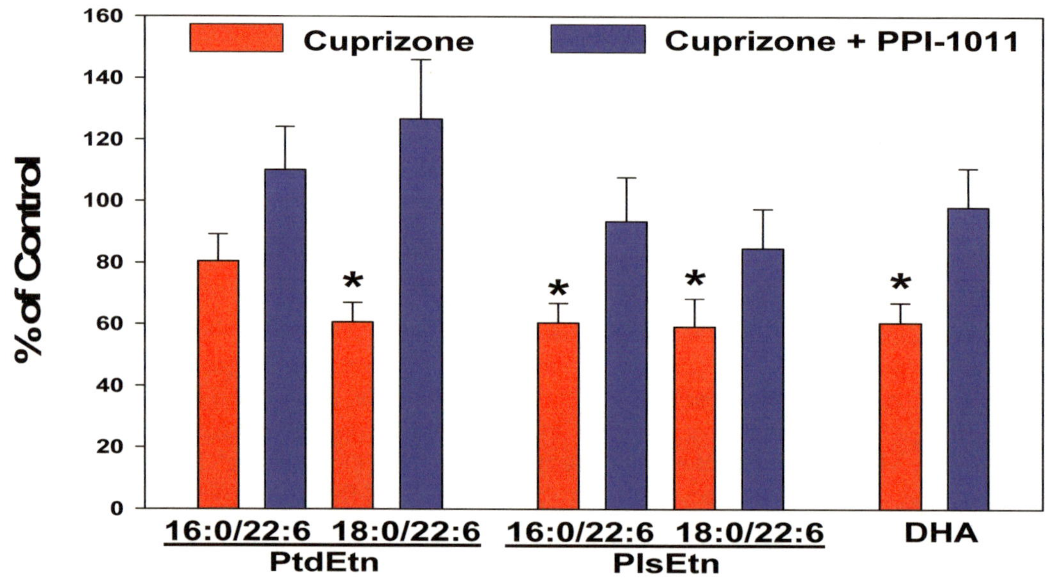

Fig. 15. Plasma DHA and DHA-containing PtdEtns and PlsEtns in mice maintained on a 0.3% cuprizone diet for 7 weeks. One group of cuprizone mice was treated with PPI-1011 (100 mg/kg, po) for weeks 6 and 7. Mean ± SEM; N=6 -7. * $p < 0.05$ vs. control.

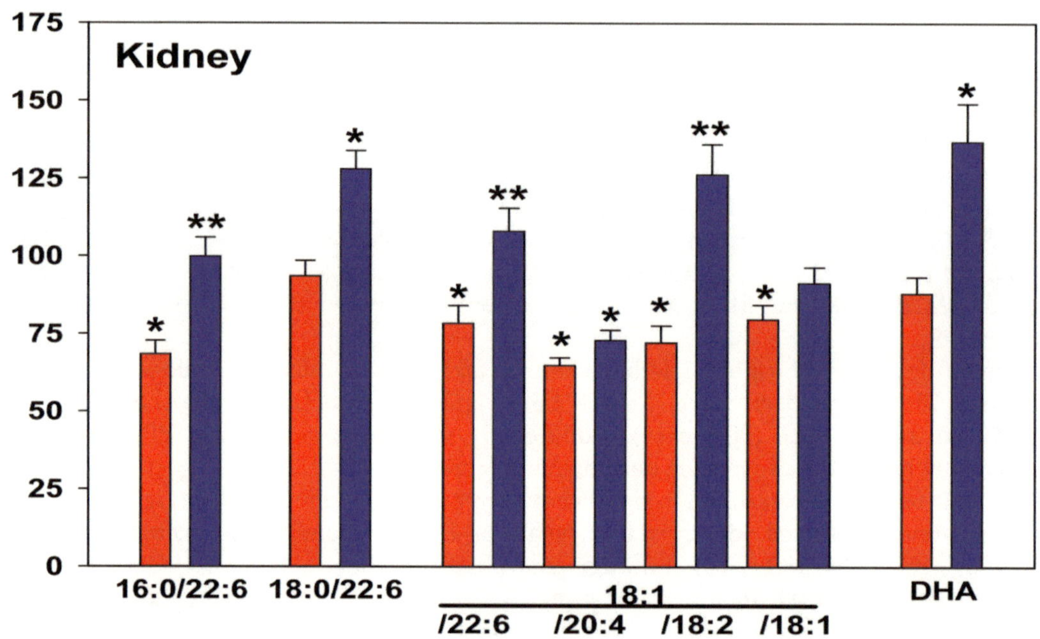

Fig. 16. Kidney PlsEtns and DHA in mice maintained on a 0.3% cuprizone diet for 7 weeks ± PPI-1011 treatment (100 mg/kg, po) for weeks 6 and 7. Mean ± SEM; N=6 -7. * $p < 0.01$ vs. control; **, $p < 0.05$ vs. cuprizone.

Analysis of neocortical ethanolamine phospholipids demonstrated selective and large reductions in white matter plasmalogens (PlsEtn). These included the 16:0/18:1 and 16:0/18:2 plasmalogens (Figure 17- B) as well as the 18:0/18:1, 18:0/18:2 PlsEtns (Figure 17-D). There were also significant reductions in the 18:0/18:1, 18:0/18:2 phosphatidylethanolamines (PtdEtn; Figure 17-C). With PlsEtn precursor treatment (PPI-1011), the decrements in the 16:0/18:2 (Figure 17-B) and 18:0/18:2 (Figure 17-D) PlsEtns and the 18:0/18:2 PtdEtns (Figure 17-C) were significantly reversed. PPI-1011 treatment also significantly augmented PtdEtn 16:0/18:2 in cuprizone treated mice (Figure 17-A). PPI-1011 did not alter PlsEtns with oleic acid (18:1) at sn-2 (Figure 17).

The marked ability of PPI-1011 to restore linoleic (18:2 at sn-2)-containing PlsEtn and phosphatidylethanolamines in both kidney and neocortex, suggests that PPI-1011 stimulates/induces a reacylation mechanism that favors 18:2 addition at sn-2.

To evaluate the potential benefits of plasmalogen replacement on myelin function, we examined the established myelin markers cholesterol, myo-inositol, myelin basic protein mRNA and 2',3'-cyclic-nucleotide 3'-phosphodiesterase mRNA. These markers were all reduced by 20 to 40% with 7 weeks of cuprizone treatment (Figure 18) and were significantly reversed by treatment with PPI-1011 for weeks 6 and 7 (Figure 18). PPI-1011 also induced reelin expression, an extracellular matrix glycoprotein involved in nerve regeneration (Figure 18). These increases in neocortical cholesterol, myo-inositol, myelin basic protein and 2',3'-cyclic-nucleotide 3'-phosphodiesterase and reelin (May et al., 2005) suggest that plasmalogen restoration may stimulate remyelination. Since cholesterol transport is dependent upon plasmalogens (Munn et al., 2003), PPI-1011 replenishment of plasmalogens may also contribute to restoration of cholesterol levels.

These data are relevant to AD in that AD pathology involves extensive hypomyelination as demonstrated by dramatic decrements in a number of myelin markers including plasmalogens (Han et al., 2001) sulfatides (Han et al., 2002); myelin basic protein (Wang et al., 2004) and 2',3'-cyclic nucleotide-3'-phosphodiesterase (Vlkolinsky et al., 2001), in autopsy studies of AD neocortex. Imaging studies also suggest that this process occurs in mild cognitive impairment (MCI) patients, consistent with the observations that myelin plasmalogens decrease early in the disease process (Han et al., 2001). Decrements in myelin and neuronal plasmalogens may well be responsible for the shrinkage in AD neurons that precedes final neuronal cell death (Scott et al., 1992; Stark et al., 2005; Vogels et al., 1990; Artaco-Perula and Insausti, 2007; Vereecken et al., 1994). Our data support previous studies indicating that myelin basic protein mRNA, 2',3'-cyclic-nucleotide 3'-phosphodiesterase mRNA, and plasmalogens with oleic acid and linoleic acid at sn-2 are reliable markers of myelin loss.

Our data for the first time also demonstrate that myelin decrements are reflected by decreases in neocortical phosphatidylethanolamines with oleic acid and linoleic acid at sn-2. With regard to therapeutic implications, these data indicate that plasmalogen precursors have the potential to correct brain plasmalogen and phosphatidylethanolamines deficits in leukodystrophies, multiple sclerosis and Alzheimer's disease.

4.4 PPI-1011: Safety

While PPI-1011 is not an endogenous molecule, it is rapidly cleaved in the gut to yield two endogenous molecules, an alkyl-acyl-glycerol and lipoic acid. Previous human experience indicates that 1-o-octadecyl-sn-glycerol is consumed in the diet up to 100 mg/day and that supplementation with this ether lipid (5 to 10 mg/kg/day for 2 to 4 years) was not associated with any toxicity in children with peroxisomal disorders (Das et al., 1992)

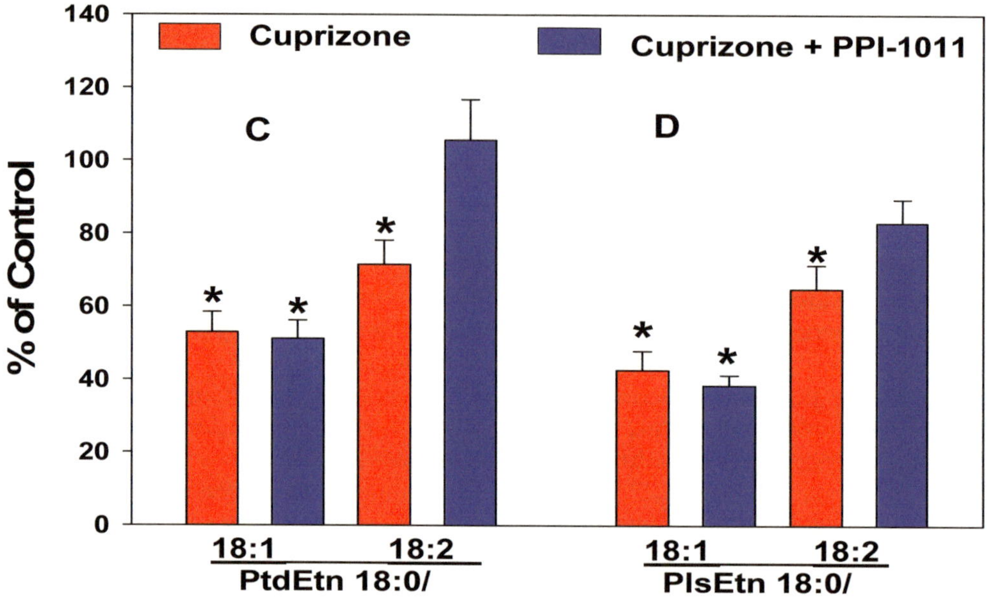

Fig. 17. Neocortical PtdEtns and PlsEtns in mice maintained on a 0.3% cuprizone diet for 7 weeks ± PPI-1011 treatment (100 mg/kg, po) for weeks 6 and 7. Mean ± SEM; N=6 -7. * $p < 0.01$ vs. control.

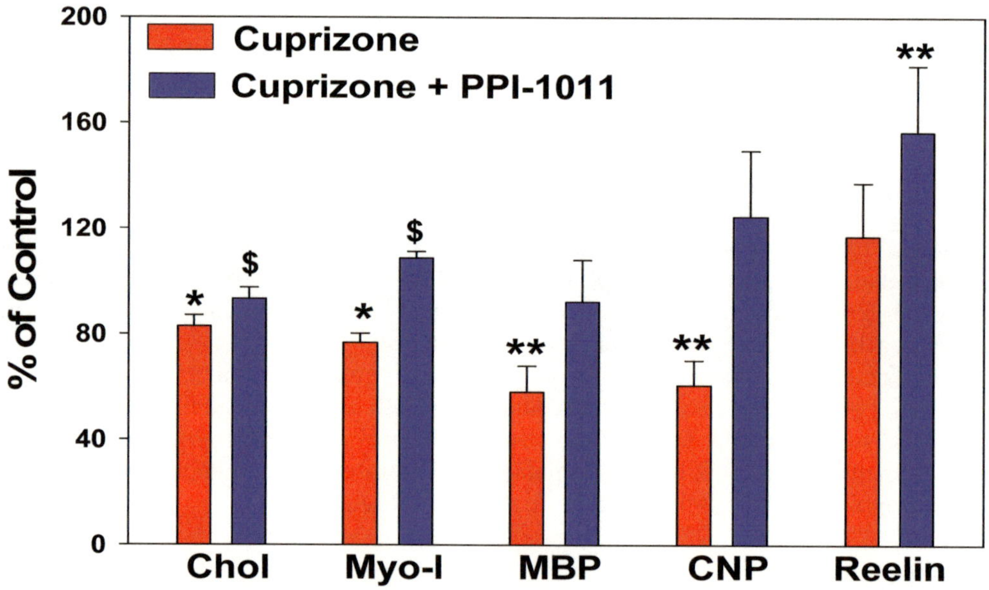

Fig. 18. Neocortical cholesterol (Chol) and myoinositol (Myo-I) levels and mRNA levels for myelin basic protein (MBP), 2',3'-cyclic-nucleotide 3'-phosphodiesterase (CNP) and reelin. Mice were maintained on a 0.3% cuprizone diet for 7 weeks ± PPI-1011 treatment (100 mg/kg, po) for weeks 6 and 7. Mean ± SEM; N=6 -7. * $p < 0.01$ vs. control; ** $p < 0.05$ vs. control; $, $p < 0.01$ vs. cuprizone alone.

AD patients treated with 1.72 g DHA/day for 12 months also have demonstrated no toxicity. Gastrointestinal side effects resulted in several drop-outs (Freund-Levi et al., 2008; Kotani et al., 2006); and 3) AD patients have been dosed with 600 mg of lipoic acid daily for 48 month with no toxicity (Maczurek et al., 2008). Lipoic acid (600 mg) also is an approved therapy for treating diabetic neuropathy, in Germany. These data suggest that PPI-1011 is a safe plasmalogen precursor that should restore neuronal membrane function. This should result in enhanced cholinergic transmission and improve the ADAS-cog scores of AD patients at least as well as a cholinesterase inhibitor. Furthermore, restoring membrane function should halt amyloid deposition and other ongoing pathological processes. PPI-1011 has the potential to be a first-in-class disease-modifying agent for AD.

4.5 PPI-1011: Formulation and stability

PPI-1011 is unstable as an oil but is stable in organic solvents (eg. dichloromethane) and in Neobee. The main impurity is the sulfoxide form of lipoic acid at sn-3. This impurity appears to be minimized by addition of the antioxidant thioglycerol to the formulation. We currently have 14 months of accelerated stability on this formulation.

5. Conclusions

In summary, our data support previous histochemical and biochemical studies demonstrating decrements in markers of neocortical myelin in the cuprizone mouse model (Skripuletz et al., 2008). However, ours is the first data to show that an orally administered plasmalogen precursor is capable of restoring some of these plasmalogens in the brain and that this can also result in remyelination as indicated by increases in cholesterol, myoinositol, myelin basic protein and 2',3'-cyclic nucleotide-3'-phosphodiesterase. Our data suggest that orally bioavailable plasmalogen precursors may offer a new therapeutic approach for neurodegenerative disorders. It has long been known that peripheral sources of DHA lipids are critical for brain and retinal function (Scott and Bazan, 2007). The importance of these observations has been highlighted by recent reports of decreased liver synthesis (Astarita et al., 2010) and circulating levels (Goodenowe et al., 2007) of DHA and DHA phospholipids in Alzheimer's disease, which correlate with cognitive decline and brain decrements in DHA-containing plasmalogens (Han et al., 2001; Goodenowe et al., 2007; Wood et al., 2010). Clearly a next step is to define the site or sites of phospholipid remodeling that allow restoration of myelin plasmalogens and phosphatidylethanolamines. Labeled PPI-1011 is hoped to answer some of these questions. However, there are multiple anatomical sites and multiple enzymes that may participate in phospholipid remodeling processes. The gut, liver, brain and associated endothelial cell populations are all rich in remodeling enzymes. These include: i) the 1-acyl hydrolases, phospholipase A1 (EC 3.1.1.32), lysophospholipase (EC 3.1.1.5), acylglycerol lipase (EC 3.1.1.23); lipoprotein lipase (EC 3.1.1.34) and triacylglycerol lipase (EC 3.1.1.3); ii) the 2-acyl hydolases, phospholipase A2 (EC 3.1.1.4) and acylglycerol lipase (EC 3.1.1.23); iii) the 1-alkenyl hydrolase, alkenylglycerophosphoethanolamine hydrolase (EC 3.3.2.5); iv) the phosphethanolamine hydrolase, phospholipase C (EC 3.1.4.3); and v) the 2-acyltransferases, acylglycerophosphcholine o-acyltransferase (EC 2.3.1.23) and acyl Co-A:lyso-phosphatidylethanolamine acyltransferase (LPEAT2) (Cao et al., 2008). It remains to be defined if these remodeling enzymes can augment plasmalogens with oleic acid (18:1) at sn-2, after longer term dosing with PPI-1011.

6. Acknowledgement

We thank Dr. D.A. Bennett from the Rush Alzheimer's Disease Center, Rush University Medical Center, Chicago, IL, for the human brain samples collected with support from National Institute on Aging grant R01AG17917.

7. References

Andre, A., Juaneda, P., Sebedio, J.L. and Chardigny, J.M.: Plasmalogen metabolism-related enzymes in rat brain during aging: influence of n-3 fatty acid intake. Biochimie 2006, 88: 103-111.

Artacho-Pérula, E. and Insausti, R.: Quantitative estimations of the entorhinal cortex in Alzheimer's disease. Anal. Quant. Cytol. Histol. 2007, 29:1-16.

Astarita, G., Jung, K.M., Berchtold, N.C., Nguyen, V.Q., Gillen, D.L., Head, E., Cotman, C.W. and Piomelli, D.: Deficient liver biosynthesis of docosahexaenoic acid correlates with cognitive impairment in Alzheimer's disease. PLoS One. 2010, 5:e12538.

Bachman, D.L., Wolf, P.A., Linn, R., Knoefel, J.E., Cobb, J., Belanger, A., D'Agostino, R.B. and White, L.R.: Prevalence of dementia and probable senile dementia of the Alzheimer type in the Framingham study. Neurology 1992, 42: 115-119.

Bartzokis, G.: Age-related myelin breakdown: a developmental model of cognitive decline and Alzheimer's disease. J. Neurobiol. Aging 2004, 25:5-18.

Behl, P., Lanctot, K.L., Streiner, D.L., Guimont, I. and Black, S.E.: Cholinesterase inhibitors slow decline in executive functions, rather than memory, in Alzheimer's disease: a 1-year observational study in the Sunnybrook dementia cohort. Curr. Alzheimer Res. 2006, 3: 147-156.

Bennett, D.A., Schneider, J.A., Arvanitakis, Z., Kelly, J.F., Aggarwal, N.T., Shah, R.C. and Wilson, R.S.: Neuropathology of older persons without cognitive impairment from two community-based studies. Neurology 2006, 66: 1837-1844.

Braak, H. and Braak, E.: Frequency and stages of Alzheimer-related lesions in different age categories. J. Neurobiol. Aging 1997, 18:351-357.

Braak, H. and Del Tredici, K.: Poor and protracted myelination as a contributory factor to neurodegenerative disorders. J. Neurobiol. Aging. 2004, 25:19-23.

Cao, J., Shan, D., Revett, T., Li, D., Wu, L., Liu, W., Tobin, J.F. and Gimeno, R.E.: Molecular identification of a novel mammalian brain isoform of acyl-CoA:lysophospholipid acyltransferase with prominent ethanolamine lysophospholipid acylating activity, LPEAT2. J. Biol. Chem. 2008, 283:19049-57.

Chauhan, N.B.: Membrane dynamics, cholesterol homeostasis, and Alzheimer's disease. J. Lipid Res. 2003, 44: 2019-2029.

Cordy, J.M., Hussain, I., Dingwall, C., Hooper, N.M. and Turner, A.J.: Exclusively targeting beta-secretase to lipid rafts by GPI-anchor addition up-regulates beta-site processing of the amyloid precursor protein. Proc. Nat. Acad. Sci. U.S.A. 2003, 100: 11735-11740.

Cutler, R.G., Kelly, J., Storie, K., Pedersen, W.A., Tammara, A., Hatanpaa, K., Troncoso, J.C. and Mattson, M.P.: Involvement of oxidative stress-induced abnormalities in ceramide and cholesterol metabolism in brain aging and Alzheimer's disease. Proc. Nat. Acad. Sci. U.S.A. 2004, 101: 2070-2075.

Das, A.K., Holmes, R.D., Wilson, G.N. and Hajra, A.K.: Dietary ether lipid incorporation into tissue plasmalogens of humans and rodents. Lipids 1992, 27:401-5.

DeKosky, S.T., Harbaugh, R.E., Schmitt, F.A., Bakay, R.A., Chui, H.C., Knopman, D.S., Reeder, T.M., Shetter, A.G., Senter, H.J. and Markesbery, W.R.: Cortical biopsy in Alzheimer's disease: diagnostic accuracy and neurochemical, neuropathological, and cognitive correlations. Intraventricular Bethanecol Study Group. Annals of neurology 1992, 32: 625-632.

Drachman, D.A: Memory and cognitive function in man: does the cholinergic system have a specific role? Neurology 1977, 27: 783-790.

Etienne, P., Robitaille, Y., Wood, P., Gauthier, S., Nair, N.P. and Quirion, R.: Nucleus basalis neuronal loss, neuritic plaques and choline acetyltransferase activity in advanced Alzheimer's disease. 1986, Neuroscience 19, 1279-1291.

Farber, S.A., Savci, V., Wei, A., Slack, B.E. and Wurtman, R.J.: Choline's phosphorylation in rat striatal slices is regulated by the activity of cholinergic neurons. Brain Res. 1996, 723: 90-99.

Favreliere, S., Stadelmann-Ingrand, S., Huguet, F., De Javel, D., Piriou, A., Tallineau, C. and Durand, G.: Age-related changes in ethanolamine glycerophospholipid fatty acid levels in rat frontal cortex and hippocampus. Neurobiol. Aging 2000, 21: 653-660.

Ferguson, S.M., Savchenko, V., Apparsundaram, S., Zwick, M., Wright, J., Heilman, C.J., Yi, H., Levey, A.I. and Blakely, R.D.: Vesicular localization and activity-dependent trafficking of presynaptic choline transporters. J. Neurosci. 2003, 23: 9697-9709.

Ferguson, S. M. and Blakely, R.D.: The choline transporter resurfaces: new roles for synaptic vesicles? Mol. Interv. 2004, 4: 22-37.

Freund-Levi, Y., Basun, H., Cederholm, T., Faxén-Irving, G., Garlind, A., Grut, M., Vedin, I., Palmblad, J., Wahlund, L.O. and Eriksdotter-Jönhagen, M.: Omega-3 supplementation in mild to moderate Alzheimer's disease: effects on neuropsychiatric symptoms. Int. J. Geriatr. Psychiatry. 2008, 23:161-169.

Glaser, P.E. and Gross, R.W.: Plasmenylethanolamine facilitates rapid membrane fusion: a stopped-flow kinetic investigation correlating the propensity of a major plasma membrane constituent to adopt an HII phase with its ability to promote membrane fusion. Biochemistry 1994, 33: 5805-5812.

Glaser, P. E. and Gross, R. W.: Rapid plasmenylethanolamine-selective fusion of membrane bilayers catalyzed by an isoform of glyceraldehyde-3-phosphate dehydrogenase: discrimination between glycolytic and fusogenic roles of individual isoforms. Biochemistry 1995, 34: 12193-12203.

Goodenowe, D.B., Cook, L.L., Liu, J., Lu, Y., Jayasinghe, D.A., Ahiahonu, P.W., Heath, D., Yamazaki, Y., Flax, J., Krenitsky, K.F., Sparks, D.L., Lerner, A., Friedland, R.P., Kudo, T., Kamino, K., Morihara, T., Takeda, M. and Wood, P.L.: Peripheral ethanolamine plasmalogen deficiency: a logical causative factor in Alzheimer's disease and dementia. J. Lipid Res. 2007, 48:2485-98.

Guttman, C.R.., Jolesz, F.A., Kikinis, R., Killiany, R.J., Moss, M.B., Sandor, T. and Albert, M.S.: White matter changes with normal aging. Neurology 1998, 50: 972-978.

Haining, J.L. and Legan, J. S.: Catalase turnover in rat liver and kidney as a function of age. Exp. Gerontol. 1973, 8: 85-91.

Han, X.L. and Gross, R.W.: Plasmenylcholine and phosphatidylcholine membrane bilayers possess distinct conformational motifs. Biochemistry 1990, 29: 4992-4996.

Han, X.L. and Gross R.W.: Proton nuclear magnetic resonance studies on the molecular dynamics of plasmenylcholine/cholesterol and phosphatidylcholine/cholesterol bilayers. Biochim. Biophys. Acta. 1991, 1063: 129-136.

Han, X., Holtzman, D.M. and McKeel, D.W.Jr: Plasmalogen deficiency in early Alzheimer's disease subjects and in animal models: molecular characterization using electrospray ionization mass spectrometry. J. Neurochem. 2001, 77: 1168-1180.

Han, X, Holtzman, D.M., McKeel, D.W.Jr., Kelley. J. and Morris, J.C.: Substantial sulfatide deficiency and ceramide elevation in very early Alzheimer's disease: potential role in disease pathogenesis. J. Neurochem. 2002, 82:809-18.

Hegner, D.: Age-dependence of molecular and functional changes in biological membrane properties. Mech. Ageing Dev. 1980, 14: 101-118.

Heinrich, C., Nitta, N., Flubacher, A., Muller, M., Fahrner, A., Kirsch, M., Freiman, T., Suzuki, F., Depaulis, M., Frotscher. M. and Haas, C.A.: Reelin deficiency and displacement of mature neurons, but not neurogenesis, underlie the formation of granule cell dispersion in the epileptic hippocampus. J. Neurosci. 2006, 26: 4701-4713.

Hiratsuka, S., Koizumi, K., Ooba, T. and Yokosgoshi, H.: Effects of dietary docosahexaenoic acid connecting phospholipids on the learning ability and fatty acid composition of the brain. J. Nutr. Sci. Vitaminol. 2009, 55:374-380.

Hoppel, C.L. and Tandler, B.: Biochemical effects of cuprizone on mouse liver and heart mitochondria. Biochem. Pharmacol. 1973, 22:2311-8.

Horrocks, L.A. and Sharma, M.: Plasmalogens and O-alkyl glycerophospholipids. Phospholipids. Hawthorne, J.N. and Ansell, G.B., editors. Elsevier, Amsterdam. 1982, 51-93.

Kojro, E., Gimpl, G., Lammich, S., Marz, W. and Fahrenholz, F.: Low cholesterol stimulates the nonamyloidogenic pathway by its effect on the alpha -secretase ADAM 10. Proc. Nat. Acad. Sci. U.S.A. 2001, 98: 5815-5820.

Kotani, S., Sakaguchi, E., Warashina, S., Matsukawa, N., Ishikura, Y., Kiso, Y., Sakakibara, M., Yoshimoto, T., Guo, J. and Yamashima, T.: Dietary supplementation of arachidonic and docosahexaenoic acids improves cognitive dysfunction. Neurosci. Res. 2006, 56:159-64.

Lohner, K., Balgavy, P., Hermetter, A., Paltauf, F. and Laggner, P.: Stabilization of non-bilayer structures by the etherlipid ethanolamine plasmalogen. Biochim. Biophys. Acta 1991, 1061: 132-140.

Lohner, K.: Is the high propensity of ethanolamine plasmalogens to form non-lamellar lipid structures manifested in the properties of biomembranes? Chem. Phys. Lipids 1996, 81: 167-184.

Mack, J.T., Beljanski, V., Soulika, A.M., Townsend, D.M., Brown, C.B., Davis, W. and Tew, K.D.: "Skittish" Abca2 knockout mice display tremor, hyperactivity, and abnormal myelin ultrastructure in the central nervous system. Mol. Cell. Biol. 2007, 27:44-53.

Maire, J.C. and Wurtman, R.J.: Effects of electrical stimulation and choline availability on the release and contents of acetylcholine and choline in superfused slices from rat striatum. J. Physiol. (Paris) 1985, 80: 189-195.

Maczurek, A., Hager, K., Kenklies, M., Sharman, M., Martins, R., Engel, J., Carlson, D.A. and Münch, G. : Lipoic acid as an anti-inflammatory and neuroprotective treatment for Alzheimer's disease. Adv. Drug Deliv. Rev. 2008, 60: 1463-70.

Mandel, H., Sharf, R., Berant, M., Wanders, R.J., Vreken, P. and Aviram, M.: Plasmalogen phospholipids are involved in HDL-mediated cholesterol efflux: insights from investigations with plasmalogen-deficient cells. Biochem. Biophys. Res. Commun. 1998, 250: 369-373.

Mankidy, R., Ahiahonu, P.W., Ma, H., Jayasinghe, D., Ritchie, S.A., Khan, M.A., Su-Myat, K.K., Wood, P.L. and Goodenowe, D.B.: Membrane plasmalogen composition and cellular cholesterol regulation: a structure activity study. Lipids Health Dis. 2010, 9:62.

Martinez, M.: Severe deficiency of docosahexaenoic acid in peroxisomal disorders: a defect of delta 4 desaturation? Neurology 1990, 40: 1292-1298.

May, P., Herz, J. and Bock, H.H.: Molecular mechanisms of lipoprotein receptor signalling. Cell Mol Life Sci. 2005, 62:2325-38.

Meier-Ruge, W., Ulrich, J. and Meier, E.: Age-related white matter atrophy in the human brain. Ann. N.Y. Acad. Sci. 1992, 673:260-269.

Munn, N.J., Arnio, E., Liu, D., Zoeller, R.A. and Liscum, L.: Deficiency in ethanolamine plasmalogen leads to altered cholesterol transport. J. Lipid Res. 2003, 44: 182-192.

Nagan, N., Hajara, A.K., Larkins, L.K., Lazarow, P., Perdue, P.E., Rizzo, W.B. and Zoeller, R.A.: Isolation of a Chinese hamster fibroblast variant defective in dihydroxyacetonephosphate acyltransferase activity and plasmalogen biosynthesis: use of a novel two-step selection protocol. J.Biochem. 1998, 32: 273-27.

Nagan, N. and Zoeller, R.A.: Plasmalogens: biosynthesis and functions. Prog. Lipid Res. 2001, 40: 199-229.

Perichon, R. and Bourre J.M.: Peroxisomal beta-oxidation activity and catalase activity during development and aging in mouse liver. Biochimie 1995, 77: 288-293.

Perichon, R., Moser, A.B., Wallace, W.C., Cunningham, S.C., Roth, G.S. and Moser, H.W.: Peroxisomal disease cell lines with cellular plasmalogen deficiency have impaired muscarinic cholinergic signal transduction activity and amyloid precursor protein secretion. Biochem. Biophys. Res. Commun. 1998, 248: 57-61.

Perry, E.K., Tomlinson, B.E., Blessed, G., Bergmann, K., Gibson, P.H. and Perry R.H.: Correlation of cholinergic abnormalities with senile plaques and mental test scores in senile dementia. Br. Med. J. 1978, 2: 1457-1459.

Pratico, D., Uryu, K., Leight, S., Trojanoswki, J.Q. and Lee, V.M.: Increased lipid peroxidation precedes amyloid plaque formation in an animal model of Alzheimer amyloidosis. J. Neurosci. 2001, 21: 4183-4187.

Puglielli, L., Tanzi, R.E. and Kovacs, D.M.: Alzheimer's disease: the cholesterol connection. Nat. Neurosci. 2003, 6: 345-351.

Rao, G., Xia, E. and Richardson, A.: Effect of age on the expression of antioxidant enzymes in male Fischer F344 rats. Mech. Ageing Dev. 1990, 53: 49-60.

Refolo, L.M., Malester, B., LaFrancois, J., Bryant-Thomas, T., Wang, R., Tint, G.S., Sambamurti, K., Duff, K. and Pappolla, M.A.: Hypercholesterolemia accelerates the Alzheimer's amyloid pathology in a transgenic mouse model. Neurobiol. Dis. 2000, 7: 321-331.

Scott, B.L., and Bazan, N.G.: Membrane docosahexaenoate is supplied to the developing brain and retina by the liver. Proc. Natl. Acad. Sci. U.S.A. 1989, 86: 2903-2907.

Scott, S.A., DeKosky, S.T., Sparks, D.L., Knox, C.A. and Scheff, S.W.: Amygdala cell loss and atrophy in Alzheimer's disease. Ann. Neurol. 1992, 32:555-63.

Skripuletz,T., Lindner, M., Kotsiari, A., Garde, N., Fokuhl, J., Linsmeier, F., Trebst, C. and Stangel, M.: Cortical demyelination is prominent in the murine cuprizone model and is strain-dependent. Am. J. Pathol. 2008, 172:1053-61.

Stark, A.K., Pelvig, D.P., Jørgensen, A.M., Andersen, B.B. and Pakkenberg, B.: Measuring morphological and cellular changes in Alzheimer's dementia: a review emphasizing stereology. Curr. Alzheimer Res. 2005, 2:449-81.

Ulus, I.H., Wurtman, R.J., Mauron, C. and Blusztajn, J.K.: Choline increases acetylcholine release and protects against the stimulation-induced decrease in phosphatide levels within membranes of rat corpus striatum. Brain research 1989, 484: 217-227.

Vereecken, T.H., Vogels, O.J. and Nieuwenhuys, R.: Neuron loss and shrinkage in the amygdala in Alzheimer's disease. Neurobiol. Aging. 1994, 15:45-54.

Vlkolinský, R., Cairns, N., Fountoulakis, M. and Lubec, G.: Decreased brain levels of 2',3'-cyclic nucleotide-3'-phosphodiesterase in Down syndrome and Alzheimer's disease. Neurobiol. Aging. 2001, 22:547-53.

Voss, A., Reinhart, M., Sankarappa, S. and Sprecher, H.: The metabolism of 7,10,13,16,19-docosapentaenoic acid to 4,7,10,13,16,19-docosahexaenoic acid in rat liver is independent of a 4-desaturase. J. Biol. Chem. 1991, 266: 19995-20000.

Vogels, O.J., Broere, C.A., ter Laak, H.J., ten Donkelaar, H.J., Nieuwenhuys, R. and Schulte, B.P.: Cell loss and shrinkage in the nucleus basalis Meynert complex in Alzheimer's disease. Neurobiol. Aging. 1990, 11:3-13.

Wang, D.S., Bennett, D.A., Mufson, E.J., Mattila, P., Cochran, E. and Dickson, D.W.: Contribution of changes in ubiquitin and myelin basic protein to age-related cognitive decline. Neurosci ,Res. 2004, 48:93-100.

Wilcock, G.K., Esiri, M.M., Bowen, D.M. and Smith, C.C.: Alzheimer's disease. Correlation of cortical choline acetyltransferase activity with the severity of dementia and histological abnormalities. J. Neurol. Sci. 1982, 57: 407-417.

Wood, P.L., Mankidy, R., Ritchie, S., Heath, D., Wood, J.A., Flax, J. and Goodenowe, D.B.: Circulating plasmalogen levels and Alzheimer Disease Assessment Scale-Cognitive scores in Alzheimer patients. J. Psychiatry Neurosci. 2010, 35:59-62.

Zoeller, R.A., and Raetz, C.R.: Isolation of animal cell mutants deficient in plasmalogen biosynthesis and peroxisome assembly. Proc. Natl. Acad. Sci. U.S.A. 1986, 83: 5170-5174.

25

Gangliosides as a Double-Edged Sword in Neurodegenerative Disease

Akio Sekigawa[1], Masayo Fujita[1], Kazunari Sekiyama[1], Yoshiki Takamatsu[1], Jianshe Wei[2] and Makoto Hashimoto[1]
[1]*Division of Chemistry and Metabolism, Tokyo Metropolitan Institute for Neuroscience*
[2]*Division of Molecular and Cellular Neurodegeneration, Department of Biology, Henan University*
[1]*Japan*
[2]*China*

1. Introduction

Gangliosides are sialic acid-containing glycolipids that are mainly localized in the outer leaflet of the plasma membrane of vertebrate cells and are involved in diverse physiological functions such as cell growth, differentiation, and cell-cell recognition(Hakomori, 1990). In the nervous system, gangliosides are highly expressed in neurons and are implicated in neurite outgrowth, synaptogenesis, and modulation of synaptic transmission(Posse de Chaves and Sipione, 2010). In this context, gangliosides have been proposed to act as co-receptors for growth factors (e.g. fibroblast growth factor) and neurotransmitters (e.g. serotonin)(Posse de Chaves and Sipione, 2010). Gangliosides are also localized in some glial cells in both gray and white matter, thereby affecting myelin sheath stability through association with myelin-associated glycoprotein(Schnaar, 2010).

There is immense large body of knowledge on the biosynthesis and catabolism of gangliosides. In brief, gangliosides are synthesized by sequential addition of single sugars catalyzed by multiple glycosyltransferases (Fig. 1). The profiles of ganglioside components in neurons and glia are developmently regulated(Yamamoto et al., 1996; Yu et al., 2009). For instance, the dominant pathway in neurons during the neonate stage is pathway "a", which starts from GM3 and leads to GT1a via GM1 and GD1a. In adult human brain, four gangliosides (GM1, GD1a, GD1b and GT1b) are mainly produced, and these make up the majority (> 66 %) of gangliosides in the brain(Ando et al., 1978). It is also believed that each ganglioside has a specific function in the brain and is not merely an intermediate metabolite in the synthesis of more prevalent gangliosides(Yamamoto et al., 1996; Yu et al., 2009).

Gangliosides are in turn degraded by various lysosomal hydrolases with the aid of sphingolipid activator proteins. If a specific hydrolase required for this process is partially or totally missing due to a genetic deficit, gangliosides accumulate in the lysosomes and result in lysosomal dysfunction, which manifests as a lysosomal storage diseases (LSD)(Jalanko and Braulke, 2009; Vitner et al., 2010). Furthermore, it has been shown that gangliosides are secondarily upregulated in many other sphingolipidoses(Vitner et al.,

2010). In this review, we do not describe the details of LSDs, but we refer to the linkage of LSDs and neurodegenerative diseases in a later section.

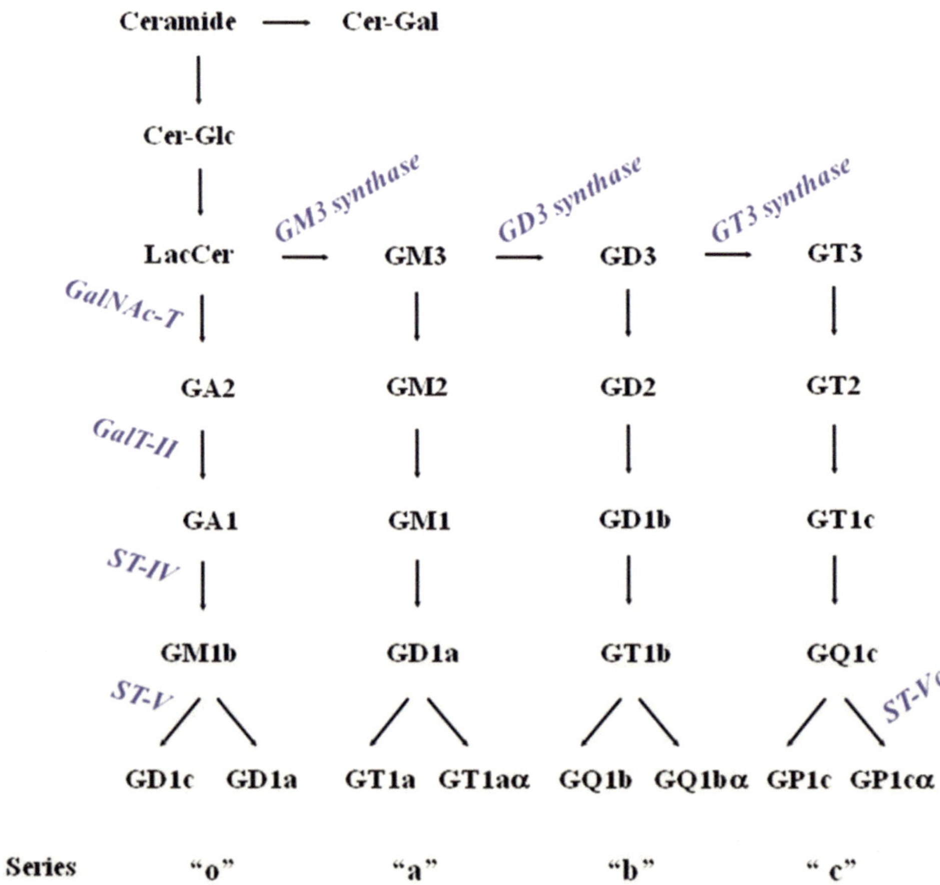

Fig. 1. Schemes of ganglioside synthesis

Synthesis is depicted starting with lactosylceramide (LacCer). GalNAc-T, GA2/GM2/GD2/GT2 synthase; GalT-II, GA1/GM1/GD1b/GT1c synthase; ST-IV, GM1b/GD1a/GT1b/GQ1c synthase; ST-V, GD1c/GT1a/GQ1b/GP1c synthase; ST-Vα, GD1a/GT1aα/GQ1bα/GP1cα synthase.

Beyond LSDs, gangliosides have been implicated in various pathologies. In particular, evidence has accumulated to suggest a role of gangliosides in age-associated neurodegenerative diseases such as Alzheimer's disease (AD) and Parkinson's disease (PD). To date, the effect of gangliosides on the pathogenesis of AD is a controversial issue. Many studies suggest that gangliosides stimulate fibrillogenesis of amyloid β-protein (Aβ) in the early stage of pathogenesis(Yanagisawa et al., 1995), whereas others have shown that GM1 ganglioside has a beneficial effect on early onset AD, presumably through the sequestration of Aβ(Matsuoka et al., 2003; Svennerholm, 1994). A limited number of reports also suggest that gangliosides are protective against the pathogenesis of PD(Hadjiconstantinou et al., 1986; Wei et al., 2009b). With this background, the main objective of this review is to outline what is known about the roles of gangliosides in neurodegenerative diseases, including AD and PD. We also examine the linkage of these neurodegenerative diseases to LSDs.

2. Gangliosides stimulate amyloidogenesis in AD

2.1 Aggregation of Aβ in AD

AD is a progressive degenerative disease of the brain with loss of memory and cognition, and is characterized by the two neuropathological hallmarks of senile plaques and neurofibrillary tangles. The former are mainly composed of aggregated Aβ derived from amyloid precursor protein (APP), while the latter consist of paired helical filaments containing hyperphosphorylated tau(Yankner, 2000).

It is well characterized that amyloidogenic Aβ is generated by the consecutive cleavage of two proteases: β- and γ-secretase(Selkoe, 2008). Consistent with biochemical studies demonstrating that Aβ42 is more amyloidogenic compared to Aβ40 and other Aβ forms, it has been shown genetically that increased Aβ42 production is associated with inherited familial AD. In contrast, alternative cleavage of Aβ at amino acid 17 by α-secretase releases sAPPα and excludes production of Aβ. The predominant cleavage product is sAPPα, serving to prevent production of Aβ.

The mechanism of neurotoxicity caused by Aβ is incompletely understood. However, it is generally believed that aggregation of Aβ results in formation of neurotoxic protofibrils and deposition of amyloid plaques(Yankner, 2000). Thus, factors regulating Aβ aggregation and secretion are very important for the etiology of AD.

2.2 Ganglioside interactions with Aβ

Considerable attention has been focused on the roles of gangliosides in the development of AD, since a number of *in vitro* studies have shown that GM1 ganglioside has a high affinity for Aβ and accelerates Aβ assembly, which leads to amyloid fibril formation. In this regard, Yanagisawa and Ihara reported that Aβ adopts an altered conformation through binding to GM1 in brain, which subsequently facilitates the assembly of soluble Aβ by acting as an endogenous seed, GAβ (GM1-Aβ) (Fig. 2A)(Yanagisawa et al., 1995). Subsequently, Yanagisawa and colleagues developed a monoclonal antibody against purified GAβ from AD brain(Hayashi et al., 2004). Notably, the antibody inhibits Aβ assembly *in vitro* through binding to GAβ and Aβ. In addition, this antibody potently inhibits the assembly of Aβ40 and Aβ42 *in vitro*. Furthermore, peripheral administration of Fab fragments of the antibody to transgenic mice expressing a mutant APP resulted in marked suppression of Aβ deposition in the brain(Yamamoto et al., 2005b), thus suggesting that targeting of the endogenous seed could be a therapeutic strategy. Similar results have been obtained by other groups(Ariga et al., 2008; Choo-Smith et al., 1997; Matsuzaki and Horikiri, 1999; McLaurin and Chakrabartty, 1996).

It is of particular interest that several Aβ mutations in familial AD and hereditary cerebral amyloid angiopathy show distinct ganglioside affinity (Fig. 3A). Aβ with the Arctic-type mutation (E22G) rapidly assembles in the presence of GM1, similarly to wild type Aβ(Yamamoto et al., 2007). In contrast, Aβ with the Dutch-type mutation (E22Q) assembles in the presence GM2 or GM3(Yamamoto et al., 2005a), and Aβ with the Flemish-type mutation (A21G) assembles in the presence GD3(Yamamoto et al., 2005a). The pathological meaning of these phenomena is unknown.

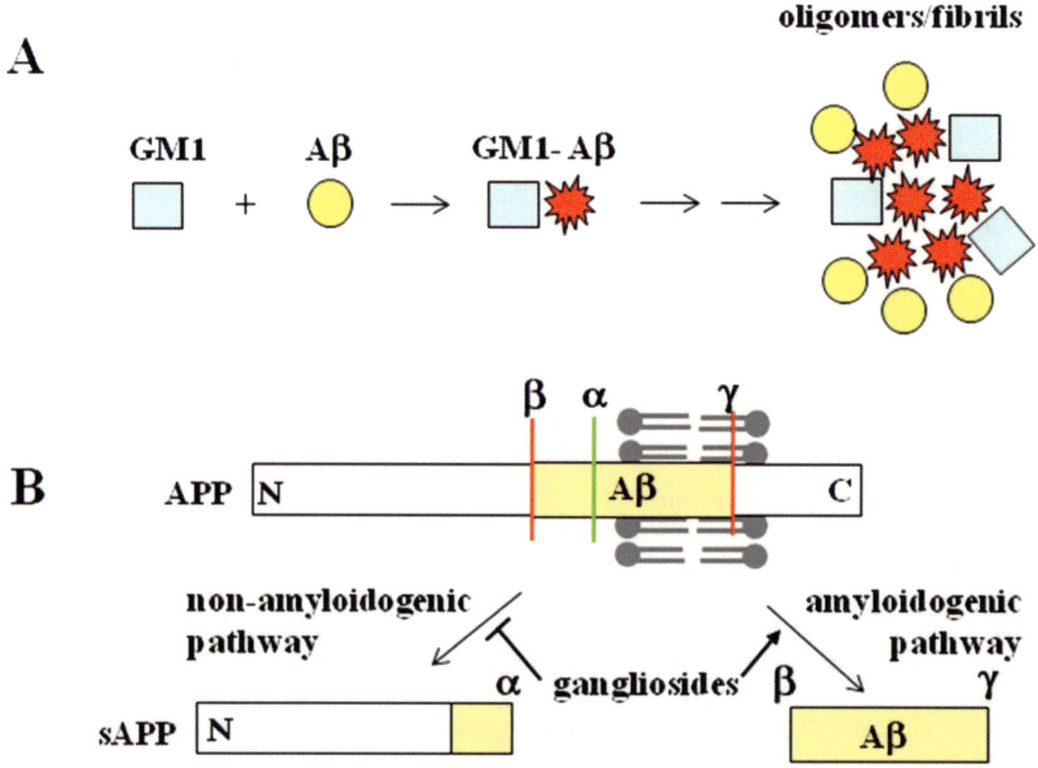

Fig. 2. Mechanism of the stimulatory effects of GM1 on Aβ aggregation.
A) Aβ adopts an altered conformation through binding to GM1, which subsequently facilitates the assembly of soluble Aβ by acting as an endogenous seed, GAβ (GM1-Aβ), leading to amyloid fibril formation.
B) GM1 regulates the processing of APP by inhibition of α-secretase and stimulation of β- and/or γ-secretase activity, leading to increased secretion of Aβ.

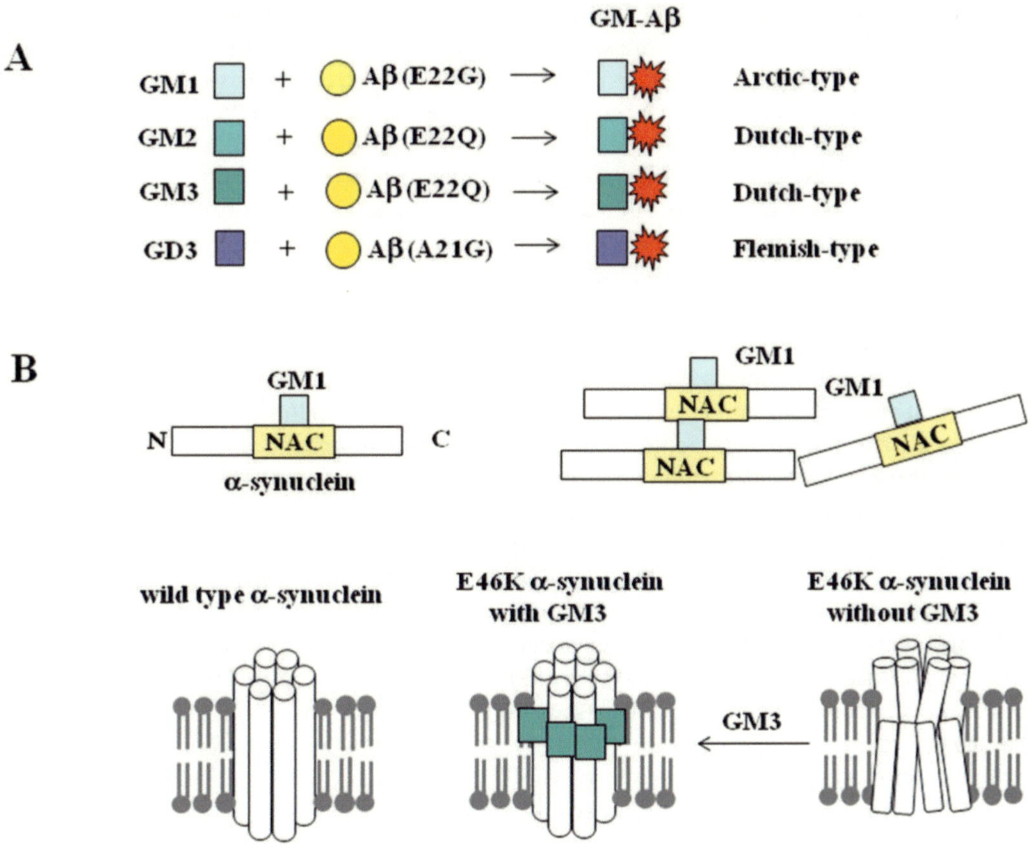

Fig. 3. Affinity of gangliosides to amyloidogenic proteins.
A) GM1, GM2/GM3 and GD3 stimulates assembly of E22G (Arctic-type mutation), E22Q (Dutch-type mutation) and A21G (Flemish-type mutation), respectively.
B) GM1 strongly inhibits α-synuclein fibrillation through binding to the NAC region, while channel formation by the DLB-linked E46K mutant of α-synuclein is corrected by GM3.

2.3 Regulatory roles of gangliosides on APP processing

Besides a direct interaction with Aβ, gangliosides might also dysregulate APP processing associated with increased secretion of Aβ, which could ultimately lead to enhanced aggregation of Aβ (Fig. 2B). In support of this view, exogenous addition of GM1 in cultured neurons enhances Aβ production in parallel with inhibition of sAPPα secretion(Zha et al., 2004). These results suggest that GM1 regulates processing of APP by regulating the activity of secretases. There are two potential mechanisms for the inhibition of α-secretase cleavage by GM1(Zha et al., 2004). First, stiffening of the membrane due to GM1 loading may decrease sAPPα by inhibiting lateral movement and preventing the required contact between the enzyme and substrate. Second, since GM1 has been reported to have an inhibitory action on PKC, and sAPPα is positively regulated by PKC activation, GM1 may inhibit sAPPα secretion by inhibiting PKC activity. Both hypotheses require examination in further experimental work.

It is also possible that GM1 could increase β- and/or γ-secretase activity directly or indirectly. Indeed, since these secretases are thought to be localized to rafts, there might be as yet unknown biological functions underlying the connection between gangliosides and the secretases. Such a view may fit with a recent suggestion that amyloidogenic processing of APP depends on lipid rafts(Vetrivel and Thinakaran, 2010). Rafts are lateral assemblies of sphingolipids and cholesterol within the membrane. In this context, both gangliosides and cholesterol have been shown to bind to Aβ and facilitate amyloid fibril formation(Kakio, 2001). Taken together, these results suggest that processing of APP and generation of Aβ can be modulated depending on the cellular content of gangliosides.

2.4 Gangliosides and tau

Currently, only a few reports have suggested a role of gangliosides in tau aggregation and NFT formation. McGeer and co-workers showed that the monoclonal antibody A2B5, which recognizes neuronal surface gangliosides, was strongly immunopositive for many NFTs, neuropil threads, and dystrophic neurites in AD(Tooyama et al., 1992). Similar strong immunoreactivities were observed in globose-type NFTs in cases of progressive supranuclear palsy cases and in Pick bodies in Pick's disease(Yasuhara et al., 1995). Takahashi et al. showed that fetal antigens such as the C-series gangliosides and microtubule-associated protein 5 immunostained dystrophic neurites of senile plaques, NFTs and neuropil threads in the cerebral cortex in AD brain, with similar immunostaining patterns to those of tau(Takahashi et al., 1991). These results suggest that regeneration or sprouting of neurons is ongoing in association with the re-induction of gene expression characteristics in the AD brain in the early stage of development. Further studies are required to investigate the interesting possibility that gangliosides bind with tau, and that this leads to formation of NFTs and other histopathologies in AD.

2.5 Glial activation by gangliosides

It has been well characterized that gangliosides are involved in regulation of glial activation(Cammer and Zhang, 1996). In this context, recent clinical reports show that reactive astrocytes have ganglioside GD3, unlike protoplasmic astrocytes, in patients with Creutzfeldt-Jakob disease and cerebral infarction(Kawai et al., 1999). Thus, it is likely that expression and localization of individual ganglioside subtypes in neurons and glia might change under the neurodegenerative conditions of AD and PD.

3. Amelioration of the neuropathology of AD by gangliosides

As described above, many studies have shown a role for gangliosides as stimulators of Aβ amyloidogenesis in the early stage of AD. However, some studies have focused on the beneficial effects of gangliosides in treatment of AD. Svennerholm and Gottfries showed that the ganglioside content is reduced in early-onset or familial AD to 58-70% of that of control brains in gray matter and to 81% in frontal white matter(Svennerholm and Gottfries, 1994). Notably, both GT1b and GQ1b were significantly decreased, while GD3 was increased, suggesting that metabolism of gangliosides may be dysregulated in AD. Furthermore, given the neurotrophic activities of gangliosides(Fusco et al., 1993), it seems likely that loss of gangliosides is correlated with the severity of AD. Based on this idea, Svennerholm performed intraventricular infusion of GM1 for AD brains and concluded that

GM1 treatment was effective for early onset AD, presumably through sequestration of Aβ by GM1(Svennerholm, 1994). More recently, Matsuoka et al. found that PS/APP mice administered peripherally with gelsolin or GM1 showed a substantial decrease in aggregated Aβ40 and Aβ42 in the brain. The result is reminiscent of the "sink effect" leading to reduction of Aβ accumulation in the brain following passive immunization with anti-Aβ antibodies(DeMattos et al., 2002). Based on this result, a novel therapeutic strategy was proposed using derivatives that are structurally related to gangliosides for specific targeting of pathogenic peptides in the periphery.

4. Roles of gangliosides in the pathogenesis of PD and related disorders

4.1 Synucleinopathies

PD is a progressive degenerative disorder of dopaminergic neurons in the substantia nigra. PD manifests clinically as movement disorder, including tremor, rigidity, and gait disturbance, while non-motor type symptoms such as cognitive difficulties and sleep problems may arise in advanced stages(Hashimoto and Masliah, 1999; Trojanowski et al., 1998). Because the pathology of PD is characterized by accumulation of α-synuclein into inclusions called Lewy bodies in neurons, the disease is classified as a synucleinopathy. This spectrum of diseases also includes dementia with Lewy bodies (DLB), multiple system atrophy, and neurodegeneration with brain iron accumulation type I(Hashimoto and Masliah, 1999; Trojanowski et al., 1998).

α-Synuclein is a presynaptic protein of unknown function that is characterized by a natively unfolded structures, with highly conserved N-termini and divergent C-terminal acidic regions in the synuclein family of peptides, which has two other members: β- and γ-synuclein(Hashimoto and Masliah, 1999). Importantly, α-synuclein is distinct from other members of the synuclein family in that it possesses a highly hydrophobic central region that has been identified as a non-amyloid β component in Alzheimer disease(Ueda et al., 1993). Since the discovery of the linkage of two missense mutations (A53T and A30P) to familial PD(Kruger et al., 1998; Polymeropoulos et al., 1997), numerous histopathological studies have shown that α-synuclein fibrils are the major constituent in Lewy bodies and glial cell inclusions in synucleinopathies(Hashimoto and Masliah, 1999). Furthermore, another missense mutation, E46K, was recently identified for DLB(Zarranz et al., 2004). All the mutant proteins have a greater propensity for self-association and aggregation compared with wild-type α-synuclein, suggesting that aggregation and protofibril formation of α-synuclein has a causative role in stimulation of neurodegenerative disorders.

4.2 Gangliosides bind with α-synuclein

Among various modulators, gangliosides may be particularly important as endogenous molecules that negatively regulate α-synuclein aggregation. In this regard, Fink and colleagues investigated the interactions between various brain sphingolipids and α-synuclein and found that α-synuclein specifically bound to ganglioside GM1(Martinez et al., 2007). Furthermore, GM1 strongly inhibited α-synuclein fibrillation, whereas total brain gangliosides, GM2, GM3, and asialo-GM1 had weak inhibitory effects on α-synuclein fibrillation and induced some α-helical structure(Martinez et al., 2007). Given the immunoreactivity of α-synuclein in rafts, it is possible that α-synuclein is recruited by GM1 to lipid raft regions in presynaptic membranes. In this context, perturbation of GM1/raft association could induce changes in α-synuclein that contribute to the pathogenesis of PD. It is also noteworthy that GM3 may have a protective effect against channelopathy caused by α-synuclein(Lashuel et al., 2002). The ability of α-synuclein oligomers to form ionic channels was postulated as a channelopathy mechanism in human brain. Di Pasquale et al. identified a ganglioside-binding domain in the N-terminal region of α-synuclein (aa 34-50) and showed that altered ion channel formation by the DLB-linked E46K mutant of α-synuclein was corrected by GM3, but not by GM1 ganglioside(Di Pasquale et al., 2010). This result suggests that GM3, a minor brain ganglioside that is increasingly expressed with aging, might play a critical role in the neurotoxicity of α-synuclein. It is also an intriguing possibility that gangliosides might have affinity for α-synuclein mutations, as is the case for Aβ mutations (Fig. 3B).

4.3 Protective effects of gangliosides on lysosomal pathology of synucleinopathies

Results in cell-free systems indicate that gangliosides may protect against synucleinopathies, and we have shown that changes in endogenous ganglioside levels affect lysosomal pathology in a cellular model of synucleinopathy(Wei et al., 2009a; Wei et al., 2007). In this work, DLB-linked P123H β-synuclein neuroblastoma cells transfected with α-synuclein were used as a model system because these cells have extensive formation of lysosomal inclusion bodies. Treatment of the cells with D-threo-1-phenyl-2-decanoylamino-3-morpholino-1-propanol (PDMP), an inhibitor of glycosyl ceramide synthase, resulted in various features of lysosomal pathology, including compromised lysosomal activity, enhanced lysosomal membrane permeabilization, and increased cytotoxicity (Fig. 4). Consistent with these findings, expression levels of lysosomal membrane proteins, ATP13A2 and LAMP-2, were significantly decreased, and electron microscopy demonstrated alterations in the lysosomal membrane structures. Furthermore, accumulation of P123H β-synuclein and α-synuclein was significant in PDMP-treated cells because of the suppressive effect of PDMP on the autophagy pathway. Finally, the detrimental effects of PDMP on the lysosomal pathology were significantly ameliorated by addition of gangliosides to the cultured cells. These data suggest that endogenous gangliosides have protective roles against lysosomal pathology of synucleinopathies.

4.4 Protective effects of gangliosides in an MPTP model

There are few reports on the roles of gangliosides in synucleinopathies *in vivo*, but many studies have documented the beneficial effects of GM1 in drug-induced Parkinsonian models in animals, including those induced by treatment with 1-methyl-4-phenyl-1,2,3,6-tetrahydropyridine (MPTP) and 6-hydroxydopamine(Hadjiconstantinou et al., 1986; Jonsson et al., 1984). Mitochondrial dysfunction and oxidative stress are induced by these drugs, and it is possible that such oxidative stress is mitigated by gangliosides, similarly to suppression of oxidative stress induced by α-synuclein aggregation.

Despite the protective effects of gangliosides on drug-induced Parkinsonism, clinical trials of gangliosides for treatment of PD have been suspended because of the occasional development of an acute motor neuropathy (e.g. Guillain-Barré syndrome). Therefore, new derivatives of gangliosides are required that might efficiently sequester α-synuclein without causing neuropathy and other side effects.

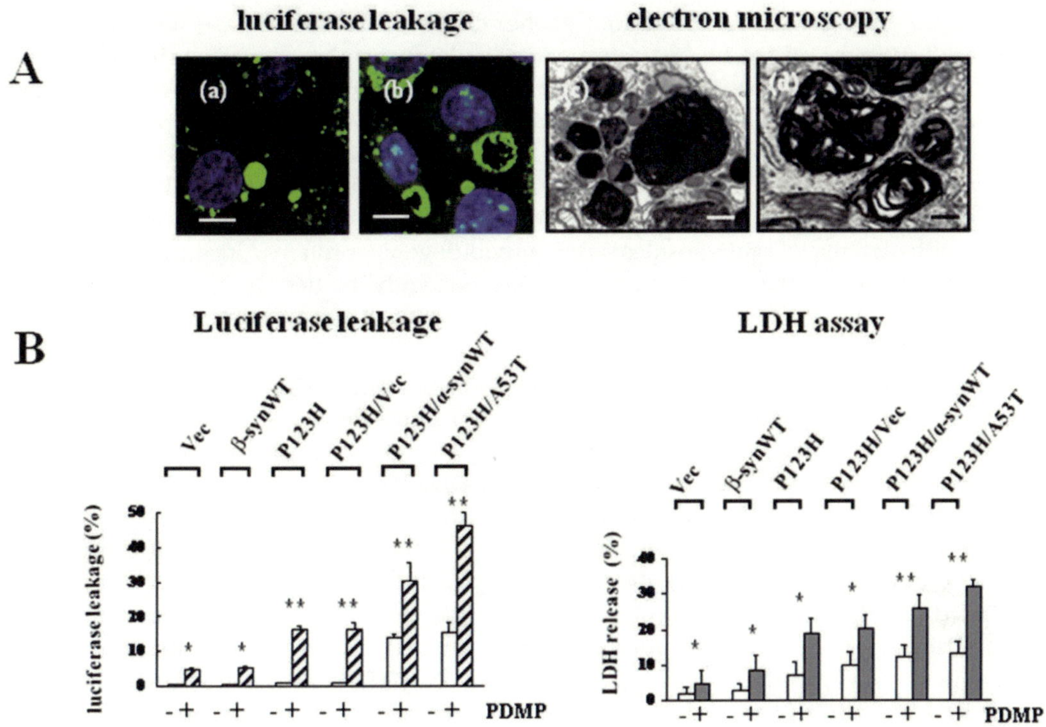

Fig. 4. Protective effects of gangliosides on lysosomal pathology in the DLB-linked cellular model.

A) Immunofluorescence showed that the fluorescence of Lucifer Yellow in P123H β-synuclein-overexpressing B103 rat neuroblastoma cells transfected with A53T α-synuclein was significantly increased by PDMP treatment (25 μmol/L, 24 hrs) (b) compared to PDMP-untreated cells (a). Ultrastructurally, some large electron-dense inclusions were composed of various types of giant autophagosomes (c, d), the membrane integrities of which were loosened by PDMP treatment (d). Scale bars: 10 μm (a, b) or 1 μm (c, d)

B) Quantifications of Lucifer Yellow redistribution and LDH assay. In addition to P123H β-synuclein-overexpressing cells transfected with vector, wild-type α-synuclein, or A53T α-synuclein, vector-transfected cells, wild-type β-synuclein-overexpressing cells, and P123H β-synuclein-overexpressing cells were also analyzed. The number of Lucifer Yellow-positive cells in their cytosols at 48 hours of PDMP treatment was calculated as a percentage of the total number of cells (left panel). LDH assay was performed under the same conditions (right panel). Data are shown as means ± SD (n = 4). $^{*}P < 0.05$, $^{**}P < 0.01$ versus PDMP-untreated cells. (Reprinted with permission from *Am J Pathol*, Wei et al, 2009, 174(5):1891-1909.)

5. Common pathology between neurodegenerative diseases and LSDs

5.1 LSDs are associated with Lewy bodies and NFTs

In the previous sections, we have described how gangliosides might be involved in the pathogenesis of neurodegenerative disorders such as AD and PD. Conversely, accumulating evidence suggests that LSDs, including Gaucher disease, Sandhoff disease, Nieman-Pick C1 disease, Tay-Sachs disease, metachromatic leukodystrophy, β-galactosialidosis, and adrenoleukodystrophy, are associated with neuropathologies such as Lewy bodies and NFT(Saito et al., 2004; Suzuki et al., 2003; Suzuki et al., 2007). Furthermore, a recent study suggested that LSDs and neurodegenerative diseases are characterized by disorder of the autophagy-lysosomal pathway(Settembre et al., 2008; Tamboli et al., 2011). The overlapping pathology between the two disease spectrums might be attributable to direct and/or indirect interactions of gangliosides with amyloidogenic proteins, including Aβ and α-synuclein. However, the two disease types are currently treated as completely separate entities, which may mainly be due to the differences in onset age and clinical symptoms.

5.2 Genetic link between neurodegenerative diseases and LSDs

Emerging genetic evidence suggests that the distinction between the two disease types should be reconsidered. In this regard, several cohort studies of screening for the glucocerebrosidase gene in patients with PD and DLB have identified a high frequency of mutations(Hruska et al., 2006; Mitsui et al., 2009; Sidransky, 2004), suggesting that mutation of this gene is a risk factor for α-synucleinopathies. Furthermore, the affinity of gangliosides for amyloidogenic proteins raises the intriguing possibility that the two disease spectrums are linked to each other more closely than previously thought. GM1 associates with the β-sheet structure of α-synuclein (probably with the central NAC region), while GM3 preferentially binds to the N-terminus of α-synuclein. GM2 is abundantly accumulated in Sandhoff disease and Tay-Sachs disease, both of which have a Lewy body pathology(Suzuki et al., 2003), and this raises the question of how GM2 interacts with α-synuclein. Furthermore, other sphingolipids may have affinity for α-synuclein, given the accumulation of α-synuclein in other types of LSDs.

6. Conclusion

In summary, gangliosides may be involved in the pathogenesis of AD, either by stimulating the seeding step of amyloidogenesis or through deregulation of the processing of APP. On the other hand, addition of gangliosides may be a useful strategy to sequester Aβ, leading to suppression of extracellular deposits of Aβ. In a similar context, the sequestering effects of gangliosides on α-synuclein may protect against an α-synuclein pathology, such as channelopathy and intracellular lysosomal inclusion. Thus, currently available data suggest that gangliosides may act as a double-edged sword in neurodegenerative diseases such as AD and PD.

However, information is still limited and further studies are required to elucidate the roles of gangliosides with respect to Aβ and α-synuclein, and also with tau and glial activation. Finally, the affinity of gangliosides to amyloidogenic proteins is an issue that may provide a key to solve as yet unknown mechanisms underlying common aspects of age-associated neurodegenerative diseases and LSDs.

7. Acknowledgements

This work was supported in part by a grant-in-aid for Science Research from the Ministry of Education, Culture, Sports, Science, and Technology, Japan. The authors have no conflict of interest to declare.

8. References

Ando, S., Chang, N.C., & Yu, R.K. (1978). High-performance thin-layer chromatography and densitometric determination of brain ganglioside compositions of several species. *Anal Biochem*, Vol. 89, No. 2, pp. 437-450, ISSN 0003-2697

Ariga, T., McDonald, M.P., & Yu, R.K. (2008). Role of ganglioside metabolism in the pathogenesis of Alzheimer's disease--a review. *J Lipid Res*, Vol. 49, No. 6, pp. 1157-1175, ISSN 0022-2275

Cammer, W., & Zhang, H. (1996). Ganglioside GD3 in radial glia and astrocytes in situ in brains of young and adult mice. *J Neurosci Res*, Vol. 46, No. 1, pp. 18-23, ISSN 0360-4012

Choo-Smith, L.P., Garzon-Rodriguez, W., Glabe, C.G., & Surewicz, W.K. (1997). Acceleration of amyloid fibril formation by specific binding of Abeta-(1-40) peptide to ganglioside-containing membrane vesicles. *J Biol Chem*, Vol. 272, No. 37, pp. 22987-22990, ISSN 0021-9258

DeMattos, R.B., Bales, K.R., Cummins, D.J., Paul, S.M., & Holtzman, D.M. (2002). Brain to plasma amyloid-beta efflux: a measure of brain amyloid burden in a mouse model of Alzheimer's disease. *Science*, Vol. 295, No. 5563, pp. 2264-2267, ISSN 0036-8075

Di Pasquale, E., Fantini, J., Chahinian, H., Maresca, M., Taieb, N., & Yahi, N. (2010). Altered ion channel formation by the Parkinson's-disease-linked E46K mutant of alpha-synuclein is corrected by GM3 but not by GM1 gangliosides. *J Mol Biol*, Vol. 397, No. 1, pp. 202-218, ISSN 0022-2836

Fusco, M., Vantini, G., Schiavo, N., Zanotti, A., Zanoni, R., Facci, L., & Skaper, S.D. (1993). Gangliosides and neurotrophic factors in neurodegenerative diseases: from experimental findings to clinical perspectives. *Ann N Y Acad Sci*, Vol. 695, pp. 314-317, ISSN 0077-8923

Hadjiconstantinou, M., Rossetti, Z.L., Paxton, R.C., & Neff, N.H. (1986). Administration of GM1 ganglioside restores the dopamine content in striatum after chronic treatment with MPTP. *Neuropharmacology*, Vol. 25, No. 9, pp. 1075-1077, ISSN 0028-3908

Hakomori, S. (1990). Bifunctional role of glycosphingolipids. Modulators for transmembrane signaling and mediators for cellular interactions. *J Biol Chem*, Vol. 265, No. 31, pp. 18713-18716, ISSN 0021-9258

Hashimoto, M., & Masliah, E. (1999). Alpha-synuclein in Lewy body disease and Alzheimer's disease. *Brain pathology (Zurich, Switzerland)*, Vol. 9, No. 4, pp. 707-720, ISSN 1015-6305

Hayashi, H., Kimura, N., Yamaguchi, H., Hasegawa, K., Yokoseki, T., Shibata, M., Yamamoto, N., Michikawa, M., Yoshikawa, Y., Terao, K., *et al.* (2004). A seed for Alzheimer amyloid in the brain. *J Neurosci*, Vol. 24, No. 20, pp. 4894-4902, ISSN 0270-6474

Hruska, K.S., Goker-Alpan, O., & Sidransky, E. (2006). Gaucher disease and the synucleinopathies. *J Biomed Biotechnol*, Vol. 2006, No. 3, pp. 78549, ISSN 1110-7243

Jalanko, A., & Braulke, T. (2009). Neuronal ceroid lipofuscinoses. *Biochim Biophys Acta*, Vol. 1793, No. 4, pp. 697-709, ISSN 0006-3002

Jonsson, G., Gorio, A., Hallman, H., Janigro, D., Kojima, H., Luthman, J., & Zanoni, R. (1984). Effects of GM1 ganglioside on developing and mature serotonin and noradrenaline neurons lesioned by selective neurotoxins. *J Neurosci Res*, Vol. 12, No. 2-3, pp. 459-475, ISSN 0360-4012

Kakio, A. (2001). Cholesterol-dependent Formation of GM1 Ganglioside-bound Amyloid beta -Protein, an Endogenous Seed for Alzheimer Amyloid. *Journal of Biological Chemistry*, Vol. 276, No. 27, pp. 24985-24990, ISSN 1083-351X

Kawai, K., Watarai, S., Takahashi, H., Ishizu, H., Fukai, K., Tanabe, Y., Yokota, O., & Kuroda, S. (1999). Demonstration of ganglioside GD3 in human reactive astrocytes. *Psychiatry Clin Neurosci*, Vol. 53, No. 1, pp. 79-82, ISSN 1323-1316

Kruger, R., Kuhn, W., Muller, T., Woitalla, D., Graeber, M., Kosel, S., Przuntek, H., Epplen, J.T., Schols, L., & Riess, O. (1998). Ala30Pro mutation in the gene encoding alpha-synuclein in Parkinson's disease. *Nat Genet*, Vol. 18, No. 2, pp. 106-108, ISSN 1061-4036

Lashuel, H.A., Hartley, D., Petre, B.M., Walz, T., & Lansbury, P.T., Jr. (2002). Neurodegenerative disease: amyloid pores from pathogenic mutations. *Nature*, Vol. 418, No. 6895, pp. 291, ISSN 0028-0836

Martinez, Z., Zhu, M., Han, S., & Fink, A.L. (2007). GM1 specifically interacts with alpha-synuclein and inhibits fibrillation. *Biochemistry*, Vol. 46, No. 7, pp. 1868-1877, ISSN 0006-2960

Matsuoka, Y., Saito, M., LaFrancois, J., Gaynor, K., Olm, V., Wang, L., Casey, E., Lu, Y., Shiratori, C., Lemere, C., & Duff, K. (2003). Novel therapeutic approach for the treatment of Alzheimer's disease by peripheral administration of agents with an affinity to beta-amyloid. *J Neurosci*, Vol. 23, No. 1, pp. 29-33, ISSN 0270-6474

Matsuzaki, K., & Horikiri, C. (1999). Interactions of amyloid beta-peptide (1-40) with ganglioside-containing membranes. *Biochemistry*, Vol. 38, No. 13, pp. 4137-4142, ISSN 0006-2960

McLaurin, J., & Chakrabartty, A. (1996). Membrane disruption by Alzheimer beta-amyloid peptides mediated through specific binding to either phospholipids or gangliosides. Implications for neurotoxicity. *J Biol Chem*, Vol. 271, No. 43, pp. 26482-26489, ISSN 0021-9258

Mitsui, J., Mizuta, I., Toyoda, A., Ashida, R., Takahashi, Y., Goto, J., Fukuda, Y., Date, H., Iwata, A., Yamamoto, M., *et al.* (2009). Mutations for Gaucher disease confer high susceptibility to Parkinson disease. *Arch Neurol*, Vol. 66, No. 5, pp. 571-576, ISSN 0003-9942

Polymeropoulos, M.H., Lavedan, C., Leroy, E., Ide, S.E., Dehejia, A., Dutra, A., Pike, B., Root, H., Rubenstein, J., Boyer, R., *et al.* (1997). Mutation in the alpha-synuclein gene identified in families with Parkinson's disease. *Science*, Vol. 276, No. 5321, pp. 2045-2047, ISSN 0036-8075

Posse de Chaves, E., & Sipione, S. (2010). Sphingolipids and gangliosides of the nervous system in membrane function and dysfunction. *FEBS Letters*, Vol. 584, No. 9, pp. 1748-1759, ISSN 0014-5793

Saito, Y., Suzuki, K., Hulette, C.M., & Murayama, S. (2004). Aberrant phosphorylation of alpha-synuclein in human Niemann-Pick type C1 disease. *J Neuropathol Exp Neurol*, Vol. 63, No. 4, pp. 323-328, ISSN 0022-3069

Schnaar, R.L. (2010). Brain gangliosides in axon–myelin stability and axon regeneration. *FEBS Letters*, Vol. 584, No. 9, pp. 1741-1747, ISSN 0014-5793

Selkoe, D.J. (2008). Biochemistry and molecular biology of amyloid beta-protein and the mechanism of Alzheimer's disease. *Handb Clin Neurol*, Vol. 89, pp. 245-260, ISSN 0072-9752

Settembre, C., Fraldi, A., Jahreiss, L., Spampanato, C., Venturi, C., Medina, D., de Pablo, R., Tacchetti, C., Rubinsztein, D.C., & Ballabio, A. (2008). A block of autophagy in lysosomal storage disorders. *Hum Mol Genet*, Vol. 17, No. 1, pp. 119-129, ISSN 0964-6906

Sidransky, E. (2004). Gaucher disease: complexity in a "simple" disorder. *Mol Genet Metab*, Vol. 83, No. 1-2, pp. 6-15, ISSN 1096-7192

Suzuki, K., Iseki, E., Katsuse, O., Yamaguchi, A., Katsuyama, K., Aoki, I., Yamanaka, S., & Kosaka, K. (2003). Neuronal accumulation of alpha- and beta-synucleins in the brain of a GM2 gangliosidosis mouse model. *Neuroreport*, Vol. 14, No. 4, pp. 551-554, ISSN 0959-4965

Suzuki, K., Iseki, E., Togo, T., Yamaguchi, A., Katsuse, O., Katsuyama, K., Kanzaki, S., Shiozaki, K., Kawanishi, C., Yamashita, S., *et al.* (2007). Neuronal and glial accumulation of alpha- and beta-synucleins in human lipidoses. *Acta Neuropathol*, Vol. 114, No. 5, pp. 481-489, ISSN 0001-6322

Svennerholm, L. (1994). Gangliosides--a new therapeutic agent against stroke and Alzheimer's disease. *Life Sci*, Vol. 55, No. 25-26, pp. 2125-2134, ISSN 0024-3205

Svennerholm, L., & Gottfries, C.G. (1994). Membrane lipids, selectively diminished in Alzheimer brains, suggest synapse loss as a primary event in early-onset form (type I) and demyelination in late-onset form (type II). *J Neurochem*, Vol. 62, No. 3, pp. 1039-1047, ISSN 0022-3042

Takahashi, H., Hirokawa, K., Ando, S., & Obata, K. (1991). Immunohistological study on brains of Alzheimer's disease using antibodies to fetal antigens, C-series gangliosides and microtubule-associated protein 5. *Acta Neuropathol*, Vol. 81, No. 6, pp. 626-631, ISSN 0001-6322

Tamboli, I.Y., Hampel, H., Tien, N.T., Tolksdorf, K., Breiden, B., Mathews, P.M., Saftig, P., Sandhoff, K., & Walter, J. (2011). Sphingolipid storage affects autophagic metabolism of the amyloid precursor protein and promotes Abeta generation. *J Neurosci*, Vol. 31, No. 5, pp. 1837-1849, ISSN 0270-6474

Tooyama, I., Yamada, T., Kim, S.U., & McGeer, P.L. (1992). Immunohistochemical study of A2B5-positive ganglioside in postmortem human brain tissue of Alzheimer disease, amyotrophic lateral sclerosis, progressive supranuclear palsy and control cases. *Neurosci Lett*, Vol. 136, No. 1, pp. 91-94, ISSN 0304-3940

Trojanowski, J.Q., Goedert, M., Iwatsubo, T., & Lee, V.M. (1998). Fatal attractions: abnormal protein aggregation and neuron death in Parkinson's disease and Lewy body dementia. *Cell Death Differ*, Vol. 5, No. 10, pp. 832-837, ISSN 1350-9047

Ueda, K., Fukushima, H., Masliah, E., Xia, Y., Iwai, A., Yoshimoto, M., Otero, D.A., Kondo, J., Ihara, Y., & Saitoh, T. (1993). Molecular cloning of cDNA encoding an unrecognized component of amyloid in Alzheimer disease. *Proc Natl Acad Sci U S A*, Vol. 90, No. 23, pp. 11282-11286, ISSN 0027-8424

Vetrivel, K.S., & Thinakaran, G. (2010). Membrane rafts in Alzheimer's disease beta-amyloid production. *Biochim Biophys Acta*, Vol. 1801, No. 8, pp. 860-867, ISSN 0006-3002

Vitner, E.B., Platt, F.M., & Futerman, A.H. (2010). Common and uncommon pathogenic cascades in lysosomal storage diseases. *J Biol Chem*, Vol. 285, No. 27, pp. 20423-20427, ISSN 0021-9258

Wei, J., Fujita, M., Nakai, M., Waragai, M., Sekigawa, A., Sugama, S., Takenouchi, T., Masliah, E., & Hashimoto, M. (2009a). Protective role of endogenous gangliosides for lysosomal pathology in a cellular model of synucleinopathies. *The American Journal of Pathology*, Vol. 174, No. 5, pp. 1891-1909, ISSN 0002-9440

Wei, J., Fujita, M., Nakai, M., Waragai, M., Watabe, K., Akatsu, H., Rockenstein, E., Masliah, E., & Hashimoto, M. (2007). Enhanced lysosomal pathology caused by beta-synuclein mutants linked to dementia with Lewy bodies. *J Biol Chem*, Vol. 282, No. 39, pp. 28904-28914, ISSN 0021-9258

Wei, J., Fujita, M., Sekigawa, A., Sekiyama, K., Waragai, M., & Hashimoto, M. (2009b). Gangliosides' protection against lysosomal pathology of synucleinopathies. *Autophagy*, Vol. 5, No. 6, pp. 860-861, ISSN 1554-8627

Yamamoto, A., Haraguchi, M., Yamashiro, S., Fukumoto, S., Furukawa, K., Takamiya, K., Atsuta, M., & Shiku, H. (1996). Heterogeneity in the expression pattern of two ganglioside synthase genes during mouse brain development. *J Neurochem*, Vol. 66, No. 1, pp. 26-34, ISSN 0022-3042

Yamamoto, N., Hirabayashi, Y., Amari, M., Yamaguchi, H., Romanov, G., Van Nostrand, W.E., & Yanagisawa, K. (2005a). Assembly of hereditary amyloid beta-protein variants in the presence of favorable gangliosides. *FEBS Letters*, Vol. 579, No. 10, pp. 2185-2190, ISSN 0014-5793

Yamamoto, N., Matsubara, E., Maeda, S., Minagawa, H., Takashima, A., Maruyama, W., Michikawa, M., & Yanagisawa, K. (2007). A ganglioside-induced toxic soluble Abeta assembly. Its enhanced formation from Abeta bearing the Arctic mutation. *J Biol Chem*, Vol. 282, No. 4, pp. 2646-2655, ISSN 0021-9258

Yamamoto, N., Yokoseki, T., Shibata, M., Yamaguchi, H., & Yanagisawa, K. (2005b). Suppression of Abeta deposition in brain by peripheral administration of Fab fragments of anti-seed antibody. *Biochem Biophys Res Commun*, Vol. 335, No. 1, pp. 45-47, ISSN 0006-291X

Yanagisawa, K., Odaka, A., Suzuki, N., & Ihara, Y. (1995). GM1 ganglioside-bound amyloid beta-protein (A beta): a possible form of preamyloid in Alzheimer's disease. *Nat Med*, Vol. 1, No. 10, pp. 1062-1066, ISSN 1078-8956

Yankner, B.A. (2000). The pathogenesis of Alzheimer's disease. Is amyloid beta-protein the beginning or the end? *Ann N Y Acad Sci*, Vol. 924, pp. 26-28, ISSN 0077-8923

Yasuhara, O., Matsuo, A., Tooyama, I., Kimura, H., McGeer, E.G., & McGeer, P.L. (1995). Pick's disease immunohistochemistry: new alterations and Alzheimer's disease comparisons. *Acta Neuropathol*, Vol. 89, No. 4, pp. 322-330, ISSN 0001-6322

Yu, R.K., Nakatani, Y., & Yanagisawa, M. (2009). The role of glycosphingolipid metabolism in the developing brain. *J Lipid Res*, Vol. 50 Suppl, pp. S440-445, ISSN 0022-2275

Zarranz, J.J., Alegre, J., Gomez-Esteban, J.C., Lezcano, E., Ros, R., Ampuero, I., Vidal, L., Hoenicka, J., Rodriguez, O., Atares, B., *et al.* (2004). The new mutation, E46K, of alpha-synuclein causes Parkinson and Lewy body dementia. *Ann Neurol*, Vol. 55, No. 2, pp. 164-173, ISSN 0364-5134

Zha, Q., Ruan, Y., Hartmann, T., Beyreuther, K., & Zhang, D. (2004). GM1 ganglioside regulates the proteolysis of amyloid precursor protein. *Mol Psychiatry*, Vol. 9, No. 10, pp. 946-952, ISSN 1359-4184

26

Structure Based 3D-QSAR Studies on Cholinesterase Inhibitors

Zaheer ul Haq and Reaz Uddin
Dr. Panjwani Center for Molecular Medicine and Drug Research, International Center for Chemical and Biological Sciences, University of Karachi
Pakistan

1. Introduction

Alzheimer's disease (AD) is a slowly progressive neurodegenerative disorder of the elderly. It is characterized by widespread loss of central cholinergic neuronal function (Butters et al., 1995). The only symptomatic treatment proven to be effective to date is the use of cholinesterase inhibitors (ChEI) to augment surviving cholinergic activity (Giacobini, 2003, Terry & Buccafusco, 2003). Two types of ChE enzyme are found in the Central Nervous System (CNS), acetylcholinesterase (AChE; EC 3.1.1.7) and butyrylcholinesterase (BuChE; EC 3.1.1.8).

AChE and BuChE share 65% amino acid sequence homology despite being encoded by different genes on human chromosomes 7(7q22) and 3(3q26), respectively (Soreq & Zaku, 1993). Acetylcholinesterase is responsible for the hydrolysis of acetylcholine at the synaptic cleft and the neuromuscular junction in response to nerve action potential (Massoulie et al., 1993) while the BuChE preferentially acts on butyrylcholine, but also hydrolyzes acetylcholine (Cokugras, 2003). In addition, both AChE and BuChE seem to be involved in roles that are independent of their catalytic activities, such as cell differentiation and development (Behra et al., 2002, Meshorer et al., 2002). BuChE and AChE are able to catalyze the hydrolysis of acetylcholine (ACh) at a rate of >10,000 molecules per second (Bazelyansky et al., 1986).

Because BuChE is relatively abundant in plasma (about 3 mg/liter), and can degrade a large number of ester-containing compounds, it plays important pharmacological and toxicological roles (Lockridge & Masson, 2000). For instance, BuChE is a potential detoxifying enzyme to be used as a prophylactic scavenger against neurotoxic organophosphates such as the nerve gas soman (Lockridge & Masson, 2000, Massoulie et al., 1993, Xie et al., 2000).

Previously, the relative contribution of BuChE to the regulation of ACh levels was largely ignored presumably due to unclear physiological function of BuChE (Chatonnet & Lockridge, 1989, Mack & Robitzki, 2000, Massoulie, Pezzementi, 1993, Xie, Stribley, 2000). However, there is growing evidence that both enzymes regulate ACh levels and may also play a part in the development and progression of AD (Greig et al., 2001).

In the normal brain, AChE represents approximately 80% of ChE activity with BuChE comprising the remainder (Giacobini, 1964). In advanced AD, however, AChE activity may be reduced to 55-67% of normal levels in specific brain regions, while BuChE activity increases (Giacobini, 1964, Greig, Utsuki, 2001, Mack & Robitzki, 2000). Cytochemical studies have revealed that in certain neuronal pathways of some species, BuChE replaces AChE (Graybiel & Ragsdale, 1982). The BuChE may also have a role in the aggregation of β-amyloid protein (Aβ) that occurs in the early stages of senile plaque formation in AD (Guillozet et al., 1997). Selective inhibition of BuChE versus AChE derives from an ability to utilize the additional space present in the gorge of BuChE.

From the resolved 3D structures of various cholinesterases, it is known that the active sites residues of these enzymes lay at the bottom of a 20 Å deep hydrophobic gorge (Bourne et al., 1995, Doorn et al., 2001, Harel et al., 1992, Nachon et al., 2005, Nachon et al., 2005, Nicolet et al., 2003, Sussman et al., 1991, Tormos et al., 2005). Due to a large cavity of this gorge BuChEs accept in comparison to AChEs, broader variety of substrates and inhibitors (Radic et al., 1993, Saxena et al., 1999, Saxena et al., 1997). For instance they metabolize butyrylcholine, the choline ester with large acyl moiety whose hydrolysis by vertebrate AChEs is negligible.

Although a similar peripheral site has been described for human BuChE but site-directed mutagenesis and photo-affinity labeling studies showed that its location and the response upon ligand binding differ significantly from those of AChE (Graybiel & Ragsdale, 1982, Perry et al., 1978).

Structure-activity analysis is the foundation for understanding the structural features of both the inhibitors and the target receptors involved in particular biological process and thus helps to design more effective inhibitors (Cho et al., 1996). It appears relatively difficult to find a reliable predictive model based on the calculated energies obtained by docking (Donini & Kollman, 2000, Tame, 1999). To overcome this problem, highly predictive QSAR i.e., CoMFA (Cramer Iii et al., 1988) and CoMSIA (Klebe et al., 1994) modeling techniques have been developed by using the technique of structure-based alignments of the substrates. These models can be used to identify important protein-ligand interactions and are found to be consistent with the crystal structure of the protein-ligand complex (Prathipati et al., 2005). The availability of X-ray crystal coordinates of inhibitors bound with the receptor have contributed to formulate effective predictive 3D-QSAR models based on (1) identification of possible conformations of related inhibitors in the active site and (2) understanding of the interactions of the inhibitors with the receptor in three-dimension (Debnath, 1999). A 3D-QSAR experiment performs two functions: the derivation of a statistically significant and highly predictive model that is used to estimate and rank new compounds for planned synthesis and the provision of an easily interpretable graphical tool which can identify a particular physicochemical property for increased affinity and selectivity (Klebe, 1998). These physicochemical properties include steric bulk, partial charge, local hydrophobicity, or hydrogen bond donor and acceptor (Bohm et al., 1999).

The level-dependent contouring of usual CoMFA-field contributions highlights those regions in space where the aligned molecules would favourably or unfavourably interact with a possible environment. The CoMSIA field contributions identify those areas within the region occupied by the ligand that "favour" or "dislike" the presence of a group with a particular physicochemical property. This association of required properties with a possible ligand shape is a more direct indicator to check whether all features important for a particular activity are present in the structures under consideration (Klebe, Abraham, 1994).

The discovery of natural cholinesterase inhibitors has been a very challenging area of drug development due to the involvement of cholinesterases in Alzheimer's disease and other related dementias. We have previously reported a number of new natural inhibitors of cholinesterases (AChE and BuChE) isolated from indigenous medicinal plants (Atta ur et al., 2000, Atta ur et al., 2004, Atta ur et al., 2004, Atta ur et al., 2002, Kalauni et al., 2001). The steady state inhibition kinetics, pharmacological profiles, SAR and molecular docking studies have been conducted on a similar series of compounds for AChE inhibition (Khalid et al., 2004, Khalid et al., 2004, Zaheer-Ul-Haq et al., 2003, Zaheer ul et al., 2003).

In the present study, two 3D-QSAR methods, CoMFA and CoMSIA, were applied and evaluated in order to accurately predict the inhibitory activity. For this reason a set of structurally similar cholinesterase inhibitors (both BuChE and AChE) were used to create a predictive model. The results from this study will be helpful for the design of new and more potent cholinesterase inhibitors.

Docking is one method in which the binding of an inhibitor to a receptor can be explored (Dominguez et al., 2003, Jain, 2003, Johnson et al., 2003, Sabnis et al., 2003, Todorov et al., 2003, Vicker et al., 2003, Wang et al., 2003, Wu et al., 2003, Zhou et al., 2003). In CoMFA or other 3D-QSAR studies, the molecule alignment and conformation determination are so important that they affect the success of a model. In the present case, a bound complex of steroidal alkaloid with cholinesterase was not available, and therefore, a computational method has to be implemented to determine possible conformations and alignment of a set of molecules so that 3D-QSAR can be carried out. Several strategies have been used in the past, to determine the conformation and alignment of molecules. Of them, docking is an attractive way to align molecules for CoMFA and/or CoMSIA. Several applications of docking alignment with CoMFA have been reported (Buolamwini & Assefa, 2002, Hu & Stebbins, 2005, Medina-Franco et al., 2004, Pan et al., 2006, Wei et al., 2005).

Recently, we used FlexX and FRED (FRED, 2007) to successfully dock a set of steroidal alkaloid inhibitors into the active site gorge of cholinesterase. A 3D-QSAR model was developed based on the docked conformation of the most active compound. In this paper we have performed CoMFA modeling utilizing the genetic algorithm (GA) in the selection of the ligand conformations. Previously this GA strategy has been utilized by Yuan and Zaheer ul Haq et al (Yuan et al., 2004, Yuan & Petukhov, 2006, Zaheer ul et al., 2008) and found that this is very efficient in terms of the reliability of the CoMFA models. GA is inspired by natural selection in evolution (Holland, 1975). GA approaches the optimum of a given function in the same way nature selects the individual fittest for the environment. The GA uses a blind search strategy, requiring no knowledge of the properties of the function to be optimized, thus enabling the algorithm to be applied to a variety of optimization problems from robot behavior to drug design (Fogel et al., 1966, Forrest, 1993, Goldberg, 1989).

2. Materials and methods

2.1 Biological data

The cholinesterase inhibitory activities, represented by IC_{50} (μM), were obtained from recently published data (Atta ur, Choudhary, 2000, Atta ur, Feroz, 2004, Atta ur et al., 2003, Atta ur et al., 1997, Atta ur, Zaheer ul, 2004, Atta ur, Zaheer ul, 2002, Kalauni, Choudhary, 2001, Khalid, Zaheer ul, 2004) (Table 1). The structures of inhibitors are presented in Table 2. The pIC_{50} (-$logIC_{50}$) values were used to derive 3D-QSAR models. From a total of forty compounds, a training set was created with thirty five compounds (with the case of BuChE) and thirty three compounds (with the case of AChE) while other 5 compounds were used as the test set (Table 1). This test set was used to validate the predictive ability of the training set.

S. No.	Comp. No.	Compound Name	IC_{50} (μM) BuChE	IC_{50} (μM) AChE	pIC_{50} BuChE	pIC_{50} AChE
1	SAR01	Isosarcodine	1.89±0.06	10.31±0.13	5.72	2.99
2	SAR02	Iso-*N*-formylchoneformine	4.07±0.11	6.36±0.22	5.39	3.20
3	SAR03	Saracodinine	12.51±0.06	40.04±0.13	4.9	2.40
4	SAR04	Sarcorine	10.33±0.02	69.99±0.056	4.99	2.15
5	SAR05	N_a-Demethylsaracodine	16.55±0.20	204.2±4.951	4.78	1.69
6	SAR06	Saracocine	3.86±0.01	20±1.30	5.41	2.70
7	SAR07	Sarcodine	18.31±0.74	49.77±1.26	4.74	2.30
8	SAR08	Salignenamide-A	4.63±0.07	50.64±0.930	5.33	2.30
9	SAR09	Vaganine-A	2.32±0.06	8.59±0.155	5.63	3.07
10	SAR10	Saligcinnamide	4.84±0.12	19.99±0.123	5.32	2.70
11	SAR11	Salignenamide-C	38.36±0.74	61.3±2.02	4.42	2.21
12	SAR12	5,6-Dehydrosarconidine	1.89±0.06	20.29±1.82	5.72	2.69
13	SAR13	Salignamine	25.7±0.63	249±10.23	4.59	1.60
14	SAR14	Salignenamide-D	23.78±0.15	185.2±7.66	4.62	1.73
15	SAR15	Salignenamide-E	3.65±0.02	6.21±0.234	5.44	3.21
16	SAR16	Salignenamide-F	4.07±0.11	6.357±0.224	5.39	3.20
17	SAR17	2*β*-Hydroxyepipachysamine-D	28.96±0.01	78.2±2.325	4.54	2.11
18	SAR18[a]	Salonine-B	4.50±0.07	-------	5.35	-------
19	SAR19	Salonine-A	32.70±1.20	33.4±3.21	4.49	2.48
20	SAR20	Salonine-C	32.20±0.50	7.8±0.5	4.49	3.11
21	SAR21	Salignarine-F	1.90±0.20	30.2±2.0	5.72	2.52
22	SAR22	16-Dehydrosarcorine	3.95±0.53	12.5±0.01	5.4	2.90
23	SAR23	Axillarine-C	17.99±0.22	227.92±8.677	4.74	1.64
24	SAR24	Axillarine-F	18.24±0.01	182.4±5.542	4.74	1.74
25	SAR25	Dictyophlebine	3.65±0.02	6.21±0.23	5.44	3.21
26	SAR26	Sarsalignenone	4.29±0.03	5.83±0.070	5.37	3.23
27	SAR27	Nepapakistamine	25.00±0.79	50.1±1.35	4.6	2.30
28	SAR28	Sarcoveganin-C	1.50±0.02	187.8±0.71	5.82	1.73
29	SAR29	Salignarine-C	1.25±0.01	19.7±0.05	5.9	2.71
30	SAR30	Sarsalignone	2.18±0.04	7.02±0.007	5.66	3.15
31	SAR31	*N*-Methylformamidesalonine-B	10.50±0.30	48.6±2.7	4.98	2.31
32	SAR32[a]	5,14-dehydro-N_a-demethylsaracodine	25.00±0.60	-------	4.6	-------
33	SAR33	Axilliridine-A	2.49±0.06	5.21±0.105	5.6	3.28
34	SAR34	14-Dehydro- N_a-demtehylsaracodine	10.10±0.15	183.1±2.60	5	1.74
35	SAR35[t]	Vaganine-D	10.00±0.120	46.89±1.94	5	2.33
36	SAR36[t]	2-Hydroxysalignarin E	6.91±0.06	15.99±0.13	5.16	2.80
37	SAR37[t]	Epipachysamine-D	2.82±0.02	28.93±0.54	5.55	2.54
38	SAR38[t]	2-Hydroxysalignamine	20.95±3.20	82.5±2.22	4.68	2.08
39	SAR39[t]	2,3-Dehydrosarsalignone	32.20±0.50	7.0±0.1	4.49	3.15
40	SAR40	Alkaloid C	22.13±0.14	42.2±0.26	2.65	2.37

[t] = test set

[a] = not included in AChE modelling

Table 1. Inhibitory Activities of the Compounds

2.2 Modeling tools

All molecular modeling and comparative molecular field evaluations were performed using SYBYL 7.2 (Sybyl, 2007), running on AMD Athlon (tm) workstation. The aliphatic amine groups of all compounds were considered protonated. Geometry optimizations were performed using the Tripos forcefield (Clark et al., 1989) with a distance-dependent dielectric and the Powell conjugate gradient algorithm. Gasteiger Huckel charges were used. All water molecules, sulfate and chloride anions, glycerol, fucose, *N*-acetyl-*D*-glucosamine and 2-(*N*-morpholino)-ethanesulfonic acids were removed from the original protein data bank file.

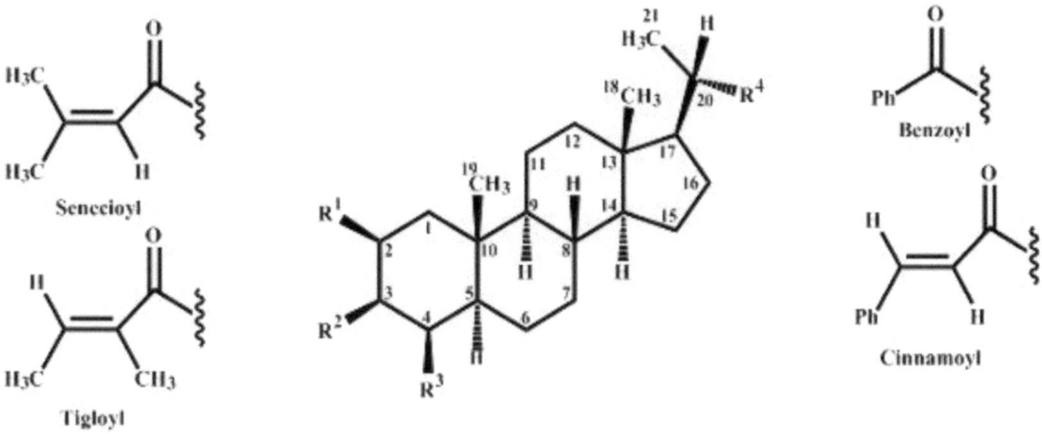

Comp. No.	R¹	R²	R³	R⁴	Unsaturation
SAR01	H	NCH_3Ac	H	$N(CH_3)_2$	
SAR02	H	$N(CH_3)_2$	H	NHCHO	
SAR03	H	$N(CH_3)_2$	H	$N(CH_3)_2$	$\Delta^{5,6}$
SAR04	H	NHAc	H	$N(CH_3)_2$	
SAR05	H	$NHCH_3$	H	NCH_3Ac	
SAR06	H	$N(CH_3)_2$	H	NCH_3Ac	$\Delta^{5,6}$
SAR07	H	$N(CH_3)_2$	H	NCH_3Ac	
SAR08	H	$NHCOCH{=}CCH_3CH(CH_3)_2$	H	$N(CH_3)_2$	
SAR09	H	HN-Senecioyl	OAc	$N(CH_3)_2$	
SAR10	H	CH_3N-Cinnamoyl	H	$N(CH_3)_2$	
SAR11	OH	HN-Tigloyl	OAc	$N(CH_3)_2$	$\Delta^{14,15}$
SAR12	H	$NHCH_3$	H	$N(CH_3)_2$	$\Delta^{16,17}$
SAR13	H	OCH_3	H	$NHCH_3$	$\Delta^{5,6}$ & $\Delta^{16,17}$
SAR14	*a*-OH	HN-Tigloyl	H	$N(CH_3)_2$	$\Delta^{4,5}$ & $\Delta^{16,17}$
SAR15	H	$N(CH_3)COCH{=}C(CH_3)CH(CH_3)_2$	H	$N(CH_3)_2$	$\Delta^{16,17}$
SAR16	H	$N(CH_3)COCH{=}C(CH_3)CH(CH_3)_2$	H	$N(CH_3)_2$	
SAR17	OH	HN-Benzoyl	H	$N(CH_3)_2$	
SAR18	H	OCH_3	H	$N(CH_3)_2$	$\Delta^{5,6}$ & $\Delta^{16,17}$
SAR19	OH	HN-Tigloyl	OH	$N(CH_3)_2$	$\Delta^{14,15}$
SAR20	H	HN-Tigloyl	H	$N(CH_3)_2$	$\Delta^{4,5}$ & $\Delta^{14,15}$

SAR21	H	HN-Tigloyl	OH	$N(CH_3)_2$	$\Delta^{5,6}$
SAR22	H	$NHCOCH_3$	H	$N(CH_3)_2$	$\Delta^{16,17}$
SAR23	OH	HN-Benzoyl	OAc	$N(CH_3)_2$	
SAR24	OH	HN-Tigloyl	OAc	$N(CH_3)_2$	
SAR25	H	$NHCH_3$	H	$N(CH_3)_2$	
SAR27	OAc	HN-Tigloyl	OAc	$NHCH_3$	$\Delta^{16,17}$
SAR29	OH	HN-Senecioyl	H	$N(CH_3)_2$	$\Delta^{5,6}$
SAR31	H	OCH_3	H	$NCH_3(CHO)$	$\Delta^{5,6}$ & $\Delta^{16,17}$
SAR32	H	$NHCH_3$	H	NCH_3Ac	$\Delta^{5,6}$ & $\Delta^{14,15}$
SAR34	H	$NHCH_3$	H	NCH_3Ac	$\Delta^{14,15}$
SAR35	H	HN-Senecioyl	OAc	$N(CH_3)_2$	$\Delta^{16,17}$
SAR36	OH	HN-Tigloyl	H	$N(CH_3)_2$	$\Delta^{4,5}$
SAR37	H	HN-Benzoyl	H	$N(CH_3)_2$	
SAR38	OH	OCH_3	H	$N(CH_3)_2$	$\Delta^{5,6}$ & $\Delta^{16,17}$
SAR40					

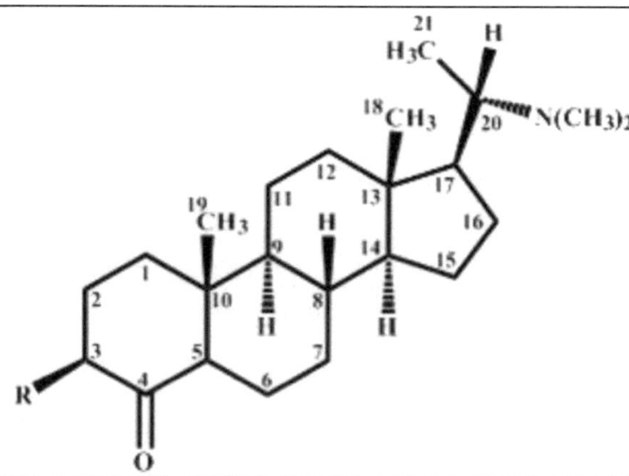

Comp. No.	R	Unsaturation
SAR26	HN-Tigloyl	$\Delta^{5,6}$ & $\Delta^{14,15}$
SAR28	HN-Tigloyl	$\Delta^{2,3}$ & $\Delta^{16,17}$
SAR30	HN-Tigloyl	$\Delta^{5,6}$
SAR33	HN-Benzoyl	$\Delta^{2,3}$
SAR39	HN-Tigloyl	$\Delta^{2,3}$ & $\Delta^{5,6}$

Table 2. Chemical Structures of the Compounds

2.3 Docking

FlexX, incremental construction algorithm (Rarey et al., 1996), was used to choose the appropriate binding conformations of the steroidal alkaloids inhibitors into the BuChE binding pocket. The crystal structure of human BuChE (pdb code: 1P0I) was used. One of the most active compound, SAR29 (see Table 2), was docked into the binding pocket and the best conformation was used as a template to align rest of the compounds. The FlexX scoring function was used to select the best conformation. Prior to dock the inhibitors with protein crystal structure, a re-docking of co-crystallized ligand with 1P0I was performed to validate the docking protocol. The top most docked solution was found in good agreement with the crystal structure of the co-crystallized ligand. The RMSD between the docking solution and the crystal structure was 1.53 Å.

Molecular docking with AChE was carried out using FRED docking program. FRED (Fast Rigid Exhaustive Docking) is a protein-ligand docking program, which takes a multiconformer library/database and receptor file as input and output molecules of the input database most likely to bind to the receptor (FRED, 2007, McGann et al., 2003).

First stage in FRED docking is a shape fitting process, which takes a set of ligand conformers as input and tests them against a "bump map" (a Boolean grid with true values where ligand atoms can potentially be placed). Orientations that clash with the protein or are distant from the active site are rejected. The crude docking solutions are further tested against a pharmacophore feature if specified and any poses that do not fit in the pharmacophore criteria are rejected. Poses surviving the shape fitting routine can then be passed through up to three scoring function filters in the screening process. Available scoring functions in FRED are ChemScore, PLP, ScreenScore, and Gaussian shape fitting (McGann, Almond, 2003).

2.4 Conformational sampling and alignment

The selected poses for SAR29 (one of the most active compound against BuChE) and SAR33 (one of the most active compound against AChE) were used as templates in structure alignment for all molecules in the respective series. For BuChE, this step was performed by using an incremental construction algorithm and a scoring function based on intermolecular interactions and overlapping density functions implemented in the Flexible Superposition (FlexS) technique (Lemmen et al., 1998). The minimum volume overlap was set at 0.6 and the number of alignments per ligand was used initially as 30 (default) but was changed for the cases where optimum alignment was not obtained. The Gasteiger Huckel charges were calculated during conformational alignment with FlexS. A top-ranked conformer for each compound was initially utilized for CoMFA modeling and then the ten best conformations were used in order to explore all possible conformational space for each compound. The ten best poses were selected based on the following:

1. FlexS ranks and
2. If the pose is correctly oriented on the template.

The Figure 1a represents the alignment of the molecules using SAR29 as a template for BuChE modeling.

In the case of AChE, the superimposition was performed using the ROCS from openeyes (OE ROCS, 2008). The ROCS is a Rapid Overlay on Crystal Structures (ROCS). ROCS method has a number of applications in virtual screening, lead hopping and in 3D-QSAR. ROCS can be utilized as an alignment method in order to produce the conformations which subsequently can be utilized in conformations sensitive 3D-QSAR i.e. CoMFA. The ROCS was used with its default settings except the maximum numbers of conformations and numbers of best hits to be saved were 30 and 1000, respectively. ROCS overlays the multiconformer compound's database in shape and chemistry with respect to the reference ligand. The overlays can be performed very quickly based on a description of the molecules as atom-centered Gaussian functions. ROCS maximizes the shared volume between a query molecule and a single conformation of a database molecule. Figure 1b represents the alignment of the molecules using SAR33 as a template for AChE modeling.

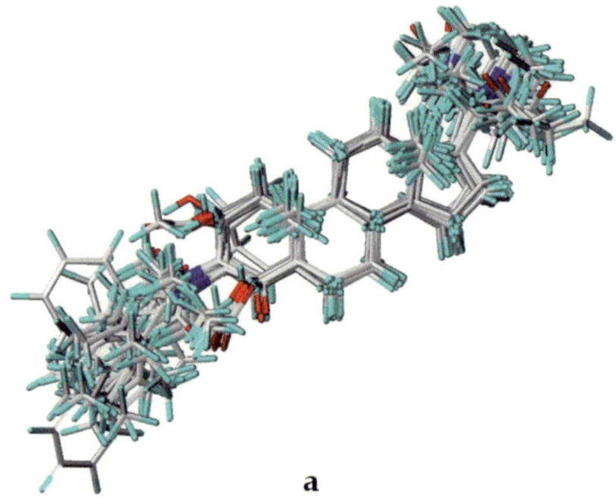

a

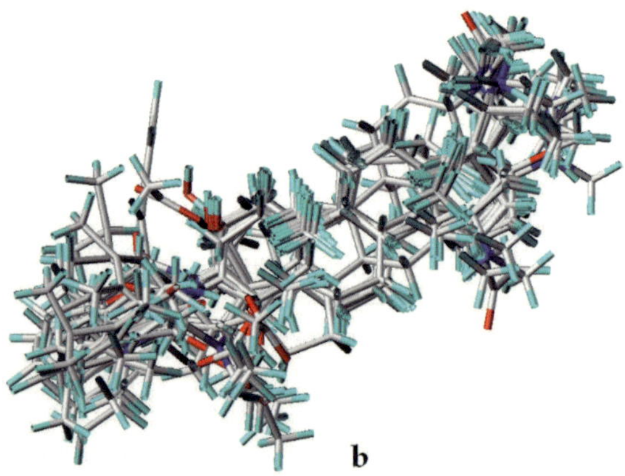

b

Fig. 1. Superposition of all studied inhibitors: **a**) BuChE using SAR29 as template **b**) AChE using SAR 33 as template

2.5 CoMFA modeling based on genetic algorithm

The overall strategy for CoMFA GA modeling is shown as a scheme in Figure 2. A brief description of the procedure is outlined here. To explore the multiple conformations of the ligands, a genetic algorithm analysis was applied in the selection of ligand's conformations for CoMFA. The genetic algorithm consisted of the following steps:

Initialization: This step generates an initial population P_i of CoMFA models using one randomly selected conformation among pre-filtered conformations of each ligand. The population size was set to 100.

Iterations:

Crossover: Exchange the conformations of corresponding ligands for any two models in the population P_i. The crossover ratio was set to 50:50.

Mutation: For randomly selected ligands, replace the conformations obtained in step 1 with randomly selected conformations in the database. Store the results as a temporary population P_{tmp}. The mutation rate was set to 0.05.

Selection: Generate new CoMFA models for P_{tmp}. Compare their q^2 values with those generated for population P_i and keep the best models in population P_{i+1}.

Until: The 100 generations limit is reached or the best model remains unchanged for 10 consecutive generations.

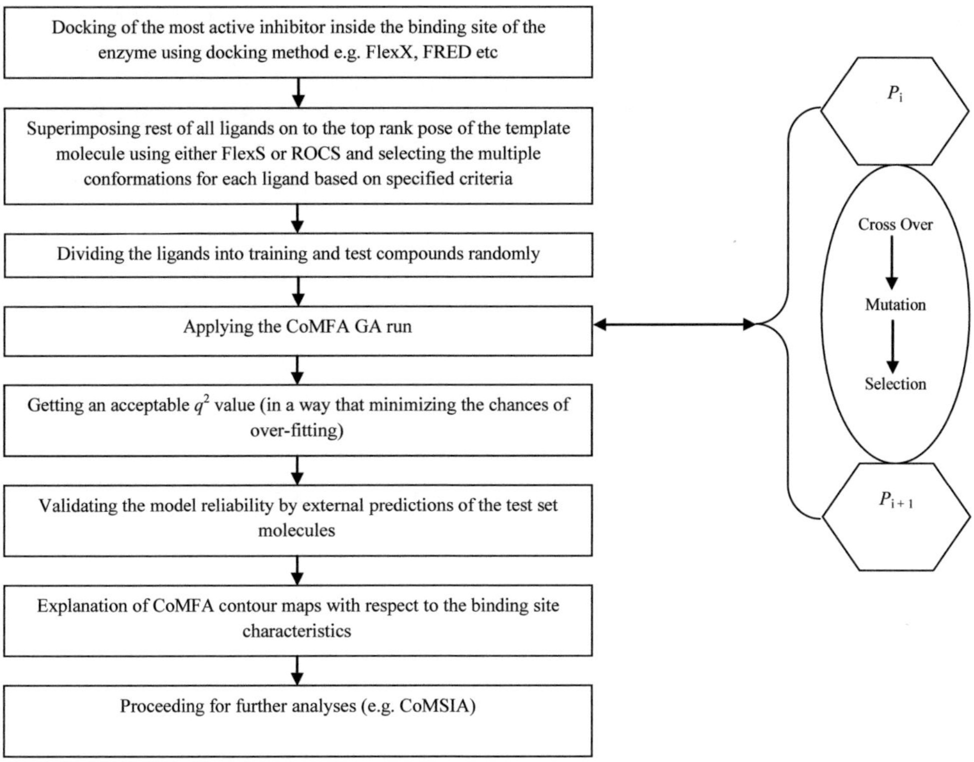

Fig. 2. Scheme for overall procedure applied during GA based 3D-QSAR modeling

2.6 CoMFA fields

Training sets of, thirty five compounds (with the case of BuChE) and thirty three compounds (with the case of AChE; see Table 1), were selected from the existing database, representing the diversity of structures and activities. After alignment, the molecules were inserted as rows of a QSAR table along with their respective IC_{50} values (as pIC_{50}). CoMFA steric and electrostatic fields were calculated as described below and entered as columns in the QSAR table. Standard steric and electrostatic CoMFA field energies of each inhibitor were calculated using an sp^3 probe atom with a +1 charge at all intersections in regularly spaced (2.0 Å) grids surrounding each molecule. Lennard Jones 6-12 potential and coulumbic potential functions, within the Tripos forcefield (Clark, Cramer, 1989) and a distance dependent (1/r) dielectric constant were used in the calculation. The grid box dimensions were determined by the "create automatically" features in the CoMFA module within the "SYBYL" program. The same grid box was used in all calculations. An energy cutoff of 30 kcal/mol for both steric and electrostatic contributions was set as threshold and the electrostatic terms were dropped within regions of steric maximum i.e., 30 kcal/mol. Five additional inhibitors (Table 1) were selected as a predictive set to test the robustness of the resulting model. They were aligned with template structures using the same alignment protocol as described earlier and finally their activities were predicted.

2.7 CoMSIA fields

Another 3D-QSAR procedure, CoMSIA can avoid some inherent deficiencies arising from the functional forms of Lennard-Jones and Coulumb potentials used in CoMFA. In CoMSIA, a distance dependent Guassian-type functional form has been introduced. This can avoid singularities at the atomic positions and the dramatic changes of potential energy due to grids in the proximity of the surface. Meanwhile, no arbitrary definition of cut-off limits is required in CoMSIA and the contour maps of the relative spatial contributions of the different fields can be substantially improved. This is essential for the interpretation in terms of separate property fields. The procedures of getting a 3D-QSAR model from a CoMSIA can be summarized into following three steps.

First, all molecules are structure-based or field-based aligned.

Then, an evenly-spaced rectangular grid is generated to enclose the molecular aggregate. A probe atom is placed at every lattice point to measure the electrostatic, steric, hydrophobic, and H-bond donor or acceptor fields.

Finally, the results from the field samplings are combined with the biological activities from the tested compounds are put into a table and partial least squares (PLS) fitting is applied to obtain the final CoMSIA model.

To choose the appropriate components and to check the statistical significance of the models, leave-one-out cross-validations were used by PLS. Then, the final 3D-QSAR model was derived from no cross-validation calculations. The CoMSIA results are finally interpreted graphically by field contribution maps using the field type "stdev*coeff".

Similar to the usual CoMFA approach, a data table has been constructed from similarity indices (Klebe, 1998) calculated via a common probe atom that is placed at the intersections of a regularly spaced lattice. A grid spacing of 2 Å has been used throughout this study. Similarity indices $A_{F,K}$ between the compounds of interest and a probe atom, systematically placed at the intersections of the lattice, have been calculated according to equation 1 (e.g., at grid point q for molecule j of the data set).

$$A_{FK}^{q}(j) = -\sum_{i} \omega_{probe,k}\omega_{ik}(e_{iq}^{-\alpha r})^2 \quad (1)$$

Where i = summation index over all atoms of the molecule j under investigation; ω_{ik} = actual value of the physicochemical property k of atom i; $\omega_{probe,k}$ = probe atom with charge +1, a = attenuation factor; and r_{iq} = mutual distance between probe atom at grid point q and atom i of the test molecule. Large values of a will result in a strong attenuation of the distance-dependent consideration of molecular similarity. Accordingly, there is little averaging of local feature matches of the molecules being compared. With small values of a, also remote parts of each molecule will be experienced by the probe and the global molecular features become more important. In the present study the a has been set at 0.3. With this selection, at a given lattice point the property value of an atom of the molecule under investigation (e.g., the partial atomic charge) is experienced in 1 Å distance by 74.1%, in 2 Å by 30.1% and in 3 Å by 6.7% of its total value. This permits a reasonable "local smearing" of the molecular similarity indices and should help to avoid extreme dependencies on small changes of the mutual alignments (Bohm, St rzebecher, 1999). In the present study five physicochemical properties k (steric, electrostatic, hydrophobic and hydrogen bond donor and acceptor) were evaluated, using a common probe atom with 1 Å radius and charge, hydrophobicity and hydrogen-bond property of +1. Steric property fields were expressed by the third power of the atomic radii. Local hydrophobicities were associated using atom-based parameters developed by Viswanadhan et al (Viswanadhan et al., 1989).

2.8 Statistical analysis/PLS

Correlations were derived using the method of Partial Least Squares (PLS) (Geladi & Kowalski, 1986) and cross validated to reduce the probability of obtaining chance correlations. As used in this report, the cross-validated q^2 refers to the squared correlation coefficient of the equation derived from the cross-validation of the training set to determine the optimum number of principal components. The conventional r^2 is the fitted correlation of the training set using the optimum number of principal components with no cross validation. The predictive *r*-squared was calculated by the equation 2.

$$predictive\ r - squared = \frac{SSD - PRESS}{SSD} \qquad (2)$$

Where SSD is sum of squared deviations and PRESS is predictive residual sum of squares.

3. Results and discussion

3.1 Docking

The best docking poses for SAR29 and SAR33 inside the binding pockets of BuChE and AChE are shown in Figure 3a and 3b, respectively. The poses indicated that the ligands were

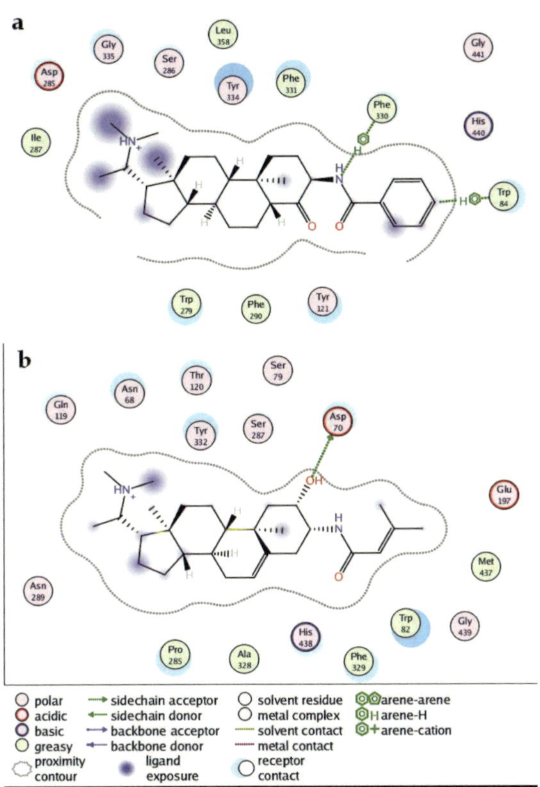

Fig. 3. Docked poses of most active compound **a**) SAR29 for BuChE and **b**) SAR33 for AChE within the surrounding binding site residues. The figures are rendered by MOE Ligand interaction

accommodated well inside the binding sites. The compound enters the cavity preferably by ring A. This might contribute highly to the stabilization of the complex since the steroid backbone of the ligand is highly hydrophobic due to its aliphatic character and therefore, not well hydrated. The main hydrophobic interactions between the hydrocarbon skeleton of the inhibitors and the cholinesterases binding sites were observed with the most common residues i.e. Thr, Tyr, Trp, Ala, and Phe.

3.2 3D-QSAR of inhibitors

3.2.1 Model selection

The CoMFA based on GA, resulted in several models and among them, the final model selection is an important issue. With the case of BuChE, four different models have been selected based on q^2 values. Among them, models 72 and 80 were obtained with the cutoff $q^2 \geq 0.65$; and the other two models 9 and 21, with the cutoff $q^2 \geq 0.90$ (Table 3).

Parameters	Model9	Model21	Model72	Model80
q^2 [a]	0.902	0.911	0.730	0.701
r^2 [b]	0.998	0.998	0.994	0.979
SEE [c]	0.022	0.020	0.040	0.072
F-value [d]	2326.92	2957.134	738.562	264.356
No. of Components [e]	6	6	6	5
Fraction [f]				
Steric	0.499	0.484	0.500	0.531
Electrostatic	0.501	0.516	0.500	0.469
Predictive r-Squared [g]	0.441	0.523	0.311	0.682
PRESS [h]	0.384	0.328	0.475	0.218

[a] Cross-validated correlation coefficient.
[b] Noncross-validated correlation coefficient.
[c] Standard error of estimate.
[d] F-test value.
[e] Optimum number of components obtained from cross-validated PLS analysis and same used in final non-cross-validated analysis.
[f] Field contributions.
[g] Correlation coefficient for test set predictions.
[h] Predicted residual sum of squares.

Table 3. Summary of Statistics and Field Contributions for the Top Four CoMFA Models with the case of BuChE

The external predictivity of the CoMFA model is extremely important in terms of the applicability of the CoMFA model. Therefore, it was decided to use the predictive-r^2 as a criterion for final selection of the one best model. As reflected by the Table 3, model 80 has the highest predictive-r^2 value and hence the lowest PRESS value for the test set predictions. Therefore, model 80 was selected as the best CoMFA model. In addition, to study the effect of charges on 3D-QSAR studies, different methods were employed to calculate the charges on ligands included in this study. Quantitative comparisons of the charges calculated by different methods are reported in Table 4. Different charges resulting from different

calculation methods may influence the results of CoMFA as well as CoMSIA, but there is no significant effects of charges observed during our study for this particular steroidal class of compounds.
With the case of AChE, another way of model selection was done. In each case of GA run the predictive- r^2 was also calculated and compared it with each generation's top model. The default settings of 100 individuals and 100 generations were used but the GA resulted in early termination with 28th generation due to achieving the cutoff value of fitness function (i.e. $q^2 = 0.80$). The graphical representation is presented in Figure 4. The generation number six (highlighted in circle in Figure 4) was the first in identifying the acceptable q^2 as well as the predictive r^2. Hence, the model number six was utilized for further analysis with the case of AChE.

S.No.	Charges Method	CoMFA			CoMSIA		
		q^2	r^2	Components	q^2	r^2	Components
1	Gasteiger Marsilli	0.696	0.989	6	0.636	0.980	5
2	Gasteiger Huckel	0.701	0.979	5	0.627	0.982	5
3	Huckel	0.673	0.988	5	0.637	0.981	5
4	MMFF94	0.716	0.993	6	0.669	0.986	4
5	Pullman	0.697	0.989	6	0.630	0.981	5
6	Delre	0.680	0.987	5	0.634	0.980	6

Table 4. Influence of Different Charges on BuChE Predictive Model

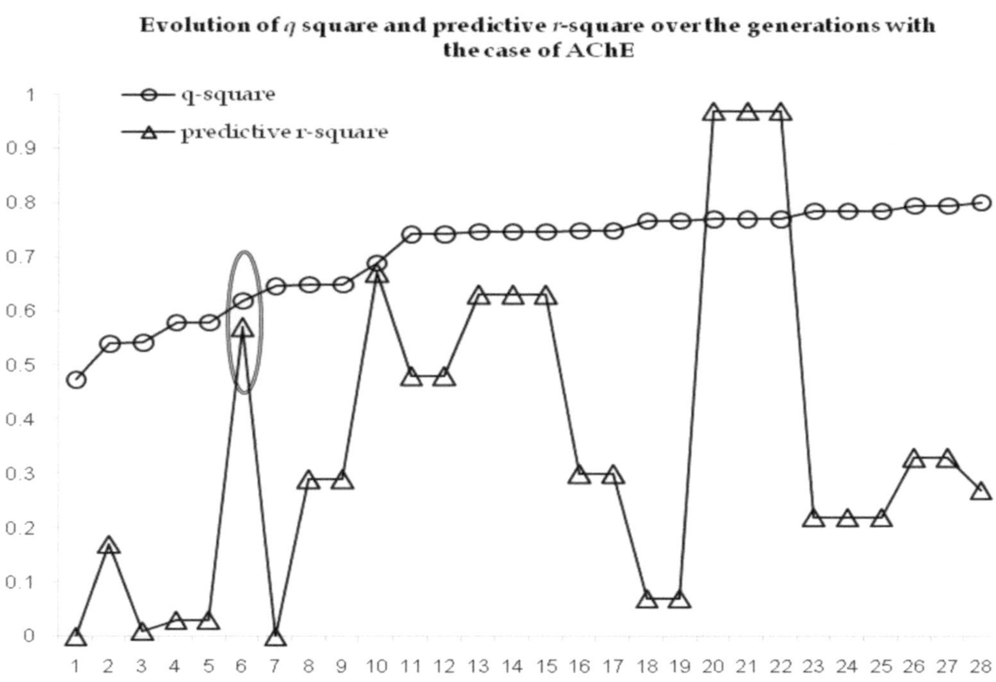

Fig. 4. Comparison between q^2 and predictive $-r^2$ over the generations with AChE modeling

3.2.2 Predictive power of the 3D-QSAR model

The final results of CoMFA and CoMSIA analysis in both cases (i.e. BuChE and AChE) with 2.0 Å grid spacing are shown in Table 5 and Table 6, respectively. PLS analysis yielded consistent results. The optimal components that produce the best cross-validation linear regression coefficient were used to produce the non-cross-validated model. The inhibitory activities (pIC_{50}) and the calculated activities using CoMFA and CoMSIA models for training set and test set are listed in Table 7. Graphic representation of observed vs calculated inhibitory activity is shown in the Figure 5. Best selected 3D-QSAR models showed good prediction for five tested compounds, which reflects that the derived models were satisfactory enough in respect to statistical significance and actual predictive ability.

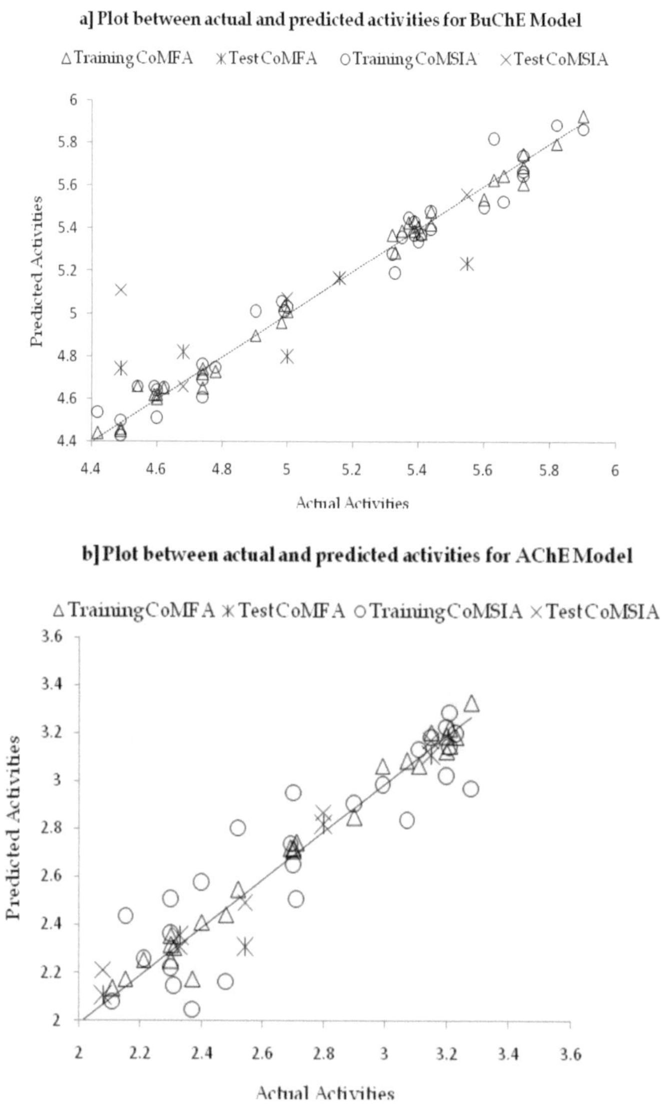

Fig. 5. Plots of the predicted versus experimental activity data of 3D-QSAR from both CoMFA and CoMSIA for training and test compounds **a**) BuChE and **b**) AChE

Parameters	CoMFA	CoMSIA				
	S, E (h)	S, E, H, D, A (h)	S, E (h)	S, E, H (h)	S, E, H, A (h)	S, E, H, D (h)
q^2 [a]	0.701	0.627	0.382	0.444	0.386	0.615
SEP [b]	0.273	0.305	0.393	0.373	0.392	0.310
No. of Components [c]	5	5	5	5	5	5
r^2 [d]	0.979	0.982	0.880	0.927	0.924	0.967
SEE [e]	0.072	0.085	0.174	0.135	0.138	0.090
Field Contributions	0.531, 0.469	0.064, 0.173, 0.135, 0.373, 0.255	0.330, 0.670	0.211, 0.393, 0.396	0.122, 0.237, 0.251, 0.390	0.102, 0.246, 0.197, 0.456
F-value [f]	264.356	185.867	40.877	70.649	68.035	166.192
Predictive *r*-squared [g]	0.682	0.453	0.228	0.529	0.048	0.774

[a] Cross-validated correlation coefficient.
[b] Standard error of predictions.
[c] Optimum number of components obtained from cross-validated PLS analysis and same used in final non-cross-validated analysis.
[d] Noncross-validated correlation coefficient.
[e] Standard error of estimate.
[f] *F*-test value.
[g] Correlation coefficient for test set predictions.
[h] CoMFA and CoMSIA with different field contributions such as steric (S), electrostatic (E), hydrophobic (H), donor (D), and acceptor (A) fields.

Table 5. Results of CoMFA and CoMSIA Analyses for Compounds Used in Training Set (BuChE modeling)

Parameters	CoMFA	CoMSIA				
	S, E [(h)]	S, E, H, D, A [(h)]	S, E [(h)]	S, E, H [(h)]	S, E, H, A [(h)]	S, E, H, D [(h)]
q^2 [a]	0.632	0.630	0.661	0.641	0.650	0.636
SEP [b]	0.374	0.355	0.359	0.370	0.358	0.359
No. of Components [c]	6	3	6	6	5	4
r^2 [d]	0.989	0.909	0.979	0.984	0.966	0.947
SEE [e]	0.066	0.176	0.090	0.078	0.111	0.136
Field Contributions	0.524, 0.476	0.066, 0.237, 0.114, 0.307, 0.276	0.201, 0.799	0.139, 0.568, 0.293	0.095, 0.349, 0.160, 0.396	0.087, 0.341, 0.172, 0.401
F-value [f]	377.882	96.415	220.40	269.126	154.86	125.930
Predictive *r*-squared [g]	0.964	0.985	0.877	0.917	0.954	0.888

[a] Cross-validated correlation coefficient.
[b] Standard error of predictions.
[c] Optimum number of components obtained from cross-validated PLS analysis and same used in final non-cross-validated analysis.
[d] Noncross-validated correlation coefficient.
[e] Standard error of estimate.
[f] *F*-test value.
[g] Correlation coefficient for test set predictions.
[(h)] CoMFA and CoMSIA with different field contributions such as steric (S), electrostatic (E), hydrophobic (H), donor (D), and acceptor (A) fields.

Table 6. Results of CoMFA and CoMSIA Analyses for Compounds Used in Training Set (AChE modeling)

S.No.	Compound	Actual pIC_{50} *BuChE*	CoMFA Predicted pIC_{50} *BuChE*	CoMSIA Predicted pIC_{50} *BuChE*	Actual pIC_{50} *AChE*	CoMFA Predicted pIC_{50} *AChE*	CoMSIA Predicted pIC_{50} *AChE*
Training set							
1	SAR01	5.72	5.61	5.65	2.99	3.07	2.98
2	SAR02	5.39	5.44	5.43	3.2	3.13	3.23
3	SAR03	4.90	4.90	5.01	2.4	2.41	2.58
4	SAR04	4.99	5.04	5.01	2.15	2.18	2.44
5	SAR05	4.78	4.73	4.75	1.69	1.69	1.75
6	SAR06	5.41	5.38	5.37	2.70	2.71	2.65
7	SAR07	4.74	4.72	4.76	2.30	2.32	2.36
8	SAR08	5.33	5.29	5.19	2.30	2.25	2.51
9	SAR09	5.63	5.63	5.82	3.07	3.09	2.84
10	SAR10	5.32	5.37	5.28	2.70	2.72	2.95
11	SAR11	4.42	4.44	4.54	2.21	2.25	2.26
12	SAR12	5.72	5.75	5.67	2.69	2.72	2.74
13	SAR13	4.59	4.62	4.66	1.60	1.76	1.72
14	SAR14	4.62	4.65	4.65	1.73	1.68	1.71
15	SAR15	5.44	5.42	5.48	3.21	3.15	3.14
16	SAR16	5.39	5.39	5.37	3.20	3.19	3.02
17	SAR17	4.54	4.66	4.66	2.11	2.13	2.08
18	SAR18[a]	5.35	5.39	5.36	-------	-------	-------
19	SAR19	4.49	4.45	4.43	2.48	2.44	2.17
20	SAR20	4.49	4.46	4.50	3.11	3.07	3.14
21	SAR21	5.72	5.69	5.74	2.52	2.55	2.81
22	SAR22	5.40	5.41	5.34	2.90	2.85	2.91
23	SAR23	4.74	4.74	4.69	1.64	1.60	1.79
24	SAR24	4.74	4.65	4.61	1.74	1.71	1.89
25	SAR25	5.44	5.48	5.40	3.21	3.22	3.29
26	SAR26	5.37	5.43	5.45	3.23	3.19	3.20
27	SAR27	4.60	4.62	4.64	2.30	2.36	2.22
28	SAR28	5.82	5.80	5.89	1.73	1.74	1.89
29	SAR29	5.90	5.93	5.87	2.71	2.74	2.51
30	SAR30	5.66	5.65	5.53	3.15	3.20	3.19
31	SAR31	4.98	4.96	5.06	2.31	2.30	2.14
32	SAR32[a]	4.60	4.60	4.51	-------	-------	-------
33	SAR33	5.60	5.54	5.50	3.28	3.33	2.97
34	SAR34	5.00	5.01	5.03	1.74	1.77	1.58
35	SAR40	2.65	2.613	2.620	2.37	2.18	2.05
Test set							
36	SAR35	5.00	4.80	5.07	2.33	2.35	2.31
37	SAR36	5.16	5.17	5.17	2.80	2.82	2.87
38	SAR37	5.55	5.24	5.56	2.54	2.31	2.49
39	SAR38	4.68	4.82	4.66	2.08	2.10	2.21
40	SAR39	4.49	4.74	5.11	3.15	3.11	3.17

[a] = not included in AChE modeling

Table 7. Comparisons of Experimental and Calculated Biological Activities of the Compounds by Using CoMFA and CoMSIA Analyses

3.2.3 Graphical interpretation of the results (CoMFA)

3.2.3.1 BuChE

CoMFA steric and electrostatic fields from the final non-cross-validated analysis were plotted as three-dimensional colored contour maps in Figure 6a. The field energies at each lattice point were calculated as the scalar results of the coefficient and the standard deviation associated with a particular column of the data table (stdev*coeff), plotted as the percentage of contribution to the CoMFA equation. These maps show regions where differences in molecular fields are associated with differences in biological activity.

The steric interactions are represented by green and yellow colors while electrostatic interactions are represented by red and blue colors (Figure 6a). In the green regions of steric contour plot, bulky substituent enhances biological activity while bulky substituent in the yellow region is likely to decrease activity. The green steric contour near the substituent at C20 of the D ring indicates that any bulky substituent is preferred at this position. This may provide more possibilities to establish hydrophobic interactions with peripheral site of the target protein. This observation is consistent with the experimental findings as compound SAR13 is less active than SAR38 because SAR13 is having less bulky substituent at C20 than SAR38.

In electrostatic contour map blue-colored contours represent regions where electropositive groups increase activity whereas red colored regions represent areas where electronegative groups enhance activity. The electrostatic contour plot on the set of compounds showed that there is a red-colored region situated close to the substituent at C3 that is to say, the negative charges at this region are in a high demand for ligand binding and a charge withdrawing group linked to this position will enhance the biological activity. This observation also correlates with the experimental determinations, for example, the compound SAR37 is more active than compound SAR17. The only difference in both of them is the presence of a hydroxyl group at C-2 in compound SAR17 which makes SAR17 less active than SAR37 since C2 position is covered by the blue contour map. On the other hand a negative group at C-4 position makes compound SAR26, SAR28, SAR30, and SAR33 the most active compounds among the listed compounds. The presence of a double bond between C-5 and C-6 makes compound SAR06 more active than compound SAR07, which has otherwise identical structure.

3.2.3.2 AChE

In Figure 7a it is possible to observe two well-defined zones (close to the substituent at position C-4 and side chain at C-3 position) in which the presence of negative density favors an increase of AChE inhibitory activity. Furthermore, the presence of a double bond in ring B, between C-5 and C-6, also increases the activity. Small zones near C-2 have an opposite effect, that is, a negative density decreases the activity: for example, the only difference between compounds SAR17 and SAR37 is the presence of a hydroxyl group at C-2, which makes compound SAR17 less active than SAR37, on the other hand a negative group at C-4 position makes compounds SAR33, SAR30 and SAR26 the most active compounds in our study. Similarly, the presence of a double bond between C-5 and C-6 makes compound SAR06 more active than compound SAR07 which has an otherwise identical structure. Figure 7a displays two big zones near position C-4 and near the side chain at C-3, where the presence of bulky substituents decreases the activity. The region between C14 and C15 is also not favorable for bulky groups, which assigns a further role to the presence of the double bond in ring D as it means the lack of a further substitution. This difference can be easily seen by comparing compounds SAR30 and SAR26.

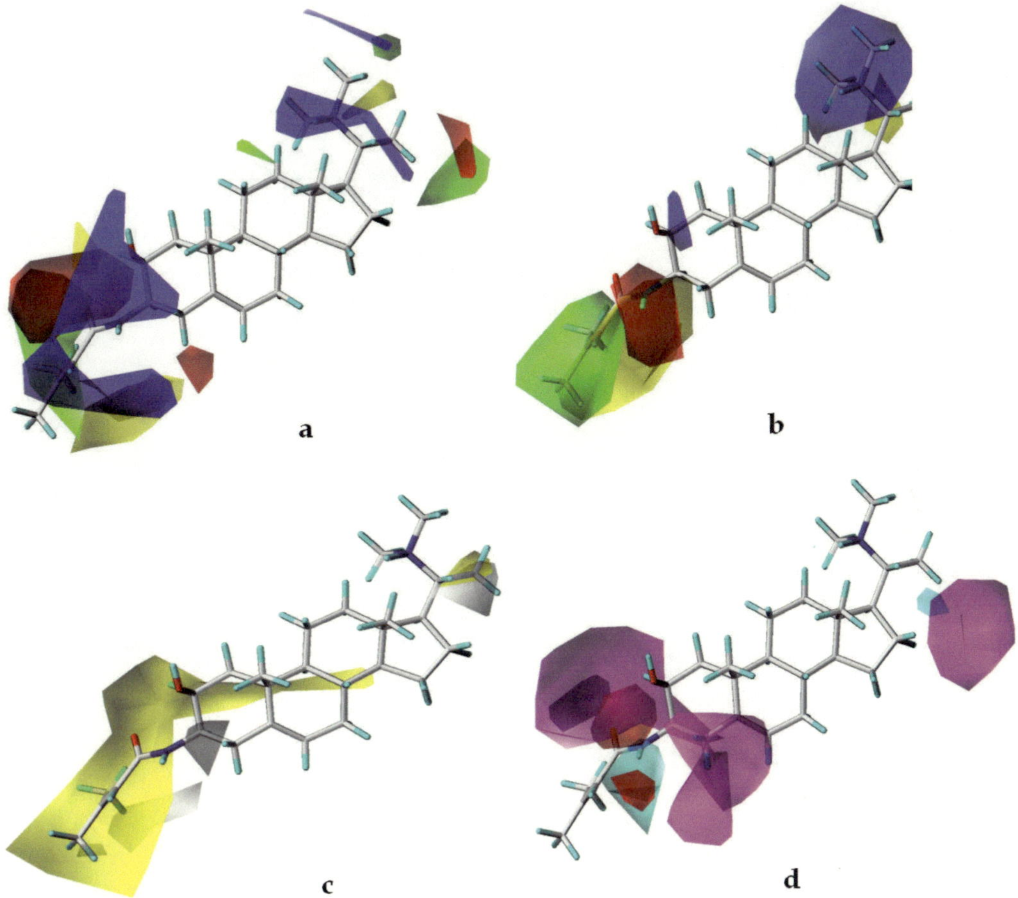

Fig. 6. **a**) The CoMFA (stdev*coeff) steric and electrostatic contour plots for BuChE modeling. The favorable steric areas in green; disfavored steric areas in yellow. The positive potential favored area in blue; positive potential disfavored areas in red. The most active compound in the series (SAR29) is shown as the reference compound. **b**) The CoMSIA (stdev*coeff) steric and electrostatic contour plots. Color scheme same as in figure 6a. The most active compound in the series (SAR29) is shown as the reference compound. **c**) The CoMSIA (stdev*coeff) hydrophobic contour plots. The favorable hydrophobic areas indicated by yellow color, whereas the disfavored hydrophobic areas are shown by white color. The most active compound (SAR29) is shown as the reference compound. **d**) The contour plots of the CoMSIA (stdev*coeff) H-bond donor and acceptor fields. The favorable H-bond donor in cyan; unfavorable H-bond donor in purple. The favorable H-bond acceptor in magenta; unfavorable H-bond acceptor in red. The most active compound (SAR29) is shown as the reference compound

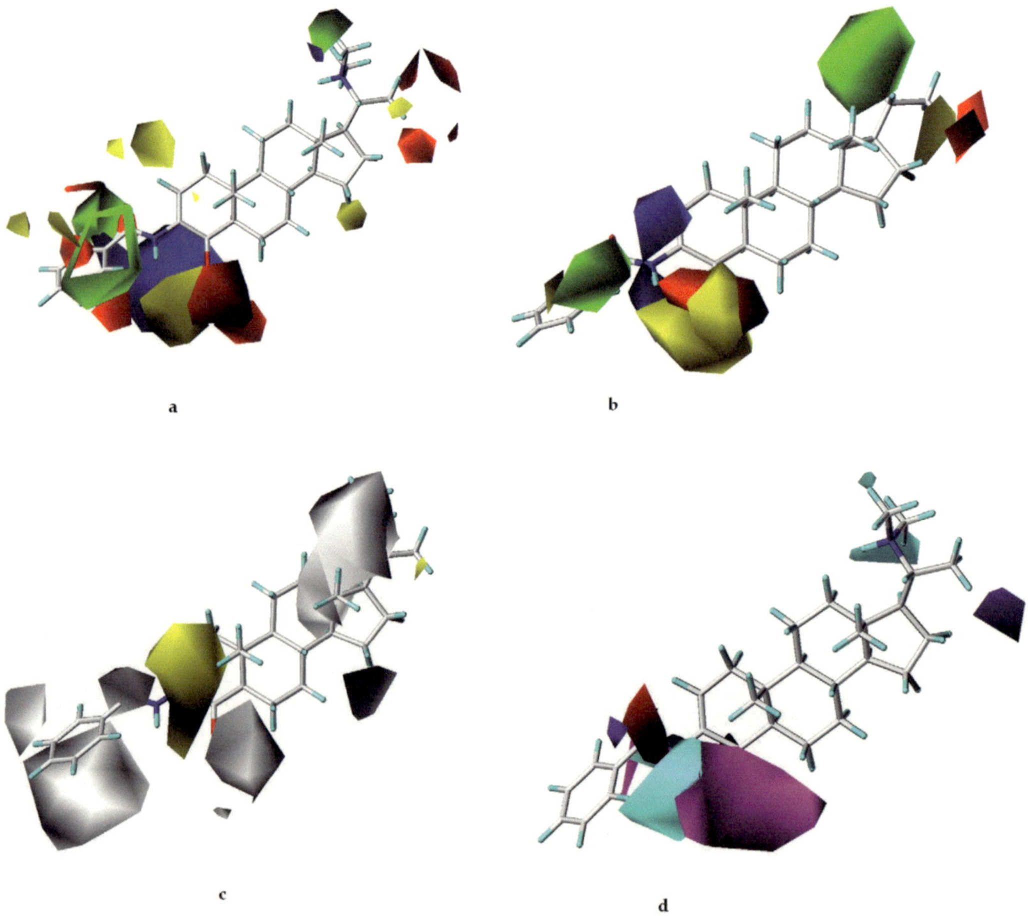

Fig. 7. **a**) The CoMFA (stdev*coeff) steric and electrostatic contour plots for AChE modeling. The favorable steric areas in green; disfavored steric areas in yellow. The positive potential favored area in blue; positive potential disfavored areas in red. The most active compound in the series (SAR33) is shown as the reference compound. **b**) The CoMSIA (stdev*coeff) steric and electrostatic contour plots. Color scheme same as in figure 7a. The most active compound in the series (SAR33) is shown as the reference compound. **c**) The CoMSIA (stdev*coeff) hydrophobic contour plots. The favorable hydrophobic areas indicated by yellow color, whereas the disfavored hydrophobic areas are shown by white color. The most active compound (SAR33) is shown as the reference compound. **d**) The contour plots of the CoMSIA (stdev*coeff) H-bond donor and acceptor fields. The favorable H-bond donor in cyan; unfavorable H-bond donor in purple. The favorable H-bond acceptor in magenta; unfavorable H-bond acceptor in red. The most active compound (SAR33) is shown as the reference compound

3.2.4 Graphical interpretation of the results (CoMSIA)

3.2.4.1 BuChE

The CoMSIA steric and electrostatic fields based on PLS analyses are represented as 3D contour plots in Figure 6b. In the electrostatic contour map, positive charge can be appeared closer to the regions of positive coefficients (blue) and negative charge can be moved closer to the regions of negative coefficients (red). A close inspection of the electrostatic contour plots (Figure 6b), reveals that for the tested molecules the electropositive groups are more preferred and appearance of the blue regions near R4 zone, indicate that more positive charge group substituted at this zone on the parent skeleton will enhance the biological activity.

In the steric contour map, it can be seen that, the areas (green contour) correspond to regions where steric occupancy with bulky groups are preferred and the areas encompassed by yellow contour should be sterically avoided. For the studied compounds on ring A, there exist two contour areas, a larger favorable area near the group substituted at the C3 on the ring A, and at the opposite site, a relatively smaller unfavorable area. Due to the steric complementarity between receptor and inhibitor, the positions which are encompassing the green region are sterically preferred to produce good steric interactions with the receptor and hence increasing the inhibitory activity. By observing the steric contour map with the compound SAR29 (one of the most active compound; Table 2), it can be readily seen that the green contour covered the whole carbonyl and double bond region at the senecioyl group while the terminal substituent on double bond in senecioyl group is covered by yellow contour. The green area is indicating that bulky substituent at double bond but adjacent to the carbonyl position will enhance the biological activity. Similarly, a smaller terminal substituent on the double bond will enhance the inhibitory activity. For example, the structure of the compound SAR12 has relatively small substituent, in the form of -NHCH3, at C3, while SAR35 has a bulky substituent in the form of senecioyl group, shows less inhibitory activity than compound SAR12. The same is observed if we compare the compound SAR25 with SAR35.

The contour map of hydrophobic properties indicates (Figure 6c) one distinct hydrophobically favorable site, a larger region near the R2 zone, which means that groups with high hydrophobicity (indicated by yellow contour in Figure 6c) will favor biological activity. It can be reasonably presumed that ring A combined with a substituent on it, is composed of a large hydrophobic core, and will produce a strong hydrophobic interaction with the receptor. This observation is also consistent with the CoMFA steric contour map (Figure 6a) in which the sterically more crowded substituent is necessary to enhance the biological activity at the same R2 zone (see Figure 8 for R zones descriptions).

The graphical interpretations of the field contributions of the H-bond properties are shown in Figure 6d as both H-bond donor and H-bond acceptor fields. In principle, they should highlight the areas beyond the ligands where putative hydrogen partners in the enzyme can form H-bonds that influence binding affinity. The hydrogen bond donor and acceptor fields showed the favorable (cyan) area near the amido group and the H-bond acceptor field showed the favorable (magenta) area around the oxygen atom in amido group (Figure 6d). This may be due to the involvement of hydrogen bonding during interaction with target.

Superimposition of the CoMFA and CoMSIA coefficient contour maps on the ligand in the active site of BuChE (Figure 9a and 9b) additionally supports the result that most of the interactions are hydrophobic in nature and the residues nearby the hydrophobic favorable area are mostly consisting of hydrophobic amino acids (i.e., Gly, Val, and Leu). As depicted in the figures 9a and 9b, the substituents at position R2 is placed in the hydrophobic pocket formed by Leu286, Gly116, Gly117, Val288, and Ala199. A green color contour map of CoMFA model (Figure 6a) and similarly of green contour of CoMSIA (Figure 6b) is appeared at this position suggesting for bulky substituents at this position. Another yellow color CoMSIA contour near the same R2 region suggesting the favorable hydrophobic interaction with the receptor hydrophobic pocket which is formed by the same amino acid residues. Most of the amino acid residues near the yellow contour regions are in hydrophobic in nature e.g., Gly, Val, and Leu. The same is true when comparing the CoMFA and CoMSIA contour maps within the active site residues of acetylcholinesterase (Figure 9c and 9d)

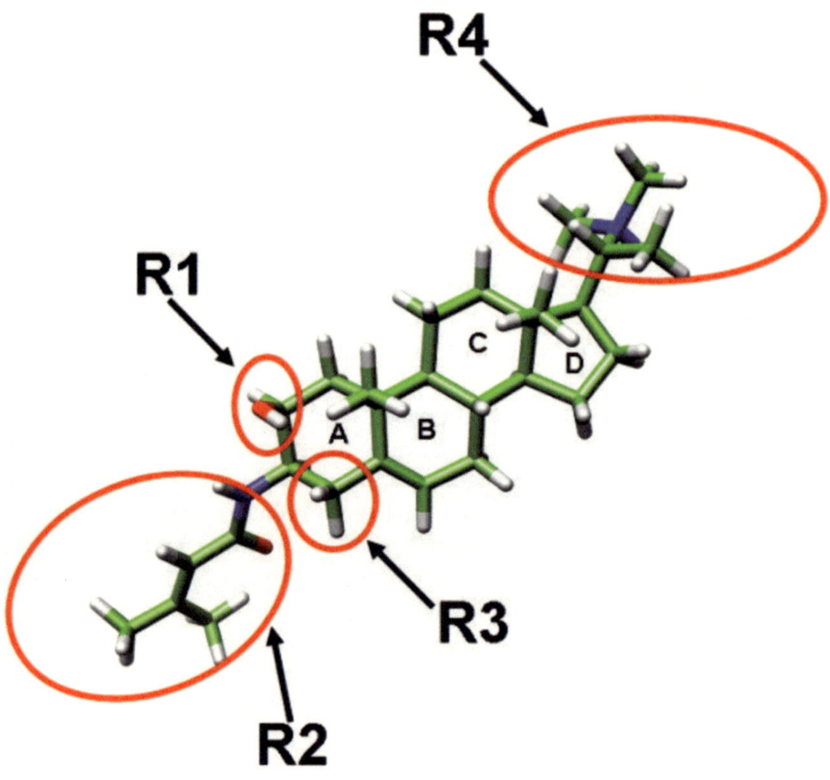

Fig. 8. An example of representative compound; showing important regions of the parent skeleton; circled here, as R1, R2, R3 and R4

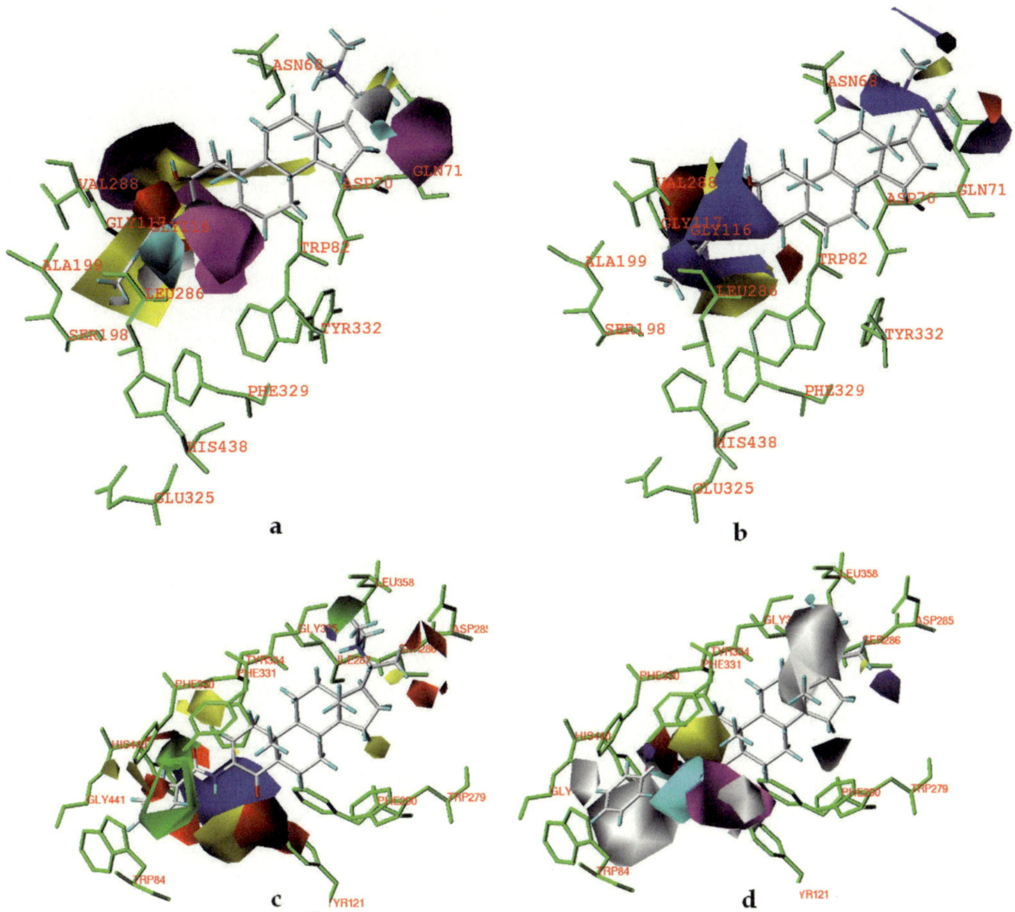

Fig. 9. **a**) CoMSIA contour plots superimposed within the active site of BuChE with compound SAR29 **b**) CoMFA contour plots superimposed within the active site of BuChE with compound SAR29 **c**) CoMFA contour plots superimposed within the active site of AChE with compound SAR33 **d**) CoMSIA contour plots superimposed within the active site of AChE with compound SAR33

3.2.4.2 AChE

The CoMSIA steric and electrostatic descriptors (Figure 7b) for the set of AChE inhibitors remain similar as the CoMFA and hence not described further. The CoMSIA hydrophobic descriptors are presented as contour maps in Figure 7c. The contour map of hydrophobic properties indicates a favourable region around the substituents as R2 (yellow contours in Figure 7c), pointing the hydrophobic groups is advantageous for the AChE inhibitory activity. The graphical interpretations of the H-bond properties are shown in Figure 7d. The contours present in the Figure 7d signify the importance of H-bond donor and acceptor characters in the region. In principle, almost all compounds have amide group present in the region and hence presence of these contours is correlated with potentially donor and acceptor amide group.

4. Conclusion

Present study correlates the cholinesterase inhibitory activities of isolated natural compounds with the steric, electrostatic and hydrophobicity parameters. Statistically significant 3D-QSAR models of the steroidal alkaloids inhibitors were designed by exploring multiple conformations of each ligand using the genetic algorithm. An alignment technique scheme was generated from the docking results and it yielded highly predictive 3D-QSAR models. The good correlation observed in all cases of 3D-QSAR supports the proposed method of alignment and selection of conformers.

Final models were validated by the prediction of inhibitory activities of the test set compounds. In terms of external predictions, CoMSIA and CoMFA both performed great. A comparison of the 3D-QSAR PLS coefficient contour maps with the structural and functional features of the binding sites also showed good correlation. It is evident from the contour plots of both analyses that the hydrophobic effect plays main contribution to the cholinesterase inhibitory activity and it's quite in agreement with the fact that the cholinesterases are having a wide active site gorge lining with hydrophobic amino acid residues. Also, bulky groups in the side chain at R2 position generally cause the increase in activity but at the same time the bulkier substituent at position R3 resulted in decreasing the activity. This R3 position is covered by a yellow steric contour and hence the bulkiness at this region is detrimental to the activity. The preference for bulky group at position R2 as described in CoMFA, seems to be correlated in CoMSIA with increased hyrdrophobicity expected at the same region. As an attempt to exploiting the cholinesterase inhibitors for 3D-QSAR approach combined with all detailed information obtained by 3D-QSAR models, we strongly believe that this study can help to design novel molecules with improved activity in near future.

The results, together with the good correlations between the actual and predicted inhibitory activities, demonstrate the power of combined docking/QSAR approach to explore the probable binding conformations of compounds at the active sites of the protein target. Additionally, present study also demonstrates that charges resulting from different calculation methods may influence the results of CoMFA as well as CoMSIA, although in our case this effect has not been significant. This is evident from the q^2 values calculated for different charge calculation methods (Table 4).

5. Acknowledgment

Financial support from Higher Education Commission, Pakistan to Uddin, R., under Split PhD program is highly acknowledged. The authors are thankful to Dr. Michael A Brunsteiner, Dr. Hongbin Yuan and Dr. Pavel A Petukhov from University of Illinois at Chicago for their help in developing the GA scripts in SPL and Perl languages. Authors are also thankful to S. T. Moin for assisting during the calculation runs. Authors are grateful to the Pakistan Science Foundation (PSF) for financial support to develop computational chemistry software facilities at the ICCBS.

Authors are also thankful to the OpenEye for providing us free academic license.

6. References

Atta ur, R.; Choudhary, M. I.; Khan, M. R.; Anjum, S.; Farooq, A. & Iqbal, M. Z. (2000). New Steroidal Alkaloids from Sarcococca saligna. *Journal of Natural Products*, Vol.63, No.10, (October 2000), pp. 1364-8, ISSN 0163-3864

Atta ur, R.; Feroz, F.; Naeem, I.; Zaheer ul, H.; Nawaz, S. A.; Khan, N.; Khan, M. R. & Choudhary, M. I. (2004). New Pregnane-type Steroidal Alkaloids from Sarcocca saligna and their Cholinesterase Inhibitory Activity. *Steroids*, Vol.69, No.11-12, (October-November 2004), pp. 735-41, ISSN 0039-128X

Atta ur, R.; Feroz, F.; Zaheer ul, H.; Nawaz, S. A.; Khan, M. R. & Choudhary, M. I. (2003). New Steroidal Alkaloids from Sarcococca saligna. *Natural Product Research*, Vol.17, No.4, (August 2003), pp. 235-41, ISSN 1478-6419

Atta ur, R.; Nasreen, A.; Akhtar, F.; Shekhani, M. S.; Clardy, J.; Parvez, M. & Choudhary, M. I. (1997). Antifungal Diterpenoid Alkaloids from Delphinium denudatum. *Journal of Natural Products*, Vol.60, No.5, (May 1997), pp. 472-474, ISSN 0163-3864

Atta ur, R.; Zaheer ul, H.; Feroz, F.; Khalid, A.; Nawaz, S. A.; Khan, M. R. & Choudhary, M. I. (2004). New Cholinesterase-Inhibiting Steroidal Alkaloids from Sarcococca saligna. *Helvetica Chimica Acta*, Vol.87, No.2, (February 2004), pp. 439, ISSN 1522-2675

Atta ur, R.; Zaheer ul, H.; Khalid, A.; Anjum, S.; Khan, M. R. & Choudhary, M. I. (2002). Pregnane-type Steroidal Alkaloids of Sarcococca saligna: A New Class of Cholinesterases Inhibitors. *Helvetica Chimica Acta*, Vol.85, No.2, (Februay 2002), pp. 678-688, ISSN 1522-2675

Bazelyansky, M.; Robey, E. & Kirsch, J. F. (1986). Fractional diffusion-limited component of reactions catalyzed by acetylcholinesterase. *Biochemistry*, Vol.25, No.1, (January 1986), pp. 125-30, ISSN 0006-2960

Behra, M.; Cousin, X.; Bertrand, C.; Vonesch, J. L.; Biellmann, D.; Chatonnet, A. & Strahle, U. (2002). Acetylcholinesterase is Required for Neuronal and Muscular Development in the Zebrafish Embryo. *Nature Neuroscience*, Vol.5, No.2, (February 2002), pp. 111-8, ISSN 1097-6256

Bohm, M.; St rzebecher, J. & Klebe, G. (1999). Three-Dimensional Quantitative Structure-Activity Relationship Analyses using Comparative Molecular Field Analysis and Comparative Molecular Similarity Indices Analysis to Elucidate Selectivity Differences of Inhibitors Binding to Trypsin, Thrombin, and Factor Xa. *Journal of Medicinal Chemistry*, Vol.42, No.3, (Febraury 1999), pp. 458-77, ISSN 0022-2623

Bourne, Y.; Taylor, P. & Marchot, P. (1995). Acetylcholinesterase Inhibition by Fasciculin: Crystal Structure of the Complex. *Cell*, Vol.83, No.3, (November 1995), pp. 503-12, ISSN 0092-8674

Buolamwini, J. K. & Assefa, H. (2002). CoMFA and CoMSIA 3D QSAR and Docking Studies on Conformationally-Restrained Cinnamoyl HIV-1 Integrase Inhibitors: Exploration of a Binding Mode at the Active Site. *Journal of Medicinal Chemistry*, Vol.45, No.4, (February 2002), pp. 841-852, ISSN 0022-2623

Butters, N.; Delis, D. C. & Lucas, J. A. (1995). Clinical Assessment of Memory Disorders in Amnesia and Dementia. *Annual Review of Psychology*, Vol.46, (February 1995), pp. 493-523, ISSN 0066-4308

Chatonnet, A. & Lockridge, O. (1989). Comparison of Butyrylcholinesterase and Acetylcholinesterase. *The Biochemical Journal*, Vol.260, No.3, (June 1989), pp. 625-34, ISSN 0264-6021

Cho, S. J.; Garsia, M. L.; Bier, J. & Tropsha, A. (1996). Structure-Based Alignment and Comparative Molecular Field Analysis of Acetylcholinesterase Inhibitors. *Journal of Medicinal Chemistry*, Vol.39, No.26, (December 1996), pp. 5064-71, ISSN 0022-2623

Clark, M.; Cramer, R. D. & Van Opdenbosch, N. (1989). Validation of the General Purpose Tripos 5. 2 Force Field. *Journal of Computational Chemistry*, Vol.10, No.8, (December 1989), pp. 982-1012, ISSN 1096-987X

Cokugras, A. N. (2003). Butyrylcholinesterase: Structure and Physiological Importance. *Turkish Journal of Biochemistry*, Vol.28, No.2, (October 2003), pp. 54-61, ISSN 0250-4685

Cramer Iii, R. D.; Patterson, D. E. & Bunce, J. D. (1988). Comparative Molecular Field Analysis (CoMFA). 1. Effect of Shape on Binding of Steroids to Carrier Proteins. *Journal of the American Chemical Society*, Vol.110, No.18, (August 1988), pp. 5959-5967, ISSN 0002-7863

Debnath, A. K. (1999). Three-Dimensional Quantitative Structure-Activity Relationship Study on Cyclic Urea Derivatives as HIV-1 Protease Inhibitors: Application of Comparative Molecular Field Analysis. *Journal of Medicinal Chemistry*, Vol.42, No.2, (January 1999), pp. 249-59, ISSN 0022-2623

Dominguez, C.; Boelens, R. & Bonvin, A. M. (2003). HADDOCK: A Protein-Protein Docking Approach Based on Biochemical or Biophysical Information. *Journal of American Chemical Society*, Vol.125, No.7, (Feb 19), pp. 1731-7, ISSN 0002-7863

Donini, O. A. & Kollman, P. A. (2000). Calculation and Prediction of Binding Free Energies for the Matrix Metalloproteinases. *Journal of Medicinal Chemistry*, Vol.43, No.22, (November 2000), pp. 4180-8, ISSN 0022-2623

Doorn, J. A.; Talley, T. T.; Thompson, C. M. & Richardson, R. J. (2001). Probing the Active Sites of Butyrylcholinesterase and Cholesterol Esterase with Isomalathion: Conserved Stereoselective Inactivation of Serine Hydrolases Structurally Related to Acetylcholinesterase. *Chemical Research in Toxicology*, Vol.14, No.7, (July 2001), pp. 807-13, ISSN 0893-228X

Fogel, L. J.; Owens, A. J. & Walsh, M. J. (1966). *Artificial Intelligence Through Simulated Evolution*, Wiley, New York

Forrest, S. (1993). Genetic Algorithms: Principles of Natural Selection Applied to Computation. *Science*, Vol.261, No.5123, (August 1993), pp. 872, ISSN 0036-8075

FRED (2007). FRED, version 2.2.3, OpenEye Scientific Software, Inc., Santa Fe, NM, USA, www.eyesopen.com, 2007. pp.

Geladi, P. & Kowalski, B. R. (1986). Partial Least Squares: A Tutorial. *Analytica Chimica Acta*, Vol.185, (July 1986), pp. 1-17, ISSN 0003-2670

Giacobini, E. (2003). Cholinesterases: New Roles in Brain Function and in Alzheimer's Disease. *Neurochemical Research*, Vol.28, No.3-4, (April 2003), pp. 515-22, ISSN 0364-3190

Giacobini, E. (1964). Metabolic Relations Between Glia and Neurons Studied in Single Cells, In: *Morphological and Biochemical Correlates of Neural Activity*, pp. 15-38, Harper & Row, ISBN 978-006-1406-40-9, New York, USA

Goldberg, D. E. (1989). *Genetic Algorithm in Search, Optimization and Machine Learning*, Addison-Wesley Professional, ISBN 978-020-1157-673, Reading, MA

Graybiel, A. M. & Ragsdale, C. W., Jr. (1982). Pseudocholinesterase Staining in the Primary Visual Pathway of the Macaque Monkey. *Nature*, Vol.299, No.5882, (September 1982), pp. 439-42, ISSN 0028-0836

Greig, N. H.; Utsuki, T.; Yu, Q.; Zhu, X.; Holloway, H. W.; Perry, T.; Lee, B.; Ingram, D. K. & Lahiri, D. K. (2001). A New Therapeutic Target in Alzheimer's Disease Treatment:

Attention to Butyrylcholinesterase. *Current Medical Research and Opinion*, Vol.17, No.3, pp. 159-65, ISSN 0300-7995

Guillozet, A. L.; Smiley, J. F.; Mash, D. C. & Mesulam, M. M. (1997). Butyrylcholinesterase in the Life Cycle of Amyloid Plaques. *Annals of Neurololgy*, Vol.42, No.6, (December 1997), pp. 909-18, ISSN 0364-5134

Harel, M.; Sussman, J. L.; Krejci, E.; Bon, S.; Chanal, P.; Massoulie, J. & Silman, I. (1992). Conversion of Acetylcholinesterase to Butyrylcholinesterase: Modeling and Mutagenesis. *Proceedings of the National Academy of Sciences of the United States of America*, Vol.89, No.22, (November 1992), pp. 10827-31, ISSN 0027-8424

Holland, J. H. (1975). *Adaptation in Natural and Artificial Systems*, University of Michigan press, ISBN 978-026-2581-11-0, Ann Arbor, MI

Hu, X. & Stebbins, C. E. (2005). Molecular Docking and 3D-QSAR Studies of Yersinia Protein Tyrosine Phosphatase YopH Inhibitors. *Bioorganic and Medicinal Chemistry*, Vol.13, No.4, (February 2005), pp. 1101-9, ISSN 0968-0896

Jain, A. N. (2003). Surflex: Fully Automatic Flexible Molecular Docking using a Molecular Similarity-Based Search Engine. *Journal of Medicinla Chemistry*, Vol.46, No.4, (February 2003), pp. 499-511, ISSN 0022-2623

Johnson, M. A.; Hoog, C. & Pinto, B. M. (2003). A Novel Modeling Protocol for Protein Receptors Guided by Bound-Ligand Conformation. *Biochemistry*, Vol.42, No.7, (February 2003), pp. 1842-53, ISSN 0006-2960

Kalauni, S. K.; Choudhary, M. I.; Shaheen, F.; Manandhar, M. D.; Atta ur, R.; Gewali, M. B. & Khalid, A. (2001). Steroidal Alkaloids from the Leaves of Sarcococca coriacea of Nepalese Origin. *Journal of Natural Products*, Vol.64, No.6, (June 2001), pp. 842-4, ISSN 0163-3864

Khalid, A.; Zaheer ul, H.; Anjum, S.; Khan, M. R.; Atta ur, R. & Choudhary, M. I. (2004). Kinetics and Structure-Activity Relationship Studies on Pregnane-Type Steroidal Alkaloids that Inhibit Cholinesterases. *Bioorganic and Medicinal Chemistry*, Vol.12, No.9, (May 1), pp. 1995-2003, ISSN 0968-0896

Khalid, A.; Zaheer ul, H.; Ghayur, M. N.; Feroz, F.; Atta ur, R.; Gilani, A. H. & Choudhary, M. I. (2004). Cholinesterase Inhibitory and Spasmolytic Potential of Steroidal Alkaloids. *Journal of Steroid Biochemistry and Molecular Biology*, Vol.92, No.5, (December 2004), pp. 477-84, ISSN 0960-0760

Klebe, G. (1998). Comparative Molecular Similarity Indices Analysis: CoMSIA, In: *3D QSAR in Drug Design: Recent Advances*, pp. 87-104, Kluwer Academic Publishers, ISBN 978-904-8149-35-3, London

Klebe, G.; Abraham, U. & Mietzner, T. (1994). Molecular Similarity Indices in a Comparative Analysis (CoMSIA) of Drug Molecules to Correlate and Predict their Biological Activity. *Journal of Medicinal Chemistry*, Vol.37, No.24, (November 1994), pp. 4130-46, ISSN 0022-2623

Lemmen, C.; Lengauer, T. & Klebe, G. (1998). FLEXS: A Method for Fast Flexible Ligand Superposition. *Journal of Medicinal Chemistry*, Vol.41, No.23, (October 1998), pp. 4502-4520, ISSN 0022-2623

Lockridge, O. & Masson, P. (2000). Pesticides and Susceptible Populations: People with Butyrylcholinesterase Genetic Variants may be at Risk. *Neurotoxicology*, Vol.21, No.1-2, (February-April 2000), pp. 113-26, ISSN 0161-813X

Mack, A. & Robitzki, A. (2000). The Key Role of Butyrylcholinesterase during Neurogenesis and Neural Disorders: An Antisense-5'Butyrylcholinesterase-DNA Study. *Progress in Neurobiology*, Vol.60, No.6, (April 2000), pp. 607-28, ISSN 0301-0082

Massoulie, J.; Pezzementi, L.; Bon, S.; Krejci, E. & Vallette, F. M. (1993). Molecular and Cellular Biology of Cholinesterases. *Progress in Neurobiology*, Vol.41, No.1, (July 1993), pp. 31-91, ISSN 0301-0082

Massoulie, J.; Sussman, J.; Bon, S. & Silman, I. (1993). Cholinergic Function and Dysfunction: Structure and Functions of Acetylcholinesterase and Butyrylcholinesterase, In: *Progress in Brain Research*, pp. 139-46, ISBN 978-044-4897-17-6,

McGann, M. R.; Almond, H. R.; Nicholls, A.; Grant, J. A. & Brown, F. K. (2003). Gaussian Docking Functions. *Biopolymers*, Vol.68, No.1, pp. 76-90, ISSN 1097-0282

Medina-Franco, J. L.; Rodríguez-Morales, S.; Juárez-Gordiano, C.; Hernández-Campos, A. & Castillo, R. (2004). Docking-Bbased CoMFA and CoMSIA Studies of Non-Nucleoside Reverse Transcriptase Inhibitors of the Pyridinone Derivative Type. *Journal of Computer-Aided Molecular Design*, Vol.18, No.5, (July 2004), pp. 345-360, ISSN 0920-654X

Meshorer, E.; Erb, C.; Gazit, R.; Pavlovsky, L.; Kaufer, D.; Friedman, A.; Glick, D.; Ben-Arie, N. & Soreq, H. (2002). Alternative Splicing and Neuritic mRNA Translocation Under Long-Term Neuronal Hypersensitivity. *Science*, Vol.295, No.5554, (January 2002), pp. 508-12, ISSN 0036-8075

Nachon, F.; Asojo, O. A.; Borgstahl, G. E.; Masson, P. & Lockridge, O. (2005). Role of Water in Aging of Human Butyrylcholinesterase Inhibited by Echothiophate: The Crystal Structure Suggests Two Alternative Mechanisms of Aging. *Biochemistry*, Vol.44, No.4, (February 2005), pp. 1154-62, ISSN 0006-2960

Nachon, F.; Nicolet, Y. & Masson, P. (2005). Butyrylcholinesterase: 3D structure, Catalytic Mechanisms. *Annales Pharmaceutiques Francaises*, Vol.63, No.3, (June 2005), pp. 194-206, ISSN 0003-4509

Nicolet, Y.; Lockridge, O.; Masson, P.; Fontecilla-Camps, J. C. & Nachon, F. (2003). Crystal Structure of Human Butyrylcholinesterase and of Its Complexes with Substrate and Products. *Journal of Biological Chemistry*, Vol.278, No.42, (October 2003), pp. 41141-7, ISSN 0021-9258

OE ROCS, v. (2008). OpenEye Scientific Software, Inc., Santa Fe, NM, USA, www.eyesopen.com, 2008. pp.

Pan, X.; Tan, N.; Zeng, G.; Han, H. & Huang, H. (2006). 3D-QSAR and Docking Studies of Aldehyde Inhibitors of Human Cathepsin K. *Bioorganic and Medicinal Chemistry*, Vol.14, No.8, (April 2006), pp. 2771-2778, ISSN 0968-0896

Perry, E. K.; Tomlinson, B. E.; Blessed, G.; Bergmann, K.; Gibson, P. H. & Perry, R. H. (1978). Correlation of Cholinergic Abnormalities with Senile Plaques and Mental Test Scores in Senile Dementia. *British Medical Journal*, Vol.2, No.6150, (November 1978), pp. 1457-1459, ISSN 1759-2151

Prathipati, P.; Pandey, G. & Saxena, A. K. (2005). CoMFA and Docking Studies on Glycogen Phosphorylase a Inhibitors as Antidiabetic Agents. *Journal of Chemical Information and Modeling*, Vol.45, No.1, (Jan-Feb 2005), pp. 136-45, ISSN 1549-9596

Radic, Z.; Pickering, N. A.; Vellom, D. C.; Camp, S. & Taylor, P. (1993). Three Distinct Domains in the Cholinesterase Molecule Confer Selectivity for Acetyl- and

Butyrylcholinesterase Inhibitors. *Biochemistry*, Vol.32, No.45, (November 1993), pp. 12074-84, ISSN 0006-2960

Rarey, M.; Kramer, B.; Lengauer, T. & Klebe, G. (1996). A Fast Flexible Docking Method Using an Incremental Construction Algorithm. *Journal of Molecular Biology*, Vol.261, No.3, (August 1996), pp. 470-489, ISSN 0022-2836

Sabnis, Y. A.; Desai, P. V.; Rosenthal, P. J. & Avery, M. A. (2003). Probing the Structure of Falcipain-3, A Cysteine Protease from Plasmodium falciparum: Comparative Protein Modeling and Docking Studies. *Protein Science*, Vol.12, No.3, (March 2003), pp. 501-9, ISSN 0961-8368

Saxena, A.; Redman, A. M.; Jiang, X.; Lockridge, O. & Doctor, B. P. (1999). Differences in Active-Site Gorge Dimensions of Cholinesterases Revealed by Binding of Inhibitors to Human Butyrylcholinesterase. *Chemico-Biological Interactions*, Vol.119-120, (May 1999), pp. 61-9, ISSN 0009-2797

Saxena, A.; Redman, A. M.; Jiang, X.; Lockridge, O. & Doctor, B. P. (1997). Differences in Active Site Gorge Dimensions of Cholinesterases Revealed by Binding of Inhibitors to Human Butyrylcholinesterase. *Biochemistry*, Vol.36, No.48, (December 1997), pp. 14642-51, ISSN 0006-2960

Soreq, H. & Zaku, H. (1993). *Human Cholinesterases and Anticholinesterases*, Academic Press, ISBN 978-012-6552-90-4, San Diego, USA

Sussman, J. L.; Harel, M.; Frolow, F.; Oefner, C.; Goldman, A.; Toker, L. & Silman, I. (1991). Atomic Structure of Acetylcholinesterase from Torpedo californica: A Prototypic Acetylcholine-Binding Protein. *Science*, Vol.253, No.5022, (August 1991), pp. 872-9, ISSN 0036-8075

Sybyl, V. (2007). 7.3, Tripos Inc, St. *Louis, MO*, pp.

Tame, J. R. (1999). Scoring Functions: A View from the Bench. *Journal of Computer-Aided Molecular Design*, Vol.13, No.2, (March 1999), pp. 99-108, ISSN 0920-654X

Terry, A. V., Jr. & Buccafusco, J. J. (2003). The Cholinergic Hypothesis of Age and Alzheimer's Disease-Related Cognitive Deficits: Recent Challenges and their Implications for Novel Drug Development. *The Journal of Pharmacology and Experimental Therapeutics*, Vol.306, No.3, (September 2003), pp. 821-27, ISSN 0022-3565

Todorov, N. P.; Mancera, R. L. & Monthoux, P. H. (2003). A New Quantum Stochastic Tunnelling Optimisation Method for Protein-Ligand Docking *Chemical Physics Letters*, Vol.369, No.3-4, (February 2003), pp. 257-263, ISSN 0009-2614

Tormos, J. R.; Wiley, K. L.; Seravalli, J.; Nachon, F.; Masson, P.; Nicolet, Y. & Quinn, D. M. (2005). The Reactant State for Substrate-Activated Turnover of Acetylthiocholine by Butyrylcholinesterase is a Tetrahedral Intermediate. *Journal of the American Chemical Society*, Vol.127, No.42, (October 2005), pp. 14538-9, ISSN 0002-7863

Vicker, N.; Ho, Y.; Robinson, J.; Woo, L. L.; Purohit, A.; Reed, M. J. & Potter, B. V. (2003). Docking Studies of Sulphamate Inhibitors of Estrone Sulphatase in Human Carbonic Anhydrase II. *Bioorganic Medicinal Chemistry Letters*, Vol.13, No.5, (March 2003), pp. 863-5, ISSN 0960-894X

Viswanadhan, V. N.; Ghose, A. K.; Revankar, G. R. & Robins, R. K. (1989). Atomic Physicochemical Parameters for Three Dimensional Structure Directed Quantitative Structure-Activity Relationships. 4. Additional Parameters for Hydrophobic and Dispersive Interactions and their Application for an Automated Superposition of

Certain Naturally Occurring Nucleoside Antibiotics. *Journal of Chemical Information and Computer Sciences*, Vol.29, No.3, (August 1989), pp. 163 - 172, ISSN 1549-9596

Wang, L.; Merz, A. J.; Collins, K. M. & Wickner, W. (2003). Hierarchy of Protein Assembly at the Vertex Ring Domain for Yeast Vacuole Docking and Fusion. *Journal of Cell Biology*, Vol.160, No.3, (February 2003), pp. 365-74, ISSN 0021-9525

Wei, H. Y.; Tsai, K. C. & Lin, T. H. (2005). Modeling Ligand- Receptor Interaction for Some MHC Class II HLA-DR4 Peptide Mimetic Inhibitors Using Several Molecular Docking and 3D QSAR Techniques. *Journal of Chemical Information and Modeling*, Vol.45, No.5, (September-October 2005), pp. 1343-1351, ISSN 1549-9596

Wu, X.; Milne, J. L.; Borgnia, M. J.; Rostapshov, A. V.; Subramaniam, S. & Brooks, B. R. (2003). A Core-Weighted Fitting Method for Docking Atomic Structures into Low-Resolution Maps: Application to Cryo-Electron Microscopy. *Journal of Structural Biology*, Vol.141, No.1, (January 2003), pp. 63-76, ISSN 1047-8477

Xie, W.; Stribley, J. A.; Chatonnet, A.; Wilder, P. J.; Rizzino, A.; McComb, R. D.; Taylor, P.; Hinrichs, S. H. & Lockridge, O. (2000). Postnatal Developmental Delay and Supersensitivity to Organophosphate in Gene-Targeted Mice Lacking Acetylcholinesterase. *Journal of Pharmacology and Experimental Therapeutics*, Vol.293, No.3, (June 2000), pp. 896-902, ISSN 0022-3565

Yuan, H.; Kozikowski, A. P. & Petukhov, P. A. (2004). CoMFA Study of Piperidine Analogues of Cocaine at the Dopamine Transporter: Exploring the Binding Mode of the 3 Alpha-Substituent of the Piperidine Ring Using Pharmacophore-Based Flexible Alignment. *Journal of Medicinal Chemistry*, Vol.47, No.25, (December 2004), pp. 6137-43, ISSN 0022-2623

Yuan, H. & Petukhov, P. A. (2006). Improved 3D-QSAR CoMFA of the Dopamine Transporter Blockers with Multiple Conformations Using the Genetic Algorithm. *Bioorganic and Medicinal Chemistry Letters*, Vol.16, No.24, (December 2006), pp. 6267-72, ISSN 0960-894X

Zaheer-Ul-Haq; Wellenzohn, B.; Liedl, K. R. & Rode, B. M. (2003). Molecular Docking Studies of Natural Cholinesterase-Inhibiting Steroidal Alkaloids from Sarcococca saligna. *Journal of Medicinal Chemistry*, Vol.46, No.23, (November 2003), pp. 5087-90, ISSN 0022-2623

Zaheer ul, H.; Uddin, R.; Yuan, H.; Petukhov, P. A.; Choudhary, M. I. & Madura, J. D. (2008). Receptor-based modeling and 3D-QSAR for a quantitative production of the butyrylcholinesterase inhibitors based on genetic algorithm. *Journal of Chemical Information and Modeling*, Vol.48, No.5, pp. 1092-1103, ISSN 1549-9596

Zaheer ul, H.; Wellenzohn, B.; Tonmunphean, S.; Khalid, A.; Choudhary, M. I. & Rode, B. M. (2003). 3D-QSAR Studies on Natural Acetylcholinesterase inhibitors of Sarcococca saligna by comparative molecular field analysis (CoMFA). *Bioorg Med Chem Lett*, Vol.13, No.24, (Dec 15), pp. 4375-80, ISSN 0960-894X

Zhou, Z.; Fisher, D.; Spidel, J.; Greenfield, J.; Patson, B.; Fazal, A.; Wigal, C.; Moe, O. A. & Madura, J. D. (2003). Kinetic and Docking Studies of the Interaction of Quinones with the Quinone Reductase Active Site. *Biochemistry*, Vol.42, No.7, (February 2003), pp. 1985-94, ISSN 0006-2960

Part 7

Potential Therapeutic Strategies

27

Tau Oligomers as Potential Drug Target for Alzheimer Disease (AD) Treatment

Rakez Kayed
University of Texas Medical Branch
USA

1. Introduction

The microtubule-associated protein tau is required for microtubule assembly, axonal transport, neurite outgrowth, and stability of microtubules (Binder *et al.* 1985). Tau self-assembly, aggregation, and accumulation in neurofibrillary tangles (NFTs) are major pathological hallmarks of Alzheimer disease (AD) and other neurodegenerative diseases (Lee *et al.* 2001, Alonso *et al.* 2008). Although the importance of tau in AD and other tauopathies is well established (Iqbal *et al.* 2009, Ballatore *et al.* 2007, Haroutunian *et al.* 2007) still unanswered is whether NFTs are the primary neurotoxic factor (Brunden *et al.* 2008, Marx 2007, Kayed & Jackson 2009).

Despite the poor correlation between NFTs and disease progression, and evidence showing, that neuronal loss in AD actually precedes NFTs formation research until recently focused on them and other large meta-stable inclusions composed of aggregated hyperphosphorylated tau protein. Lately, the significance and toxicity of NFTs have been challenged and new aggregated tau entity has emerged as the true pathogenic species in tauopathies and a possible mediator of Aβ toxicity in AD. Tau intermediate aggregate (tau oligomers; aggregates of an intermediate that is between monomers and NFTs in size) can cause neurodegeneration and memory impairment in the absence of Aβ. This exciting body of evidence includes results from human brain samples, transgenic mouse and cell-based studies, thus tau oligomers present a new and novel drug target for AD treatment.

In this chapter, we summarize the characterization and toxicity of tau oligomers; discuss the evidence supporting their critical role in AD pathogenesis, and the potential and challenges for targeting them by immunotherapy and drug discovery as a novel approach for AD treatment

2. Tau oligomer formation

A key early finding about tau in NFTs accumulated in AD and non-AD tauopathies was the fact that it is abnormally phosphorylated (Spires-Jones *et al.* 2009, Grundke-Iqbal *et al.* 1986). The sequence of early tau phosphorylation suggests that there are events prior to NFT formation that are specific to particular phosphorylated tau epitopes, leading to conformational changes and cytopathological alterations. Using phosphorylation dependent tau antibodies, three stages of NFT development were introduced: *(1)* pre-NFT, *(2)* intra-, and *(3)* extra-neuronal NFT. The pre-NFT state, in which neurons display nonfibrillar, punctate regions in the cytoplasm, dendrites, somata, and nuclei, was observed especially with phospho-tau antibodies TG3 (pT231), pS262, and pT153. Intraneuronal NFTs were homogeneously stained with fibrillar tau structures, which were most prominently stained with pT175/181, 12E8 (pS262/pS356), pS422, pS46, pS214 antibodies. Extracellular NFTs, which contain substantial filamentous tau, are most prominently stained with AT8 (pS199/pS202/pT205), AT100 (pT212/pS214), and PHF-1 (pS396/pS404) antibodies, which also stain intracellular NFT. Moreover, the severity of AD and neuronal loss correlates with the patterns of tau phosphorylation in NFT(Augustinack *et al.* 2002, Trinczek *et al.* 1995).

Tau hyperphosphorylation is thought to be an early event in the cascade leading from soluble to insoluble tau protein, but evidence demonstrating that hyperphosphorylation is sufficient for filament formation is lacking. Why does hyperphosphorylation promote aggregation of tau proteins into abnormal filaments? One possibility is that the negative charge imparted by phosphorylation neutralizes the basic charges of tau, thus facilitating intermolecular interaction and aggregation (Alonso *et al.* 2001a, Alonso *et al.* 2001b). An alternative explanation is that hyperphosphorylation detaches tau from microtubules, thus increasing the pool of unbound tau. Unbound, hyperphosphorylated tau may compete with microtubules for binding to normal tau and other microtubule associated proteins, thereby sequestering them and enhancing disassembly of microtubules (Alonso et al. 2001a). As compared to microtubule-bound tau, this unbound tau may be more degradation-resistant and more likely to aggregate. Reduced proteolysis of hyperphosphorylated tau may also increase the pool of soluble tau available for formation of paired helical filaments (PHF). Thus, abnormal phosphorylation of tau may result in an increase in the total cellular pool of tau, and may change its solubility, thus negatively regulating stability of microtubules (Litersky & Johnson 1992, Litersky & Johnson 1995, Litersky *et al.* 1993).

One important contributor to tau phosphorylation and NFT formation may be amyloid. The "amyloid cascade" hypothesis holds that the accumulation of Aβ peptides in senile plaques results in the formation of NFTs and neuronal cell death (Busciglio *et al.* 1995). In primary neuronal cultures, Aβ is capable of inducing tau phosphorylation (Busciglio et al. 1995). Aβ42 fibrils induced formation of neurofibrillary tangles in P301L tau transgenic mice (Gotz *et al.* 2001), and pre-aggregated Aβ42 induced PHF formation mediated by distinct phospho-epitopes of tau in cells overexpressing wild-type and mutant forms of human tau (Ferrari *et al.* 2003, Pennanen & Gotz 2005). Aβ oligomers, but not the soluble or fibrillar forms of Aβ, induced tau hyperphosphorylation in cells overexpressing human tau(De Felice *et al.* 2008); this phenomenon is not Aβ-specific, but rather conformation specific, as demonstrated by the ability of soluble oligomers from a non-disease related protein, hen egg white lysozyme, to mimic tau hyperphosphorylation induced by Aβ aggregates(Vieira *et al.* 2007).

Amyloid formation is a complex process that involves many morphologically and conformationally distinct species. The critical role of soluble amyloid oligomers in neurodegeneration has become generally accepted for multiple neurodegenerative diseases (Haass & Selkoe 2007, Brunden et al. 2008, Glabe 2006, Glabe 2008). Very little is known about tau oligomers, because reliable methods for preparing homogeneous populations of tau oligomers are lacking, which prevents researchers from studying them and testing chemical and other approaches to combating their formation and toxicity.

Unlike Aβ peptide,which is highly prone to aggregation and spontaneously forms amyloid in vitro, tau is an unfolded, soluble protein. In vitro aggregation of tau into filaments can be achieved using high concentrations and via the addition of promoters (Avila *et al.* 2004,

Barghorn *et al.* 2005, Barghorn & Mandelkow 2002). Mechanistic studies of full-length tau protein aggregation and filament formation in vitro have revealed striking similarities to Aβ aggregation; tau aggregates via either a nucleation-dependent mechanism (Congdon & Duff 2008) or the formation of intermediates (Xu *et al.*). In vitro, amyloid fibrils can accelerate the aggregation of the same protein via a nucleation-dependent mechanism, i.e., "seeding" (Jarrett *et al.* 1993, Kelly 2000). Seeding refers to the addition of a substoichiometric amount of fibrils, intact or sonicated, to a monomeric solution of the same protein, thus increasing the rate of conversion to amyloid fibrils. Lately, we and others have reported methods for preparing homogeneous Aβ and α-synuclein amyloid species (e.g., oligomers and fibrils) (Kayed *et al.* 2003, Kayed *et al.* 2007). These techniques provide an opportunity to test the effectiveness of different amyloid species as seeds. We have observed that amyloid oligomers similar to fibrils, can seed and induce monomer aggregation and oligomer formation (Kayed et al. 2007, Kayed & Glabe 2006). As we mentioned above it is well established that aggregated Aβ makes an important contribution to tau phosphorylation and aggregation in animal models and cell cultures. These experiments have used aggregated Aβ, which is likely to contain different prefibrillar and fibrillar Aβ aggregates. We recently demonstrated that Aβ42 and α-synuclein oligomer seeds induce the conversion of unstructured,monomeric human recombinant tau into β-sheet rich toxic tau oligomers(Lasagna-Reeves *et al.* 2010). This study show the ability of oligomer to cross-seed in vitro and induce tau aggregation

Tau oligomers prepared by this novel method were largely SDS-stable apparent trimers and display a spherical morphology similar to oligomers formed by other amyloidogenic proteins (Kayed & Glabe 2006, Kayed *et al.* 2004). When shaken in PBS buffer for longer periods of time, tau oligomers prepared by this method continue to aggregate and eventually form tau filaments. Biophysical characterization of tau oligomers demonstrates that tau oligomers are β-sheet rich with minimal ellipticity as compared with the natively unfolded monomeric tau, which shows a random coil with minimal ellipticity(Lasagna-Reeves et al. 2010).

Dynamic oligomers represent a toxic amyloid species that is conformationally distinct from fibrils and monomers. Targeting oligomers is a challenge that requires reliable protocols and reagents. Further investigations and analysis are needed to elucidate the synergy between different oligomer species and the contribution of amyloid oligomers to the induction of tau aggregation and to understand fully the role of tau oligomers in tauopathies.

2.1 Tau oligomers toxicity in vivo

The correlation between NFT in the brains of AD patients the disease progression remains contentious. Many studies have shown corelation between NFT and disease progresstion (Braak & Braak 1991, Delacourte & Buee 2000, Morsch *et al.* 1999, Bretteville & Planel 2008, Congdon & Duff 2008, Arriagada *et al.* 1992, Bird *et al.* 1999, Hernandez & Avila 2008, Rankin & Gamblin 2008, Cash *et al.* 2003, Tabaton *et al.* 1989). Other stereological studies show that neuronal loss actually exceeds NFT formation (Gomez-Isla et al. 1997, Terry 2000, van de Nes *et al.* 2008, Vogt *et al.* 1998). This and the exciting data published in the last half decade, emerging from biochemical, cell-based and transgenic mouse studies suggest that pre-filament forms of tau may be the most toxic and pathologically significant form of tau aggregates (Brunden et al. 2008, Marx 2007, Kayed *et al.* 2009, Meraz-Rios *et al.* 2009). This evolutionary transition was overdue in the tau field and similar to the transition witnessed for Aβ in the last 15 years driven by the characterization of Aβ intermediate species and their crucial role in Aβ-mediated toxicity (Harper *et al.* 1997, Roher *et al.* 1993, Walsh & Selkoe 2004, Walsh & Selkoe 2007).

Analogous to Aβ oligomers, tau oligomers have been shown to be neurotoxic when applied extracellularlly to cultured neuronal cells (Lasagna-Reeves et al. 2010) and to provoke an increase in intracellular calcium levels (Gomez-Ramos *et al.* 2006, Gomez-Ramos *et al.* 2008). Detailed characterization of newly developed tau animal models suggests that tau oligomers play a key role in eliciting neurodegeneration and behavioral impairments. These phenotypes are concurrent with accumulation of soluble aggregated tau species and dissociated from the accumulation of NFT (Brunden et al. 2008). Cell death and synaptic lesions occurred independently of NFT formation (h-tau mice) expressing non-mutant human tau (Andorfer et al. 2005, Polydoro et al. 2009); hippocampal synapse loss, impaired synaptic function and microgliosis precede the formation of NFT in the P301S mutant human tau transgenic mouse model (P301S Tg) (Yoshiyama et al. 2007), similar resuls were found in (Tau(RD)/deltaK280) mouse model, (Mocanu *et al.* 2008), fly model (Wittmann *et al.* 2001) and zebra fish model (Paquet *et al.* 2009). Tau oligomers were biochemically characterized in JNPL3 mice expressing human tau with the P301L mutation, and the conditional model (rTg4510) expressing the same P301L human tau mutant; surprisingly, the accumulation of oligomeric tau correlated best with neuronal loss and behavioral deficits in these models, whereas NFT did not. These findings suggest that the accumulation of tau oligomers, behavioral deficits and neuronal loss precede the formation NFT (Berger et al. 2007, Spires et al. 2006). Tau oligomers were biochemically characterized in post mortem human brain, and a correlation between disease progression and the accumulation of granular tau oligomers in the brains of AD patients was reported. Moreover, increased levels of tau oligomers detected in the frontal cortex at very early stage of the disease (Braak stage I), when clinical symptoms of AD and NFT are believed to be absent. This finding suggests that an increase in tau oligomer levels occurs before NFT formation and before individuals manifest clinical symptoms of AD (Maeda et al. 2007, Maeda et al. 2006). Tau-positive fine granules (TFGs) resembling tau oligomers were found in the cerebral white matter of post mortem tissue from the parkinsonism-dementia complex of guam (PDC) tauopathy (Yamazaki et al. 2005). The data discussed here support the notion that soluble oligomers of amyloid proteins including tau are the acutely toxic structures of these proteins, rather than insoluble aggregates such as plaques and tangles. This concept has become more generally accepted for multiple neurodegenerative diseases including AD and tauopathies (Haass & Selkoe 2007, Brunden et al. 2008).

Recently, we investigated the neurotoxiciy of different forms of tau in vivo by injecting well characterized oligomers , fibrils, or monomers of full length recombinant h-tau-441 (2N4R) into the hippocampus of C57BL/6 wild-mice. We found that the mice injected with tau oligomers presented with memory deficits in their performance of the novel-object recognition task, (Lasagna-Reeves 2010) which is widely used for evaluating memory in AD mouse models (Huang et al., 2006; Mouri et al., 2007; Scholtzova et al., 2008; Zhang et al., 2006). These observations correlate with previous studies in humans and primates that have shown hippocampal lesions to result in impaired object recognition (Reed and Squire, 1997; Zola et al., 2000).We also showed the loss of synaptic-related proteins and mitochondrial respiratory chain components in conjunction with the activation of the mitochondrial dysfunction markers and the pro-apoptotic protein caspase-9. Our results strongly suggest that tau oligomers result in learning impairment through the disruption of synaptic and mitochondrial functions. If we take into consideration these studies and the novel data presented above, we can postulate that tau oligomers generated intracellularly could be released either by binding and local rupture of the membrane, or after cell death. The oligomers in the extracellular space could be taken up by healthy neurons in the vicinity disrupt normal activity like lysosomal function and stimulate further aggregation of functional monomeric tau. Thus, understanding the negative impact of tau oligomers in neuronal damage, specifically in reference to important cellular mechanisms, such as mitochondrial and synaptic function, will likely be of great importance to understanding the relevant disease processes and progression in AD and other tauopathies.

2.1.1 Tau based therapies

The important role of tau in neurodegenerative diseases, supports tau as a potential target for the development of disease modifying therapeutics. Therapeutic approaches targeting tau include, (1) interference with the splicing machinery to decrease the four-repeat tau isoforms, (2) activation of proteolytic or proteasomal degradation pathways, (3) prevention/reduction of tau hyperphosphorylation using inhibitors of tau kinases, (4) pharmacological stabilization of microtubule networks, (5) inhibition of tau aggregation by small molecules, and (6) tau-directed immunotherapy (Schneider & Mandelkow 2008).

Inhibition of tau hyperphosphorylation: This approach to treat AD was first introduced in 1998 (Gong & Iqbal 2008). Although a kinase inhibitor was shown to reduce tau hyperphosphorylation and the formation of soluble aggregated tau and to prevent motor deficits in mice expressing mutant human tau (Iqbal & Grundke-Iqbal 1998), a major drawback to targeting kinases is that these enzymes are commonly found throughout the body playing normal physiological roles and their inhibition may have unwanted side effects.

Activation of proteolytic or degradation pathway: Tau was found to be sensitive to calpain protolysis (Johnson *et al.* 1989). Recently, puromycin-sensitive aminopeptidase (PSA), which was identified by a genetic screen as a modifier of tau pathology (Abazov *et al.* 2006), was shown to be effective in degrading both recombinant and PHF tau purified from AD brain(82)

Stabilization of microtubules: Microtubule-binding drugs could be beneficial in treating tauopathies by functionally substituting for the MT-binding protein tau (Trojanowski *et al.* 2005). Paclitaxel, a drug know to bind and stabilize microtubule, was tested in transgenic mice and showed to be effective in restoring axonal transport and ameliorating motor impairments (Zhang *et al.* 2005)

Inhibition of tau aggregation by small molecules: The last decade has witnessed a renaissance of interest in inhibitors of tau aggregation as potential disease-modifying drugs. A search for non-toxic, cell penetrant inhibitors of tau aggregation capable of crossing the blood-brain barrier (BBB) was performed using a high throughput screen, which resulted in the identification of more than 139 hits (Pickhardt *et al.* 2005, Larbig *et al.* 2007). This and the recent report of a phase-II clinical trial with the tau aggregation inhibitor MTC (ma ethylene blue derivative) could hold promise for the validation of the concept. The research on tau aggregation inhibitors was recently reviewed (Bulic et al. 2009).

Tau clearance by immunotherapy: Tau immunotherapy is a new concept (Sigurdsson 2009). A few reports of tau immunotherapy in animal models have been published, all using active vaccination (Boimel *et al.* , Asuni *et al.* 2007, Boutajangout *et al.* 2010). In these reports, the authors used tau fragments phosphorylated at positions commonly associated with NFT, such as Ser396 and Ser404. Behavioral analysis showed improved performance after immunization as compared to controls, biochemical and immunohistochemical i analyses showed reduction of both soluble and insoluble tau species, moreover the studies showed reduction of phosphorylated NFTs in the brains of these animals. One study clearly demonstrated that antibodies were able to cross the blood-brain barrier and bind to phosphorylated tau (Asuni et al. 2007). Although the use of phosphorylated tau antigens seems promising for vaccination studies, such an approach mainly targets NFTs, rather than pre-filament tau species (tau oligomers) which form at early stages of NFT development (Kayed & Jackson 2009, Kayed 2010).

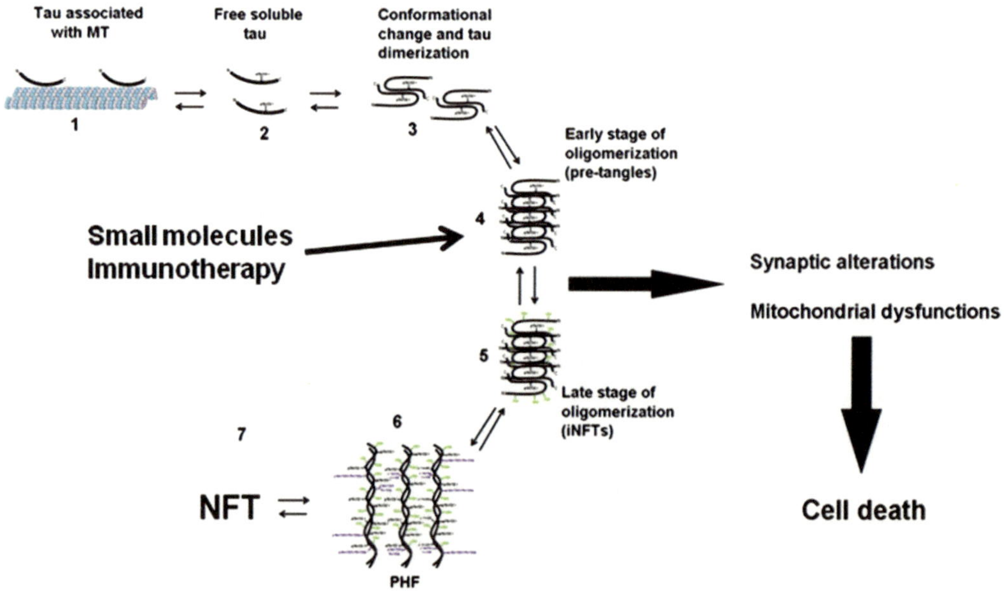

Fig. 1. Schematic presentation of tau aggregation, and the potential therapeutic approaches targeting tau oligomers.

3. Conclusion

Despite extensive efforts to develop anti amyloid treatments the results have, been disappointing. This led to the resurgence of tau as a potential therapeutic target for the treatment of AD. The question remains, which form of tau is the best target? The elegant studies over the past decade argue that soluble tau oligomers represent the primary pathological species of tau, therefore elucidating the pathways and mechanisms triggering their formation and understanding their mechanisms of toxicity are of immense importance. Studies focused on developing anti tau therapies must dissect the targets and better illuminate mechanisms of action for such approaches on each tau entity. As a starting point, it is important to evaluate the effects of immunotherapy and other therapeutic approaches on tau oligomers, this will be helpful for optimization of these approaches and may lead to the development of disease modifying therapies for AD and other neurodegenerative diseases.

4. Acknowledgment

Supported by the Cullen Trust, the Alzheimer`s Drug Discovery foundation (ADDF), and the Mitchell Center to Neurodegenerative Diseases. I am grateful for Dr. Cristian Lasagna-Reeves, and Prof. George Jackson for their helpful suggestions.

5. References

Abazov, V. M., Abbott, B., Abolins, M. et al. (2006) Search for neutral Higgs bosons decaying to tau pairs in pp[over] collisions at sqrt[s]=1.96 TeV. *Phys Rev Lett,* 97, 121802.

Alonso, A., Zaidi, T., Novak, M., Grundke-Iqbal, I. and Iqbal, K. (2001a) Hyperphosphorylation induces self-assembly of tau into tangles of paired helical filaments/straight filaments. *Proc Natl Acad Sci U S A,* 98, 6923-6928.

Alonso, A. C., Li, B., Grundke-Iqbal, I. and Iqbal, K. (2008) Mechanism of tau-induced neurodegeneration in Alzheimer disease and related tauopathies. *Curr Alzheimer Res,* 5, 375-384.

Alonso, A. D., Zaidi, T., Novak, M., Barra, H. S., Grundke-Iqbal, I. and Iqbal, K. (2001b) Interaction of tau isoforms with Alzheimer's disease abnormally hyperphosphorylated tau and in vitro phosphorylation into the disease-like protein. *J Biol Chem,* 276, 37967-37973.

Andorfer, C., Acker, C. M., Kress, Y., Hof, P. R., Duff, K. and Davies, P. (2005) Cell-cycle reentry and cell death in transgenic mice expressing nonmutant human tau isoforms. *J Neurosci,* 25, 5446-5454.

Arriagada, P. V., Growdon, J. H., Hedley-Whyte, E. T. and Hyman, B. T. (1992) Neurofibrillary tangles but not senile plaques parallel duration and severity of Alzheimer's disease. *Neurology,* 42, 631-639.

Asuni, A. A., Boutajangout, A., Quartermain, D. and Sigurdsson, E. M. (2007) Immunotherapy targeting pathological tau conformers in a tangle mouse model reduces brain pathology with associated functional improvements. *J Neurosci,* 27, 9115-9129.

Augustinack, J. C., Schneider, A., Mandelkow, E. M. and Hyman, B. T. (2002) Specific tau phosphorylation sites correlate with severity of neuronal cytopathology in Alzheimer's disease. *Acta Neuropathol,* 103, 26-35.

Avila, J., Perez, M., Lucas, J. J., Gomez-Ramos, A., Santa Maria, I., Moreno, F., Smith, M., Perry, G. and Hernandez, F. (2004) Assembly in vitro of tau protein and its implications in Alzheimer's disease. *Curr Alzheimer Res,* 1, 97-101.

Ballatore, C., Lee, V. M. and Trojanowski, J. Q. (2007) Tau-mediated neurodegeneration in Alzheimer's disease and related disorders. *Nat Rev Neurosci,* 8, 663-672.

Barghorn, S., Biernat, J. and Mandelkow, E. (2005) Purification of recombinant tau protein and preparation of Alzheimer-paired helical filaments in vitro. *Methods Mol Biol,* 299, 35-51.

Barghorn, S. and Mandelkow, E. (2002) Toward a unified scheme for the aggregation of tau into Alzheimer paired helical filaments. *Biochemistry,* 41, 14885-14896.

Berger, Z., Roder, H., Hanna, A. et al. (2007) Accumulation of pathological tau species and memory loss in a conditional model of tauopathy. *J Neurosci,* 27, 3650-3662.

Binder, L. I., Frankfurter, A. and Rebhun, L. I. (1985) The distribution of tau in the mammalian central nervous system. *J Cell Biol,* 101, 1371-1378.

Bird, T. D., Nochlin, D., Poorkaj, P. et al. (1999) A clinical pathological comparison of three families with frontotemporal dementia and identical mutations in the tau gene (P301L). *Brain,* 122 (Pt 4), 741-756.

Boimel, M., Grigoriadis, N., Lourbopoulos, A., Haber, E., Abramsky, O. and Rosenmann, H. Efficacy and safety of immunization with phosphorylated tau against neurofibrillary tangles in mice. *Exp Neurol,* 224, 472-485.

Boutajangout, A., Quartermain, D. and Sigurdsson, E. M. (2010) Immunotherapy targeting pathological tau prevents cognitive decline in a new tangle mouse model. *J Neurosci,* 30, 16559-16566.

Braak, H. and Braak, E. (1991) Neuropathological stageing of Alzheimer-related changes. *Acta Neuropathol,* 82, 239-259.

Bretteville, A. and Planel, E. (2008) Tau aggregates: toxic, inert, or protective species? *J Alzheimers Dis,* 14, 431-436.

Brunden, K. R., Trojanowski, J. Q. and Lee, V. M. (2008) Evidence that non-fibrillar tau causes pathology linked to neurodegeneration and behavioral impairments. *J Alzheimers Dis,* 14, 393-399.

Bulic, B., Pickhardt, M., Schmidt, B., Mandelkow, E. M., Waldmann, H. and Mandelkow, E. (2009) Development of tau aggregation inhibitors for Alzheimer's disease. *Angew Chem Int Ed Engl,* 48, 1740-1752.

Busciglio, J., Lorenzo, A., Yeh, J. and Yankner, B. A. (1995) beta-amyloid fibrils induce tau phosphorylation and loss of microtubule binding. *Neuron,* 14, 879-888.

Cash, A. D., Aliev, G., Siedlak, S. L. et al. (2003) Microtubule reduction in Alzheimer's disease and aging is independent of tau filament formation. *Am J Pathol,* 162, 1623-1627.

Congdon, E. E. and Duff, K. E. (2008) Is tau aggregation toxic or protective? *J Alzheimers Dis,* 14, 453-457.

De Felice, F. G., Wu, D., Lambert, M. P. et al. (2008) Alzheimer's disease-type neuronal tau hyperphosphorylation induced by A beta oligomers. *Neurobiol Aging,* 29, 1334-1347.

Delacourte, A. and Buee, L. (2000) Tau pathology: a marker of neurodegenerative disorders. *Curr Opin Neurol,* 13, 371-376.

Ferrari, A., Hoerndli, F., Baechi, T., Nitsch, R. M. and Gotz, J. (2003) beta-Amyloid induces paired helical filament-like tau filaments in tissue culture. *J Biol Chem,* 278, 40162-40168.

Glabe, C. G. (2006) Common mechanisms of amyloid oligomer pathogenesis in degenerative disease. *Neurobiol Aging,* 27, 570-575.

Glabe, C. G. (2008) Structural classification of toxic amyloid oligomers. *J Biol Chem,* 283, 29639-29643.

Gomez-Isla, T., Hollister, R., West, H., Mui, S., Growdon, J. H., Petersen, R. C., Parisi, J. E. and Hyman, B. T. (1997) Neuronal loss correlates with but exceeds neurofibrillary tangles in Alzheimer's disease. *Ann Neurol,* 41, 17-24.

Gomez-Ramos, A., Diaz-Hernandez, M., Cuadros, R., Hernandez, F. and Avila, J. (2006) Extracellular tau is toxic to neuronal cells. *FEBS Lett,* 580, 4842-4850.

Gomez-Ramos, A., Diaz-Hernandez, M., Rubio, A., Miras-Portugal, M. T. and Avila, J. (2008) Extracellular tau promotes intracellular calcium increase through M1 and M3 muscarinic receptors in neuronal cells. *Mol Cell Neurosci,* 37, 673-681.

Gong, C. X. and Iqbal, K. (2008) Hyperphosphorylation of microtubule-associated protein tau: a promising therapeutic target for Alzheimer disease. *Curr Med Chem,* 15, 2321-2328.

Gotz, J., Chen, F., van Dorpe, J. and Nitsch, R. M. (2001) Formation of neurofibrillary tangles in P301l tau transgenic mice induced by Abeta 42 fibrils. *Science,* 293, 1491-1495.

Grundke-Iqbal, I., Iqbal, K., Tung, Y. C., Quinlan, M., Wisniewski, H. M. and Binder, L. I. (1986) Abnormal phosphorylation of the microtubule-associated protein tau (tau) in Alzheimer cytoskeletal pathology. *Proc Natl Acad Sci U S A,* 83, 4913-4917.

Haass, C. and Selkoe, D. J. (2007) Soluble protein oligomers in neurodegeneration: lessons from the Alzheimer's amyloid beta-peptide. *Nat Rev Mol Cell Biol,* 8, 101-112.

Haroutunian, V., Davies, P., Vianna, C., Buxbaum, J. D. and Purohit, D. P. (2007) Tau protein abnormalities associated with the progression of alzheimer disease type dementia. *Neurobiol Aging,* 28, 1-7.

Harper, J. D., Wong, S. S., Lieber, C. M. and Lansbury, P. T. (1997) Observation of metastable Abeta amyloid protofibrils by atomic force microscopy. *Chem Biol,* 4, 119-125.

Hernandez, F. and Avila, J. (2008) Tau aggregates and tau pathology. *J Alzheimers Dis,* 14, 449-452.

Iqbal, K. and Grundke-Iqbal, I. (1998) Tau phosphatase activity as a therapeutic target for AD. *Drug News Perspect,* 11, 10-14.

Iqbal, K., Liu, F., Gong, C. X., Alonso, A. D. and Grundke-Iqbal, I. (2009) Mechanisms of tau-induced neurodegeneration. *Acta Neuropathol,* 118, 53-69.

Jarrett, J. T., Berger, E. P. and Lansbury, P. T., Jr. (1993) The carboxy terminus of the beta amyloid protein is critical for the seeding of amyloid formation: implications for the pathogenesis of Alzheimer's disease. *Biochemistry,* 32, 4693-4697.

Johnson, G. V., Jope, R. S. and Binder, L. I. (1989) Proteolysis of tau by calpain. *Biochem Biophys Res Commun,* 163, 1505-1511.

Kayed, R. (2010) Anti-tau oligomers passive vaccination for the treatment of Alzheimer's disease. *Hum Vaccin,* 6, 47-51.

Kayed, R. and Glabe, C. G. (2006) Conformation-dependent anti-amyloid oligomer antibodies. *Methods Enzymol,* 413, 326-344.

Kayed, R., Head, E., Sarsoza, F. et al. (2007) Fibril specific, conformation dependent antibodies recognize a generic epitope common to amyloid fibrils and fibrillar oligomers that is absent in prefibrillar oligomers. *Mol Neurodegener,* 2, 18.

Kayed, R., Head, E., Thompson, J. L., McIntire, T. M., Milton, S. C., Cotman, C. W. and Glabe, C. G. (2003) Common structure of soluble amyloid oligomers implies common mechanism of pathogenesis. *Science,* 300, 486-489.

Kayed, R. and Jackson, G. R. (2009) Prefilament tau species as potential targets for immunotherapy for Alzheimer disease and related disorders. *Curr Opin Immunol,* 21, 359-363.

Kayed, R., Pensalfini, A., Margol, L., Sokolov, Y., Sarsoza, F., Head, E., Hall, J. and Glabe, C. (2009) Annular protofibrils are a structurally and functionally distinct type of amyloid oligomer. *J Biol Chem,* 284, 4230-4237.

Kayed, R., Sokolov, Y., Edmonds, B., McIntire, T. M., Milton, S. C., Hall, J. E. and Glabe, C. G. (2004) Permeabilization of lipid bilayers is a common conformation-dependent activity of soluble amyloid oligomers in protein misfolding diseases. *J Biol Chem,* 279, 46363-46366.

Kelly, J. W. (2000) Mechanisms of amyloidogenesis. *Nat Struct Biol,* 7, 824-826.

Larbig, G., Pickhardt, M., Lloyd, D. G., Schmidt, B. and Mandelkow, E. (2007) Screening for inhibitors of tau protein aggregation into Alzheimer paired helical filaments: a ligand based approach results in successful scaffold hopping. *Curr Alzheimer Res,* 4, 315-323.

Lasagna-Reeves, C. A., Castillo-Carranza, D. L., Guerrero-Muoz, M. J., Jackson, G. R. and Kayed, R. (2010) Preparation and characterization of neurotoxic tau oligomers. *Biochemistry,* 49, 10039-10041.

Lasagna-Reeves, C. A. C.-C., D.L. Clos, A.L. Sengupta, U. Jackson, G.R. Kayed. R. (2010) Tau oligomers impair memory and induce synaptic and mitochondrial dysfunction in wild type mice. *Society for Neuroscience, San Diego, USA. November 2010.*

Lee, V. M., Goedert, M. and Trojanowski, J. Q. (2001) Neurodegenerative tauopathies. *Annu Rev Neurosci,* 24, 1121-1159.

Litersky, J. M. and Johnson, G. V. (1992) Phosphorylation by cAMP-dependent protein kinase inhibits the degradation of tau by calpain. *J Biol Chem,* 267, 1563-1568.

Litersky, J. M. and Johnson, G. V. (1995) Phosphorylation of tau in situ: inhibition of calcium-dependent proteolysis. *J Neurochem,* 65, 903-911.

Litersky, J. M., Scott, C. W. and Johnson, G. V. (1993) Phosphorylation, calpain proteolysis and tubulin binding of recombinant human tau isoforms. *Brain Res,* 604, 32-40.

Maeda, S., Sahara, N., Saito, Y. et al. (2007) Granular tau oligomers as intermediates of tau filaments. *Biochemistry,* 46, 3856-3861.

Maeda, S., Sahara, N., Saito, Y., Murayama, S., Ikai, A. and Takashima, A. (2006) Increased levels of granular tau oligomers: an early sign of brain aging and Alzheimer's disease. *Neurosci Res,* 54, 197-201.

Marx, J. (2007) Alzheimer's disease. A new take on tau. *Science,* 316, 1416-1417.

Meraz-Rios, M. A., Lira-De Leon, K. I., Campos-Pena, V., De Anda-Hernandez, M. A. and Mena-Lopez, R. (2009) Tau oligomers and aggregation in Alzheimer's disease. *J Neurochem.*

Mocanu, M. M., Nissen, A., Eckermann, K. et al. (2008) The potential for beta-structure in the repeat domain of tau protein determines aggregation, synaptic decay, neuronal loss, and coassembly with endogenous Tau in inducible mouse models of tauopathy. *J Neurosci,* 28, 737-748.

Morsch, R., Simon, W. and Coleman, P. D. (1999) Neurons may live for decades with neurofibrillary tangles. *J Neuropathol Exp Neurol,* 58, 188-197.

Paquet, D., Bhat, R., Sydow, A. et al. (2009) A zebrafish model of tauopathy allows in vivo imaging of neuronal cell death and drug evaluation. *J Clin Invest,* 119, 1382-1395.

Pennanen, L. and Gotz, J. (2005) Different tau epitopes define Abeta42-mediated tau insolubility. *Biochem Biophys Res Commun,* 337, 1097-1101.

Pickhardt, M., von Bergen, M., Gazova, Z., Hascher, A., Biernat, J., Mandelkow, E. M. and Mandelkow, E. (2005) Screening for inhibitors of tau polymerization. *Curr Alzheimer Res,* 2, 219-226.

Polydoro, M., Acker, C. M., Duff, K., Castillo, P. E. and Davies, P. (2009) Age-dependent impairment of cognitive and synaptic function in the htau mouse model of tau pathology. *J Neurosci,* 29, 10741-10749.

Rankin, C. A. and Gamblin, T. C. (2008) Assessing the toxicity of tau aggregation. *J Alzheimers Dis,* 14, 411-416.

Roher, A. E., Palmer, K. C., Yurewicz, E. C., Ball, M. J. and Greenberg, B. D. (1993) Morphological and Biochemical Analyses of Amyloid Plaque Core Proteins Purified from Alzheimer Disease Brain Tissue. *Journal of Neurochemistry,* 61, 1916-1926.

Schneider, A. and Mandelkow, E. (2008) Tau-based treatment strategies in neurodegenerative diseases. *Neurotherapeutics,* 5, 443-457.

Sigurdsson, E. M. (2009) Tau-focused immunotherapy for Alzheimer's disease and related tauopathies. *Curr Alzheimer Res,* 6, 446-450.

Spires-Jones, T. L., Stoothoff, W. H., de Calignon, A., Jones, P. B. and Hyman, B. T. (2009) Tau pathophysiology in neurodegeneration: a tangled issue. *Trends Neurosci,* 32, 150-159.

Spires, T. L., Orne, J. D., SantaCruz, K., Pitstick, R., Carlson, G. A., Ashe, K. H. and Hyman, B. T. (2006) Region-specific dissociation of neuronal loss and neurofibrillary pathology in a mouse model of tauopathy. *Am J Pathol,* 168, 1598-1607.

Tabaton, M., Cammarata, S., Manetto, V., Perry, G. and Mancardi, G. (1989) Tau-reactive neurofibrillary tangles in cerebellar cortex from patients with Alzheimer's disease. *Neurosci Lett,* 103, 259-262.

Terry, R. D. (2000) Do neuronal inclusions kill the cell? *J Neural Transm Suppl,* 59, 91-93.

Trinczek, B., Biernat, J., Baumann, K., Mandelkow, E. M. and Mandelkow, E. (1995) Domains of tau protein, differential phosphorylation, and dynamic instability of microtubules. *Mol Biol Cell,* 6, 1887-1902.

Trojanowski, J. Q., Smith, A. B., Huryn, D. and Lee, V. M. (2005) Microtubule-stabilising drugs for therapy of Alzheimer's disease and other neurodegenerative disorders with axonal transport impairments. *Expert Opin Pharmacother,* 6, 683-686.

van de Nes, J. A., Nafe, R. and Schlote, W. (2008) Non-tau based neuronal degeneration in Alzheimer's disease -- an immunocytochemical and quantitative study in the supragranular layers of the middle temporal neocortex. *Brain Res,* 1213, 152-165.

Vieira, M. N., Forny-Germano, L., Saraiva, L. M., Sebollela, A., Martinez, A. M., Houzel, J. C., De Felice, F. G. and Ferreira, S. T. (2007) Soluble oligomers from a non-disease related protein mimic Abeta-induced tau hyperphosphorylation and neurodegeneration. *J Neurochem,* 103, 736-748.

Vogt, B. A., Vogt, L. J., Vrana, K. E., Gioia, L., Meadows, R. S., Challa, V. R., Hof, P. R. and Van Hoesen, G. W. (1998) Multivariate analysis of laminar patterns of neurodegeneration in posterior cingulate cortex in Alzheimer's disease. *Exp Neurol,* 153, 8-22.

Walsh, D. M. and Selkoe, D. J. (2004) Oligomers on the brain: the emerging role of soluble protein aggregates in neurodegeneration. *Protein Pept Lett,* 11, 213-228.

Walsh, D. M. and Selkoe, D. J. (2007) A beta oligomers - a decade of discovery. *J Neurochem,* 101, 1172-1184.

Wittmann, C. W., Wszolek, M. F., Shulman, J. M., Salvaterra, P. M., Lewis, J., Hutton, M. and Feany, M. B. (2001) Tauopathy in Drosophila: neurodegeneration without neurofibrillary tangles. *Science,* 293, 711-714.

Xu, S., Brunden, K. R., Trojanowski, J. Q. and Lee, V. M. Characterization of tau fibrillization in vitro. *Alzheimers Dement,* 6, 110-117.

Yamazaki, M., Hasegawa, M., Mori, O., Murayama, S., Tsuchiya, K., Ikeda, K., Chen, K. M., Katayama, Y. and Oyanagi, K. (2005) Tau-positive fine granules in the cerebral white matter: a novel finding among the tauopathies exclusive to parkinsonism-dementia complex of Guam. J Neuropathol Exp Neurol, 64, 839-846.

Yoshiyama, Y., Higuchi, M., Zhang, B. et al. (2007) Synapse loss and microglial activation precede tangles in a P301S tauopathy mouse model. Neuron, 53, 337-351.

Zhang, B., Maiti, A., Shively, S. et al. (2005) Microtubule-binding drugs offset tau sequestration by stabilizing microtubules and reversing fast axonal transport deficits in a tauopathy model. Proc Natl Acad Sci U S A, 102, 227-231.

28

In Silico Design of Preventive Drugs for Alzheimer's Disease

Arpita Yadav and Minakshi Sonker
University Institute of Engineering and Technology, CSJM University, India

1. Introduction

Alzheimer's disease is a debilitating dementia occurring in the elderly. Its pathological symptoms include forgetfulness and memory loss (Mattson, 2004). Disease imposes financial burden on family and society. Current line of treatment only provides symptomatic relief (Davis & Powchik 1995; Sugimoto et al., 1995). Drugs of purely curative or preventive type are still not marketed. Commonly used drugs are Acetylcholine esterase inhibitors (Sugimoto et al., 1995) which temporarily alleviate symptoms by raising levels of neurotransmitter Acetylcholine and thus improving cognitive behavior. These drugs are associated with a number of adverse side effects as well (Davis & Powchik, 1995). The aim of this chapter is to discuss strategies and hurdles in the design of preventive drugs. In the following section we briefly discuss causes behind onset and progression of disease as it is imperative to understand these issues.

1.1 Generation of amyloid beta peptides and pathological condition of AD

This disease is characterized by production of amyloid beta (Aβ) plaques and intracellular neurofibrillary tangles in the brain (cf. fig.1). Amyloid plaques are formed by aggregation of Aβ peptide (Glenner & Wong, 1984) and neurofibrillary tangles are composed of hyper phosphorylated Tau protein (Alonso et al., 2001). 42 amino acid form of Aβ has been identified as the predominant constituent of plaques (Yin et al., 2007). Therefore preventive and curative strategies deal with reduction in Aβ 42 production. Aβ peptides are generated by successive cleavages of amyloid precursor protein (APP) by β and γ secretase (Potter & Dressal, 2000) enzyme. Aβ can also be cleaved by α secretase enzyme. Cleavage by α followed by γ secretase leads to formation of another truncated form of Aβ called P3. Aβ 42 is produced by cleavages taking place in Golgi (Hartman et al., 1997) apparatus. Cleavage of APP giving rise to different forms of Aβ is shown in fig.2. Discovery and isolation of these enzymes has provided us the benefit of a target for preventive drug designing. β secretase being the key enzyme involved has been assigned several popular names out of which β amyloid precursor protein cleaving enzyme (BACE 2) is the most frequently used. BACE is a transmembrane protein with aspartyl protease family catalytic motif as in pepsin (Yan et al., 2001). It is a homologous protein and interestingly not expressed in brain (Bennett et al., 2000). It is still an important enzyme target as transgenic mice lacking BACE gene produce little or no Aβ (Luo et al., 2003).

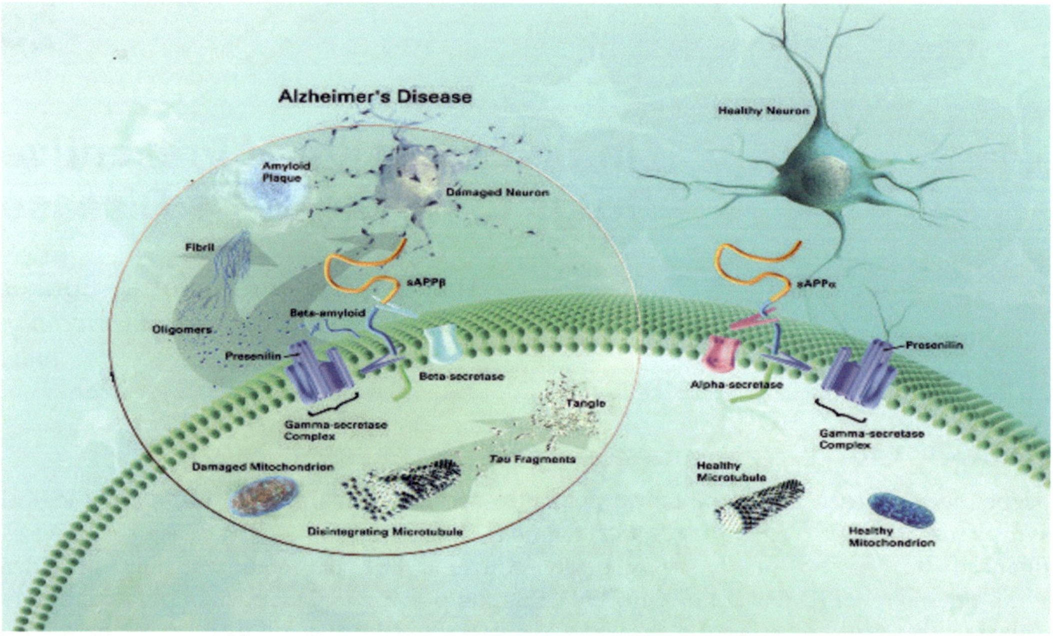

Damaged neuron in Alzheimer's Disease

Fig. 1. Shows a healthy neuron and presence of various enzymes. Encircled region shows formation of amyloid plaques and how they damage a healthy neuron

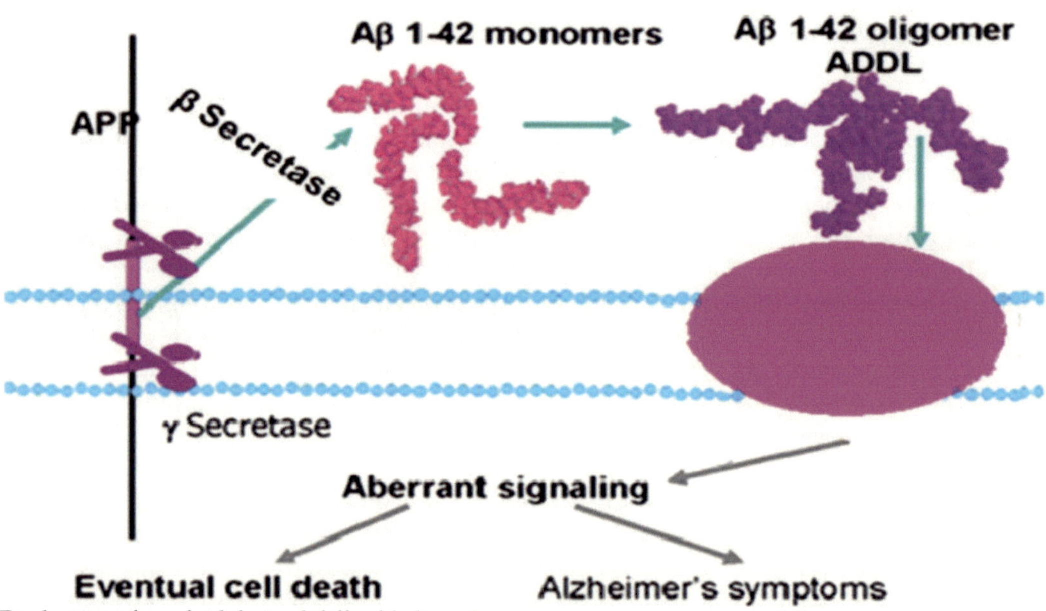

Production of amyloid derived diffusible ligands

Fig. 2. Shows formation of Aβ 42 monomers, their subsequent oligomerization to form diffusible ligands and generation of Alzheimer's symptoms

1.2 Past strategies for design of preventive drugs

Researchers involved in developing drugs for AD have employed numerous strategies to combat this disease. Most of the techniques involved interfere in formation of Aβ at some stage.

1.2.1 Secretase inhibition

Secretase enzyme is the most promising target. Inhibitors of β secretase as well as γ secretase have been synthesized. Both type of inhibitors stop formation of toxic Aβ. Chemical structures for some of these potency values (Kazikowsky et al., 1996; Harel et al., 1996; Camps et al., 1999; Weihofen et al., 2003) are shown in fig.3. Despite numerous efforts these preventive drugs have not been able to reach our markets due to their poor pharmacodynamics and bioavailability problems. These problems have been largely associated with peptidic nature of BACE inhibitors and failure to design low molecular weight inhibitors. These compounds also show inhibitory effect on other signal transduction pathways and are hence undesirable from this point of view as well.

1.2.2 Metal chelation

Aβ aggregation has been observed to be induced by several metal species including aluminum, iron, zinc and copper (Barnham et al., 2004). Therefore, apart from secretase inhibition anti aggregatory agents like metal chelators have been used which will remove metal ion thus reducing aggregation of Aβ peptide. Clioquinol, Deferriprone, Curcumin etc are such drugs (Hanson et al., 2007) (c. f. fig. 4). Although metal chelators lead to behavioral improvements but they have not emerged as preventive alternatives. Energetic aspects related to inefficiency of these drugs have been studied in this chapter.

1.2.3 NMDA receptor antagonism

Persistent activation of CNS NMDA receptor has been hypothesized in AD patients. Therefore, NMDA receptor antagonists have also been tried out as possible AD drugs (Kemp & Mc Kernan 2002). Memantine (c.f. fig. 4) is such a recent FDA approved drug for AD. It protects neuro cells against excess glutamate by partially blocking NMDA receptor.

1.2.4 MAO inhibitor

Monoamine oxidase (MAO) inhibitors have shown neuroprotective activities; For example, selegiline, TVP1022, rasagiline (Sano et al., 1997; Ridderer et al., 2004; Yaudin & Buccafusco 2005; Huang et al., 1999) (cf. fig 5) have shown delayed progression of AD. MAO inhibition has also been considered as a strategy for controlling AD.

1.2.5 Dual inhibition for synergistic effects

In this strategy either two compounds are joined together to achieve better inhibition at a receptor (c. f. dual tacrine in fig. 5) or two compounds showing inhibitory activity at different receptors are joined to produce synergistic effects. Such examples include AChE/SERT dual inhibitors (Bolognesi et al., 2005; Camps et al., 2005; Rosini et al., 2005; Kogen et al., 2002; Toda et al., 2002; Abe et al., 2003; Toda et al., 2003) (c. f. fig. 5).

The aim of this chapter is to explain energetics involved in self aggregation of Aβ. In silico design of a preventive drug based on understanding of underlying energetic aspects has been explored. A possible explanation for failures encountered in design of low molecular weight BACE 2 inhibitors has been provided. Design of low molecular weight preventive drugs is attempted.

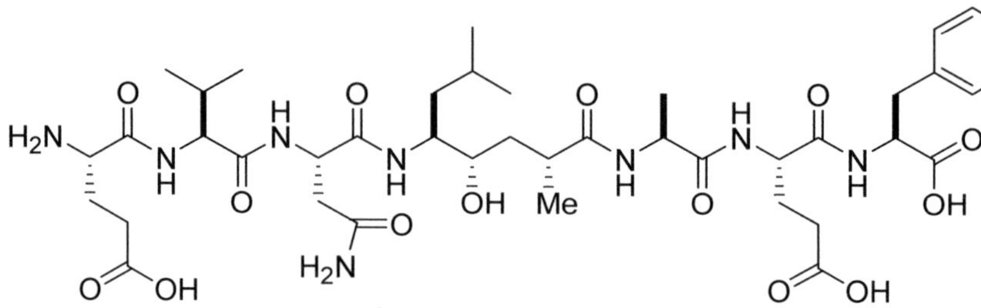

OM-992, Ki = 1.6 nM

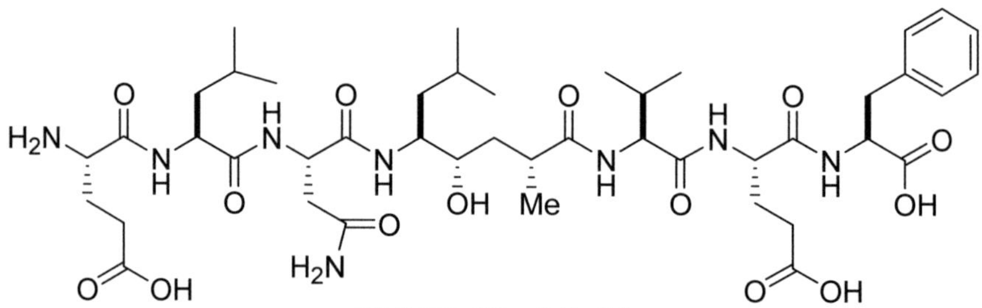

OM-003, Ki = 0.3 nM

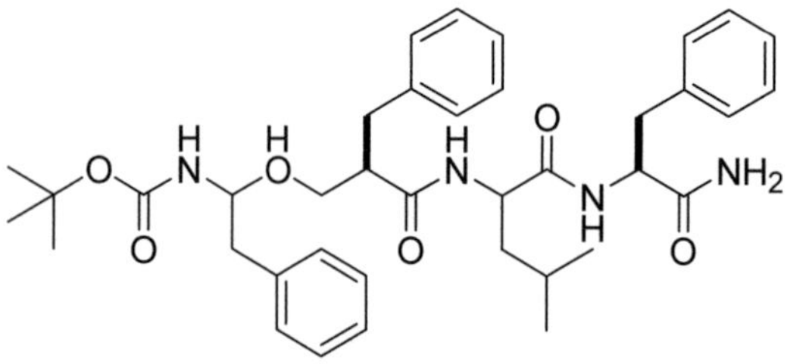

L-685,458, IC50 = 0.46µM

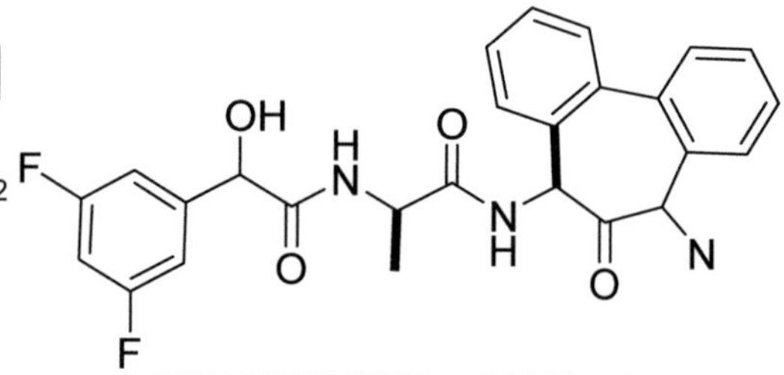

MLY411757, IC50 = 0.00004µM

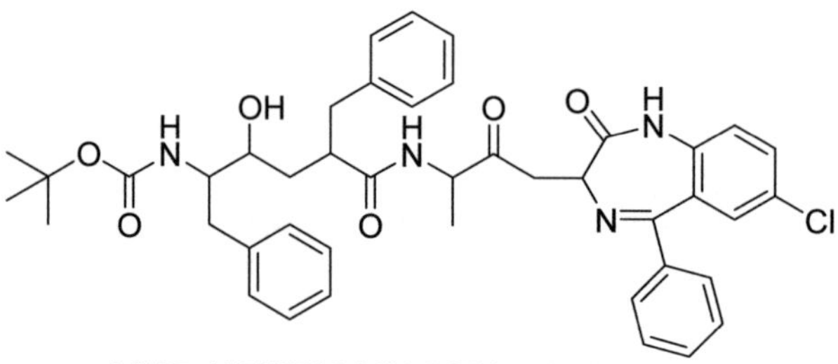

NVP-AHW700-NX, IC50 = 0.62µM

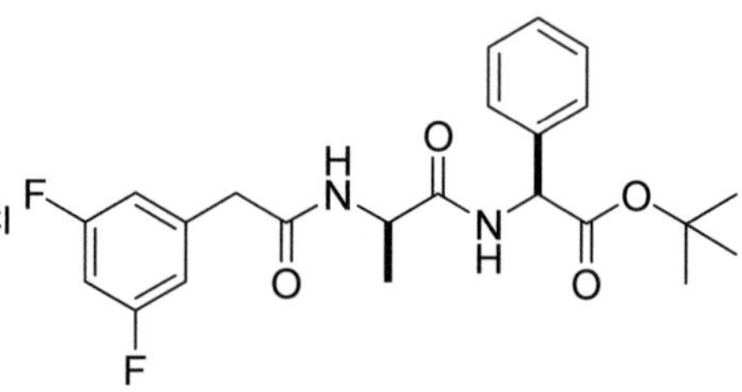

DAPT, IC50 = 0.17µM

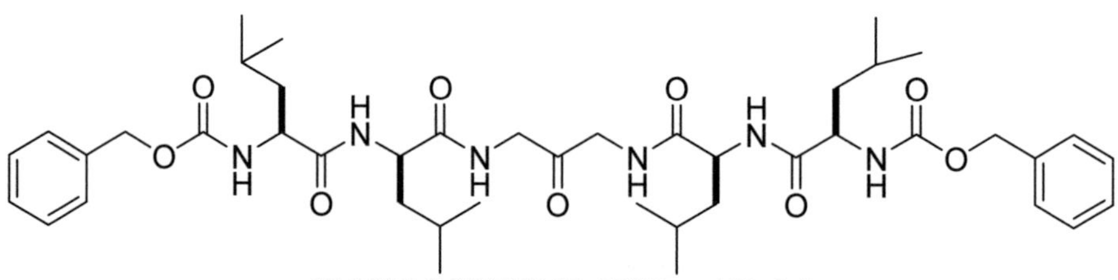

(Z-LL)2 2-KETONE, IC50 =>100µM

Secretase inhibitors

Fig. 3. Shows chemical structures of some β and γ-secretase inhibitors

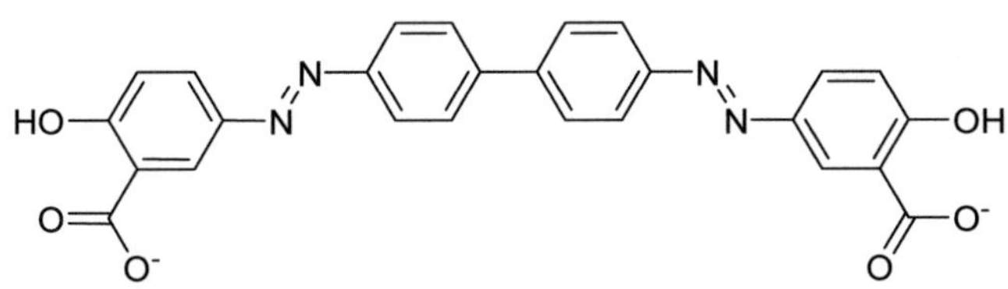

Chrysamine G

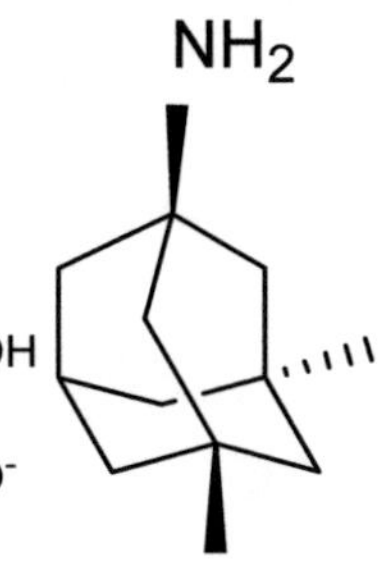

Memantine

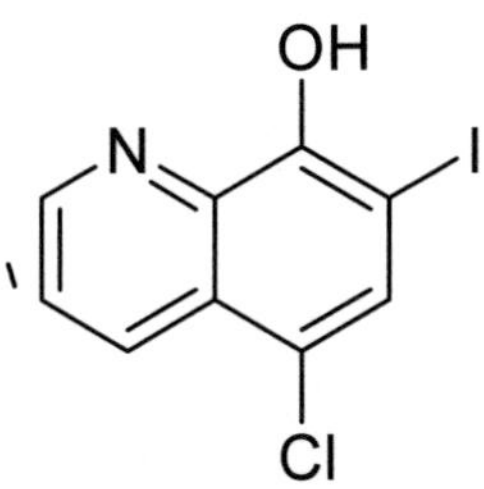

Clioquinol

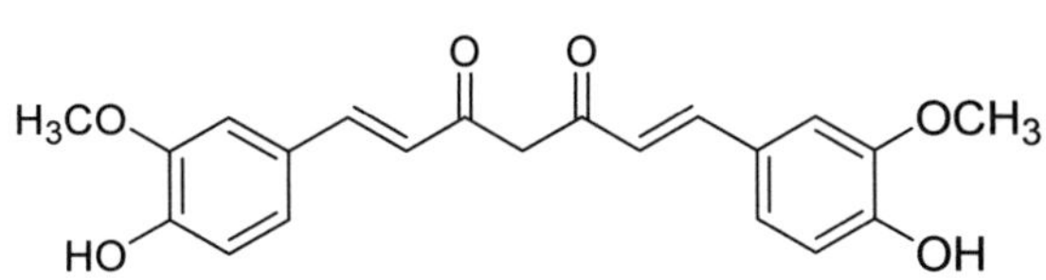

Curcumin

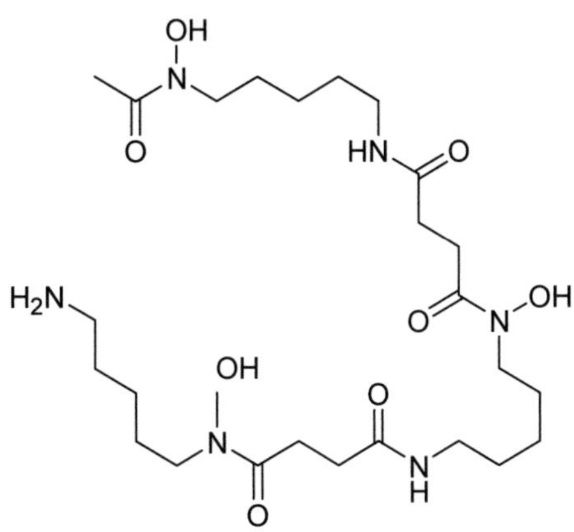

Desferrioxamine (DFO)

Metal chelators

Fig. 4. Shows chemical structures for some selected metal chelators

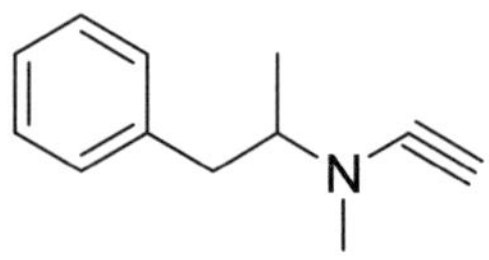

Selegiline

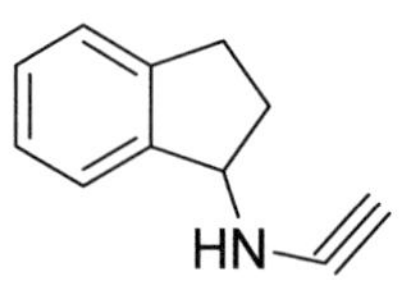

Rasgline

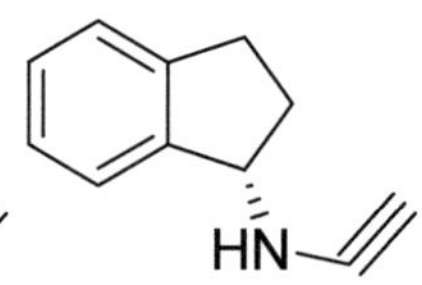

TVP1022

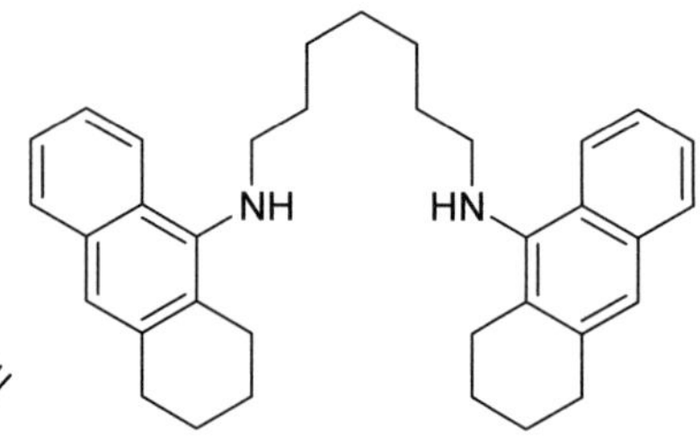

Dual Tacrine

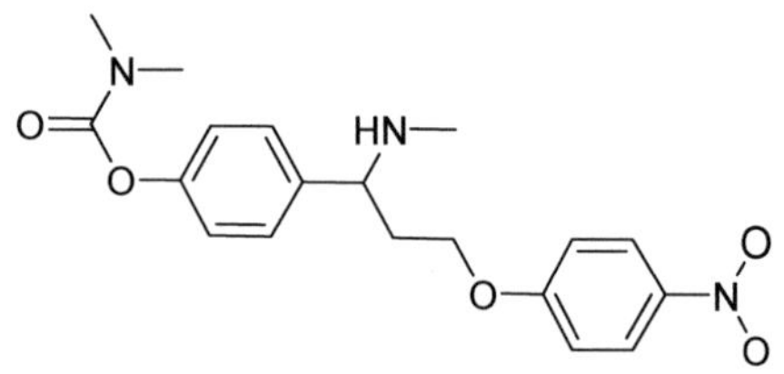

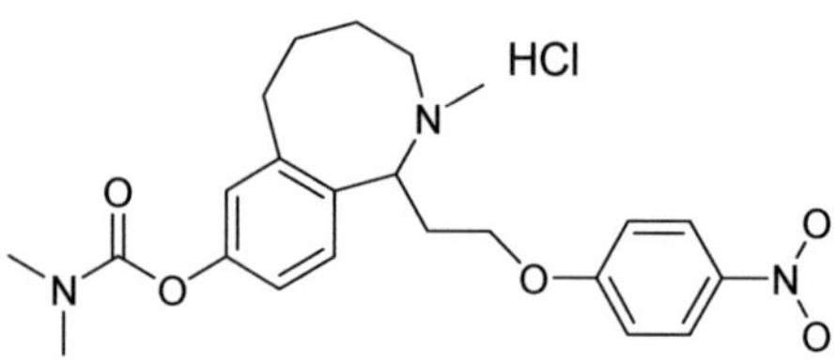

AChE/SERT dual inhibitor

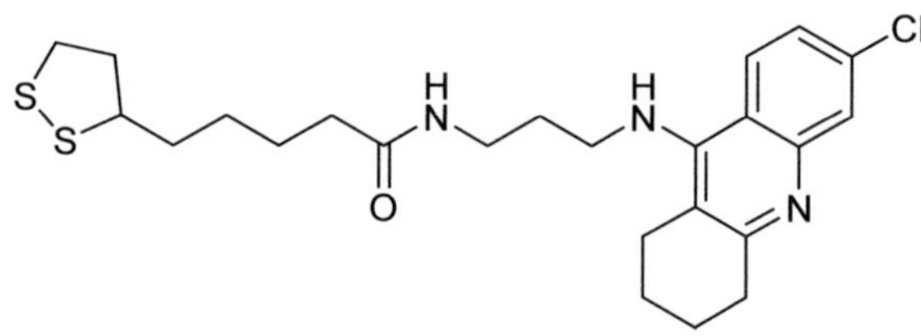

Lipocrin

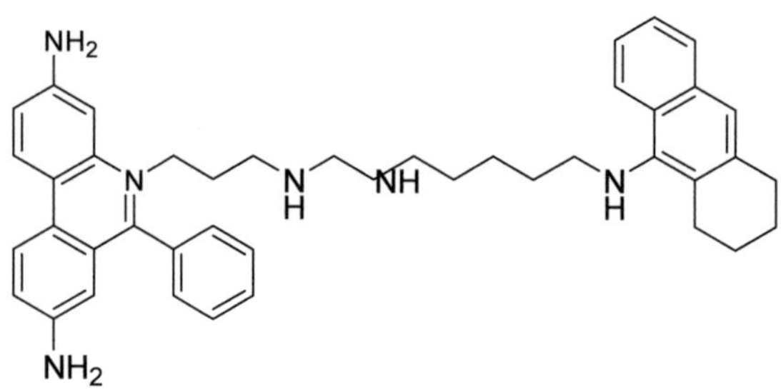

Prodium-tacrine heterodimer

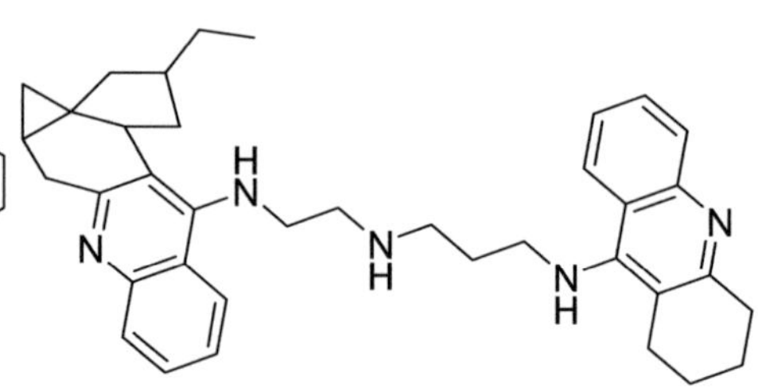

Huprine-tacrine heterodimer

Dual inhibitors

Fig. 5. Shows dual inhibitors which inhibit two targets (AChE/ SERT dual inhibitor) or show enhanced activity at single target (Huprine-tacrine heterodimer-enhanced activity at acetylcholinesterase enzyme)

2. Methodology

Ab initio molecular orbital calculations in conjunction with intermolecular interaction calculations and docking studies have been performed to study energetics involved in self aggregation of Aβ and drug……Aβ interactions. Automated docking tools provided in Glide have been used for flexible ligand docking studies and generating poses for drug interacting with Aβ or BACE. The whole procedure in brief may be summarized as follows. Aβ solution structure was taken and minimized using Macromodel. Middle portion of Aβ was taken for accurate ab initio calculations. Drugs and ions were docked in different poses (500 poses were generated) using GLIDE. Interaction energies were calculated ab initio for relevant poses using supermolecule calculations. All calculations have been carried out utilizing MAESTRO module of SCHRODINGER software (Maestro, 2010).

3. Results and discussion

Foremost Aβ solution structure has been minimized keeping ionizable residues in ionized form. Middle piece of Aβ (c.f. fig.6) was extracted to study Aβ……ion interactions and possibility of self aggregation.

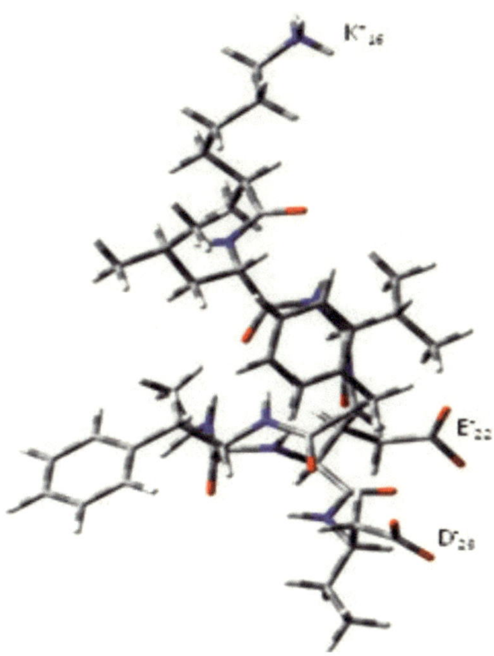

Middle piece of Aβ (16-23 residues)

Fig. 6. Depicts optimized conformation of middle portion of amyloid peptide at physiological pH

3.1 Energetics of self aggregation of Aβ

It is not clear from literature whether self aggregation of Aβ is metal induced or not. However, Zn^{2+} ions are known to play the dual role of neuroprotection as well as being neurotoxic. To understand neurotoxic role of Zn^{2+} ions we have studied affinity of Aβ for

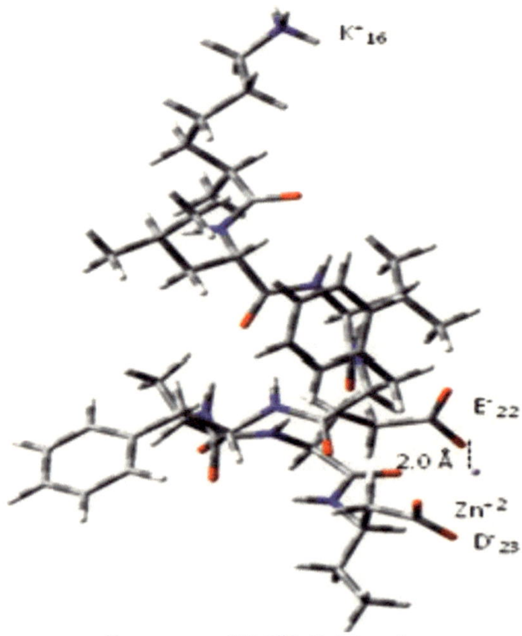

Int.en. =--499.70kCal/mol

Affinity of Aβ for Zn^{2+} ion

Fig. 7. Depicts that amyloid beta peptide has great affinity for zinc ions.

these ions and tendency for aggregation in presence of these ions. Fig. 7 indicates highly favored metal induced aggregation tendency.

3.2 Role of an anti aggregatory compound

Any compound may act as anti aggregatory in two possible ways –

1. By removing toxic metal ions from brain
2. By intercalating on to Aβ and masking its portion actively involved in aggregation.

Any attempt at designing anti aggregatory compound is bound to succeed if we first try to understand why metal chelator drugs used for removal of metal toxicity in the past are not so effective in present case. For a compound to be an efficient anti aggregation agent, it must be sufficiently competitive with metal ion for interaction at Aβ. Curcumin and Chrysamine G are known to possess anti aggregation property as well as brain permeability. To understand their mode of action we have studied their metal chelation property and intercalative power. Fig. 8 depicts that both the drugs can remove metal toxicity. However, Curcumin will not be sufficiently competitive with Aβ for metal ions. Chrysamine G can competitively inhibit metal induced aggregation by removing metal ion toxicity. Exploration of intercalative property of these compounds indicates that Curcumin cannot intercalate and Chrysamine G intercalates poorly. Therefore, it is understood that efficiency of preventive drugs depends on their ability to compete with Aβ for metal ions which is extremely difficult as Aβ has very high affinity for metal ions especially the middle piece. On the basis of this understanding we have tried to design a preventive compound that can compete with metal ions for Aβ and can also intercalate to Aβ.

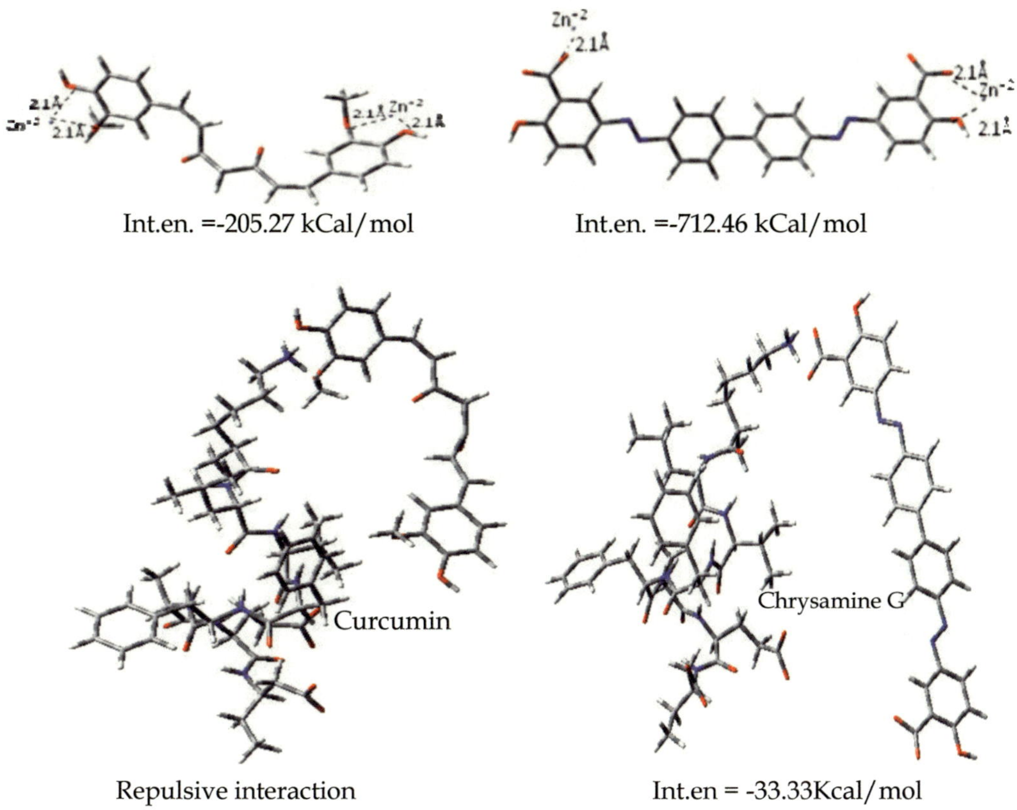

Metal chelation and intercalation of Aβ by Curcumin and Chrysamine G

Fig. 8. Shows possible modes of action for known anti aggregatory agents

3.3 Design of an intercalative preventive drug

A peptidomimetic lead compound has been designed keeping in mind charge complementarity and conformational aspects of middle piece of Aβ. A peptidomimetic compound has been designed to exploit peptide……peptide interactions for intercalation and to bring about specificity with the help of same. This compound contains peptide bonds in backbone here and there and substituents similar to amino acid residues toned according to needs to achieve good charge and conformational complementarity with Aβ. Design of compound is based on visual examination of length required for intercalation and anionic / cationic sites required for interaction to middle portion of Aβ.

Optimized conformation of lead compound and calculation of its metal removal efficiency are shown in fig. 9. Calculated metal interaction energies indicate that the compound will efficiently remove metal ions from brain. To study intercalative property of compound, flexible ligand docking studies have been performed. Drug……Aβ interaction energies have been calculated in various poses and results of best poses are shown in fig. 10. Some of the important energetically filtered poses are shown in fig. 11. Calculated Aβ……lead compound interaction energies clearly indicate that designed lead compound can compete with metal ions for Aβ. At the same time it will also reduce concentration of metal ions from brain due to its metal ion removal efficiency.

Intercalation is not through covalent linkage so that it does not bring about physical or chemical changes in the state of Aβ peptide. The availability and concentration of metal ions in brain will decide on exact role of compound. This strategy of designing a curative drug is superior as compared to previous efforts where researchers have tried to break down aggregated Aβ into smaller soluble Aβ fragments as they only increase concentration of amyloid derived diffusible ligands (ADDLs). ADDLs have also been reported to cause certain problems due to their diffusible nature and high permeability. Our designed compound not only avoids aggregation of Aβ 42 it also avoids ADDLs from diffusing inside brain as they would increase molecular weight of ADDLs by intercalation. Pharmacokinetic aspects of lead compound can also be judged by considering compliance with rule of five.

Designed compound has molecular weight slightly above 500, less than 5 hydrogen bond donor groups and less than 10 hydrogen bond acceptor groups. Thus it is expected to show sufficiently good pharmacokinetics. Being peptidomimetic it may show moderate bioavailability. Synthetic considerations and associated efficacy remain to be experimentally verified. This work emphasizes need for energetics based designing to attain desired efficacy.

3.4 Design of a low molecular weight BACE inhibitor

As mentioned in introduction BACE catalyzes cleavage of APP leading to formation of neurotoxic Aβ peptide. Therefore, it is an obvious target for development of preventive drugs. Compounds inhibiting this enzyme are expected to block extracellular first cleavage of APP that subsequently leads to formation of Aβ. BACE being an aspartyl protease catalyzes cleavage of APP assisted by two active site aspartyl residues which operate cooperatively with a net charge of -1. Most of the BACE inhibitors are transition state analogs derived from natural product pepstatin. Statine isostere has been derived from pepstatin and used to design transition state analogs for BACE that engage catalytic aspartics with a hydroxyl group. Some peptidic BACE inhibitors employing statine isostere are shown in fig. 12. These compounds have shown activity in enzymatic preparations but do not show appreciable activity in cellular assays. This attribute has been associated with the fact that they are peptides. The aim of this study is to understand mechanistic aspects of BACE

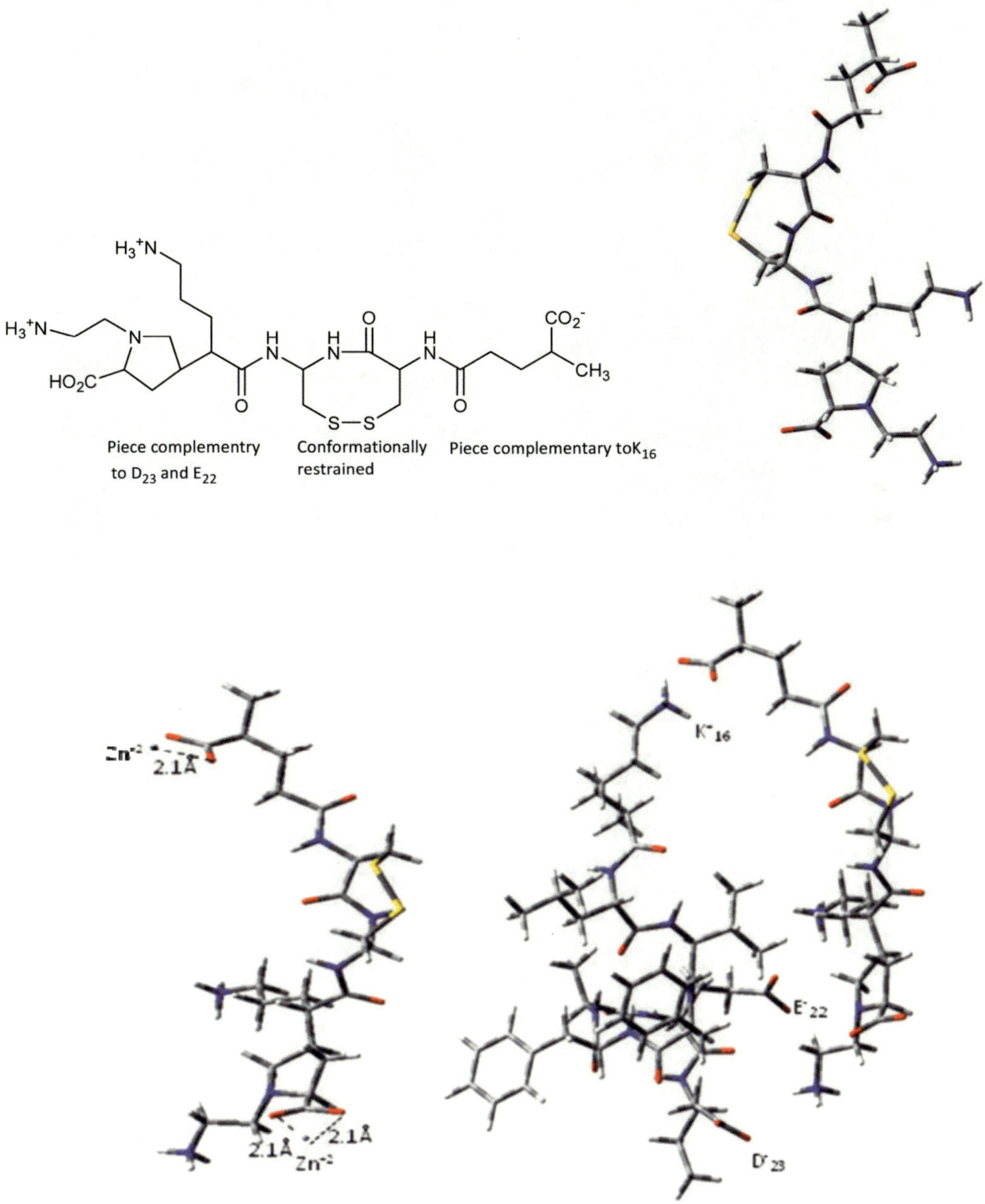

Int. en. = -405.53 kCal/mol Int. en. = -173.39 kCal/mol

Metal chelation and intercalation of Aβ by designed lead compound

Fig. 9. Shows predicted modes of action of designed lead compound

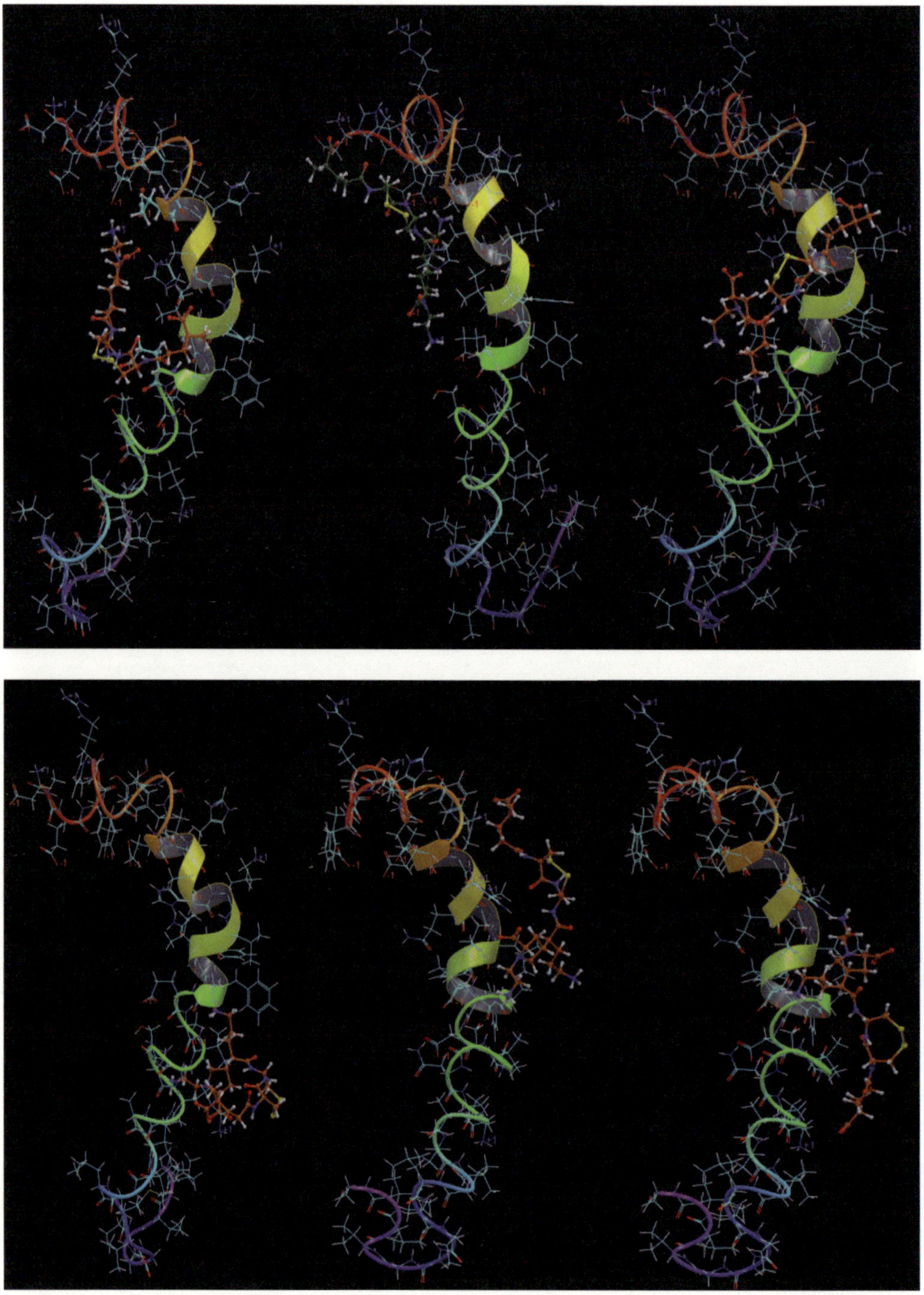

Various poses for designed lead compound intercalating Aβ 42

Fig. 10. Shows automated flexible ligand docking results for designed lead compound

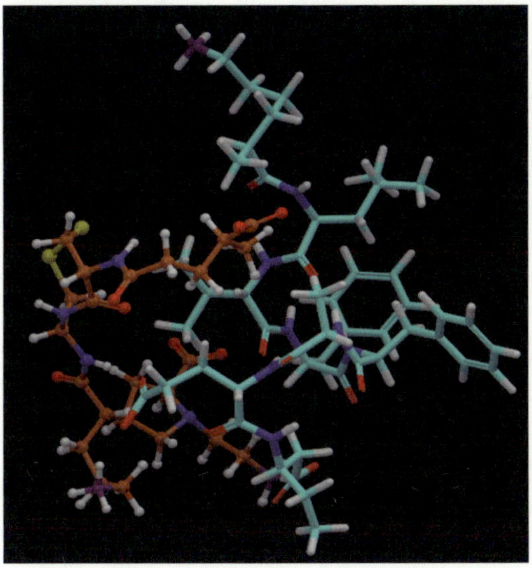

Int.en. = -259.76 kCal/mol

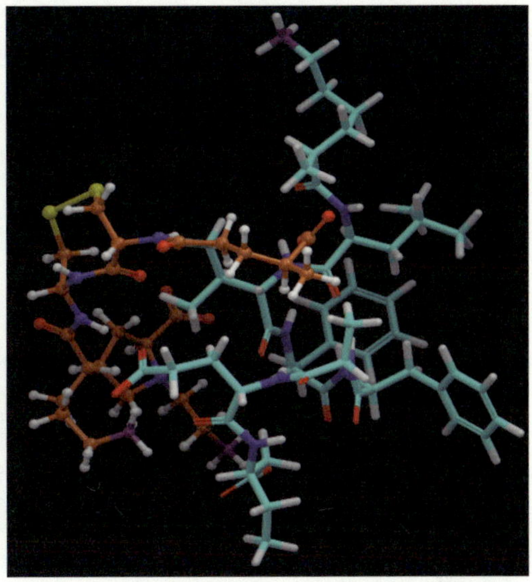

Int.en. = -249.83 kCal/mol

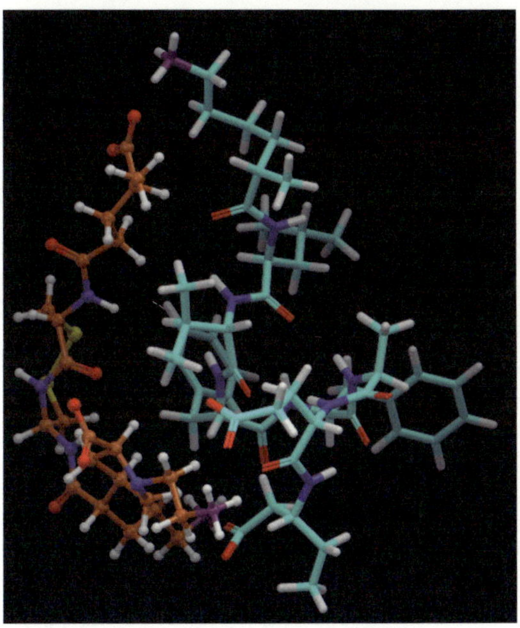

Int.en. = -223.39 kCal/mol

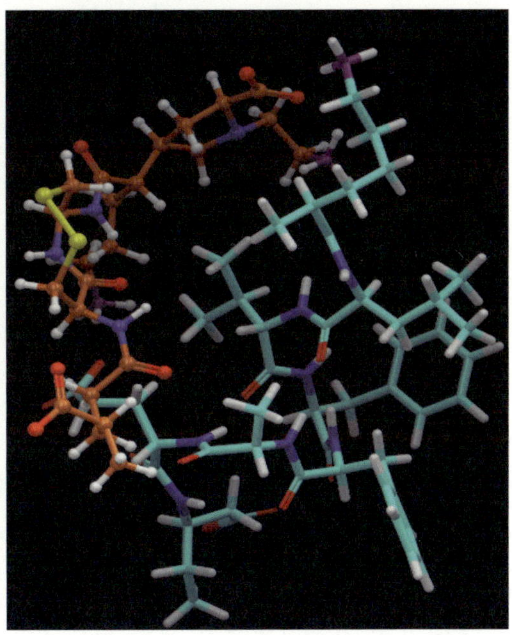

Int.en. = -136.32 kCal/mol

Interaction energies for designed lead compound masking middle portion of Aβ 42

Fig. 11. Shows preferred mode of action of designed lead compound

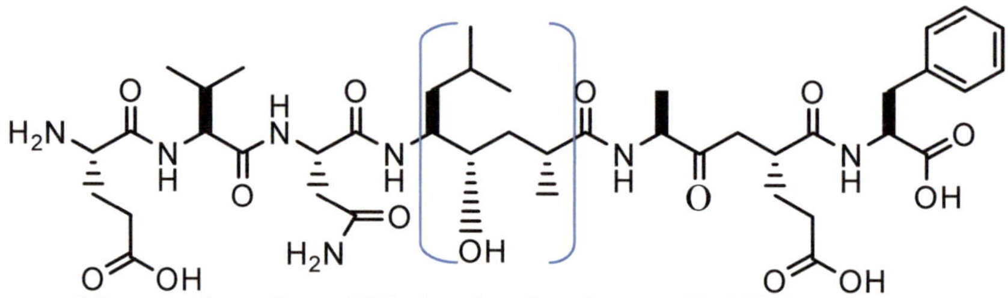

N-term-glu-val-asn-HE-ala-glu-phe-C-term OM 99-2, K_i = 1nM

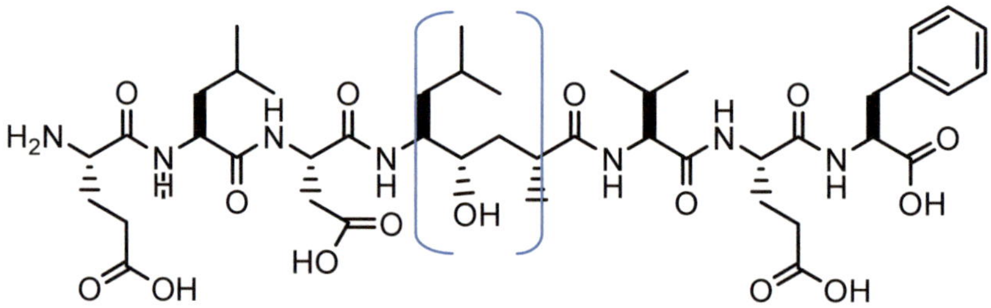

N-term-glu-leu-asp-HE-val-glu-phe-C-term OM 003, K_i = 1nM

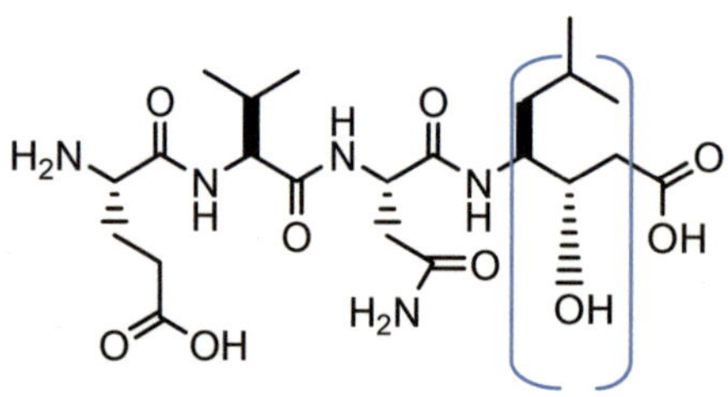

N-term-glu-val-asn-statine Statine analog Peptide B IC_{50} =>91 μM

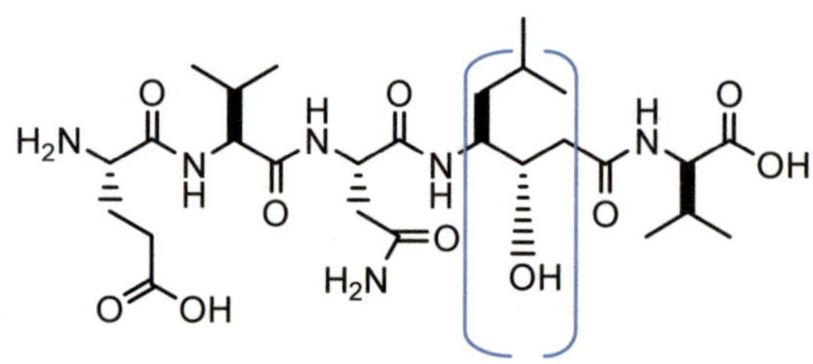

N-term-glu-val-asn-statine-val Statine analog Peptide A IC_{50} = 9.4 μM

Peptidic inhibitors of BACE 2

Fig. 12. Shows chemical structures of some peptidic inhibitors and their potencies

inhibitors through molecular docking studies and intermolecular interaction calculations. Aim being to design reduced molecular weight compound with more 'drug like features'. We first try to understand why low molecular weight peptide inhibitors have not been successful so far and why truncation of amino acid residues on either side of isostere leads to drastic loss in potency.

3.4.1 Mechanistic aspects of small statine analog inhibitor of BACE

Peptide inhibitors containing hydroxyethylene isostere or statine isostere show significant variation in potency from μM to nM range (c.f. fig. 12). Calculations and docking studies have been performed on Peptide A to understand causes of loss in activity. Peptides possess conformational flexibility. A number of conformations (c.f. fig. 13) for Peptide A were generated using Ligprep module of SCHRODINGER. These conformations were energetically filtered for docking studies. Energetically filtered conformations were cyclic as small peptides (typically less than 10 amino acids) cannot attain stabilization through secondary structure that is β-turn etc. Therefore, they possess greater tendency to cyclize and attain stabilization. To understand bioactive conformation and perform docking studies a model of BACE 2 active site has been prepared utilizing X- ray crystallography data for OM003 complexed in human BACE 2 (1M4H. pdb). This model covers 8Å environment around active site. All amino acid residues are taken in their normal occurring ionization states. For example, asp, glu, are negatively charged and lys, arg are positively charged. All possible protonation states of catalytic motif have been tried out in search of best mechanistic option. Best interaction energies obtained for peptide A conformation 1 and 2 are shown in figs. 14 and 15. Flexible ligand, rigid protein dockings have been carried out. Asp 228 has been kept in ionized form in these calculations. Fig. 14 clearly indicates that the inhibitor cannot fit properly in the active site so as to interact efficiently with catalytic motif. In fact transition state isostere is oriented away from catalytic motif. The transition state isostere does not come in contact with catalytic motif. Interactions with asp 228 have been completely lost. There is no utilization of enhanced binding interactions that is, interacting residues in pockets of enzyme close to catalytic motif. Fig. 15 depicts docking results with conformation 2 of peptide A. Conformation 2 is still worse in terms of interactions with active site residues. Inhibitor can fit in active site only at distances 6 and 8Å from catalytic motif due to its conformation. At these distances very little interaction with catalytic motif can be achieved. Interaction with asp 228 becomes impossible due to highly spatially constrained active site of BACE 2 and the conformational aspects of inhibitor.

These docking results when compared with X-ray crystallography data for OM003 complexed in BACE 2 reveal that low molecular weight peptide inhibitors show conformationally controlled mechanistic aspects leading to decrease in their potency. Cyclic type conformations impart stability to small peptides but render them unsuitable for spatial requirements of BACE 2 active site leading to drastic reduction in activity. This understanding led us to design conformationally stable low molecular weight lead compound.

3.5 Design of low molecular weight BACE inhibitor

Designing has been strategically and systematically pursued. Peptide backbone has been replaced with peptidomimetic backbone to control conformational problems. Residues similar to natural substrate have been retained for specificity. Drug has been designed to be a competitive inhibitor as opposed to transition state analog. Transition state isostere containing hydroxyl group to engage catalytic aspartic dyad has been replaced with a positive site to electrostatically interact with ionized asp 228 of active site for binding interactions (c.f. fig. 16). Conformational aspect is not an issue in this case. Designed compound was subjected to in silico testing that is, docking studies were performed to judge its activity. Best results of docking studies are shown in fig. 16. Designed lead compound can fit in active site and interact with catalytic motif. Fig. 16 shows that interaction energy predicted is not particularly attractive but indicates that lead compound may bind with retention of conformation leading to perhaps enhanced bioavailability and good potency.

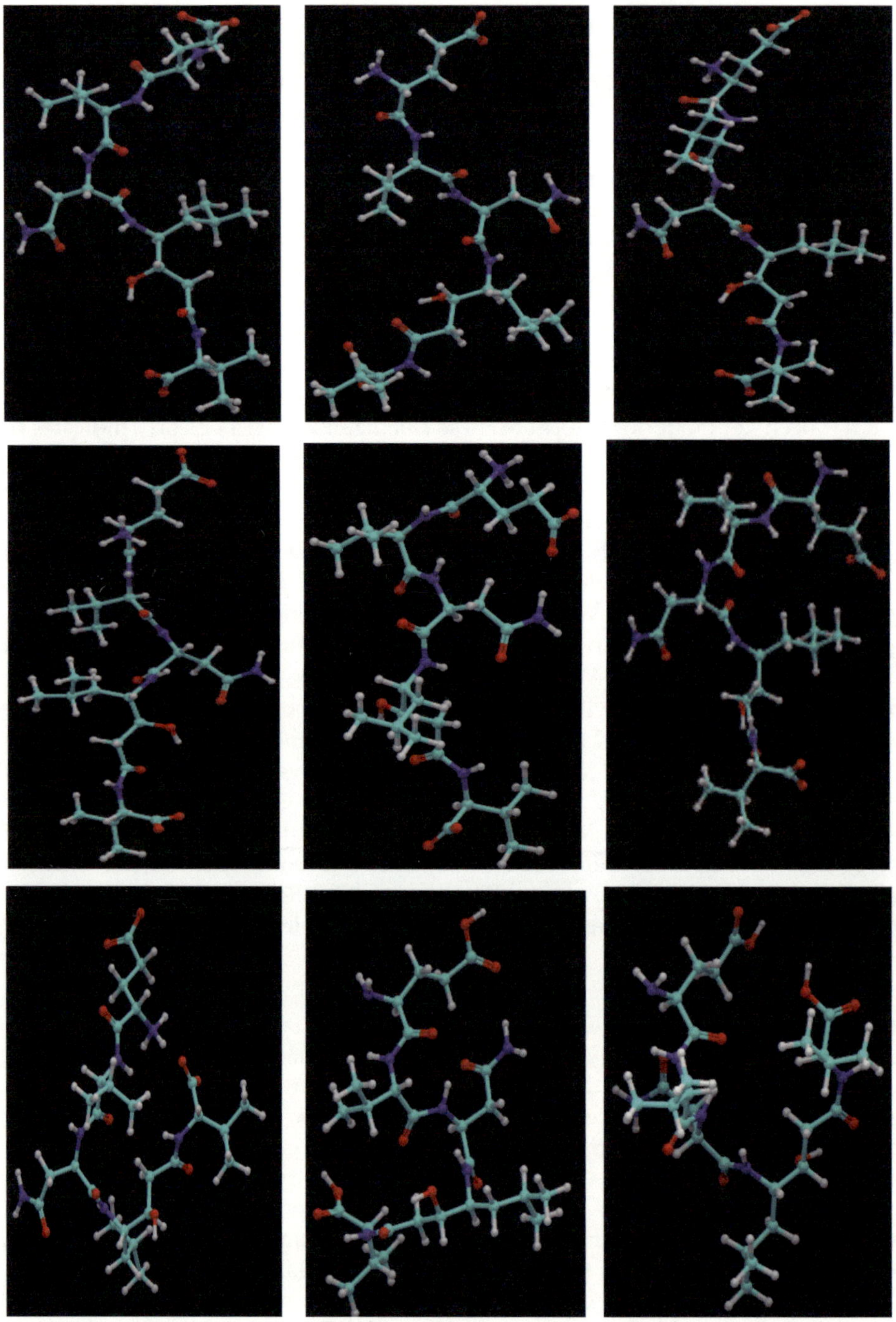

Conformation 1 Conformation 2

Energetically filtered conformations of Statine isostere containing Peptide A

Fig. 13. Shows bioactive conformations of peptide A

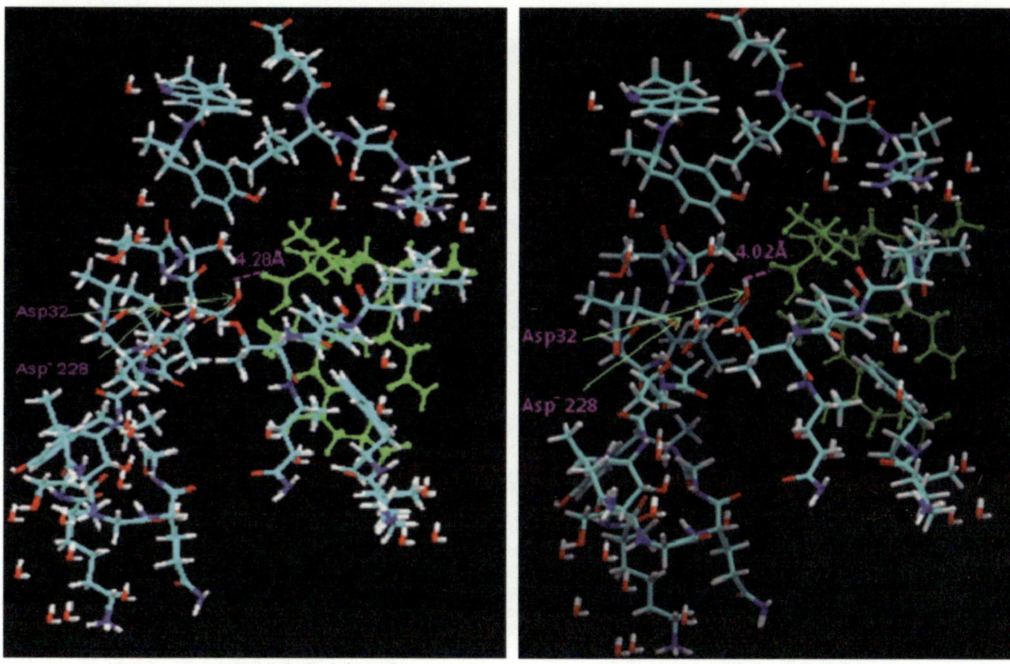

Int.en. = -17.93 kCal/mol   Int.en. = -17.71 kCal/mol

Peptide A (conformation 1) interacting with BACE 2 catalytic motif

Fig. 14. Shows mode of action of a small peptidic inhibitor of BACE 2

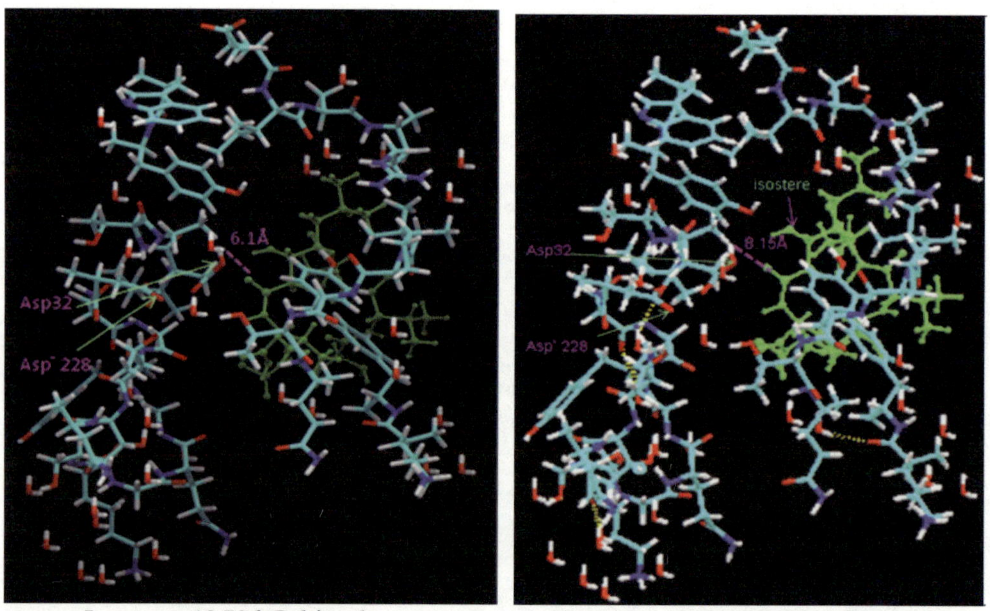

Int.en. = -10.58 kCal/mol   Int.en. = -12.18 kCal/mol

Peptide A (conformation 2) interacting with BACE 2 catalytic motif

Fig. 15. Shows mode of action of a small peptidic inhibitor of BACE 2

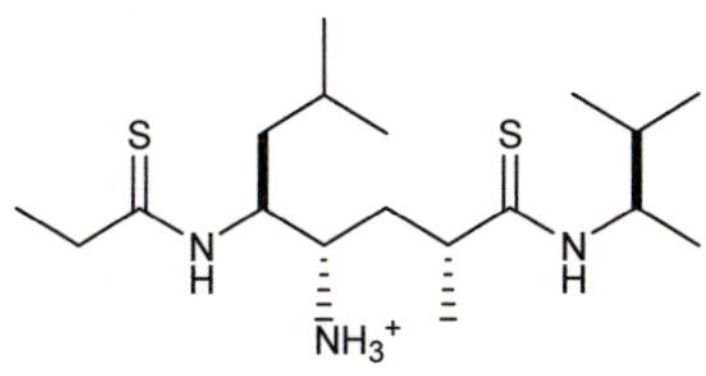

(Reduced molecular weight, conformationally locked)

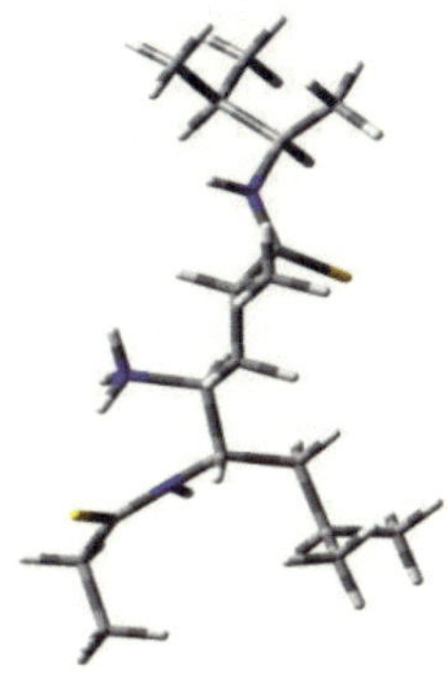

Int. en. = -9.95 kCal/mol

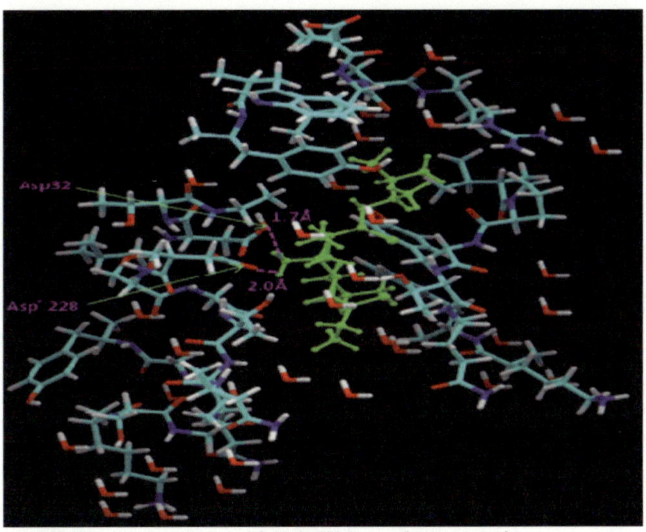

Designed competitive inhibitor interacting with BACE 2 catalytic motif

Fig. 16. Shows predicted mode of action of a designed compound as competitive inhibitor of BACE 2

4. Conclusions

This chapter describes ab initio Hartree Fock molecular orbital calculations combined with docking tools and intermolecular interaction calculations on amyloid beta peptide. Energetics involved in metal ion induced self aggregation of amyloid beta peptide has been studied. Study indicates that metal induced self assemblage of Aβ is highly favored. Any compound can act as an anti aggregatory agent if it can compete with Aβ for metal ions. To be competitive it must have an interaction energy of ~500 kCal/mol with metal ions like Zn^{2+} ion. Intercalative and metal detoxification properties are desired in prospective preventive drug for AD. A peptidomimetic lead compound with these properties has been designed and tested in silico.

Mechanistic aspects of peptide inhibitors of BACE 2 have been studied in detail. Mode of action of peptide transition state analog drugs has been highlighted. Conformationally controlled mechanistic aspects of low molecular weight peptide inhibitors have been discussed. Low molecular weight peptide inhibitors tend to possess cyclic type conformation which is not suitable for interactions with catalytic motif. Large peptide inhibitors on the other hand show bioavailability problems due to their poor pharmacokinetics and membrane permeability problems. An attempt has been made at designing conformationally stable, reduced molecular weight lead compound that follows Lipinski's rule and is expected to cross cell membranes. Designed compound is competitive inhibitor as opposed to transition state analog. Designed lead compound is reduced molecular weight and is expected to retain specificity as it utilizes same sequence of amino acid residues as in natural substrate APP. Designed compound is expected to overcome conformational complications, bioavailability however remains to be asserted by experimental studies.

5. Acknowledgment

We gratefully acknowledge financial support by Department of Science and Technology (DST), New Delhi, India project number SR/S1/PC-19/2008. Minakshi Sonker gratefully acknowledges DST for Senior Research Fellowship.

6. References

Abe, Y.; Aoyagi, A.; Hara, T.; Abe, K.; Yamazaki, R.; Kumagae, Y.; Naruto, S.; Koyama, K.; Marumoto, S.; Tago, K.; Toda, N.; Takami, K.; Yamada, N.; Ori, M.; Kogen, H.& Kaneko, T.(2003) Pharmacological Characterization of RS-1259, an Orally Active Dual Inhibitor of Acetylcholinesterase and Serotonin Transporter, in Rodents: Possible Treatment of Alzheimer's Disease, *J. Pharmacol. Sci.*, 93, 95-105.

Alonso, A.; Zaidi, T.; Novak, M.; Grundke-Iqbal, I.; Iqbal, K.; (2001)Hyper phosphorylation induce self-assembly of τ into tangles of paired helical filaments/straight filaments, *Proc. Natl. Acad. Sci.* USA, 98 (12), 6923-6928.

Barmham, K. J. Masters, C. L.& Bush, A. I.; (2004) Clioquinol down-regulates mutant huntingtin expression *in vitro* and mitigates pathology in a Huntington's disease mouse model, *Nat. Rev. Drug Dis.* 3, 205-214.

Bennett, B. D.; Babu-Khan, S.; Loeloff, R.; Louis, J. C.; Curran, E.; Citron, M. & Vassar, R.,(2000) Expression Analysis of BACE2 in Brain and Peripheral Tissues. *J. Biol. Chem.*, 275, 20647-20651.

Bolognesi, M.L.; Andrisano, V.; Bartolini, M.; Bazi, R.& Melchiorre, C.J.(2005) Propidium-Based Polyamine Ligands as Potent Inhibitors of Acetylcholinesterase and Acetylcholinesterase-Induced Amyloid-β Aggregation *J. Med. Chem.*, 48, 24-27.

Camps, P.; Formosa, X.; Munoz-Torrero, D.; Petrignet, J.; Badia, A.& Clos, M.V.(2005) Synthesis and Pharmacological Evaluation of Huprine−Tacrine Heterodimers: Subnanomolar Dual Binding Site Acetylcholinesterase Inhibitors, *J. Med. Chem.*, 48, 1701-1704.

Davis, K. L.; Powchik, P. (1995) Tacrine, *Lancet*, 345, 625-630.

Glenner, G. G. & Wong, C.W. (1984) Alzheimer's disease: initial report of the purification and characterization of a novel cerebrovascular amyloid protein. *Biochem. Biophys. Res.Comm.*, 120, 885-890.

Hanson, L.R.; Fine, J. M.; Tuttle, N.J.; Marti, D. L.; Matthews, R.B.; Nguyen, T.M.; Svitak, A.L.; Panter, S. S.; Frey II, W.H.; Oral 02-05-01: *Intervention and Treatments* 3, S 195, (2007).

Harel, M.; Quin, D. M.; Nair, H. K.; Silman, L. & Sussman, J. L.(1996) The X-ray Structure of a Transition State Analog Complex Reveals the Molecular Origins of the Catalytic Power and Substrate Specificity of Acetylcholinesterase, *J. Am. Chem. Soc.* , 118, 2340-2346.

Hartman, T.; Bieger, S. C.; Bruhl, B.; Tienari, P.J.; Ida, N.; Allsop, D.; Roberts, G. W. ; Masters, C. L.; Dotti, C. G.; Unsicker, K.& Beyreuther, K.(1997) Distinct sites of intracellular production for Alzheimer's disease Aβ40/42 amyloid peptides, *Nature (Medicine)*, 3, 1016-1020.

Huang, W.; Chen, Y.; Shohami, E. & Weinstock, M. (1999) Neuroprotective effect of rasagiline, a selective monoamine oxidase-B inhibitor, against closed head injury in the mouse, *Eur. J. Pharmacol.*, 366, 127-135.

Kazikowsky, A. P.; Compiani, G. L.; Sun, O.; Wang, S.; Saxena, A.& Doctor, B. P.; (1996) Identification of a More Potent Analogue of the Naturally Occurring Alkaloid Huperzine A. Predictive Molecular Modeling of Its Interaction with AChE, *J. Am. Chem. Soc.*, 118,11357-11362.

Kemp, J. A. & Kernan, R. M. Mc, (2002) NMDA receptor pathways as drug targets, *Nature Neurosci.*, 5, 1039-1042.

Kogen, H.; Toda, N.; Tago, K.; Marumoto, S.; Abe, K.; Yamazaki, R.; Hara, T.; Aoyagi, A.; Abe, Y.& Kaneko, T. (2002) Design and Synthesis of Dual Inhibitors of Acetylcholinesterase and Serotonin Transporter Targeting Potential Agents for Alzheimer's Disease, *Org. Lett.*, 4, 3359-3362.

Luo, Y.; Bolon, B.; Damore, M. A.; Fitzpatrick, D.; Liu, H.; Zhang J. et al, (2003) BACE 1 knock out mice do not acquire compensatory gene expression changes or develop neural lesions over time, *Neurobiol. Dis.*, 14, 81-88.

Mattson, M. P.; (2004) Pathways towards and away from Alzheimer's Disease, *Nature, 430, 631-639.*

Potter H. & Dresslar, D. (2000) The potential of BACE inhibitors for Alzheimer's therapy, *Natural Biotech.* , 18, 125-126.

Riedderer, P.; Danielczyk, W. & Grunblatt, E. (2004) Monoamine Oxidase-B inhibition in Alzheimer's Disease, *Neurotoxicology*, 25, 271-277.

Rosini, M.; Andrisano, V.; Bartolini, M.; Bolognesi, M. L.; Hrelia, P.; Minarini, A.; Tarozzi, A. & Melchirre, C.(2005) Rational Approach To Discover Multipotent Anti-Alzheimer Drugs, *J. Med. Chem.*, 48, 360-363.

Sano, M.; Ernesto, C.; Thomas, R.G.; Klauber, M.R.; Schafer, K.; Grundman, M.; Woodbury, P.; Growdow, J.; Cotman, C.W.& Feiffer, E. P. (1997) A controlled trial of Selegiline, Alpha-Tocopherol or both as treatment for Alzheimer's Disease, *New Eng. J. Med.*, 336, 1216-1222.

Sugimoto, H.; Iimura, Y.; Yamanishi, Y. & Yamatsu, K. (1995) Synthesis and Structure-Activity Relationships of Acetylcholinesterase Inhibitors: 1-Benzyl-4-[(5,6-

dimethoxy-1-oxoindan-2-yl)methyl]piperidine Hydrochloride and Related Compounds, *J. Med. Chem.* , 38, 4821-4829.

Toda, N.; Tago, K.; Marumoto, S.; Takami, K.; Ori, M.; Yamada, N.; Koyama K.; S.; Naruto, Abe, K.; Yamazaki, R.; Hara, T.; Aoyagi, A.; Abe, Y.; Kaneko, T. & Kogen, H.(2003) Design, synthesis and structure–Activity relationships of dual inhibitors of acetylcholinesterase and serotonin transporter as potential agents for Alzheimer's disease, *Bioorg. Med. Chem.*, 11, 1935 - 1955.

Toda, N.; Tago, K.; Marumoto, S.; Takami, K.; Ori, M.; Yamada, N.; Koyama, K.; Naruto, S.; Abe, K.; Yamazaki, R.; Hara, T.; Aoyagi, A.; Abe, Y.; Kaneko, T.& Kogen, H.(2003) A conformational restriction approach to the development of dual inhibitors of acetylcholinesterase and serotonin transporter as potential agents for Alzheimer's disease, *Bioorg. Med. Chem.*, 11, 4389-4415.

Weihofen, A.; Lemberg, M.K.; Friedmann, E.; Rueeger, H.; Schmitz, A.; Paganetti, P.; Rovelli G. & B. Martoglio, (2003) Targeting Presenilin-type Aspartic Protease Signal PeptidePeptidase with γ-Secretase Inhibitors. *J. Biol. Chem.*, 278, 16528-16533.

Yan, R.; Han, P.; Miao, H.; Greengard, P.& Xu, H.(2001) The Transmembrane Domain of the Alzheimer's β-Secretase(BACE1) Determines Its Late Golgi Localization and Access to β-Amyloid Precursor Protein (APP) Substrate. *J. Biol. Chem.*, 276, 36788-36796.

Yin, Y. I.; Bassit, B.; Zhu, L.; Yang, X.; Wang, C. & Li, Y. M.(2007) Secretase Substrate Concentration Modulates theAβ42/Aβ40 Ratio. *IMPLICATIONS FOR ALZHEIMER DISEASE, J. Biol Chem.*, 282 (32), 23639-23644.

Yaudin, M.B.H. & Buccafusco, J. J. (2005) Multi functional drugs for various CNS targets in the treatment of neurodegenerative disorders, *Trends Pharmacol. Sci.*, 26, 27-35.

Maestro, version 9.1, Schrödinger, LLC, New York, NY, (2010).

29

Protective Roles of the Incretin Hormones Glucagon-Like Peptide-1 and Glucose-Dependent Insolinotropic Polypeptide Hormones in Neurodegeneration

Christian Hölscher
Ulster University, Neuroscience department, School of Biomed Sci, Northern Ireland, United Kingdom

1. Introduction

Alzheimer's disease is a sporadic disease with very few risk gene links associated with it. Therefore, it is very difficult to assess what the underlying causes of this diseases are, and what the initial triggering mechanisms may be. As the disease can only be diagnosed when it has already developed, very little is known what those early phase processes are that initiate the sequence of events that evenutally lead to neurodegeneration. Another approach to investigate the contributing factors is the correlation with other conditions that increase the risk of developing AD. Several such risk factors have been identified, and interestingly, type 2 diabetes is one of these. In type 2 diabetes mellitus (T2DM), insulin is no longer able to reduce the levels of blood sugar after a meal. In fact, ensulin levels may even be increased as an attempt by the body to overcome the reduced effectiveness of insulin in the periphery, which may be caused by insulin receptor desensitisation. Due to the change of lifelstyle in the industrialised nations, an unhealthy diet in combination with lack of exercise, levels of T2DM are on the rise. This may increase the rate of AD cases in the future. A lot of research is currently conducted in developing novel treatments of T2DM (Dailey 2008, Frias & Edelman 2007, Pi-Sunyer 2008, Scheen 2008). Since insulin effectiveness is reduced in diabetes, research into other signalling pathways that support insulin actions or that reduce blood glucose independently is ongoing. One of these strategies focus on the use of the incretins, a class of peptide hormones that helps to normalise insulin signaling and also improves blood sugar levels. Incretins increase the release of insulin during high blood sugar levels, the so-called 'incretin effect'. They have little effect on normal blood sugar levels and therefore are suitable for treating non-diabetics. In addition, incretins have a range of other effects that help regulate physiological lipid and glucose levels, eg. they increase the uptake of lipids and glucose in cells that express the receptor (Baggio & Drucker 2007, Drucker & Nauck 2006, D. E. Green 2007).

T2DM has been identified as a risk factor for AD, indicating that insulin signaling impairment may be a factor in initiating or accelerating the development of AD. Epidemiological studies found a clear correlation between T2DM and the risk of developing AD or other neurodegenerative disorders at a later stage (Haan 2006, Luchsinger, Tang, Shea, & Mayeux 2004, Ristow 2004, Strachan 2005). For example, a study of patient databases of the Mayo clinic showed a clear correlation between T2DM and AD. In this study, 85% of AD patients also had T2DM or increased fasting glucose levels, compared to only 42% in the control group. T2DM was clearly identified as a risk factor that doubled the chance of developing AD (Janson et al. 2004). Reduced insulin sensitivity and efficacy is also observed in the majority of elderly people and contributes to the development of AD (Carro & Torres-Aleman 2004, Hoyer 2004). It was also shown that insulin receptors in the brain are desensitised in AD patients, which has been named 'type 3 diabetes' (Lester-Coll et al. 2006, Steen et al. 2005). A recent study reported that insulin receptor levels are downregulated in the brains of patients with AD. Insulin receptors were found to be internalised in neurons, and the second messengers IRS1 and IRS2 were reduced in total levels but had increased levels of inactivated phospho^{Ser312} (Moloney et al. 2010). This unexpected connection between T2DM and AD opened up novel research avenues to investigate what the underlying mechanisms for this may be. Insulin is a hormone that has a range of functions in the body. Its general physiological profile is that of a growth factor (see fig. 1). Insulin is crucial for cell growth and survival. Neurons also carry insulin receptors, and activating these induces dendritic sprouting, neuronal stem cell activation, and general cell growth, repair and neuroprotection (Holscher 2005, Hoyer 2004, L. Li & Hölscher 2007, Stockhorst, de Fries, Steingrueber, & Scherbaum 2004, van Dam & Aleman 2004). Furthermore, insulin has potent neuroprotective factors, and also regulates GSK3ß, the main kinase that phosphorylates Tau, which is the major component of neurofibrillary tangles found in the brains of AD (Carro & Torres 2004, L. Li & Hölscher 2007). Insulin also improves brain activity such as attention, memory formation and cognition in humans (Okereke et al. 2008, Reger, Watson, Green, Baker et al. 2008, Watson & Craft 2004, W. Q. Zhao, Chen, Quon, & Alkon 2004). Nasal application of insulin, an application route where it enters the brain more directly, had clear effects on attention and memory formation (S. Craft 2007, Reger, Watson, Green, Baker et al. 2008, Reger, Watson, Green, Wilkinson et al. 2008). A recent phase II clinical trial showed that nasal application of insulin improves memory in patients with mild cognitive impairments and early AD patients, improves the CSF amyloid1-40/1-42 ratio, showed enhancement of cortical activation in PET scans, and also showed improvement in cognitive tasks (S Craft 2010).

In animal models, a decrease in insulin receptor signalling produces cognitive impairments and a reduction in hippocampal synaptic neurotransmission and synaptic plasticity, a mechanism that may be linked to memory formation (Biessels, De Leeuw, Lindeboom, Barkhof, & Scheltens 2006, C. Hölscher 2001, Trudeau, Gagnon, & Massicotte 2004). Diabetic mice show clear imprairments in spatial learning and synaptic plasticity (LTP) in the hippocampus. Treatment with incretins effectively prevented or reversed these impairments (V. A. Gault, Porter, Flatt, & Holscher 2010, Porter, Kerr, Flatt, Holscher, & Gault 2010). People with T2DM also have cognitive impairments, and effective treatment with diabetes medication improves these impairments (Gispen & Biessels 2000, Hoyer 2004). Conversely, insulin injected into the brain can improve performance in memory tasks in animals (Stockhorst et al. 2004). Treatments of diabetic animals with insulin also rescues the impairment in synaptic plasticity (Biessels, Bravenboer, & Gispen 2004, Gispen & Biessels 2000). The basis for this neuroprotective effect is that activation of neuronal insulin receptors has been shown to induce dendritic sprouting, neuronal stem cell activation, and general cell growth, repair, and additional neurotropic effects (Holscher 2005, Hoyer 2004, L. Li & Hölscher 2007, Stockhorst et al. 2004, van Dam & Aleman 2004). Therefore it is not surprising that insulin also improves brain function such as attention, memory and cognition in humans (Okereke et al. 2008, Reger, Watson, Green, Baker et al. 2008, Watson & Craft 2004, W. Q. Zhao et al. 2004).

In conclusion, the impairment of insulin signalling in the brain appears to play a role in the development of neurodegenerative disorders, as it leaves neurons more vulnerable to cytotoxic influences (S. Craft 2005, 2007, Hallschmid & Schultes 2009, Holscher 2005, Hoyer 2004).

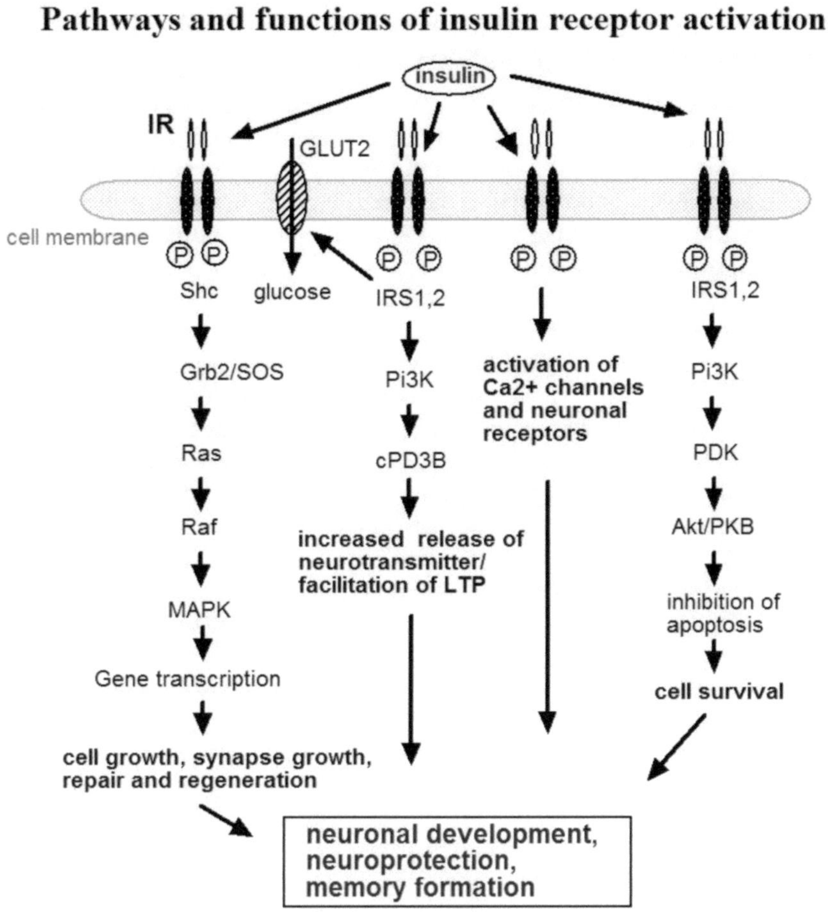

Fig. 1. An overview of some of the roles and functions of insulin receptors (IR). Traditionally, insulin is associated with its blood glucose lowering activity. This is achieved by activating a glucose uptake transporter, eg. GLUT-2. This function is only one of many of the IR. Recent research has uncovered a number of important roles in neuronal growth, synaptic development, and direct control of neurotransmitter release. During neuronal activity, insulin is released and binds to the a-subunit of the receptor. This activates the tyrosine kinase phosphorylation of the b-subunit. Then, several second messenger pathways can be activated:

1. Activation of the insulin receptor-Shc-MAP kinase pathway activates gene expression. These code for proteins that are required for cell growth, synapse growth, and for cell repair and maintenance (Biessels et al. 2006, Hoyer 1997).

2. IR activation has a direct effect on neurotransmission, and primes synapses for induction of long-term potentiation of neuronal transmission (LTP) (Biessels et al. 2004). This pathway most likely involves binding of insulin receptor substrate-1 (IRS1) and insulin receptor substrate-2 (IRS2) to phosphatidylinositol 3-kinase (PI3K). Then, the cyclic nucleotide phosphodiesterase 3B (cPD3B) is activated (A. Z. Zhao et al. 2000). This would prime the synapse for increased neurotransmitter vesicle release (de la Monte & Wands 2006). Modulation of neurotransmission will influence memory formation, information processing, and cognitive processes (C Hölscher 1999).

2. The incretins hormones: Glucagon-like Peptide-1 (GLP-1) and Glucose-dependent Insolinotropic Polypeptide (GIP)

As insulin receptors are desensitised in T2DM and in AD, and injection of insulin itself can have dangerous effects on blood sugar levels and loses its effectiveness over time, scientist in the field are investigating different strategies how to improve blood glucose level maintenance. In addition, it is not sensible to treat AD patients with insulin that do not have diabetes. However, other signalling pathways exist that also modulate blood glucose levels, eg. the incretin hormone signalling pathways - in particular GLP-1 and GIP (Frias & Edelman 2007, V. A. Gault, McClean et al. 2007).

GLP-1 is an endogenous 30-amino acid peptide hormone (fig 3a), which is released by intestinal L and K-cells after a meal. It has several physiological roles in the body to control cell metabolism (fig. 2). GLP-1 is a product of the glucagons gene which encodes the precursor peptide proglucagon. This peptide contains three glucagon-like peptides: glucagon, glucagon-like peptide 1 and glucagon-like peptide 2 (Baggio & Drucker 2007, B. D. Green et al. 2004). The GLP-1 receptor belongs to the class B family of G-protein coupled receptors. The receptors for glucagon, GLP-2 and GIP also belong to this group. Activation of the receptor activates an adenylate cyclase, increases IP3 levels, increases intracellular Ca^{2+} and affects levels of other second messengers (Baggio & Drucker 2007, Holscher 2010). GLP-1 receptor stimulation enhances beta-cell proliferation in the pancreas by activating stem cell proliferation, facilitates glucose-dependent insulin secretion and lowers blood glucose in patients with T2DM (B. D. Green et al. 2006, Lovshin & Drucker 2009).

GIP is a 42-amino acid incretin hormone which activates pancreatic islets to enhance insulin secretion and to help reduce postprandial hyperglycaemia, similar to GLP-1 (V. A. Gault, Flatt, & O'Harte 2003; Fig 3b). GIP also has been shown to promote pancreatic beta-cell growth, differentiation, proliferation and cell survival, documenting its growth-hormone properties (V. A. Gault et al. 2003). Therefore, research is ongoing to develop GIP as an therapeutic tool for T2DM treatment (Irwin et al. 2006) (see fig. 3b). GIP is a member of the vasoactive intestinal peptide seretin/glucagon family of neuroregulatory polypeptides which also include the pituitary adenylate cyclase activating peptide and the growth hormone releasing factor. It is expressed in pancreatic alpha cells, endocrine K and L cells, and also in neurons (Nyberg et al. 2005). Apart from the incretin effect of enhancing insulin release under hyperglycaemic conditions, GIPR activity in bone tissues enhances bode density, uptake of fat into adipose cells, and stem cell or neuronal progenitor cell proliferation (Baggio & Drucker 2007, Figueiredo et al. 2010). GIPR KO mice show a decrease in neuronal stem cell proliferation, and GIP analogues activate neuronal stem cells (E Faivre, McClean, & Hölscher 2010, Nyberg, Jacobsson, Anderson, & Eriksson 2007).

2.1 Incretins also play important roles in the brain

GLP-1 receptors are found on neurons in the brains of rodents and humans (Goke, Larsen, Mikkelsen, & Sheikh 1995, Perry & Greig 2005). They are predominately expressed on large size neurons, on the cell bodies and also on dendrites, indicating that they are located on the synapse (A Hamilton & Holscher 2009). Similar to insulin, GLP-1 is predominately known for its action on blood sugar levels. However, just as insulin, GLP-1 is principally a growth factor and has the main properties of all growth factors (Holscher & Li 2010). GLP-1 increases cell growth, proliferation and repair, and inhibits apoptosis (A. Hamilton, Patterson, Porter, Gault, & Holscher 2011, Perfetti, Zhou, Doyle, & Egan 2000). In the brain,

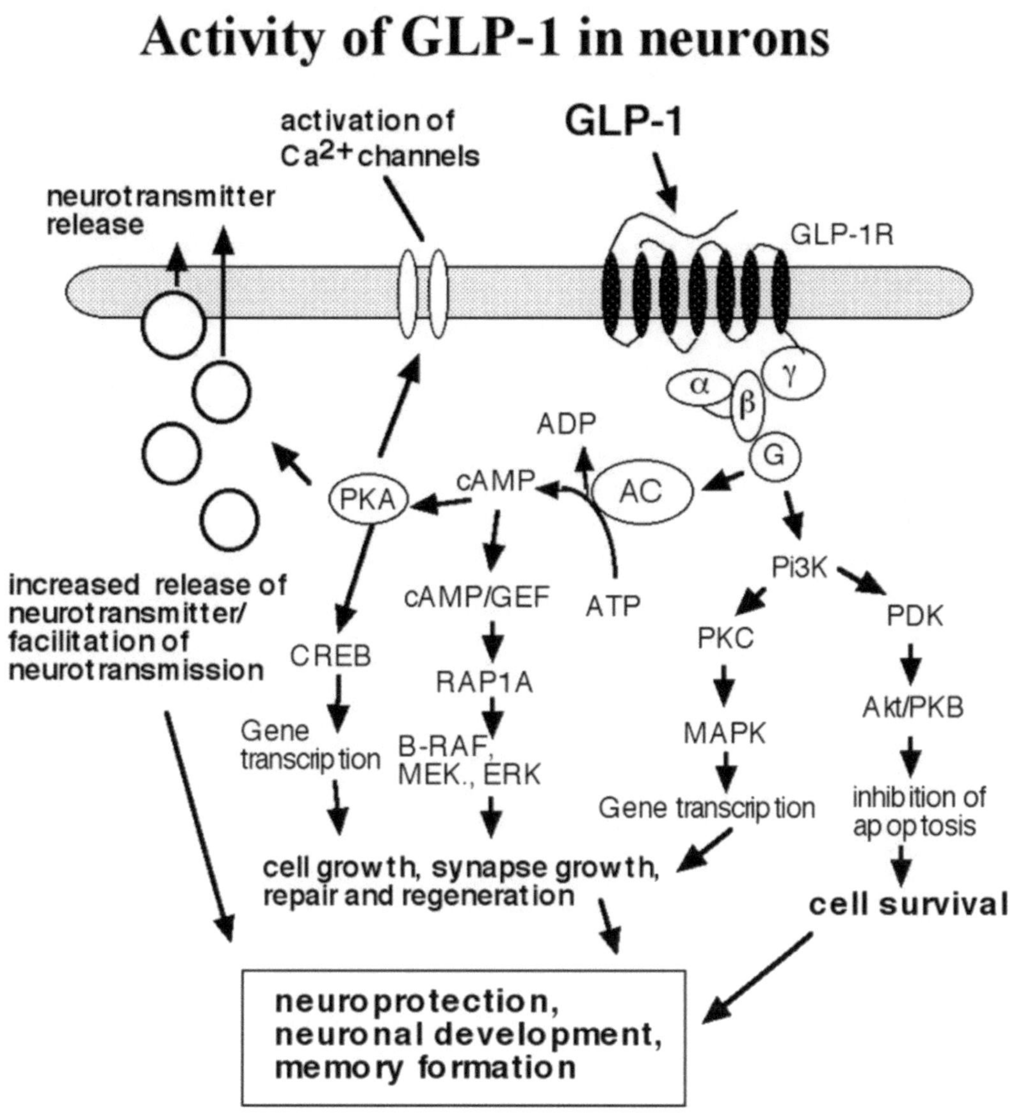

Fig. 2. Overview of the main pathways induced by GLP-1 in neurons. As compared to fig. 1, the overall mechanisms are very similar. The main physiological effects of GLP-1 on cell growth, proliferation, regeneration and inhibition of apoptosis are identical. Differences can be seen in the control of vesicle release, which is glucose-dependent in ß-cells but not in neurons. For more details see (Holscher 2010, Holscher & Li 2010).

GLP - 1 sequences

Native GLP - 1
HAEGTFTSDVSSYLEGQAAKEFIAWLVKGR

Asp(7)GLP - 1
DAEGTFTSDVSSYLEGQAAKEFIAWLVKGR

Val(8)GLP - 1
HVEGTFTSDVSSYLEGQAAKEFIAWLVKGR

Pro(9)GLP - 1
HAPGTFTSDVSSYLEGQAAKEFIAWLVKGR

Exendin - 4
HGEGTFTSDLSKQMEEEAVRLFIEWLKNGGPSSGAPPPS

Lixisenatide
HGEGTFTSDLSKQMEEEAVRLFIEWLKNGGPSSGAPPSKKKKKK - NH2

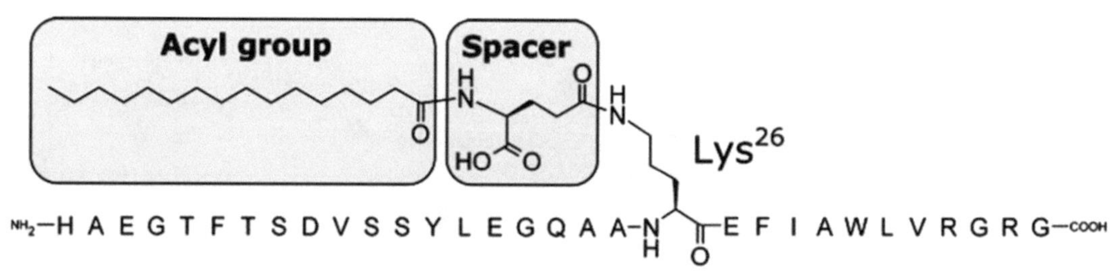

Liraglutide

Fig. 3. a. Shown are the amino acid sequences of the native GLP-1 peptide and also of some modifications of GLP-1 designed to prevent degradation by the DPP-IV protease. Shown are amino acid substitutions at position 7, 8, or 9 (Holscher 2010), and a fatty acid addition to a modified GLP-1 peptide (liraglutide). Liraglutide has the amino acid sequence of native GLP-1 with one modification, Arg34, and are derivatised at position 26 with a spacer and an acyl group (Madsen et al. 2007). The natural GLP-1 analogue exendin-4 sequence is shown. This peptide is found in the saliva of the reptile Gila monster. A derivative of this sequence is Lixisenatide, which is a long-acting GLP-1 analogue currently in clinical trials as a treatment of T2DM (Christensen, Knop, Holst, & Vilsboll 2009).

GIP sequences

Native GIP
MVATKTFALLLLSLFLAVGLGEKKEGHFSALPSLPVGSHAKV

*d*Ala(2)GIP
MAATKTFALLLLSLFLAVGLGEKKEGHFSALPSLPVGSHAKV

Pro(3)GIP
MVPTKTFALLLLSLFLAVGLGEKKEGHFSALPSLPVGSHAKV

Fig. 3. b. Shown are the amino acid sequences of the native GIP peptide and also of some of the modifications of GIP to prevent degradation by the DPP-IV protease. Shown are amino acid substitutions at position 2 and 3. The analogue D-ALA(2)GIP acts as an agonist to the receptor, while the analogue Pro(3)GIP has antagonistic properties (V. Gault et al. 2005, V. A. Gault & C. Holscher 2008, V. A. Gault, Hunter et al. 2007).

GLP-1 has been documented to induce neurite outgrowth and to protect against excitotoxic cell death and oxidative injury in cultured neuronal cells (Perry et al. 2002, Perry et al. 2003). Neurons were found to be protected against cell death induced by beta-amyloid 1-42, the peptide that aggregates in the brains of Alzheimer patients, and against oxidative stress and membrane lipid peroxidation caused by iron (Perry & Greig 2005). In addition to this, mice that overexpress GLP-1 receptors in the hippocampus showed increased neurite outgrowth and improved spatial learning. Enhanced progenitor cell proliferation in the brain was also found in this study (During et al. 2003). The novel GLP-1 analogue Liraglutide also increases the division of neuronal progenitor cells in the brain, and even increases neuronal neogenesis in the brains of a mouse model of AD (P. McClean, Parthsarathy, Faivre, & Hölscher 2011) (see fig 4). These properties are typical growth factor effects, and by activating neuronal progenitor cell proliferation and neurogenesis it may be possible to regenerate parts of the lost brain tissue and to regain some of the lost cognitive functions in patients with AD (Sugaya et al. 2007).

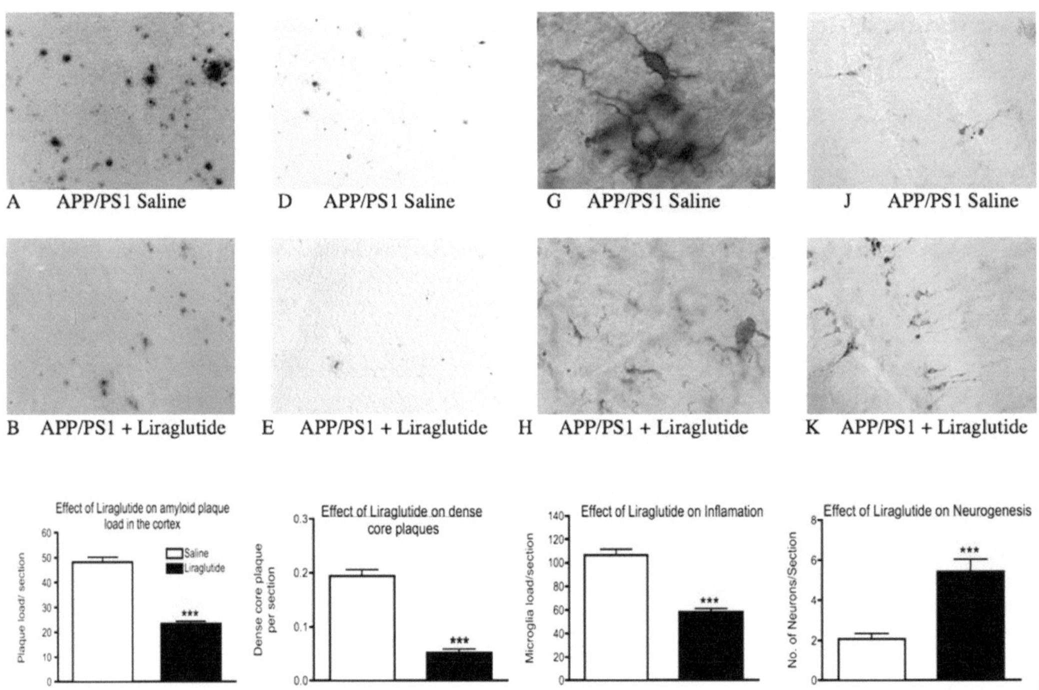

Fig. 4. Histological hallmarks of AD are improved with Liraglutide. Histological analysis of the liraglutide-injected APP/PS1 mice showed a reduction in the number of plaques in the cortex and hippocampus of Liraglutide-treated APP/PS1 mice was halved (A, B, C). The number of Congo-red positive dense core plaques was reduced to 25% (D, E, F). The inflammatory response, as shown by activated glia (IBA-1stain), was also halved (G, H, I). Mice treated with Liraglutide also had a significant increase in neurogenesis (Doublecortin positive cells) compared with saline treated animals (J, K, L). Sample micrographs show saline-treated on top, Liraglutide below, and overall quantification at bottom. ***P<0.001, (student's t-test), n=6) (P. McClean et al. 2011).

GIP is expressed in neurons and used as a neurotransmitter, and GIP receptors are also found in the brain (V. A. Gault & C. Holscher 2008, Nyberg et al. 2005, Nyberg et al. 2007). Even less is known about the roles of GIP in the brain than about the roles of GLP-1. GIP enhances neuronal progenitor proliferation in the dentate gyrus and affects learning, as discussed below (E. Faivre, Gault, Thorens, & Holscher 2011, E Faivre & Hölscher 2011).

2.2 Effects of incretins on synaptic transmission

Insulin as well as the incretins not only have growth-factor like properties in the brain, but also modulate synaptic activity. Neurons communicate via synaptic activity, and this activity can be enhanced for longer periods of time (long-term potentiation of synaptic transmission, LTP (C Hölscher 1999). One study showed that the injection of GLP-1 into the basal ganglia increased the synaptic release of the neurotransmitter glutamate (Mora, Exposito, Sanz, & Blazquez 1992). GLP-1 also increased the spontaneous firing rate of pyramidal neurons in the hippocampus (J. I. Oka, Goto, & Kameyama 1999). Interestingly, beta-amyloid fragments can directly affect synaptic transmission and impair the use-dependent upregulation of synaptic transmission (LTP). Since such a mechanism could be a used for storing information in the brain (C. Hölscher 2001), this amyloid-induced block of LTP may be in part responsible for impaired memory formation in patients with AD (Freir, Holscher, & Herron 2001, C Hölscher, Gengler, Gault, Harriott, & Mallot 2007). In addition, a recent study has shown that soluble beta-amyloid fragments directly bind to and decrease insulin receptor densities on neuronal dendrites (Xie et al. 2002, W. Q. Zhao et al. 2008). This may be a mechanism how insulin signalling in the brain becomes impaired in people with AD.

Further studies showed that direct injection of GLP-1 or long-lasting GLP-1 analogues into the brain markedly enhanced LTP in the hippocampus, a brain area that is involved in memory formation. Agonists such as Val^{8}-GLP-1 showed a clear upregulation of LTP, while the selective GLP-1 antagonist exendin(9-36) blocked LTP (V. Gault & C. Holscher 2008). The novel GLP-1 analogue liraglutide that has been released onto the market as a treatment for T2DM also upregulated LTP (P. L. McClean, Gault, Harriott, & Holscher 2010). Importantly, GLP-1 analogues were able to prevent the impairment of LTP that was induced by beta-amyloid fragments (V. Gault & C. Holscher 2008, Gengler, McClean, McCurtin, Gault, & Holscher 2010, P. McClean et al. 2011). These effects are most impressive and underline the fact that beta-amyloid has numerous independent effects on cell physiology; some of which may occur very early on in AD, long before amyloid aggregates appear and neuronal death is observed (Gong et al. 2003, Townsend, Shankar, Mehta, Walsh, & Selkoe 2006). Moreover, GLP-1, liraglutide and exendin-4 have been shown to reduce endogenous levels of beta-amyloid in a mouse model of AD, and to reduce levels of beta-amyloid precursor protein (APP) in neurons (P. McClean et al. 2011, Perry et al. 2003). In contrast, the elimination of the GLP-1R in a KO mouse model severely impaired learning abilities and also strongly reduced synaptic plasticity (Abbas, Faivre, & Hölscher 2009). Interestingly enough, spatial learning and synaptic plasticity is also impaired in mouse models of diabetes, and exendin-4 is able to reverse these impairments (V. A. Gault et al. 2010). These results suggest that treatment with GLP-1 or long-lasting analogues beneficially affect a number of the therapeutic targets associated with AD, such as impaired memory, impaired neuronal synaptic transmission, increased neurodegenerative processes and reduced neuronal regeneration.

Interestingly, GIP receptors are also expressed in the brain and are found on larger neurons such as the pyramidal cortical neurons (Nyberg et al. 2005), which is similar to the pattern of expression of GLP-1 receptors (A Hamilton & Holscher 2009). The peptide GIP is also expressed in neurons and serves as a neuronal transmitter (Nyberg et al. 2007). Stable analogues such as D-ala^{2}-GIP or N-glyc-GIP facilitate synaptic plasticity in the hippocampus, while the antagonist Pro^{3}-GIP impairs LTP (V. A. Gault & C. Holscher 2008). Impressively, GIP analogues can prevent the LTP impairment that beta-amyloid fragments induce on synaptic transmission in the brain (V. A. Gault & C. Holscher 2008). In a GIPR-KO mouse strain, LTP was also much reduced, and paired-pulse facilitation showed an effect on the presynapse, indicating that the release of synaptic vesicles is reduced (E. Faivre et al. 2011). The long-lasting GIP analogue D-Ala^{2}-GIP also had neuroprotective effects in an APP/PS1 mouse model of AD. In 12 months old mice, synaptic plasticity in area CA1 of the hippocampus and spatial memory formation was impaired in control APP/PS1 mice but was unimpaired in D-Ala^{2}-GIP treated APP/PS1 mice. In addition, the amyloid plaque load was much reduced, showing impressive effects in reducing the main hallmarks of AD (E Faivre & Hölscher 2011). This suggests that these analogues have neuroprotective properties in AD and protect synapses from the detrimental effects of beta-amyloid. The receptor distribution in the brain and also the effects of analogues on LTP is very similar when comparing GLP-1 analogues with GIP analogues. This would suggest that the physiological roles of these incretins may also be very similar. However, the clear results in impairing LTP (and learning) in the GLP-1R KO or GIPR KO mice show that one incretin cannot compensate the impairment or receptor loss of the another. This suggests that both incretins play distinctive roles that we currently know very little about, but also show very similar growth-factor-like effects.

2.3 Effects of incretins on memory formation

GLP-1 and longer acting analogues that can cross the BBB have beneficial effects on cognition. A behavioural study showed that the GLP-1 analogue exendin-4 can prevent the learning impairments induced by the injection of beta-amyloid fragments (J. Oka, Suzuki, & Kondo 2000). The GLP-1 analogue Val^{8}-GLP-1 also prevented the detrimental effect of beta-amyloid injected icv. has on learning a water maze task (Wang et al. 2010). Another study showed that GLP-1 when injected *icv.* can enhance memory formation. The study also showed that the GLP-1 analogue Ser(2)exendin(1-9) can enhance learning of a spatial task when injected *ip.*, indicting that this analogue crosses the BBB (During et al. 2003). The overexpression of the GLP-1 receptor also enhanced learning of a spatial task, while the deletion of GLP-1 receptor in KO mice impaired learning (During et al. 2003). In a different study, GLP-1 receptor KO mice were impaired in learning spatial and recognition tasks, while LTP in the hippocampus was severely impaired (Abbas et al. 2009). These results show that GLP-1 receptors do play an important role in cognitive processes in the brain, and that GLP-1 analogues can enhance learning even when injected *ip*.

Recent studies have shown that stable GIP analogues such as D-ala^{2}-GIP or Pro^{3}-GIP cross the BBB and also enhance neuronal stem cell proliferation in the brain (E Faivre et al. 2010). Furthermore, GIP analogues have clear effects on memory formation, with the GIP receptor agonist D-Ala^{2}GIP facilitating memory, and the GIP receptor antagonist Pro^{3}-GIP impairing memory (E Faivre et al. 2010). GIP analogues also have clear effects on synaptic plasticity in the brain. They enhance synaptic plasticity in the hippocampus, a mechanism considered by some to represent the cellular level of memory formation. Importantly, beta-amyloid impairs synaptic plasticity, and injection of GIP analogues protect synapses from the detrimental effects of beta-amyloid(25-35) (V. A. Gault & C. Holscher 2008). In another study, icv. infusion of Abeta1-40 in mice produced impairments in a water maze test, and the infusion of GIP icv. prevented the amyloid induced impairment in spatial learning (Figueiredo et al. 2010).

These properties make GIP analogues a promising target for the development of novel treatments of AD. As described earlier, spatial and non-spatial learning was greatly impaired in a GIPR- KO mouse strain, showing that the lack of GIP signalling plays an important role in memory formation, and cannot be compensated for by the still functioning insulin and GLP-1 signalling pathways (E. Faivre et al. 2011).

2.4 Novel incretin analogues have neuroprotective effects in mouse models of AD

As an important pre-clinical test, novel analogues of GLP-1 have shown neuroprotective properties in mouse models of AD. In one study, the GLP-1 analogue Val^8-GLP-1 had neuroprotective effects in a mouse model of AD that overexpresses the human Swedish mutated form of APP and a human mutated form of presenelin-1. The mice develop high densities of beta-amyloid plaques in the cortex and hippocampus, starting at 3 months of age (Radde et al. 2006). When injecting Val^8-GLP-1 chronically ip. at a dose of 25nmol/kg *ip.* once-daily for 3 weeks, synaptic plasticity in the hippocampus was protected from the effects of plaque formation and did not differ from littermate wildtype control mice. LTP was completely protected even at 18 months of age. In addition, the number of Congo red positive dense-core amyloid plaques in the brain was reduced. LTP was also improved in 18 month old *wild-type* mice when compared to controls, indicating that GLP-1 analogues also protect the brain to some degree from age-related synaptic degenerative processes (Gengler et al. 2010). Furthermore, the GLP-1 analogue exendin-4 which is currently on the market as a treatment of T2DM (Byetta®) had been tested in a triple transgenic mouse model of AD. This model also expresses the Swedish mutated form of human APP and a PS-1, and in addition expresses a mutated form of tau protein. The mice develop plaques at around 12-14 months. They also show hyperphosphorylated tau, similar to humans with AD. Exendin-4 was applied subcutaneously via osmotic pumps. To test the effects of a combination of diabetes and AD, a group of transgenic mice were made diabetic by injection of streptozotocin. The main findings were that in the diabetic mouse model of AD, beta-amyloid production had increased and plaque formation in the brain was enhanced. The treatment with exendin-4 treated the diabetes, reduced beta-amyloid production and plaque formation (Y. Li et al. 2010).

In another study, the novel GLP-1 analogue liraglutide that is also on the market as a T2DM treatment (Victoza®) enhanced memory formation and synaptic plasticity in the brains of APP/PS1 mice after ip. injection (25nmol/kg bw, once daily) for 8 weeks, at a dose that is comparable to the dose given to T2DM patients (0.9-1.8 mg subcutaneously once-daily). The learning impairments observed in untreated AD mice were reversed by liraglutide (fig. 5), and the impairment of hippocampal synaptic plasticity that develops over time in untreated mice was also prevented. More importantly, amyloid plaque formation was reduced to 50%, and the formation of Congo-red dense core plaques was reduced to 30%. In addition, the inflammation response (activated microglia) was also halved. Furthermore, increased neurogenesis was observed in the dentate gyrus of these mice, normalising the number of young neurons when compared to wild type controls (fig. 4). The level of soluble amyloid-oligomers was also greatly reduced (P. McClean et al. 2011).

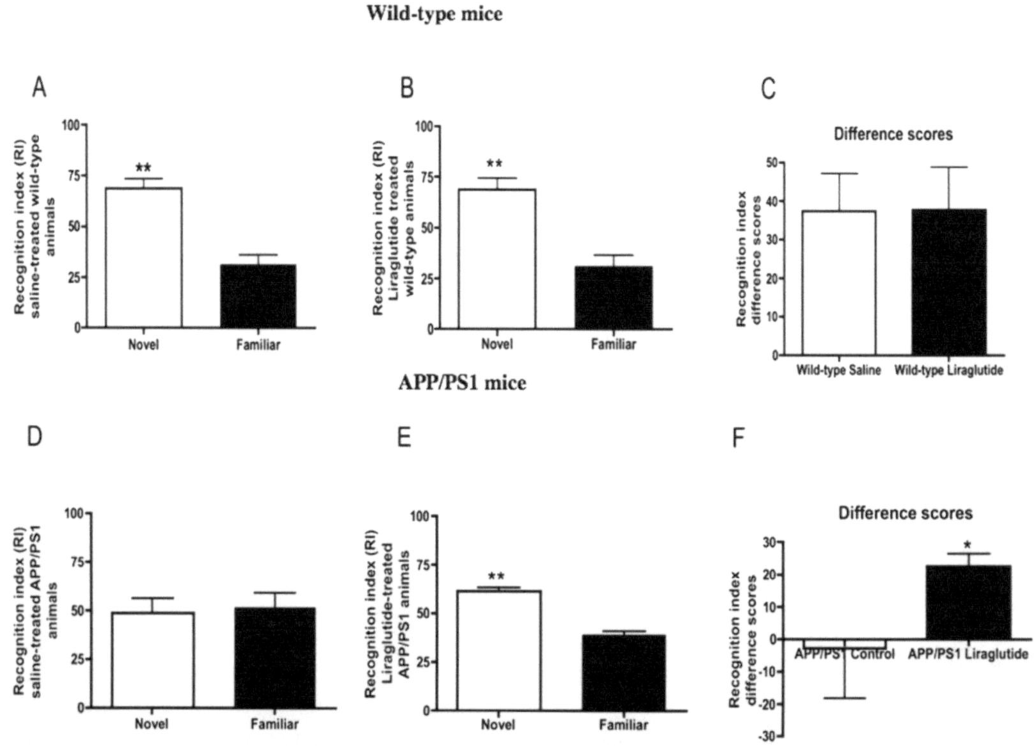

Fig. 5. Effect of the diabetes drug Liraglutide on recognition memory in APP/PS1 mice. In the object recognition task two identical objects were shown to mice for 10min, after 56 days treatment with either 0.9% Saline or Liraglutide (25nm/kg bw). After a 3h interval mice were exposed to one novel and one familiar object. Shown is the recognition index (RI) which is the % time spent exploring the novel object vs. the overall exploration time. Liraglutide treatment made no difference to the learning ability of wild-type mice (A, B), with overall difference scores comparable (C). In contrast Liraglutide rescued the recognition memory of APP/PS1 mice (E), with controls unable to discriminate between novel and familiar objects (D). Overall difference scores were significantly increased in APP/PS1 Liraglutide-treated mice. (F, student's t-test, *$p<0.05$, **$p<0.01$; all groups n=12) (P. McClean et al. 2011).

GIP analogues have shown similar effects in a APP/PS1 mouse model of AD. Injection of the GIP peptide ip. had protective effects on spatial learning in memory tasks and also reduced plaque formation and amyloid load (Figueiredo et al. 2010). In 12 months old APP/PS1 mice, spatial memory formation and object recognition memory as well as LTP was impaired in control APP/PS1 mice but was unimpaired in D-Ala^2-GIP treated APP/PS1 mice. In addition, the amyloid plaque load was much reduced, showing clear effects in reducing the main hallmarks of AD. The numer of neuronal progenitor cells in the dentate gyrus was also increased by D-Ala^2-GIP (E Faivre & Hölscher 2011).

These findings confirm that incretin analogues cross the BBB when injected peripherally and have pronounced neuroprotective effects on the main hallmarks and symptoms of AD as observed in these mouse models. This suggest that treating AD patients with novel stable

GLP-1 analogues has the potential to prevent or prolong the early phase of neurodegeneration, and potentially prevent the late phase of degeneration altogether. Since two such GLP-1 analogues are already on the market as T2DM treatment, the use of such drugs to treat neurodegenerative conditions is most promising. Importantly, clinical trials of the effects of exendin-4 in patients with Parkinson's disease (UCL, London, UK) have been started, and clinical trials in patients with MCI or early-phase AD are on their way (NIH/NIA, USA) (see an update on www.clinicaltrials.gov).

3. Acknowledgement

Dr Holscher is supported by the Alzheimer Research Trust, UK, and the Alzheimer Society, UK.

4. References

Abbas, T., Faivre, E. & Hölscher, C. (2009) Impairment of synaptic plasticity and memory formation in GLP-1 receptor KO mice: interaction between type 2 diabetes and Alzheimer's disease. *Behav Brain Res 205*: 265-271.

Baggio, L. L. & Drucker, D. J. (2007) Biology of incretins: GLP-1 and GIP. *Gastroenterology 132*(6): 2131-2157.

Biessels, G. J., Bravenboer, B. & Gispen, W. H. (2004) Glucose, insulin and the brain: modulation of cognition and synaptic plasticity in health and disease: a preface. *Eur J Pharmacol 490*(1-3): 1-4.

Biessels, G. J., De Leeuw, F. E., Lindeboom, J., Barkhof, F. & Scheltens, P. (2006) Increased cortical atrophy in patients with Alzheimer's disease and type 2 diabetes mellitus. *J Neurol Neurosurg Psychiatry 77*(3): 304-307.

Carro, E. & Torres, A. I. (2004) The role of insulin and insulin-like growth factor I in the molecular and cellular mechanisms underlying the pathology of Alzheimer's disease. *Eur J Pharmacol 490*(1-3): 127-133.

Carro, E. & Torres-Aleman, I. (2004) Insulin-like growth factor I and Alzheimer's disease: therapeutic prospects? *Expert Rev Neurother 4*(1): 79-86.

Christensen, M., Knop, F. K., Holst, J. J. & Vilsboll, T. (2009) Lixisenatide, a novel GLP-1 receptor agonist for the treatment of type 2 diabetes mellitus. *IDrugs 12*(8): 503-513.

Craft, S. (2005) Insulin resistance syndrome and Alzheimer's disease: age- and obesity-related effects on memory, amyloid, and inflammation. *Neurobiol Aging 26 Suppl 1*: 65-69.

Craft, S. (2007) Insulin resistance and Alzheimer's disease pathogenesis: potential mechanisms and implications for treatment. *Curr Alzheimer Res 4*(2): 147-152.

Craft, S. (2010). A randomized, placebo-controlled trial of intranasal insulin in amnestic MCI and early Alzheimer's, *ICAD conference* (pp. abstr. P3-455.). Hawaii, USA.

Dailey, G. (2008) Beyond insulin replacement: addressing the additional needs of the diabetes patient. *Diabetes Obes Metab 10 Suppl 2*: 83-97.

de la Monte, S. M. & Wands, J. R. (2006) Molecular indices of oxidative stress and mitochondrial dysfunction occur early and often progress with severity of Alzheimer's disease. *J Alzheimers Dis 9*(2): 167-181.

Drucker, D. J. & Nauck, M. A. (2006) The incretin system: glucagon-like peptide-1 receptor agonists and dipeptidyl peptidase-4 inhibitors in type 2 diabetes. *Lancet 368*(9548): 1696-1705.

During, M. J., Cao, L., Zuzga, D. S., Francis, J. S., Fitzsimons, H. L., Jiao, X., Bland, R. J., Klugmann, M., Banks, W. A., Drucker, D. J. & Haile, C. N. (2003) Glucagon-like peptide-1 receptor is involved in learning and neuroprotection. *Nat Med 9*(9): 1173-1179.

Faivre, E., Gault, V. A., Thorens, B. & Holscher, C. (2011) Glucose-dependent insulinotropic polypeptide receptor knockout mice are impaired in learning, synaptic plasticity, and neurogenesis. *J Neurophysiol.*

Faivre, E. & Hölscher, C. (2011). DAla2-GIP improves memory, synaptic plasticity and decreases amyloid plaques and inflammation in APP/PS1 transgenic mice, *AR-UK*. Leeds.

Faivre, E., McClean, P. & Hölscher, C. (2010). *Novel GIP analogues cross the BBB and have effects on cognitive processes and synaptic plasticity in the hippocampus.* Paper presented at the Annual conference of the Alzheimer Research Trust UK, Southampton.

Figueiredo, C. P., Pamplona, F. A., Mazzuco, T. L., Aguiar, A. S., Jr., Walz, R. & Prediger, R. D. (2010) Role of the glucose-dependent insulinotropic polypeptide and its receptor in the central nervous system: therapeutic potential in neurological diseases. *Behav Pharmacol 21*: 394-408.

Freir, D. B., Holscher, C. & Herron, C. E. (2001) Blockade of Long-Term Potentiation by beta-Amyloid Peptides in the CA1 Region of the Rat Hippocampus In Vivo. *J Neurophysiol 85*(2): 708-713.

Frias, J. P. & Edelman, S. V. (2007) Incretins and their role in the management of diabetes. *Curr Opin Endocrinol Diabetes Obes 14*(4): 269-276.

Gault, V. & Holscher, C. (2008) GLP-1 agonists facilitate hippocampal LTP and reverse the impairment of LTP induced by beta-amyloid. *Eur J Pharmacol 587*: 112-117.

Gault, V., Irwin, N., Green, B., McCluskey, J., Greer , B., Bailey, C., Harriott, P., O'Harte, F. & Flatt, P. (2005) Chemical ablation of gastric inhibitory polypeptide receptor action by daily (Pro3)GIP administration improves glucose tolerance and ameliorates insulin resistance and abnormalities of islet structure in obesity-diabetes. *Diabetes 54*: 2436-2446.

Gault, V. A., Flatt, P. R. & O'Harte, F. P. (2003) Glucose-dependent insulinotropic polypeptide analogues and their therapeutic potential for the treatment of obesity-diabetes. *Biochem Biophys Res Commun 308*(2): 207-213.

Gault, V. A. & Holscher, C. (2008) Protease-resistant glucose-dependent insulinotropic polypeptide agonists facilitate hippocampal LTP and reverse the impairment of LTP induced by beta-amyloid. *J Neurophysiol 99*(4): 1590-1595.

Gault, V. A., Hunter, K., Irwin, N., Green, B. D., Greer, B., Harriott, P., O'Harte, F. P. & Flatt, P. R. (2007) Characterisation and biological activity of Glu3 amino acid substituted GIP receptor antagonists. *Arch Biochem Biophys 461*(2): 263-274.

Gault, V. A., McClean, P. L., Irwin, N., Power, G. J., McCluskey, J. T. & Flatt, P. R. (2007) Effects of subchronic treatment with the long-acting glucose-dependent insulinotropic polypeptide receptor agonist, N-AcGIP, on glucose homeostasis in streptozotocin-induced diabetes. *Pancreas 35*(1): 73-79.

Gault, V. A., Porter, W. D., Flatt, P. R. & Holscher, C. (2010) Actions of exendin-4 therapy on cognitive function and hippocampal synaptic plasticity in mice fed a high-fat diet. *Int J Obes (Lond) 34*: 1341-1344.

Gengler, S., McClean, P., McCurtin, R., Gault, V. & Holscher, C. (2010) Val(8)GLP-1 rescues synaptic plasticity and reduces dense core plaques in APP/PS1 mice. *Neurobiol Aging DOI*: 10.1016/j.neurobiolaging.2010.1002.1014.

Gispen, W. H. & Biessels, G. J. (2000) Cognition and synaptic plasticity in diabetes mellitus. *Trends Neurosci 23*(11): 542-549.

Goke, R., Larsen, P. J., Mikkelsen, J. D. & Sheikh, S. P. (1995) Distribution of GLP-1 binding sites in the rat brain: evidence that exendin-4 is a ligand of brain GLP-1 binding sites. *Eur J Neurosci 7*(11): 2294-2300.

Gong, Y., Chang, L., Viola, K. L., Lacor, P. N., Lambert, M. P., Finch, C. E., Krafft, G. A. & Klein, W. L. (2003) Alzheimer's disease-affected brain: Presence of oligomeric A beta ligands (ADDLs) suggests a molecular basis for reversible memory loss. *Proc Natl Acad Sci U S A 100*(18): 10417-10422.

Green, B. D., Gault, V. A., Flatt, P. R., Harriott, P., Greer, B. & O'Harte, F. P. (2004) Comparative effects of GLP-1 and GIP on cAMP production, insulin secretion, and in vivo antidiabetic actions following substitution of Ala8/Ala2 with 2-aminobutyric acid. *Arch Biochem Biophys 428*(2): 136-143.

Green, B. D., Lavery, K. S., Irwin, N., O'Harte F, P., Harriott, P., Greer, B., Bailey, C. J. & Flatt, P. R. (2006) Novel GLP-1 analogue (Val8)GLP-1 results in significant improvements of glucose tolerance and pancreatic beta cell function after 3 weeks daily administration in obese diabetic (ob/ob) mice. *J Pharmacol Exp Ther 318*(2): 914-921.

Green, D. E. (2007) New therapies for diabetes. *Clin Cornerstone 8*(2): 58-63; discussion 64-55.

Haan, M. N. (2006) Therapy Insight: type 2 diabetes mellitus and the risk of late-onset Alzheimer's disease. *Nat Clin Pract Neurol 2*(3): 159-166.

Hallschmid, M. & Schultes, B. (2009) Central nervous insulin resistance: a promising target in the treatment of metabolic and cognitive disorders? *Diabetologia 52*(11): 2264-2269.

Hamilton, A. & Holscher, C. (2009) Receptors for the insulin-like peptide GLP-1 are expressed on neurons in the CNS. *Neuroreport 20*: 1161-1166.

Hamilton, A., Patterson, S., Porter, D., Gault, V. A. & Holscher, C. (2011) Novel GLP-1 mimetics developed to treat type 2 diabetes promote progenitor cell proliferation in the brain. *J Neurosci Res 89*(4): 481-489.

Holscher, C. (2005) Development of beta-amyloid-induced neurodegeneration in Alzheimer's disease and novel neuroprotective strategies. *Rev Neurosci 16*(3): 181-212.

Holscher, C. (2010) Incretin Analogues that have been Developed to Treat Type 2 Diabetes Hold Promise as a Novel Treatment Strategy for Alzheimer's Disease. *Recent Pat CNS Drug Discov 5*: 109-117.

Hölscher, C. (1999) Synaptic plasticity and learning and memory: LTP and beyond. *J Neurosci Res 58*: 62-75.

Hölscher, C. (Ed.). (2001). *Long-term potentiation induced by stimulation on the positive phase of theta rhythm: a better model for learning and memory?* Cambridge: Cambridge University Press.

Hölscher, C., Gengler, S., Gault, V., Harriott, P. & Mallot, H. (2007) Soluble beta-amyloid[25-35] reversibly impairs hippocampal synaptic plasticity and spatial learning. *Eur J Pharmacol 561*: 85-90.

Holscher, C. & Li, L. (2010) New roles for insulin-like hormones in neuronal signalling and protection: New hopes for novel treatments of Alzheimer's disease? *Neurobiol Aging 31*: 1495-1502.

Hoyer, S. (1997) Models of Alzheimer's disease: cellular and molecular aspects. *J Neural Transm 49*(11): 11-21.

Hoyer, S. (2004) Glucose metabolism and insulin receptor signal transduction in Alzheimer disease. *Eur J Pharmacol 490*(1-3): 115-125.

Irwin, N., O'Harte F, P., Gault, V. A., Green, B. D., Greer, B., Harriott, P., Bailey, C. J. & Flatt, P. R. (2006) GIP(Lys(16)PAL) and GIP(Lys(37)PAL): Novel Long-Acting Acylated Analogues of Glucose-Dependent Insulinotropic Polypeptide with Improved Antidiabetic Potential. *J Med Chem 49*(3): 1047-1054.

Janson, J., Laedtke, T., Parisi, J., O'Brien, P., Petersen, R. & Butler, P. (2004) Increased risk of type 2 diabetes in Alzheimer disease. *Diabetes 53*: 474-481.

Lester-Coll, N., Rivera, E. J., Soscia, S. J., Doiron, K., Wands, J. R. & de la Monte, S. M. (2006) Intracerebral streptozotocin model of type 3 diabetes: relevance to sporadic Alzheimer's disease. *J Alzheimers Dis 9*(1): 13-33.

Li, L. & Hölscher, C. (2007) Common pathological processes in Alzheimer Disease and Type 2 Diabetes: a review. *Brain Res Rev 56*: 384-402.

Li, Y., Duffy, K., Ottinger, M., Ray, B., Bailey, J., Holloway, H., Tweedie, D., Perry, T., Mattson, M., Kapogiannis, D., Sambamurti, K., Lahiri, D. & Greig, N. (2010) GLP-1 Receptor Stimulation Reduces Amyloid-beta Peptide Accumulation and Cytotoxicity in Cellular and Animal Models of Alzheimer's Disease. *J Alzheimers Dis 19*: 1205-1219.

Lovshin, J. A. & Drucker, D. J. (2009) Incretin-based therapies for type 2 diabetes mellitus. *Nat Rev Endocrinol 5*(5): 262-269.

Luchsinger, J. A., Tang, M. X., Shea, S. & Mayeux, R. (2004) Hyperinsulinemia and risk of Alzheimer disease. *Neurology 63*(7): 1187-1192.

Madsen, K., Knudsen, L. B., Agersoe, H., Nielsen, P. F., Thogersen, H., Wilken, M. & Johansen, N. L. (2007) Structure-activity and protraction relationship of long-acting glucagon-like peptide-1 derivatives: importance of fatty acid length, polarity, and bulkiness. *J Med Chem 50*(24): 6126-6132.

McClean, P., Parthsarathy, V., Faivre, E. & Hölscher, C. (2011) The diabetes drug Liraglutide prevents degenerative processes in a mouse model of Alzheimer's disease. *J Neurosci* 31: 6587-6594.

McClean, P. L., Gault, V. A., Harriott, P. & Holscher, C. (2010) Glucagon-like peptide-1 analogues enhance synaptic plasticity in the brain: A link between diabetes and Alzheimer's disease. *Eur J Pharmacol 630*: 158-162.

Moloney, A. M., Griffin, R. J., Timmons, S., O'Connor, R., Ravid, R. & O'Neill, C. (2010) Defects in IGF-1 receptor, insulin receptor and IRS-1/2 in Alzheimer's disease indicate possible resistance to IGF-1 and insulin signalling. *Neurobiol Aging 31*(2): 224-243.

Mora, F., Exposito, I., Sanz, B. & Blazquez, E. (1992) Selective release of glutamine and glutamic acid produced by perfusion of GLP-1 (7-36) amide in the basal ganglia of the conscious rat. *Brain Res Bull 29*(3-4): 359-361.

Nyberg, J., Anderson, M. F., Meister, B., Alborn, A. M., Strom, A. K., Brederlau, A., Illerskog, A. C., Nilsson, O., Kieffer, T. J., Hietala, M. A., Ricksten, A. & Eriksson, P. S. (2005)

Glucose-dependent insulinotropic polypeptide is expressed in adult hippocampus and induces progenitor cell proliferation. *J Neurosci 25*(7): 1816-1825.

Nyberg, J., Jacobsson, C., Anderson, M. F. & Eriksson, P. S. (2007) Immunohistochemical distribution of glucose-dependent insulinotropic polypeptide in the adult rat brain. *J Neurosci Res 85*: 2099-2119.

Oka, J., Suzuki, E. & Kondo, Y. (2000) Endogenous GLP-1 is involved in beta-amyloid protein-induced memory impairment and hippocampal neuronal death in rats. *Brain Res 878*(1-2): 194-198.

Oka, J. I., Goto, N. & Kameyama, T. (1999) Glucagon-like peptide-1 modulates neuronal activity in the rat's hippocampus. *Neuroreport 10*(8): 1643-1646.

Okereke, O. I., Selkoe, D. J., Pollak, M. N., Stampfer, M. J., Hu, F. B., Hankinson, S. E. & Grodstein, F. (2008) A profile of impaired insulin degradation in relation to late-life cognitive decline: A preliminary investigation. *Int J Geriatr Psychiatry 24*: 177-182.

Perfetti, R., Zhou, J., Doyle, M. E. & Egan, J. M. (2000) Glucagon-like peptide-1 induces cell proliferation and pancreatic-duodenum homeobox-1 expression and increases endocrine cell mass in the pancreas of old, glucose-intolerant rats. *Endocrinology 141*(12): 4600-4605.

Perry, T. & Greig, N. H. (2005) Enhancing central nervous system endogenous GLP-1 receptor pathways for intervention in Alzheimer's disease. *Curr Alzheimer Res 2*(3): 377-385.

Perry, T., Lahiri, D. K., Chen, D., Zhou, J., Shaw, K. T., Egan, J. M. & Greig, N. H. (2002) A novel neurotrophic property of glucagon-like peptide 1: a promoter of nerve growth factor-mediated differentiation in PC12 cells. *J Pharmacol Exp Ther 300*(3): 958-966.

Perry, T., Lahiri, D. K., Sambamurti, K., Chen, D., Mattson, M. P., Egan, J. M. & Greig, N. H. (2003) Glucagon-like peptide-1 decreases endogenous amyloid-beta peptide (Abeta) levels and protects hippocampal neurons from death induced by Abeta and iron. *J Neurosci Res 72*(5): 603-612.

Pi-Sunyer, F. X. (2008) The effects of pharmacologic agents for type 2 diabetes mellitus on body weight. *Postgrad Med 120*(2): 5-17.

Porter, D. W., Kerr, B. D., Flatt, P. R., Holscher, C. & Gault, V. A. (2010) Four weeks administration of Liraglutide improves memory and learning as well as glycaemic control in mice with high fat dietary-induced obesity and insulin resistance. *Diabetes Obes Metab 12*(10): 891-899.

Radde, R., Bolmont, T., Kaeser, S. A., Coomaraswamy, J., Lindau, D., Stoltze, L., Calhoun, M. E., Jaggi, F., Wolburg, H., Gengler, S., Haass, C., Ghetti, B., Czech, C., Holscher, C., Mathews, P. M. & Jucker, M. (2006) Abeta42-driven cerebral amyloidosis in transgenic mice reveals early and robust pathology. *EMBO Rep 7*(9): 940-946.

Reger, M. A., Watson, G. S., Green, P. S., Baker, L. D., Cholerton, B., Fishel, M. A., Plymate, S. R., Cherrier, M. M., Schellenberg, G. D., Frey, W. H., 2nd & Craft, S. (2008) Intranasal insulin administration dose-dependently modulates verbal memory and plasma amyloid-beta in memory-impaired older adults. *J Alzheimers Dis 13*(3): 323-331.

Reger, M. A., Watson, G. S., Green, P. S., Wilkinson, C. W., Baker, L. D., Cholerton, B., Fishel, M. A., Plymate, S. R., Breitner, J. C., DeGroodt, W., Mehta, P. & Craft, S. (2008) Intranasal insulin improves cognition and modulates beta-amyloid in early AD. *Neurology 70*(6): 440-448.

Ristow, M. (2004) Neurodegenerative disorders associated with diabetes mellitus. *J Mol Med 82*(8): 510-529.

Scheen, A. J. (2008) New therapeutic approaches in type 2 diabetes. *Acta Clin Belg 63*(6): 402-407.

Steen, E., Terry, B. M., Rivera, E., Cannon, J. L., Neely, T. R., Tavares, R., Xu, X. J., Wands, J. R. & de la Monte, S. M. (2005) Impaired insulin and insulin-like growth factor expression and signaling mechanisms in Alzheimer's disease - is this type 3 diabetes? *J Alzheimers Dis 7*(1): 63-80.

Stockhorst, U., de Fries, D., Steingrueber, H. J. & Scherbaum, W. A. (2004) Insulin and the CNS: effects on food intake, memory, and endocrine parameters and the role of intranasal insulin administration in humans. *Physiol Behav 83*(1): 47-54.

Strachan, M. W. (2005) Insulin and cognitive function in humans: experimental data and therapeutic considerations. *Biochem Soc Trans 33*(Pt 5): 1037-1040.

Sugaya, K., Kwak, Y., Ohmitsu, O., Marutle, A., Greig, N. & Choumrina, E. (2007) Practical issues in stem cell therapy for Alzheimer's disease. *Curr Alzheimer Res 4*: 370-377.

Townsend, M., Shankar, G. M., Mehta, T., Walsh, D. M. & Selkoe, D. J. (2006) Effects of secreted oligomers of amyloid beta-protein on hippocampal synaptic plasticity: a potent role for trimers. *J Physiol 572*(Pt 2): 477-492.

Trudeau, F., Gagnon, S. & Massicotte, G. (2004) Hippocampal synaptic plasticity and glutamate receptor regulation: influences of diabetes mellitus. *Eur J Pharmacol 490*(1-3): 177-186.

van Dam, P. & Aleman, A. (2004) Insulin-like growth factor-I, cognition and brain aging. *Eur J Pharmacol 490*(1-3): 87-95.

Wang, X. H., Li, L., Holscher, C., Pan, Y. F., Chen, X. R. & Qi, J. S. (2010) Val8-glucagon-like peptide-1 protects against Abeta1-40-induced impairment of hippocampal late-phase long-term potentiation and spatial learning in rats. *Neuroscience 170*(4): 1239-1248.

Watson, G. S. & Craft, S. (2004) Modulation of memory by insulin and glucose: neuropsychological observations in Alzheimer's disease. *Eur J Pharmacol 490*(1-3): 97-113.

Xie, L., Helmerhorst, E., Taddei, K., Plewright, B., Van, B. W. & Martins, R. (2002) Alzheimer's beta-amyloid peptides compete for insulin binding to the insulin receptor. *J Neurosci 22*(10): RC221.

Zhao, A. Z., Shinohara, M. M., Huang, D., Shimizu, M., Eldar-Finkelman, H., Krebs, E. G., Beavo, J. A. & Bornfeldt, K. E. (2000) Leptin induces insulin-like signaling that antagonizes cAMP elevation by glucagon in hepatocytes. *J Biol Chem 275*(15): 11348-11354.

Zhao, W. Q., Chen, H., Quon, M. J. & Alkon, D. L. w. (2004) Insulin and the insulin receptor in experimental models of learning and memory. *Eur J Pharmacol 490*(490): 71-81.

Zhao, W. Q., De Felice, F. G., Fernandez, S., Chen, H., Lambert, M. P., Quon, M. J., Krafft, G. A. & Klein, W. L. (2008) Amyloid beta oligomers induce impairment of neuronal insulin receptors. *Faseb J 22*: 246-260.